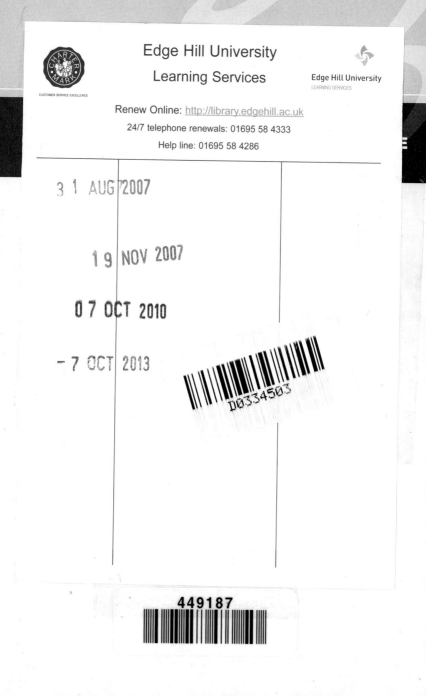

MANUAL OF INTENSIVE CARE MEDICINE

MANUAL OF INTENSIVE CARE MEDICINE
Fourth Edition

Edited By

Richard S. Irwin, M.D.
Professor of Medicine and Nursing
University of Massachusetts Medical School and Graduate School of Nursing;
Chief, Division of Pulmonary, Allergy, and Critical Care Medicine
UMass Memorial Health Care
Worcester, Massachusetts

James M. Rippe, M.D.
Associate Professor of Medicine (Cardiology)
Tufts University School of Medicine
Boston, Massachusetts;
Founder and Director
Rippe Lifestyle Institute
Shrewsbury, Massachusetts

This Edition is Based on *Irwin and Rippe's Intensive Care Medicine*, Fifth Edition, edited by Richard S. Irwin and James M. Rippe.

 LIPPINCOTT WILLIAMS & WILKINS
A **Wolters Kluwer** Company
Philadelphia · Baltimore · New York · London
Buenos Aires · Hong Kong · Sydney · Tokyo

Acquisitions Editor: Brian Brown
Developmental Editor: Nancy Winter
Production Manager: Bridgett Dougherty
Senior Manufacturing Manager: Benjamin Rivera
Marketing Manager: Angela Panetta
Design Coordinator: Terry Mallon
Production Services: Nesbitt Graphics, Inc.
Printer: R.R. Donnelley and Sons

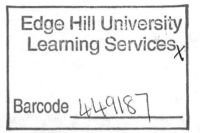

© 2006 by Lippincott Williams & Wilkins

530 Walnut Street
Philadelphia, PA 19106 USA
LWW.com

Printed in the USA

0-7817-5497-6
Library of Congress Cataloging-in-Publication Data
Available upon request

Care has been taken to confirm the accuracy of the information presented and to describe generally accepted practices. However, the authors, editors, and publisher are not responsible for errors or omissions or for any consequences from application of the information in this book and make no warranty, expressed or implied, with respect to the currency, completeness, or accuracy of the contents of the publication. Application of this information in a particular situation remains the professional responsibility of the practitioner.

The authors, editors, and publisher have exerted every effort to ensure that drug selection and dosage set forth in this text are in accordance with current recommendations and practice at the time of publication. However, in view of ongoing research, changes in government regulations, and the constant flow of information relating to drug therapy and drug reactions, the reader is urged to check the package insert for each drug for any change in indications and dosage and for added warnings and precautions. This is particularly important when the recommended agent is a new or infrequently employed drug.

Some drugs and medical devices presented in this publication have Food and Drug Administration (FDA) clearance for limited use in restricted research settings. It is the responsibility of the health care provider to ascertain the FDA status of each drug or device planned for use in their clinical practice.

To purchase additional copies of this book, call our customer service department at (800) 639-3030 or fax orders to (301) 824-7390. International customers should call (301) 714-2324.

Visit Lippincott Williams & Wilkins on the Internet: at LWW.com. Lippincott Williams & Wilkins customer service representatives are available from 8:30 am to 6pm, EST.

10 9 8 7 6 5 4 3 2

CONTENTS

I: PROCEDURES AND TECHNIQUES
Editor—Stephen O. Heard

II: CARDIOVASCULAR PROBLEMS AND CORONARY CARE
Editor—Patrick O'Gara

III: PULMONARY PROBLEMS IN THE INTENSIVE CARE UNIT
Editor—J. Mark Madison

IV: RENAL PROBLEMS IN THE INTENSIVE CARE UNIT
Editor—David M. Clive

*Deceased

IX: PHARMACOLOGY, OVERDOSES AND POISONINGS
Editor—Christopher H. Linden

XII: NEUROLOGIC PROBLEMS IN THE INTENSIVE CARE UNIT
Editors—David A. Drachman and David Paydarfar

XVI: MORAL, ETHICAL, LEGAL ISSUES AND PUBLIC POLICY IN THE INTENSIVE CARE UNIT
Co-Editors—James M. Rippe aand Richard S. Irwin

CONTRIBUTING AUTHORS

Thomas Abbruzzese, M.D.
Resident in General Surgery, Clinical
Fellow, Surgical Critical Care, Brigham
and Women's Hospital; Harvard Medical
School, Boston, Massachusetts

Gerard Abood, M.D.
Loyola University Medical Center,
Department of Surgery, Maywood, Ilinois

Payam Aghassi, M.D.
Pulmonary and Critical Care Medicine
Fellow, UMass Memorial Health Care,
Worcester, Massachusetts

David Ahrenholz, M.D.
Loyola University Medical Center,
Department of Surgery, Maywood, Ilinois

Joshua M. Ammerman, M.D.
Inova Regional Trauma Center, Falls
Church, Virginia

Gustavo G. Angaramo, M.D.
Instructor in Surgery and Cardiothoracic
Surgery, University of Massachusetts
Medical School, Worcester, Massachusetts

Neil Aronin, M.D.
Chief, Division of Endocrinology;
Professor, Department of Endocrinology,
UMass Memorial Medical Center,
Worcester, Massachusetts

Reza Askari, M.D.
Inova Regional Trauma Center, Falls
Church, Virginia

Gerard P. Aurigemma, M.D.
Professor of Medicine and Radiology,
Division of Cardiology, University of
Massachusetts Medical School Worcester,
MA; Director, Mom-Invasive Cardiology,
Division of Cardiology, UMass Memorial
Medical Center, Worcester, Massachusetts

Riad Azar, M.D.
Assistant Professor of Medicine,
Washington University School of Medicine;
Gastroenterology Division, Department of
Internal Medicine, Barnes-Jewish Hospital
–North Campus, St. Louis, Missouri

Karen K. Ballen, M.D.
Assistant Professor, Department of
Medicine, Harvard Medical School;
Director, Leukemia Program, Division of
Hematology/Oncology, Massachusetts
General Hospital, Boston, Massachusetts

Daniel Baran, M.D.
National Scientific Director, Merck & Co.,
Inc., West Point, Pennsylvania; Adjunct
Professor, Orthopedics and Medicine,
UMass Memorial Health Care, Worcester,
Massachusetts

Julie L. Barone, M.D.
Loyola University Medical Center,
Department of Surgery, Maywood, Illinois

Pamela S. Becker, M.D., Ph.D.
Associate Professor, Department of
Medicine, Division of Hematology,
University of Washington; Attending
Physician, Department of Medicine,
Division of Hematology, University of
Washington Medical Center, Seattle,
Washington

Richard C. Becker, M.D.
Director, Cardiovascular Thrombosis
Center, Duke Clinical Research Institute,
Duke University Medical Center; Professor
of Medicine, Division of Cardiology, Duke
University School of Medicine, Durham,
North Carolina

Joshua A. Beckman, M.D.
Associate Attending, Division of
Cardiovascular Medicine, Brigham and
Women's Hospital, Boston, Massachusetts

Isabelita R. Bella, M.D.
Associate Professor, Department of
Neurology, UMass Memorial Medical
Center , Worcester, Massachusetts

Michael F. Bellamy, M.D., MRCP
Consultant Cardiologist, Hammersmith
Hospital, London, UK

Steven B. Bird, M.D.
Assistant Professor, Department of
Emergency Medicine, Division of
Toxicology , University of Massachusetts,
Worcester, Massachusetts

Suzanne F. Bradley, M.D.
Associate Professor, Department of
Internal Medicine, University of Michigan;
Staff Physician, Medicine Service, VA Ann
Arbor Healthcare System, Ann Arbor,
Michigan

D. Eric Brush, M.D.
Assistant Professor, Department of
Emergency Medicine, Division of
Toxicology, UMass Medical Center,
Worcester, Massachusetts

John G. Byrne, M.D.
William S. Stoney Professor and Chairman,
Department of Cardiac Surgery, Vanderbilt
University Medical Center, Nashville,
Tennessee

Hugh G. Calkins, M.D.
Department of Cardiology, Johns Hopkins
Medicine, Baltimore, Maryland

Christopher P. Cannon, M.D.
TIMI Study Group, Cardiovascular
Division, Brigham and Women's Hospital;
Associate Professor of Medicine, Harvard
Medical School, Boston, Massachusetts

Karen C. Carroll, M.D.
Associate Professor, Pathology, The Johns
Hopkins University School of Medicine;
Director, Microbiology Laboratory, The
Johns Hopkins Hospital, Baltimore,
Maryland

David A. Chad, M.D.
Professor, Department of Neurology,
UMass Memorial Medial Center,
Worcester, Massachusetts

Sarah H. Cheeseman, M.D
Professor, Department of Internal
Medicine, Pediatrics, Molecular Genetics
and Microbiology, Division of Infectious
Diseases, UMass Medical Center,
Worcester, Massachusetts

David Clive, M.D.
Associate Professor, Division of Renal
Medicine, UMass Memorial Health Care,
Worcester, Massachusetts

Ray E. Clouse, M.D.
Professor of Medicine and Psychiatry ,
Division of Gastroenterology, Washington
University; Physician, Department of
Medicine, Barnes-Jewish Hospital, St.
Louis, Missouri

Sean P. Collins, M.D.
Assistant Professor, Department of
Emergency Medicine, University of
Cincinnati, Cincinnati, Ohio

Elifce O. Cosar, M.D.
Assistant Professor, Department of
Anesthesiology, UMass Memorial Medical
Center, Worcester, Massachusetts

Oliver Court, M.D.
Inova Regional Trauma Center, Falls
Church, Virginia

Michael A. Coyne, M.D.
ER Department , Berkshire Medical Center,
Pittsfield, Massachusetts

Kara Criswell, M.D.
Loyola University Medical Center,
Department of Surgery, Maywood, Illinois

Jonathan Critchlow, M.D.
Assistant Professor of Surgery, Beth Israel
Hospital Deaconess Center, West Campus,
Boston, Massachusetts

Frederick J. Curley, M.D.
Associate Professor, Department of
Medicine, UMass Mass Medical School;
Medical Director, Department of
Pulmonary and Critical Care, Milford
Regional Hospital, Milford, Massachusetts

Bruce S. Cutler, M.D.
Chief, Division of Vascular Surgery;
Professor, Department of Surgery, UMass
Memorial Medical Center, Worcester,
Massachusetts

Jennifer Daly, M.D.
Professor, Department of Medicine, Division of Infectious Diseases and Immunology, University of Massachusetts Medical School, UMass Memorial Health Care, Worcester, Massachusetts

Raul E. Davaro, M.D.
Assistant Professor, Department of Infectious Disease, UMass Memorial Medical Center, Worcester, Massachusetts

G. William Dec, M.D.
Chief, Division of Cardiology, Massachusetts General Hospital; Professor of Medicine, Department of Medicine, Harvard Medical School, Boston, Massachusetts

James A. de Lemos, M.D.
Associate Professor of Medicine, Department of Cardiology, UT Southwestern Medical Center; Coronary Care Unit Director, Parkland Memorial Hospital, Dallas, Texas

Paul F. Dellaripa, M.D.
Assistant Clinical Professor of Medicine, Tufts University School of Medicine, Boston, MA; Chairman, Department of Rheumatology, Lahey Clinic, Burlington, Massachusetts

E. Patchen Dellinger, M.D.
Professor and Vice Chairman, Department of Surgery, University of Washington School of Medicine; Associate Medical Director and Chief of General Surgery, Department of Surgery, University of Washington Medical Center, Seattle, Washington

Mark Dershwitz, M.D., Ph.D.
Vice Chair, Department of Anesthesiology; Professor, Department of Anesthesiology, UMass Memorial Medical Center, Worcester, Massachusetts

Josh R. Doll, M.D.
Fellow, Department of Medicine, Division of Cardiology, The Medical University of South Carolina, Charleston, South Carolina

David Drachman, M.D.
Professor and Chairman, Department of Neurology, UMass Memorial Medical Center, Worcester, Massachusetts

Ty Dunn, M.D.
Instructor, Department of Surgery, University of Minnesota, Minneapolis, Minnesota

Kevin Dushay, M.D., FCCP
Assistant Professor, Division of Biology and Medicine, Brown University; Pulmonary, Critical Care and Sleep Disorder Medicine, Rhode Island Hospital, Providence, Rhode Island

Kevin M. Dwyer, M.D.
Inova Regional Trauma Center, Falls Church, Virginia

Richard T. Ellison III, M.D.
Hospital Epidemiologist; Professor, Division of Infectious Disease, UMass Memorial Health Care, Worcester, Massachusetts

Charles Emerson, M.D.
Professor of Medicine, Division of Endocrinology and Metabolism, University of Massachusetts Medical School, Worcester, Massachusetts

Maurice Enriquez-Sarano, M.D., FACC, FAHA
Professor of Medicine, Mayo College of Medicine; Director, Valvular Heart Disease Clinic, Cardiovascular Diseases and Internal Medicine, Mayo Clinic, Rochester, Minnesota

Laurence M. Epstein, M.D.
Director Electrophysiology and Pacing Laboratory; Chief, Cardiac Arrhythmia Service, Brigham and Women's Hospital, Cardiovascular Division, Boston, Massachusetts

Samir Fakhry, M.D.
Chief, Trauma and Surgical Critical Care Services, Inova Regional Trauma Center, Falls Church, Virginia

Khaldoun Faris, M.D.
Assistant Professor, Department of Anesthesiology, UMass Memorial Medical Center, Worcester, Massachusetts

Alan Farwell, M.D.
Associate Professor of Medicine, Division of Endocrinology and Metabolism, University of Massachusetts Medical School, Worcester, Massachusetts

Paola Fata, M.D.
Inova Regional Trauma Center, Falls Church, Virginia

Thomas W. Felbinger, M.D.
Department of Anesthesiology, Perioperative and Pain Medicine, Brigham and Woman's Hospital and Harvard Medical School, Boston, Massachusetts

Philip Fidler, M.D.
Medical Director, Andrew J Panettieri Burn Center, Bridgeport Hospital, Bridgeport, Connecticut; Assistant Professor, General Surgery and Plastic Surgery, Yale School of Medicine, New Haven, Connecticut

Marc Fisher, M.D.
Professor, Department of Neurology, UMass Memorial Medical Center, Worcester, Massachusetts

Nancy M. Fontneau, M.D.
Associate Professor, Department of Neurology, UMass Memorial Medical Center, Worcester, Massachusetts

Cynthia T. French, NP, MS
Department of Pulmonary Medicine, UMass Memorial Health Care, Worcester, Massachusetts

Brian J. Gallay, M.D., Ph.D.
Assistant Professor, Department of Medicine, University of California, Davis; Medical Director, Kidney and Pancreas Transplant, University of California, Davis Medical Center, Sacramento, California

Nelson M. Gantz, M.D.
Chief, Department of Infectious Disease, Boulder Community Hospital, Boulder, Colorado

Leonard I. Ganz, M.D.
Assistant Professor of Medicine, Department of Electrophysiology, Allegheny University of the Health Sciences, Allegheny University Hospitals, Pittsburgh, Pennsylvania

Jonathan Gates, M.D.
Assistant Professor of Surgery, Director of Trauma, Division of Burns, Trauma, and Critical Care; Associate Vascular Surgeon, Division of Vascular Surgery, Brigham and Women's Hospital, Harvard Medical School, Boston, Massachusetts

Eli V. Gelfand, M.D.
Fellow in Cardiovascular Diseases, Beth Israel Deaconess Medical Center; Clinical Fellow in Medicine, Harvard Medical School, Boston, Massachusetts

Edith S. Geringer, M.D.
Massachusetts General Hospital, Wang Ambulatory Care Center, Boston, Massachusetts

Terry Gernsheimer, M.D.
Associate Professor of Medicine, Department of Medicine, Division of Hematology, University of Washington School of Medicine; Director, Medical Transfusion Services, Seattle Cancer Care Alliance, Seattle, Washington

Laura L.Gibson, M.D.
Assistant Professor, Department of Infectious Disease, Worcester, Massachusetts

Michael Givertz, M.D.
Co-Director, Cardiomyopathy and Heart Failure Program, Brigham and Women's Hospital; Assistant Professor of Medicine, Harvard Medical School, Boston, Massachusetts

Richard H. Glew, M.D.
Professor, Department of Medicine, Molecular Genetics and Microbiology, University of Massachusetts Medical School; Associate Chair, Department of Medicine and Director, Division of Infectious Diseases and Immunology, UMass Memorial Health Care, Worcester, Massachusetts

Jack Gluckman
Professor and Chairman, Department of Otolaryngology – Head and Neck Surgery, University of Cincinnati College of Medicine, Cincinnati , Ohio

Michael R. Gold, M.D., Ph.D.
Chief, Division of Cardiology, Medical University Hospital; Professor, Department of Medicine, Division of Cardiology, Medical University of South Carolina, Charleston, South Carolina

Heather Gornik, M.D.
Vascular Medicine Section, Cardiovascular Division, Department of Medicine, Brigham and Women's Hospital, Boston, Massachusetts

Gopal S. Grandhige, M.D.
Bridgeport Hospital, Bridgeport,
Connecticut

Barth A. Green, M.D.
Professor and Chairman, Department of
Neurological Surgery, University of Miami
School of Medicine,Lois Pope LIFE Center,
Miami, Florida

Rainer W. G. Gruessner, M.D., FACS
Professor of Surgery, Department of
Surgery, University of Minnesota,
Minneapolis, Minnesota

Stephen O. Heard, M.D.
Professor and Chair, Department of
Anesthesiology , UMass Memorial Medical
Center, Worcester, Massachusetts

Stephan Heckers, M.D.
Medical Director of Bipolar and Psychotic
Disorders, McLean Hospital, Belmont,
Massachusetts

Helen M. Hollingsworth, M.D.
Associate Professor, Department of
Medicine, Pulmonary Center, Boston
University School of Medicine; Director,
Adult Asthma and Allergy Services,
Department of Medicine, Boston Medical
Center, Boston, Massachusetts

Donough Howard, M.D.
Department of Rheumatology, Lahey
Clinic, Burlington, Massachusetts

Eric Iida, M.D.
Department of Medicine, Division of
Renal Medicine, UMass Medical School,
Worcester, Massachusetts

Richard S. Irwin, M.D.
Professor of Medicine and Nursing; Chief,
Pulmonary, Allergy and Critical Care
Medicine Division, UMass Memorial
Medical Center,
of Pulmonary Medicine, Worcester,
Massachusetts

Olga Ivanov, M.D.
Resident in General Surgery, Loyola
University Medical Center, Maywood,
Illinois

Jaroslaw Jac, M.D.
Baylor College of Medicine; Hematology-
Oncology, VA Medical Center, Houston,
Texas

Andrew Jea, M.D.
Resident, Department of Neurological
Surgery, University of Miami School of
Medicine, Lois Pope LIFE Center, Miami,
Florida

Carol Kaufman, M.D.
Divisions of Infectious Diseases and
Geriatrics, VA Ann Arbor Healthcare
System, Ann Arbor, Michigan

Shubjeet Kaur, M.D.
Clinical Vice-Chair Department of
Anesthesiology; Medical Director, Peri-
Operative Services; Associate Professor,
Department of Anesthesiology, UMass
Memorial Medical Center, Department of
Anesthesiology, Worcester, Massachusetts

Renée Killian, RN, MPH
Puget Sound Blood Center, Seattle,
Washington

John Kitzmiller, M.D.
Associate Professor, Department
of Surgery, Division of Plastic and
Reconstructive, University of Cincinnati
Medical Center, Cincinnati, Ohio

Bruce A. Koplan, M.D.
Associate Physician, Department
of Cardiac Arrhythmia Service and
Cardiovascular Division, Brigham and
Women's Hospital, Boston, Massachusetts

Kevin Korenblat, M.D.
Assistant Professor of Medicine,
Washington University School of Medicine,
Gastroenterology Division, St. Louis,
Missouri

Michael H. Kroll, M.D.
Associate Professor of Medicine,Molecular
Physiology and Biophysics, Baylor College
of Medicine; Hematology-Oncology, VA
Medical Center, Houston, Texas

Lawrence Labbate, M.D.
Associate Professor of Psychiatry and
Behavioral Sciences, Ralph H. Johnson
VA Medical Center , Charleston, South
Carolina

Ivan E. Liang, M.D.
Emergency Medicine Residency Program,
University of Massachusetts Medical
School, Worcester, Massachusetts

Christopher H. Linden, M.D. FACEP
Associate Professor, Emergency Medicine, Milford Regional, Milford, Massachusetts

Michael L. Linenberger, M.D.
Medical Director, Apheresis and Cellular Therapy, Seattle Cancer Care Alliance; Associate Professor, Department of Medicine, University of Washington, Seattle, Washington

Carol F. Lippa, M.D.
Department of Neurology, Medical College of Pennsylvania, Hahnemann University, Philadelphia, Pennsylvania

N. Scott Litofsky, M.D.
Associate Professor, Division of Neurosurgery, UMass Medical School, Worcester, Massachusetts

Randall R. Long, M.D., Ph.D.
Professor of Clinical Neurology, UMass Health Care, Worcester, Massachusetts

*Christopher Longcope, M.D.
(Deceased)

Samuel D. Luber, M.D., MPH
Instructor, Department of Surgery, Division of Emergency Medicine, University of Texas Southwestern Medical Center, Parkland Memorial Hospital, Dallas, Texas

Fred A. Luchette M.D., FACS, FCCM
The Ambrose and Gladys Bowyer Professor of Surgery; Director, Division of Trauma/Critical Care/Burns, Department of Surgery, Burn Shock Trauma Institute, Maywood, Illinois

J. Mark Madison, M.D.
Associate Professor, Department of Medicine and Physiology, Pulmonary, Allergy, and Critical Care Medicine, UMass Medical School, Worcester, Massachusetts

Brian Mady, M.D.
Associate Professor, Division of Infectious Diseases, UMass Memorial Medical Center, Worcester, Massachusetts

William H. Maisel, M.D.
Associate Physician, Department of Cardiac Arrhythmia Service and Cardiovascular Division, Brigham and Women's Hospital, Boston, Massachusetts

Michael D. Mancenido, D.O.
Fellow, Division of Infectious Disease, UMass Memorial Health Care, Worcester, Massachusetts

Deborah H Markowitz, M.D.
Assistant Professor of Medicine, Pulmonary, Allergy and Critical Care Medicine Division, UMass-Memorial Health Care, Worcester, Massachusetts

Raimis Matulionis, M.D.
Assistant Professor, Department of Anesthesiology, University of Massachusetts; Cardiovascular Anesthesiologist, Surgical Intensive Care Attending, Department of Anesthesiology, UMass Memorial Health Care, University Campus, Worcester, Massachusetts

Ata Mazaheri, M.D.
Loyola University Medical Center, Department of Surgery, Maywood, Illinois

Savant Mehta, M.D.
Medical Director, Liver Transplant Program; Assistant Professor, Division of Gastroenterology, Department of Internal Medicine, UMass Memorial Medical Center, Worcester, Massachusetts

Glenn Meininger, M.D.
Division of Cardiology, Johns Hopkins Hospital, Baltimore, Maryland

Robert M. Mentzer, Jr., M.D.
Chair, Department of Surgery, Frank C. Spencer Professor of Surgery, University of Kentucky, Lexington, Kentucky

Christopher P. Michetti, M.D., FACS
Trauma/Surgical Critical Care, Associate Surgical Clerkship Director, Inova Fairfax Hospital; Assistant Professor, Department of Surgery, Virginia Commonwealth University School of Medicine, Inova Campus; Trauma/Critical Care Surgeon, Department of Surgery, Trauma Services, Inova Fairfax Hospital, Falls Church, Virginia

Marco Mielcarek, M.D.
Assistant Professor, Medical Oncology, Fred Hutchinson Cancer Research Center, Seattle, Washington

Ann Linda Mitchell, M.D.
Associate Professor, Department of Neurology, UMass Memorial Medical Center, Worcester, Massachusetts

Majaz Moonis, M.D.
Director, Stroke Prevention Clinic; Associate Professor, Department of Neurology, UMass Memorial Medical Center, Worcester, Massachusetts

John P. Mordes, M.D.
Professor, Department of Diabetes, University of Massachusetts Hospital, Worcester, Massachusetts

Kapil Moza, M.D.
Resident, Department of Neurological Surgery, University of Miami School of Medicine, Lois Pope LIFE Center, Miami, Florida

W. Garrett Nichols, M.D., MS
Associate in Clinical Research, Program in Infectious Diseases, Fred Hutchinson Cancer Research Center, Seattle, Washington

Dominic J. Nompleggi, M.D., Ph.D.
Chief , Division of Gastroenterology, UMass Memorial Health Care; Associate Professor, Department of Medicine, University of Massachusetts Medical School, Worcester, Massachusetts

Patrick T. O'Gara, M.D.
Director, Clinical Cardiology and Vice Chairman, Clinical Affairs, Department of Medicine, Brigham and Women's Hospital, Boston, Massachusetts

Paulo Oliveira, M.D.
Pulmonary and Critical Care Medicine Fellow, UMass Memorial Health Care, Worcester, Massachusetts

Anil A. Panackal, M.D.
Fellow, Infectious Diseases/Clinical Research, Fred Hutchinson Cancer Research Center; Fellow, Internal Medicine, University of Washington, Seattle, Washington

Nereida A. Parada, M.D.
Clinical Associate Professor of Medicine, Tulane University Health Sciences Center, School of Medicine, Section of Pulmonary Diseases and Critical Care Medicine, New Orleans, Louisiana

John Paraskos, M.D.
Professor of Medicine, University of Massachusetts, Worcester, Massachusetts

John J. Paris, S.J., Ph.D.
Walsh Professor of Bioethics, Theology Department, Boston College, Chestnut Hill, Massachusetts; Clinical Professor of Family Medicine, Family Medicine and Community Health, Tufts Medical School, Boston, Massachusetts

Jateen Patel, M.D.
Loyola University Medical Center, Department of Surgery, Maywood, Illinois

Marie Pavini, M.D.
Assistant Professor, Division of Critical Care, Rutland Regional Medical Center, Rutland, Vermont

David Paydarfar, M.D.
Associate Professor, Department of Neurology, UMass Memorial Medical Center, Worcester, Massachusetts

Catherine A. Phillips M.D.
Associate Professor, Department of Neurology, UMass Memorial Medical Center, Worcester, Massachusetts

Mark H. Pollack, M.D.
Director, MGH Anxiety Program, Massachusetts General Hospital, Wang Ambulatory Care Center, Boston, Massachusetts

Chandra Prakash, M.D., MRCP
Assistant Professor of Medicine, Division of Gastroenterology, Washington University School of Medicine; Faculty Gastroenterologist, Division of Gastroenterology, Barnes-Jewish Hospital, St. Louis, Missouri

John Querques, M.D.
Instructor, Psychiatry, Harvard Medical School; Department of Psychiatry, Beth Israel Deaconess Medical Center, Boston, Massachusetts

Asimah Quyyum, MD
UMass Memorial Health Care, Worcester, Massachusetts

Paula D. Ravin, M.D.
Associate Professor, Department of Neurology, UMass Memorial Medical Center, Worcester, Massachusetts

Frank E. Reardon, J.D.
Hassan & Reardon, Boston, Massachusetts

Lawrence Recht, M.D.
Professor of Neurology and Clinical
Neurosciences, Stanford University
Medical Center, Palo Alto, California

Harvey S. Reich, MD, FACP, FCCP
Director of Critical Care Medicine,
Rutland Regional Medical Center; Clinical
Associate Professor of Medicine, University
of Vermont College of Medicine, Rutland,
Vermont

Peter E. Rice, M.D.
Professor of Surgery, New York, New York

James M. Rippe, M.D.
Associate Professor of Medicine
(Cardiology), Tufts University School of
Medicine, Boston, Massachusetts; Founder
and Director, Rippe Lifestyle Institute,
Shrewsbury, Massachusetts

Mark J. Rosen, M.D.
Chief, Department of Pulmonary and
Critical Care Medicine, Beth Israel Medical
Center; Professor of Medicine, Albert
Einstein College of Medicine, New York,
New York

Ido A. Rossini, M.D.
Chief, Department of Diabetes, UMass
Memorial Medical Center, Worcester,
Massachusetts

Alan L. Rothman, M.D.
Associate Professor, Department of
Medicine, Molecular Genetics and
Microbiology, University of Massachusetts
Medical School; Attending Physician,
Department of Medicine, UMass Memorial
Health Care, Worcester, Massachusetts

John L. Sapp, Jr., M.D., FRCPC
Director, Cardiac Electrophysiology,
Division of Cardiology, Queen Elizabeth II
Health Sciences Centre; Assistant Professor,
Department of Medicine, Dalhousie
University, Halifax, Nova Scotia, Canada

Diane M. F. Savarese, M.D.
Clinical Instructor in Medicine, Harvard
Medical School; Division of Hematology
Oncology, Department of Medicine, Beth
Israel Deaconess Medical Center, Boston,
Massachusetts; Deputy Editor, Oncology,
Up To Date, Waltham, Massachusetts

Gregory S. Sayuk, M.D.
Fellow in Gastroenterology, Department
of Medicine, Washington University
School of Medicine, St. Louis, Missouri

David W. Scaff, D.O.
Instructor of Surgery, Division of
Traumatology and Surgical Critical Care,
University of Pennsylvania, Philadelphia,
Pennsylvania

Jim Scanlon, M.D.
Inova Regional Trauma Center, Falls
Church, Virginia

Oren P. Schaefer, M.D.
Director, Pulmonary and Critical Care
Medicine Fellowship Program, UMass
Memorial Medical Center; Associate
Professor of Clinical Medicine, Department
of Medicine, University of Massachusetts
Medical School, Worcester, Massachusetts

Paul Schalch, M.D.
Loyola University Medical Center,
Department of Surgery, Maywood, Illinois

Benjamin M. Scirica, M.D.
Cardiovascular Division, Brigham and
Women's Hospital, Boston, Massachusetts

Hani Seoudi, M.D.
Inova Regional Trauma Center, Falls
Church, Virginia

Kenneth Serio, M.D.
University of California, San Diego, San
Diego, California

Mark L. Shapiro, M.D.
Associate Director, Adult Trauma,
Department of Surgery, UMass Memorial
Medical Center; Assistant Professor,
Department of Surgery, University of
Massachusetts Medical School, Worcester,
Massachusetts

Vibha Sharma, M.D.
UMass Memorial Health Care, Worcester,
Massachusetts

Michael J. Singh, M.D.
Assistant Professor, Department of
Vascular Surgery, UMass Memorial
Medical Center, Worcester, Massachusetts

Nicholas A. Smyrnios, M.D., FACP, FCCP
Associate Professor of Medicine, Department of Medicine, University of Massachusetts Medical School; Associate Chief of Pulmonary, Allergy, and Critical Care Medicine, Department of Medicine, UMass Memorial Medical Center, Worcester, Massachusetts

Piotr Sobieszczyk, M.D.
Vascular Medicine Section, Cardiovascular Division, Department of Medicine, Brigham and Women's Hospital, Boston, Massachusetts

Joseph Solomkin, M.D.
Professor of Surgery, University of Cincinnati College of Medicine, Cincinnati, Ohio

Michael L. Steer, M.D.
Professor of Surgery, Anatomy and Cellular Biology, Tufts University School of Medicine; Chief, General Surgery, Tufts–New England Medical Center, Boston, Massachusetts

Antine Stenbit, M.D.
University California, San Diego, San Diego, California

Theodore Stern, M.D.
Chief, Psychiatry Consultation Service, Associate Professor of Psychiatry, Harvard Medical School; Massachusetts General Hospital, Department of Psychiatry, Boston, Massachusetts

Donald S. Stevens, M.D.
Director, Center for Pain Management, Marlborough Hospital, Marlborough, Massachusetts

William Stevenson, M.D.
Cardiovascular Division, Bringham and Women's Hospital, Boston, Massachusetts

F. Marc Stewart, M.D.
Medical Director, Seattle Cancer Care Alliance, Member, Fred Hutchinson Cancer Research Center, Seattle, Washington

Peter H. Stone, M.D.
Associate Professor of Medicine, Harvard Medical School; Co-Director, Samuel A. Levine Cardiac Unit; Director, Clinical Trials CVD Division, Department of Medicine; Director, Clinical Trials Center, Brigham and Women's Hospital, CV Division, Boston, Massachusetts

Alan B. Storrow, M.D.
Associate Professor, Department of Emergency Medicine, University of Cincinnati, Cincinnati, Ohio

Arash Tabaee, M.D.
Clinical Instructor, Division of Medicine, New York University School of Medicine; Attending Physician, Department of Medicine, New York University Medical Center, New York, New York

George E. Tesar, M.D.
Chairman of Department of Psychiatry and Psychology, The Cleveland Clinic Foundation, Cleveland, Ohio

Aneetha Thirumalai, M.D.
UMass Memorial Health Care, Worcester, Massachusetts

Arthur Thompson, M.D.
Professor of Medicine, University of Washington; Director of Hemophilia Care and Coagulation Laboratories, Puget Sound Blood Center, Seattle, Washington

Michael J. Thompson, M.D.
Associate Professor, Department of Diabetes, UMass Memorial Medical Center, Worcester, Massachusetts

Dennis A. Tighe, M.D.
Associate Director, Noninvasive Cardiology, Department of Cardiovascular Medicine, UMass Memorial Health Care; Associate Professor, Department of Medicine, University of Massachusetts Medical School, Worcester, Massachusetts

Arthur L. Trask, M.D., FACS
Department of Trauma, Professor of Surgery, Uniformed Services, University for Health Sciences, Bethesda Maryland; Past Chief Trauma Services, Inova Regional Trauma Center, Falls Church, Virginia

Christoph Troppmann, M.D., FACS
Associate Professor, Division of Transplantation, Department of Surgery, University of California, Davis Medical Center, Sacramento, California

Thomas W. Wallace, M.D.
Chief Medical Resident, Department of Internal Medicine, The University of Texas Southwestern Medical Center, Dallas, Texas

J. Matthias Walz, M.D.
Assistant Professor, Department of Anesthesiology, UMass Memorial Medical Center, Worcester, Massachusetts

John P. Weaver, M.D.
Division Chief, Department of Neurosurgery; Associate Professor, Department of Neurosurgery, UMass Memorial Medical Center, Worcester, Massachusetts

Gregory Webster, M.D.
Clinical Instructor, Department of Pediatrics, University of California, San Francisco, San Francisco, California

Mark Meredith Wilson, M.D.
Associate Director of Medical Intensive Care Unit, Department of Medicine, UMass Memorial Health Center; Associate Professor of Medicine, University of Massachusetts Medical School, Worcester, Massachusetts

Robert Witherspoon, M.D.
Medical Director, Outpatient Transplant Department; Associate Professor, Medicine, Fred Hutchinson Cancer Research Center, Seattle, Washington

Dietmar H. Wittmann, M.D.
Professor of Surgery, Colonna Institute for Surgical Research and Therapy, Nokomis, Florida

Mary Wolfe, M.D.
Loyola University Medical Center, Department of Surgery, Maywood, Illinois

Catherine Yu, M.D.
University of Massachusetts Medical School, Department of Medicine, Worcester, Massachusetts

David D. Yuh, M.D.
Assistant Professor of Surgery and Director, Cardiac Surgical Research, Division ofCardiac Surgery, The Johns Hopkins Hospital, Baltimore, Maryland

Iva Zivna, M.D.
UMass Memorial Health Care, Worcester, Massachusetts

$\mathcal{W}$e are happy to present the fourth edition of the *Manual of Intensive Care Medicine*. Previous editions established this *Manual* as a leading source of information in the diverse and complicated field of critical care and intensive care medicine. The practical format and user-friendly, portable size of the *Manual* have made it a particularly valuable addition to the bedside practice of intensive care and a valuable reference for students, interns, residents, fellows and others practicing critical care medicine no matter in which environment critically ill patients are cared for.

Just as in the previous edition of this work, the fourth edition of the *Manual* is intended to parallel our major textbook *Irwin* and *Rippe's Intensive Care Medicine*. This latter, hardcover book is now in its fifth edition and continues to be a leading source of intensive care knowledge both in the United States and throughout the world.

Readers of the current edition of our *Manual* will immediately notice a significant change in format. We have adopted a more user-friendly, outline format to try to give busy house officers more direct and immediate access to the information they need to manage the complex and time-sensitive issues of the practice of critical care medicine. As with the previous edition, we have challenged the authors to emphasize critical concepts and pare down chapters to the key clinically relevant points. Annotated references are provided to guide the interested reader through key articles in the relevant literature.

The *Manual of Intensive Care Medicine* opens with an extensive section on Procedures and Techniques. The next seven sections are divided according to organ system. In each chapter, discussions of key entities that present in the intensive care or coronary care unit environment appear together with targeted discussions focusing on treatment.

Section IX presents a review of key Pharmacology, Overdoses, and Poisonings considerations recognizing that these remain important issues in intensive care. This section has been pared down from the previous edition of our *Manual*. We recognize this area as being so important that we have co-edited, along with our colleague, toxicologist Dr. Christopher Linden, an entire *Manual of Overdoses and Poisonings*, which can be used in conjunction with the current edition of the *Manual of Intensive Care Medicine*.

As in the previous edition, there are extensive sections on surgical issues in critical care as well as shock and trauma. The *Manual* closes with sections on Neurology; Transplantation; Rheumatology and Immunology; Psychiatry; and Moral, Ethical, Legal and Public Policy Issues in Intensive Care all of which are crucial to a comprehensive view of adult intensive care medicine.

We wish to acknowledge that many of the chapter authors for the current *Manual* have also made major contributions to our larger format textbook, *Irwin and Rippe's Intensive Care Medicine*. Although the *Manual of Intensive Care Medicine* has been edited and revised with the expert guidance of many section editors, many of the chapters were developed based on the expert knowledge of the original textbook contributors and reorganized and rewritten in a style necessary for the scope of this portable text.

We also wish to once again thank a number of individuals without whose able assistance the fourth edition of this *Manual* would not have been possible. First and foremost, Dr. Rippe's Editorial Director, Elizabeth Porcaro Grady, has done her usual superb job in organizing and expediting all aspects of manuscript preparation. Without Beth's superb editorial skills, projects such as this would not be possible. Karen Barrell, Dr. Irwin's Administrative Assistant, has provided important assistance in managing his complex clinical and academic endeavors. Carol Moreau, Executive Assistant to Dr. Rippe, expertly juggles the diverse aspects of his clinical, research, and travel calendar to carve out time for efforts of this magnitude. A special word of thanks to the editorial team at Lippincott Williams & Wilkins, who, as with all of our medical editing projects, have supported the process every step of the way. We wish to particularly thank our editor, Brian Brown, for multiple helpful suggestions and support throughout the process of writing this book.

We wish to especially thank the Section Editors for the *Manual*, each of whom contributed long hours and the expert guidance necessary to ensure that the *Manual* would contain up-to-date, user-friendly, and practical information.

Finally, we wish to thank our families Diane and Rebecca Irwin; Rachel, Andrew, and Truman Koh; Sara, John, Benjamin, Jacob, and Isaac Dilorio; Catherine, Andrew, and Emmett McIntosh; and Stephanie, Hart, Jaelin, Devon, and Jamie Rippe who continue to love and support us in all of our efforts, both personal and academic, and make it all worthwhile.

James M. Rippe, M.D.
Richard S. Irwin, M.D.

Procedures and Techniques

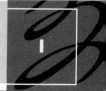

I

AIRWAY MANAGEMENT AND ENDOTRACHEAL INTUBATION

Elifce Cosar

1

I. GENERAL PRINCIPLES

A. Maintenance of the airway is the first step to the successful resuscitation of a compromised patient. The vital role of airway management of the critical care patient demands thoughtful consideration.

B. Critical care physicians should be familiar with the equipment and the techniques to maintain and secure the airway.

II. ANATOMY. The normal upper airway begins functionally at the nares or mouth and extends to the cricoid cartilage. The upper airway is functionally divided into the nose, the pharynx and the larynx.

A. Nose

The nasal mucosa remains well vascularized throughout the nasal cavity. Trauma during nasal intubations can result in brisk bleeding.

B. Larynx

1. The laryngeal skeleton consists of thyroid, cricoid, epiglottic, arytenoid, corniculate, and cuneiform cartilages.

2. The cricoid cartilage is the only structure that completely encircles the airway. Two nerves that are branches of the vagus innervate the larynx.

a. The external branch of superior laryngeal nerve supplies the motor innervation to the cricothyroid muscle. The internal branch supplies the sensory innervation above the vocal cords.

b. The recurrent laryngeal nerve supplies all other motor innervation to the laryngeal musculature and also provides sensory innervation to the larynx below the vocal cords.

C. Trachea

1. The adult trachea begins at the cricoid cartilage. It is 10 to 20 cm long and 12 mm in diameter.

2. It divides into right and left main bronchi at the level of fourth and fifth thoracic vertebrae. In the adult, the right main bronchus is wider and shorter and takes off at a less acute angle than the left, thus making right main bronchus intubation more likely.

III. EVALUATION OF THE AIRWAY

A. The ability to rapidly evaluate the patient's airway before endotracheal intubation is very important. A difficult airway in some patients will remain undetected despite the most careful preoperative airway examination.

B. If possible, the airway should be evaluated while the patient is sitting upright. Several clinical criteria can be assessed.

1. Mouth opening (interincisor gap should be greater than 4 cm)

2. Mallampati classification (Fig. 1-1)

3. Head and neck movement

4. Ability to prognath (i.e., to bring the lower incisors in front of the upper incisors)

5. Thyromental distance (should be greater than 6.5 cm)

6. Body weight

7. Previous history of difficult intubation

C. The presence of cervical collars, halo devices, trauma to the mandible or neck, morbid obesity and obstructive sleep apnea may signal a difficult airway.

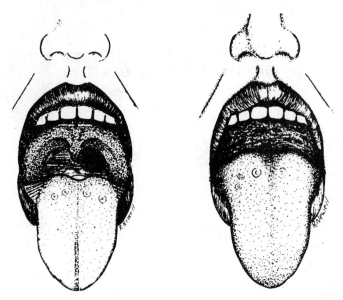

Figure 1-1. Mallampati classification: class I airway, faucial pillars, soft palate, and uvula can be visualized (*left*); class II airway, faucial pillars and soft palate can be visualized but the uvula is masked by the base of the tongue; class III airway, only the soft palate can be visualized. The patient on the right has a class III airway, which is one of the predictors of difficult orotracheal intubation. (From Mallampati SR, Gatt SP, Gugino LD, et al. A clinical sign to predict difficult tracheal intubation: a prospective study. Can Anaesth Soc J 1985;32:420, with permission.)

   D. History of snoring, facial hair, edentulous patients, patients with age greater than 56 and body mass index greater than 26 are preoperative clinical predictors for difficult mask ventilation.

IV. AIRWAY EQUIPMENT
   A. A source of oxygen, face masks of different sizes, a bag-valve ventilation device, tonsillar suction and suction source with canister and tubing.
   B. Oral and nasopharyngeal airways (Fig 1-2).
   C. Laryngoscope blades and handle. Two basic types of laryngoscope blades are available: the curved blade (Macintosh) and the straight blade (Miller). The Miller blade is more useful in patients who have a cephalad and anterior laryngeal inlet (Fig. 1-3).
   D. Various sizes of endotracheal tubes with stylets. The selection of proper tube diameter is very important. In adults, endotracheal tube sizes 7.0 to 8.0 mm internal diameter are commonly used for women, while sizes 8.0 to 9.0 mm internal diameter tubes are used for men.
   E. A device to detect end-tidal carbon dioxide: colorimetric detector or capnograph.
   F. The required size of the endotracheal tubes used in children may be based on this formula: Endotracheal tube size (mm)=[16 + age (yr)] / 4
   G. Laryngeal mask airways (LMAs) can be used to provide a temporary airway until a more definite airway can be achieved. The LMA is contraindicated in patients at risk of aspiration due to the presence of a full stomach (Fig. 1-4).

V. AIRWAY OBSTRUCTION
   A. The hallmark of upper airway obstruction is diminished or absent airflow in the presence of continued respiratory effort.

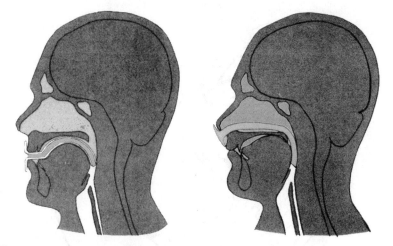

Figure 1-2. *Left:* The proper position of the oropharyngeal airway. *Right:* The proper position of the nasopharyngeal airway. (Reprinted with permission from Dorsch JA, Dorsch SE: *Understanding Anesthesia*. Williams & Wilkins, Baltimore, 1984.)

    B. Airway obstruction can be complete or partial. Partial obstruction will be accompanied by snoring during expiration or with stridor during inspiration. Breath sounds will be absent during complete obstruction.

VI. TREATMENT

    A. The head tilt is the simplest airway maneuver. The head is tilted back by placing one hand under the neck and pushing down on the forehead. This approach should not be used in patients with a fractured neck or extensive cerebrovascular disease.

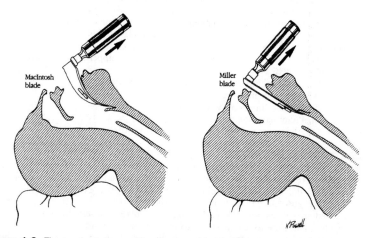

Figure 1-3. The two basic types of laryngoscope blades, MacIntosh (left) and Miller (right). The MacIntosh blade is curved. The blade tip is placed in the vallecula, and the handle of the laryngoscope pulled forward at a 45-degree angle. This maneuver allows visualization of the epiglottis. The Miller blade is straight. The tip is placed posterior to the epiglottis, thus pinning the epiglottis between the base of the tongue and the straight laryngoscope blade. The motion on the laryngoscope handle is the same as that used with the MacIntosh.

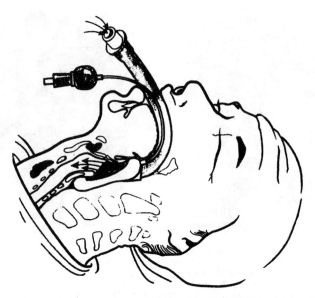

Figure 1-4. Correct position of the laryngeal mask airway. (From Maltby JR, Loken RG, Watson NC, et al. The laryngeal mask airway: clinical appraisal in 250 patients. Can J Anaesth 1990;37:509, with permission.)

    B. The second maneuver (jaw thrust) displaces the jaw forward by applying anterior pressure on the angle of the mandible. This procedure should not be done in patients with a dislocated or fractured jaw.

    C. The triple airway maneuver (combination of head tilt, jaw thrust and opening the mouth) is the most reliable manual method to establish airway patency.

    D. When airway maneuvers are inadequate to establish airway patency, airway aids such as an oral or nasopharyngeal airway should be used (see Fig. 1-2).

    E. Applying positive pressure to the airway throughout the respiratory cycle via the mask-bag-valve device can also be used to relieve the upper airway obstruction.

        1. PROCEDURE

           a. Endotracheal intubation achieves four main goals:

              (1) Airway protection

              (2) Provides upper airway patency

              (3) Pulmonary hygiene

              (4) Allows mechanical positive pressure ventilation

VII. OROTRACHEAL INTUBATION

    A. Successful orotracheal intubation requires alignment of oral, pharyngeal, and laryngeal axes (Fig. 1-5). The optimal position is the "sniffing" position: the head is extended about the atlanto-occipital joint and the neck is extended.

    B. The laryngoscope handle is held in the left hand while the patient's mouth is opened as wide as possible. The laryngoscope blade is inserted into the right side of the mouth, the tongue is swept to the left and the blade is advanced forward toward the base of the tongue. Clear the lips if they are caught between the blade and teeth.

    C. The curved blade is advanced into the vallecula and upward force at a 45-degree angle is used to raise the epiglottis. The straight blade is advanced and the tip of the blade is positioned beneath the epiglottis and upward force is applied in the same manner as with the curved blade. Do not rotate the blade back onto the teeth.

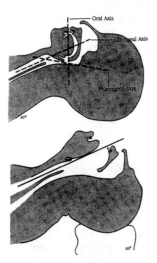

Figure 1-5. Top: In the supine patient, the axes of the mouth, pharynx, and the larynx lie in divergent directions. To facilitate intubation, the axes of these three regions must be brought into close approximation. Bottom: With the patient's head in the proper position and with the use of the laryngoscope, the axes of the mouth, pharynx, and larynx can be brought into approximation, thus allowing easy visualization of the opening to the larynx.

D. Once the glottic opening is visualized, the endotracheal tube is advanced through the vocal cords until the cuff just disappears. The cuff is inflated with enough air to prevent leak during positive-pressure ventilation.

E. Determine that the tube is in the trachea. Signs of tracheal intubation consist of presence of CO_2 in the exhaled breath, breath sounds over the chest, lack of breath sounds over the stomach, lack of gastric distention and respiratory gas moisture in the endotracheal tube.

F. Insertion of the tube to 23 cm at the incisors in males, and 21 cm in females generally provides optimal endotracheal tube position.

G. In the unconscious patient who is considered to have a full stomach, laryngoscopy should be preformed with cricoid pressure (Sellick maneuver). Cricoid pressure should be applied by using the thumb and forefinger together to push downward on the cricoid cartilage. This maneuver can prevent passive regurgitation of stomach contents into the trachea during intubation.

VIII. NASOTRACHEAL INTUBATION

A. The nasal approach generally provides the easier route for intubation.

B. Topical vasoconstrictors such as phenylephrine or cocaine (4%) should be applied to the nares to minimize nasal bleeding.

C. A well-lubricated, warmed tube with the cuff fully deflated should be inserted via either prepared nostril. Once the tube is beyond the nasopharynx, both blind and direct laryngoscopy techniques can be used to accomplish nasotracheal intubations.

D. Nasotracheal intubation is contraindicated in basilar skull fractures, coagulopathies and intranasal abnormalities.

IX. FLEXIBLE ENDOSCOPY AND ALTERNATIVE TECHNIQUES OF AIRWAY MANAGEMENT

A. Flexible endoscopy is useful in suspected spine injury, known or anticipated difficult airway, morbid obesity, and in patients with high risk of aspiration.

B. It may be used in both awake and anesthetized patients via oral or nasal route.

C. It may be useful in critically ill patients to evaluate the endotracheal tube patency and position and to change endotracheal tubes in patients with difficult airways.

D. The LMA or its variants are other alternative devices to manage the patient with a difficult airway.

E. Needle cricothyrotomy and percutaneous dilatational tracheostomy can be done for emergent airway access.

X. COMPLICATIONS OF ENDOTRACHEAL INTUBATION
A. During intubation,
   1. Laryngospasm
   2. Laceration
   3. Bruising of lips or tongue
   4. Damage to teeth
   5. Aspiration
   6. Endobronchial or esophageal intubation
   7. Perforation of oropharynx, trachea or esophagus
   8. Epistaxis
B. Postextubation
   1. Laryngospasm, sore throat, hoarseness, stridor, glottic or subglottic edema
   2. Long-term intubation may result in tracheal stenosis, tracheomalacia, tracheal mucosal ulceration

XI. EXTUBATION
A. Should be done in the patient who is fully awake and can protect his airway.
B. Oropharyngeal secretions should be suctioned, head of the bed should be elevated and endotracheal tube should be removed after a cuff leak test.
C. In patients with a known difficult airway, extubation using a flexible broncho-scope or airway exchange catheter should be considered.
D. Supplemental oxygen should be provided and patient should be observed in a monitoring setting.
E. Emergency airway equipment should be available to manage postextubation problems.

Selected Readings
Behringer EC. Approaches to managing the upper airway. *Anesth Clin North Am* 2002;20: 813–832.
   Detailed and organized article about managing upper airway.

Benumof JL. *Airway management principles and practice.* 1996; St. Louis: Mosby-Year Book.
   The classic textbook in airway management.

Ganzouri E. Preoperative airway assessment: Predictive value of a multivariate risk index. *Anesth Analg* 1996;82:1197–1204.
   Good article about applying a multivariable composite airway risk index in predicting preoperative difficult airways.

Hall CE. Nasotracheal intubation for head and neck surgery. *Anaesthesia* 2003;58:249–256.
   Review article about nasotracheal intubations.

Hillman DR. The upper airway during anaesthesia. *Brit J Anaesth* 2003;91:31–9.
   A description of airway obstruction and treatment modalities.

Itani M. New airway techniques. *Semin Anesth* 2003;22:3–10.
   A review of recent advances in managing the difficult airway.

Langeron O. Prediction of difficult mask ventilation. *Anesthesiology* 2000;92:1229–1236.
   First organized and detailed study evaluating the predictors for difficult mask ventilation.

Moore KL. *Clinically oriented anatomy.* 1999: Baltimore: Williams & Wilkins.
   A very useful anatomy text for the clinician.

Rosenblatt WH. Preoperative planning of airway management in critical care patients. *Crit Care Med* 2004;32:(suppl)186–192.
   Review article about defining the importance of preoperative evaluation in critically ill patients.

CENTRAL VENOUS CATHETER

Shubjeet Kaur and Stephen O. Heard

2

I. GENERAL PRINCIPLES
A. Catheter types
1. Single lumen
2. Multilumen (double, triple or quad)
3. Introducer
4. Double-lumen dialysis catheters
B. Site selection
1. Major sites
   a. Internal jugular vein (IJV)
   b. Subclavian vein (SCV)
   c. External jugular (EJV)
   d. Femoral vein
   e. Antecubital vein (peripherally inserted central catheters).
2. Depends on skill of operator: greater risk of pneumothorax with subclavian approach
3. Risk of infection: femoral > internal jugular > subclavian
C. Methods to reduce risk of catheter infection
1. Education program
2. Use chlorhexidine prep solution
3. Use subclavian site
4. Use of maximum barrier precautions: cap, mask, sterile gloves and gown, sterile drape that covers entire patient
5. Use of antimicrobial impregnated catheters

II. INDICATIONS
1. Monitoring of fluid status
2. Administration of irritant medications or vasoactive substances
3. Total parenteral nutrition
4. Hemodialysis
5. Placement of a temporary transvenous pacing wire
6. Procurement of venous access when peripheral vein cannulation is not possible
7. Aspiration of air in surgical procedures considered high risk for venous air embolism (e.g., posterior fossa craniotomy with the patient in the sitting position).

III. PROCEDURE
A. Antecubital approach (Fig. 2-1A)
1. Patient's arm at the side
2. Basilic vein may be found with aid of ultrasound
3. The antecubital fossa is prepared and draped with strict aseptic technique.
4. A tourniquet is placed proximally to distend the vein.
5. Basilic vein is entered proximal to crease at a 45-degree angle with the needle bevel pointing upward and cephalad.
6. When free backflow of blood is confirmed, the tourniquet is released, a guidewire is inserted through the needle, and the needle is removed.
7. A vessel dilator is threaded over the guidewire if necessary.
8. The dilator is removed and the catheter is advanced over the guidewire.

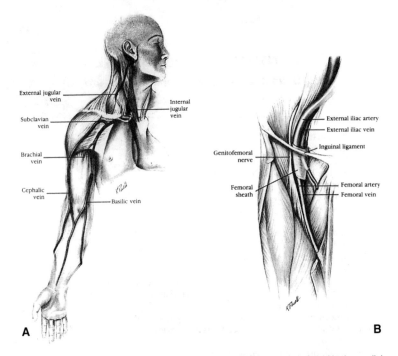

Figure 2-1. (A) Venous anatomy of the upper extremity. The basilic vein is found in the medial part of the antecubital fossa and joins the brachial vein in the upper arm to form the axillary vein. The EJV is formed by the union of the posterior auricular and retromandibular veins, anterior and caudal to the ear; courses obliquely across the anterior surface of the sternocleidomastoid muscle (SCM); pierces the deep fascia posterior to the SCM and joins the subclavian vein at a sharp acute angle behind the medial third of the clavicle. (B) Anatomy of the femoral vein. The femoral vein is a direct continuation of the popliteal vein and becomes the external iliac vein at the inguinal ligament. At the ligament, it lies in the femoral sheath medial to the femoral artery and nerve.

9. The length of insertion is estimated by measuring the distance from the venipuncture site to the manubriosternal junction.

10. The guidewire is removed and the catheter is sutured into place.

11. The first-pass success rate is 70% with the basilic vein approach.

B. Internal jugular vein (IJV) approach

1. Approaches to IJV cannulation are the anterior, central, and posterior (Fig. 2-2).

2. Central

a. The patient is placed in a 15-degree Trendelenburg position and the head is turned to the contralateral side.

b. Using maximum barrier precautions, after infiltration of local anesthetic, the operator punctures the skin with a 22-gauge "finder" needle with an attached syringe at the apex of the triangle formed by the two muscle bellies of the sternocleidomastoid (SCM) and the clavicle. The internal carotid artery pulsation is usually felt 1 to 2 cm medial to this point.

c. The finder needle is directed at a 45-degree angle toward the ipsilateral nipple while the operator applies constant aspiration on the syringe. After successful venipuncture with the finder needle, the large-bore needle is introduced in the identical plane.

d. After cannulation, the guidewire is then inserted through the large needle. Depth of insertion is limited to 15 to 20 cm to avoid arrhythmias.

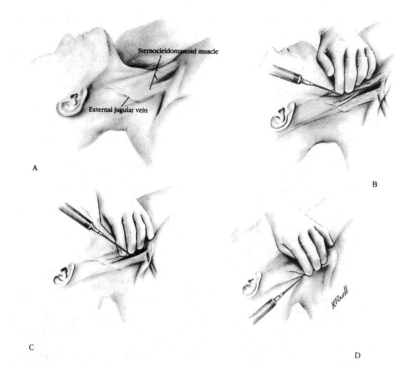

Figure 2-2. Surface anatomy and various approaches to cannulation of the internal jugular vein. *(A)* Surface anatomy. The internal jugular vein emerges from the base of the skull and enters the carotid sheath dorsally with the internal carotid artery, courses posterolaterally to the artery beneath the sternocleidomastoid muscle (SCM), lies medial to the anterior portion of the SCM in its upper part and beneath the triangle formed by the two heads of the muscle in the lower part, and enters the superior vena cava near the medial border of the anterior scalene muscle and beneath the sternal border of the clavicle. *(B)* Anterior approach. *(C)* Central approach. *(D)* Posterior approach. To provide greater clarity of the anatomical landmarks,the sterile drape has been omitted from the figure.

    e. The central venous cathether (CVC) is then threaded over the guide wire after using a scalpel to make a larger skin incision if needed and a dilator to dilate the subcutaneous tract.
  3. Anterior approach (see Fig. 2-2). Initial needle insertion is 0.5 to 1 cm. lateral to the carotid artery pulsation at the midpoint of the sternal head of the SCM.
  4. Posterior approach.
    a. The EJV is the key landmark.
    b. The needle is inserted 1 cm dorsal to the point where the EJV crosses the posterior border of the SCM or 5 cm cephalad from the clavicle along the clavicular head of the SCM and is directed caudally and ventrally toward the suprasternal notch at an angle of 45 degrees from the sagittal plane and with a 15-degree upward angulation.
C. External jugular vein approach (see Fig. 2-1A)
  1. The patient is placed in a slight Trendelenburg position, with arms by the side and face turned to the contralateral side.
  2. After sterile preparation, the venipuncture is performed with a 16-gauge catheter over the needle, using the operator's left index finger and thumb to distend and anchor the vein.
  3. The needle is advanced in the axis of the vein at 20 degrees to the frontal plane. When free backflow of blood is established, the needle is advanced a few millimeters further, and the catheter is threaded into the vein over the needle.

    4. A guidewire can be introduced through this catheter, and a CVC can be advanced over the guidewire.

    5. Abduction of the ipsilateral arm and anteroposterior pressure exerted on the clavicle may help the guidewire to negotiate the angle formed at the junction of the EJV with the SCV.

    6. The EJV can be successfully cannulated in 80% of patients.

D. Femoral vein approach (see Fig. 2-1B)

    1. The patient is placed supine, the groin is prepared and draped, and the venipuncture is made 1 to 1.5 cm medial to the femoral arterial pulsation.

    2. The femoral arterial pulsation is usually found at the junction of the medial and middle third of a line joining the anterior superior iliac spine and the pubic tubercle.

    3. An 18-gauge thin-walled needle attached to a syringe is inserted at a 45-degree angle pointing cephalad and 2 to 3 cm inferior to the inguinal ligament to minimize the risk of a retroperitoneal hematoma in the event of an arterial puncture.

    4. Once venous blood return is established, the syringe is depressed to skin level and free aspiration of blood is reconfirmed.

    5. A guidewire and subsequently a dilator are advanced, and the catheter is finally threaded over the guidewire after the dilator has been removed.

E. Subclavian vein approach (Fig. 2-3)

    1. The patient is placed in a 15- to 30-degree Trendelenburg position, with a small bedroll between the scapulae.

    2. The patient's head is turned to the contralateral side, and arms are by the side.

    3. Infraclavicular approach

        a. Skin puncture is made with an 18-gauge thin-wall needle attached to a syringe, 2 to 3 cm caudal to the midpoint of the clavicle and directed toward the suprasternal notch until it abuts the clavicle.

        b. The needle is "walked" down the clavicle until the inferior edge is cleared.

        c. As the needle is advanced, it is kept as close to the inferior edge of the clavicle as possible to avoid puncturing the dome of the pleura.

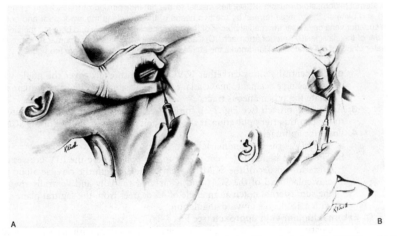

A   B

Figure 2-3. *(A)* Patient positioning for subclavian cannulation. The subclavian vein (SCV) is a direct continuation of the axillary vein, beginning at the lateral border of the first rib and extending 3 to 4 cm along the undersurface of the clavicle to join the ipsilateral internal jugular vein behind the sternoclavicular articulation to become the brachiocephalic vein. The SCV is bordered by muscles anteriorly, the subclavian artery and brachial plexus posteriorly, and the first rib inferiorly. *(B)* Cannulation technique for the supraclavicular approach. To provide greater clarity of the anatomical landmarks, the sterile drape has been omitted from the figure.

    d. When blood return is established, the needle bevel (initially facing upward) is turned 90 degrees toward the heart, the syringe is removed, the guidewire is inserted, the needle is removed, and a dilator is advanced over the guidewire and removed.

    e. The CVC is advanced over the guidewire to the appropriate depth.

  4. Supraclavicular approach

    a. The skin puncture is just above the clavicle and is lateral to the insertion of the clavicular head of the SCM.

    b. The needle is advanced toward the contralateral nipple, just under the clavicle, and it should enter the jugular subclavian at a depth of 1 to 4 cm.

    c. A 90% to 95% success rate can be achieved with this approach.

IV. POSTPROCEDURE CONSIDERATIONS

  A. A chest radiograph is required to confirm proper position of the catheter and to ensure absence of a pneumothorax.

    1. Positioning of the catheter tip within the right atrium or right ventricle may result in perforation of the cardiac wall and tamponade.

    2. Arrhythmias from mechanical irritation may also result from catheter tip malposition. The caval atrial junction is approximately 13 to 17 cm from the right-sided SCV or IJV insertion sites and 15 to 20 cm for left-sided insertions.

  B. Complications

    1. Vascular erosions

      a. Hemothorax or hydrothorax

      b. Cardiac tamponade

      c. Air and catheter embolism

        (1) Hematoma

        (2) Infection

        (3) Arterial puncture

        (4) Pneumothorax

Selected Readings

Keenan SP. Use of ultrasound to place central lines. *J Crit Care* 2002;17:126–137.
Review of the utility of ultrasound to insert central venous catheters.

McGee DC, Gould MK. Preventing complications of central venous catheterization. *N Engl J Med* 2003;348:1123–1133.
Concise review of the mechanical and infectious complications associated with central venous catheterization.

O'Grady NP, Alexander M, Dellinger EP, et al. Guidelines for the prevention of intravascular catheter-related infections. *Infect Control Hosp Epidemiol* 2002;23:759–769.
Comprehensive review of and recommendations to prevent intravascular catheter—related infections.

Seneff MG. Central venous catheters. In: Irwin RS, Rippe JM, Curley FJ, et al., eds. *Procedures and techniques in intensive care medicine,* 3rd ed. Philadelphia: Lippincott Williams and Wilkins, 2003.
More detailed description of the techniques used to insert central venous catheters.

ARTERIAL LINE PLACEMENT AND CARE
Khaldoun Faris

I. GENERAL PRINCIPLES
A. Cannulation sites
1. Radial artery
2. Dorsalis pedis artery
3. Brachial artery
4. Femoral artery
5. Axillary artery

B. Anatomy
1. The radial artery is one of two final branches of the brachial artery. It lies just lateral to the flexor carpi radialis at the wrist (Fig. 3-1). The anastomoses between radial and ulnar arteries provide excellent collateral flow to the hand. A

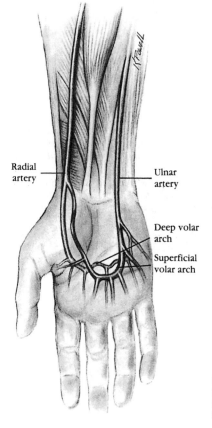

Radial artery

Ulnar artery

Deep volar arch

Superficial volar arch

Figure 3-1. Anatomy of the radial artery. Note the collateral circulation to the ulnar artery through the deep volar arterial arch and dorsal arch.

competent superficial or deep arch must be present to ensure adequate collateral flow.

2. The dorsalis pedis artery runs from the level of the ankle to the great toe. It lies very superficially and just lateral to the tendon of the extensor hallucis longus.

3. The brachial artery lies in the antecubital fossa, medial to the tendon of the biceps, and in close proximity to the median nerve.

4. The common femoral artery courses under the inguinal ligament near the junction of the ligament's medial and middle thirds (Fig. 3-2).

5. The axillary artery begins at the lateral border of the first rib and ends at the inferior margin of the teres major muscle. The artery is mostly superficial and covered only by skin and fasciae.

C. Site selection

1. The ideal artery should have extensive collateral circulation that will maintain the viability of distal tissues if thrombosis occurs.

2. The site should be comfortable for the patient, accessible for nursing care, and close to the monitoring equipment.

3. Sites involved by infection or disruption in the epidermal barrier should be avoided.

4. Larger arteries and catheters provide more accurate (central aortic) pressure measurements. Distal artery recordings yield higher systolic values than central artery recordings, but the mean pressures are similar.

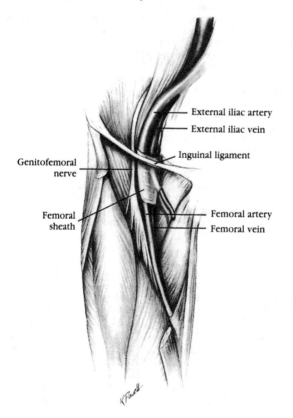

External iliac artery

External iliac vein

Inguinal ligament

Genitofemoral nerve

Femoral sheath

Femoral artery

Femoral vein

Figure 3-2. Anatomy of the femoral artery and adjacent structures. The artery is cannulated below the inguinal ligament.

II. INDICATIONS

A. Hemodynamic monitoring
  1. Beat-to-beat changes
  2. Waveform inspection
  3. The effect of arrhythmia on perfusion

B. Frequent arterial blood gas sampling (more than two measurements per day)

C. Arterial administration of drugs such as thrombolytics

D. Intraaortic balloon pump use

III. PROCEDURE

A. Equipment

1. The equipment necessary to display and measure arterial waveform includes:
  a. An appropriate intravascular catheter
  b. Fluid-filled noncompliant tubing with stopcocks
  c. A transducer
  d. A constant flushing device
  e. Electronic monitoring equipment consisting of a connecting cable, a monitor with amplifier, a display screen, and a recorder

2. Sources of error
  a. Improper zeroing of the system is the single most important source of error.
  b. Calibration of the system is usually not necessary because of standardization of the disposable transducer.
  d. If the zero referencing and calibration are correct, a fast-flush test will assess the system's dynamic response.
  d. An optimum fast-flush test results in an undershoot followed by a small overshoot, then settles to the patient's waveform (Fig. 3-3).
  e. Overdamped tracings are usually caused by air bubbles, kinks, clot formation, compliant tubing, loose connections, a deflated pressure bag, or anatomic factors. All these problems are usually correctable.
  f. Underdamped tracings are caused by long tubing or an increased inotropic or chronotropic state.

B. Technique

1. Radial artery cannulation
  a. Modified Allen test
    (1) The modified Allen test is sometimes used to assess the degree of collateral flow.
    (2) To perform this test, the examiner compresses both radial and ulnar arteries and asks the patient to clench and unclench the fist repeatedly until pallor of the palm is produced. One artery is then released, and the time to blushing of the palm is noted. The procedure is repeated with the other artery.

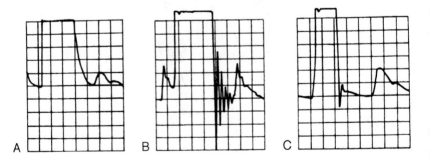

A   B   C

Figure 3-3. Fast-flush test. (A) Overdamped system. (B) Underdamped system. (C) Optimal damping.

(3) Normal palmar blushing is complete before 7 seconds (positive test), 8 to 14 seconds is considered equivocal, and a result of 15 or more seconds is abnormal (negative test).

(4) Hyperextension of the hand is avoided, because it may cause a false-negative result.

(5) The modified Allen test does not necessarily predict the presence of collateral circulation, and some centers have abandoned its use as a routine screening procedure.

b. Percutaneous insertion

(1) The hand is placed in 30 to 60 degrees of dorsiflexion. The volar aspect of the wrist is prepared and draped using the sterile technique and lidocaine is infiltrated through a 25-gauge needle.

(2) A 20-gauge, Teflon 1.5- to 2-inch catheter-over-needle apparatus is used for the puncture. Entry is made at a 30- to 60-degree angle to the skin approximately 3 cm proximal to the distal wrist crease.

(3) The needle and cannula are advanced until arterial blood return is noted in the hub (Fig. 3-4). A small amount of further advancement is necessary for the cannula to enter the artery as well.

(4) With this accomplished, needle and cannula are brought flat to the skin and the cannula is advanced to its hub with a firm, steady rotary action.

(5) Correct positioning is confirmed by pulsatile blood return on removal of the needle.

(6) The cannula is then secured firmly and attached to the transducer tubing. Aseptic ointment is applied and the site is bandaged

c. Special catheter

(1) Catheters with self-contained guidewires to facilitate passage of cannula into the artery are available.

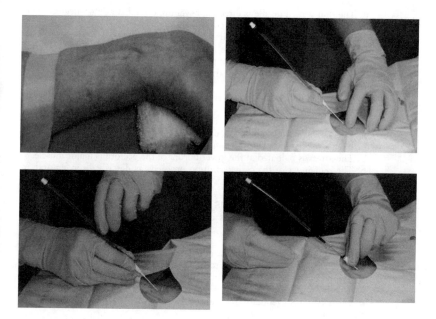

Figure 3-4. Cannulation of the radial artery. *(A)* A towel is placed behind the wrist, and the hand is immobilized with tape. The radial artery is fixated with a 20-gauge angiocatheter connected to a 5-mL syringe (optional). *(B)* The angiocatheter is withdrawn until pulsatile blood return is noted. *(C)* The trocar is withdrawn as the Teflon catheter is simultaneously advanced.

       (2) Percutaneous puncture is made in the same manner, but when blood return is noted in the catheter hub, the guidewire is passed through the needle into the artery to serve as a stent for subsequent catheter advancement.

       (3) The guidewire and needle are then removed and placement is confirmed by pulsatile blood return.

  2. Dorsalis pedis artery cannulation

    a. The patient's foot is placed in plantar flexion and is prepared in the usual fashion.

    b. Vessel entry is obtained approximately halfway up the dorsum of the foot.

    c. Advancement is the same as with cannulation of the radial artery.

    d. Systolic pressure readings are usually 5 to 20 mm Hg higher with dorsalis pedis catheters than with radial artery catheters, but mean pressure values are generally unchanged.

  3. Brachial artery cannulation

    a. Brachial artery cannulation is infrequently performed because of concern regarding the lack of effective collateral circulation.

    b. The median nerve lies in close proximity to the brachial artery in the antecubital fossa and may be punctured in 1% to 2% of cases.

    c. Cannulation of the brachial artery can be performed with a 2-inch catheter over-the-needle apparatus as described for radial artery catheterization.

  4. Femoral artery cannulation

    a. The artery is cannulated using the Seldinger technique and any one of several available prepackaged kits.

    b. The patient lies supine with the leg extended and slightly abducted.

    c. Skin puncture should be made a few centimeters caudal to the inguinal ligament to minimize the risk of retroperitoneal hematoma or bowel perforation.

    d. The thin-walled needle is directed, bevel up, cephalad at a 45-degree angle. When arterial blood return is confirmed, the needle and syringe are brought down against the skin to facilitate guidewire passage.

    e. The guidewire is inserted, the needle is withdrawn, and a stab incision is made with a scalpel at the skin puncture site.

    f. The catheter is threaded over the guidewire to its hub, and the guidewire is withdrawn.

    g. The catheter is then sutured securely to the skin and is connected to the transducer tubing.

  5. Axillary artery cannulation

    a. The patient's arm is abducted, externally rotated, and flexed at the elbow by having the patient place the hand under his or her head.

    b. The artery is palpated at the lower border of the pectoralis major muscle.

    c. The remainder of the catheterization proceeds as described for femoral artery cannulation.

IV. POSTPROCEDURE CONSIDERATIONS

  A. Complications. The complications associated with arterial catheterization are listed in Table 3-1.

    1. Thrombosis

      a. Thrombosis is the single most common complication of intraarterial catheters with an incidence of 5% to 25%.

      b. Symptomatic occlusion requiring surgical intervention occurs in less than 1% of cases.

      c. Most patients eventually recanalize, generally by 3 weeks after removal of the catheter.

      d. If evidence of ischemia persists after catheter removal, thrombolytic therapy, radiologic or surgical embolectomy, or cervical sympathetic blockade is a treatment option.

TABLE 3-1	Complications Associated with Arterial Cannulation
Site	**Complication**
All sites	Pain and swelling
	Thrombosis
	Asymptomatic
	Symptomatic
	Embolization
	Hematoma
	Hemorrhage
	Limb ischemia
	Catheter-related infection
	Local
	Systemic
	Diagnostic blood loss
	Pseudoaneurysm
	Heparin-associated thrombocytopenia
Radial artery	Cerebral embolization
	Peripheral neuropathy
Femoral artery	Retroperitoneal hemorrhage
	Bowel perforation
	Arteriovenous fistula
Axillary artery	Cerebral embolization
	Brachial plexopathy
Brachial artery	Median nerve damage
	Cerebral embolization

2. Cerebral embolization
   a. Factors that increase the risk for retrograde passage of air into the cerebral circulation are patient size and position (air travels up in a sitting patient), injection site, and flush rate.
   b. The risk is minimized by clearing all air from tubing before flushing, opening the flush valve for no more than 2 to 3 seconds, and avoiding overaggressive manual flushing of the line.
3. Diagnostic blood loss (DBL)
   a. In patients with frequent arterial blood gas determinations, DBL can be substantial and result in a transfusion requirement.
   b. DBL can be minimized in several ways, including tubing systems that use a reservoir for blood sampling, continuous intraarterial blood gas monitoring, point of care microchemistry analysis, and the use of pediatric collection tubes.
4. Infection
   a. Infectious sequelae are the most important clinical complications associated with arterial cannulation.
   b. Operators must wash their hands and wear sterile gloves during insertion and care of the catheter.
   c. Nursing personnel should follow strict guidelines when drawing blood samples or manipulating tubing.
   d. Daily inspection of the site is mandatory, and the catheter should be removed promptly if signs of infection are noted.
   e. It is no longer necessary to change arterial catheters routinely, because studies of catheters remaining in place a week or longer have not demonstrated a higher rate of clinically important infection.

Selected Readings

Ejrup B, Fischer B, Wright IS. Clinical evaluation of blood flow to the hand: the false-positive Allen test. *Circulation* 1966;33:778.
More detail about the Allen test.

Gardner RM. Accuracy and reliability of disposable pressure transducer coupled with modern pressure monitors. *Crit Care Med* 1996;24:879.
Good material to read for understanding of equipment used to monitor arterial pressure invasively.

Mann S, Jones RI, Miller-Craig MW, et al. The safety of ambulatory intraarterial pressure monitoring: a clinical audit of 1000 studies. *Int J Cardiol* 1984;5:585.
Details about complications related to brachial artery cannulation.

Seneff MG. Arterial line placement and care. In: Irwin RS, Rippe JM, eds. *Irwin and Rippe's intensive care medicine, 5th ed*. Philadelphia: Lippincott Williams and Wilkins, 2003;36–45.
Thorough and detailed chapter about arterial lines.

Slogoff S, Keats AS, Arlund C. On the safety of radial artery cannulation. *Anesthesiology* 1983;59:42.
Good review about the safety of radial artery cannulation.

Wilkins RG. Radial artery cannulation and ischemic damage: a review. *Anesthesia* 1985; 40:896.
This article provides more detail about safety of this procedure.

PULMONARY ARTERY CATHETERS
Khaldoun Faris

I. GENERAL PRINCIPLES
A. Objectives
1. Assess left ventricular (LV) or right ventricular (RV) function
2. Monitor hemodynamic status
3. Guide treatment
4. Provide prognostic information

B. Types
1. Standard pulmonary artery (PA) catheter
2. Pacing PA catheter
3. Continuous cardiac output PA catheter
4. Continuous mixed venous O_2 PA catheter
5. RV ejection fraction PA catheter

II. INDICATIONS
A. Cardiovascular disease
1. Myocardial infarction, associated with cardiogenic shock, mechanical complications or right heart failure
2. Severe or progressive congestive heart failure
3. Primary pulmonary hypertension for diagnosis and to guide vasodilator therapy
4. Shock

B. Perioperative period
1. Cardiac surgery
2. Aortic and peripheral vascular surgery
3. Major abdominal and thoracic surgery

C. Critical illness
1. Major trauma
2. Severe sepsis and septic shock
3. Acute renal failure
4. Major burns
5. Acute respiratory distress syndrome with multiple-organ dysfunction.
6. Severe head injury with refractory intracranial hypertension
7. Cerebral vasospasm
8. Severe preeclampsia/eclampsia

III. PROCEDURE
A. Equipment
1. The standard catheter length is 110 cm, and the most commonly used external diameter is 5 or 7 French.
2. A balloon is present 1 to 2 mm from the tip; when it is inflated with air or filtered CO_2, it guides the catheter from the greater intrathoracic veins through the right heart chambers into the PA.
3. The standard PA catheter used in the ICU is a quadruple-lumen catheter, which has a lumen containing electrical leads for a thermistor positioned at the catheter surface 4 cm proximal to its tip. The thermistor measures PA blood temperature and allows thermodilution cardiac output measurements.
4. A five-lumen catheter allows passage of a specially designed 2.4-Fr bipolar pacing electrode probe through the additional lumen for intracardiac pacing.

5. Continuous mixed venous oxygen saturation measurement is clinically available using a fiberoptic five-lumen PA catheter.

6. Catheters equipped with fast-response (95 milliseconds) thermistors allow determination of right ventricle ejection fraction (RVEF) and RV systolic time intervals.

B. Technique

1. Standard PA catheter insertion procedure

a. Central venous access using the appropriate size introducer sheath must first be obtained using sterile technique (see Chapter 2).

b. Continuous monitoring of the ECG and pressure waveforms of the catheter is required as well as equipment and supplies for cardiopulmonary resuscitation.

c. Pass the catheter through the introducer sheath into the vein and advance it, using the marks on the catheter shaft indicating 10-cm distances from the tip, until the tip is in the right atrium.

d. This maneuver requires advancement of approximately 35 to 40 cm from the left antecubital fossa, 10 to 15 cm from the internal jugular vein, 10 cm from the subclavian vein, and 35 to 40 cm from the femoral vein.

e. A right atrial waveform on the monitor with appropriate fluctuations accompanying respiratory changes or cough confirms proper intrathoracic location (Fig. 4-1).

f. With the catheter tip in the right atrium, inflate the balloon with the recommended amount of air or carbon dioxide.

(1) Inflation of the balloon should be associated with a slight feeling of resistance—if it is not, suspect balloon rupture and do not attempt further inflation or advancement of the catheter until balloon integrity has been properly reevaluated.

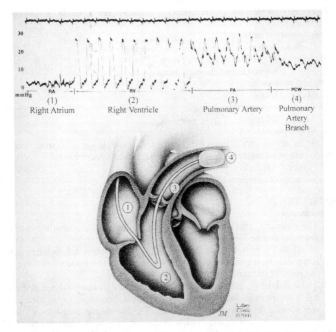

Figure 4-1. Pressure tracing recordings with corresponding locations as the pulmonary artery catheter is passed into the occlusion position. (Reprinted with permission from O'Donnell JM, Nacul FE. *Surgical intensive care medicine.* Kulwer Academic Publishers, 2001, p. 47)

(2) If significant resistance to balloon inflation is encountered, suspect malposition of the catheter in a small vessel; withdraw the catheter and re-advance it to a new position.

(3) Do not use liquids to inflate the balloon because they may be irretrievable and could prevent balloon deflation.

g. With the balloon inflated, advance the catheter until an RV pressure tracing is seen. Continue advancing the catheter until the diastolic pressure tracing rises above that observed in the RV center, thus indicating PA placement. Raising the head of the bed and tilting the patient to the right will facilitate passage of the catheter through the RV and reduce the risk of arrhythmias.

h. Advancement beyond the PA position results in a fall on the pressure tracing from the levels of systolic pressure noted in the RV and PA. When this is noted, record the pulmonary artery occlusion pressure (PAOP) and deflate the balloon.

i. Phasic PA pressure should reappear on the pressure tracing when the balloon is deflated. If it does not, pull back the catheter with the deflated balloon until the PA tracing appears.

(1) Carefully record the balloon inflation volume needed to change the PA pressure tracing to the PAOP tracing.

(2) If the inflation volume is significantly lower than the manufacturer's recommended volume, or if subsequent PAOP determinations require decreasing balloon inflation volumes as compared with an initial appropriate volume, the catheter tip has migrated too far peripherally and should be pulled back immediately.

j. Most introducers have a valve that can be tightened to secure the catheter in the correct PA position. To avoid catheter kinkage, the valve should not be tightened too much..

k. Order a chest radiograph to confirm the catheter's position; the catheter tip should appear no more than 3 to 5 cm from the midline.

2. Paceport PA catheter insertion procedure

a. The Paceport catheter has an additional lumen 19 cm from the catheter tip (the RV port), which allows passage of a specially designed 2.4-Fr pacemaker wire (probe).

b. The catheter is inserted as described for a standard PA catheter.

c. Connect the RV port to a pressure transducer to verify the location of the orifice in the RV. Ideally, the RV orifice is positioned 1 to 2 cm distal to the tricuspid valve.

(1) To achieve this after initial placement, pull the catheter back until a right atrial pressure tracing is recorded from the RV port.

(2) Advance the catheter (with balloon inflated) until an RV pressure tracing is first obtained. At this point, the opening of the RV port is at the level of the tricuspid valve; simply advancing the catheter an additional 1 to 2 cm will place the opening in the desired position.

(3) A special package enables sterile introduction of the pacemaker probe. Attach the tip of the pacemaker probe introducer package to the hub of the RV port.

(4) Advance the 2.4-Fr pacing probe gently through the Paceport lumen. Passage of the probe is facilitated by keeping the extravascular portion of the PA catheter as straight as possible and by keeping the probe on its packaging spool during insertion.

(5) Allow the spool to spin slowly as the probe is advanced. When the marker on the probe reaches the 0 marking on the external part of the RV lumen, the tip of the probe is at the lumen opening.

(6) Connect the distal electrode of the probe to the V lead of an ECG and advance it until ST-segment elevation occurs, thereby indicating contact with the endocardium.

(7) Connect the probe to a pacemaker generator and check the thresholds.

(8) Obtain a chest radiograph to ensure proper probe placement at the RV apex.

IV. POSTPROCEDURE CONSIDERATIONS
A. Pressure and waveform interpretation
1. Normal resting right atrial pressure is 0 to 6 mm Hg.
2. The normal resting RV pressure is 17 to 30/0 to 6 mm Hg.
3. The RV systolic pressure should equal the PA systolic pressure (except in cases of pulmonic stenosis or RV outflow tract obstruction).
4. The RV pressure should equal the mean right atrial pressure during diastole when the tricuspid valve is open.
5. Normal resting PA pressure is 15 to 30/5 to 13 mm Hg with a normal mean pressure of 10 to 18 mm Hg.
6. The normal resting PAOP is 2 to 12 mm Hg and averages 2 to 7 mm Hg below the mean PA pressure.
7. Wedge position may be confirmed by measuring an oxygen saturation of 95% or more from blood withdrawn from the distal lumen.
8. PAOP should be measured at end expiration because pleural pressure returns to baseline at the end of passive deflation.

B. Cardiac output measurement
1. Most PA catheters are equipped with a thermistor 4 cm from the tip that allows calculation of cardiac output using the thermodilution principle.
2. In practice, a known amount of cold or room temperature solution (typically 10 mL of normal saline in adults and 5 mL of normal saline in children) is injected into the right atrium through the catheter's proximal port.
3. The thermistor allows recording of the baseline PA blood temperature and subsequent temperature change.
4. Cardiac output is inversely proportional to the integral of the time-versus-temperature curve.
5. Thermodilution cardiac output is inaccurate in low-output states, tricuspid regurgitation, and atrial or ventricular septal defects.

C. Complications
1. Balloon rupture
2. Knotting
3. Pulmonary infarction (peripheral migration of the catheter with persistent undetected wedging of the catheter)
4. PA perforation
   a. Incidence is approximately 0.1% to 0.2%, although recent pathologic data suggest that the true incidence of PA perforation is higher.
   b. Risk factors include pulmonary hypertension, mitral valve disease, advanced age, hypothermia, and anticoagulant therapy.
   c. Technical factors related to PA hemorrhage are distal placement or migration of the catheter, excessive catheter manipulation, use of stiffer catheter designs, and multiple overzealous or prolonged balloon inflations.
   d. PA perforation typically presents with hemoptysis.
   e. Emergency management for significant bleeding includes:
      (1) Immediate wedge arteriography and bronchoscopy, intubation of the unaffected lung, and consideration of emergent embolization of the bleeding artery or emergency lobectomy or pneumonectomy.
      (2) PA catheter balloon tamponade resulted in rapid control of bleeding in one case report.
      (3) Application of positive end-expiratory pressure (PEEP) to intubated patients may also produce tamponade of hemorrhage caused by a PA catheter.
5. Thromboembolic complications
6. Rhythm disturbances
   a. Atrial and ventricular arrhythmias occur commonly during insertion of PA catheters.

TABLE 4-1 Hemodynamic Parameters in Commonly Encountered Clinical Situations (idealized)

	RA	RV	PA	PAWP	AO	CI	SVR	PVR
Normal	0–6	25/0–6	25/6–12	6–12	130/80	≥2.5	1,500	≤250
Hypovolemic shock	0–2	15–20/0–2	15–20/2–6	2–6	≤90/60	<2.0	>1,500	≤250
Cardiogenic Shock	8	50/8	50/35	35	≤90/60	<2.0	>1,500	≤250
Septic Shock								
Early	0–2	20–25/0–2	20–25/0–6	0–6	≤90/60	≥2.5	<1,500	<250
Late[a]	0–4	25/4–10	25/4–10	4–10	≤90/60	<2.0	>1,500	>250
Acute massive pulmonary embolish	8–12	50/12	50/12–15	≤12	≤90/60	<2.0	>1,500	>450
Cardiac tamponade	12–18	25/12–18	25/12–18	12–18	≤90/60	<2.0	>1,500	≤250
AMI without LVF	0–6	25/0–6	25/12–18	≤18	140/90	≤2.5	1,500	≤250
AMI with LVF	0–6	30–40/0–6	30–40/18–25	>18	140/90	>2.0	>1,500	>250
Biventricular failure secondary to LVF	>6	50–60/>6	50–60/25	18–25	120/80	<2.0	>1,500	>250
RVF secondary to RVI	12–20	30/12–20	30/12	<12	≤90/60	~2.0	>1,500	>250
Cor pulmonale	>6	80/>6	80/35	<12	120/80	~2.0	>1,500	>400
Idiopathic pulmonary hypertension	0–6	80–100/0–6	80–100/40	<12	100/60	<2.0	>1,500	>500
Acute VSR[b]	6	60/6–8	60/35	30	≤90/60	<2.0	>1,500	>250

RA, right atrium; RV, right ventricle; PA, pulmonary artery; PAWP, pulmonary artery wedge pressure; AO, aortic; CI, cardiac index; SVR, systemic vascular resistance; PVR, pulmonary vascular resistance; AMI, acute myocardial infarction; LVF, left ventricular failure; RVF, right ventricular failure; RVI, right ventricular infarction; VSR, ventricular septal rupture.

[a]Hemodynamic profile seen in approximately one third of patients in late septic shock.
[b]Confirmed by appropriate RA–PA oxygen saturation step-up.
Adapted from Gore JM, Albert JS, Benotti JR, et al. *Handbook of hemodynamic monitoring*. Boston: Little, Brown, 1984.

    b. Patients with preexisting left bundle branch block are at risk of developing complete heart block during catheter insertion.

    7. Intracardiac damage

    8. Catheter-related bloodstream infection and bacterial endocarditis

D. Appropriate use of pulmonary artery catheters

    1. An observational study published in 1996 by Connors et al. reported an association between the use of PA catheterization and an increased risk of death, costs, length of stay, and intensity of care.

    2. A randomized trial conducted by the Canadian Critical Care Clinical Trials Group to compare goal-directed therapy guided by a PA catheter with standard care without the use of a PA catheter in elderly, high-risk surgical patients showed no improvement in mortality.

    3. A recently published multicenter randomized controlled trial conducted in France demonstrated that the use of PA catheters in the management of shock or ARDS, or both, albeit safe, does not improve mortality or mobidity.

Selected Readings

Connors, AF, Speroff T, Dawson NV, et al. The effectiveness of right heart catheterization in the initial care of critically ill patients. *JAMA* 1996;276:889.
Prospective cohort study of 5,735 patients in an intensive care unit illustrating the need for a randomized control trial of pulmonary artery catheters.

Mark JB. *Atlas of cardiovascular monitoring.* New York: Churchill Livingstone, 1998.
Clear, concise manual for expert interpretation of hemodynamic waveforms.

O'Quin R, Marini JJ. Pulmonary artery occlusion pressure: clinical physiology, measurement, and interpretation. *Am Rev Respir Dis* 1983;128:319.
Nice discussion of possible errors made in the measurement of PAOP.

Richard C, Warszawski J, Anguel N, et al. Early use of the pulmonary artery catheter and outcomes in patients with shock and acute respiratory distress syndrome. *JAMA.* 2003;290:2713–2720.
PA catheters do not improve mortality or morbidity in the setting of shock or ARDS, or both. The study was not goal-directed, and echocardiography was used more frequently in the control group.

Sandham JD, Hull RD, Brant RF, et al. A randomized controlled trial of the use of pulmonary-artery catheters in high-risk surgical patients. *N Engl J Med* 2003;348:5–14.
There was no difference in mortality between patients monitored with pulmonary artery catheters and treated with goal-directed therapy and control patients.

Teboul JL, Zapol WM, Brun-Bruisson C, et al. A comparison of pulmonary artery occlusion pressure and left ventricular end-diastolic pressure during mechanical ventilation with PEEP in patients with severe ARDS. *Anesthesiology* 1989;70:261.
PAOP as a reliable indicator of LVEDP in adult respiratory distress syndrome with up to 20 PEEP.

Voyce SJ, McCaffree DR. Pulmonary artery catheters. In: Irwin RS, Rippe JM, eds. *Irwin and Rippe's intensive care medicine,* 5th edition. Philadelphia: Lippincott Williams and Wilkins, 2003;45–67
Thorough and detailed chapter about pulmonary artery catheters.

CARDIOVERSION AND DEFIBRILLATION

Paulo Oliveira and Deborah H. Markowitz

5

I. GENERAL PRINCIPLES. Cardioversion and defibrillation involve delivering a quantity of electrical energy to depolarize the myocardium to terminate a tachyarrhythmia.

  A. Cardioversion delivers the shock at a specific point in the electromechanical cycle, which is *synchronized* to coincide with the QRS complex of the electrocardiogram (ECG). There is a significant risk of inducing ventricular fibrillation (VFib) should the countershock fall on the "vulnerable" period of late ventricular systole marked by the T wave on the ECG. Thus, under most circumstances, emergency and elective treatment of various tachyarrhythmias requires *synchronized* cardioversion.

  B. Defibrillation delivers electrical energy in a nonsynchronized manner to terminate fibrillating rhythms, most notably VFib. Because VFib is immediately life-threatening, and because there is no well-defined QRS complex, a random electrical countershock is delivered during the cardiac cycle. Thus, by definition, defibrillation is *unsynchronized*.

  C. Biphasic defibrillation: One of the main goals of modern electric countershock therapy is to provide the lowest amount of energy to successfully terminate a tachyarrhythmia while avoiding myocardial damage from delivery of high energy. Too little energy may not eradicate the arrhythmia and may actually lead to its propagation. Pursuit of a balance of sufficient electrical energy has led to the development of new waveform technology in the form of biphasic defibrillation waveform, as opposed to monophasic waveform.

   1. Monophasic defibrillation waveforms, used in most manual defibrillators, are unipolar and deliver current in one direction through the heart.

   2. The bipolar nature of these waveforms leads to the delivery of current through the heart that reverses polarity and returns back through the myocardium. Thus, the energy needed for successful termination of tachyarrhythmias is much less when compared to monophasic waveforms. Biphasic waveform shocks of relatively low energy (150 to 200 J) are safe and have equivalent or higher efficacy for termination of VFib compared with higher energy escalating (i.e., 200, 300, 360 J) monophasic waveform shocks. This technology is now available in most automatic external defibrillators (AEDs), implantable cardioverters-defibrillators (ICDs) and many manual defibrillators.

II. TECHNICAL CONSIDERATIONS. The efficacy of the countershock depends on the size of the paddles, the skin–electrode interface, and the location of the paddles on the thorax. These relate to the concept of transthoracic impedance (the resistance to current flow through the heart), which ultimately influences cardioversion/defibrillation success and the level of electrical energy required.

  A. Paddle size. To a limit, a larger electrode size will decrease transthoracic resistance and consequently increase the current density delivered to a greater area of myocardium.

  B. Self-adhesive pads. Hand-held paddles are traditional, but self-adhesive pads are now widely available, likely more effective, and have several advantages over hand-held paddles. The operator does not come into contact with the bed and thus avoids the risk of receiving an electrical shock. The application of conductive gel is not necessary. If the defibrillator is equipped with pacing capabilities, the pads may be used for external pacing should bradycardia or asystole occur after countershocking.

C. Skin contact. Both electrode/paddle types need uniform application to the skin and the skin–electrode interface will also contribute to the overall transthoracic impedance to current flow.

D. Conductive gel. For hand-held electrodes, a layer of conductive gel is required over their entire surface to prevent skin burns. The gel must be a conductive type that contains salt; use of non–salt-containing gels, such as ultrasound gels, leads to increased impedance to flow (and thus unsuccessful cardioversion) as well as potential burn injuries.

III. CARDIOVERSION PROCEDURE

A. Patient preparation. Success for elective procedures is optimized by the following:

1. Serum electrolytes should be normalized and acidosis and hypoxemia corrected for greater success in maintaining normal sinus rhythm after cardioversion.
2. Digoxin level should be normal to prevent proarrhythmic side effects.
3. Fasting for 8 hours or more may help prevent aspiration.
4. A 12-lead ECG should be obtained before and after the procedure.
5. An intravenous catheter should be placed in case antiarrhythmic medications or pressors need to be infused on an emergency basis.
6. Vital signs, rhythm, and respiratory status should be monitored continuously.

B. Anesthesia. Short-acting sedatives, such as midazolam, should be carefully titrated to avoid respiratory depression and the need for mechanical ventilation.

C. Paddle positioning. Unsuccessful countershocks are due mostly to incorrect electrode placement. It is important to maximize the amount of myocardium in the electrical pathway.

1. **Anterolateral.** Place the anterior paddle just to the left of the patient's sternum and below the sternomanubrial joint and the lateral paddle over the cardiac apex.
2. **Anteroposterior.** Position the anterior paddle over the left precordium and the posterior paddle just below the tip of the left scapula. Less energy is required and the success rate is higher with this position, particularly for atrial fibrillation.

D. Electrical discharge. For cardioversion, before each electrical discharge the monitor should be checked to ensure synchronization. Discharge should occur during patient exhalation to minimize the distance between the electrode and the heart, thereby decreasing transthoracic impedance. Prior to discharge, ensure that no assisting personnel are in contact with the patient or the bed, because the electrical energy may be transmitted.

IV. CARDIOVERSION FOR SPECIFIC ARRHYTHMIAS

A. Atrial fibrillation (AFib). In the general population, the most common indication for cardioversion is AFib. Cardioversion in AFib should be performed in the hemodynamically unstable patient or under elective circumstances to attempt reversion to normal sinus rhythm. Elective cardioversion for stable AFib may become less common. Recent data (AFFIRM Trial) have demonstrated that overall outcome may be more dependent on rate control and anticoagulation than rhythm normalization.

1. Before the procedure, consider the duration of AFib, the embolic risk, and the likelihood of maintaining sinus rhythm after countershocking. In general, large atrial size (larger than 45 mm), long-standing arrhythmia (more than 1 year's duration), previous unsuccessful attempts, and intolerance to antiarrhythmic medications are believed to predict unsuccessful cardioversion.
2. For elective cardioversion of AFib of undetermined onset or AFib lasting more than 48 hours, anticoagulation is recommended for 3 weeks before and 4 weeks after cardioversion to minimize the risk of subsequent embolic events.
3. Alternatively, transesophageal echocardiography may determine the safety of early cardioversion, given its ability for accurately detecting atrial thrombi.

The ACUTE Trial demonstrated that if atrial thrombi can be excluded, early cardioversion can be performed safely without the need for prior prolonged anticoagulation.

4. Anticoagulation after cardioversion for an additional 4 weeks is still indicated irrespective of transesophageal ultrasound evaluation because residual electromechanical instability persists, despite the emergence of normal conduction.

5. The starting dose is usually 100 J. If conversion does not occur, then each successive dose should be increased by 100 J to a maximum dose of 360 J.

B. Atrial flutter. Because it is a more organized and localized tachyarrhythmia in terms of its reentrant characteristics as compared to AFib, starting cardioversion doses are lower than for AFib at 25 to 50 J. Anticoagulation in atrial flutter to prevent thromboembolic events is controversial. Because atrial flutter may also be associated with unstable atrial electromechanical process after cardioversion, anticoagulation is recommended.

C. Supraventricular tachycardia (SVT). The success rate for cardioverting SVT is high, approximately 75% to 80%. But medications, especially adenosine, can also be used effectively. Increasing ventricular ectopy after low-dose shocks suggests the presence of digoxin toxicity, and further attempts at cardioversion should be abandoned.

D. Wolff-Parkinson-White syndrome (WPW). In WPW, an accessory pathway, bypasses the atrioventricular node. Supraventricular tachycardia reentrant circuits may develop involving the atrioventricular node and the accessory pathway. Cardioversion may be beneficial for supraventricular tachycardias in WPW because countershocking breaks the reentrant circuit.

1. Cardioversion is the treatment of choice for unstable AFib in WPW syndrome.

2. Most medications used to control ventricular rate in AFib slow the atrioventricular (AV) node. However, blocking the AV node directs all the depolarizing atrial waves down the accessory path, which has a shorter refractory property than the AV node and bombards the ventricle with depolarizations, risking VFib.

3. For hemodynamically stable patients, procainamide may also be used, which stabilizes the myocardium and prolongs refractoriness of the accessory pathway.

E. Ventricular tachycardia (VT). Cardioversion is one of the leading therapeutic options for monomorphic VT. A starting energy dose required to convert VT is typically 100 J, with a success rate of about 95% to 100%. Cardioversion of VT in the synchronized mode is preferable. In emergencies, with hemodynamic compromise and insufficient time for synchronization, *unsynchronized* countershocking is warranted. In ventricular flutter, where tall T waves may be mistaken for QRS complexes, unsynchronized cardioversion is also used.

V. DEFIBRILLATION

A. Defibrillation is the essential and critical treatment of choice for VFib and pulseless VT.

B. Early, rapid and prompt delivery of defibrillation is the single most important intervention that improves survival from adult cardiac arrest. Survival for victims of cardiac arrest caused by VFib declines by 7% to 8% for every minute that defibrillation is delayed.

C. Treat VFib with three sequential monophasic unsynchronized shocks, beginning with 200 J. If VFib persists, a second shock at 300 J should be given. The dose of the third and all subsequent shocks should be 360 J. The three shocks should be delivered sequentially before other therapies are initiated because the transthoracic impedance decreases immediately after the initial countershock. Consequently, subsequent shocks may be effective even when the initial shock is unsuccessful.

D. If the third shock fails to restore the rhythm, then continue cardiopulmonary resuscitation and follow the Advanced Cardiac Life Support (ACLS) protocol, with administration of vasopressin and/or epinephrine and possibly amiodarone for refractory VFib.

VI. CARDIOVERSION AND DEFIBRILLATION UNDER SPECIAL CIRCUMSTANCES

A. Pediatric population. The energy level needed to revert any arrhythmia should be reduced for the pediatric patient. The recommended starting dose for defibrillation is 2 J/kg, which should be doubled on the second countershock to 4 J/kg. Adult-sized paddles/pads can be used in children older than 1 year old weighing more than 10 kg. VFib is uncommon in pediatric patients and should prompt vigorous correction of acidosis and hypoxia.

B. Pacemakers. Permanent pacemakers are susceptible to dysfunction after exposure to countershocks. Potential complications include lead dislodgment, especially for newly implanted devices, acute or chronic impairment of pacing and sensing capabilities, reprogramming of pacing modes, and general damage to the electrical circuitry. If a pacemaker is present, use the lowest possible defibrillation energy dose and place the electrodes as far away from the pulse generator as possible (>10 cm). Alternatively, placing a magnet over the implantable device may deactivate it prior to delivering shocks. A backup pacing system should always be available in case a malfunction of pacing capabilities develops after a delivered countershock.

C. Implantable cardioverter-defibrillators (ICDs). ICDs are also susceptible to damage after exposure to a countershock. If elective cardioversion is planned, inactivate the device before the procedure. In patients with epicardial ICD patches higher energies may be necessary because of increased transthoracic impedance. Place the electrodes perpendicular to the orientation of the epicardial patches. Always recheck or interrogate the ICD after countershocking.

D. Accidental hypothermia. Ventricular arrhythmias and asystole may be refractory to conventional therapy until the patient has been rewarmed due to sensitization of the myocardium associated with hypothermia. Cardiac arrest in this situation should be managed with an initial attempt at defibrillation and use of appropriate pharmacologic therapy. If unsuccessful, aggressive rewarming should continue and further attempts at defibrillation held until the core temperature reaches 30° to 32°C. Animal studies suggest bretylium is the antiarrhythmic drug of choice in this setting, but definitive therapy for arrhythmias associated with hypothermia centers around patient rewarming.

VII. COMPLICATIONS

A. Thermal burns to the chest.

B. Risk of thromboembolic events, particularly when cardioverting AFib or atrial flutter.

C. Countershocks can induce tachyarrhythmias different from the original rhythm, bradycardias, or asystole, which require prompt recognition and treatment, either with another shock or with medications, as necessary.

D. Defibrillation in asystole should always be avoided because excessive vagal response may suppress intrinsic nodal activity. Yet, one should always consider the possibility that VFib with small-amplitude waves ("fine VFib") may mimic asystole. Check more than one lead before assuming a diagnosis of asystole.

E. Depolarizing the myocardium may inhibit the recovery of ventricular escape beat and may lead to worsening intrinsic pacemaker failure in individuals with underlying sinoatrial node disease or other baseline conduction abnormalities.

F. Applying countershocks to patients with digoxin toxicity may be proarrhythmogenic and could induce serious ventricular dysrhythmias such as VFib. This is not usually an issue with normal serum digoxin and potassium levels prior to cardioversion/defibrillation.

Selected Readings

American Heart Association guidelines 2000 for cardiopulmonary resuscitation and emergency cardiovascular care. *Circulation* 2000;102:I-63.

A comprehensive presentation of guidelines for cardiopulmonary resuscitation, published over numerous supplements.

The Atrial Fibrillation Follow-up Investigation of Rhythm Management Investigators. A comparison of rate control and rhythm control in patients with atrial fibrillation. *N Engl J Med* 2002;347:1825–1833.
One of several studies that have demonstrated that the management of atrial fibrillation with the rhythm-control strategy offers no survival advantage over the rate-control strategy setting.

Danzl DF, Pozos RS. Accidental hypothermia. *N Engl J Med* 1994;331:1756–1760.
Discussion of resuscitation recommendations for hypothermic patients.

DiMarco JP. Medical progress: implantable cardioverter-defibrillators. *N Engl J Med* 2003; 349:1836–1847.
A current review of implantable defibrillators including resuscitation in patients with these devices in place.

Falk RH. Medical progress: atrial fibrillation. *N Engl J Med* 2001;344:1067–1078.
An excellent review of the topic of atrial defibrillation including a useful algorithm to guide its management.

Klein GJ, Bashore TM, Sellers TD, et al. Ventricular fibrillation in the Wolff-Parkinson-White syndrome. *N Engl J Med* 1997;301:1080.
An electrophysiologic study on the risk factors for the development of ventricular fibrillation in the WPW syndrome.

Klein AL, Grimm RA, Murray RD, et al. Use of transesophageal echocardiography to guide cardioversion in patients with atrial fibrillation. *N Engl J Med* 2001;344:1411–1420.
Also known as the ACUTE Trial, this article formed the basis for the current atrial fibrillation protocols, which use transesophageal echocardiography to help guide the management of elective cardioversion.

Peberdy MA. Defibrillation. *Cardiol Clin* 2002;20:13–21.
A concise review on the topic of defibrillation with an emphasis on the use and implementation of automatic external defibrillators.

Schneider T, Martens PR, Paschen H, et al. Multicenter, randomized, controlled trial of 150-J biphasic shocks compared with 200-360-J monophasic shocks in the resuscitation of out-of hospital cardiac arrest victims. *Circulation* 2000;102;1780–1787.
This study demonstrated that a biphasic waveform was more successful in converting VFib at lower energy levels when compared to a traditional monophasic defibrillation waveform.

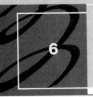

6 PERICARDIOCENTESIS

Payam Aghassi and Deborah H. Markowitz

I. GENERAL PRINCIPLES

A. Pericardiocentesis is a procedure whereby a needle is inserted into the space between the visceral and parietal pericardium for the purpose of sampling or draining pericardial fluid.

B. Diagnostic versus therapeutic pericardiocentesis

1. Diagnostic pericardiocentesis is performed to obtain small amounts of pericardial fluid for culture, cytologic study, or other fluid analyses.

2. Therapeutic pericardiocentesis is intended to drain fluid from the pericardial space and to relieve pressure that limits diastolic filling.

3. Diagnostic and therapeutic pericardiocenteses are best performed electively, under controlled circumstances, with echocardiographic or fluoroscopic support.

4. Occasionally, pericardiocentesis needs to be performed on an emergency basis to treat cardiac tamponade, and, as a consequence, the risk of complications such as pneumothorax and myocardial puncture increases.

C. Pericardial anatomy. Normally, there is only 10 to 15 mL of clear fluid in that space, with composition similar to that of plasma ultrafiltrate.

1. Visceral pericardium is composed of a single layer of mesothelial cells covering the myocardium and is loosely adherent to the underlying muscle by a network of blood vessels, lymphatics, and connective tissue.

2. Parietal pericardium is composed of a thick layer of fibrous connective tissue surrounding another mesothelial monolayer. This fibrous capsule is relatively nondistensible. Effusions that develop rapidly, over minutes to hours, are limited by this noncompliant fibrous parietal pleura, thus placing the fluid under tension

D. Diseases affecting the pericardium

1. Several disease states lead to inflammation of the pericardium and subsequent fluid accumulation including infections, malignancy, diffuse rheumatologic disorders, uremia, myocardial infarction, and myocardial rupture.

2. The composition of the fluid may become exudative, purulent, or frank blood, depending on the underlying cause.

E. Tamponade. Abrupt accumulation 250 mL or more may lead to the clinical signs and symptoms of tamponade, with equalization of pressures in all four cardiac chambers. However, if the effusion develops slowly, the parietal pericardium is able to stretch and significantly larger amounts of fluid (>2 L) may accumulate without hemodynamic compromise.

II. PROCEDURE

A. General considerations

1. If the procedure is performed on an emergency basis, then hemodynamic compromise is implied. Aggressive resuscitation measures should be ongoing, with infusion of fluids, blood products, or vasopressors as indicated.

2. If time allows, a coagulation profile should be checked and corrected.

B. Material preparation

1. *Site preparation:* 10% providone-iodine solution; sterile drapes, gowns, gloves; 1% lidocaine (without epinephrine), atropine, and code cart to bedside

2. *Procedure:* a pericardiocentesis kit or an 18-gauge, 8-cm thin-walled needle with blunt tip; No. 11 blade; multiple syringes (20 to 60 mL); electrocardiograph

(ECG); hemostat; sterile alligator clip; specimen collection tubes; pericardial drain if indicated

   3. *Postprocedure:* sterile gauze, dressings, and sutures

C. Patient preparation

   1. The patient should be placed in a comfortable supine position with the head of the bed elevated to approximately 45 degrees or more.

   2. The fully upright position may be necessary for extremely dyspneic patients. This position allows free-flowing effusions to collect inferiorly and anteriorly where they are easiest to access through the subxiphoid approach.

D. Pericardiocentesis needle preparation

   1. Attaching an ECG lead to the pericardiocentesis needle helps prevent advancing the needle through the myocardium.

   2. This lead substitutes for a precordial V lead on the ECG recording and allows for continuous monitoring throughout the procedure.

   3. ST-segment elevation occurs if the needle contacts cardiac muscle or the epicardium.

   4. Sterile leads are preferable and are available in some pericardiocentesis kits or from the cardiac catheterization laboratory.

   5. Attach the alligator clamp close to needle hub to allow maximum needle penetration.

   6. The distance between the skin and the parietal pericardium is typically between 6.0 and 7.5 cm, but it may be more in obese patients or in those with a protuberant abdomen.

   7. The clinician should attach the needle to a 10-mg syringe, approximately half filled with 1% lidocaine. This technique permits one to anesthetize the subcutaneous tissues and pericardium during needle entry while still allowing sufficient space in the syringe for withdrawal of pericardial fluid.

E. Needle entry site selection

   1. Inspection and palpation help locate the xiphoid process and the left costal margin.

   2. The needle entry site should be 0.5 cm lateral to the left border of the xiphoid process and 1.0 cm inferior to the costal margin.

   3. The pericardial space may be entered at various points along the anterior thorax but the subxiphoid approach is preferred, particularly in an emergency.

F. Site preparation

   1. Strict sterile technique should be followed at all times. A wide area of the skin in the xiphoid region is prepared with a 10% povidone-iodine solution, and the area is draped with sterile towels while leaving the subxiphoid area exposed.

   2. The patient's skin is anesthetized with 1% lidocaine without epinephrine.

   3. A small skin incision is made at the entry site with a scalpel to facilitate inserting the blunt needle through the skin; the pericardiocentesis needle does not have a beveled edge, to minimize the risk of myocardial puncture.

G. Needle insertion

   1. When passing through the skin, the angle of entry should be 45 degrees. Direct the needle superiorly, aiming for the patient's left shoulder.

   2. Always remember to draw back on the plunger of the syringe while advancing the needle and before injecting the lidocaine.

   3. The posterior edge of the bony thorax is usually between 1.0 and 2.5 cm below the skin, but it may be more in obese patients. If the bony thorax is hit during needle entry, reposition the needle so that it may be advanced under the costal margin.

   4. Once the needle has passed beyond the posterior border of the bony thorax, one should reduce the angle that the needle makes with the skin to 15 degrees. This angle is maintained while the needle is still directed at the patient's left shoulder.

H. Needle advancement

   1. Move the needle only in a straight trajectory from front to back. Moving the needle side to side may injure epicardial blood vessels and lymphatics.

2. Remember to aspirate whenever advancing the needle, then pause to inject the subcutaneous tissue with lidocaine at periodic intervals.
3. A "give" is felt on entry into the pericardial space and as fluid is aspirated.
4. A vasovagal response can occur when the pericardium is breached and may need intravenous atropine or saline infusion to reverse bradycardia and hypotension.
5. Should the ECG tracing from the precordial needle lead demonstrate new ST-segment elevations or premature ventricular contractions, immediately and carefully withdraw the needle.
6. Continue to aspirate on the syringe while withdrawing the needle.
7. Rapid entry may cause the needle to go through the pericardial space unknowingly, and correct positioning may be identified with slow extraction.
8. If unsuccessful in isolating the pericardial space, completely withdraw the needle, reposition, and try again.

I. Fluid evacuation. A large-volume pericardial effusion may be evacuated by attaching a 50-mL syringe onto the pericardiocentesis needle with repeated aspiration attempts. Alternatively, a pericardial drain may be placed by passing a catheter over a guidewire, as in the Seldinger technique.

J. Tamponade. If the procedure was performed to relieve tamponade, the patient's hemodynamic status should improve promptly. Such improvement may be observed after the evacuation of only 50 to 100 mL of fluid. Clinical signs that tamponade has been alleviated include an increase in systemic blood pressure and cardiac output with a fall in right atrial pressure and resolution of pulsus paradoxus.

III. POSTPROCEDURE CONSIDERATIONS

A. Monitoring. After pericardiocentesis, close monitoring is required to gauge the rate of pericardial effusion reaccumulation and the potential return of tamponade.

B. Chest radiograph. All patients should have an end-expiratory chest radiograph immediately after the procedure to detect the presence of a pneumothorax.

C. A transthoracic echocardiogram should be obtained within several hours of the pericardiocentesis to confirm adequacy of pericardial drainage.

D. Potential complications Cardiac puncture with or without hemopericardium or myocardial infarction; pneumothorax; ventricular tachycardia; bradycardia; abdominal organ trauma; cardiac arrest; coronary artery laceration; infection; fistula formation; pulmonary edema.

E. Complications are most likely when the effusion is small (<250 mL), is located posteriorly, or is loculated or if the maximum anterior pericardial space is less than 10 mm as determined by echocardiography, because the margin for error is greater.

F. Unguided pericardiocenteses, performed under emergency conditions, are also associated with higher complication rates, so ultrasound guidance is recommended.

G. Samples of the pericardial fluid should be sent according to the suspected disease process.

H. Diagnostic studies to perform on pericardial fluid: White count with differential; hematocrit; glucose, total protein, lactate dehydrogenase; Gram stain and culture for bacteria, fungi, and acid-fast bacilli; cytology; amylase; cholesterol; antinuclear antibody, rheumatoid factor; total complement; C3; viral or parasite studies.

Selected Readings

Kirkland LL, Taylor RW. Pericardiocentesis. *Crit Care Clin* 1992;8:699.
   A review of the pathophysiology of pericardial effusions and the pericardiocentesis procedure.

Lovell BH, Braunwald E. Pericardiocentesis. In: Braunwald EF, ed. *Heart disease: a textbook of cardiovascular medicine.* Philadelphia: WB Saunders, 1992:1479.
   A comprehensive guide to pericardiocentesis.

Meyers DG, Meyers RE, Prendergast TW. The usefulness of diagnostic tests on pericardial fluid. *Chest* 1997;111:1213.
A comprehensive treatise on the prognostic value of various biochemical tests for pericardial fluid analysis; probably the definitive article at this time.

Prager RL, Wilson CH, Bender HW. The subxiphoid approach to pericardial disease. *Ann Thorac Surg* 1982;34:6.
An earlier review of 25 subxiphoid pericardiocenteses.

Scheinman MM. Pericardiocentesis. In: *Cardiac emergencies*. Philadelphia: WB Saunders, 1984:264.
A practical guide to performing pericardiocentesis.

Spodick DH. Technique of pericardiocentesis. In: *The pericardium: a comprehensive textbook*. New York: Marcel Dekker, 1997:145.
A practical guide to the diagnostic and treatment benefits of pericardiocentesis and the relevant discussion of pericardial anatomy.

Tsang TS, Freeman WK, Sinak LJ, et al. Echocardiographically guided pericardiocentesis: evolution and state-of-the-art technique. *Mayo Clin Proc* 1998;73:647.
An extensive review of the procedure with emphasis on echocardiographic guidance.

Wong B, Murphy J, Chang CJ, et al. The risk of pericardiocentesis. *Am J Cardiol* 1979;44:1110.
A review of the outcomes and complications from a series of 52 pericardiocenteses at one institution.

THE INTRAAORTIC BALLOON AND COUNTERPULSATION

Michael Singh and Bruce S. Cutler

7

I. GENERAL PRINCIPLES
  A. The intraaortic balloon (IAB) pump is designed to assist an ischemic ventricle through improvement in coronary artery perfusion and reduction in systemic afterload by counterpulsation.

  B. Counterpulsation increases myocardial oxygen supply by diastolic augmentation of coronary perfusion, and it decreases myocardial oxygen requirements through afterload reduction. Counterpulsation causes an increase in cerebral and peripheral blood flow but no significant alteration of renal perfusion.

II. INDICATIONS
  A. Cardiogenic shock. The IAB was developed with the hope of reversing cardiogenic shock after myocardial infarction. Counterpulsation should be initiated as soon as it is determined that the shock state is not responsive to intravascular volume manipulation and drug therapy. The ideal candidate for IAB placement should have a reversible anatomic or functional derangement responsible for the shock state.

  B. Reversible mechanical defects. Counterpulsation is effective in the initial stabilization of patients with mechanical intracardiac defects complicating myocardial infarction, such as acute mitral regurgitation and ventricular septal perforation, while preparations for definitive intervention are under way.

  C. Unstable angina. Counterpulsation is indicated for ongoing myocardial ischemia in the face of maximal medical therapy.

  D. Weaning from cardiopulmonary bypass

  E. Preoperative use: for high-risk patients such as those with critical stenosis of coronary arteries or severely depressed left ventricular function.

  F. Bridge to transplantation. Provide mechanical support for patients in congestive heart failure who are awaiting cardiac transplantation.

  G. Other indications. Control unstable angina before and during coronary angioplasty and atherectomy. Counterpulsation may be lifesaving after a failed angioplasty, to support the myocardium until emergency aortocoronary revascularization can be performed. The IAB has also been used during interhospital transfers of unstable patients, for treatment of heart failure after myocardial trauma, and for perioperative support for high-risk noncardiac surgery.

  H. Contraindications. Aortic valvular insufficiency, aortic dissection, and severe aortoiliac disease are absolute contraindications to counterpulsation. Because of the need for anticoagulation during use of the IAB, gastrointestinal bleeding, thrombocytopenia, and other bleeding diatheses are relative contraindications to counterpulsation.

III. PROCEDURE
  A. Equipment
    1. The balloon is made from a thin film of polyurethane because of its strength and antithrombotic properties.

    2. IABs are available in variable sizes, with different balloon volumes and catheter diameters.

    3. The catheter itself has two concentric lumina. The central lumen is used to pass a guidewire during insertion and to monitor central aortic pressure. The outer lumen is the passageway for gas exchange and is connected to a console that controls balloon operation as well as having a monitoring function. Helium is used as the driving gas.

4. The following equipment is needed:
   a. A manufacturer-supplied sterile insertion kit
   b. Portable fluoroscope or transesophageal echocardiography (TEE)
   c. Povidone-iodine prep solution, sterile drapes, gown, gloves, and towel clips
   d. 1% Lidocaine with syringe and 22-gauge, 1.5-inch needle
   e. Sterile gauze pads
   f. No. 11 scalpel and handle
   g. Dilute heparin solution (10,000 units in 500 mL of 0.9% saline)
   h. Two 0 silk sutures on curved cutting needles, needle holder
   i. 5,000 units of heparin and a10-mL syringe

5. After careful assessment of the patient, the side with the best circulation is chosen for IAB insertion. The procedure should be performed with the patient supine on a bed or table that permits the use of fluoroscopy. Both inguinal areas are prepared and draped in sterile fashion. Maximum barrier precautions are used. The instructions for preparing the IAB should be followed closely because the technique varies with the manufacturer.

6. Lidocaine (1%) is instilled subcutaneously and subdermally over the femoral artery pulse. The puncture site should be 1 cm below the inguinal crease directly over the femoral pulsation (Fig. 7-1).

7. After cannulation of the artery, a J-guidewire is passed and advanced under fluoroscopy until the tip is in the thoracic aorta (Fig. 7-2). At this point, the patient should be intravenously anticoagulated with 5,000 units of heparin.

8. A small incision is made at the puncture site to allow passage of dilators and the sheath (Fig. 7-3). The IAB is advanced over the guidewire so that its radiopaque tip is positioned 2 cm distal to the ostium of the left subclavian artery (Fig. 7-4).

9. When the IAB is properly positioned, the central lumen is aspirated and then is flushed with heparinized saline and used to monitor intraaortic pressure and to time counterpulsation. The IAB and sheath are secured with sutures.

10. Alternatively, the IAB may be inserted without the use of the sheath, a technique that reduces the intraluminal arterial obstruction and may decrease the risk of ischemic complications to the lower limb.

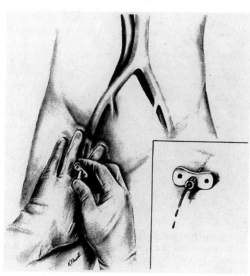

Figure 7-1. The Potts-Cournand needle is inserted at a 45-degree angle into the common femoral artery. *Inset:* Pulsatile jet of blood indicates that the needle is properly located in the center of the arterial lumen.

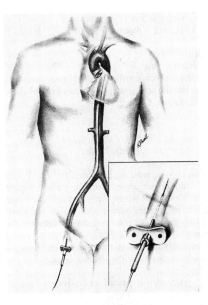

Figure 7-2. When the Potts-Cournand needle is properly placed in the artery, the guidewire is advanced under fluoroscopic control until the tip is in the thoracic aorta (*inset*).

11. Anticoagulation with a heparin infusion is recommended to reduce the risk of thromboembolic complications related to the IAB. When anticoagulation is contraindicated, an infusion of low-molecular-weight dextran may be used. Prophylactic antibiotics effective against skin flora are recommended.

12. As soon as the IAB is in position, the circulatory status of the limb should be checked by assessing pulses, Doppler ankle pressures, or the ankle-arm index.

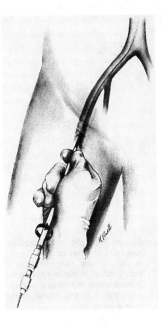

Figure 7-3. A 9.5-Fr dilator with overlying Teflon sheath is passed over the guidewire. A rotary motion and firm pressure are necessary to enter the lumen of the femoral artery.

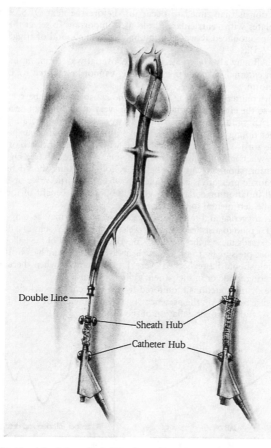

Double Line

Sheath Hub

Catheter Hub

Figure 7-4. The tip of the intraaortic balloon is positioned 2 cm distal to the orifice of the left subclavian artery. The balloon must be inserted to the level of the double line to be sure the entire membrane has emerged from the sheath. *Inset:* The sheath seal is pushed over the sheath hub to control bleeding. The sheath and catheter hubs are sutured in place.

While the device is in position, the circulatory status must be monitored every 2 to 4 hours.

IV. POSTPROCEDURE CONSIDERATIONS

   A. Acute limb ischemia may occur anytime after initiation of counterpulsation, but it is most likely to occur immediately after IAB placement. Initial management is conservative if the ischemia is mild, but severe ischemia requires prompt treatment, which may involve placement of the IAB at another site or even a vascular bypass procedure in IAB-dependent patients.

   B. Triggering and timing of the intraaortic balloon pump

   1. Proper timing of the inflation-deflation cycle of the balloon is crucial to the optimal functioning of the IAB.

   2. The R wave of the patient's electrocardiogram (ECG) is the most common means of triggering balloon deflation. The IAB is initially set so inflation occurs at the peak of the T wave, which corresponds approximately with closure of the aortic valve.

3. Deflation is then timed to occur just before the next QRS complex, which correlates with ventricular systole. It is important to select the lead with the most pronounced R wave to minimize the likelihood of triggering problems (Fig. 7-5).
4. The IAB may also be triggered by the arterial waveform, or, in an emergency, by an external pacemaker if triggering cannot be effected by ECG or arterial waveform.
5. When counterpulsation is initiated, the console should be set to a 1:2 assist ratio so the effects of augmentation on every other beat can be analyzed.
6. The IAB should be inflated initially to one half the operating volume until proper timing is effected. Ideally, IAB inflation should occur just after closure of the aortic valve, which corresponds with the dicrotic notch of the aortic root pulse when it is measured through the lumen of the IAB (see Fig. 7-5).
7. Deflation should occur just before systole and thus should be timed so the intraaortic pressure is at a minimum when the aortic valve opens. Improperly timed inflation or deflation negates the potential benefit of the IAB and may even be detrimental to the patient.
8. When triggering and timing are satisfactory, the IAB may be fully inflated and set to a 1:1 ratio to assist each cardiac cycle. IAB inflation results in a diastolic pressure that exceeds the systolic pressure. Conversely, deflation of the balloon reduces end-diastolic pressure by 15 to 20 mm Hg and systolic pressure by 5 to 10 mm Hg.
9. Timing should be rechecked every 1 to 2 hours or when there is a change in triggering mode or in the patient's clinical status.
10. Some of the functions monitored by the IAB console include the volume and pressure in the IAB, the presence of gas leaks, the loss of ECG or arterial trigger signal, and improper deflation of the IAB.

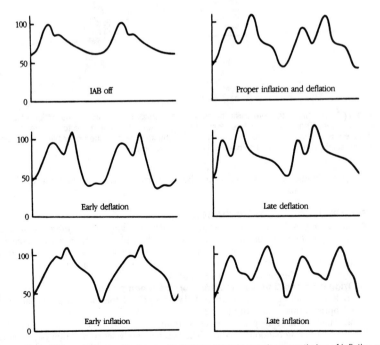

Figure 7-5. Slide switches on the intraaortic balloon console permit proper timing of inflation and deflation during the cardiac cycle.

C. Weaning from counterpulsation

1. Cessation of counterpulsation involves two steps: weaning and IAB removal. The patient may be weaned by progressively reducing the assist ratio or IAB volume. Usually, a period of 1 to 2 hours is required to establish stability at each new assist level. When the patient has been weaned to 1:3 and has been stable, the IAB may be removed.

2. The heparin infusion should be stopped 2 hours before IAB removal. The operator should not attempt to withdraw the balloon into the sheath. The IAB and sheath are removed as a unit, and prolonged pressure is applied to the puncture site. The use of sandbags is not recommended. Rarely, surgical management is required to control ongoing bleeding from the insertion site.

D. Complications of counterpulsation. The overall complication rate for percutaneous IAB is about 15%.

1. **Complications during insertion.** The most common complication related to insertion is failure of the IAB to pass the iliofemoral system because of atherosclerotic occlusive disease. The reported failure rate ranges from 5% to 7%. Other complications of IAB insertion include aortic dissection and arterial perforation, with a reported incidence of 1% to 2%. Arterial perforation is an acute emergency requiring surgical intervention.

2. **Complications while the intraaortic balloon is in place**
   a. Limb ischemia is the most common complication of counterpulsation and is sufficiently severe to require removal of the IAB in 11% to 27% of patients. Several large reviews suggest that the most important risk factors for limb ischemia are the female gender, insulin-dependent diabetes, and significant peripheral vascular occlusive disease.
   b. Infection, thrombocytopenia, and embolization of platelet aggregates or atherosclerotic debris have been reported.
   c. Rupture of the IAB occurs in 2% to 4% of patients and may cause gas embolization. Blood in the connecting tubing is a hallmark of rupture, and its presence requires immediate cessation of counterpulsation and IAB removal.

3. **Complications during or after removal.** Arterial perfusion of the limb should be checked soon after removal of the IAB by palpation of pulses and measurement of the ankle-arm index. The puncture site should be examined for hematoma, false aneurysm formation, and arteriovenous fistula.

Selected Readings

Cutler BS, Singh MJ: The intraaortic balloon and counterpulsation. In: Irwin RS and Rippe JM (eds). *Irwin and Rippe's intensive care medicine,* 5th ed. Philadelphia, PA: Lippincott Williams & Williams, 2003.
A more in-depth description of balloon pump insertion.

Eltchaninoff H, Dimas AP, Whitlow PL. Complications associated with percutaneous placement and use of intraaortic balloon counterpulsation. *Am J Cardiol* 1993;71:328.
A report of 231 cases of IAB use that suggests predictors of limb ischemia.

Kantrowitz A, Wasfie T, Freed PS, et al. Intraaortic balloon pumping 1967 through 1982: analysis of complications in 733 patients. *Am J Cardiol* 1986;57:976.
A good review of complications of IAB.

Katz ES, Tunick PA, Kronzon I. Observations of coronary flow augmentation and balloon function during intraaortic balloon counterpulsation using transesophageal echocardiography. *Am J Cardiol* 1992;69:1635.
A report of six patients studied with transesophageal echocardiography while assisted with IAB; it suggests that transesophageal echocardiography can be used to evaluate IAB positioning and to monitor coronary artery flow augmentation during counterpulsation.

O'Murchu B, Foreman RD, Shaw RE, et al. Role of intraaortic balloon pump counterpulsation in high risk coronary rotational atherectomy. *J Am Coll Cardiol* 1995;26:1270.
A retrospective review of elective use of IAB in high-risk patients before coronary rotational atherectomy.

8

CHEST TUBE INSERTION AND CARE
Gustavo G. Angaramo

I. GENERAL PRINCIPLES. Chest tube insertion (tube thoracostomy) involves the placement of a sterile tube into the pleural space to evacuate air or fluid into a closed collection system to restore negative intrathoracic pressure, promote lung expansion, and prevent lethal levels of pressure from developing in the thorax.

II. ANATOMY AND PHYSIOLOGY OF THE PLEURAL SPACE
   A. The pleural space is a closed, serous sac surrounded by two separate layers of mesothelial cells, the parietal and visceral pleura. Normally there is a negative intrapleural pressure of -2 to -5 cm of water.
   B. The pleural layers are in close apposition and under normal physiologic conditions allow free expansion of the lung in a lubricated environment.

III. INDICATIONS
   A. Pneumothorax
      1. Accumulation of air in the pleural space is the most common indication for chest tube placement.
      2. Diagnosis is often confirmed by chest radiography.
      3. The risk of a recurrent ipsilateral spontaneous pneumothorax is as high as 50% and the risk of a third episode is 60% to 80%.
   B. Hemothorax
      1. Accumulation of blood in the pleural space can be classified as spontaneous, iatrogenic or traumatic.
   C. Empyema
      1. Empyemas are pyogenic infections of the pleural space that may result from:
         a. Necrotizing pneumonia
         b. Septic pulmonary emboli
         c. Spread of intraabdominal infections
         d. Inadequate drainage of a traumatic hemothorax.
   D. Pleural effusion
      1. Treatment of transudative pleural effusions is aimed at controlling the underlying cause (congestive heart failure, nephrotic syndrome, cirrhosis). Tube thoracostomy is uncommonly indicated.
      2. Exudative effusions, however, often require tube drainage depending on whether the fluid is free or loculated.

IV. CONTRAINDICATIONS
   A. There are no absolute contraindications to chest tube insertion.
   B. There are many *relative* contraindications:
      1. Anticoagulation
      2. Prior ipsilateral thoracic surgery
      3. Extensive bullous lung disease
   C. The most obvious contraindication to chest tube insertion seems obvious: lack of pneumothorax or of a fluid collection in the pleural space.

V. PROCEDURE
A. Preparation
1. Sterile technique including maximum barrier precautions is mandatory whether the procedure is performed in the operating room, the intensive care unit, or the emergency room.
2. Obtain a detailed informed consent.
3. Careful titration of parenteral opioids or benzodiazepines (if necessary) and injection of a local anesthetic to provide a relatively painless procedure.
4. Standard large-bore drainage tubes are made of either Silastic or rubber.
   a. Rubber tubes elicit more pleural inflammation, have fewer drainage holes, and are not easily identified on chest radiograph.
   b. Silastic chest tubes are either right angled or straight, have multiple holes, and contain a radiopaque stripe with a gap to mark the most proximal drainage holes.
   c. Sizes are available from 6 to 40 Fr, with size selection dependent on the patient population and the type of collection being drained .

B. Technique
1. To properly insert a chest tube, the following steps are suggested:
   a. Examine the x-ray carefully.
   b. Gather all the necessary equipment:
      (1) A scalpel
      (2) Two Kelly clamps
      (3) A suture
      (4) Local anesthesia (10 mL of 1 % lidocaine)
      (5) Needles (25-gauge for the skin and a 22-gauge for deeper lawyers)
      (6) Syringes (10 mL), dressings, tape and a filled drainage apparatus (Pleur-Evac)
   c. **Prepare the patient.**
      (1) Position the patient with the operative side up, in the lateral decubitus position.
      (2) Mark out the 4th or 5th intercostal space in the anterior axillary line by landmarks (chest tubes are occasionally inserted in the second intercostal space for pneumothoraces only!) (Fig. 8-1).

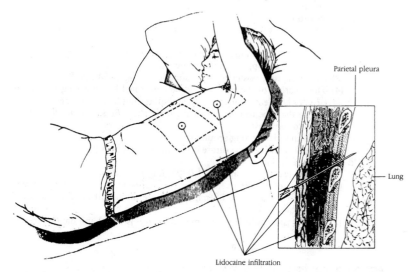

Figure 8-1. Proper patient positioning for chest tube insertion. (From Lancey RA. Chest tube insertion and care. In: Irwin RS, Rippe JM, eds. *Irwin and Rippe's intensive care medicine*, 5th ed. Philadelphia: Lippincott Williams & Wilkins, 2003, with permission.)

d. Prepare and drape the surgical site.
  (1) The area is prepared under sterile conditions with 10% povidone-iodine solution.
  (2) The area is draped to include the ipsilateral nipple as a landmark.

e. Anesthetize the area.
  (1) Include the skin over the incision site, periosteum above and below ribs, and the pleura.
  (2) Use 10 mL of 1% lidocaine, but have a syringe full in reserve if the patient needs supplementary medication during the procedure.
  (3) Tunnel the chest tube slightly to avoid air leak on removal. Therefore, the actual entry point into the pleura will not be directly under the skin incision.

f. Make a skin incision.
  (1) This should be no larger than the index finger (2 cm), because this is the actual "instrument" that will insert into the chest.

g. Make the subcutaneous tunnel.
  (1) This should be done with *spreading* motions only using a Kelly clamp.
  (2) *Do not cut any tissue.* This will greatly decrease bleeding and will make a tract that will collapse on tube removal and seal off.
  (3) Spread along the interspace, going posteriorly for about 2 to 3 cm. This will place the tube in the posterior-superior direction, which will drain air and fluid well.

h. Enter the pleural space.
  (1) Using the tips of a Kelly clamp closed, holding the body of the clamp with two hands, preventing uncontrolled entry and possible damage to underlying structures.
  (2) Once entered, spread the pleura with the tips of the clamp and do not insert the clamp into the chest (Fig. 8-2A).

i. Digitally explore the pleural space.
  (1) A finger is inserted into the pleural space to explore the anatomy and confirm proper location and lack of pleural symphysis (Fig. 8-2B).
  (2) If the space is not free, *do not insert the tube.* Suture the skin hole closed. The lung will not collapse if the lung and pleura are adherent to the chest wall!

j. Insert the tube.
  (1) The easiest way to do this is to have the tip of the tube clamped in the Kelly clamp.
  (2) Push the Kelly clamp and the tip of the chest tube into the pleural space, release the clamp, and continue inserting the tube.
  (3) Direct the tube posteriorly and superiorly (Fig. 8-3A and B).
  (4) The location of the tube should be confirmed by observing flow of air (seen as condensation within the tube) or fluid from the tube.
  (5) Suture the tube to the skin to avoid slippage. *Be sure that all the holes are into the chest.*
  (6) The suture is left long around the tube.
  (7) To seal the tunnel, the suture is tied when the tube is pulled out (Fig. 8-4).

k. Connect to the PleurEvac.
  (1) *Do not evacuate more than 1,000 mL of fluid at a time.*
  (2) In a case of a massive hemothorax or effusion, allow the lung to reexpand for about 15 to 30 minutes before taking off another 1,000 mL maximum.
  (3) Reexpansion pulmonary edema (*ex vacuo*) is a real and dangerous phenomenon.

l. Order a chest radiograph.

VI. POSTPROCEDURE CONSIDERATIONS

  A. Complications. Insertion alone is usually accompanied by a 1% to 2% incidence of complications, even when performed by experienced personnel.

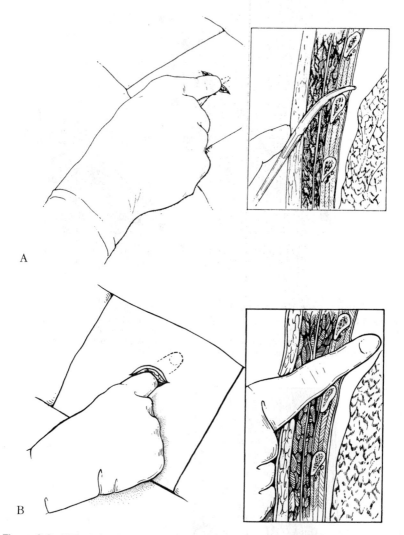

A

B

Figure 8-2. *(A)* Enter the pleural space. *(B)* Digitally explore the pleural space. (From Lancey RA. Chest tube insertion and care. In: Irwin RS, Rippe JM, eds.: *Irwin and Rippe's intensive care medicine,* 5th ed. Philadelphia: Lippincott Williams & Wilkins, 2003, with permission.)

1. Unintentional placement of the tube through the intercostals vessels or into the lung, heart, liver, or spleen can result in considerable morbidity and possible mortality.
2. Malposition of the tube within the pleural space limits its effectiveness.
3. Residual pneumothorax may follow removal of the tube as a result of a persistent air leak or due to entry of air through the tube site during or after removal.
4. Secondary infection of the pleural space following chest tube insertion is infrequent. Several investigations suggested benefit of prophylactic antibiotic regimens directed against *Staphylococcus aureus* only in patients undergoing tube thoracostomy in a trauma setting.

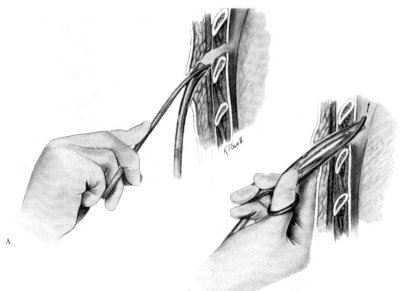

Figure 8-3 A: The end of the chest tube is grasped with a Kelly clamp and guided through the chest incision. B: The chest tube is oriented toward the apex. (From Lancey RA. Chest tube insertion and care. In: Irwin RS, Rippe JM, eds.: *Irwin and Rippe's intensive care medicine*, 5th ed. Philadelphia: Lippincott Williams & Wilkins, 2003, with permission.)

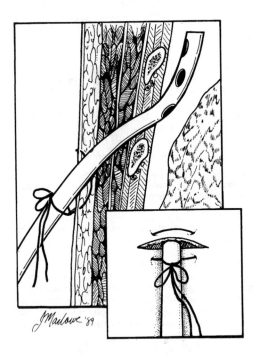

Figure 8-4. The tube is securely sutured to the skin with a 1-0 or 2-0 silk suture. The suture is left long, wrapped around the tube. To seal the tunnel, the suture is tied when the tube is pulled out. (From Lancey RA. Chest tube insertion and care. In: Irwin RS, Rippe JM, eds.: *Irwin and Rippe's intensive care medicine*, 5th ed. Philadelphia: Lippincott Williams & Wilkins, 2003, with permission.)

B. Chest tube management and care

1. The tube and drainage system must be checked daily for adequate functioning.
2. Suction is routinely established at 15 to 20 cm H_2O.
3. Connection between the tube and the drainage system should be tightly fitted and securely taped.
4. Dressing changes should be performed every 2 to 3 days or as needed.
5. Serial chest radiographs should be obtained to evaluate the result of drainage.
6. Chest tubes can be pulled back but not *readvanced* into the pleural space, and if a tube is to be replaced, it should always be at a different site rather than the same hole.

C. Chest tube removal

1. Indications for removal of chest tubes include:
   a. Resolution of the pneumothorax or fluid accumulation in the pleural space, or both.
   b. For a pneumothorax, the drainage system is left on suction until the air leak stops. If an air leak persists, brief clamping of the chest tube can be performed to confirm that the leak is from the patient and not the system. When the leak has ceased for more than 24 to 48 hours (or if no fluctuation is seen in the underwater seal chamber), the drainage system is placed on water seal by disconnecting the wall suction, followed by a chest film several hours later.
   c. If no pneumothorax is present and no air leak appears in the system with coughing and reestablishment of suction, the tube can be removed.
   d. For fluid collections, the tube can be removed when drainage is minimal.
2. Tube removal is often preceded by oral or parenteral analgesia.
3. The suture holding the tube to the skin is cut.
4. As the patient takes deep breaths, the tube is removed and the hole is simultaneously covered with petrolatum gauze dressing at peak inspiration, at which point only positive pressure can be generated into the pleural space.
5. A chest x-ray is performed to check for a pneumothorax and is repeated 24 hours later to rule out accumulation of air or fluid.

Selected Readings

Advanced Trauma Life Support student manual. Chicago: American College of Surgeons, 1993, p.138.
Methods of tube thoracostomy in emergency situations.

Bauman, MH, Strange C, Heffner JE, et al. Management of spontaneous pneumothorax: An American College of Chest Physicians delphi consensus statement. *Chest* 2001; 112:590–602.
Expert-based consensus recommendations for the management of adults with primary and secondary spontaneous pneumothoraces in an emergency and inpatient hospital setting.

Daly RC, Mucha P, Pairolero PC, et al. The risk of percutaneous chest tube thoracostomy for blunt thoracic trauma. *AnnEmerg Med* 1985;14:865.
Complications of percutaneous tube thoracostomy in victims of blunt trauma.

DeMeester TR, Lafontaine E: The pleura In: Sabiston DC, Spencer FC, eds. *Surgery of the chest.* Philadelphia. WB Saunders, 1990:444.
Detailed description of the pleural anatomy.

Evans JT, Green JD, Carlin PE, et al. Meta-analysis of antibiotics in tube thoracostomy. *Am Surg* 1995;61:215.
Benefit of prophylactic antibiotic regimens directed against Staphylococcus aureus in patients undergoing tube thoracostomy in a trauma setting.

Hurford W. Thoracic surgery. In: Hurford W, Bigatello L, Haspel K, et al., eds. Critical *care handbook of the Massachusetts General Hospital,* 3rd ed. Philadelphia: Lippincott Williams & Wilkins: 2000, pp. 613–617.
This chapter gives a precise description of the technique of chest tube insertion from the standpoint of a critical care physician.

Miller JI Jr. Infections of the pleura. In: Shields TW, ed.: *General thoracic surgery.* Philadelphia, Lea & Febiger, 1989, p. 633.
Detailed management of empyema.

Millikan JS, Moore EE, Steiner E, et al. Complications of tube thoracostomy for acute trauma. *Am J Surg* 1980; 140:738.
Tube thoracostomy is both diagnostic and therapeutic in trauma patients. There is a 4% technical complication rate in tube thoracostomy in the emergency room.

I. GENERAL PRINCIPLES
  A. Definition. The endoscopic examination of the bronchial tree.
  B. Can be performed with either flexible or rigid bronchoscope.
  C. Compared with rigid bronchoscopy, flexible bronchoscopy is more comfortable and safer for the patient, allows visualization of the entire tracheobronchial tree, and does not require general anesthesia or an operating room.

II. DIAGNOSTIC INDICATIONS
  ### A. Hemoptysis
  1. To localize the bleeding site and diagnose its cause.
  2. With active bleeding the site and origin are disclosed in approximately 90%. The yield is 50% after bleeding stops.
  ### B. Atelectasis.
  To rule out endobronchial obstruction by malignancy or foreign body; mucus plugging, however, is most common.
  ### C. Diffuse parenchymal disease
  1. Transbronchial lung biopsy and bronchoalveolar lavage (BAL) can offer information about parenchymal processes.
  2. BAL is an aid in diagnosing opportunistic infections in the immunocompromised host.
  3. Lung biopsy with fluoroscopy can improve localization and minimize pneumothorax.
  ### D. Acute inhalation injury
  1. To identify the anatomic level and severity of injury after smoke inhalation.
  2. Upper airway obstruction may develop within 24 hours after inhalation injury.
  3. Acute respiratory failure is more likely with mucosal change at segmental or lower levels.
  ### E. Blunt chest trauma.
  To rule out airway fracture after blunt trauma, suggested by hemoptysis, lobar atelectasis, pneumomediastinum, or pneumothorax.
  ### F. Assessment of intubation damage.
  To assess laryngeal or tracheal damage from endotracheal tubes.
  ### G. Cultures
  1. To identify organisms that colonize the respiratory tract when a patient is unable to expectorate sputum.
  2. Protected specimen brush with quantitative culture improves accuracy of routine bronchoscopic culture.
  3. Aspirates obtained from the bronchoscope in an unintubated patient are no more predictive than cultures obtained by expectorated sputum. Both are associated with high false-positive and false-negative rates.
  ### H. Diagnosis of ventilator-associated pneumonia (VAP)
  1. To provide a specimen for culture.
  2. Purulent secretions surging from distal bronchi during exhalation may be predict VAP.

III. THERAPEUTIC INDICATIONS
  ### A. Excessive secretions/atelectasis
  1. Lobar atelectasis not responding to chest physical therapy, incentive spirometry, and cough.

   2. Instillation of N-acetylcysteine (NAC) may help liquefy inspissated mucus.
   3. NAC may induce bronchospasm; pretreatment with albuterol is recommended in asthmatics.
B. Foreign bodies
   1. Rigid bronchoscopy is the procedure of choice to remove aspirated foreign bodies.
   2. Devices are available to help remove foreign bodies with the flexible scope.
C. Endotracheal intubation. The bronchoscope, used as an obturator, with an endotracheal tube passed over it, can help place the endotracheal tube transnasally or orally.
D. Hemoptysis
   1. Endobronchial tamponade can stabilize the patient to allow for more definitive therapy.
   2. Tamponade can be achieved with an inflated balloon-tipped catheter wedged in the lobar orifice.
   3. Massive hemoptysis can be controlled with iced saline lavage.
E. Central airway obstructing lesions. Laser photoresection or stenting of obstructing lesions of the larynx, trachea, and major bronchi.
F. Closure of bronchopleural fistula
   1. To visualize a proximal or localize a more distal bronchopleural fistula.
   2. Materials injected through the bronchoscope may seal the fistula.

IV. COMPLICATIONS
   A. When performed by a trained specialist, routine flexible bronchoscopy is extremely safe.
   B. Mortality should not exceed 0.1%.
   C. Death results from excessive premedication or topical anesthesia, respiratory arrest from hemorrhage, laryngospasm or bronchospasm, cardiac arrest from acute myocardial infarction.
   D. Overall complication rate is less than 8.0%.
   E. Nonfatal complications: fever, pneumonia, vasovagal reactions, laryngospasm and bronchospasm, hypotension, cardiac arrhythmia, pneumothorax, anesthesia-related problems, and aphonia.

V. CONTRAINDICATIONS
   A. Poorly experienced physician
   B. Uncooperative patient
   C. Unable to maintain adequate oxygen tension
   D. Coagulopathy in patients whom biopsy specimens (brush or forceps) will be taken
   E. Unstable cardiac patients
   F. Untreated, symptomatic asthmatic patients
   G. Severe, chronic obstructive pulmonary disease with associated hypercapnea (premedication, sedation, and supplemental oxygen must be used with caution)
   H. Elevated intracranial pressure (anesthetize using a combination of medications for cerebral protection, paralysis to prevent cough, and monitor to ensure adequate cerebral perfusion pressure)

VI. PROCEDURAL CONSIDERATIONS
A. Preprocedural
   1. Presence of underlying disease, such as asthma, cardiovascular disease, uremia, bleeding diathesis should be assessed.
   2. Presence of drug allergies or medication that interferes with coagulation should be assessed.
   3. Has the patient had a chest radiograph, electrocardiogram, and assessment of oxygenation?
   4. Has the patient fasted before the procedure?
   5. Has informed consent been obtained?

6. Has premedication been ordered?
7. Does the patient have intravenous access?

B. Procedural

1. Local anesthesia is achieved by nebulized lidocaine and topical lidocaine jelly.
   a. Lidocaine is absorbed through mucous membranes, and significant, even toxic, blood levels can be reached after topical administration.
   b. Levels in the low therapeutic range are achieved if a total of less than 200 mg is used.
   c. Sudden change in mental status, hallucinations, increased sedation, or hypotension should suggest lidocaine toxicity.
2. Unintubated patients: transnasal or transoral passage of the bronchoscope
3. Intubated patients:
   a. The bronchoscope is passed through a swivel adapter with a rubber diaphragm that prevents loss of the delivered tidal volume. Use a bite block to prevent damage to the bronchoscope.
   b. Consider the following before and during bronchoscopy:
      (1) Endotracheal tube 8 mm or greater internal diameter for delivery of adequate tidal volume
      (2) Positive end-expiratory pressure of 20 cm H_2O may develop with bronchoscopy, with the risk of barotrauma.
      (3) PEEP already being delivered should be discontinued.
      (4) Inspired oxygen concentration must be increased to 100%.
      (5) Expired volumes should be constantly measured; tidal volume usually has to be increased by 40% to 50%.
      (6) Suctioning will decrease delivered tidal volume and should be minimized.
4. During bronchoscopy, continuous oxygen therapy, oximetry, electrocardiography, and blood pressure monitoring are necessary.

C. Postprocedural

1. Obtain a chest radiograph to rule out pneumothorax.
   a. After transbronchial biopsy in the nonintubated patient
   b. After routine bronchoscopy in the intubated, mechanically ventilated patient.
2. Return the ventilated patient to preprocedure ventilator settings.
3. In unintubated patients, supplemental oxygen is continued for 4 hours.
4. Frequent vital signs until the patient is stable for at least 2 hours.
5. Patients must not eat or drink until local anesthesia has worn off, about 1 to 2 hours.
6. Fever after the procedure is common; fever lasting more than 24 hours raises concern for postbronchoscopy pneumonia.

Selected Readings

Cavaliere S, Foccoli P, Farina PL. Nd: YAG laser bronchoscopy: a five-year experience with 1,396 applications in 1,000 patients. *Chest* 1988;94:15.
Laser bronchoscopy was found to be a safe and effective method in the treatment of obstructive lesions of the tracheobronchial tree.

Conlan AA, Hurwitz SS. Management of massive hemoptysis with the rigid bronchoscope and cold saline lavage. *Thorax* 1980;35:901.
The authors describe the technique of iced saline lavage to control hemorrhage.

Dellinger RP. Fiberoptic bronchoscopy in adult airway management. *Crit Care Med* 1990; 18:882.
The author provides an in-depth review of the use of the flexible bronchoscope in management of the airway: intubation with single- and double-lumen endotracheal tubes, tube changes and extubation, and other aspects of airway management.

Imgrund SP, Goldberg SK, Walkenstein MD, et al. Clinical diagnosis of massive hemoptysis using the fiberoptic bronchoscope. *Crit Care Med* 1985;13:438.
Illustrative cases are presented with a review of the use of the flexible bronchoscope in the evaluation and treatment of massive hemoptysis.

Jolliet PH, Chevrolet JC. Bronchoscopy in the intensive care unit. *Intensive Care Med* 1992;18:160.
Bronchoscopy in the intensive care unit, including its effects on respiratory mechanics, gas exchange, and hemodynamics, and performing the procedure in high-risk patients is reviewed.

Pisani RJ, Wright AJ. Clinical utility of bronchoalveolar lavage in immunocompromised hosts. *Mayo Clin Proc* 1992;67:221.
The sensitivity and specificity of BAL were found to be 82% and 53%, respectively. The strengths and weaknesses of BAL in this patient population are discussed.

Silver MR, Balk RA. Bronchoscopic procedures in the intensive care unit. *Crit Care Clin* 1995;11:97–109.
Review of the application of bronchoscopy for the critical care specialist.

Timsit J-F, Misset B, Azoulay E, et al. Usefulness of airway visualization in the diagnosis of nosocomial pneumonia in ventilated patients. *Chest* 1996;110:172.
Direct visualization of the bronchial tree by bronchoscopy was found to predict nosocomial pneumonia accurately in ventilated patients.

Torres A, Bellacasa JP, Xauber A, et al. Diagnostic value of quantitative cultures of bronchoalveolar lavage and telescoping plugged catheters in mechanically ventilated patients with bacterial pneumonia. *Am Rev Respir Dis* 1989;140:306.
The diagnostic value of quantitative cultures of BAL and telescoping plugged catheter samples in 34 immunocompetent patients suspected of having bacterial pneumonia was studied. Both techniques were found to diagnose pneumonia with similar accuracy.

Turner JS, Willcox PA, Hayhurst MD, et al. Fiberoptic bronchoscopy in the intensive care unit—a prospective study of 147 procedures in 107 patients. *Crit Care Med* 1994; 22:259–264.
Safety and benefit of the procedure performed in 107 critically ill patients.

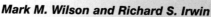

THORACENTESIS

Mark M. Wilson and Richard S. Irwin

10

I. GENERAL PRINCIPLES

A. Thoracentesis is the introduction of a needle, cannula, or trocar into the pleural space to remove accumulated fluid or air.

B. History (cough, dyspnea, or pleuritic chest pain) and examination (dullness to percussion, decreased breath sounds, and decreased tactile fremitus) suggest that an effusion is present.

C. Chest radiograph (CXR) or ultrasonic examination is essential to confirm the clinical suspicion.

D. Analysis of pleural fluid yields clinically useful information in more than 90% of cases.

E. Thoracentesis may be performed for diagnostic (generally 50 to 100 mL) or therapeutic (evacuation of air or more than 100 mL fluid) reasons.

F. The most common causes of pleural effusions are congestive heart failure, parapneumonic, malignancy, and postoperative sympathetic effusions.

II. INDICATIONS AND CONTRAINDICATIONS

A. Consider thoracentesis for pleural effusions in patients with pleurisy, who are febrile or are suspect for infection, whose clinical presentation is atypical for congestive heart failure, or whose course does not progress as anticipated.

B. Relative contraindications include those settings in which a complication from the procedure may prove catastrophic (i.e., known underlying bullous disease, the presence of positive end-expiratory pressure, a patient with only one functional lung).

C. Absolute contraindications include an uncooperative patient, the inability to identify the top of the rib at the planned puncture site clearly, operator inexperience with the procedure, and coagulopathy that cannot be corrected.

III. PROCEDURE

A. Technique for diagnostic (needle-only) thoracentesis

1. Obtain a lateral decubitus CXR to confirm a free-flowing pleural effusion.
2. Obtain informed written consent for the procedure.
3. With the patient sitting, arms at side, mark the inferior tip of the scapula on the side to be tapped. This approximates the eighth intercostal space, the lowest level punctured unless previous sonography determined that a lower interspace can safely be entered.
4. Position the patient sitting at the edge of the bed, leaning forward over a pillow-draped, bedside table and with arms crossed in front to elevate and spread the scapulae. An assistant should stand in front of the table to prevent any unexpected movements.
5. Percuss the patient's posterior chest for the highest point of the effusion. The interspace below this should be entered in the posterior axillary line. Mark the superior aspect of the rib with your fingernail (the inferior border of each rib contains an intercostal artery and should be avoided).
6. Using sterile technique, cleanse and drape the area surrounding the puncture site.
7. Anesthetize the superficial skin with 2% lidocaine using a 25-gauge needle. Use an 18- to 22-gauge needle to anesthetize the deeper soft tissues, aiming for the top of the rib. Always aspirate as the needle is advanced and before instilling lidocaine to ensure that the needle is not in a vessel or the pleural

space. Fluid enters the syringe on reaching the pleural space. The patient may experience discomfort as the needle penetrates the well-innervated parietal pleura. Be careful not to instill anesthetic into the pleural space; it is bactericidal for most organisms, including *Mycobacterium tuberculosis*. Estimate the required depth of insertion and remove the needle.

8. Attach a three-way stopcock to a 20-gauge, 1.5-inch needle and to a 50-mL syringe.

9. Insert the 20-gauge needle along the anesthetic tract, always aspirating through the syringe as the needle is slowly advanced. When pleural fluid is obtained, fill a heparinized blood gas syringe from the side port of the three-way stopcock, express all air from the sample, cap it, and place in a bag containing iced slush for immediate transport to the laboratory.

10. Fill the 50-mL syringe and transfer its contents into appropriate collection tubes and containers. Always maintain a closed system during the procedure to prevent room air from entering the pleural space.

11. When the thoracentesis is complete, remove the needle from the patient's chest. Apply pressure to the wound for several minutes, and apply a sterile bandage.

12. Obtain a postprocedure upright end-expiratory CXR if a pneumothorax is suspected. Immediately after the procedure, draw venous blood for total protein and lactate dehydrogenase determinations. These are necessary to interpret pleural fluid values.

B. Technique for therapeutic thoracentesis

1. Follow steps 1 to 7 as described previously.

2. Removal of more than 100 mL of pleural fluid involves placement of a catheter into the pleural space. Commercial kits are widely available, each with specific instructions for performing this procedure. Operators should be thoroughly familiar with the recommended procedure and should receive appropriate supervision from an experienced operator before performing therapeutic thoracentesis on their own.

C. Technique for removal of freely moving pneumothorax

1. Position the patient supine with the head of the bed elevated 30 to 45 degrees.

2. Prepare the anterior second or third intercostal space in the midclavicular line (to avoid the more medial internal mammary artery).

3. Have the bevel of the needle facing upward, and direct the needle superiorly so the catheter can be guided to the superior aspect of the hemithorax.

4. Air may be actively withdrawn by syringe or pushed out when intrapleural pressure is supraatmospheric (e.g., during a cough), as long as the catheter is intermittently open to the atmosphere. Air can leave but not reenter the pleural space if a one-way valve apparatus (Heimlich valve) is attached or if the catheter is put to underwater seal.

5. If a tension pneumothorax is known or suspected and a chest tube is not readily available, quickly insert a 14-gauge angiocatheter according to the foregoing technique. If a tension pneumothorax is present, air will escape under pressure. When the situation has been stabilized, replace the catheter with a sterile chest tube.

IV. POSTPROCEDURE CONSIDERATIONS

A. The overall complication rate from thoracentesis is as low as 5% when performed by experienced intensivists but may be as high as 50% to 78% when performed by those less experienced.

B. Major, possibly life-threatening complications may occur in up to 15% to 19% and include pneumothorax, hemorrhage, hypotension, reexpansion pulmonary edema, venous or cerebral air embolism (rare), and sheared catheter fragments left in the pleural space (rare).

C. The risk of pneumothorax varies depending on baseline patient characteristics (e.g., presence or absence of chronic obstructive pulmonary disease), operator experience, and the method used to perform the procedure.

D. Minor complications also depend on the method used and occur in 16% to 63%, including dry tap, anxiety, dyspnea, cough, pain, and subcutaneous hematoma or seroma.

V. INTERPRETATION OF PLEURAL FLUID ANALYSIS

A. A transudate is biochemically defined by meeting *all* the following criteria: pleural fluid-to-serum ratio for total protein less than 0.5, pleural fluid-to-serum ratio for lactate dehydrogenase (LDH) less than 0.6, and an absolute pleural fluid LDH less than two thirds the upper limits of normal of the serum LDH. If a transudate is present, then generally no further tests on pleural fluid are indicated.

B. An exudate is present when any of the criteria for transudate are not met. Further evaluation is usually warranted.

1. A pleural fluid pH lower than 7.20, narrows the differential diagnosis to systemic acidemia, empyema or parapneumonic effusion, malignancy, rheumatoid or lupus effusion, extrapulmonary tuberculosis, ruptured esophagus, or urinothorax. These effusions are potentially sclerotic and require consideration for chest tube drainage.

2. Pleural fluid glucose levels less than 50% of the serum level may be found with empyema, malignancy, rheumatoid or lupus effusion, extrapulmonary tuberculosis, or ruptured esophagus.

3. Although not diagnostic, pleural fluid white blood cell counts exceeding 50,000/mm^3 strongly suggest bacterial pneumonia or empyema but may also be seen in effusions associated with rheumatoid arthritis. Pleural fluid lymphocytosis is nonspecific, but when greater than 80% of cells, suggests tuberculosis or malignancy.

4. Grossly bloody effusions contain more than 100,000 cells/mm^3 and are most commonly seen in trauma, malignancy, or pulmonary infarction. Hemothorax is defined by a pleural fluid hematocrit of 50% or greater of the serum hematocrit.

5. If initial cytologic results are negative for malignancy and a strong clinical suspicion exists, additional pleural fluid samples can increase the chance of a positive result. The addition of a pleural biopsy increases the yield a modest amount over cytology on two separate specimens. Cytologic examination may also definitively diagnose rheumatoid pleuritis.

Selected Readings

Bowditch HI. Paracentesis thoracis. *Am J Med Sci* 23:105, 1852.
The first description of thoracentesis.

Collins TR, Sahn SA. Thoracentesis: clinical value, complications, technical problems, and patient experience. *Chest* 1987; 91:817.

Grogan D, Irwin RS, Channick R, et al. Complications associated with thoracentesis: a prospective randomized study comparing three different methods. *Arch Intern Med* 1990;150:873.
The foregoing two articles provide an excellent overview of the complications and pitfalls associated with thoracentesis.

Good JT, Taryle DA, Maulitz RM, et al. The diagnostic value of pleural fluid pH. *Chest* 1980;78:55.

Light RW, Ball WC. Glucose and amylase in pleural effusions. *JAMA* 1973;225:257.

Sahn SA. The differential diagnosis of pleural effusions. *West J Med* 1982;137:99.

Heffner JE, Brown LK, Barbieri CA. Diagnostic value of tests that discriminate between exudative and transudative pleural effusions. *Chest* 1997;111:970.
The preceding four readings provide a good review of the use of biochemical testing in the evaluation of pleural effusions.

Light RW, MacGregor MI, Luchsinger PC, et al. Pleural effusions: the diagnostic separation of transudates and exudates. *Ann Intern Med* 1972;77:507.
A must-read classic article!

11

THE TRACHEOSTOMY
Mark L. Shapiro

I. GENERAL PRINCIPLES
A. Invasive procedure usually performed by surgeons in most centers
B. Patients who warrant tracheostomy have a high mortality rate (2% to 5%)
    1. Secondary to comorbid disease states
C. Can be performed in almost any setting safely
    1. Emergency department
    2. Intensive care unit
    3. Operating room
D. Variety of techniques
    1. Open
    2. Semiopen
    3. Percutaneous

II. ANATOMY
A. Distal continuation of the larynx
B. Much shorter in pediatric population than adults
C. Thyroid cartilage
    1. Easily palpable
    2. Most superior cartilage
D. Cricothyroid membrane
    1. Exists between thyroid cartilage and cricoid cartilage
    2. Access for emergent cricothyrotomy
    3. Palpable indentation between the two cartilages
    4. Do not perform emergent cricothyrotomy in children less than 9 years old.
        a. Emergent tracheotomy is procedure of choice.
E. Cricoid cartilage is the only continuous ring of the trachea.
F. Occupies neck and thorax
G. Immediately anterior to the esophagus
H. Divides into right and left principal bronchi and subsequently into lobar bronchi
    1. Principal bronchi originate behind the aorta, to the right and just below the arch.
    2. Carina (bifurcation) at the level of seventh thoracic vertebra

III. INDICATIONS
A. Airway obstruction
    1. Thyroid tumors
    2. Pharyngeal abscess
    3. Granulation tissue from prolonged intubation/irritation
    4. Severe inflammation
        a. Asthma
        b. Trauma
        c. Anaphylaxis
B. Prolonged mechanical ventilation
    1. Head injuries
    2. Severe chronic obstructive pulmonary disease (COPD)
    3. Quadriplegia
    4. High spine injuries
    5. Improved pulmonary toilet but does not decrease incidence of pneumonia

C. Prophylaxis
   1. Facial reconstruction
   2. Esophageal reconstruction
D. Comfort
   1. Decreased work of breathing
   2. Decrease risk of sinus infection (nasotracheally intubated)
   3. Easier to wean from mechanical ventilation
E. Contraindications
   1. Recent surgical procedures
      a. Contamination of wound
         (1) Anterior cervical spine surgery
         (2) Median sternotomy

IV. PROCEDURE

A. Considerations
   1. In elective tracheotomies, ensure that the patient is not coagulopathic.
      a. Liver disease
      b. Therapeutic anticoagulation
   2. Obese patient needs
      a. Extra long cannula—*very important*
      b. May need a headlight
      c. Liberal incision
   3. Patients on moderate amounts of positive end-expiratory pressure (PEEP)
      a. Caution on patients responsive to PEEP
      b. If PEEP is greater than 10 cm H_2O, consider delaying the procedure.
         (1) Derecruitment of alveoli may occur.
            (a) Hypoxemia
            (b) Acute lung injury
   4. Closed head injured with increased intracranial pressure (ICP)
      a. Inappropriate for tracheostomy while ICP is elevated or uncontrolled
      b. Percutaneous tracheostomy may increase ICP when facilitated with bronchoscopy
      c. Elevated $PaCO_2$ during bronchoscopy
B. Open
   1. General anesthesia
   2. Inspect the surgery technician's table for needed equipment
   3. Test cuff
   4. Ensure that 6.5 mm internal diameter endotracheal tube (ET) is available
   5. Make sure that anesthesiologist has released the ET tube holder and all tape is ready for removal on request.
   6. If cervical spine injury, do not extend or flex neck, but maintain neutral attitude.
   7. Do not overextend neck because 2nd and 3rd tracheal rings may be displace too far superiorly.
   8. Prepare neck with chlorhexidine gluconate with alcohol or povidone-iodine with alcohol from the chin to below nipples.
   9. Infiltrate area of anticipated incision with 1% lidocaine with epinephrine.
   10. Longitudinal or transverse incision is acceptable.
      a. Longitudinal to avoid anterior jugular veins and facilitate speed of procedure
      b. Transverse for cosmetic purposes
      c. Make incision below cricoid ring and above 3rd tracheal ring
   11. Combination of blunt dissection and electrocautery through to midline raphae and then down to pretracheal fascia
   12. Thyroid often obstructs view
      a. Very vascular
      b. Cautious electrocautery or suture ligation and divide, or use cricoid hook to elevate gland out of the way by inserting into membrane just inferior to cricoid cartilage

     13. Continuous assessment and palpation to maintain midline integrity

     14. Identify trachea, cricoid cartilage, 3rd tracheal ring

     15. Extirpate partial anterior portion 3rd tracheal ring

     16. Tracheal dilators to dilate tracheostomy

     17. Anesthesiologist to retract endotracheal tube under surgeons request

     18. Place tracheostomy catheter into surgical wound gently following curve of cannula and anatomy of trachea.

     19. Attach breathing circuit to tracheostomy cannula.

     20. Inflate balloon.

     21. Observe for end-tidal carbon dioxide on monitor.

     22. Suture in place with four-point fixation and trachea ties

C. Percutaneous technique

     1. Prepare neck as above.

     2. Respiratory therapist presence to maintain minute volume and ventilation during procedure

     3. Use flexible bronchoscope to visualize tracheal tree.

     4. Retract ET tube slowly.

     5. Transilluminate 2nd or 3rd tracheal ring.

     6. Anesthetize area with 1% lidocaine with epinephrine.

     7. Pull bronchoscope into lumen of ET tube to protect scope from percutaneous catheter placement.

     8. Insert percutaneous needle into lumen of trachea perpendicular to skin under direct visualization via bronchoscope to avoid perforating the posterior aspect of the trachea and entering esophagus.

     9. Place guidewire through needle into trachea, then remove needle.

     10. Over the guidewire, pass dilator(s)—kits vary—until able to pass trachea cannula easily.

     11. Suture into place

D. Semiopen

     1. Variation of the two above techniques

     2. Higher risk of tracheoesophageal fistula

     3. Ultrasound may be advantageous

V. CONSIDERATIONS

A. Postprocedure chest radiography (CXR)

     1. Often the standard of care, recently controversial in the literature

     2. Several studies demonstrate that this is not cost effective.

     3. CXR for those who are symptomatic only

     4. Look for bronchial plugging and pneumothorax.

B. Tracheal stenosis

     1. Older literature suggests stenosis occurs more frequently with open procedures.

     2. Occurred more frequently in the past with ET tubes with high-pressure/low-volume cuffs. Modern cuffs are high-volume/low-pressure.

C. Tracheoinnominate artery fistula

     1. Rare event and rapidly fatal even when recognized early

     2. Prototypical patient is female; long, gracile neck; and slender.

     3. Etiology is often placement of tracheostomy below the 3rd tracheal ring.

       a. Can be due to percutaneous needle placement into innominate artery directly through trachea.

       b. Caution with overextension of neck because it retracts thoracic airway cephalad.

Selected Readings

Beiderlinden M, Karl Walz M, Sander A, et al. Complications of bronchoscopically guided percutaneous dilational tracheostomy: beyond the learning curve. *Intensive Care Med* 2002;28:59–62.

    Percutaneous dilational tracheostomy (PDT) complications are attenuated with omission of routine tracheostomy tube changes not the type of kit used.

Byhahn C, Wilke HJ, Lischke V, et al. Translaryngeal tracheostomy: two modified techniques versus the basic technique—early experience in 75 critically ill adults. *Intensive Care Med* 2000;26:457–461.

Modified technique did not have as many complications of retrograde passage of guidewire; yet, no difference in gas exchange or perioperative complications.

Dollner R, Verch M, Schweiger P, et al. Long-term outcome after Griggs tracheostomy. *J Otolaryngol* 2002;31:386–389.

Bronchoscopy should be used for percutaneous dilational tracheostomy to ensure adequate placement and attenuate possibility of stenosis.

Ernst A, Critchlow J: Percutaneous tracheostomy—special considerations. *Clin Chest Med* 2003; 24:409–412.

Nice review of percutaneous tracheostomies. This institution claims a less than 5% open tracheostomy rate.

Freeman BD, Isabella K, Lin N, et al. A meta-analysis of prospective trials comparing percutaneous and surgical tracheostomy in critically ill patients. *Chest* 2000;118:1412–1418.

In appropriately selected ICU patients, percutaneous tracheostomy is a safe, simple, cost-effective means of establishing a tracheostomy over an open procedure.

Kerwin AJ, Croce MA, Timmons SD, et al. Effects of fiberoptic bronchoscopy on intracranial pressure in patients with brain injury: a prospective clinical study. *J Trauma* 2000;48:878–882.

Bronchoscopy may increase the ICP in the head-injured despite chemical sedation and paralysis; however, no secondary brain injury was identified in 26 bronchoscopies.

Melloni G, Muttini S, Gallioli G, et al. Surgical tracheostomy versus percutaneous dilatational tracheostomy. A prospective-randomized study with long-term follow-up. *J Cardiovasc Surg* (Torino) 2002;43:113–121.

Randomized, prospective, controlled trial demonstrating PDT has a lower early complication rate, and not a statistically different late complication rate.

Pryor JP, Reilly PM, Shapiro MB. Surgical airway management in the intensive care unit. *Crit Care Clin* 2000;16:473–488.

Nice review complimenting percutaneous tracheostomies for their cost effectiveness.

Sugerman HJ, Wolfe L, Pasquale MD, et al. Multicenter, randomized, prospective trial of early tracheostomy. *J Trauma* 1997;43:741–747.

No difference in early versus late tracheostomy in 157 patients. Study flawed by physician bias and head-injured patients. Caution in interpreting these data.

Tyroch AH, Kaups K, Lorenzo M, et al. Routine chest radiograph is not indicated after open tracheostomy: a multicenter perspective. *Am Surg* 2002;68:80–82.

In uncomplicated open tracheostomies, routine chest radiography is not indicated or cost effective.

12 GASTROINTESTINAL ENDOSCOPY
Savant Mehta

I. **GENERAL PRINCIPLES.** This chapter reviews the indications, contraindications, techniques, and complications of gastrointestinal endoscopy in critically ill patients.

  A. Charged couple device chip technology and video monitors have replaced fiberoptic bundles on newer instruments, although fiberoptic and rigid endoscopes are still in use.

  B. Wheels and buttons on the handle of the flexible instrument control tip deflection, suction, and air and water insufflation.

II. **INDICATIONS.** Although cardiopulmonary complications of gastrointestinal endoscopy are infrequent, the procedure should be performed only when the tangible benefits clearly outweigh the risks. Gastrointestinal endoscopy in patients with clinically insignificant bleeding or minimally troublesome gastrointestinal complaints should be postponed until the medical-surgical illnesses improve. All endoscopists performing diagnostic gastrointestinal procedures should be competent in endoscopic therapy.

  A. Upper gastrointestinal endoscopy

  1. Upper gastrointestinal bleeding. Patients with evidence of hemodynamic instability, continuing need for transfusions or suspected variceal bleeding should undergo urgent upper endoscopy with plans for appropriate endoscopic therapy.

  2. Caustic ingestion

  3. Foreign body ingestion

  4. Percutaneous endoscopic gastrostomy (PEG) placement

  B. Endoscopic retrograde cholangiopancreatography (ECRP)

  1. ERCP is used only occasionally in the intensive care unit (ICU).

  2. Indications

    a. Cholangitis unresponsive to medical therapy

    b. Acute gallstone pancreatitis complicated by cholangitis or jaundice

    c. Severe gall stone pancreatitis within the first 24 hours.

  C. Lower gastrointestinal endoscopy

  1. Acute lower gastrointestinal bleeding, but this procedure is technically difficult. Colonoscopy appears to have the highest yield in diagnosing and sometimes treating lower gastrointestinal bleeding. It is safe when appropriate resuscitation has been performed. Technetium-labeled erythrocyte scanning and angiography are other methods commonly used for localizing a bleeding site.

  2. Endoscopic colonic decompression has been advised in critically ill patients with acute adynamic ileus when the diameter of the right colon exceeds 12 cm. Other studies suggest that the colonic dilation may not progress to life-threatening complications and decompression is unnecessary. Decompression by colonoscopy should not be first-line therapy for pseudoobstruction. Nasogastric and rectal tube placement, discontinuation of offending medications (opioids and phenothiazines), treatment of underlying illness, and frequent repositioning (every 2 hours) of debilitated patients in the ICU often allows resolution of pseudoobstruction. In patients who have not had a response to conservative therapy, treatment with neostigmine should be tried.

III. **CONTRAINDICATIONS**

  A. GI perforation. Endoscopy (and the associated air insufflation) should be avoided in patients with known or suspected gastrointestinal perforation and those known to be at high risk of perforation.

B. Hemodynamic instability is a relative contraindication for endoscopy, but the benefit of therapeutic endoscopy may outweigh the risks in critically ill patients.

C. Coagulopathy. The risk of a bleeding complication of endoscopic sphincterotomy is higher in patients with gross coagulopathy, and ERCP may be delayed while the coagulopathy is corrected.

D. Aspiration. Endotracheal intubation and heavy sedation or general anesthesia may be necessary to facilitate the procedure. Patients with acute upper gastrointestinal bleeding who are confused or stuporous should have their airway protected with an endotracheal tube before endoscopy is performed.

IV. COMPLICATIONS

A. Bleeding. Most bleeding is minimal and self-limited, but repeat endoscopy and surgery may be necessary to control recurrent bleeding. Angiography can assist in localizing the bleeding source in postendoscopy bleeding.

B. Perforation. Perforation of the bowel may result, and antibiotics and intravenous fluids should be given; surgery may be required. If duodenal perforation is encountered after endoscopic sphincterotomy, early medical therapy and stabilization of the patient may preclude the need for surgery.

C. Cardiopulmonary complications. Aspiration of stomach contents and blood in acute upper gastrointestinal bleeding can be minimized by protecting the airway with endotracheal intubation in patients with severe bleeding or an altered mental state.

D. Infections. Infectious complications can be minimized by appropriate use of prophylactic antibiotics in high-risk patients (with prosthetic mechanical valves or grafts) or high-risk procedures (prior to PEG placement, dilation, sclerotherapy, ERCP).

E. Other. Sedative medications have their own complications, usually as a consequence of medication-induced hypoxemia (2 to 5/1,000 cases). Other complications can occur, including apnea, hypotension, and, rarely, death (0.3 to 0.5/1,000 cases).

V. TECHNIQUES

A. Upper gastrointestinal endoscopy

1. Fluid resuscitation and optimal treatment of hypoxemia should precede all endoscopic examinations.

2. Endotracheal intubation should be considered in obtunded patients with severe bleeding and those undergoing foreign-body removal. Nasogastric or orogastric lavage with a large-bore tube (greater than 40 Fr) should be performed to evacuate blood and clots from the stomach before endoscopy is performed in a patient with acute gastrointestinal bleeding.

3. Upper gastrointestinal bleeding is the most common indication for upper endoscopy in the ICU. Patients with continued or recurrent upper gastrointestinal bleeding should have urgent upper endoscopy as early as possible, certainly within 6 to 8 hours after presentation. In patients with massive hemorrhage, endoscopy may be performed in the operating room in anticipation of surgical therapy.

4. The team consists of an experienced endoscopist, a specially trained endoscopy assistant, and a nurse skilled in monitoring patients undergoing endoscopy. A topical anesthetic is applied to the patient's pharynx to reduce the gag reflex. Intravenous anxiolytics and/or opioids are used (see Chapter 20).

5. Proper patient monitoring is needed, with frequent (every 5 minutes) blood pressure and pulse measurements and continuous measurement of oxygen saturation by pulse oximetry.

6. Endoscopy is performed with a "therapeutic" instrument, equipped with a large operating channel to allow suctioning of blood, and hemostatic therapy. The endoscope is passed, and the upper gastrointestinal tract is rapidly surveyed to locate the site of bleeding and to facilitate surgical therapy if endoscopic therapy fails. If an active bleeding site is found, hemostatic therapy may be attempted immediately.

7. In patients with significant recent bleeding and endoscopic evidence of recent hemorrhage (a visible vessel or adherent clot on an ulcer), hemostatic therapy to prevent recurrent bleeding should be strongly considered.

8. Actively bleeding lesions in the upper gastrointestinal tract can be treated by injection therapy, mechanical clipping devices, band ligation, argon plasma coagulation, heater probe therapy, or monopolar and bipolar electrocoagulation.

   a. Injection therapy is simple and inexpensive, requiring only a needle catheter and various liquid media to effect hemostasis, including absolute ethanol, sclerosants (sodium morrhuate), or vasoconstrictors (epinephrine). Injection therapy may be less effective in briskly bleeding ulcers or in bleeding esophageal varices. Injection therapy using epinephrine, absolute alcohol, or sclerosants (sodium morruhate, ethanolamine) allows treatment of lesions even when seen tangentially. Injection therapy generally begins on the periphery of the lesion, with injections in all four quadrants. Variceal sclerotherapy involves a direct or paravariceal injection of 1 to 4 mL of sclerosant.

   b. A newer method of banding esophageal varices is superior to sclerotherapy in terms of overall complications, recurrent bleeding, and mortality. Banding of varices is performed with an endoscopic adaptor that allows placement of small rubber bands directly onto a varix.

   c. Heater probes generate heat using electrical current delivered to the tip of the catheter, whereas bipolar electrocautery delivers electrical currently directly to the tissue and causes coagulation necrosis. Because hemostatic therapy with the heater probe or bicap equipment requires an *en face* view; lesions seen tangentially may be difficult to treat with these methods

B. Lower gastrointestinal endoscopy

   1. Lower gastrointestinal endoscopy can be extremely difficult to perform in critically ill patients with colonic hemorrhage.

   2. Instruments available for the examination of the lower gastrointestinal tract include the following:

   a. Anoscope, which is useful mainly to evaluate for hemorrhoids or fissures

   b. Sigmoidoscope

   c. Colonoscope

   3. Colonoscopy

   a. Colonoscopes are generally 140 to 180 cm long and are necessary to reach colonic lesions situated proximal to the splenic flexure.

   b. Patient preparation for colonoscopy usually consists of a gallon of nonabsorbed polyethylene glycol given by mouth over 4 to 6 hours or by nasogastric tube 12 hours before examination. Magnesium citrate may be used over 24 to 48 hours in patients who have been taking clear liquids.

   C. Abdominal pressure that is applied by an assistant during colonoscopy may assist in advancing the colonoscope.

Selected Readings

Fan S, Lai E, Mok F, et al. Early treatment of acute biliary pancreatitis by endoscopic papillotomy. *N Engl J Med* 1993;328:228.
   A controversial article that ERCP is indicated in the early treatment of patients with acute pancreatitis.

Freeman ML, Cass OW, Peine CJ, et al. The non-bleeding visible vessel versus the sentinel clot: natural history and risk of rebleeding. *Gastrointest Endosc* 1993;39:3.
   An evaluation of the stigmata of ulcers and the need for early surgical intervention.

Hirschowitz BI. Development and application of endoscopy. *Gastroenterology* 1993;104:337.
   An excellent review of the development of GI endoscopy from the use of rigid tubes and candlelight to the charge couple device chip and sophisticated flexible instruments.

Laine L. Refining the prognostic value of endoscopy in patients with bleeding ulcers. *Gastrointest Endosc* 1993;39:436.
   A good review supporting the efficacy of early endoscopy of ICU GI bleeders.

Lin HJ, Perng CL, Lee FY, et al. Endoscopic injection for the arrest of peptic ulcer hemorrhage: final results of a prospective, randomized comparative trial. *Gastrointest Endosc* 1993;39:1.

A review of the two treatment options of UGI bleed and their efficacy.

Ponec RJ, Saunders MD, Kimmey MB. Neostigmine for the treatment of acute colonic pseudoobstruction. *N Engl J Med* 1999;341:137.

The usefulness of neostigmine was shown in the randomized, placebo controlled study.

Sloyer AF, Panella VS, Demas BE, et al. Olgivie's syndrome: successful management without colonoscopy. *Dig Dis Sci* 1988;33:1391.

An outline of the noninvasive management of pseudoobstruction.

13

DIAGNOSTIC PERITONEAL LAVAGE AND PARACENTESIS
Mark L. Shapiro

I. GENERAL PRINCIPLES
A. Introduction
1. Diagnostic peritoneal lavage (DPL)
2. Often performed emergently in the traumatically injured
   a. Ease of conduct
   b. Expedites patient disposition
   c. Versatile: blunt and penetrating trauma
   d. Rapid
   e. Cost effective compared to CT scan, laparoscopy, laparotomy
   f. Relatively simple

II. ACCURACY
A. Can detect as little as 20 mL of blood
B. Sensitivity approximates 85% to 98%
   1. Dependent on facility of surgeon and intraperitoneal injuries
   2. Cannot diagnose contained retroperitoneal structures
C. Specificity approximates 93% to 97%
D. Blunt trauma
   1. Positive DPL
      a. 10 mL Gross blood on initial aspiration
      b. Greater than 100,000 RBC/mm^3 in lavage fluid
      c. WBC greater than 500/mm^3
      d. Amylase higher than 175 U/dL
      e. Presence of food, particulate matter, stool, bile
      f. Cannot read the print on the side of the liter bag of crystalloid because of turbidity of fluid return
   2. Negative DPL
      a. Often considered negative when the above criteria are not present
      b. Multiple reasons for equivocal findings (i.e., 50,000 to 99,000 RBCs, 400 WBCs, etc.); leave catheter in and repeat in 2 to 3 hours if patient remains stable.
      c. If the print on the side of a liter bag of crystalloid is legible, it is reasonably safe to say the DPL is negative.
E. Penetrating trauma
   1. Positive DPL
      a. Same criteria as blunt with the exception of RBC count
         (1) RBC count of 10,000 is commonly accepted as positive.
         (2) Some institutions desire 1,000 as positive.
         (3) Sensitivity is variable when these lower values are used.
            i. Sensitivity ranges from 67% to 100%.
            ii. Accuracy ranges from 97% to 98%.
         (4) Nontherapeutic laparotomy rate is 10% to 15%.
   2. Negative DPL: not satisfying the above criteria

III. INDICATIONS
A. Clinical judgment supersedes overall.
B. Note: the surgeon must decide whether to perform the DPL because he or she is the one who will operate or not operate and follow these patients. Without surgical presence, the patient must be transferred to a trauma center.

C. Most commonly accepted indication: hypotension and unstable patient
   1. Hemorrhagic shock
   2. Intoxication
      a. Ethanol
      b. Illicit drugs
   3. Associated head injury
D. Other acceptable criteria include
   1. Multitrauma patients who will undergo general anesthesia
   2. Penetrating injuries suspected of invading multiple body cavities (e.g., transdia-phragmatic)
   3. CT scanner is unavailable

IV. CONTRAINDICATIONS
A. Absolute
   1. Predetermined exploratory laparotomy (e.g., penetrating abdominal wound with evisceration)
B. Relative
   1. Multiple previous abdominal operations
   2. Grossly distended abdomen
      a. Tympanitic
      b. Gravid uterus
   3. Abdominal wall hematomas (high false-positive rate)

V. OPTIONS
A. CT scan
   1. Study of choice in the *stable* patient
      a. Can visualize the retroperitoneum simultaneously
      b. Upper cuts visualize the heart and base of lungs
      c. May differentiate between solid organ injury
      d. Assess vascular integrity
   2. Disadvantages
      a. Extraordinarily dangerous if patient becomes unstable in the CT scanner
      b. Costly
      c. Early CT may miss pancreatic and duodenal injuries
      d. Contrast nephropathy
      e. Anaphylaxis
      f. Labor intensive
      g. Risks of extubation, loss of venous access
B. FAST (focused abdominal sonography for trauma)
   1. Reliability
      a. 90% to 98% accurate
      b. 88% to 98% sensitive
      c. 93% to 97% specific
   2. Wide variation in reliability is accounted for by the size of studies, grade of organ injury, different types of fluid in abdomen (blood, bile, pus, succus)
   3. Advantages
      a. Noninvasive
      b. Portable
      c. Rapid, real-time images
      d. Repeatable
      e. Cost effective
      f. Easily used on patients with prior abdominal operations
      g. Also provides pericardial visualization
   4. Disadvantages
      a. Poor visualization with subcutaneous emphysema
      b. Unreliable with pleural effusions
      c. Poor visualization of the retroperitoneal structures
      d. Not indicated in penetrating abdominal injuries, but one exception is the

pericardial view.
  e. Learning curve
    (1) Need about 25 to 50 FAST examinations to be proficient. If not profi-
        cient by then, literature suggests that FAST examination may not be the
        study of choice for that individual.
  C. Diagnostic laparoscopy
    1. Advantages
      a. Direct visualization of solid organs and most of bowel
      b. Can lead to early diagnosis when under way
      c. Can be therapeutic as well as diagnostic
      d. If nontherapeutic, patient can be discharged from PACU barring other issues.
    2. Disadvantages
      a. Time-consuming
      b. Different levels of comfort for mobilizing structures and running the bowel
      c. Costly
      d. Occupies an operating room most often
      e. Risk of general anesthesia
      f. Possible delay in diagnosis
      g. Higher risk of iatrogenic injuries related to laparoscopy
        (1) Bowel perforation
        (2) Cautery burns
  D. Local wound exploration
    1. For penetrating abdominal injuries only
    2. Check for invasion of anterior fascia
      a. If positive, to operating room
      b. If negative, done
    3. Can be cumbersome if overlying muscle or bleeding skin
  E. Celiotomy
    1. Advantages
      a. Direct visualization
      b. Palpate areas in question
      c. Therapeutic
      d. Very low missed injury rate
      e. Can be performed rapidly, with quick control
    2. Disadvantages
      a. General anesthesia
      b. Occupies an operating room
      c. Larger, painful incision
      d. Can be costly
      e. Nontherapeutic laparotomy rates: 10% to 15%

VI. PROCEDURE
  A. Control the situation and environment
  B. Think clearly
  C. Decompress hollow viscus
    1. Nasogastric/orogastric decompression
      a. Salem sump
      b. Often distended by aggressive bag valve mask ventilation, anxiety with aero-
         phagia, esophageal intubation, or oral contrast
    2. Urinary bladder decompression: Foley catheter
  D. Decide to incise above or below the umbilicus
    1. Above the umbilicus for those patients with:
      a. Pelvic fractures
        (1) Large retroperitoneal bleeding
        (2) Stay above arcuate line
      b. Gravid uterus
        (1) Perforate the uterus

(2) Increases morbidity and mortality of fetus and mother
2. Below the umbilicus for most others
  a. Unless a previous surgery obviates this choice
  b. Ease of placing the catheter into proper anatomic space
E. Infiltrate with 1% lidocaine with epinephrine for length of incision (2 cm)
  1. Epinephrine to decrease skin bleeding, which may obstruct view or confound results
F. Choose open, semiopen, blind technique
  1. Based on experience mostly
  2. All can be performed rapidly
  3. Blind technique has marginally, but significantly more complications
  4. Most often performed is the semiopen technique
G. Semiopen technique
  1. Incision made through the skin to expose the fascia
  2. Two penetrating towel clips placed in closed position placed into surgical wound facing each other
  3. Clamps opened at same time in the surgical wound
  4. Clamps are closed while pressing downward grasping the fascia
  5. Clamps and fascia are raised anteriorly through the surgical wound
  6. Anterior fascia is incised
  7. Peritoneal dialysis catheter placed at 45 to 60 degrees to the vertical aimed toward the pelvis
  8. Two distinct "pops" should be appreciated as catheter enters peritoneum
  9. Fenestrated catheter advanced via Seldinger technique into place
  10. One liter (or 25 mL/kg) of crystalloid infused into peritoneal cavity (can use pressure bag) via two-way intravenous tubing
  11. Once in, bag is placed on floor to dependent drainage
  12. At least 200 to 300 mL should be collected into the bag before 70 mL is sent for laboratory analysis and quantification
  13. Catheter may be removed and skin stapled shut, or keep the site sterile and repeat if necessary in 3 hours

VII. GENERAL PRINCIPLES OF PARACENTESIS
  A. Is performed as an adjunctive study for a variety of medical and sometimes surgical conditions
  B. Patients should have documentation of ascites prior to paracentesis with the exception of the DPL for trauma by history, physical examination, or radiographically.

VIII. INDICATIONS
  A. Therapeutic
    1. Removal of ascitic fluid to alleviate cardiovascular or pulmonary embarrassment
  B. Diagnostic
    1. Etiology of ascites
      a. Diagnostic peritoneal lavage in trauma
      b. Hepatorenal syndrome
      c. Spontaneous bacterial peritonitis
      d. Neoplastic process
      e. Heart failure

IX. CONTRAINDICATIONS
  A. Gravid uterus
  B. Gross distension of hollow viscus
  C. Organomegaly
  D. Multiple prior abdominal surgeries
  E. Localized infection at percutaneous site

X. PROCEDURE
  A. For added accuracy and decreased risk of complications use ultra-sonography.

| TABLE 13-1 | Common Laboratory Studies with Findings in the Diagnostic Paracentesis |

	Gram stain	Albumin$_{S/A}$*	Glucose	Specific gravity	Cytology	Total protein
Spontaneous bacterial peritonitis	+	1.1	>50	>1.016 if purulent	−	<1.0
Cirrhosis	−	>1.1	−	<1.016	−	<2.5
Congestive heart failure	−	>1.1	−	Variable <1.016	−	>2.5
Neoplastic process	−	<1.1 >1.1 with Hepatic Mets	NL to low	Variable >1.016	+	>2.5 Can be <3.0 if liver replaced with Mets
Nephrosis	−	<1.1	−	<1.016	−	<2.5

*Serum albumin/ascites albumin gradient.

    B. Prepare skin with alcohol–chlorhexidine solution (e.g., Dura-Prep)
    C. Select site
        1. Midline approximately 3 cm from umbilicus
        2. Lateral to rectus muscles in the lower quadrant
    D. Anesthetize with 1% lidocaine with epinephrine and make a skin wheel
    E. Retract skin gently (creates a Z-track) to attenuate risk of leaking ascitic fluid at completion of procedure
    F. Under sterile conditions, percutaneously insert paracentesis catheter via Seldinger technique into peritoneal cavity
    G. If paracentesis kit is unavailable or constant drainage is not indicated, an 18- to 22-gauge needle may be used. This can be connected to a negative pressure specimen bottle.
    H. Approximately 50 mL is all that is needed for most diagnostic studies.
    I. Place sterile dressing over procedure site.

XI. DIAGNOSTIC STUDIES
    A. Gram stain, AFB smear, culture, and sensitivity
    B. Cytology
    C. Cell count, LDH, total protein, glucose, amylase, triglyceride
    D. Specific gravity
    E. Albumin for determination serum albumin/ascites albumin gradient

XII. COMPLICATIONS
    A. Bleeding
    B. Infection
    C. Perforation of bowel, bladder, stomach or vessel
    D. Exacerbation of encephalopathy, renal failure, electrolyte disturbance, hypotension

Selected Readings
Bansal S, Kaur K, Bansal AK. Diagnosing ascitic etiology on a biochemical basis. *Hepato-gastroenterology* 1998;45:1673–1677.
    Paracentesis is useful in cirrhotic patients for guiding further diagnostic studies instead of ordering a broad panel in hopes of obtaining a diagnosis.

Blendis L, Wong F. The natural history and management of hepatorenal disorders: from pre-ascites to hepatorenal syndrome. *Clin Med* 2003; 3:154–159.
Transjugular intrahepatic portasystemic shunt (TIPS) may prevent onset or even reverse hepatorenal syndrome. Repeat paracentesis does not.

Dittrich S, Yordi LM, de Mattos AA. The value of serum-ascites albumin gradient for the determination of portal hypertension in the diagnosis of ascites. *Hepatogastroenterology* 2001;48:166–168.
Serum-ascites albumin gradient is a reliable indicator of portal hypertension and its relationship with the origin of ascites.

Fabian TC, Croce MA, Stewart RM, et al. A prospective analysis of diagnostic laparoscopy in trauma. *Ann Surg* 1993;217:557–564.
Early paper demonstrating cost effectiveness of diagnostic laparoscopy in trauma in a major trauma center.

Feliciano DV, Bitondo-Dyer CG. Vagaries of the lavage white blood cell count in evaluating abdominal stab wounds. *Am J Surgery* 1994;168:680–683.
Small study demonstrating the significant amount of false positives in WBC count when evaluating bowel injury by DPL.

Gonzalez RP, Ickler J, Gachassin P. Complementary roles of diagnostic peritoneal lavage and computed tomography in the evaluation of blunt abdominal trauma. *J Trauma* 2001;51:1128–1134.
Randomized prospective investigation in blunt trauma using diagnostic peritoneal lavage (DPL) as a screening tool for operation or CT and subsequent evaluation in relation to sensitivity and cost effectiveness.

Gonzalez RP, Turk B, Falimirski ME, et al. Abdominal stab wounds: diagnostic peritoneal lavage criteria for emergency room discharge. *J Trauma* 2001;51:939–943.
Prospective study using DPL with RBC counts lower than 1,000 RBC/mm³ to decide on sending patients home. Observation of hemodynamically stable patients decreases nontherapeutic laparotomies.

McKenney MG, McKenney KL, Hong JJ, et al. Evaluating blunt abdominal trauma with sonography: a cost analysis. *Am Surg* 2001;67:930–934.
FAST examination decreases significant cost by decreasing DPL rates eightfold and CT twofold in blunt trauma.

Nagy KK, Roberts RR, Joseph KT, et al. Experience with over 2500 diagnostic peritoneal lavages. *Injury* 2000;31:479–482.
Large investigation of blunt and penetrating trauma patients demonstrating the safety and accuracy, specificity and sensitivity of the DPL.

Prall JA, Nichols JS, Brennan R, et al. Early definitive abdominal evaluation in the triage of unconscious normotensive blunt trauma patients. *J Trauma* 1994;37:792–797.
Retrospective analysis of 290 blunt trauma patients suggesting that if unconscious and normotensive, immediate DPL is warranted.

Rozycki GS, Ochsner MG, Schmidt JA, et al. A prospective study of surgeon-performed ultrasound as the primary adjuvant modality for injured patient assessment. *J Trauma* 1995;39:492–498.
Original paper demonstrating the accuracy and specificity and cost effectiveness of the FAST examination in a large trauma center.

Runyon BA, Montano AA, Akriviadis EA, et al. The serum-ascites albumin gradient is superior to the exudate-transudate concept in the differential diagnosis of ascites. *Ann Internal Med* 1992;117:215–220.
Although the serum-ascites albumin gradient is superior to ascitic total fluid protein concentration (AFTP), the AFTP is a useful test for the differential diagnosis of ascites.

Saab S, Nieto J, Ly D, et al. TIPS versus paracentesis for cirrhotic patients with refractory ascites. *Cochrane Database Syst Rev* 2004; 3:CD004889.
Although patients with TIPS suffered more encephalopathy, ascitic fluid was removed more effectively by TIPS than by paracentesis with no increase in complications.

14 GASTROESOPHAGEAL BALLOON TAMPONADE FOR ACUTE VARICEAL HEMORRHAGE
Marie T. Pavini

I. GENERAL PRINCIPLES
  A. Definitions
   1. Esophageal variceal hemorrhage: an acute, severe, dramatic complication of the patient with portal hypertension that carries a high mortality and significant incidence of recurrence.
   2. Gastroesophageal balloon tamponade: a multilumenal tube with esophageal and gastric inflatable cuffs that can be inflated to compress esophageal varices and gastric cardia submucosal veins.

II. ALTERNATIVE PROCEDURES AND THERAPEUTICS
  A. Sclerotherapy is an example of first-line therapy offering a lower incidence and severity of complications and greater success in controlling bleeding.
  B. Band ligation is also first-line therapy carrying a more desirable complication and success profile.
  C. Combined vasoactive pharmacologic therapy and balloon tamponade can control hemorrhage in 90% of cases.
  D. Octreotide or combination vasopressin and nitroglycerin diminish portal vein pressure while emergency endoscopy is performed to confirm the diagnosis.
  E. Percutaneous transhepatic embolization is recommended in poor-risk patients who do not stop bleeding despite other measures.
  F. Esophageal devascularization with gastroesophageal stapling can be performed for patients without cirrhosis as well as for low-risk patients with cirrhosis.
  G. Transjugular intrahepatic portosystemic shunt (TIPS) is used as a bridge to transplant.
  H. Esophageal transection is an extreme measure used to control bleeding.

III. INDICATIONS
  A. Therapeutic and diagnostic
   1. Gastroesophageal balloon tamponade is indicated in patients with a diagnosis of esophageal variceal hemorrhage in whom neither sclerotherapy nor band ligation is technically possible, readily available, or has failed.
   2. With use of the infragastric balloon suction port, it is possible to differentiate bleeding from esophageal and gastric varices.

IV. CONTRAINDICATIONS
  A. Balloon tamponade is contraindicated in patients with recent esophageal surgery or esophageal stricture.
  B. Some authors do not recommend balloon tamponade when a hiatal hernia is present, although there are reports of successful hemorrhage control in some patients (Fig. 14-1).

V. PROCEDURE
  A. Preprocedure considerations
   1. Endotracheal intubation
    a. Any patient who will undergo balloon tamponade should have the trachea intubated.
    b. Suctioning of pulmonary secretions and blood accumulated in the hypopharynx is facilitated in patients with endotracheal intubation.

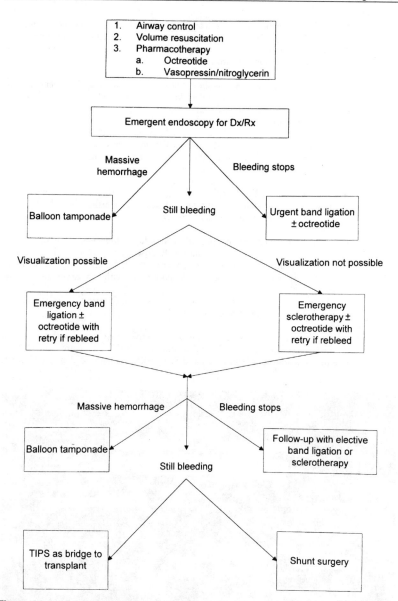

Figure 14-1. Management of esophageal variceal hemorrhage. Dx: diagnosis; Rx: therapy; TIPS: transjugular intrahepatic portosystemic shunt. (From Pavini MT, Puyana JC. Management of acute esophageal variceal hemorrhage with gastroesophageal balloon tamponade. In: Irwin RS, Rippe JM, eds.: *Irwin and Rippe's intensive care medicine*, 5th edition. Philadelphia: Lippincott Williams & Wilkins, 2003, with permission.)

    c. Administration of sedatives and analgesics in intubated patients is safer and may be required often because these tubes are poorly tolerated in most patients.

    d. The incidence of pulmonary complications is significantly lower when endotracheal intubation is routinely used.

2. Hemodynamics and resuscitation

    a. Adequate intravenous access should be obtained with large-bore venous catheters and fluid resuscitation undertaken with crystalloid and colloid fluids.

    b. A central venous catheter or pulmonary catheter may be required to monitor intravascular filling pressures, especially in patients with severe cirrhosis, advanced age, or underlying cardiac and pulmonary disease.

    c. Four to six units of packed red cells should always be available in case of severe recurrent bleeding, which commonly occurs in these patients.

    d. Coagulopathy should be treated with fresh frozen plasma and platelets.

3. Diagnostic endoscopy and gastric lavage

    a. Placement of an Ewald tube and aggressive lavage and suctioning of the stomach and duodenum facilitates endoscopy, diminishes the risk of aspiration and may help control hemorrhage from causes other than esophageal varices.

    b. The diagnostic endoscopic procedure should be done as soon as the patient is stabilized after basic resuscitation. Endoscopy is performed in the intensive care unit or operating room under controlled monitoring and with adequate equipment and personnel. An endoscope with a large suction channel should be used.

    c. Octreotide or combination vasopressin and nitroglycerin should be administered as part of initial resuscitation.

B. Equipment

    1. Although several studies have published combined experience with tubes such as the Linton and Nachlas tube, the techniques described here are limited to the use of the Minnesota (Fig. 14-2) and Sengstaken-Blakemore (Fig. 14-3) tubes.

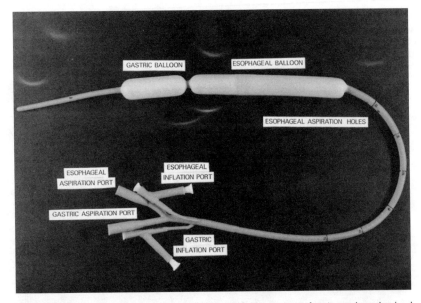

Figure 14-2. Minnesota tube. (From Pavini MT, Puyana JC. Management of acute esophageal variceal hemorrhage with gastroesophageal balloon tamponade.. In: Irwin RS, Rippe JM, eds.: *Irwin and Rippe's intensive care medicine*, 5th edition. Philadelphia: Lippincott Williams & Wilkins, 2003, with permission.)

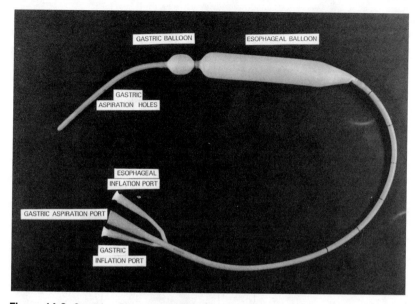

Figure 14-3. Senstaken-Blakemore tube. (From Pavini MT, Puyana JC. Management of acute esophageal variceal hemorrhage with gastroesophageal balloon tamponade. In: Irwin RS, Rippe JM, eds.: *Irwin and Rippe's intensive care medicine*, 5th edition. Philadelphia: Lippincott Williams & Wilkins, 2003, with permission.)

When using a Sengstaken-Blakemore tube, a No. 18 Salem sump is attached above the esophageal balloon and inserted through the mouth as originally described by Boyce. Suctioning above the esophageal balloon and hypopharynx diminishes, but does not eliminate, the risk of aspiration pneumonia.

2. The Minnesota tube has a fourth lumen that allows intermittent suctioning of saliva, blood, and pulmonary secretions in the hypopharynx (see Fig. 14-2).

C. Technique

1. All lumens should be patent, and the balloons should be inflated and checked for leaks. If using the Sengstaken-Blakemore tube, a No. 18 Salem sump should be secured above the esophageal balloon with surgical ties. The tube should be generously lubricated with lidocaine jelly.

2. The tube can be inserted through the nose or mouth; however, the nasal route is not recommended in patients with coagulopathy. The tube is passed into the stomach (Fig. 14-4).

3. Auscultation in the epigastrium while air is injected through the gastric lumen verifies the position of the tube, but the position of the gastric tube must be confirmed radiologically at this time.

4. The gastric balloon is inflated with no more than 80 mL of air, and a portable radiograph is obtained that includes the upper abdomen and lower chest.

5. When it is documented that the gastric balloon is below the diaphragm, it should be further inflated slowly to a volume of 250 to 300 mL. The gastric balloon of the Minnesota tube can be inflated to 450 mL. Tube inlets should be clamped with rubber shod hemostats after insufflation.

6. Hemorrhage is frequently controlled with insufflation of the gastric balloon alone without applying traction; but, in patients with torrential hemorrhage, it is necessary to apply traction (*vide infra*). If the bleeding continues, the esophageal balloon should be inflated to a pressure of approximately 45 mm Hg (bedside manometer).

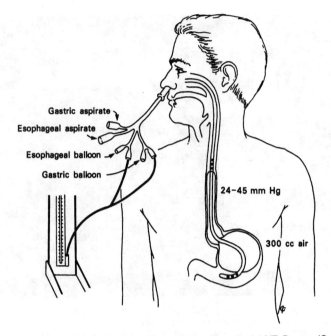

Figure 14-4. Proper positioning of the Minnesota tube. (From Pavini MT, Puyana JC. Management of acute esophageal variceal hemorrhage with gastroesophageal balloon tamponade. In: Irwin RS, Rippe JM, eds.: *Irwin and Rippe's intensive care medicine*, 5th edition. Philadelphia: Lippincott Williams & Wilkins, 2003, with permission.)

This pressure should be monitored and maintained. Some authors advocate inflation of the esophageal balloon immediately after insertion (see Complications).

7. When the nasal route is used, traction should not be applied against the nostril because this can easily cause skin and cartilage necrosis. When traction is required, the tube should be attached to a cord that is passed over a pulley in a bed with an overhead orthopedic frame and aligned directly as it comes out of the nose to avoid contact with the nostril. This system allows maintenance of traction with a known weight (500 to 1500 g) that is easily measured and constant.

8. When the tube is inserted through the mouth, traction is better applied by placing a football helmet on the patient and attaching the tube to the face mask of the helmet after a known weight (500 to 1,500 g) is applied for tension. Pressure sores can occur in the head and forehead when the helmet does not fit properly or when it is used for a prolonged period of time. Several authors recommend overhead traction for oral insertions as well as for nasal insertions.

9. The gastric lumen is placed on intermittent suction. The Minnesota tube has an esophageal lumen that can also be placed on low intermittent suction. If the Sengstaken-Blakemore tube is used, then the Salem sump (see Equipment) should be set to continuous suction.

VI. POSTPROCEDURE CONSIDERATIONS

A. Monitoring

1. The tautness and inflation of the balloons should be checked an hour after insertion and periodically by experienced personnel.

2. The position of the tube should be monitored radiographically every 24 hours (Fig. 14-5) or sooner if there is suspicion of tube displacement. A pair of scissors should be

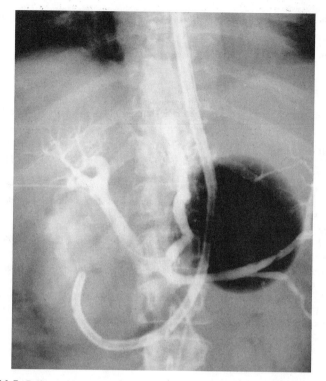

Figure 14-5. Radiograph showing correct position of the tube; the gastric balloon is below the diaphragm. (Courtesy of Ashley Davidoff, MD.) (From Pavini MT, Puyana JC. Management of acute esophageal variceal hemorrhage with gastroesophageal balloon tamponade. In: Irwin RS, Rippe JM, eds.: *Irwin and Rippe's intensive care medicine*, 5th edition. Philadelphia: Lippincott Williams & Wilkins, 2003, with permission.)

at the bedside in case the balloon port needs to be cut for rapid decompression because the balloon can migrate and acutely obstruct the airway.

B. Weaning and removal

   1. The tube should be left in place a minimum of 24 hours. The gastric balloon tamponade can be maintained continuously up to 48 hours. The esophageal balloon, however, must be deflated for 30 minutes every 8 hours.

   2. Once hemorrhage is controlled, the esophageal balloon is deflated first; the gastric balloon is left inflated for an additional 24 to 48 hours. If there is no evidence of bleeding, the gastric balloon is deflated, and the tube is left in place 24 hours longer. If bleeding recurs, the appropriate balloon is reinflated. The tube is removed if no further bleeding occurs.

C. Complications

   1. The incidence of complications that are a direct cause of death in published reports ranges from 0% to 20%.

   2. Tube migration (inadequate gastric balloon inflation or excessive traction)

      a. Acute laryngeal obstruction

      b. Tracheal rupture.

   3. Perforation of the esophagus

   4. Aspiration pneumonia (0% to 12%)

   5. Mucosal ulceration of the gastroesophageal junction is related to prolonged traction time (greater than 36 hours).

6. Impaction—inability to deflate the balloon. Occasionally, surgery is required to remove the balloon.
7. Necrosis of the nostrils
8. Nasopharyngeal bleeding

Acknowledgments

The authors wish to thank Charles F. Holtz and Susan A. Bright, Medical Media Service, West Roxbury Veterans Administration Medical Center, West Roxbury, MA for the photographs in this chapter; and Marguerite Eckhouse, UMass Memorial Medical Center, Worcester, MA for her secretarial support.

Selected Readings

Boyce HW. Modification of the Sengstaken-Blakemore balloon tube. *N Engl J Med* 1962; 267:195.
A classic article describing the evolution of the gastroesophageal balloon tube.

Cook D, Laine L. Indications, technique and complications of balloon tamponade for variceal gastrointestinal bleeding. *J Intensive Care Med* 1992;7:212.
An overall look at the various aspects of balloon tamponade.

Pasquale MD, Cerra FB. Sengstaken-Blakemore tube placement. *Crit Care Clin* 1992;8:743.
A description of a technique for placement of the Sengstaken-Blakemore tube.

Stein C, Korula J. Variceal bleeding: what are the options? *Postgrad Med* 1995;98:143.
A paper that puts the role of esophageal balloon tamponade into perspective.

Terblanche J, Krige JE, Bornman PC. The treatment of esophageal varices. *Annu Rev Med* 1992;43:69.
A good review of the therapeutic options for the management of esophageal varices.

I. GENERAL PRINCIPLES

A. Introduction

1. Enteral nutrition (EN) in the critically ill patient is superior to parenteral nutrition:

    a. EN maintains the integrity of the intestinal mucosal barrier thereby preventing intestinal bacterial translocation.

    b. EN decreases infectious morbidity and improves wound healing.

    c. EN is less expensive.

B. Classification

1. Administration of EN can be distinguished according to anticipated duration or anatomic location of the feeding tube:

    a. Short-term administration (less than 4 weeks)

      (1) It can be applied via nasogastric (polyvinylchloride tube, 16- or 18-Fr) or nasoduodenal or nasojejunal fine-bore tubes (silicone or polyurethane feeding tube, 6 to 14 Fr)

      (2) Multilumen tubes allow gastric decompression while delivering feeding formula into the jejunum.

    b. Long-term administration (longer than 4 weeks)

      (1) Access routes for long-term EN include esophagostomy, gastrostomy, duodenostomy, and jejunostomy.

2. Anatomic location of the feeding tube:

    a. Gastric feeding is a physiologic route for enteral nutrition, but is often poorly tolerated due to gastric dysmotility with delayed emptying.

    b. Feeding into the duodenum decreases the occurrence of regurgitation; infusion into the jejunum is associated with the lowest risk of aspiration.

C. Routes of insertion of feeding tubes

1. Nasoenteric tubes are inserted blindly or endoscopically, or with fluoroscopy, magnetic guidance, or endoscopy.

2. Options for the creation of a gastrostomy, duodenostomy or jejunostomy include:

    a. Open surgery or laparoscopy

    b. Percutaneously using endoscopy (PEG), ultrasonography, fluoroscopy (PFG), or CT guidance.

3. Advancing jejunal tubes through an existing PEG tube (PEGJ, G to J-tube) is also possible (sizes range from 20 to 28 Fr).

D. Contraindications for tube placement

1. Absolute contraindications include coagulopathy, strictures of pharynx or esophagus, (contraindication for placement of gastroscope), and abdominal wall infections.

2. Relative contraindications include severe ascites, gastric cancer, and gastric ulcer.

E. Contraindications for tube feeding

1. Absolute contraindications include intestinal obstruction, severe upper gastrointestinal hemorrhage and severe mesenteric ischemia.

2. Relative contraindications include:

    a. Gastric feeding in patients with increased risk of pulmonary aspiration

    b. Enteral feeding proximal to the jejunum during acute severe pancreatitis

    c. Entero-cutaneous fistulas, severe inflammatory bowel disease, severe malabsorption and severe short gut syndrome

II. PROCEDURE

A. Placement of nasoenteral feeding tubes

1. Appropriate length of the feeding tube: stomach, 30 to 36 in.; duodenum, 43 in.; jejunum, at least 48 in. (most tubes are radiopaque and have a tungsten-weighted tip or a stylet to facilitate passage into the duodenum).

2. With the patient in the right lateral decubitus position (if not contraindicated), the tube is lubricated and advanced through the patient's nose into the stomach.

3. Once the tube is in position, air is insufflated through the tube during auscultation (presence of gurgling abdominal sounds suggest gastric positioning).

4. A prokinetic agent like erythromycin (500 mg IV) may facilitate passage of the tube into the small bowel. Metoclopramide has been shown to be ineffective.

5. The tube is securely taped to the patient's forehead or cheek without tension.

6. If the tube is placed for duodenal or jejunal feeding, a loop 6 to 8 in. long may be left extending from the nose, and the tube may be advanced one to 2 in. every hour.

7. If the tube does not migrate into the duodenum over several hours, endoscopic assistance or fluoroscopic guidance can be attempted:

    a. After sedation and topical anesthesia, a nasoenteric feeding tube (43 to 48 in.) with an inner wire stylet is passed transnasally into the stomach.

    b. The endoscope is then advanced into the gastric lumen and endoscopy forceps are passed through the biopsy channel to grasp the tip of the enteral feeding tube.

    c. The endoscope, along with the enteral feeding tube is advanced into the duodenum as far as possible, the endoscopy forceps and feeding tube remain in position as the endoscope is withdrawn back into the stomach.

    d. The forceps are opened and withdrawn carefully back into the stomach. The feeding tube is usually lodged in the second portion of the duodenum.

    e. The portion of the feeding tube that is redundant in the stomach is advanced slowly into the duodenum with the endoscopy forceps.

B. Placement of percutaneous feeding tubes

1. Percutaneous endoscopic gastrostomy (PEG). The three methods for placement of PEG-tubes are pull-, push- and introducer-technique.

    a. Pull technique (supine position):

       (1) After adequate sedation and prophylactic antibiotics (e.g. first-generation cephalosporin), the posterior pharynx is anesthetized and a flexible gastroscope is inserted into the stomach which is insufflated with air.

       (2) Digital pressure to the patient's anterior abdominal wall in the left subcostal area (2 cm below costal margin) identifies the area of brightest transillumination.

          i. The indentation in the stomach created by digital pressure must be identified endoscopically, otherwise, another site should be chosen.

       (3) A polypectomy snare is introduced through the endoscope.

          i. After prepping, local anesthesia and skin incision, a large-bore catheter-needle-stylet assembly is advanced into the stomach and through the snare.

          ii. The snare is tightened securely around the catheter.

       (4) After removal of the stylet, a looped insertion wire is introduced through the catheter into the stomach.

       (5) The cannula is withdrawn slowly, so the snare grasps the wire.

       (6) The gastroscope is removed from the stomach and the end of the transgastric wire exiting the patient's mouth is tied to a gastrostomy tube.

       (7) The wire exiting from the abdominal wall is pulled while the endoscopist guides the lubricated gastrostomy tube into the stomach and then out through the abdominal wall.

       (8) The gastroscope is reinserted into the stomach to confirm adequate placement and to rule out bleeding (the intraluminal portion of the tube should contact the mucosa, but excessive tension on the tube should be avoided).

       (9) The tube is sutured to the abdominal wall.

b. Push technique:

(1) The gastroscope is inserted into the stomach pointing towards the anterior abdominal wall.

(2) A short straight guidewire is introduced into the stomach and dilators of increasing size are advanced over the wire into the stomach to create a large enough stoma to accommodate the gastrostomy tube.

(3) A gastrostomy tube with a tapered end is "pushed" over the guidewire into the stomach and sutured into place.

c. Introducer (peel-away) technique:

(1) The gastroscope is inserted into the stomach, and an appropriate position for placement of the tube is identified.

(2) After infiltration of the skin with local anesthetic, a 16- or 18-gauge needle is advanced into the stomach.

(3) A J-tipped guidewire is inserted into the stomach, and the needle is withdrawn.

(4) Using a twisting motion, a 16-Fr introducer with a peel-away sheath is passed over the guidewire into the gastric lumen.

(5) The guidewire and introducer are removed, leaving in place the sheath that allows placement of a 14-Fr Foley catheter.

(6) The sheath is peeled away after inflating the balloon (10 mL of normal saline).

2. Percutaneous endoscopic jejunostomy (PEJ)

a. The PEJ tube allows for simultaneous gastric decompression and duodenal or jejunal enteral feeding if a small feeding tube is attached and passed through the gastrostomy tube and advanced endoscopically into the duodenum or jejunum.

b. When the PEG is in position, a guidewire is passed through the PEG, grasped using endoscopy forceps, and passed into the duodenum as distally as possible.

c. The jejunal tube is then passed over the guidewire through the PEG into the distal duodenum and is advanced into the jejunum, and the endoscope is withdrawn.

III. POSTPROCEDURE CONSIDERATIONS

A. Safety measures

1. A chest radiograph ideally including the upper abdominal segments for nasoenteric tubes and an abdominal film for PEG/PEJ should be obtained to confirm the position of the tube before feedings are started (intra-bronchial positioning of feeding tubes can cause a pneumothorax; capnography can be useful to avoid this complication).

2. Inspect all cuffs to rule out malfunction prior to initiation of feeding.

B. Daily care of feeding tubes

1. Daily irrigation of feeding tubes with normal saline or distilled water may avoid occlusion.

2. Should occlusion occur, tubes could be cleared by irrigation with warm saline, carbonated liquid or digestive enzymes (Viokase and Pancrease).

C. Delivering the feeding formula

1. EN via nasoenteric feeding tubes may be initiated immediately after radiographic confirmation of correct tube position.

2. EN via PEG/PEJ tubes can be started as early as one hour after the procedure if the placement was uncomplicated.

3. Jejunal feeding may be instituted as early as 12 to 24 hours post operatively because small bowel motility and absorption capacity may recover within 24 hours after surgery or trauma.

4. Continuous pump infusion is the preferred method for the delivery of enteral nutrition in critically ill patients, which results in decreased abdominal distention, less diarrhea, and lower gastric residuals when compared to bolus administration.

D. Administration of medications through feeding tubes

1. Ensure compatibility of drugs with each other and with the enteral formula.

2. Administration of medications in an elixir formulation through enteral feeding tubes is preferable to prevent occlusion (tubes should always be flushed with 20 mL of saline after administration of medications).

   E. Complications associated with nasoenteric or percutaneous feeding tubes

   1. Possible complications include local infection, peritonitis, significant hemorrhage, dislocation, necrosis (pressure ulcer), enterocutaneous fistula and pneumoperitoneum.

Selected Readings

Gopalan S, Khanna S. Enteral nutrition delivery technique. *Curr Opin Clin Nutr Metab Care* 2003;6(3):313–317.
Good review article on currently employed delivery techniques for enteral nutrition.

McClave SA, Marsano LS, Lukan JK. Enteral access for nutritional support: rationale for utilization. *J Clin Gastroenterol* 2002;35(3):209–213.
Nice review article about clinical benefits of nutritional support in critically ill patients.

Moore FA, Feliciano DV, Andrassy RJ, et al. Early enteral feeding, compared with parenteral, reduces postoperative septic complications: the results of a meta-analysis. *Ann Surg* 1992;216;172.
This meta-analysis showed that septic complications were reduced in high-risk surgical patients who received early enteral nutritional support.

Silva CC, Saconato H, Atallah AN. Metoclopramide for migration of naso-enteral tube. *Cochrane Database Syst Rev* 2002;(4):CD003353.
A meta-analysis of four prospective studies found that neither parenteral nor enteral metoclopramide was more effective than placebo in facilitating transpyloric migration of feeding tube.

Stone SJ, Pickett JD, Jesurum JT. Bedside placement of postpyloric feeding tubes. *AACN Clin Issues* 2000;11(4):517–530.
A discussion of various bedside techniques is presented in this review article.

CEREBROSPINAL FLUID ASPIRATION

Raimis Matulionis

16

I. GENERAL PRINCIPLES

A. Cerebral spinal fluid (CSF) test profile includes glucose and protein values, a cell count, stains, cultures, a pressure reading, and special tests

 1. CSF glucose
  a. Normally equivalent to two thirds of serum glucose
  b. Lags behind blood levels by about 2 hours
  c. Increased CSF glucose is nonspecific and usually reflects hyperglycemia.
  d. Decreased levels are the result of any inflammatory or neoplastic meningeal disorder.

 2. CSF protein
  a. Content is normally less than 0.5% of that in plasma.
  b. Nonspecific
  c. Elevated level in the CSF is an indicator of central nervous system (CNS) pathology.
  d. Low levels are seen in healthy children younger than 2 years of age and in patients with pseudotumor cerebri, acute water intoxication, and leukemia.

 3. CSF cell count
  a. Normal count includes no erythrocytes and a maximum of 5 leukocytes/mm^3.
  b. Greater numbers are normally found in children (up to 10/mm^3, mostly lymphocytes).
  c. Helpful in identifying cells from CNS primary or metastatic tumors and differentiation from inflammatory disorders

II. INDICATIONS

A. CSF access for diagnostic purposes

 1. Hemorrhage
  a. A lumbar puncture (LP) is indicated if the head computed tomographic (CT) scan is not diagnostic and the clinical history and presentation are atypical.
  b. LP should not be performed without prior CT if the patient has any focal neurologic deficits because transtentorial herniation may occur.

 2. Infection
  a. CSF evaluation is the most important aspect of the laboratory diagnosis of meningitis.
  b. Includes a Gram stain, cell count with differential, protein and glucose levels, and aerobic and anaerobic cultures with antibiotic sensitivities
  c. If tuberculosis or fungal infection is suspected, the fluid is analyzed by acid-fast stain, India ink preparation, or cryptococcal antigen and then is cultured in appropriate media.
  d. For rapid diagnosis and early specific treatment
   (1) Immunoprecipitation tests to identify bacterial antigens for *Streptococcus pneumoniae*, *Streptococcus* group B, *Haemophilus influenzae*, *Neisseria meningitidis* (meningococcus)
   (2) Viral cultures or polymerase chain reaction tests for herpes, varicella zoster, CMV, Epstein-Barr virus, *Toxoplasma*, *Mycobacterium tuberculosis*.

 3. Shunt system failure (CSF accessed through shunt system)
 4. Benign intracranial hypertension (pseudotumor cerebri)

5. Neoplasms
6. Other neurologic disorders
  a. Multiple sclerosis
  b. Alzheimer's disease
  c. Guillain-Barré syndrome
B. CFS access for therapeutic intervention
  1. Fistulas
    a. Cause
      (1) Skull fractures
      (2) Nontraumatic
        i. Resection of skull base tumors (dural or bony defects)
        ii. Lumbar surgery
        iii. Myelography
    b. Diagnosis—clinical examination
    c. If clinical examination uncertain
      (1) Testing for glucose might be misleading because glucose is present in nasal secretions.
      (2) Interpretation of higher chloride level compared to blood levels is not accurate.
      (3) Identification of β_2-transferrin—the most accurate diagnostic for CSF. β_2-transferrin is produced by neuraminidase in the brain and is uniquely found in the spinal fluid and perilymph.
    d. Treatment
      (1) Postural drainage by keeping the patient's head elevated for several days
      (2) Nonoperative approaches should conservative therapy fail
        i. Lumbar drainage catheter—controversial due to risk of infection
        ii. Daily LPs can be useful.
  2. Intracranial hypertension
    a. Access to intracranial CSF space can be diagnostic and therapeutic.
    b. Most common intracranial pressure (ICP) monitor used for measurement of ICP and for treatment of intracranial hypertension by CSF drainage is ventriculostomy.
    c. Indications
      (1) Head trauma
      (2) Ischemic cerebral insults
      (3) Obstructive hydrocephalus
      (4) Aneurysmal subarachnoid hemorrhage (SAH)
      (5) Spontaneous cerebral hematoma
C. Drug therapy
  1. Intrathecal injections of various agents via LP or intraventricular injections via an implanted reservoir for treatment of lymphoma or leukemia
  2. Intrathecal chemotherapy in attempt to minimize agent neurotoxicity
  3. Intrathecal antibiotics in addition to systemic therapy

III. PROCEDURE
A. Lumbar puncture (LP)
  1. LP is a common procedure that rarely requires radiologic or other assistance.
  2. Contraindications
    a. Skin infection at the entry site
    b. Anticoagulation
    c. Blood dyscrasias
    d. Known spinal subarachnoid block
    e. Known spinal cord arteriovenous malformations
    f. Papilledema in the presence of supratentorial masses
    g. Posterior fossa lesions
  3. Procedure (Figs. 16-1 and 16-2)
    a. The patient is placed in the lateral knee-chest position or is sitting while leaning forward over a table at the bedside.

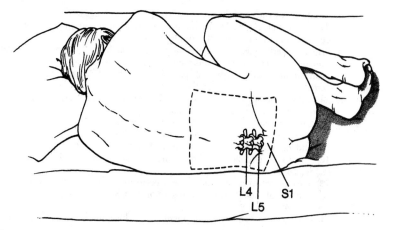

Figure 16-1. The patient is in the lateral decubitis position with the back at the edge of the bed and the knees, hips, back, and neck flexed. (From Vander Salm TJ, Cutler BS, Wheeler HB, eds. *Atlas of bedside procedures*, 2nd ed. Boston: Little, Brown, 1988, with permission.)

b. The point of access is midline between the spinous processes of L3–L4, at the level of the superior iliac crests.

c. The area is prepped with 10% povidone-iodine solution and draped.

d. Local anesthetic is injected subcutaneously using a 25- or 27-gauge needle.

e. A 1.5-in. needle is then inserted through the skin wheal, and additional local anesthetic is injected along the midline.

f. The spinal needle (18- to 25-gauge) is advanced with the stylet or obturator in place.

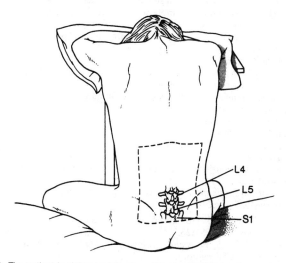

Figure 16-2. The patient is sitting on the edge of the bed and is leaning on the bedside stand. (From Vander Salm TJ, Cutler BS, Wheeler HB, eds. *Atlas of bedside procedures*, 2nd ed. Boston: Little, Brown, 1988, with permission.)

g. The bevel of the needle should be parallel to the longitudinal fibers of the dura or to the spinal column and oriented rostrally at an angle of about 30 degrees to the skin—virtually aiming toward the umbilicus

h. When properly oriented, the needle passes through the following structures: skin → superficial fascia → supraspinous ligament → interspinous ligament → ligamentum flavum → epidural space with its fatty areolar tissue and internal vertebral plexus → dura → arachnoid membrane.

i. The total depth varies from less than 2.5 cm in the extremely young patient to as much as 12 cm in the obese adult

j. An 18- to 20-gauge spinal needle should be used for pressure measurement

    (1) The opening pressure is best measured with the patient's legs relaxed and extended partly from the knee-chest position.

    (2) Once CSF is collected, the closing pressure is measured before needle withdrawal.

    (3) Measurements are not accurate if performed while the patient is sitting because of the hydrostatic pressure of the CSF column.

4. Complications

  a. Hemorrhage is uncommon but possible with bleeding disorders and anticoagulation.

  b. Spinal subarachnoid hemorrhage (SAH) can result in blockage of CSF outflow, with subsequent back and radicular pain with sphincter disturbances and even paraparesis.

  c. Spinal subdural hematoma is similarly infrequent, but it is associated with significant morbidity; clot evacuation must be prompt.

  d. Infection by introduction of skin flora in the subarachnoid spaces causing meningitis is uncommon and preventable if aseptic techniques are used.

  e. Postdural puncture headache is the most common post-LP complication.

    (1) Reported frequency varies from 1% to 70%.

    (2) A smaller needle, parallel orientation to the dural fibers, and a paramedian approach are associated with a decreased risk of this complication.

    (3) Atraumatic (pencil point) needles are associated with a lower risk.

    (4) Typically develops within 72 hours and lasts 3 to 5 days

    (5) Conservative treatment consisting of bed rest, hydration, and analgesics

    (6) Antiemetics are administered if the headache is associated with nausea.

    (7) If the symptoms are more severe, methylxanthines (caffeine or theophylline) may be successful in up to 85% of patients.

    (8) If the headache persists or is unaffected, an epidural blood patch is then recommended.

B. Aspiration from other sites

  1. CSF may be aspirated from C1–C2 (lateral cervical puncture)

  2. Cisternal punctures via cisterna magna

  3. Inline subcutaneous reservoirs such as Ommaya reservoirs, ventriculostomies, ventriculoperitoneal shunts

  4. Lumboperitoneal shunts

  5. Lumbar catheters

Selected Readings

Agrillo U, Simonetti G, Martino V. Postoperative CSF problems after spinal and lumbar surgery: general review. *J Neurosurg Sci* 1991;35:93.
Good review of the etiopathology, the symptomatology, the diagnosis and treatment of early and delayed CSF problems.

Bigner SH. Cerebrospinal fluid cytology: current status and diagnostic applications. *J Neuropathol Exp Neurol* 1992;51:235.
A review of the clinical features and cytologic presentation of common conditions that can be diagnosed by CSF cytology.

Davidson RI. Lumbar puncture. In: Vander Salm TJ, Cutler BS, Wheeler HB, eds. *Atlas of bedside procedures*, 2nd ed. Boston: Little, Brown, 1988.

A classic literature describing multitude of bedside procedures and recommended ways of safe performance.

Leibold RA, Yealy DM, Coppola M, et al. Post-dural puncture headache: characteristics, management and prevention. *Ann Emerg Med* 1993;22:1863.
The classic paper describing how prompt recognition of the clinical syndrome, followed by supportive and corrective actions, can decrease the morbidity in those afflicted.

Nandapalan V, Watson ID, Swift AC. Beta$_2$-Transferrin and CSF rhinorrhea. *Clin Otolaryngol* 1996;21:259.
Good article describing why betaTP (a noninvasive, highly sensitive, quick, and inexpensive method) can be used for the detection of CSF rhinorrhea in nasal secretions.

Wood J. Cerebrospinal fluid: techniques of access and analytical interpretation. In: Wilkins R, Rengachary S, eds. *Neurosurgery*, 2nd ed. New York: McGraw-Hill, 1996:165.
Classic reading material, good for references on neurosurgical issues.

NEUROLOGIC AND INTRACRANIAL PRESSURE MONITORING
Raimis Matulionis

17

I. GENERAL PRINCIPLES

A. The brain uses more oxygen and glucose per 100 g of tissue than any large organ.

B. The brain is completely dependent on uninterrupted cerebral blood flow (CBF) (i.e., it has no appreciable reserves of oxygen and glucose).

C. Clinical monitoring is directed toward early detection and reversal of potentially dangerous conditions.

D. Neurologic monitoring falls into two distinct categories:
  1. Electroencephalography (EEG) and evoked potentials (EPs) define a qualitative threshold consistent with the onset of cerebral ischemia.
  2. Monitoring of intracranial pressure (ICP), CBF, and cerebral metabolism provides quantitative physiologic information.

E. Cerebral ischemia is defined as cerebral oxygen delivery (CDO_2) insufficient to meet metabolic needs.
  1. CDO_2 components
    a. CBF
    b. Hemoglobin concentration
    c. Arterial hemoglobin saturation (S_aO_2).

II. TECHNIQUES

A. Systemic monitoring
  1. Pulse oximetry and blood pressure provide clues about the adequacy of global brain oxygenation.
  2. Cerebral perfusion pressure (CPP = mean arterial pressure [MAP] − ICP) does not alter CBF over a range of pressures of about 50 to 150 mm Hg.
  3. P_aCO_2 regulates cerebral vascular resistance over a range of 20 to 80 mm Hg.
  4. CBF is acutely halved if P_aCO_2 is halved, and it is doubled if P_aCO_2 is doubled.
  5. A decreasing C_aO_2, resulting from a decrease in hemoglobin or in S_aO_2, normally causes CBF to increase.

B. Neurologic examination
  1. Neurologic examination quantifies three key characteristics:
    a. Level of consciousness
    b. Focal brain dysfunction
    c. Trends in neurologic function
  2. The Glasgow Coma Scale (GCS), originally developed as a prognostic tool, has become popular as a quick, reproducible *estimate* of level of consciousness (Table 17-1).

C. Neuroimaging
  1. Cerebral computed tomographic (CT) scans obtained at the time of the patient's admission provide valuable prognostic information about ultimate neurologic outcome and about the risk of subsequent intracranial hypertension; however, they provide static, infrequent information about brain structure rather than function.
  2. Magnetic resonance imaging provides better resolution than CT, but powerful magnets are incompatible with ferrous material (a frequent component of life support systems).

D. Cerebral blood flow monitoring
  1. Xenon-133 clearance and CT

TABLE 17-1	Glasgow Coma Score	

Component	Response	Score
Eye opening	Spontaneously	4
	To verbal command	3
	To pain	2
	None	1
	Subtotal: 1—4	
Motor response	Obeys verbal command	6
(best extremity)	Localizes pain	5
	Exhibits flexion-withdrawal	4
	Exhibits flexor response	3
	(decorticate posturing)	
	Exhibits extensor response	2
	(decerebrate posturing)	
	Shows no response (flaccid)	1
	Subtotal: 1—6	
Best verbal response	Oriented and converses	5
	Disoriented and converses	4
	Uses inappropriate words	3
	Makes incomprehensible sounds	2
	Has no verbal response	1
	Subtotal: 1—5	
	Total: 3—15	

    a. Intracarotid, intravenous, or inhaled administration of xenon-133 uses gamma detectors to generate washout curves for the tracer; the rate of clearance is inversely proportional to CBF.

    b. Clinical use is limited because of cumbersome regulations governing the administration of radionuclides, the technically demanding nature of the measurements, and the sustained stable conditions (5 to 15 minutes) required to perform a single measurement.

  2. Transcranial Doppler flow velocity

    a. In most patients, arterial flow velocity (but not actual CBF) can be readily measured in intracranial vessels, especially the middle cerebral artery (MCA).

    b. Velocity is a function not only of blood flow rate but also of vessel diameter; if it remains constant, changes in velocity are proportional to changes in CBF.

    c. Used to identify vasospasm after traumatic and nontraumatic subarachnoid hemorrhage.

  3. Thermal diffusion

    a. If the brain surface adjacent to a thermal detector is slightly heated, the rate at which the added thermal energy is dissipated can be used to calculate local blood flow.

    b. The device determines CBF in one small region of cortex; it could be a useful monitor of global CBF or of a specific region at risk of ischemia.

    c. The necessity of surgical placement and maintenance of an invasive intracranial device carries a risk of infection.

E. Intracranial pressure monitoring

  1. ICP functions as the outflow pressure for the cerebral circulation.

  2. Although CBF cannot be directly inferred from MAP and ICP, severe increases in ICP reduce both CPP and CBF.

  3. ICP monitoring has been used for surveillance and goal-directed therapy.

4. The Brain Trauma Foundation and the American Association of Neurologic Surgeons have published guidelines for the management of traumatic brain injury, including standards, guidelines, and options for the use of ICP monitoring.
   a. ICP monitoring is appropriate:
      (1) In patients with an abnormal admission CT scan and severe head injury (GCS score of 3 to 8) after cardiopulmonary resuscitation.
      (2) In patients with severe head injury and a normal CT scan if two or more of the following are noted at admission: age greater than 40 years, unilateral or bilateral motor posturing, and systolic blood pressure less than 90 mm Hg.
      (3) Not indicated in patients with mild or moderate head injury.
      (4) However, a physician may choose to monitor ICP in certain conscious patients with traumatic mass lesions.
   b. Treatment of ICP should begin at a threshold of 20 to 25 mm Hg and should be corroborated by frequent clinical examination and CPP data.
   c. Types of ICP monitors
      (1) Intraventricular monitors
      (2) Parenchymal catheter tip transducers
      (3) Subdural, catheter tip transducers and fluid-coupled catheters
      (4) Subarachnoid fluid-coupled devices
      (5) Epidural devices.
   d. In addition to intracranial hypertension, other data that may prompt concern:
      (1) Widening of the pulse ICP (indicating diminishing intracranial compliance)
      (2) Plateau waves (cyclic increases in ICP, often 50 mm Hg or greater and lasting as long as 15 to 30 minutes)
5. Complications of ICP monitoring include
   a. Aggravation of cerebral edema
   b. Intracranial hemorrhage
   c. Cortical damage
   d. Infection
   e. Device-related malfunction and injuries
6. Cerebral oxygen extraction
   a. Jugular venous saturation
      (1) Jugular venous bulb oxygenation reflects the balance between C_{DO_2} and cerebral metabolic rate of oxygen (CMRO)
      (2) Experience with tissue oxygen pressure (P_{O_2}) monitoring in traumatic brain injury suggests a correlation between poor outcome and tissue hypoxia.
      (3) Mortality doubles with a single episode of jugular venous desaturation.
      (4) Jugular venous bulb monitoring can detect excessive hyperventilation and may also distinguish between vasospasm or hyperemia.
      (5) Retrograde cannulation of the jugular bulb is a low-risk, technically simple procedure.
   b. Near-infrared spectroscopy
      (1) Determines the relative concentrations of oxygenated and deoxygenated hemoglobin in brain tissue
      (2) Extensive preclinical and clinical data demonstrate the sensitivity of the technique for the detection of qualitative changes in brain oxygenation.
   c. Neurochemical monitoring
      (1) Microdialysis—new technique
      (2) Fluid is infused and withdrawn through a catheter inserted into the brain parenchyma.
      (3) Recovered dialysate can be analyzed for neurotransmitters or metabolic intermediates such as lactate, pyruvate, and adenosine.
7. Electrophysiologic monitoring
   a. Used to detect potentially damaging cerebral hypoperfusion, isolated seizures, and status epilepticus and to define the depth or type of coma
   b. Has limited value as a precise diagnostic tool

c. Quantitative EEG monitoring used to identify delayed ischemic deficits after subarachnoid hemorrhage, occasionally before clinical deterioration

d. Sensory EPs, which include somatosensory evoked potentials (SSEPs), brainstem auditory evoked potentials (BAEPs), and visual evoked potentials (VEPs), can be used as qualitative threshold monitors to detect severe neural ischemia by evaluating characteristic waveforms to specific stimuli.

e. Obliteration of EPs occurs only under conditions of profound cerebral ischemia or mechanical trauma. EP monitoring is one of the most specific ways in which to assess neurologic integrity.

f. EPs are insensitive to less severe deterioration of cerebral or spinal cord oxygen availability and are modified by sedatives, narcotics, and anesthetics.

Selected Readings

Brain Trauma Foundation, American Association of Neurological Surgeons, Joint Section on Neurotrauma and Critical Care. Guidelines for the management of severe head injury. *J Neurotrauma* 2000;17:507–511.
Very useful guidelines for the management of severe head injury.

Gopinath SP, Robertson CS, Contant CS, et al. Jugular venous desaturation and outcome after brain injury. *J Neurol Neurosurg Psychiatry* 1994;57:717–723.
Jugular venous desaturation was associated with a poor neurologic outcome.

Martin NA, Doberstein C, Zane C, et al.:Posttraumatic cerebral arterial spasm: transcranial Doppler ultrasound, cerebral blood flow, and angiographic findings. *J Neurosurg* 1992;77:575–583.
Vasospasm is an important secondary posttraumatic insult that is potentially treatable.

Rosner MJ, Rosner SD, Johnson AH. Cerebral perfusion pressure: management protocol and clinical results. *J. Neurosurg* 1995;83:949–962.
Authors of this article attempt to refine management techniques directed at CPP maintenance.

Smith DS, Levy W, Maris M, et al. Reperfusion hyperoxia in brain after circulatory arrest in humans. *Anesthesiology* 1990;73:12–13.
This article depicts differences in reperfusion mechanisms of the brain and muscle.

Teasdale GM, Pettigrew LE, Wilson JT, et al. Analyzing outcome of treatment of severe head injury: a review and update on advancing the use of the Glasgow Outcome Scale. *J Neurotrauma* 1998;15:587–597.
This review considers limitations recognized in the use of the GOS.

18 PERCUTANEOUS SUPRAPUBIC CYSTOSTOMY
Kevin M. Dushay

I. GENERAL PRINCIPLES
Percutaneous cystostomy is an invasive procedure for gaining entry through the skin to the urinary bladder to allow drainage of urine.

II. ANATOMY
  A. The urinary bladder is located anterior and inferior to the peritoneal cavity and posterior to the pubic symphysis.
    1. When distended with urine, the bladder dome rises above the pubic symphysis.
  B. The anterior superior midline of the external surface of the urinary bladder is generally free of major blood vessels.
    1. Major arterial supply to the anterior and superior surface is from branches of the internal iliac arteries; they enter the lateral walls of the bladder.
    2. Venous drainage flows inferiorly and laterally to branches of the internal iliac veins.

III. ALTERNATIVES TO PERCUTANEOUS SUPRAPUBIC CYSTOSTOMY
  A. Urethral catheterization
    1. Indwelling—utilizes Foley balloon–tipped urinary catheter
    2. Intermittent—utilizes straight catheter for bladder drainage followed by catheter withdrawal
    3. Passing filiform and follower (catheter or bougie) to dilate urethral stricture may allow successful urethral catheterization.
    4. Urology consultation may permit bedside flexible cystoscopy with passage of guidewire followed by urethral catheter insertion using Seldinger technique.

IV. INDICATIONS
See Table 18-1.

V. CONTRAINDICATIONS
  A. Urethral catheterization may be contraindicated in the setting of:
    1. Severe urethritis, prostatitis, or epididymitis, because of the risk of inducing bacteremia
    2. Pelvic trauma with possible urethral laceration
  B. Contraindications to percutaneous suprapubic cystostomy are listed in Table 18-2.

VI. PROCEDURE
  A. Equipment—a number of kits and devices are available
    1. Chiou SP Tube Introducer Set and O'Brien Suprapubic Peel-Away Access Set
      a. Both use Seldinger technique following guidewire insertion into the bladder to place dilator(s) and a peel-away sheath through which a Foley or other catheter may be inserted.
    2. Stamey Percutaneous Suprapubic catheter set and Rutner Percutaneous Suprapubic Balloon catheter sets
      a. Both use catheter-over-trocar to place catheter in the bladder.
    3. In addition to kits listed above, the operator may need to supply razor, prep solution, gauzes, sterile gloves, sterile field, local anesthetic, syringes and needles, dressing sponges, adhesive tape, and urinometer/collection device.

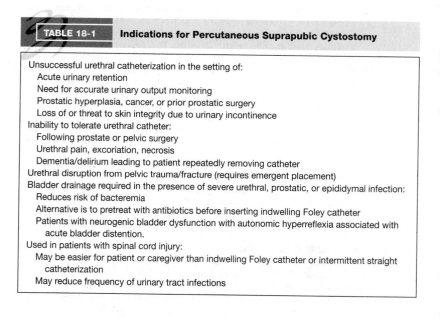

TABLE 18-1	Indications for Percutaneous Suprapubic Cystostomy

Unsuccessful urethral catheterization in the setting of:
  Acute urinary retention
  Need for accurate urinary output monitoring
  Prostatic hyperplasia, cancer, or prior prostatic surgery
  Loss of or threat to skin integrity due to urinary incontinence
Inability to tolerate urethral catheter:
  Following prostate or pelvic surgery
  Urethral pain, excoriation, necrosis
  Dementia/delirium leading to patient repeatedly removing catheter
Urethral disruption from pelvic trauma/fracture (requires emergent placement)
Bladder drainage required in the presence of severe urethral, prostatic, or epididymal infection:
  Reduces risk of bacteremia
  Alternative is to pretreat with antibiotics before inserting indwelling Foley catheter
  Patients with neurogenic bladder dysfunction with autonomic hyperreflexia associated with acute bladder distention.
Used in patients with spinal cord injury:
  May be easier for patient or caregiver than indwelling Foley catheter or intermittent straight catheterization
  May reduce frequency of urinary tract infections

  B. Technique
   1. Be sure bladder is sufficiently full to allow localization and needle entry to bladder cavity without risk of trauma to adjacent structures.
      a. If available, bedside ultrasound localization and/or guidance is recommended and has been shown to reduce complication rate.
      b. Ideal entry site for catheter is dome of bladder.
   2. Place patient in supine position, shave entry site if needed, prep, and drape. Check catheter balloon to be sure it is intact.
   3. Use 1% or 2% lidocaine to make skin wheal 2 to 4 cm above the pubic symphysis, then anesthetize on a 10- to 20-degree angle toward the pelvis, including subcutaneous tissues and rectus abdominis muscle fascia, using a 22-gauge 7.75 cm spinal needle. Bladder puncture confirmed by aspirating urine into syringe.
   4. For catheter-over-trocar kits:
      a. Use No. 11 scalpel to make stab wound, then insert catheter–trocar combination along same course used with finder needle, grasping device close to skin surface.

TABLE 18-2	Contraindications to Percutaneous Suprapubic Cystostomy

Nonpalpable bladder
Previous lower abdominal surgery
Bladder cancer
Coagulopathy
Blood clot retention in bladder
Lower abdominal wall cellulitis

(Not recommended as first-line treatment for prostatic obstruction.)

   b. Once position is again confirmed by aspirating urine into syringe, the catheter is advanced forward and the trocar is withdrawn.
   c. Catheter is then secured by self-deploying struts or mushroomlike structure at its tip, inflating balloon with 10 mL air/water/saline, or suturing to skin.
5. For Seldinger technique kits (continuing from VII.B.3, omitting VII.B.4 above):
   a. Syringe is removed and flexible J-tipped guidewire is inserted through needle into bladder. Needle is then backed out, leaving guidewire in place.
   b. Scalpel used to make stab incision along axis of the guidewire. Peel-away sheath preloaded on dilator is then passed as a unit over guidewire into the bladder.
      (1) Hold dilator close to skin to supply necessary pressure without bending it.
      (2) Some kits may use several dilators to create tract to bladder before sheath is inserted.
   c. Guidewire and dilator are removed, leaving peel-away sheath in place in the bladder; pinching sheath will prevent urine backflow onto field.
   d. Preselected catheter is then passed through peel-away sheath into bladder. Return of urine through catheter confirms proper placement. Balloon inflated with 10 mL of air, water, or saline. Peel-away sheath is removed by gradually withdrawing it over catheter as its two halves are drawn apart.

VII. POSTPROCEDURE CONSIDERATIONS
A. Complications—see Table 18-3.
   1. Bladder spasms are the most common complication.
   a. Avoid them by pulling cystostomy tube against the bladder wall immediately after placement, then advancing tube 2 cm into the bladder to allow for movement.
   b. Severe bladder spasms can be treated with oxybutynin.
      (1) Medication must be withdrawn before suprapubic tube is removed to avoid urinary retention.
   2. Misplaced catheter complications
   a. Attempt procedure only on well-distended bladders using midline approach no more than 4 cm above the pubis.
   b. If available, portable ultrasound visualization of bladder is proven to reduce complications

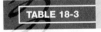 **TABLE 18-3**	**Complications of Percutaneous Suprapubic Cystostomy**

Bladder spasms
Hematuria
Retropubic bleeding
Bowel perforation
Rectal, uterine, or vaginal injury
Peritoneum perforation with intraperitoneal urine extravasation
Extraperitoneal urine extravasation
Ureteral catheterization
Catheter dislodgment
Infection:
   Cellulitis
   Deep wound infection
   Cystitis, pyelonephritis, secondary bacteremia
Postobstructive diuresis
Hypotension
Retained catheter fragment
Bladder stones

(1) Helpful in patients with prior abdominal or pelvic surgery or older women with bladder prolapse, to rule out entrapped bowel or abnormal location of bladder

(2) Recommended for less-experienced operators

3. Hypotension treated with intravenous fluids

4. Postobstructive diuresis may require fluid replacement for its management.

Selected Readings

Aguilera PA, Chan J. Ultrasound-guided vs. the blinded landmark technique for the placement of percutaneous suprapubic cystostomy catheter placement in the emergency department. *Acad Emerg Med* 2004;11:583 (abstract).
  Prospective evaluation of ultrasound-guided versus blind technique, demonstrating the advantage of the former even in experienced hands.

Ayvazian PJ. Percutaneous suprapubic cystostomy. In: Irwin RS, Rippe JM, eds. *Irwin and Rippe's intensive care medicine*, 5th edition. Philadelphia: Lippincott Williams & Wilkins, 2003, pp. 210–213.
  Excellent review of the subject.

Lawrentschuk N, Lee D, Marriott P, et al. Suprapubic stab cystostomy: a safer technique. *Urology* 2003; 62:932–934.
  Additional recommendation for ultrasound guidance in performing this procedure.

MacDiarmid SA, Arnold EP, Palmer NB, et al. Management of spinal cord injured patients by indwelling suprapubic catheterization. *J Urol* 1995;154:492–494.
  Retrospective review of 44 spinal cord injury patients requiring indwelling suprapubic cystostomy catheters for over 1 year.

Percutaneous suprapubic cystostomy. In: Roberts JR, Hedges JR, Chanmugam AS, et al., eds. Clinical procedures in emergency medicine, 4th edition [electronic resource available through MDConsult (http://home.mdconsult.com)]. St. Louis, MO: Mosby, 2004, pp. 1100–1103.
  Another good review of the subject with step-by-step instructions and accompanying illustrations.

Walsh PC, Retik AB, Vaughan ED Jr, et al., eds. *Campbell's urology*, 8th edition. Philadelphia: WB Saunders, 2002; 114,3728, 3732.
  Standard textbook of urology.

19

ASPIRATION OF JOINTS
Harvey S. Reich

I. GENERAL PRINCIPLES
A. Overview
1. Arthrocentesis involves the introduction of a needle into a joint space to remove synovial fluid.
2. It is an essential diagnostic technique for the evaluation of arthritis of unknown cause.
3. The presentation of conditions, such as septic arthritis and crystalline arthritis, may be similar, yet treatment may be different.
4. Arthrocentesis and synovial fluid analysis are important for accurate diagnosis.
5. Arthritis can involve a single joint (monoarthritis).
6. Arthritis can involve multiple joints (oligoarthritis).

II. INDICATIONS
A. Principles
1. Arthrocentesis is performed for both diagnostic and therapeutic reasons.
2. The evaluation of arthritis of unknown cause is the main indication for arthrocentesis.
3. In the intensive care unit, arthrocentesis is most commonly performed to rule out septic arthritis in a patient with acute monoarthritis or oligoarthritis.
4. Before performing arthrocentesis, one must be certain that a true joint space inflammation with effusion is present rather than a periarticular inflammatory process, such as bursitis, tendinitis, or cellulitis.
5. In the knee, the presence of an effusion may be confirmed by the bulge test or patella tap.
   a. Bulge test—milk fluid from the suprapatellar pouch into the joint, slide the hand down the lateral aspect of the joint line and watch for a bulge medial to the joint.
   b. Patellar tap—apply pressure to the suprapatellar pouch while tapping the patella against the femur to determine whether the patella is ballottable, which indicates an effusion.
6. Arthrocentesis may also be used therapeutically, as in the serial aspiration of a septic joint for drainage and monitoring of the response to treatment.
7. Arthrocentesis allows for injection of corticosteroid preparations into the joint space, a form of therapy useful for various forms of inflammatory and noninflammatory arthritis.
B. Etiology of inflammatory arthritis
1. Rheumatoid arthritis
2. Spondyloarthropathies
3. Crystal-induced arthritis
4. Infectious arthritis
5. Connective tissue diseases
6. Hypersensitivity
C. Etiology of noninflammatory arthritis
1. Osteoarthritis
2. Trauma/internal derangement
3. Avascular necrosis
4. Hemarthrosis

       5. Malignancy

       6. Benign tumors

D. Contraindications

    1. Absolute contraindications to arthrocentesis include infection of the overlying skin or periarticular structures and severe coagulopathy.

    2. If septic arthritis is suspected in the presence of severe coagulopathy, efforts to correct the bleeding diathesis should be made prior to joint aspiration.

    3. Therapeutic anticoagulation is not an absolute contraindication.

    4. Although known bacteremia is a contraindication to arthrocentesis given the potential for joint space seeding, joint aspiration is nonetheless indicated if septic arthritis is the presumed source of the bacteremia.

    5. Articular damage and instability constitute relative contraindications to arthrocentesis.

III. PROCEDURE

  A. Arthrocentesis equipment

    1. Skin preparation

      a. Iodophor or chlorhexidine solution

      b. Alcohol swab

      c. Ethyl chloride spray

    2. Local anesthesia:

      a. 1% lidocaine; 25-gauge, 1-in. needle; 22-gauge, 1.5-in. needle; 5-mL syringe

      b. Sterile sponge/cloth

    3. Arthrocentesis

      a. Gloves

      b. 10- to 60-mL syringe (depending on size of effusion)

      c. 18- to 20-gauge, 1.5-in. needle

      d. Sterile sponge/cloth

      e. Sterile clamp

      f. Adhesive bandage (Band-Aid)

    4. Collection

      a. 15-mL anticoagulated tube (with sodium heparin or EDTA)

      b. Sterile tubes for routine cultures

  B. Technique

    1. Joint aspiration requires knowledge of the relevant joint and periarticular anatomy and strict adherence to aseptic technique.

    2. Joints other than the knee should probably be aspirated by an appropriate specialist, such as a rheumatologist or an orthopedic surgeon.

    3. Aspiration of some joints, such as the hip or sacroiliac joints, may require fluoroscopic or computed tomographic guidance.

    4. The technique for knee aspiration is as follows:

      a. Confirm the presence of an effusion with the patient supine and the knee extended.

      b. Obtain written informed consent from the patient or legal guardian if feasible.

      c. Collect the items required for the procedure (see Arthrocentesis equipment).

    5. The superior and inferior borders of the patella are landmarks for needle placement.

    6. Entry should be halfway between these borders just inferior to the undersurface of the patella, either from a medial or lateral approach, the former being more commonly used and preferable with small effusions.

    7. Cleanse the area with an iodine-based or chlorhexidine antiseptic solution. Allow the area to dry, then wipe once with an alcohol swab.

    8. Local anesthesia can be achieved either with sterile ethyl chloride spray or infiltration of local anesthetic solution (e.g., 1% lidocaine) into the subcutaneous and deeper tissues.

    9. To enter the knee joint, use an 18- to 20-gauge, 1.5-in. needle with a sterile 20- to 60-mL syringe.

10. Use a quick thrust through skin and capsule.

11. Avoid periosteal bone to minimize pain.

12. Aspirate fluid to fill the syringe. If the fluid appears purulent or hemorrhagic, try to tap the joint dry.

13. Drainage of large effusions may require additional syringes, which may be exchanged for the original one while leaving the needle in place.

14. When the fluid has been obtained, the needle is removed, and pressure is applied to the puncture site with sterile gauze.

15. Apply an adhesive bandage after cleaning the area with alcohol. Apply prolonged pressure if the patient has a bleeding diathesis of any type.

16. Document the amount, color, clarity, and viscosity of the fluid. Send the fluid for cell count with differential, Gram stain, routine culture; cultures for gonococcus, mycobacteria, and fungi, if indicated, and polarized microscopic examination for crystal analysis.

17. Anticoagulated tubes are needed for accurate assessment of fluid for cell count and crystal analysis.

18. Sodium heparin and ethylenediamine tetraacetic acid (EDTA) are appropriate anticoagulants.

19. Fluid may be sent for Gram stain and culture in the syringe or in a sterile red-top tube.

20. Other tests, including glucose and complement levels, are generally not helpful.

C. Synovial fluid analysis: see Table 19-1.

D. Viscosity

    1. The viscosity of synovial fluid is a measure of the hyaluronic acid content.

    2. Degradative enzymes result in a thinner, less viscous fluid.

    3. The string sign is a bedside measure of viscosity.

    4. Normal synovial fluid forms at least a 6 cm continuous string when a drop of fluid is allowed to fall from the needle or syringe.

    5. Inflammatory fluid drips like water and will not form a string.

    6. A good, tenacious mucin clot (produced by mixture of synovial fluid and 5% acetic acid) forms only with normal, noninflammatory fluid.

E. Crystals

    1. Fluid is examined for crystals using a compensated polarized light microscope.

    2. The presence of intracellular monosodium urate (needle shaped, negatively birefringent) or calcium pyrophosphate dihydrate (CPPD; small rhomboid, weakly positive birefringent) crystals confirms the diagnosis of gout or pseudogout, respectively.

| **TABLE 19-1** | **Joint Fluid Characteristics** | | | |

	Normal	Noninflammatory	Inflammatory	Septic
Color	Clear	Yellow	Yellow or opalescent	Variable; may be purulent
Clarity	Transparent	Transparent	Transparent	Opaque
Viscosity	Very high	High	Low	Typically low
Mucin clot	Firm	Firm	Friable	Friable
WBC/mm^3	<200	200–2,000	2,000–100,000	>50,000, often >100,000
PNM %	<25	<25	>50	>75
Culture	Negative	Negative	Negative	Usually positive

WBC, white blood count; PNM %, polymorphonuclear leukocyte %.

F. Gram stain and culture
   1. Synovial fluid should routinely be cultured for aerobic and anaerobic organisms. Additional cultures for fungi and mycobacteria should be sent in some circumstances, such as in chronic monoarticular arthritis.
   2. Special growth media are required when disseminated gonorrhea is suspected.
   3. A positive culture confirms septic arthritis.

IV. POSTPROCEDURE CONSIDERATIONS
   A. Complications
      1. The major complications of arthrocentesis are bleeding and iatrogenically induced infection.
      2. These complications are exceedingly rare with strict adherence to aseptic technique and with correction of significant coagulopathy prior to joint aspiration.
      3. Direct cartilaginous damage by the needle is difficult to quantitate and likely is minimized by avoidance of excessive needle movement or complete drainage of the joint, as well as avoiding advancement of the needle any deeper than needed to obtain fluid.

Selected Readings

Doherty M, Hazelman BL, Hutton CL, et al. *Rheumatology examination and injection techniques.* London: WB Saunders, 1992.
   Detailed description of the Bulge test in determining a joint effusion.

Gatter RA, Schumacher HR. *A practical handbook of joint fluid analysis.* Philadelphia: Lippincott Williams & Williams, 1991.
   Classic reference on all aspects if arthrocentesis and synovial fluid analysis.

Hollander JL, Jessar RA, McCarty DJ. Synovianalysis: an aid in arthritis diagnosis. *Bull Rheum Dis* 1961;12:263.
   Classic article on the categorization of different types of arthritis.

Ruddy S, Sledge CB, Harris ED et al. *Kelley textbook of rheumatology,* 6th ed. Philadelphia: WB Saunders, 2000.
   A standard, comprehensive text of rheumatology.

20 ANESTHESIA FOR BEDSIDE PROCEDURES
J. Matthias Walz and Mark Dershwitz

I. GENERAL PRINCIPLES
  #### A. Managing pain in critical illness
   1. Anesthesia for bedside procedures in the ICU is accomplished with total intravenous anesthesia (TIVA).
   2. Selecting the proper dose of an analgesic to administer is challenging because of:
      a. Difficulty in assessing the effectiveness of pain relief (delirium, obtundation, endotracheal intubation)
      b. Pharmacokinetic (PK) differences between critically ill and other patients
      c. Physiologic changes associated with aging (decrease in lean body mass, increase in volume of distribution of lipid soluble drugs, decrease in drug clearance rates, increased sensitivity to hypnotics and analgesics)
  #### B. Pharmacokinetic considerations
   1. PK behavior in critically ill patients is unlike that in normal subjects for several reasons:
      a. Intensive care unit (ICU) patients frequently have renal and/or hepatic dysfunction, therefore, drug metabolism and elimination may be significantly impaired
      b. Hypoalbuminemia, common in critical illness, decreases protein binding and increases free (active) drug concentration
   2. The doses of medications used for TIVA must therefore be individualized for a particular, critically ill patient (for more detailed pharmacokinetic considerations please refer to Dershwitz, 2003 in the Selected Readings.)

II. INDICATIONS
  #### A. Selection of agent
   1. Procedures performed in the ICU can be differentiated according to their associated levels of discomfort in:
      a. Mild to moderately uncomfortable (esophagogastroscopy, paracentesis)
      b. Moderately to severely uncomfortable (endotracheal intubation, thoracostomy bronchoscopy)
      c. Extremely painful (rigid bronchoscopy, orthopedic manipulations, tracheotomy)
   2. Specific disease states should be considered so that safety and effectiveness are maximized:
      a. Head trauma.
         (1) Effective, yet brief anesthesia is desirable so that the capacity to assess neurologic status is not lost for extended periods.
         (2) The technique should not adversely affect cerebral perfusion pressure.
         (3) If the effects of the medications dissipate too rapidly, undesirable episodes of agitation and increased intracranial pressure may occur.
      b. Coronary artery disease: sufficient analgesia is necessary during and after invasive procedures to minimize tachycardia (which is a major determinant of ischemia) and reduce plasma catecholamine and stress hormone levels.
      c. Renal or hepatic failure:
         (1) The risk of an adverse drug reaction is at least three times higher in azotemic patients compared to those with normal renal function.

TABLE 20-1	Characteristics of Intravenous Hypnotic Agents			
	Propofol	**Etomidate**	**Ketamine**	**Midazolam**
Bolus dose (mg/kg)	1−2	0.2−0.3	1−2	0.05−0.1
Onset	Fast	Fast	Fast	**Intermediate**
Duration	Short	Short	Intermediate	Intermediate
Cardiovascular effects	↓	**None**	↑	Minimal
Respiratory effects	↓	↓	**Minimal**	↓
Analgesia	None	None	**Profound**	None
Amnesia	Mild	Mild	**Profound**	**Profound**

The listed doses should be reduced 50% in elderly patients.
Entries in bold type indicate noteworthy differences among the drugs.

(2) Liver failure alters the volume of distribution of many drugs by impairing synthesis of albumin and α_1-acid glycoprotein.

(3) Reductions in hepatic blood flow and hepatic enzyme activity decrease drug clearance rates.

III. PROCEDURE

A. Hypnotics

1. The characteristics of commonly used hypnotics are listed in Table 20-1.

B. Propofol

1. Propofol is an extremely popular hypnotic agent for the following reasons:

a. Propofol is associated with pleasant emergence and little hangover.

b. It is readily titratable and has more rapid onset and offset kinetics than midazolam.

c. The rapid recovery of neurologic status makes propofol a good sedative in ICU patients, especially those with head trauma.

d. Spontaneously breathing patients anesthetized with propofol may maintain normal end-tidal carbon dioxide values during minor surgical procedures.

2. Maintenance infusion rates of 100 to 200 μg/kg/min are adequate in younger subjects, which should be reduced by 20% to 50% in elderly individuals.

3. Adverse effects of propofol administration include:

a. Depressed ventricular systolic function and decreased afterload.

b. In patients with coronary artery disease, propofol administration may be associated with a reduction in coronary perfusion pressure.

c. The emulsion used as the vehicle for propofol supports bacterial growth; iatrogenic contamination leading to septic shock is possible.

d. Hyperlipidemia with prolonged infusions can occur, particularly in infants and small children.

4. Serum zinc levels should be measured daily during continuous propofol infusions (chelation of trace metals, particularly zinc, by ethylenediaminetetraacetic acid, bacteriostatic agent in one formulation).

C. Etomidate

1. Etomidate has onset and offset PK characteristics similar to those of propofol and lacks significant effects on myocardial contractility (even in the setting of cardiomyopathy).

2. Etomidate depresses cerebral oxygen metabolism and blood flow in a dose-dependent manner without changing the intracranial volume–pressure relationship.

3. Etomidate is particularly useful in patients with:

a. Hypovolemia

b. Multiple trauma victims with closed head injury

    c. Patients with low ejection fraction, severe aortic stenosis, left main coronary artery disease, or severe cerebrovascular disease

  4. Prolonged infusion is not recommended because of adrenocortical suppression.

D. Ketamine

1. Ketamine is unique among the hypnotic agents in that it has analgesic, sedative, and amnestic effects.

2. Ketamine has a slower onset and offset as compared to propofol or etomidate following intravenous (IV) infusion, and stimulates the cardiovascular system (i.e. raises heart rate and blood pressure by direct stimulation of the central nervous system [CNS]).

3. Ketamine may be safer than other hypnotics or opioids in unintubated patients because it depresses airway reflexes and respiratory drive to a lesser degree.

4. In the usual dosage, ketamine decreases airway resistance.

5. The administration of ketamine can be associated with disorientation, sensory and perceptual illusions, and vivid dreams; these effects have been termed *emergence phenomena*. To avoid emergence phenomena after ketamine administration, pretreatment or concurrent treatment with a benzodiazepine or propofol should be considered.

6. The combination of ketamine with a benzodiazepines and/or an opioid is useful in patients with coronary artery disease to avoid myocardial ischemia (the use of ketamine alone increases myocardial oxygen consumption).

7. Ketamine is relatively contraindicated in patients with increased ICP.

E. Midazolam

1. Administration of midazolam produces anxiolysis, amnesia, and relaxation of skeletal muscle (ideally suited for brief, relatively painless procedures as well as for prolonged sedation).

2. Midazolam is highly (95%) protein bound, and recovery is prolonged in obese and elderly patients and after continuous infusion because it accumulates significantly.

3. In patients with renal failure, active conjugated metabolites of midazolam may accumulate and delay recovery.

4. Midazolam (0.15 mg/kg IV) causes respiratory depression and blunts the ventilatory response to hypoxia.

5. Midazolam has a stable cardiovascular profile and causes dose-dependent reductions in cerebral metabolic rate and cerebral blood flow.

F. Opioids

1. Opioids blunt pain by
    a. Inhibiting pain processing by the dorsal horn of the spinal cord
    b. Decreasing transmission of pain by activating descending inhibitory pathways in the brainstem
    c. Altering the emotional response to pain by actions on the limbic cortex

G. Morphine

1. Morphine is an agonist at μ, κ, and δ receptors.

2. Morphine causes significant histamine release after IV bolus injection.

3. Adverse effects of morphine include
    a. Gastrointestinal:
      (1) Constipation, nausea, and/or vomiting
      (2) Reduced gastric emptying and bowel motility
    b. Cardiovascular: hypotension, especially if it is given rapidly (i.e., 5 to 10 mg/min)
    c. Respiratory:
      (1) Morphine decreases the ventilatory response to CO_2 and hypoxia
      (2) Exaggerated ventilatory depression in patients with renal failure is possible because of the active metabolite, morphine-6-glucuronide

H. Fentanyl and related drugs

1. Fentanyl, alfentanil, sufentanil, and remifentanil enter and leave the CNS much more rapidly than morphine (much faster onset of effect after IV administration).

2. They are selective μ-opioid receptors agonists (the only significant difference among these agents is their PK behavior).

3. Fentanyl may be useful when given by intermittent bolus injection (50 to 100 µg), but when given by infusion its duration becomes prolonged.

4. Remifentanil owes its extremely short duration to rapid metabolism by tissue esterases (primarily in skeletal muscle); its PK behavior is unchanged in the presence of severe hepatic or renal failure.

5. Sufentanil infusion for TIVA may be initiated with a 0.5 to 1.5 µg/kg bolus followed by an infusion at 0.01 to 0.03 µg/kg/min.

6. Remifentanil infusion for TIVA may be initiated with a 1 to 2 µg/kg bolus followed by an infusion at 0.25 to 1 µg/kg/min.

I. Neuromuscular blocking agents

1. Succinylcholine

a. Succinylcholine 1 mg/kg IV will result in excellent intubating conditions in less than a minute. It is the drug of choice when the airway must be secured quickly (full stomach or symptomatic gastroesophageal reflux) unless there are contraindications.

b. Succinylcholine may trigger malignant hyperthermia in genetically susceptible persons.

c. Succinylcholine may cause a malignant rise in the extracellular potassium concentration in patients with major acute burns, upper or lower motor neuron lesions, prolonged immobility, massive crush injuries, and various myopathies.

J. Nondepolarizing neuromuscular blocking agents (NMB)

a. Vecuronium (0.1 mg/kg), rocuronium (0.6 to 1.2 mg/kg), and cisatracurium (0.1 to 0.2 mg/kg) are often used to facilitate intubation in persons in whom succinylcholine is contraindicated and are essentially devoid of cardiovascular effects.

b. Pancuronium (0.1 mg/kg), pipecuronium (0.09 mg/kg), and doxacurium (0.05 mg/kg) are longer-lasting NMB drugs and are commonly used to facilitate mechanical ventilation.

c. Pancuronium has a vagolytic effect that may cause tachycardia; pipecuronium and doxacurium are devoid of cardiovascular effects.

d. Use of NMB agents may cause muscle weakness persisting for months afterward: risk factors include concomitant glucocorticoid therapy or prolonged neuromuscular blockade.

Selected Readings

Barr J, Egan TD, Sandoval NF, et al. Propofol dosing regimens for ICU sedation based upon an integrated pharmacokinetic-pharmacodynamic model. *Anesthesiology* 2001;95(2):324–333.
An excellent example of theory guiding practice in the use of long-term infusions (weeks) of propofol in ICU patients.

Dershwitz M, Landow L, Joshi-Ryzewicz W. In: Irwin RS, Rippe JM, eds. *Irwin and Rippe's intensive care medicine*, 5th ed., Lippincott Williams and Wilkins, 2003.
Detailed pharmacokinetic considerations.

Dershwitz M, Rosow CE. Remifentanil: an opioid metabolized by esterases. *Exp Opin Invest Drugs* 1996;5:1361.
A comprehensive review of the pharmacology of remifentanil.

Hughes MA, Glass PSA, Jacobs JR: Context-sensitive half-time in multicompartment pharmacokinetic models for intravenous anesthetic drugs. *Anesthesiology* 1992;76:334.
The description of the new parameter, context-sensitive half-time, which represented an improved method for predicting the recovery times following infusions of lipophilic medications.

Shafer SL, Varvel JR: Pharmacokinetics, pharmacodynamics, and rational opioid selection. *Anesthesiology* 1991;74:53.
An excellent description of why PK half-lives do not describe the overall kinetic behavior of lipophilic medications.

MONITORING IN THE INTENSIVE CARE UNIT
Nicholas A. Smyrnios and Frederick J. Curley

I. TEMPERATURE MONITORING
A. Sites of measurement
1. Core temperature—true body temperature. Rectal, bladder, and tympanic temperatures are in general the most reliable sites.
2. Sublingual—convenient. Tachypnea and consumption of hot or cold substances affect result. Best for intermittent measurement.
3. Axillary—temperatures average 1.5° to 1.9°C lower than tympanic. The accuracy of axillary temperatures is affected by inability to maintain probe position.
4. Tympanic—measured with specifically designed thermometer. In theory, correlates well with core temperature. In practice, correlates poorly because of difficulty performing the technique and technical malfunctions, with a high degree of user dissatisfaction.
5. Skin—poor correlation with core temperature.
B. Standards
1. All critically ill patients should have core temperature measured at least every 4 hours.
2. Patients with a temperature above 39°C or below 36°C or those undergoing temperature-altering intervention (i.e., breathing heated air or cooling blanket) should have continuous monitoring.
3. Continuous temperature monitoring is done in great vessel, rectum, or bladder.
4. Intermittent measurements should probably be rectal.

II. ARTERIAL PRESSURE MONITORING
A. Indirect blood pressure measurement
1. Bladder width should equal 40% and length should be at least 60% of the circumference of the extremity.
2. *Auscultatory pressure* is the traditional method using a sphygmomanometer cuff. It correlates poorly with directly measured values at the extremes of pressure.
3. *Palpatory systolic pressure* is defined as the pressure when a pulse is detected in the radial artery as the cuff is deflated.
4. Automated indirect devices measure without manual inflation and deflation.
5. Oscillometric methods correlate well with group average values, but they correlate poorly with intraarterial pressures in individual patients.
6. Doppler sensing devices are slightly better but still vary quite a bit.
7. Volume clamp devices respond rapidly to changes in blood pressure and may be appropriate for use in critical care in the future.
8. Automated noninvasive monitors have a role in following trends of pressure change but are of little value in situations in which blood pressure fluctuates rapidly. Critical management decisions should not be made based on their results unless use of a direct method is impossible.
B. Direct invasive blood pressure measurement
1. Advantages of arterial catheters:
   a. measure the end-on pressure propagated by the arterial pulse
   b. detect pressures at which Korotkoff sounds are either absent or inaccurate
   c. provide beat-to-beat changes in blood pressure
   d. eliminate the need for multiple punctures when frequent blood draws needed

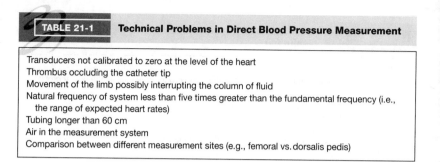

TABLE 21-1	Technical Problems in Direct Blood Pressure Measurement

Transducers not calibrated to zero at the level of the heart
Thrombus occluding the catheter tip
Movement of the limb possibly interrupting the column of fluid
Natural frequency of system less than five times greater than the fundamental frequency (i.e., the range of expected heart rates)
Tubing longer than 60 cm
Air in the measurement system
Comparison between different measurement sites (e.g., femoral vs. dorsalis pedis)

  2. Disadvantages of arterial catheters:
   a. Require invasive procedure with complications including arterial injury, ischemia, thrombus formation, infection, and blood loss, among others.
   b. Technical problems affecting invasive arterial pressure measurement are listed in Table 21-1.

III. ELECTROCARDIOGRAPHIC MONITORING
A. Arrhythmia monitoring
  1. Continuous electrocardiographic (ECG) monitoring is performed routinely in all intensive care units (ICUs). Skin electrodes detect cardiac impulses and transform them into an electrical signal, which is transmitted to the signal converter and display unit.
  2. Computerized arrhythmia detection systems are incorporated into the monitors; detects arrhythmias based on heart rate, variability, rhythm, intervals, segment lengths, complex width, and morphology
  3. Reasons for arrhythmia monitoring:
   a. Up to 95% of patients with acute myocardial infarction (AMI) have arrhythmias within 48 hours of admission.
   b. Ventricular tachycardia occurs in one third of AMI patients; monitoring enables rapid detection and increases the likelihood of survival.
   c. It improves prognosis in the post-AMI period when combined with aggressive, formalized approach to treatment.
   d. Thrombolytic therapy for AMI leads to a slight increase in arrhythmias within 8 to 12 hours after successful reperfusion.
   e. It can measure heart rate variability, which helps in risk stratification.
B. Ischemia monitoring
  1. Automated ST-segment monitoring is useful in the ICU because:
   a. Early detection of ischemic episodes could lead to early interventions.
   b. Continuous ST-segment monitoring can lead to the treatment of an expanded group of patients with thrombolytic therapy, including patients whose initial 12-lead electrocardiogram (ECG) was not diagnostic of AMI.
   c. The degree of ST-segment resolution after thrombolysis may be a marker for prognosis after AMI.
   d. ST-segment elevation may indicate ischemia acting as a barrier to weaning from mechanical ventilation.
  2. ST-monitoring systems create a "normal QRS" template and compare it to subsequent beats. Leads are chosen to represent the three major axes (anteroposterior/left-right/craniocaudal). They can be displayed individually or summed and displayed over time.
  3. Table 21-2 lists several technical and personnel issues that may impede the ability to generate and interpret high-quality ECG monitoring information in the ICU.

TABLE 21-2	Technical and Personnel Issues in Electrocardiographic Monitoring

1. Patient safety requirements
   a. All equipment in contact with patient at the same ground potential as the power ground line
   b. Insulation of exposed lead connections
   c. Use of appropriately wired three-prong plugs
2. Adequate signal size
   a. Matching of skin electrode and preamplifier impedance
   b. Good skin preparation
   c. Site selection
   d. Conducting gels
   e. High preamplifier input impedance
   f. Use of buffer amplifiers
   g. Appropriate signal "damping"
   h. Correct frequency response
   i. Unwanted ambient voltages
3. Personnel issues
   a. Initial formal training for all staff responsible for interpreting ECG monitoring
   b. Formal hospital interpretation and response protocols
   c. Physician backup available in house

ECG, electrocardiographic.

IV. RESPIRATORY MONITORING
A. Respiratory rate, tidal volume, and minute ventilation
1. Impedance monitors use ECG leads to measure changes in electrical impedance generated by the change in distance between leads. Leads must be placed at points of maximal change in thoracoabdominal contour. They are cheap when ECG monitoring is already in use, but lack the accuracy for precise measurement.
2. Respiratory inductive plethysmography (RIP) measures changes in the cross-sectional area of the chest and abdomen occurring with respiration. RIP is infrequently used because technical problems limit acceptance.
3. Most respiratory monitoring is done through the mechanical ventilator. Ventilators report respiratory rates, tidal volumes, and minute ventilation and alarm when values vary from predetermined range. Can be used when a patient is weaning from mechanical ventilation with a mode that keeps the breath flowing through the ventilator circuit (e.g., PSV or CPAP) but not if the patient is not connected to a ventilator.

B. Pulse oximetry
1. Pulse oximeters distinguish between oxyhemoglobin and reduced hemoglobin on the basis of their different absorption of light. Red light and infrared light are directed from light-emitting diodes to a photodetector across a pulsatile tissue bed and the absorption varies with the pulse. The difference between absorption in systole and diastole is due to arterialized blood.
2. Most pulse oximeters measure the saturation to within 2% of actual SaO_2.
3. Table 21-3 lists conditions that adversely affect the results of pulse oximetry.

C. Transcutaneous measurement of oxygen and carbon dioxide
1. Measure partial pressures of O_2 ($P_{tc}O_2$) and CO_2 ($P_{tc}CO_2$) that diffuse through the skin.
2. Transcutaneous values of O_2 and CO_2 are typically 10 mm Hg lower and 5 to 23 mm Hg higher than arterial values, respectively.
3. Factors that cause inaccuracy include heating of the skin by fever, hypoperfusion of the area being monitored, local variations, edema, burns, abrasions, and scleroderma.

TABLE 21-3	Conditions That adaversely Affect the Results of Pulse Oximetry

Poor signal detection
Probe malposition
Motion
Hypothermia
No pulse
Vasoconstriction
Hypotension
Falsely low S_pO_2
Nail polish
Dark skin
Ambient light
Elevated serum lipids
Methylene blue
Indigo carmine
Indocyanine green
Falsely elevated S_pO_2
Elevated carboxyhemoglobin
Elevated methemoglobin
Ambient light
Hypothermia

S_pO_2, oxyhemoglobin saturation by pulse oximetry.

4. Useful when changes in either perfusion or gas exchange are likely, but not both. When perfusion is stable, reflects gas exchange. When gas exchange is stable, it reflects perfusion.

D. Capnography

1. Involves measurement and display of expired partial pressure of CO_2(PCO_2). Is a useful adjunct for detecting unintentional extubation, ETT malposition, or absence of perfusion.

E. Arterial blood gas analysis: see Chapter 23.

Selected Readings

Carrol GC. Blood pressure monitoring. *Crit Care Clin* 1988;4:411.
  A general review of the topic of blood pressure measurement.

Clements FM, Bruijn NP. Noninvasive cardiac monitoring. *Crit Care Clin* 1988;4:435.
  A more in-depth explanation of the procedure of ischemia monitoring is described.

Kimball JT, Killip T. Aggressive treatment of arrhythmias in acute myocardial infarction: procedures and results. *Prog Cardiovasc Dis* 1968;10:483.
  A classic article validating the treatment of arrhythmias in the post-AMI period.

Levine RL. End-tidal CO_2: physiology in pursuit of clinical applications. *Intensive Care Med*; 2000; 26:1595–1597.
  Concise editorial on the utility of capnography in the intensive care unit.

New W. Pulse oximetry. *J Clin Monit* 1985;1:126.
  General review of the technique of pulse oximetry.

Parati G, Ongaro G, Bilo G, et al. Non-invasive beat-to-beat blood pressure monitoring: new developments. *Blood Press Monit* 2003; 8:31–36.
  Review of recent progress to measure blood pressure continuously and noninvasively.

Soubani AO. Noninvasive monitoring of oxygen and carbon dioxide. *Am J Emerg Med*;2001; 19:141–146.
  Recent review on pulse oximetry and capnography in the emergency setting and the intensive care unit.

22 ECHOCARDIOGRAPHY IN THE INTENSIVE CARE UNIT

Dennis A. Tighe and Gerard P. Aurigemma

I. GENERAL PRINCIPLES

   A. Echocardiography is a common technique performed on critically ill patients. The major advantages of echocardiography as a diagnostic technique relate to its portability, lack of patient exposure to ionizing radiation, and capability to provide real-time structural and functional (hemodynamic) information.

   B. Structural information is provided by transmitting ultrasound energy (2 to 10 MHz) from the echocardiograph and receiving signals returning from the cardiac structures to create real-time, two-dimensional (2D) images of the heart.

   C. Using the Doppler principle, reflected ultrasound energy can be used to determine the velocity and direction of flowing blood in the heart and great vessels, thus providing information about the hemodynamic effects of stenotic and regurgitant valve lesions and information about left heart filling pressures. Instantaneous pressure gradients can be estimated by measuring peak flow velocity (V), and, with application of the modified Bernoulli equation, the pressure gradient (P) can be estimated as $P = 4V^2$. Color-flow Doppler, a pulsed-wave Doppler technique, provides a spatial velocity map of abnormal flow within the heart and great vessels and is most useful to estimate the degree of valvular regurgitation. The recent development of tissue Doppler imaging adds to the ability to estimate left heart filling pressures.

   D. A complete echocardiographic examination includes information provided by the 2D, Doppler, color-flow, and M-mode modalities.

   E. Echocardiography methods
   1. Transducer placed directly on the patient's chest (transthoracic echocardiography [TTE])
   2. Transducer mounted on a gastroscope passed into the patient's esophagus and stomach (transesophageal echocardiography [TEE]).

II. INDICATIONS FOR ECHOCARDIOGRAPHY IN THE ICU

   A. Evaluation of left ventricular (LV) structure and function
   1. Rapid estimation of LV ejection fraction and assessment of parameters such as LV wall thickness, chamber sizes, and wall motion abnormalities.
   2. Doppler echocardiography can provide an accurate assessment of LV filling pressures.

   B. Evaluation of hypotension/shock (Tables 22-1 and 22-2)

   C. Evaluation of cardiac valves
   1. Assessment of valvular stenosis or regurgitation requires a comprehensive echocardiographic examination utilizing the 2D, pulsed-wave, and continuous-wave Doppler, and color flow Doppler modalities.
   2. Infective endocarditis (IE)
      a. TTE has a sensitivity to identify valvular vegetations of 44% to 80% among patients with suspected infective endocarditis. TTE is relatively insensitive to diagnose myocardial or aortic root abscesses and infection of prosthetic valves.
      b. TEE has a sensitivity approaching 100% for vegetations as small as 2 mm. TEE can detect complications of IE, such as fistulous tracts, perforation, and abscess formation, in 90% to 95% of cases. It is the modality of choice with suspected prosthetic valve endocarditis.

   D. Evaluation of the aorta and great vessels
   1. Aortic dissection

TABLE 22-1	Echocardiographic Features of Various Causes of Hemodynamic Compromise			
Diagnosis	**LVFAC**	**RV size and function**	**E/A ratio**	**S/D ratio**
Hyperdynamic shock	↑	Small Hyperdynamic	>/<1	>1
Cardiogenic shock	↓ or ↑	Dilated Hypokinetic	<1	>1
Hemorrhagic shock	↑	Small Hyperkinetic	<1	<1
Pulmonary embolism	↑ or ↓	Dilated Hypokinesis	<1	>1
Cardiac tamponade	↑	Small Diastolic collapse	<1	>1

E/A, ratio of mitral inflow E-wave velocity to A-wave velocity; LVFAC, left ventricular fractional area change; RV, right ventricle; S/D, systolic to diastolic ratio of pulmonary vein flow velocities.

      a. Detection of a mobile intimal flap
      b. TEE has higher sensitivity and specificity than TTE and equivalent diagnostic accuracy compared to other imaging modalities (Table 22-3).
    2. Deceleration injury to aorta/aortic trauma/valvular injuries
  E. Evaluation of hypoxemia
    1. Acute pulmonary embolism (PE)—not a first line test
    2. Right-to-left shunting via a patent foramen ovale (bubble test)
    3. Congenital heart lesions
  F. Evaluation of cardiac source of embolism

III. ECHOCARDIOGRAPHY PROCEDURE

  A. A standard TTE examination is performed by placing an ultrasound transducer on the chest and imaging from a variety of areas.
    1. In approximately 30% of critically ill patients, the image quality of TTE is inadequate, and a TEE may be required to obtain diagnostic information.
    2. Limitations of TTE relate primarily to the adequacy of the available acoustic windows: obesity, obstructive lung disease, chest wall injuries, small rib spaces, or previous sternotomy.
    3. TEE requires intubation of the esophagus. Special patient preparations are required (Table 22-4). TEE is recognized as a superior imaging modality for certain specific indications (Table 22-5).
      a. Limitations of TEE relate to factors such as cooperation, existence of a large hiatus hernia (limit the ability to acquire adequate images), and inability to intubate the esophagus.

TABLE 22-2	Estimation of Right Atrial Pressure from Assessment of Size and Respiratory Change in Diameter of the Inferior Vena Cava	
IVC size[a]	**Respiratory change**	**RA pressure (mm Hg)**
Small (<1.5 cm)	Collapse	0–5
Normal (1.5–2.5 cm)	Decrease >50%	5–10
Normal	Decrease <50%	10–15
Dilated (>2.5 cm)	Decrease <50%	15–20
Dilated with dilated hepatic veins	No change	>20

IVC, inferior vena cava; RA, right atrium
[a] Measured at RA–IVC junction

| TABLE 22-3 | Diagnostic Performance of the Various Tests for Acute Aortic Dissection | | | |

Parameter	Aortography	CT	MR	TEE
Sensitivity	++	++	+++	+++
Specificity	+++	+++	+++	+++
Site of intimal tear	++	+	+++	+++
Presence of thrombus	+++	++	+++	++
Presence of AR	+++	−	+	+++
Pericardial effusion	−	++	+++	+++
Branch vessel involvement	+++	+	++	=
Coronary artery involvement	++	−	−	++

AR, aortic regurgitation; CT, computed tomography; MR, magnetic resonance; TEE, transesophageal echocardiography.
Adapted from Cigarroa JE, Isselbacher EM, DeSanctis RW, Eagle KA. Diagnostic imaging in the evaluation of suspected aortic dissection. *N Engl J Med* 1993;328:42.

   b. Contraindications to TEE include the presence of significant esophageal pathology (strictures, varices, tumors, mediastinal radiation therapy), upper gastrointestinal bleeding, significant coagulopathy, inadequate airway, and lack of patient cooperation.
   c. Complications: untoward effects of sedation, hypoxia, bleeding, arrhythmia, angina, esophageal perforation, and death.

IV. POSTPROCEDURE CONSIDERATIONS
   A. No special postprocedure considerations are required when a TTE is performed.
   B. For TEE, postprocedure considerations include patient recovery from conscious sedation (or general anesthesia in rare instances) and care and cleaning of the probe.
      1. Monitoring for a period of no less than 30 minutes postprocedure is required for all patients receiving conscious sedation. The patient should have nothing by mouth until swallowing, cough, and gag reflexes have returned appropriately.
      2. The TEE probe should be wiped down and transported expeditiously to the area where it can be immersed in an antimicrobial solution, such as Cidex, for 10 minutes.
      3. The probe should be stored in a protective sheath in an unflexed position.

| TABLE 22-4 | Special Preparations for TEE Examination |

Nothing per mouth >4 hours
Assess for contraindications
Insert IV, nasal O_2, BP cuff, ECG monitor, saturation monitor
Topical anesthesia
Bite block
IV sedation
   narcotic
   benzodiazepine
   paralytic (endotracheally intubated patients only)
Code cart available
No requirement for infective endocarditis prophylaxis

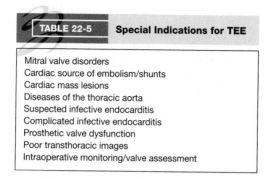

TABLE 22-5	Special Indications for TEE

Mitral valve disorders
Cardiac source of embolism/shunts
Cardiac mass lesions
Diseases of the thoracic aorta
Suspected infective endocarditis
Complicated infective endocarditis
Prosthetic valve dysfunction
Poor transthoracic images
Intraoperative monitoring/valve assessment

Selected Readings

Appelbe AF, Walker PG, Yeoh JK, et al. Clinical significance and origin of artifacts in transesophageal echocardiography of the thoracic aorta. *J Am Coll Cardiol* 1993;21:754–760.
Important article describing the significance and potential genesis of imaging artifacts involving the ascending aorta on TEE.

Burstow DJ, Oh JK, Bailey KR, et al. Cardiac tamponade: characteristic Doppler observations. *Mayo Clin Proc* 1989;64:312–324.
Study that describes the characteristic Doppler echocardiographic abnormalities in cardiac tamponade.

Cigarroa JE, Isselbacher EM, DeSanctis RW, et al. Diagnostic imaging in the evaluation of suspected aortic dissection. Old standards and new directions. *N Engl J Med* 1993;328:35–43.
Article reviewing the clinical applications, advantages, and limitations of the various imaging modalities in patients with suspected aortic dissections.

Daniel WG, Erbel R, Kasper W, et al. Safety of transesophageal echocardiography. A multicenter survey of 10,419 examinations. *Circulation* 1991;83:817–821.
A classic paper showing that TEE is associated with a very low risk of complications when performed by experienced operators.

Daniel WG, Mugge A, Martin RP, et al. Improvement in the diagnosis of abscesses associated with endocarditis by transesophageal echocardiography. *N Engl J Med* 1991;324:795–800.
Classic paper documenting the enhanced diagnostic yield of TEE for complicated infective endocarditis.

DiSalvo G, Habib G, Pergola V, et al. Echocardiography predicts embolic events in infective endocarditis. *J Am Coll Cardiol* 2001;37:1069–1076.
Recent paper documenting that vegetation size and mobility are the most important predictors of embolic events in infective endocarditis.

Dokainish H, Zoghbi WA, Lakkis NM, et al. Optimal noninvasive assessment of left ventricular filling pressures. A comparison of tissue Doppler echocardiography and B-type natriuretic peptide in patients with pulmonary artery catheters. *Circulation* 2004;109:2432–2439.
Recent article describing the utility of tissue Doppler imaging to estimate LV filling pressures.

Goldhaber SZ. Echocardiography in the management of pulmonary embolism. *Ann Intern Med* 2002;136:691–700.
Recent article reviewing the use of echocardiography in the diagnosis and management of pulmonary embolism.

Nishimura RA, Tajik AJ. Evaluation of diastolic filling of left ventricle in health and disease: Doppler echocardiography is the clinician's Rosetta stone. *J Am Coll Cardiol* 1997;30:8–18.
Important review article discussing the impact of Doppler echocardiography on the assessment of LV diastolic function. A classification of diastolic filling abnormalities and how they may be used to predict LV filling pressures is presented.

Pearson AC, Labovitz AJ, Tatineni S, Gomez CR. Superiority of transesophageal echocardiography in detecting cardiac source of embolism in patients with cerebral ischemia of uncertain etiology. *J Am Coll Cardiol* 1991;17:66–72.
Important study documenting the improved diagnostic yield of TEE versus TTE in patients with a suspected cardiac source of embolism.

Poelaret J, Schmidt C, Colardyn F. Transoesophageal echocardiography in the critically ill. *Anaesthesia* 1998;53:55–68.
Review article discussing the role and clinical impact of TEE in critically ill patients.

Reilly JP, Tunick PA, Timmermans RJ, et al. Contrast echocardiography clarifies uninterpretable wall motion in intensive care unit patients. *J Am Coll Cardiol.* 2000;35:485–490.
Important paper emphasizing that when TTEs of suboptimal image quality are obtained in ICU patients, the use of harmonic imaging with contrast echocardiography can significantly improve the assessment of chamber volumes and left ventricular wall motion analysis.

Reynolds HR, Jagen MA, Tunick PA, et al. Sensitivity of transthoracic versus transesophageal echocardiography for the detection of native valve vegetations in the modern era. *J Am Soc Echocardiogr* 2003;16:67–70.
Paper demonstrating that even when using the latest generation ultrasound systems, infective vegetations may fail to be demonstrated on a disturbingly frequent basis by TTE.

Seward JB, Khandheria BK, Oh JK, et al. Transesophageal echocardiography: technique, anatomic correlation, implementation, and clinical applications. *Mayo Clin Proc* 1988;63:649–680.
Review article discussing in depth the TEE procedure and its clinical applications.

Vignon P, Gueret P, Vedrinne JM, et al. Role of transesophageal echocardiography in the diagnosis and management of traumatic aortic disruption. *Circulation* 1995;92:2959–2968.
Article documenting the diagnostic yield and effect on management of TEE in suspected traumatic aortic injury.

ARTERIAL PUNCTURE FOR BLOOD GAS ANALYSIS

Marie T. Pavini, Deborah H. Markowitz, and Richard S. Irwin

I. GENERAL PRINCIPLES
A. Technical considerations
1. Arterial blood gas (ABG) analysis requires a sample of arterial blood for measurement of pH, partial arterial carbon dioxide pressure ($PaCO_2$), partial arterial oxygen pressure (PaO_2), bicarbonate (HCO_3^-) and percent oxyhemoglobin saturation (SaO_2) to assess a patient's respiratory, metabolic, and acid–base status.
2. Given the shape of the oxyhemoglobin dissociation curve, oximetry alone for SaO_2 measurement may not be reliable because there must be a substantial fall in PaO_2 before SaO_2 is appreciably altered. However, the calculated SaO_2 from the ABG cannot be corrected for variables such as the binding characteristics of hemoglobin (Hb) and 2,3-diphosphoglycerate.
3. The HCO_3^- in an ABG is calculated in contrast to the HCO_3^- measured in venous chemistries.

B. Equipment
1. A glass syringe is the standard to which all other methods are compared. If a large enough needle is used, entry is apparent because the syringe fills spontaneously by the pressurized arterial flow of blood, without the need for applying a vacuum or using a vacuum-sealed collecting tube.
2. Other plastic ABG kits are available that have directions specific for the type of collection syringe offered (see Cautions).

C. Alternative procedures
1. A venous blood gas (VBG) is useful when oxygenation is not suspect (i.e., past ABGs have correlated well enough with oximetric saturations, and there is no suspicion of a substantial change in oxygenation [see Normal values and corrections]).
2. Arterial catheterization is an option if frequent ABG measurements are needed (see Complications).

II. INDICATIONS
A. Diagnostic
1. Abnormal acid–base and blood oxygenation can quickly lead to unresponsiveness, serious cardiac arrhythmias, and death and can alert the physician to reversible causes of tissue hypoperfusion, metabolic derangements, and respiratory demise.
2. An ABG should be obtained when there is undiagnosed altered mental status, abnormal breathing pattern, suspicion of accuracy of oximetric saturations, or abnormal HCO_3^- on chemistry laboratory tests.
3. Discrepancy between SaO_2 by oximetry and that calculated by the ABG can aid in the diagnosis of carboxyhemoglobinemia and methemoglobinemia.
4. PaO_2 from an ABG is necessary for calculation of A-a gradient in the delineation of causes of respiratory acidosis and respiratory alkalosis.
5. Values from an ABG are necessary for determination of arterial content of oxygen (CaO_2), oxygen delivery ($\dot{D}O_2$) and oxygen consumption ($\dot{V}O_2$).

III. CONTRAINDICATIONS

A. Peripheral vascular disease (PVD) renders arterial sampling more difficult.

B. Puncturing a surgically reconstructed artery may:

   1. Result in a pseudoaneurysm

   2. Compromise the integrity of the graft site

   3. Seed the foreign body, rendering it a nidus for infection

IV. PROCEDURE

A. Cautions

   1. If a plastic syringe is used, the following errors may occur:

      a. Falsely low PaO_2 as O_2 from the sample can diffuse to the atmosphere whenever PO_2 exceeds 221 mm Hg.

      b. Plastic syringes with high surface area to volume ratios (i.e., tuberculin syringes) worsen gas permeability errors compared to 3-mL syringes. For this reason, butterfly infusion kits with their long tubing should not be used.

      c. Plastic syringes tenaciously retain air bubbles and extra effort is required to remove them.

      d. Plastic impedes smooth movement of the plunger, making arterial blood behave like venous blood (i.e., low pressure flow) and raising suspicion that the sample may be venous.

      e. If plunger retraction imparts suction, gas bubbles may be pulled out of solution. If they are expelled, measured PaO_2 and $PaCO_2$ tensions may be falsely lowered.

   2. Too much heparin causes the concentration of dissolved gases to be closer to that of heparin (PO_2 150 mm Hg; PCO_2 less than 0.3 mm Hg at sea level and room temperature). There is only a 4% dilution error when 0.2 mL heparin is used for 3 to 5 mL blood, but any less heparin risks a clotted specimen. Crystalline heparin is free of dilutional error but risks clotting.

   3. If an ABG specimen is not analyzed within 1 minute of being drawn or not immediately cooled to 2°C, the PO_2 and pH fall and PCO_2 rises due to cellular respiration and consumption of O_2 by leukocytes and platelets. This is of particular concern if leukocytes are greater than 40×10^9 per liter or platelets of $1,000 \times 10^9$ per liter.

   4. Unintentional sampling of the vein will result in a report of a low arterial PO_2.

   5. Breath holding in normal subjects of 35 seconds has been associated with a fall in PaO_2 of 50 mm Hg and a pH of 0.07 and a rise in $PaCO_2$ of 10 mm Hg.

B. Site selection

   1. It is best to select an artery that has good collateral circulation so that, if spasm or clotting occur, the distal tissue is not malperfused. It is also best to select a superficial artery for ease of entry as well as to minimize pain. The radial artery is the preferred site for arterial puncture. The ulnar artery provides sufficient collateral blood flow in approximately 92% of normal adults. The Allen's test (or its modification) is not routinely necessary (see Chapter 3) before puncture to determine superficial palmar arch collateral flow.

   2. If radial artery sites are not accessible, dorsalis pedis, posterior tibial and superficial temporal (in infants), brachial and femoral arteries are alternatives (see Chapter 3).

   3. Brachial and femoral artery punctures are not advised in patients with coagulopathies because adequate vessel tamponade may not be possible.

   4. Any vessel that has been reconstructed surgically should not be punctured for fear of creating a pseudoaneurysm, compromising the integrity of a graft site, or seeding the foreign body that could become a nidus for infection.

C. Technique

   1. Observe universal precautions.

   2. Face artery to be punctured. If radial artery is the target, supinate the arm, slightly hyperflex the wrist, and palpate the artery. Secure the patient's hand (i.e., with tape) in this position such that it is rendered immobile.

3. Cleanse the site with an alcohol swab or chlorhexidine/alcohol solution.

4. With a 25-gauge needle, inject enough 1% lidocaine intradermally to raise a small wheal where the puncture will be made.

5. Attach a 22-gauge or larger needle to a glass syringe that can accept 5 mL blood. Wet the needle and syringe with a sodium heparin solution (1,000 units per mL) and express all excess solution or use a regulation ABG kit.

6. With the needle, enter the artery at an angle of approximately 30 degrees to the long axis of the vessel to avoid painful scraping of the periosteum below the artery.

7. As soon as the artery is entered, blood appears in the syringe. Obtain at least 3 mL passively in the glass syringe or the prescribed amount for the commercial ABG.

8. Immediately after obtaining the specimen, expel any tiny air bubbles to ensure that the specimen will be anaerobic and that results will be accurate. Remove the needle and cap the syringe.

9. If using the glass syringe, have an assistant roll it between both palms for 5 to 15 seconds to mix the heparin with the blood.

10. Apply pressure to puncture site for approximately 5 minutes (longer if coagulopathy). If the brachial artery is used, compress vessel so that the radial pulse cannot be palpated.

11. Immerse the capped sample in a bag of ice and water/slush. (Some kits do not require this step.) Immediately transport the sample to the blood gas analyzer. Ensure that the sample is labeled with time of draw and ventilator settings (FiO_2 if not on ventilator) as well as position of the patient.

V. POSTPROCEDURE CONSIDERATIONS

A. Complications

1. Using the conventional radial artery technique, complications are unusual. These include:

   a. Vasovagal episode (rare)
   b. Local pain with or without breath holding (rendering false results)
   c. Limited hematomas (less than 0.58% of the time)
   d. Expanding aneurysm (frequent punctures)
   e. Reflex sympathetic dystrophy (frequent punctures)
   f. Spasm
   g. Uncontrolled bleeding
   h. Clotting with possible ischemia and loss of limb

2. Brachial and femoral sites are more difficult to tamponade, making internal bleeding a possibility (especially in coagulopathy).

B. Normal values and corrections

1. pH: 7.35 to 7.45

2. $PaCO_2$: 35 to 45

3. PaO_2 (in the normal, nonsmoking, upright person aged 40 to 90): 108.75 × (0.39 × age in years)

4. Temperature: By convention, ABG specimens are analyzed at 38°C. Although no studies have demonstrated that correction for the patient's temperature is clinically necessary, ABGs drawn at temperatures greater than 39°C should be corrected because the solubility of O_2 and CO_2 increases as blood is cooled rendering hyperthermic patients more acidotic and less hypoxemic than uncorrected values would indicate.

5. When measuring electrolytes from the same arterial collection, a lithium or electrolyte-balanced heparin should be considered as the anticoagulant because sodium-heparins may artificially increase sodium levels and lower potassium levels through binding. Dilutional error may still exist if excessive amounts of anticoagulant are used.

Selected Readings

Allen E. Thromboangiitis obliterans: methods of diagnosis of chronic occlusive arterial lesions distal to the wrist, with illustrative cases. *Am J Med Sci* 1929;178:237.
The original paper describing the classic safety maneuver before arterial puncture.

Markowitz DH, Irwin RS. Arterial puncture for blood gas analysis. In: Irwin RS, Rippe JM, Curley FJ, Heard SO, eds. *Procedures and techniques in intensive care medicine,* 3rd ed. Philadelphia: Lippincott Williams and Wilkins, 2003.
A more detailed account of the method for arterial puncture.

Petty T, Bigelow B, Levine B. The simplicity and safety of arterial puncture. *JAMA* 1966; 195:181.
A classic article describing arterial puncture.

Raffin T. Indications for arterial blood gas analysis. *Ann Intern Med* 1986; 105:390.
A good review of the indications for arterial puncture.

Sasse S, Berry R, Nguyen T, et al. Arterial blood gas changes during breath-holding from functional residual capacity. *Chest* 1996;110:958.
The arterial PO_2 fell by 50 mm Hg on average after 35 seconds of breath holding.

Schmidt C, Mullert-Plathe O. Stability of PO_2, PCO_2 and pH in heparinized whole blood samples: influence of storage temperature with regard to leukocyte count and syringe material. *Eur J Clin Chem Clin Biochem* 1992;30:767.
Storage at $22°C$ results in a significant reduction in PO_2 compared to $4°C$.

I. GENERAL PRINCIPLES

A. Indirect calorimetry (IC) measures inspired and expired gas flows, volumes, and concentrations and uses those to determine energy expenditure, respiratory quotient (RQ), and other values.

B. Indirect calorimetry measures the O_2 used and CO_2 produced when carbohydrate, protein, and lipid are oxidized to produce ATP. Therefore, it is the *production* of chemical energy that is indirectly measured by gas exchange parameters. Nevertheless, the energy activity determined by IC is typically referred to as energy expenditure.

II. ENERGY CALCULATIONS

A. Energy expenditures:

1. Basal energy expenditure (BEE)—the energy used by the body at complete rest and in the postabsorptive state (no active food absorption occurring). This occurs only in deep sleep

2. Resting energy expenditure (REE)—the energy used by the body while awake at rest plus the energy used to metabolize foods. Usually this is approximately 10% more than BEE. Because IC is typically done at rest, its measurement is usually described as resting energy expenditure.

3. Total energy expenditure (TEE) is REE plus the energy used during activity.

B. Most IC systems use the modified de Weir equation to calculate REE. The de Weir equation is not experimentally determined but is mathematically derived based on our knowledge of the metabolism of carbohydrate, fat, and protein.

1. Energy expenditure = $3.9(\dot{V}O_2) - 1.1(\dot{V}CO_2) - 2.17(UN\ g/d)$ where $\dot{V}O_2$ is oxygen consumption, $\dot{V}CO_2$ is carbon dioxide production and UN is urinary nitrogen

C. Both oxygen consumption and carbon dioxide production are measured by comparing the amount of the gas going into the patient to the amount coming out. To do that, the machine needs to know the volume and concentrations of the inspired and expired airstream. The equations that describe them are:

$$\text{Oxygen consumption} = \dot{V}O_2 = \dot{V}I(FIO_2) - \dot{V}E(FEO_2)$$

$$\text{Carbon dioxide production} = \dot{V}CO_2 = \dot{V}E(FECO_2) - \dot{V}I(FICO_2)$$

where FIO_2 and FEO_2 are the inspired and expired oxygen fractions, respectively; $FICO_2$ and $FECO_2$ are the inspired and expired carbon dioxide fractions, respectively; and $\dot{V}E$ and $\dot{V}I$ are the exhaled and inhaled minute volumes, respectively. However, most systems measure only the expired airstream volume and mathematically calculate the inspired volume from that. That is done via a mathematical formula called the Haldane transformation. The exact derivation of the equation is beyond the scope of this chapter. However, the Haldane transformation is particularly vulnerable to inaccuracy in the measurement of FIO_2 and expiratory volume. Also it becomes more erroneous as the actual FIO_2 increases. Many oxygen sensors are less accurate at higher FIO_2. Therefore, IC studies are usually limited to patients on 60% O_2 or less.

D. Indirect calorimetry may be used to determine what percentage of energy expenditure comes from each of the major foodstuffs. Once CO_2 production and O_2 consumption have been measured, their relationship and a measure of protein metabolism can be used to solve mathematically for the percentage of calories burned derived from fat or carbohydrate. The equations used for these calculations are:

$$CHO \ (g) = 4.113 \ \dot{V}CO_2 - 2.907 \ \dot{V}O_2 - 2.544 \ UN \ (g/d)$$

$$FAT \ (g) = 1.689 \ (\dot{V}CO_2 - \dot{V}O_2) - 1.943 \ UN \ (g/d)$$

$$Protein \ (g) = 6.25 \ (UN + 4) \ (g/d)$$

Important items to be remembered from this exercise include:

1. The amount of protein catabolized in a day is estimated to be the sum of urine nitrogen (UN) plus daily losses from skin and stool (assumed to be 4 g/day) multiplied by 6.25.
2. The RQ is the ratio of CO_2 produced to O_2 consumed, or $\dot{V}O_2/\dot{V}CO_2$.
3. The primary foodstuffs have established RQs: fat, 0.7; protein, 0.8; and carbohydrate, 1.0. The normal range of RQ is from 0.7 to 1.0 because a combination of processes is almost always occurring. RQs greater than 1.0 indicate that the net outcome of all the reactions occurring is the synthesis of fat (lipogenesis). Values less than 0.7 may be encountered when ketones are the primary fuel.

III. INDICATIONS

A. Nutritional assessment. Studies have compared the practice of providing calories based on energy expenditure estimated by demographically based equations with the practice of providing calories based on energy expenditure determined by IC. These studies have yielded inconsistent results. Some conclude that estimates of energy expenditure routinely overestimate caloric need, others conclude that estimates of energy expenditure are inaccurate but in no consistent direction, and still others conclude that clinical estimates are as accurate as measured values. There is no clear explanation for the discrepancy between these results. In addition, there is no clear evidence that using an approach based on IC has any impact on outcomes.

B. Substrate utilization. An elevated RQ may indicate excessive levels of carbohydrate metabolism or net lipogenesis due to excess calorie intake. Although the impact of altering substrate composition has not been shown in most diseases, in complicated cases of hepatic or renal failure an analysis of substrate utilization may be used quickly to assess the efficacy of a change in diet.

IV. PROCEDURE

A. Methods of measurement

1. Oxygen sensors in commercially available systems are either zirconium or differential paramagnetic sensors. These analyzers typically have an accuracy of ±0.02% and a response time of 130 msec or less.
2. Most carbon dioxide analyzers are nondispersed infrared devices. These analyzers have an accuracy of ±0.02% with a response time of 110 msec. Some systems measure both inspired and expired carbon dioxide and some measure only expired, assuming the inspired value to be negligible.
3. Volume is measured by measuring flow and integrating the result over time to obtain volume. Flow can be measured with a Pneumotach or a mass flow sensor or generated by the device and kept constant in response to changes in ventilation.
4. Gas concentrations are measured using one of three techniques: mixing chamber, breath by breath, or dilution.
   a. Mixing chamber is the best-established method. A mixing chamber mixes expired gases over a predetermined interval and provides the material to be sampled. A sample of mixed gas is withdrawn from the chamber, the gas concentrations analyzed, and the sample returned to the chamber. The concentrations of inspiratory gas are sampled from the inspiratory side of a mouthpiece or a ventilator circuit. A computer compares mixed expired versus inspired concentrations and multiplies by volume to yield a measure of consumption or production. The results reflect the values of gases mixed

over time and are reported as values per time interval of measurement (e.g., milliliters of oxygen consumed per minute).

b. Breath-by-breath method. The collection and analysis of gases in the breath-by-breath method is similar to that in the mixing chamber technique, but each breath is analyzed. A sample of gases is taken for analysis from each inspiration and expiration. These samples are coupled with flow measurements for each breath to calculate $\dot{V}O_2$, $\dot{V}CO_2$, and REE. The crucial component in these measurements is the alignment of various signals. Instruments that use breath-by-breath analysis align the signals automatically by computer. Improper alignment can render the measurements useless.

c. Dilution method. The dilution method is the only technique that can be used in intubated patients as well as those nonintubated patients who cannot use a mouthpiece. A predetermined flow of gas of known oxygen and carbon dioxide concentration passes through a face shield mask or a hoodlike canopy. The exhaled gases are diluted into the stream of gas. The amount of gas the machine puts into the stream is adjusted to keep the flow constant as the patient alters his or her own ventilation. Samples of the diluted gases are removed for analysis and the values obtained multiplied by the flow rate to yield a measure of volume. Oxygen consumption and carbon dioxide production are calculated by comparing concentrations in and out of the system.

B. Factors affecting accuracy

   1. All connections to the metabolic cart and in the ventilator circuit must be checked for leaks.

   2. An error in measuring O_2 oxygen or CO_2 concentrations leads to larger errors in the subsequently calculated values.

   3. Any change in inspired O_2 concentration during the study renders the measurements invalid until the inspired O_2 concentration is remeasured.

   4. Inspired and expired gas concentrations are typically sampled with long, narrow tubes. These can easily clog with patient secretions and invalidate the data.

   5. Most systems also somehow condition the gas from sample tubes to standardize for temperature and water vapor. Failure to follow the manufacturer's advice on desiccant change or timing of tubing change alters the accuracy of the data.

   6. Disruption of the normal ventilator circuit with inappropriately placed sampling devices may lead to ventilator malfunction or trigger alarms.

   7. The use of positive end-expiratory pressure may variably alter the ventilator circuit compressible volume, leading to errors in volume and concentration measurements.

   8. Traditionally, IC has not been performed on children because of leaks due to uncuffed endotracheal tubes, frequent use of high-frequency ventilation, and the common use of high FIO_2 and low ventilator flows.

Selected Readings

Daly JM, Heymsfield SB, Head CA, et al. Human energy requirements: overestimation by widely used prediction equation. *Am J Clin Nutr* 1985;42:1170.

Weissman C, Kemper M, Askanazi J, et al. Resting metabolic rate of the critically ill patient: measured versus predicted. *Anesthesiology* 1986;64:673.

Ferrannini E: The theoretical bases of indirect calorimetry: a review. *Metabolism* 1988;37:287.

   Provides a complete description of the fundamentals of indirect calorimetry, including mathematical derivations of important equations.

Hunter DC, Jaksic T, Lewis D, et al. Resting energy expenditure in the critically ill: estimations versus measurement. *Br J Surg* 1988;75:875.

   These three articles highlight the contrasting evidence on the relationship between indirect calorimetry and calculated estimates of energy needs.

Phang PT, Cunningham KF, Ronco JJ, et al. Mathematical coupling explains dependence of oxygen consumption on oxygen delivery in ARDS. *Am J Respir Crit Care Med* 1994;150:308.
Use of indirect calorimetry was crucial in explaining crucial aspects of hemodynamic management in critically ill patients.

Smyrnios NA, Curley FJ, Shaker KG. Accuracy of 30-minute indirect calorimetry studies in predicting 24-hour energy expenditure in mechanically ventilated, critically ill patients. *JPEN J Parenter Enteral Nutr* 1997;21:168.
Provides evidence for accuracy of 30-minute indirect calorimetry studies.

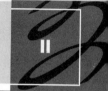

Cardiovascular Problems and Coronary Care

II

CARDIOPULMONARY RESUSCITATION

John A. Paraskos

25

I. HISTORY. The introduction of cardiopulmonary resuscitation (CPR) has changed the definitions of life and death. Although sporadic accounts of attempted resuscitations are recorded from antiquity, until the advent of CPR, no rational quarrel could be found with the sixth century BCE poetic fragment of Ibycus, "You cannot find a medicine for life once a man is dead."

II. EFFICACY. CPR does not appear to promise more than the short-term sustaining of viability until definitive therapy such as defibrillation can be administered. Data from prehospital care systems in Seattle showed that 43% of patients found to be in ventricular fibrillation are discharged from the hospital if CPR (i.e., basic life support [BLS]) is provided within 4 minutes and defibrillation as part of advanced cardiac life support [ACLS] is administered within 8 minutes. Survival rates for patients in asystole or with pulseless electrical activity (PEA) are much lower. Even though patients experiencing cardiac arrest in the hospital can be expected to receive CPR and definitive therapy well within the 4- and 8-minute time frames, their chances of being discharged alive are in general worse than for out-of-hospital victims.

III. MECHANISMS OF BLOOD FLOW DURING RESUSCITATION
   A. Cardiac compression theory. According to this theory, during sternal compression the intraventricular pressures rise higher than other intrathoracic pressures. With each sternal compression, the semilunar valves should open and blood be ejected into the aorta and pulmonary artery. Between compressions, the semilunar valves would close and the atrioventricular valves open, allowing the heart to fill from the lungs and systemic veins. There is some echocardiographic evidence that this mechanism is operative early in the course of CPR.
   B. Thoracic pump theory. According to this theory, during CPR the heart serves only as a passive conduit. Forward flow is generated by a pressure gradient between intrathoracic and extrathoracic vascular structures. This is likely the mechanism most operative during CPR. Interposed-abdominal-compression CPR (IAC-CPR) assists in raising intrathoracic pressure and improving forward flow. IAC-CPR is now advised for in-hospital CPR when abdominal compression is not contraindicated (e.g., abdominal aneurysm). Active compression-decompression CPR (ACD-CPR) and vest CPR are optional techniques for hospital personnel adequately trained in these techniques.
   C. Open-chest CPR. Open-chest CPR involves direct cardiac compression. Patients with penetrating chest trauma are unlikely to respond to chest compression and are candidates for open-chest CPR. If open-chest CPR is to be used, it must be used early to succeed. This technique should not be attempted unless adequate facilities and trained personnel are available.
   D. Cardiopulmonary bypass for unresponsive cardiac arrest. Cardiopulmonary bypass is not a form of routine life support; however, it represents a possible adjunct to artificial circulation. It is being used more frequently for invasive procedures for sudden cardiac collapse as a bridge to emergency surgery.

IV. INFECTIOUS DISEASES AND IMPLICATIONS FOR HEALTH CARE PROFESSIONALS. Bag-valve mask devices should be made available to health-care personnel as initial ventilation equipment. Early endotracheal intubation should be encouraged when equipment and trained professionals are available. Masks with one-way valves and plastic mouth and nose covers with filtered openings provide some protection from transfer of oral fluids and aerosols. S-shaped mouthpieces, masks without one-way valves, and handkerchiefs provide little if any barrier protection and should not be considered for routine use.

A. Advanced cardiac life support in adults. The use of adjunctive equipment, more specialized techniques, and pharmacologic and electrical therapy in the treatment of cardiac or respiratory arrest is generally referred to as ACLS. These techniques and their interface with BLS and emergency medical services are taught in the American Heart Association's ACLS teaching programs (Fig. 25-1).

    1. Airway and ventilatory support. Oxygenation and optimal ventilation are prerequisites for successful resuscitation. Ventilation with the rescuer's exhaled breath at sea level provides 16% to 17% oxygen and may produce an alveolar partial pressure of oxygen (P_{AO_2}) of 80 mm Hg. Arterial hypoxemia is inevitable because of diminished pulmonary blood flow, intrapulmonary shunting, and ventilation-perfusion mismatch. Therefore, 100% supplemental oxygen should be administered as soon as it is available. Endotracheal intubation is required if the patient cannot be rapidly resuscitated or when adequate spontaneous ventilation does not resume quickly. Trained personnel should attempt intubation.

    2. Circulatory support. Chest compression should not be unduly interrupted while adjunctive procedures are instituted. The person coordinating the resuscitative effort must monitor pulses generated by the compressor. The carotid or femoral pulse should be evaluated every few minutes and compressions adjusted as needed.

    3. Defibrillation. Electrocardiographic (ECG) monitoring is necessary during CPR to guide appropriate electrical and pharmacologic therapy. Until ECG monitoring becomes available, the victim should be assumed to be in ventricular fibrillation or pulseless ventricular tachycardia (VF/VT). Most defibrillators currently marketed (including automated external defibrillators) have built-in monitoring circuitry in the paddles that guides electrical therapy. Defibrillation is the definitive therapy for most cardiac arrests. It should be attempted as early as possible and repeated frequently until ventricular fibrillation or pulseless ventricular tachycardia has terminated. Proper use of the defibrillator requires special attention to the following:

        a. Selection of proper energy levels. An initial energy of 200 joules appears to be safer than higher energies and equally effective. If 200 joules of a monophasic defibrillator has not succeeded on the second try, 300 joules (or maximum output) can be used. Biphasic defibrillators appear safer and more effective. Usually 100 joules initially and 200 maximum are recommended. Very obese victims may require higher energy levels.

        b. Proper asynchronous mode. Synchronization to the R wave must be deactivated to allow the defibrillator to fire during ventricular fibrillation. During rapid VT (rates over 150), it is best not to attempt synchronization with the R wave because this is likely to increase the chance of delivering the shock on the T wave and inducing VF.

        c. Proper position of the paddles. The anterolateral position requires that one paddle be placed to the right of the upper sternum, just below the clavicle and the other to the left of the nipple in the left midaxillary line. For the anteroposterior position, one paddle is positioned under the left scapula with the patient lying on it. The anterior paddle is positioned to the left of the left sternal border. The paddle should not be placed directly over an implanted device.

        d. Adequate contact between paddles and skin. The rescuer should hold the paddles firmly against the skin with approximately 25 pounds of pressure. Electrical contact material must be adequately, but not overly, applied to the paddle surfaces.

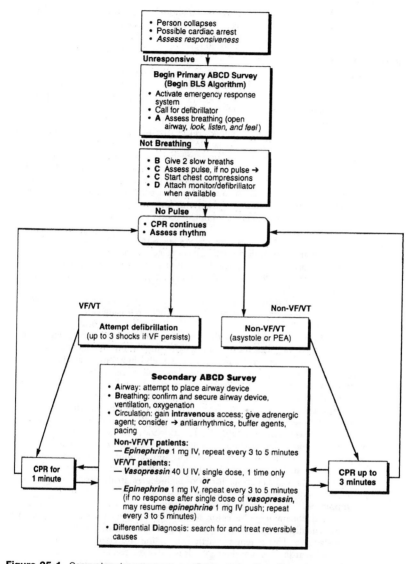

Figure 25-1. Comprehensive emergency cardiac care algorithm. (From Guidelines 2000. *Circulation* 2000;102(suppl 8):1, with permission.)

  e. **No contact with anyone other than the victim.** The rescuer must be sturdily balanced on both feet and not standing on a wet floor. The rescuer's hands should not be wet. CPR and manual ventilation must be discontinued with no one remaining in contact with the patient.
  f. **Rechecking of equipment.** If no skeletal muscle contraction is noted, the equipment, contacts, and synchronizer switch used for elective cardioversion should be checked. *Care must be taken that the synchronizer switch is in the off position.*

g. **Rhythm assessment.** The rhythm should be assessed after each counter-shock and the patient checked for a pulse at appropriate times. *This should be done before proceeding with additional therapeutic interventions.*

V. DRUG THERAPY

A. **IV access.** Venous access through a reliable intravenous route should be established early in the course of the resuscitative effort to allow administration of necessary drugs and fluids. Drugs such as epinephrine, vasopressin, and atropine can be administered by the endotracheal tube if there is a delay in achieving venous access. This route requires 2.5 times the dose and should be followed by 10 mL of saline to obtain an equivalent blood level. A sustained duration of action ("depot effect") can be expected after a return in spontaneous circulation.

B. **Correction of acidosis.** Correction of acidosis should be considered when the cardiac arrest has lasted for a prolonged period and adequate ventilation is being provided. The American Heart Association guidelines suggest that sodium bicarbonate or other buffers be avoided until a perfusing rhythm has been reestablished. Exceptions include patients with known preexisting hyperkalemia or tricyclic overdose, for whom the administration of sodium bicarbonate is recommended.

C. **Volume replacement.** Increased central volume is often required during CPR, especially if initial attempts at defibrillation have failed. Simple crystalloids, such as 5% dextrose in water, are inappropriate for rapid expansion of the intravascular space. Isotonic crystalloids (0.9% saline, Ringer's lactate), colloids, or blood is necessary for satisfactory volume expansion.

D. **Sympathomimetic drugs and vasopressors.** Sympathomimetic drugs either act directly on adrenergic receptors or act indirectly by releasing catecholamines from nerve endings.

1. **Epinephrine.** Epinephrine is the pressor agent used most frequently during CPR. It has both alpha and beta activity. Indications for its use include all forms of cardiac arrest. Its beta action is useful in asystole and bradycardiac arrest and has also been said to convert asystole to ventricular fibrillation and "fine" VF to more easily converted "course" VF. An IV bolus of 1 mg is given every 3 to 5 minutes as needed to restore a perfusing rhythm.

2. **Norepinephrine.** Norepinephrine is a potent alpha-agonist with beta activity. There is no reason to prefer it to epinephrine during cardiac arrest. It appears to be most useful in the treatment of septic shock and neurogenic shock.

3. **Isoproterenol.** This synthetic catecholamine has almost pure beta activity. Its cardiac activity includes potent inotropic and chronotropic effects. Indications for its use include atropine-resistant hemodynamically significant bradyarrhythmias as well as various forms of high-degree atrioventricular (AV) block. *It should not be used during cardiac arrest.*

4. **Dopamine.** This naturally occurring precursor of norepinephrine has alpha, beta, and dopaminergic-receptor activity. Indications for its use are primarily hemodynamically significant hypotension and cardiogenic shock.

5. **Dobutamine.** This potent synthetic beta agonist differs from isoproterenol in that tachycardia is less problematic. It is indicated primarily for the short-term enhancement of ventricular contractility in the patient with heart failure.

6. **Vasopressin.** During cardiac arrest, vasopressin has been found to be equivalent to epinephrine as a first-line agent. It may be superior to epinephrine during asystolic arrest. If it is to be used, it should be administered once (40 IU, IV) before epinephrine. If return of pulse fails, epinephrine may then be used in usual doses.

E. **Antiarrhythmic agents.** Antiarrhythmic agents play an important role in stabilizing rhythm in many resuscitative situations.

1. **Amiodarone.** Amiodarone IV has been found successful in terminating a variety of reentrant and nonreentrant supraventricular and ventricular arrhythmias. It has replaced the use of lidocaine or bretyllium during VT/VF arrest

when defibrillatory attempts have failed. An IV dose of 300 mg is administered. An additional dose of 150 mg may be considered if VT/VF persists or recurs. The maximum cumulative dose is 2.2 grams over 24 hours for recurrent VT/VF.

2. **Procainamide.** Procainamide is indicated for ventricular arrhythmias refractory to amiodarone. It is also useful in patients with supraventricular arrhythmias. An infusion is administered at 20 mg/min until the arrhythmia is suppressed, hypotension develops, or the QRS interval is lengthened by 50% from its original duration. The maximum total dose is 17 mg/kg.

3. **Adenosine.** Adenosine depresses AV nodal conduction and sinoatrial node activity. It is effective in terminating arrythmias that involve the AV node in a reentrant circuit. *It should not be used during cardiac arrest.*

4. **Verapamil and diltiazem.** These drugs are primarily useful in slowing the ventricular response during atrial fibrillation or flutter. *They should not be used during cardiac arrest.*

5. **Magnesium.** Magnesium is administered IV during VF in a patient with suspected hypomagnesemia. It also may be of value in patients with torsade de pointes. 1 to 2 grams may be diluted to 100 mL of 5% dextrose in water and given over 1 to 2 minutes.

6. **Atropine.** Atropine is a vagolytic drug of use in increasing heart rate and facilitating AV conduction by suppressing vagal tone. It is indicated in hemodynamically significant bradycardias, in which case the initial dose may be as low as 0.4 mg. It is also used in asystole and bradycardic arrests, for which 1 mg is given IV and repeated every 3 to 5 minutes, as needed, to a total dose of 0.04 mg/kg.

7. **Calcium.** Calcium is indicated only in calcium channel blocker toxicity, severe hyperkalemia, severe hypocalcemia, cardiac arrest after multiple transfusions with citrated blood, and fluoride toxicity, as well as hypotension in patients being removed from heart-lung bypass after cardioplegic arrest. *It is not indicated for routine use in cardiac arrest.*

VI. CLINICAL SETTINGS. The procedures involved in resuscitation of a victim of cardiovascular or respiratory arrest are part of a continuum progressing from initial recognition of the problem and institution of CPR to intervention with defibrillation, drugs, pacemakers, transport, and postresuscitative evaluation and care. The following sections focus on the pharmacologic and electrical interventions appropriate to various clinical settings common in cardiac arrest.

A. **Ventricular fibrillation and pulseless ventricular tachycardia.** Ventricular fibrillation is the initial rhythm encountered in 50% to 70% of prehospital cardiac arrests and in 30% to 40% of in-hospital cardiac arrests. Pulseless ventricular tachycardia is also found in a significant number of in-hospital arrests and in a smaller number of prehospital arrests. Electrical defibrillation is the most important intervention in treating these arrhythmias (Fig. 25-2). The sooner it is administered, the more likely it is to succeed. Repeated attempts are often necessary.

B. **Asystole.** Asystole is the first rhythm encountered in 30% to 40% of prehospital as well as in-hospital cardiac arrests. It is obviously the end result of any pulseless rhythm, and as such, when it is the presenting rhythm of an unwitnessed arrest it is unlikely to be reversible. Recent study suggests that vasopressin as the first pressor may have a better chance at success. Note that the algorithm for asystole developed by the American Heart Association (Fig. 25-3) does not yet recognize the potential value of vasopressin. Atropine in full vagolytic doses is also used as initial intervention.

C. **Pulseless electrical activity.** PEA occurs when an arrest victim is found to have an organized ECG rhythm unassociated with a palpable pulse and any evidence of circulation. Along with CPR and epinephrine, there must be a search and treatment for an underlying cause. Rapid IV volume expansion is warranted while a cause is sought. If PEA is associated with bradycardia, atropine is also indicated (Fig. 25-4).

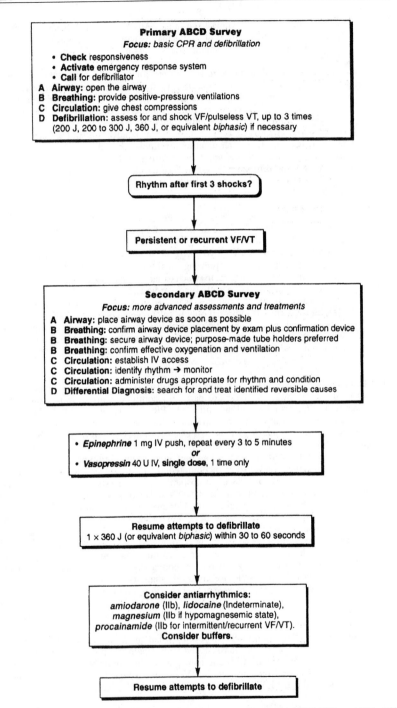

Figure 25-2. VF/VT algorithm. (From Guidelines 2000. *Circulation* 2000;102(suppl 8):1, with permission.)

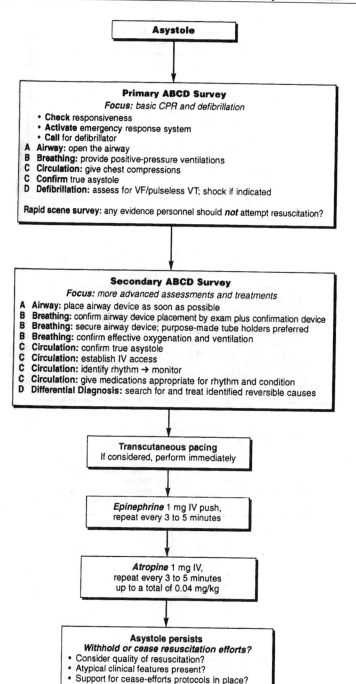

Figure 25-3. Asystole algorithm. (From Guidelines 2000. *Circulation* 2000;102(suppl 8):1, with permission.)

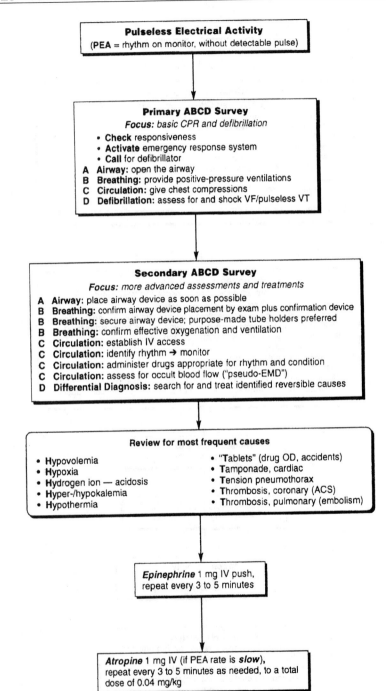

Figure 25-4. PEA algorithm. (From Guidelines 2000. *Circulation* 2000;102(suppl 8):1, with permission.)

D. Other rhythm situations addressed in ACLS programs:
1. Bradycardia with a pulse
2. Sustained ventricular tachycardia with a pulse
3. Unstable and stable supraventricular tachycardias

Selected Readings

Babbs CF, Sack JB, Kern KB. Interposed abdominal compression as an adjunct to cardiopulmonary resuscitation. *Am Heart J* 1994;127:412.
Randomized trials show that survival of patients in the hospital with IAC-CPR was improved over standard CPR.

Guidelines 2000 for cardiopulmonary resuscitation and emergency cardiovascular care. *Circulation* 2000;102 (suppl 8):1.
Supplement dedicated to the 2000 revision of guidelines for BLS and ACLS.

Kudenchuk PJ, Cobb LA, Copass MK, et al. Amiodarone for resuscitation after out-of-hospital cardiac arrest due to ventricular fibrillation. *N Engl J Med* 1999;341:871.
In patients with out-of-hospital refractory VT/VF amiodarone resulted in higher rate of survival to hospital admission, but not to hospital discharge.

Plaisance P, Lurie KG, Vicaut E, et al. A comparison of standard cardiopulmonary resuscitation and active compression-decompression resuscitation for out-of-hospital cardiac arrest. *N Engl J Med* 1999;341:569.
ACD-CPR performed during ACLS significantly improved long-term survival rates among patients with out-of-hospital cardiac arrests.

Wenzel V, Krismer AC, Arntz HR, et al. A comparison of vasopressin and epinephrine for out-of-hospital cardiopulmonary resuscitation. *N Engl J Med* 2004;350:105.
Vasopressin was as effective as epinephrine as first-line drug in out-of-hospital cardiac arrest and improved survival to hospitalization among patients initially found to be in asystole.

26 PHARMACOLOGIC MANAGEMENT OF THE HYPOTENSIVE PATIENT
Arash Tabaee and Michael M. Givertz

I. GENERAL PRINCIPLES
A. Background
1. Hypotension is frequently encountered in the intensive care setting as the final result of a heterogeneous group of disorders.
2. End-organ perfusion generally becomes compromised when the systolic arterial pressure falls below 90 mm Hg or when mean arterial pressure falls below approximately 60 mm Hg.
3. Although definitive management requires therapy directed at the underlying cause of hypotension (e.g., antibiotics for sepsis, corticosteroids for adrenal insufficiency, blood transfusion for bleeding), intravenous vasoactive agents are at times necessary to maintain perfusion to vital organs while the underlying etiology of hypotension is investigated and definitive measures have taken effect.

B. Adrenergic receptor physiology
1. With few exceptions, vasopressors and positive inotropes are sympathomimetic amines that bind to and stimulate adrenergic receptors. The characteristic hemodynamic effects of individual agents depend to a great extent on selective binding to various adrenergic receptors.
   a. α_1-Adrenergic receptors
      (1) Present in smooth muscle cells of many vascular beds, including the arterioles supplying the skin, mucosa, skeletal muscles, and kidneys, as well as peripheral venules.
      (2) Stimulation causes vasoconstriction and is the most common mechanism of vasopressor action.
      (3) Receptors in the myocardium appear to mediate a modest positive inotropic effect with little change in heart rate.
   b. β_1-Adrenergic receptors
      (1) Predominant adrenergic receptors in the heart.
      (2) Stimulation causes a positive inotropic and chronotropic response.
   c. β_2-Adrenergic receptors
      (1) Stimulation causes relaxation of smooth muscle in the bronchial tree, gastrointestinal tract, and uterus.
      (2) Mediate vasodilation of arterioles supplying skeletal muscle.
   d. Dopaminergic receptors (DA_1 and DA_2)
      (1) Mediate renal, coronary, cerebral, and mesenteric vasodilation.
      (2) Stimulate natriuresis.
2. Receptor selectivity of vasoactive drugs can be dose dependent (e.g., dopamine).
3. Overall clinical effects of a drug include both the direct sequelae of adrenergic receptor stimulation and the reflex response of homeostatic forces (e.g., norepinephrine-mediated α_1-adrenergic stimulation induces increased vagal tone, which opposes the positive chronotropic effects of β_1-adrenergic stimulation, resulting in little overall change in heart rate)

II. TREATMENT
A. Commonly used vasopressors and positive inotropes (Table 26-1)
1. Epinephrine (Adrenalin)
   a. An endogenous catecholamine that is the least selective of the vasopressor agents, and a potent agonist of α- and β-adrenergic receptors.

TABLE 26-1	**Dose Range, Receptor Activity, and Predominant Hemodynamic Effects of Vasoactive Drugs Commonly Used to Treat Hypotension**

Drug	Dose Range	DA	α_1	β_1	β_2	HR	CO	SVR
Dobutamine	2.5–20 μg/kg/min		+	+++	++	↔↑	↑↑	↑
Dopamine	1–5 μg/kg/min	+++				↔	↔	↔
	5–10 μg/kg/min	++	+	++		↑	↑↑	↔↑
	10–20 μg/kg/min	++	+++	++		↑↑	↔↑	↑↑
Epinephrine	1–10 μg/min		+++	++	++	↑↑	↑	↑↑
Norepinephrine	0.5–30 μg/min		+++	++		↔	↔	↑↑
Phenylephrine	40–180 μg/min		+++			↔	↔	↑↑
Vasopressin	0.04 units/min					↔	↔	↑↑

HR, heart rate; CO, cardiac output; SVR, systemic vascular resistance.

  b. Clinically used doses (0.5 to 10 μg per minute) result in α-mediated venous and arterial constriction and β-mediated increased heart rate and myocardial contractility. The latter effect is mitigated by increased afterload.
  c. Because of adverse effects on renal and splanchnic blood flow, and potential for inducing myocardial ischemia and tachyarrhythmias, epinephrine is considered a second-line agent in the management of hypotension secondary to septic shock.
 2. Norepinephrine (Levophed)
  a. An endogenous catecholamine with potent α_1- and β_1-adrenergic activity, but little β_2-agonism.
  b. Predominant effect is dose-dependent vasoconstriction of arterial resistance vessels and veins. Cardiac effects of β_1-stimulation are counterbalanced by increased afterload and reflex vagal activity induced by elevated systemic vascular resistance.
  c. Clinically used doses (0.5 to 30 μg per minute) result in potent vasoconstriction. Generally infused as a second-line agent in cases of severe distributive shock, but several small studies suggest that in adults with septic shock, use of norepinephrine as the initial agent is more likely to result in improved blood pressure and survival compared to dopamine.
  d. Adverse effects include increased myocardial oxygen consumption, and excessive renal and mesenteric vasoconstriction.
 3. Dopamine (Intropin)
  a. An endogenous catecholamine that functions as a central neurotransmitter and synthetic precursor to norepinephrine.
  b. Stimulates dopaminergic and adrenergic receptors in a dose-dependent manner; also stimulates release of norepinephrine from nerve terminals.
   (1) Low dose (less than 5 μg per kg per minute): predominantly stimulates dopaminergic receptors in renal, mesenteric and coronary vessels. In normal subjects, low-dose dopamine augments renal blood flow with little effect on blood pressure. The strategy of using low-dose dopamine as a renoprotective agent in critically ill patients has not been shown to be effective in controlled studies.
   (2) Moderate dose (5 to 10 μg per kg per minute): predominant effect is β_1-mediated augmentation of myocardial contractility and heart rate.
   (3) High dose (greater than 10 μg per kg per minute): overall hemodynamic effect resembles that of norepinephrine and is mediated by α_1-adrenergic receptor stimulation.

    c. As an agent with both inotropic and vasopressor activity, moderate- to high-dose dopamine has the versatility to be used as a first-line agent in hypotension of unknown etiology. However, in the setting of severe hypotension due to septic shock, a more potent α-adrenergic agonist such as norepinephrine may be more effective in restoring perfusion pressure. By itself or in combination with other inotropes, moderate-dose dopamine may be used in the management of hypotensive patients with acute decompensated heart failure.

4. Dobutamine (Dobutrex)

    a. A synthetic sympathomimetic amine that causes potent non-selective β- and mild α-adrenergic stimulation. Its mechanism of action is complex and involves two stereoisomers with distinct affinities for different adrenergic receptors (see main text).

    b. Clinically used doses (2.5 to 15 μg per kg per minute or higher) increase cardiac contractility and heart rate. The positive chronotropic effect occurs to a lesser extent than with dopamine. Systemic vascular resistance is modestly reduced or may remain unchanged.

    c. Useful in the temporary inotropic support of hypotensive patients with acute decompensated heart failure, and patients with concomitant septic shock and depressed cardiac function.

    d. In patients with marked hypotension, the initial effect on blood pressure may be unpredictable. In this setting, dobutamine should be administered with a vasopressor.

    e. As with other positive inotropic agents, increased myocardial oxygen consumption may worsen cardiac ischemia, and tachycardia or arrhythmias may limit dose titration.

5. Phenylephrine (Neosynephrine)

    a. A synthetic sympathomimetic amine that selectively stimulates α_1-adrenergic receptors, causing dose-dependent arterial vasoconstriction. Increased blood pressure activates vagal reflexes, causing slowing of the heart rate.

    b. Although there are little data regarding its relative efficacy compared to older vasopressors, phenylephrine is frequently infused at 40 to 180 μg per minute to treat vasodilatory shock. The absence of β-agonist activity at usual doses has made phenylephrine an attractive agent in clinical situations where tachycardia or tachyarrhythmias limit the use of other agents.

    c. High-dose phenylephrine can cause excess vasoconstriction, and patients with left ventricular systolic dysfunction may not tolerate the α_1-mediated increase in afterload.

6. Vasopressin (Pitressin)

    a. An endogenous antidiuretic hormone that has recently been added to the armamentarium of agents used to treat hypotension. The mechanism of pressor action has not been fully elucidated, but involves binding to V_1 receptors on vascular smooth muscle.

    b. Minimal effect on blood pressure in normal subjects, but increases blood pressure in patients with septic shock and has been shown to facilitate the tapering of adrenergic agents in this setting.

    c. It remains unclear whether hemodynamic benefits are confined to a subset of patients with relative vasopressin deficiency.

    d. Currently recommended in doses of 0.01 to 0.05 unit per minute as an adjunctive agent in the treatment of vasodilatory septic shock that is poorly responsive to traditional adrenergic agonists. Use as a stand-alone vasopressor has not been well studied.

    e. Potential adverse effects include excess vasoconstriction causing end-organ hypoperfusion including myocardial ischemia.

B. Choosing an agent (Table 26-2)

    1. There are no large adequately controlled trials to guide the pharmacologic management of hypotension. Consensus recommendations are based on animal studies and small clinical trials. The selection of an appropriate agent should be made on a case-by-case basis, with attention to the known or suspected underlying cause.

| TABLE 26-2 | Hemodynamic Profiles of Selected Causes of Hypotension and Commonly Used First-line Agents | | | |

Cause of hypotension	PAOP	CO	SVR	Preferred agent(s)
Unknown	?	?	?	Dopamine
Hypovolemia	↓	↓	↑	None
Acute decompensated heart failure	↑	↓	↑	Dopamine
				Dobutamine
Cardiogenic shock	↑↔	↓	↑	Dopamine
Hyperdynamic sepsis	↓↔	↑	↓	Norepinephrine
				Dopamine
Sepsis with depressed cardiac function	?	↓	↓	Dopamine
				Norepinephrine plus dobutamine
Anaphylaxis	?	?	↓	Epinephrine
Anesthesia-induced hypotension	?	?	↓	Phenylephrine

PAOP, pulmonary artery occlusion pressure; CO, cardiac output; SVR, systemic vascular resistance.
Volume resuscitation with intravenous fluids and/or blood products recommended.

2. Given its combined pressor and inotropic properties, moderate-dose dopamine is a reasonable choice for the initial treatment of hypotension of unknown etiology. For the treatment of severe hypotension (systolic blood pressure less than 70 mm Hg), a more potent α_1-adrenergic agonist such as norepinephrine should be considered.

3. Norepinephrine may be the pressor of choice in the treatment of vasodilatory shock related to sepsis. In cases where tachycardia, tachyarrhythmias, or both limit dose-titration of other agents, phenylephrine is a useful alternative.

4. For the mildly hypotensive patient with left ventricular systolic dysfunction, dobutamine is the drug of choice. With frank cardiogenic shock or combined vasodilation and pump failure, dopamine can be used as a single agent or in combination with other drugs such as dobutamine.

5. Vasopressin has emerged as a useful adjunctive agent for treatment of the septic patient with hemodynamic collapse resistant to traditional sympathomimetic agents.

III. COMPLICATIONS

A. Vasopressors and positive inotropes are potent agents with considerable potential for toxicity mediated by the same mechanisms that increase blood pressure. They should be used with extreme caution and at the lowest dose required to maintain end-organ perfusion.

1. Tachycardia and tachyarrhythmias result from β_1-stimulation and can limit the use of these agents in patients with underlying heart disease.

2. Depressed left ventricular systolic function may develop as a result of increased afterload or secondary to ischemia.

3. Myocardial ischemia may be caused by coronary vasoconstriction or more commonly by increased myocardial oxygen demand.

4. Excessive arterial vasoconstriction can compromise splanchnic and renal perfusion. Similarly, peripheral limb ischemia and even necrosis may occur.

B. Monitoring

1. Patients should be treated in an intensive care setting with continuous monitoring of cardiac rhythm, urine output, and arterial oxygenation.

2. Intra-arterial cannulation and direct monitoring of blood pressure is suggested during prolonged vasopressor use.

3. Fluid resuscitation and careful attention to intravascular volume are paramount as many patients with hypotension can be stabilized with fluids alone, and the administration of vasopressors to hypovolemic patients can worsen end-organ perfusion. The use of central venous or pulmonary artery catheters to monitor filling pressures can be helpful in selected cases, but the routine use of invasive hemodynamic monitoring is not necessary and may be harmful.

4. Although a mean arterial pressure of greater that 60 mm Hg is usually required to maintain autoregulatory blood flow to vital organs, some patients may require higher or lower pressures. It is essential to monitor carefully other indicators of global and regional perfusion such as mental status and urine output. The use of mixed venous oxygen saturation, serum lactate levels, and intramucosal pH monitoring by gastric tonometry can be useful, but is not advocated for routine use.

C. With few exceptions these drugs are short-acting agents with rapid onset and offset of action. They are generally initiated without a bolus and can be titrated frequently. Abrupt lowering and discontinuation of vasoactive drugs should be avoided to prevent rebound hypotension.

D. There is considerable variation in the initial dose required to restore adequate hemodynamics. Moreover, an individual patient's responsiveness to a given agent may diminish over time owing to several mechanisms including adrenergic receptor desensitization.

E. Careful attention should be paid to potential drug-drug interactions.

1. Recent or current treatment with β-adrenergic antagonists can cause resistance to the action of dobutamine and other β-agonists.

2. The administration of less selective adrenergic agonists such as epinephrine to patients treated with β-blockers can caused unopposed α-adrenergic stimulation.

3. Patients taking monoamine oxidase inhibitors will experience an exaggerated response to some catecholamines and should be treated with a very low (less than 10%) starting dose.

F. Drugs should generally be administered though central venous catheters via volumetric infusion pumps that deliver precise flow rates. In the event of vasopressor extravasation, an α_1-adrenergic antagonist (e.g., phentolamine 5 to 10 mg diluted in 10 to 15 mL of saline) can be infiltrated into the area to limit local vasoconstriction and tissue necrosis.

Selected Readings

ECC Guidelines: Part 6: Advanced Cardiovascular Life Support: Section 6: Pharmacology II: Agents to optimize cardiac output and blood pressure. *Circulation* 2000;102: I-129–I-135.
Recent consensus recommendations for the use of pressors and inotropes in emergency cardiovascular care.

Holmes CL, Patel BM, Russell JA, et al. Physiology of vasopressin relevant to management of septic shock. *Chest* 2001;120:989–1002.
A review of the mechanism of vasopressin action and its application to septic shock.

Leier CV, Heban PT, Huss P, et al. Comparative systemic and hemodynamic effects of dopamine and dobutamine in patients with cardiomyopathic heart failure. *Circulation* 1978;58:466–475.
Classic article describing the hemodynamic effects of these two inotropes in patients with systolic dysfunction.

Martin C, Viviand X, Leone M, et al. Effect of norepinephrine or dopamine on the outcome of septic shock. *Crit Care Med* 2000;28:2758–2765.
Observational study suggesting a possible survival benefit when patients with septic shock are treated initially with norepinephrine rather than dopamine.

Practice parameters for hemodynamic support of sepsis in adult patients in sepsis. Task Force of the American College of Critical Care Medicine, Society of Critical Care Medicine. *Crit Care Med* 1999;27:639–660.
Practice guidelines for the treatment of patients with sepsis by the American College of Critical Care Medicine.

THE CARDIOMYOPATHIES: DIAGNOSIS AND ICU MANAGEMENT

G. William Dec

27

I. OVERVIEW

A. Background

1. Cardiomyopathies are a diverse group of diseases characterized by primary involvement of the myocardium
2. Classified by World Health Organization by anatomic appearance and physiologic abnormality (Table 27-1):
   a. dilated cardiomyopathies (DCM)
   b. hypertrophic cardiomyopathies (HCM)
   c. restrictive cardiomyopathies (RCM)

B. Pathophysiology

1. DCM is characterized by:
   a. multichamber dilatation
   b. impaired systolic contractility
2. HCM is characterized by:
   a. marked left ventricular hypertrophy
   b. myocardial hypercontractility
   c. severely impaired diastolic relaxation and compliance
3. RCM are characterized by:
   a. abnormally stiff ventricle
   b. decreased ventricular relaxation
   c. normal contractile function
   d. biatrial enlargement

C. Diagnosis

1. Echocardiography is most useful initial test to differentiate cardiomyopathies and extent of ventricular dysfunction.

II. Dilated cardiomyopathy

A. Background

1. Cardiac enlargement (LV end-diastolic dimension greater than 55 mm) and decreased contractile function (LVEF less than 45%) are the hallmarks of the disease.
2. Reversible causes should be excluded (Table 27-2).
3. Cases with short duration of symptoms, mild ventricular dilatation, and inflammation on endomyocardial biopsy are more likely to demonstrate spontaneous improvement in ventricular function.
4. Familial pattern noted in 20% of cases; clinical clues:
   a. concomitant skeletal myopathy
   b. sensorineural hearing loss

B. Pathophysiology

1. Impaired systolic contractile function leads to ventricular dilatation via the Frank-Starling mechanism.
2. Functional mitral and/or tricuspid regurgitation are common because of annular displacement secondary to progressive left ventricular dilatation.
3. Chronic dyspnea due to elevated filling pressures is most frequent symptom. Acute pulmonary edema is uncommon except during periods of stress (e.g., infection, change in cardiac rhythm, surgical procedures).
4. Physical findings:

TABLE 27-1	Hemodynamic and Morphometric Features of the Cardiomyopathies		

Features	Dilated	Hypertrophic	Restrictive
LV ejection fraction	<45%	65%–90%	50%–70% <40% (late)
LV cavity size	Increased	Normal or decreased	Normal Increased (late)
Stroke volume	Markedly decreased	Normal or increased	Normal or Increased
Volume:mass ratio	Increased	Decreased	Markedly decreased
Diastolic compliance	Normal to decreased	Markedly decreased	Markedly decreased
Other features	Mild/moderate MR/TR are common	Dynamic obstruction	Often mimics Constrictive pericarditis

DCM: dilated cardiomyopathy; HCM, hypertrophic cardiomyopathy; LV, left ventricular; MR, mitral regurgitation; TR, tricuspid regurgitation
Adapted with permission from DeSanctis RW and Dec GW: The cardiomyopathies. Section 1, Subsection XIV, in Scientific American Medicine, Dale DC and Federman D (eds.). Copyright 1995, Scientific American, Inc. (Table 1).

TABLE 27-2	Causes of Potentially Reversible Dilated Cardiomyopathy

Toxins
Ethanol
Cocaine
Antiretroviral agents (AZT, ddI, ddC)
Phenothiazines

Metabolic abnormalities
Nutritional (thiamine, selenium, carnitine, and taurine deficiencies)
Endocrinologic (hypothyroidism, acromegaly, thyrotoxicosis, phenochromocytoma)
Electrolyte disturbances (hypocalcemia, hypophosphatemia)

Inflammatory/Infectious/Infiltrative
Infectious
  Viral (coxsackievirus, adenovirus, cytomegalovirus)
  Parasitic (toxoplasmosis)
  Spirochetal (Lyme disease)

Inflammatory/infiltrative
  Collagen vascular disorders (sarcoidosis)
  Hypersensitivity myocarditis
  Hemochromatosis
  Sarcoidosis

Miscellaneous
Tachycardia induced
Idiopathic
Peripartum

AZT, zidovudine (azidothymidine); ddI, didanosine (dideoxyinosine); ddC, zalcitabine (dideoxycytidine).

      a. jugular venous distension; hepatojugular reflux
      b. S4 and S3 gallops
      c. 1-2/6 audible mitral or tricuspid regurgitation
      d. clear lungs most commonly due to enhanced lymphatic drainage
      e. liver enlargement and peripheral edema

C. Prognosis

  1. Prognosis is highly dependent on disease etiology:
      a. idiopathic DCM: 5-year survival rate = 75%
      b. anthracycline cardiomyopathy: 5-year survival rate less than 25%
      c. Peripartum cardiomyopathy: 5-year survival rate greater than 90%

  2. Spontaneous improvement occurs in 20% to 40% of cases if symptom duration is less than 6 months.

  3. Clinical, echocardiographic, and laboratory findings can identify high-risk patients (Table 27-3).

D. Diagnosis

  1. Echocardiography is the most useful noninvasive modality because it assesses systolic and diastolic function, chamber dimensions, and ventricular wall thickness and excludes hemodynamically significant valvular disease (Table 27-4).

  2. Dobutamine stress echocardiography has a high sensitivity and specificity for assessing myocardial viability and contractile reserve.

  3. Patients with known DCM and stable symptoms require little additional diagnostic testing:

TABLE 27-3　　**High-Risk Features in Dilated Cardiomyopathy**

Clinical features
NYHA class IV symptoms on admission
Recent onset of illness (<6 months)
Active myocardial ischemia (angina or ischemic ECG abnormalities)
History of syncope
Persistent S_3 gallop
Right-sided heart failure signs
Inability to tolerate ACE inhibitors

Hemodynamic and ventriculographic findings
Left ventricular ejection fraction <20%
Right ventricular dysfunction
Pulmonary hypertension
Right atrial pressure >8 mm Hg
Pulmonary artery occlusion pressure >20 mm Hg
Cardiac index <2.0 L/min/m^2

Neurohormonal abnormalities
Hyponatremia (serum sodium <137 mmol/L)
Enhanced sympathetic tone (elevated plasma norepinephrine or resting sinus tachycardia)
Persistent elevation of BNP

Histologic features
Active lymphocytic or granulomatous myocarditis on endomyocardial biopsy

Arrhythmia pattern
History of prior cardiac arrest
Symptomatic or asymptomatic non-sustained runs of ventricular tachycardia
Second- or third-degree AV block

NYHA, New York Heart Association; S_3, third heart sound; ACE, angiotensin-converting enzyme; AV, atrioventricular.

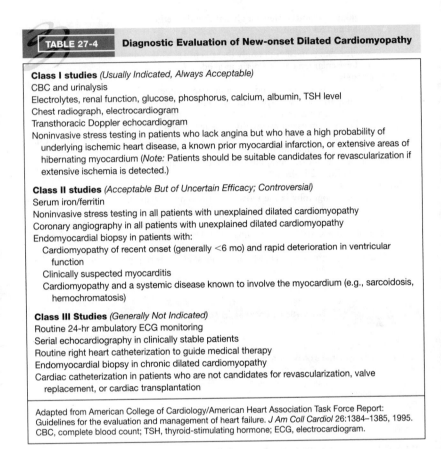

TABLE 27-4	Diagnostic Evaluation of New-onset Dilated Cardiomyopathy

Class I studies *(Usually Indicated, Always Acceptable)*
CBC and urinalysis
Electrolytes, renal function, glucose, phosphorus, calcium, albumin, TSH level
Chest radiograph, electrocardiogram
Transthoracic Doppler echocardiogram
Noninvasive stress testing in patients who lack angina but who have a high probability of
   underlying ischemic heart disease, a known prior myocardial infarction, or extensive areas of
   hibernating myocardium *(Note: Patients should be suitable candidates for revascularization if
   extensive ischemia is detected.)*

Class II studies *(Acceptable But of Uncertain Efficacy; Controversial)*
Serum iron/ferritin
Noninvasive stress testing in all patients with unexplained dilated cardiomyopathy
Coronary angiography in all patients with unexplained dilated cardiomyopathy
Endomyocardial biopsy in patients with:
   Cardiomyopathy of recent onset (generally <6 mo) and rapid deterioration in ventricular
      function
   Clinically suspected myocarditis
   Cardiomyopathy and a systemic disease known to involve the myocardium (e.g., sarcoidosis,
      hemochromatosis)

Class III Studies *(Generally Not Indicated)*
Routine 24-hr ambulatory ECG monitoring
Serial echocardiography in clinically stable patients
Routine right heart catheterization to guide medical therapy
Endomyocardial biopsy in chronic dilated cardiomyopathy
Cardiac catheterization in patients who are not candidates for revascularization, valve
   replacement, or cardiac transplantation

Adapted from American College of Cardiology/American Heart Association Task Force Report:
Guidelines for the evaluation and management of heart failure. *J Am Coll Cardiol* 26:1384–1385, 1995.
CBC, complete blood count; TSH, thyroid-stimulating hormone; ECG, electrocardiogram.

   a. serum electrolytes, Mg^{++}
   b. 12-lead ECG and CXR
   c. Preoperative echocardiography is generally unnecessary in clinically stable
      patients.
   d. Preoperative pharmacological stress testing with myocardial perfusion imaging
      should be considered for patients with ischemic cardiomyopathy and either
      worsening heart failure or anginal symptoms or in whom a major surgical pro-
      cedure is planned.

E. Treatment
   1. Elective surgery should be postponed for patients with newly diagnosed DCM
      to allow for initiation of pharmacologic therapy and time for spontaneous
      recovery of systolic function.
   2. Heart failure decompensation is the most frequent complication during hospi-
      talization.
   3. Individuals whose left ventricular ejection fraction (LVEF) is less than 20%
      are at increased risk for developing perioperative heart failure, atrial fibrilla-
      tion, ventricular arrhythmias, and inadequate renal perfusion.
   4. The cornerstones of pharmacologic therapy should include:
      a. a loop diuretic (furosemide, bumetinide, torsemide)
      b. an angiotensin-converting enzyme (ACE) inhibitor

    c. a β-blocker

    d. Digoxin and aldosterone antagonists are generally reserved for patients with advanced (NYHA class III or IV) symptoms.

5. Acute volume expansion should be avoided because it will exacerbate MR/TR and lead to decreased forward stroke volume and cardiac index.

6. Hemodynamic monitoring with a pulmonary artery catheter should be considered for major surgical procedures in DCM patients who have:

    a. recent decompensation in heart failure symptoms

    b. myocardial infarction less than 3 months previously

    c. moderate/severe stenotic valvular heart disease

7. Hemodynamic goals for DCM management in ICU setting:

    a. Pulmonary artery occlusion pressure 15 to 18 mm Hg

    b. CI greater than 2.0 L/min/m^2

8. For hemodynamically unstable patients, oral vasodilators should be replaced with short-acting intravenous agents (e.g., nitroprusside, nitroglycerin, or nesiritide). Occasionally, a β-agonist (dobutamine) or a phosphodiesterase III inhibitor (milrinone) may be required.

9. Rapid atrial fibrillation is not uncommon during hospitalization due to enhanced sympathetic tone. Acceptable agents to control heart rate may include digoxin, β-blockers, and intravenous amiodarone.

10. Intravenous heparin should be utilized to lower the risk of system or pulmonary embolism when paroxysmal or chronic atrial fibrillation exists.

11. Asymptomatic ventricular arrhythmias generally do not require pharmacologic suppression. Intravenous amiodarone and lidocaine are the agents of choice for symptomatic ventricular tachyarrhythmias.

III. HYPERTROPHIC CARDIOMYOPATHY
A. Background

1. Hereditary condition characterized by LV hypertrophy, hyperdynamic systolic function, and markedly impaired diastolic function

2. HCM must be differentiated from hypertensive concentric LVH, which is commonly seen in elderly women.

3. Clinical manifestations:

    a. dyspnea on exertion (secondary to impaired diastolic filling and elevated filling pressures)

    b. angina-like chest pain, concomitant atherosclerotic coronary artery disease may be present in older patients

    c. syncope, near-syncope (due to outflow tract obstruction, arrhythmias, inadequate diastolic filling)

B. Pathophysiology

1. HCM is inherited in more than 60% of cases as an autosomal dominant trait.

2. Specific single point mutations in genes that encode key sarcomeric contractile proteins include:

    a. α-myosin heavy chain (35%)

    b. troponin T (15%)

    c. myosin binding protein (15%)

    d. tropomyosin (less than 5%)

3. Pathologic hallmark = unexplained myocardial hypertrophy; interventricular septum >> ventricular free wall

4. HCM may have obstructive or nonobstructive physiology, depending on the presence or absence of a dynamic subaortic outflow tract pressure gradient.

5. Physical findings are dependent on the presence or absence of outflow tract obstruction, its severity, and the presence or absence of mitral regurgitation (MR).

    a. Precordial palpation typically reveals a hyperdynamic systolic apical impulse.

    b. Carotid upstoke is very rapid; if obstruction occurs, a bisferiens character (rapid upstroke, slow second carotid impulse) may be palpable.

    c. Prominent S4 gallop virtually always present.

   d. Systolic murmur(s) may be due to outflow obstruction and/or mitral regurgitation.
   e. Bedside maneuvers help differentiate HCM from aortic stenosis or MR (Table 27-5).
C. Prognosis
   1. Natural history is highly dependent on specific mutational defect
      a. Troponin T and α-tropomyosin defects produce mild hypertrophy but a high incidence of sudden cardiac death (SCD)
      b. Conversely, defects in myosin binding protein C are associated with late onset (fifth to seventh decade), moderate LV hypertrophy, and low rate of SCD.
   2. High-risk patients can be identified by clinical, ECG, and echo findings:
      a. young age (less than 30 years) at diagnosis
      b. family history of HCM and SCD
      c. syncopal history
      d. asymptomatic or symptomatic nonsustained ventricular tachycardia on ECG monitoring marked LVH (wall thickness greater than 30 mm)
D. Diagnosis
   1. ECG generally demonstrates:
      a. LVH with strain pattern
      b. "pseudo-MI pattern": QS waves due to marked LV hypertrophy
   2. Echocardiogram is the most useful diagnosis tool:
      a. asymmetrical hypertrophy of the interventricular septum with septal-to-ventricular free wall ratio equal to or greater than 1.3:1 highly suggestive
      b. varying patterns of hypertrophy may occur:
         (1) asymmetric septal hypertrophy (most common)
         (2) apical hypertrophy
         (3) concentric hypertrophy
         (4) isolated free wall hypertrophy (rare)
      c. Doppler interrogation at rest and during provocative maneuvers (premature ventricular contractions [PVCs], Valsalva) is critical to assess presence and/or severity of outflow obstruction and presence or absence of mitral regurgitation.

TABLE 27-5 **Bedside Maneuvers to Differentiate the Murmur of Obstructive Hypertrophic Cardiomyopathy from That of Valvular Heart Disease**

Maneuver	Response of murmur		
	HCM	**Aortic stenosis**	**Mitral regurgitation**
Hypovolemia Tachycardia Valsalva Venodilators (nitrates) *(Decreased LV cavity size)*	Increased	Decreased	Decreased
Volume expansion Passive leg elevation	Decreased	No change or small increase	No change or small increase
Isometric hand grip Vasopressors *(Increased cavity size)*			

HCM, hypertrophic cardiomyopathy; LV, left ventricular.

E. Treatment

1. Noncompliant LV is poorly equipped to handle sudden preload shifts.
2. Hypovolemia will worsen dynamic outflow obstruction and increase the degree of mitral regurgitation.
3. Transesophageal echocardiogram or continuous hemodynamic monitoring is recommended for patients with marked LV hypertrophy and/or significant outflow tract obstruction (greater than 50 mm Hg) undergoing surgical procedures associated with:
   a. significant blood loss
   b. decreased vascular tone
   c. need for transient inotropic support
4. Pharmacological therapy
   a. Diuretics should be used judiciously.
   b. β-blockers are most frequently utilized in patients with symptomatic HCM (Fig. 27-1)
      (1) High doses are often required.
      (2) Sustained-release preparations should be replaced with shorter-acting agents during periods of hemodynamic lability.
   c. Calcium channel blockers, particularly verapamil, are useful in patients with persistent symptoms or intolerance to β-blockers.
   d. Catecholamines, particularly β-agonists such as dobutamine, should be avoided whenever possible because they will increase dynamic outflow obstruction.
   e. Atrial fibrillation management may include:
      (1) β-blocker or calcium blocker for rate control
      (2) intravenous amiodarone
      (3) prompt cardioversion if poorly tolerated
      (4) systemic anticoagulation
   f. Surgical septal myectomy or alcohol septal ablation improves symptoms for patients with NYHA class III or IV angina or dyspnea and marked outflow tract obstruction.

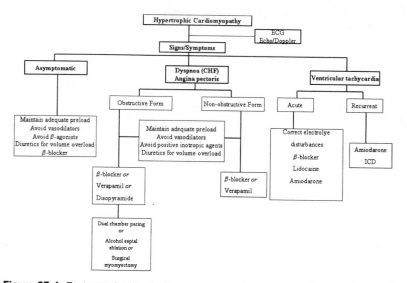

Figure 27-1. Treatment algorithm for the management of patients with known hypertrophic cardiomyopathy. CHF: congestive heart failure; ECG: electrocardiogram; ICD implantable cardioverter-defibrillator. (From Irwin JS, Rippe JM. *Irwin and Rippe's intensive care medicine*, 5th edition. 2003, page 310, with permission.)

IV. RESTRICTIVE CARDIOMYOPATHIES

A. Background

1. Least common type (less than 5%) of heart muscle disease
2. Hallmarks include:
   a. severe diastolic dysfunction
   b. normal systolic function and cavity size
   c. biatrial enlargement
3. Etiologies include (Table 27-6):
   a. infiltrative diseases (most commonly amyloidosis)
   b. diffuse myocardial fibrosis
   c. endocardial fibrosis

B. Pathophysiology

1. Ventricular myocardium is rigid and noncompliant, resulting in elevated filling pressures.
2. Clinical and hemodynamic features mimic restrictive pericardial disease.
3. Heart failure is the most common clinical manifestation.
4. Physical finding may include:
   a. increased jugular venous pressure (JVP), prominent Y descent
   b. + Kussmaul's sign
   c. moderate MR/TR murmurs

C. Natural history

1. Epidemiology and natural history depend on particular disease etiology.
2. Cardiac amyloidosis is the disease paradigm:
   a. cardiac involvement common in immunologic (AL) and transthyretin types (TT)
   b. survival less than 24 months from onset of heart failure symptoms
3. Idiopathic restrictive disease
   a. disease of elderly
   b. 5-year survival rate: 65%

TABLE 27-6	Causes of Restrictive Cardiomyopathy

Myocardial
Noninfiltrative
  Idiopathic
  Scleroderma
Infiltrative
  Amyloidosis
  Sarcoidosis
  Gaucher's disease
  Hurler's disease
Storage diseases
  Hemochromatosis
  Fabry's disease
  Glycogen storage diseases

Endomyocardial
Endomyocardial fibrosis
Hypereosinophilic syndrome
Carcinoid
Metastatic malignancies
Radiation injury
Anthracycline toxicity

From Wynne J. and Braunwald E.: Restrictive and infiltrative cardiomyopathies. *In* Braunwald E., ed.: *Heart disease,* 5th ed. Philadelphia, WB Saunders, 1997, p. 1427.

D. Diagnosis

1. Evaluation centers on differentiating RCM from constrictive disease and idiopathic origin from infiltrative disease etiologies.
2. Echocardiography will typically show: LVH, normal cardiac size, biatrial enlargement, and Doppler evidence of restrictive physiology on transmitral inflow:
   a. prominent E wave
   b. short isovolumetric relaxation time
   c. short deceleration time
3. Increased myocardial echogenicity ("speckling") suggests an infiltrative process such as amyloidosis, which can be confirmed by:
   a. rectal biopsy (70% sensitivity)
   b. abdominal fat pad biopsy (80% sensitivity)
   c. endomyocardial biopsy (greater than 99% sensitivity)
4. Cardiac MR or high-resolution CT imaging should be performed to exclude pericardial constriction if diagnosis remains uncertain based on clinical and/or hemodynamic features.
5. Hemodynamic measurement of simultaneous RV/LV pressure tracings reveals classic restrictive pattern:
   a. elevated RA, RV end-diastolic, PA end-diastolic, and pulmonary artery occlusion pressures (typically greater than 20 mm Hg)
   b. dip and plateau to RV and LV diastolic tracing
   c. prominent atrial Y descent
   d. ventricular concordance

E. Treatment

1. General measure include:
   a. diuretics to decrease "congestive" symptoms
   b. Pulmonary artery occlusion pressures should generally exceed 15 mm Hg if hemodynamic monitoring is undertaken to avoid inadequate preload during periods of instability.
   c. ACE inhibitors, β-blockers are generally ineffective but may be used if systolic dysfunction develops.
2. Cardiac amyloidosis may respond to:
   a. prednisone and melphalan immunosuppression
   b. heart transplantation followed by autologous bone marrow transplantation
3. Atrial fibrillation is poorly tolerated and may require urgent cardioversion and initiation of amiodarone or β-blocker treatment

Selected Readings

Adams HF, Baughman K, Dec GW, et al. Heart Failure Society of America. Guidelines for management of patients with heart failure caused by left ventricular systolic dysfunction-pharmacological approaches. *J Cardiac Failure* 1999;5:357–382.
Consensus guidelines based on published literature on pharmacologic therapy of chronic heart failure in adults.

American College of Cardiology/American Heart Association Task Force Report: guidelines for the evaluation and management of chronic heart failure in the adult. *Circulation* 2001;104:2996–3007.
Recently updated consensus practice guidelines on the diagnostic evaluation and pharmacologic treatment of heart failure using evidence-based methodologies.

Braunwald E, Seidman CE, Sigwart U. Contemporary evaluation and management of hypertrophic cardiomyopathy. *Circulation* 2002;106:1312–1316.
Concise summary of current management of the patient with hypertrophic cardiomyopathy.

Dec GW, DeSanctis RW. The cardiomyopathies. In: Dale DC, Federman D., eds: *Scientific American medicine*, New York, 2003, Healtheon/WebMD, pp. 333–354.
A current general review of disease etiologies, diagnosis, and evidence-based approaches to treatment.

Dec GW, Fuster V. Idiopathic dilated cardiomyopathy. *N Eng J Med* 1994; 331:1564–1575.
The definitive review of epidemiology, presenting symptoms, the role of invasive and noninvasive diagnostic techniques, and treatment strategies.

Eagle K, Berger PB, Caulkins H, et al. ACC/AHA guideline update for perioperative cardiovascular evaluation for noncardiac surgery: executive summary: a report of the American College of Cardiology/American Heart Association Task Force on Practice Guidelines (Committee to Update the 1996 Guidelines on Perioperative Cardiovascular Evaluation for Noncardiac Surgery). *J Am Coll Cardiol* 2002;105:1257–1267.
Comprehensive review of consensus practice guidelines on diagnostic evaluation, risk stratification, and management of the cardiac patient who is to undergo noncardiac surgery.

Feldman AM, McNamara D. Acute myocarditis. *N Eng J Med* 2000; 343:1388–1398.
Up-to-date review of disease pathogenesis, treatment options, and outcomes.

Griggs LE, Wiggle ED, Williams WG, et al. Transesophageal Doppler echocardiography in obstructive hypertrophic cardiomyopathy: clarification of pathophysiology and importance in intraoperative decision making. *J Am Coll Cardiol* 1992;20:42–52.
Clear summary of role of transesophageal echocardiography for intraoperative monitoring of the patient with marked hypertrophic cardiomyopathy.

Kasper EK, Agema WRP, Hutchins GM, et al. The cause of dilated cardiomyopathy: a clinicopathologic review of 673 consecutive patients. *J Am Coll Cardiol* 1994;23:586–590.
The most comprehensive single institution series of dilated cardiomyopathy with a focus on long-term natural history.

Kimmelstiel CD, Maron BJ. Role of percutaneous septal ablation in hypertrophic cardiomyopathy. *Circulation* 2004;109:452–455.
Brief summary of current indications and limitations of this technique for the treatment of symptomatic obstructive hypertrophic cardiomyopathy.

Kushwaha S, Fallon JT, Fuster V. Restrictive cardiomyopathy. *N Eng J Med* 1997;336:267–276.
Detailed review of major forms of restrictive cardiomyopathy, their natural history, diagnostic evaluation, and current management options.

Kyle RA, Gertz MA, Griepp PR, et al. A trial of three regimens for primary amyloidosis: colchicine alone, melphalan and prednisone, and melpahlan, prednisone, and colchicine. *N Eng J Med* 1997;336:1202–1207.
Comprehensive results of varied forms of immunosuppressive agents for immunologic-based cardiac amyloidosis.

Maron BJ, McKenna WJ, Danielson GK, et al. ACC/ESC clinical expert consensus document on hypertrophic cardiomyopathy: a report of the American College of Cardiology Taskforce on Clinical Expert Consensus Documents and the European Society of Cardiology Committee on Practice Guidelines (Committee to Develop and Expert Consensus Document on Hypertrophic Cardiomyopathy). *J Am Coll Cardiol* 2003;42:1687–1713.
Recently revised consensus practice guidelines on the evaluation and management (medical, catheter based, and surgical) of hypertrophic cardiomyopathy.

Nishimura RA, Holmes DR. Hypertrophic obstructive cardiomyopathy. *N Engl J Med* 2004;350:1320–1327.
Concise, lucid summary of key issues in the pathogenesis, diagnosis and therapy of hypertrophic cardiomyopathy in the current era.

Practice guidelines for pulmonary artery catheterization: a Report by the American Society of Anesthesiologists Task Force on Pulmonary Artery Catheterization. *Anesthesiology* 1993;78:380–394.
Expert recommendations on indications for hemodynamic monitoring of patients with underlying cardiovascular disease, including cardiomyopathies.

Richardson P, McKenna W, Bristow M, et al. Report of the 1995 World Health Organization International Society and Federation of Cardiology Task Force on the definition and classification of cardiomyopathies. *Circulation* 1996; 93:841–842.
The definitive classification of the cardiomyopathies based on anatomy and pathophysiology.

Roberts R, Sigwart UL. New concepts in hypertrophic cardiomyopathies, Parts 1 and II. *Circulation* 2001;104:2113–2116, 2249–2252.
Well-written summary of evolving views on molecular causes and contemporary treatment of hypertrophic disease.

VALVULAR HEART DISEASE

Michael F. Bellamy and Maurice Enriquez-Sarano

28

I. ACUTE PRESENTATION OF AORTIC STENOSIS

A. Principles: irrespective of how acute or severe its presentation, severe aortic stenosis (AS) should always be considered a surgical disease.

B. Etiology and natural history

1. **Etiology:** Mostly degenerative (atherosclerotic) on tricuspid or bicuspid valves.
2. **Progression:** constant at 0.1 cm^2 (decrease in valve area) and 7 mm Hg (increase in gradient) per year, due to calcification.
3. **Clinical natural history:** Poor once symptoms (even mild) occur

C. Pathophysiology

Increased transvalvular velocity and gradient with high afterload lead to compensatory left ventricular hypertrophy and ultimately failure due to afterload mismatch. Relief of the mechanical obstacle often reverses ventricular dysfunction.

D. Clinical presentation

1. **Acute presentation:** Mostly syncope or heart failure
2. **Clinical examination:** Harsh, loud, midsystolic murmur and decreased S2; ambiguous with minimal or absent murmur in patients with reduced ejection fraction

E. Investigations

1. **ECG and chest radiograph:** Left ventricular hypertrophy nonspecific and not always present
2. Echocardiography and Doppler
   a. **Dimensional and M-mode echocardiography** shows the calcified aortic valve and measures the LV function
   b. **Doppler echocardiography** measures the velocity, gradient and valve area (severe if 4 m/s or greater, 50 mm Hg [mean] or greater, and less than 1.0 cm^2, respectively)
   c. Low output/low gradient AS with small valve area in patients with reduced ventricular function requires dobutamine stress. With dobutamine, "true" severe AS gradient increases with unchanged valve area. Contractile reserve (greater than 20% increase in stroke volume with dobutamine) predicts better outcome.
3. Computed tomography measures the large amount of aortic valve calcium in severe AS.
4. Cardiac catheterization verifies severity of AS in difficult cases and provides preoperative coronary angiography.

F. Management

1. Intensive care unit management: support blood pressure by all means in hypotensive patients. Nitroprusside may be used for severe heart failure (if blood pressure is adequate) without delaying surgery.
2. Aortic valve replacement is the lifesaving intervention and is almost never contraindicated.
3. Percutaneous intervention with balloon valvuloplasty is rarely useful (risky and transiently effective). Percutaneous valve replacement is currently under evaluation.

II. ACUTE PRESENTATION OF AORTIC REGURGITATION

A. Etiology is most often native valve endocarditis. Aortic dissection or traumatic rupture. Chronic aortic regurgitation (AR) of any cause may present acutely with heart failure.

B. Pathophysiology: the regurgitant orifice leads to volume overload (regurgitant volume) and pressure overload (increased systolic pressure and wall stress). Acutely, AR causes reduced ventricular compliance, high filling pressures with heart failure despite low-intensity murmur.

C. Physical examination: Acutely, the diastolic murmur is often unimpressive or short, while arterial hyperpulsatility and large blood pressure differential clue to severe AR.

D. Investigations
1. ECG and chest radiograph: Acutely, pulmonary edema may contrast with normal heart size and lack of ventricular hypertrophy.
2. Echocardiography and Doppler
   Echocardiography particularly with transesophageal approach shows the aortic lesions and possible vegetations. Ventricular systolic and diastolic function is assessed.
   Doppler and color-flow imaging show the regurgitant jet. AR may be quantified by calculating the effective regurgitant orifice and regurgitant volume (severe if ≥ 30 mm^3 and ≥ 60 mL, respectively)
3. Cardiac catheterization may show AR severity by aortography, and coronary angiography may be performed in older patients (if no large vegetations).

E. Management
1. Afterload reduction is central to acute and chronic medical treatment of AR.
2. Surgical valve replacement is urgently required with heart failure. Aortic valve repair is sometimes possible. Periannular repair is necessary for abscesses.

F. Special case: combined aortic aneurysmal disease and AR
1. Clinically, may present with compression or rupture. Increased S2 is frequent. Diastolic murmur may be of low intensity
2. Investigations:
   a. quantify AR, which may be mild;
   b. assess aortic size and shape by echo (transesophageal echocardiography [TEE], if necessary), computed tomography or magnetic resonance.
3. Management of large aneurysms (≥ 5.5 or 6 cm) is surgical and urgent with signs of pre-rupture. Structurally normal aortic valve with mild AR may be preserved.

III. ACUTE PRESENTATION OF MITRAL REGURGITATION
A. Etiology and mechanism
1. **Non-ischemic, organic mitral regurgitation (MR)** due mostly to ruptured chords or perforated leaflets.
2. **Ischemic or functional MR** due rarely to ruptured papillary muscle and mostly to valve tenting secondary to chordal traction due to ventricular remodeling.

B. Pathophysiology: low compliance atrium, despite large regurgitant orifice, leads to low flow, low regurgitant volume, and low-intensity murmur but high atrial pressure and heart failure.

C. History: sudden onset of pulmonary edema isolated or in the context of myocardial infarct or endocarditis.

D. Physical examination: loud murmur in organic MR but low-intensity or nonaudible murmur in ischemic/functional MR; frequent S4 and S3.

E. Investigations
1. ECG and chest radiograph: rare atrial enlargement, no cardiomegaly.
2. Echocardiography and Doppler
   a. Two-dimensional (2D)-echocardiography: (a) etiology and mechanism (e.g., ruptured chord or papillary muscle); (b) ventricular function, global and regional.
   b. Doppler and color show the jet (TEE if necessary), direction (septal-superior for posterior leaflet, lateral for anterior leaflet, central for functional or bileaflet) and quantifies MR (effective regurgitant orifice, regurgitant volume, severe if ≥ 40 mm^2 and ≥ 60 mL, respectively). *Note:* MR is severe with effective regurgitant orifice ≥ 20 mm^2 for ischemic MR.

3. Cardiac catheterization may verify severity of MR, hemodynamics, and LV function but mostly is used to assess coronary lesions and need for revascularization.

F. Management

1. Intensive care unit management: (a) diuretics, nitrates, mechanical ventilation to control pulmonary edema; (b) vasodilators or intraaortic balloon counterpulsation to minimize MR.

2. Surgical treatment

a. Acute, organic MR: valve repair as soon as infection is controlled (earlier if hemodynamically necessary)

b. Acute, ischemic MR: Revascularization with mitral repair or replacement

c. Functional MR of dilated cardiomyopathy: maximal medical treatment and consideration of valve repair or replacement (possibly with ventricular restoration surgery) if remains severe.

IV. ACUTE PRESENTATION OF MITRAL STENOSIS (MS)

A. Etiology: mostly rheumatic

B. Pathophysiology: the fixed orifice due to commissural fusion leads to large gradient with increases in flow (pregnancy, anemia) and to heart failure

C. History: often sudden pulmonary edema

D. Physical examination: increased S1 with opening snap; loud rumble (left lateral decubitus) with high flow; sometimes inaudible rumble in low-flow MS of the elderly.

E. Investigations

1. ECG and chest radiograph: atrial enlargement often; right ventricular enlargement rarely

2. Echocardiography and Doppler

a. 2D-Echocardiography (a) rheumatic lesions; (b) reduced orifice; (c) lesion and calcifications scoring for balloon valvuloplasty

b. Doppler and color: (a) MS severity (gradient (mean) and valve area, severe if ≥ 10 mm Hg and <1.5 cm^2, respectively) at rest and with exercise; (b) associated MR; (c) hemodynamics.

c. TEE: (a)left atrial (appendage) thrombus; (b) MR presence and severity

3. Cardiac catheterization: hemodynamics and coronary angiography but mostly for balloon valvuloplasty.

F. Management

1. Intensive care unit management oxygenation, diuretics, β-blockers to control heart rate, mechanical ventilation if needed.

2. Percutaneous balloon mitral valvuloplasty is the preferred treatment with results equivalent to surgical commissurotomy; can be done in pregnant women with low risk.

3. Surgical treatment: mostly in calcified valves or with MR requiring valve replacement.

V. ACUTE PRESENTATION OF PROSTHETIC VALVE DYSFUNCTION

A. Prosthetic valve thrombosis

1. Clinical presentation: mostly stroke due to embolism or heart failure due to valve obstruction.

2. Investigations: echo, prosthetic obstruction; TEE, thrombus size and limitation of movement of mobile element (also by cine-fluoroscopy)

3. Treatment

a. Reoperation: most radical but with notable risk

b. Thrombolysis: risk of embolism and secondary recurrence. Streptokinase or r-TPA preferred. Useful for tricuspid valve thrombosis. Indication depends on size of thrombus, comorbidity, operative risk and age.

B. Prosthetic valve endocarditis

1. Clinical presentation: infection, embolism, heart failure.

2. Investigations: blood cultures and TEE are key to diagnosis. TEE also shows abscesses, fistula, intraprosthetic and periprosthetic regurgitation.

3. Treatment antibiotics: early reoperation to remove infected tissue and foreign material, especially if heart failure is present.

C. Structural failure

1. Bioprosthesis: frequent, progressive due to degeneration. Reoperation after stabilization.

2. Mechanical valve: rare, sudden due to defective material. Urgent reoperation.

D. Prosthetic regurgitation

1. Presentation: Heart failure or anemia due to hemolysis. Murmur may not be audible.

2. Investigations: Echocardiography, particularly TEE, is key to diagnosis.

3. Treatment by reoperation (urgency determined by severity of heart failure and infectious cause).

Selected Readings

Abascal VM, Wilkins GT, O'Shea JP, et al. Prediction of successful outcome in 130 patients undergoing percutaneous balloon mitral valvotomy. *Circulation* 1990;82(2):448–456.
The anatomical predictors of the results of balloon valvuloplasty.

Ben Farhat M, Ayari M, Maatouk F, et al. Percutaneous balloon versus surgical closed and open mitral commissurotomy: seven-year follow-up results of a randomized trial. *Circulation* 1998;97(3):245–250.
The similarity of surgical and percutaneous interventions for mitral stenosis.

Bonow RO, Carabello B, de Leon AC, Jr, et al. Guidelines for the management of patients with valvular heart disease: executive summary. *Circulation* 1998;98(18):1949–1984.
The official guidelines for management of valve diseases irrespective of presentation, extensively referenced.

Clouse WD, Hallett JW Jr, Schaff HV, et al. Improved prognosis of thoracic aortic aneurysms: a population-based study. *JAMA* 1998;280(22):1926–1929.
The risk associated with increasing size of thoracic aortic aneurysms.

Connolly HM, Oh JK, Schaff HV, et al. Severe aortic stenosis with low transvalvular gradient and severe left ventricular dysfunction: result of aortic valve replacement in 52 patients. *Circulation* 2000;101(16):1940–1946.
A relatively large study of patients with low gradient operated with severe aortic stenosis. Despite a high operative mortality, long-term outcome is relatively good, showing that it is almost never too late to operate on severe symptomatic aortic stenosis.

Cribier A, Eltchaninoff H, Bash A, et al. Percutaneous transcatheter implantation of an aortic valve prosthesis for calcific aortic stenosis: first human case description. *Circulation* 2002;106(24):3006–3008.
First report of percutaneous aortic valve insertion.

David TE. Current practice in Marfan's aortic root surgery: reconstruction with aortic valve preservation or replacement? What to do with the mitral valve? *J Card Surg* 1997; 12(2 suppl):147–150.
A discussion of valve surgery in Marfan syndrome.

Dujardin KS, Enriquez-Sarano M, Schaff HV, Bailey KR, Seward JB, Tajik AJ. Mortality and morbidity of aortic regurgitation in clinical practice. A long-term follow-up study. *Circulation* 1999;99:1851–1857.
The largest study of mortality associated with severe aortic regurgitation under medical management. The high risk associated with mild symptoms and specific values of left ventricular characteristics are described.

Ellis SG, Whitlow PL, Raymond RE, Schneider JP. Impact of mitral regurgitation on long-term survival after percutaneous coronary intervention. *Am J Cardiol* 2002;89(3): 315–318.
Ischemic MR is associated with poor outcome even after percutaneous revascularization.

Enriquez-Sarano M, Freeman WK, Tribouilloy CM, et al. Functional anatomy of mitral regurgitation: accuracy and outcome implications of transesophageal echocardiography. *J Am Coll Cardiol* 1999;34(4):1129–1136.

The accuracy and impact on outcome of the mitral valve anatomy defined by echocardiography.

Enriquez-Sarano M, Seward JB, Bailey KR, Tajik AJ. Effective regurgitant orifice area: a noninvasive Doppler development of an old hemodynamic concept. *J Am Coll Cardiol* 1994;23(2):443–451.
Doppler measurement of the lesion severity using the effective regurgitant orifice and its hemodynamic correlates.

Enriquez-Sarano M, Sinak LJ, Tajik AJ, Bailey KR, Seward JB. Changes in effective regurgitant orifice throughout systole in patients with mitral valve prolapse. *Circulation* 1995;92(10):2951–2958.
The variability of the mitral regurgitation severity throughout the cardiac cycle.

Enriquez-Sarano M, Tajik AJ. Clinical practice. Aortic regurgitation. *N Engl J Med* 2004; 351(15):1539–1546.
A contemporary review of aortic regurgitation management.

Gillinov AM, Cosgrove DM, Blackstone EH, et al. Durability of mitral valve repair for degenerative disease. *J Thorac Cardiovasc Surg* 1998;116(5):734–743.
The excellent results of mitral repair in degenerative disease.

Gillinov AM, Wierup PN, Blackstone EH, et al. Is repair preferable to replacement for ischemic mitral regurgitation? *J Thorac Cardiovasc Surg* 2001;122(6):1125–1141.
The lack of benefit of mitral valve repair over replacement in patients with ischemic mitral regurgitation and severe presentation.

Grigioni F, Enriquez-Sarano M, Zehr KJ, Bailey KR, Tajik AJ. Ischemic mitral regurgitation: long-term outcome and prognostic implications with quantitative Doppler assessment. *Circulation* 2001;103(13):1759–1764.
The degree of ischemic mitral regurgitation is a major predictor of mortality post MI. Severe outcome is seen with effective regurgitant orifice (ERO) of 20 mm^2 or greater.

Grunkemeier GL, Li HH, Naftel DC, et al. Long-term performance of heart valve prostheses. *Curr Probl Cardiol* 2000;25(2):73–154.
An exhaustive review of the various outcomes of prosthetic valves.

Hickey AJ, Wilcken DE, Wright JS, Warren BA. Primary (spontaneous) chordal rupture: relation to myxomatous valve disease and mitral valve prolapse. *J Am Coll Cardiol* 1985;5(6):1341–1346.
The severe clinical presentation of acute mitral regurgitation due to ruptured cords.

Iung B, Cormier B, Ducimetiere P, et al. Immediate results of percutaneous mitral commissurotomy. A predictive model on a series of 1514 patients. *Circulation* 1996;94(9):2124-
The clinical determinants of the generally good results of mitral balloon valvuloplasty.

Khot UN, Novaro GM, Popovic ZB, et al. Nitroprusside in critically ill patients with left ventricular dysfunction and aortic stenosis. *N Engl J Med* 2003;348(18):1756–1763.
Nitroprusside administration in patients with aortic stenosis and heart failure is relatively well tolerated and relieves acute failure symptoms.

Lengyel M, Fuster V, Keltai M, et al. Guidelines for management of left-sided prosthetic valve thrombosis: a role for thrombolytic therapy. Consensus Conference on Prosthetic Valve Thrombosis. *J Am Coll Cardiol* 1997;30(6):1521–1526.
A review of treatment of thrombosed prostheses.

Messika-Zeitoun D, Aubry MC, Detaint D, et al. Evaluation and clinical implications of aortic valve calcification measured by electron-beam computed tomography. *Circulation* 2004;110(3):356–362.
A large report validating the use of electron-beam computed tomography to measure valve calcifications in aortic stenosis. Diagnostic and prognostic values are also reported.

Messika-Zeitoun D, Fung Yiu S, Cormier B, et al. Sequential assessment of mitral valve area during diastole using colour M-mode flow convergence analysis: new insights into mitral stenosis physiology. *Eur Heart J* 2003;24(13):1244–1253.
The lack of valve reserve in mitral stenosis.

Mohty D, Orszulak TA, Schaff HV, et al. Very long-term survival and durability of mitral valve repair for mitral valve prolapse. *Circulation* 2001;104(12 suppl 1):I1-I7.
The 20 years' outcome of repair in mitral regurgitation due to valve prolapse. Anterior leaflet prolapse is associated with less durability, but results have improved recently.

Monin JL, Monchi M, Gest V, et al. Aortic stenosis with severe left ventricular dysfunction and low transvalvular pressure gradients: risk stratification by low-dose dobutamine echocardiography. *J Am Coll Cardiol* 2001;37(8):2101–2107.
A large Doppler study showing the good postoperative outcome associated with contractile reserve in low-gradient aortic stenosis.

Morris JJ, Schaff HV, Mullany CJ, et al. Determinants of survival and recovery of left ventricular function after aortic valve replacement. *Ann Thorac Surg* 1993;56(1):22–29; discussion 9–30.
The low-risk and good outcome of aortic valve replacement is described in a large series.

Mourvillier B, Trouillet JL, Timsit JF, et al. Infective endocarditis in the intensive care unit: clinical spectrum and prognostic factors in 228 consecutive patients. *Intensive Care Med* 2004;30:2046–2052.
The poor outcome of infective endocarditis seen in intensive care units.

Nishimura RA, Grantham JA, Connolly HM, et al. Low-output, low-gradient aortic stenosis in patients with depressed left ventricular systolic function: the clinical utility of the dobutamine challenge in the catheterization laboratory. *Circulation* 2002;106(7):809–813.
A small catheterization study showing the prognostic importance of contractile reserve in low-gradient aortic stenosis.

Omran H, Schmidt H, Hackenbroch M, et al. Silent and apparent cerebral embolism after retrograde catheterisation of the aortic valve in valvular stenosis: a prospective, randomised study. *Lancet* 2003;361(9365):1241–1246.
A report emphasizing the higher rate of subclinical cerebral infarction in patients in whom retrograde crossing of the aortic valve during catheterization is performed for hemodynamic purposes.

Otto CM, Burwash IG, Legget ME, et al. Prospective study of asymptomatic valvular aortic stenosis. Clinical, echocardiographic, and exercise predictors of outcome. *Circulation* 1997;95(9):2262–2270.
The first prospective, large (more than 100 patients) study of asymptomatic aortic stenosis outcome. Peak velocity was a major determinant or event-free survival.

Pellikka PA, Nishimura RA, Bailey KR, et al. The natural history of adults with asymptomatic, hemodynamically significant aortic stenosis. *J Am Coll Cardiol* 1990;15(5):1012–1017.
Retrospective analysis of outcome of asymptomatic severe aortic stenosis (defined as 4 m/s or greater velocity). The study shows that as long as patients remain asymptomatic, outcome is relatively good with few sudden deaths.

Roudaut R, Lafitte S, Roudaut MF, et al. Fibrinolysis of mechanical prosthetic valve thrombosis: a single-center study of 127 cases. *J Am Coll Cardiol* 2003;41(4):653–658.
The largest experience with fibrinolysis of thrombosed mechanical prosthesis: embolisms and recurrences.

Routray SN, Mishra TK, Swain S, et al. Balloon mitral valvuloplasty during pregnancy. *Int J Gynaecol Obstet* 2004;85:18–23.
The noninvasive treatment of pregnant women presenting acutely for mitral stenosis.

Skjaerpe T, Hegrenaes L, Hatle L. Noninvasive estimation of valve area in patients with aortic stenosis by Doppler ultrasound and two-dimensional echocardiography. *Circulation* 1985;72(4):810–818.
The validation of aortic valve area measurement in comparison to catheterization.

Tribouilloy CM, Enriquez-Sarano M, Bailey KR et al. Assessment of severity of aortic regurgitation using the width of the vena contracta: A clinical color Doppler imaging study. *Circulation* 2000;102(5):558–564.
The first study of the simple vena contracta measurement in aortic regurgitation.

Tribouilloy CM, Enriquez-Sarano M, Fett SL, et al. Application of the proximal flow convergence method to calculate the effective regurgitant orifice area in aortic regurgitation. *J Am Coll Cardiol* 1998;32(4):1032–1039.
The clinical quantitation of aortic regurgitation with the PISA method and its pitfalls.

Zoghbi WA, Enriquez-Sarano M, Foster E, et al. Recommendations for evaluation of the severity of native valvular regurgitation with two-dimensional and Doppler echocardiography. *J Am Soc Echocardiogr* 2003;16(7):777–802.
The recent guidelines for assessment of valve regurgitations by Doppler.

29 CRITICAL CARE OF PERICARDIAL DISEASE
Richard C. Becker

I. BACKGROUND
   A. Pericardial diseases cover a wide etiologic spectrum, including medical and surgical conditions.
   B. There are three pericardial conditions to be considered:
   1. acute pericarditis with or without pericardial effusion;
   2. cardiac tamponade; and
   3. constrictive pericarditis, including effusive-constrictive pericarditis.

II. ACUTE PERICARDITIS. Acute pericarditis most often is a strictly inflammatory fibrinous lesion without clinically recognizable pericardial fluid.
   A. Etiology. A burgeoning list of diseases, syndromes, and agents has been shown to produce pericarditis. The cause in any given case can be found in nine major categories (Table 29-1).
   B. Diagnosis
   1. Acute pericarditis may be asymptomatic, but more often the patient has central chest pain, usually sharp with a pleuritic component but sometimes with only vague precordial distress.
   2. Precordial distress may closely mimic angina, including a predominant pressure sensation.
   3. The onset is frequently sudden, particularly when it interrupts sleep, and frequently diminishes with sitting up.
   4. The pain may radiate in an anginal distribution, remain precordial, or migrate to one side of the chest; however, characteristically it radiates to the trapezius ridge.
   5. Odynophagia (pain on swallowing) occasionally occurs and may be the only symptom.
   6. The pericardial rub (friction sound) is pathognomonic of pericarditis. A fully developed rub has three components, usually distinguishable by careful auscultation even at rapid heart rates: a ventricular systolic rub, preceded by an atrial rub, and followed by an early diastolic rub.
   7. The white blood cell count, sedimentation rate, and other acute-phase reactants vary according to the etiologic agent or primary illness.
   8. Electrocardiographic (ECG) changes are of three types: typical, typical variants, and atypical (the last including no change). Of four potential ECG stages, an entirely typical stage I ECG (Fig. 29-1) is virtually diagnostic. During the evolutionary phase (stage II), all ST junctions return to baseline more or less "in phase," with little change in T waves. The T waves progressively flatten and invert in all or most of the leads that showed ST-segment elevations. In stage III, T-wave inversions appear and are not distinguishable from those of diffuse myocardial injury, myocarditis, or biventricular injury. In stage IV, the T waves return to their prepericarditic configuration. The entire ECG evolution occurs in a matter of days or weeks.
   C. Treatment
   1. The treatment of clinically noneffusive pericarditis or pericarditis without a compressing effusion is symptomatic (i.e., aimed at pain, malaise, and fever).
   2. The initial treatment begins with ibuprofen (Motrin) 600 mg every 6 hours, which sometimes relieves pain within 15 minutes to 2 hours of the first dose. Aspirin, up to 900 mg four times per day, is an acceptable treatment alternative.

TABLE 29-1	Major Etiologic Categories of Acute Pericarditis and Myopericarditis Overlapping Pathogenesis

1. Idiopathic pericarditis (syndrome)
2. Pericarditis due to living agents
3. Pericarditis in the vasculitis—connective tissue disease group
4. Immunopathic pericarditis; pericarditis in "hypersensitivity" states
5. Pericarditis in diseases of contiguous structures
6. Pericarditis in disorders of metabolism
7. Neoplastic pericarditis
8. Traumatic pericarditis
9. Pericarditis of uncertain origin or in association with syndromes of uncertain cause

3. In patients with myocardial infarction and pericarditis, indomethacin should not be used because of experimental work showing that it reduces coronary flow, increases experimental infarction size, and raises blood pressure.

4. Intractably symptomatic pericarditis can be treated with corticosteroid therapy, employed at the lowest effective dose with appropriate tapering. It should be avoided if at all possible because patients may be difficult to wean.

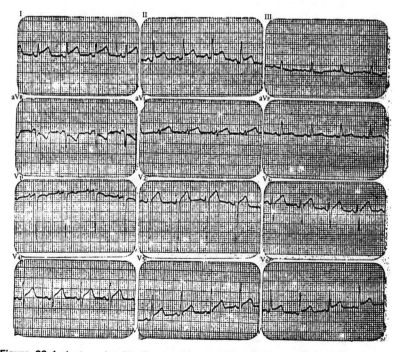

Figure 29-1. Acute pericarditis. Typical stage I electrocardiogram showing J-ST elevations in most leads (I, II, aVL, aVF, and V_3 to V_6) and J-ST depressions in leads aVF and V_1. PR segments are depressed below the TP baseline in leads I, II, aVL, aVF, and V_3 to V_6. PR-segment depression is the earliest change, occurring sooner after onset of symptoms. ST (J) elevation follows.

III. NONCOMPRESSING (LAX) PERICARDIAL EFFUSION

A. Most cases of acute pericarditis *without* tamponade probably involve some excess fluid resulting from intrapericardial exudation, with those amounting to 250 mL or more becoming clinically obvious either on physical examination or (more likely) chest radiograph.

B. Diagnosis

1. Noncompressing effusions may produce no clinical manifestations and may be the only sign of pericardial disease.

2. If a systemic or extrapericardial disease is responsible for the pericarditis, signs and symptoms of that condition may dominate the picture.

3. Extremely large noncompressing effusions may produce precordial discomfort and symptoms resulting from pressure on adjacent structures, such as dyspnea (from reduced lung capacity), cough, hoarseness, dysphagia, and hiccups. Heart sounds may be reduced with massive or rapidly developing effusions.

4. Radiography shows an enlarged cardiac silhouette and, in the absence of cardiac and pulmonary disease, clear lung fields and often a left pleural effusion.

5. The ECG may show low-voltage QRS complex and T waves (nearly always with normal P-wave voltage).

6. Echocardiography first reveals a small amount of fluid posteriorly at the left ventricular level in systole only (Table 29-2).

IV. CARDIAC TAMPONADE

A. Cardiac tamponade is defined as hemodynamically significant cardiac compression resulting from accumulating pericardial contents that evoke and defeat compensatory mechanisms (Fig. 29-2).

B. The pericardial contents may be effusion fluid, blood, pus, or gas (including air), singly or in combination, occasionally with underlying constrictive epicarditis.

C. Tamponade must be considered in any patient with cardiogenic shock and systemic congestion.

D. Pathophysiology

1. For significant cardiac compression, the pericardial contents must increase at a rate exceeding the rate of stretch of the parietal pericardium and, to some degree, the rate at which venous blood volume expands to maintain the small filling gradient to the right heart.

2. Relentlessly increasing intrapericardial pressure progressively reduces ventricular volume, producing rising diastolic pressures that resist filling to the point that even a high ejection fraction cannot avert critical reduction of stroke volume at any heart rate.

3. Beyond pericardial stretch, compensatory mechanisms for tamponade are mainly adrenergically mediated, including tachycardia, peripheral vasoconstriction, and maintained ejection fraction (in pure tamponade without heart disease, the ejection fraction is normal or increased).

4. Excessive fluid in the pericardium increases the normal pericardial effect on ventricular interaction and exaggerates the normal inspiratory decrease in systemic blood pressure, thus leading to pulsus paradoxus.

5. Although pulsus paradoxus is the hallmark of tamponade, at the bedside it must be borne in mind that pulsus is common to other disorders, including obstructive lung disease (including severe asthma), pulmonary embolism, tense ascites, obesity, mitral stenosis with right heart failure, right ventricular infarction, and hypovolemic and cardiogenic shock.

E. Diagnosis

1. Cardiac tamponade may appear insidiously as the first sign of pericardial injury or intrapericardial bleeding, especially in conditions such as neoplasia, trauma, and connective tissue disorders.

2. Patients are dyspneic and progressively feel "sicker," and with advanced cardiac compression they have pallor, tachycardia, cyanosis, impaired cerebral function, sweating, and cold acral points.

| TABLE 29-2 | Echo Doppler in Pericardial Effusion and Cardiac Tamponade[a] |

I. Pericardial effusion: M-mode and 2-D
  A. Echo-free space
    1. Posterior to LV (small to moderate effusions)
    2. Posterior and anterior (moderate to large effusions)
    3. Behind left atrium in some large to very large effusions
  B. Decreased movement of posterior pericardium-lung interface
  C. RV pulsations brisk (with anterior fluid)
  D. Aortic root movement abnormal or attenuated
  E. "Swinging heart" (large effusions)
    1. Periodicity 1:1 or 2:1 (rarely 3:1)
    2. RV and LV walls move synchronously
    3. Mitral-tricuspid pseudoprolapse (pansystolic at HR > 120 beats/min)
  F. 2-D only
    1. Loculated fluid
    2. Adhesions (fibrinous and fibrous)
II. Cardiac tamponade: M-mode and 2-D evidence of effusion plus
  A. Cardiac compression
    1. Decreased total transverse dimension (RV epicardium to LV epicardium at end diastole: may be apparent only after tap)
    2. RV diameters decreased (may be apparent only after tap), unless previous RV enlargement
    3. Early diastolic collapse of RV outflow tract with continued diastolic inward wall motion (≥ 50 msec after mitral D point)
  B. Inspiratory effects (with pulsus paradoxus)
    1. RV expands from greatly reduced expiratory end-diastolic size
    2. IV septum shifted to left
    3. LV compressed
    4. Mitral excursion-D/E amplitude and open valve area decreased
      a. E/F slope decreased or rounded
      b. Open time[b] decreased
    5. Aortic valve[b] opening decreased; premature closure
    6. Reduced increase in inferior vena cava diameter (<25%)
    7. Echocardiographic stroke volume decreased
    8. Decreased fractional shortening (short axis)
    9. Doppler: Right-sided transvalvular flows greatly exaggerated; left-sided flows greatly reduced (reversed during expiration)
  C. Notch in RV epicardium during isovolumic contraction (M-mode)
  D. Coarse oscillations of LV posterior wall (2-D echocardiography only)
  E. RA free wall indentation (buckling) during late diastole or isovolumic contraction
  F. RV indentation (buckling) during early diastole
  G. LA free wall indentation (cases with fluid behind LA)
  H. SVC and IVC dilation (unless volume depletion) and relatively fixed diameter during respiration
  I. Presystolic reflux or contrast media into IVC

[a]Sensitivities and specificities vary for each item.
[b]Often difficult to define during pericardial effusion; mitral valve may open with atrial systole only during inspiration.
HR, heart rate; IV, interventricular; IVC, inferior vena cava; LA, left atrium; LV, left ventricle; RA, right atrium; RV, right ventricle; SVC, superior vena cava; 2-D, two-dimensional.

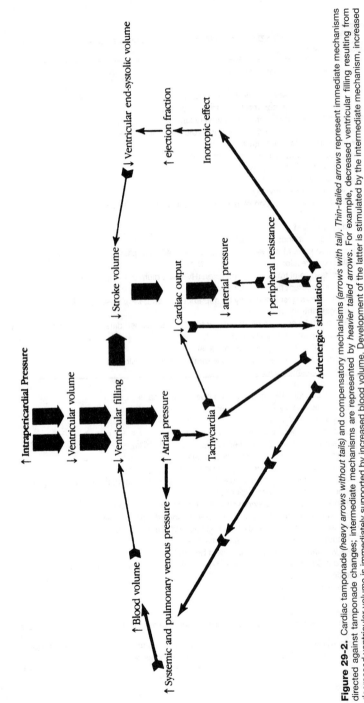

Figure 29-2. Cardiac tamponade *(heavy arrows without tails)* and compensatory mechanisms *(arrows with tail)*. *Thin-tailed arrows* represent immediate mechanisms directed against tamponade changes; intermediate mechanisms are represented by *heavier tailed arrows*. For example, decreased ventricular filling resulting from decreased ventricular volume is immediately supported by increased blood volume. Development of the latter is stimulated by the intermediate mechanism, increased venous pressures (see text).

3. Most patients are hypotensive.

4. In patients with rapid tamponade resulting from hemorrhage, as in wounds and cardiac or aortic rupture, the dominant picture is one of shock.

5. The heart sounds may be distant.

6. The neck veins are typically engorged, even with the patient sitting at 90 degrees, and sometimes there are prominent forehead, scalp, and retinal veins.

7. If the venous level can be accurately discerned, the single negative systolic phase in midsystole (x trough) is a valuable finding that may be timed while listening to the heart sounds as one watches a rapid inward darting of the neck veins between S_1 and S_2.

8. Pulsus paradoxus occurs when respiratory changes alternatively favor right and left heart filling.

9. Left ventricular hypertrophy and/or hypovolemia may minimize the likelihood of detecting pulsus paradoxus.

F. Treatment

1. Removal of pericardial fluid as soon as possible by pericardiocentesis or surgical drainage is the definitive treatment.

2. Surgical drainage is optimal for either traumatic tamponade or tamponade from pericarditis caused by pyogenic organisms.

3. Needle aspiration, using a sub-xiphoid approach under emergent conditions, can be performed with echocardiographic guidance.

V. PERICARDITIS VERSUS MYOCARDIAL INFARCTION. Special consideration must be given to differentiating acute pericarditis, with or without effusion or tamponade, from both acute myocardial infarction and acute pericarditis in the setting of (and presumably resulting from) myocardial infarction (Table 29-3).

VI. CONSTRICTIVE PERICARDITIS

A. Constrictive pericarditis is seen less in its traditional chronic form and more often in subacute and acute forms, soon after a detectable bout of acute pericarditis with or without effusion.

B. Most cases are idiopathic or follow cardiac surgery (see Table 29-1).

C. Pathophysiology

1. Like tamponade, constriction severely limits ventricular filling, with equalization of left and right heart diastolic pressures. Systolic right ventricular pressure rises, but usually to less than 50 mm Hg, and the ratio of right ventricular end-diastolic pressure to systolic pressure is usually greater than 0.3.

2. Respiratory changes in cardiac pressures are minimal, and jugular venous pressure increases during inspiration (Kussmaul's sign, also seen in right ventricular infarction, acute cor pulmonale, and tricuspid stenosis).

3. Inspiratory decrease in arterial pressure in pure constriction is slight, nearly always less than 10 mm Hg.

4. Unlike in cardiac tamponade, the heart is not compressed in early diastole and relaxes normally or abruptly (rubber bulb effect) as filling proceeds until it reaches its pericardial limit. There is, therefore, a "square-root" configuration to the diastolic pressure (not seen in tamponade, particularly when measured by manometer tip catheters).

5. Venous and atrial pressures show prominent y as well as x descents. The y descent tends to be deeper and precipitous as it corresponds to the ventricular pressure dip when the atrioventricular valves are open (Fig. 29-3).

D. Diagnosis

1. Patients have one or more of the following signs and symptoms of systemic congestion (usually with clear lung fields) and a normal or slightly enlarged (rarely small) cardiac size:

a. easy fatigability;

b. dyspnea on exertion, usually without orthopnea;

c. pedal edema, ascites, or both;

d. hepatomegaly (and, in some chronic cases, splenomegaly); and

TABLE 29-3   **Differential Diagnosis of Acute Pericarditis**

Finding	Acute pericarditis	Acute ischemia
Pain		
Onset	More often sudden	Usually gradual, crescendo
Main location	Substernal or left precordial	Same or confined to zones of radiation
Radiation	May be same as ischemic, also trapezius ridges	Shoulders, arms, neck back; not trapezius ridges
Quality	Usually sharp; stabbing, "background" ache	Usually "heavy" or "burning"
Inspiration	Worse	No effect unless with infarct in pericarditis
Duration	Persistent; may wax and wane	Usually intermittent
Electrocardiogram		
J-ST	Diffuse elevation usually concave, without reciprocal depressions	Localized deviation usually convex (with reciprocal infarction)
PR segment depressions	Frequent	Rarely
Abnormal Q waves	None unless with infarction	Common with infarction ("Q wave" infarcts)
T waves	Inverted after J points return to baseline	Inverted while St still elevated (infarct)
Myocardial enzymes	Normal or elevated	Elevated (infarct)
Pericardial friction	Rub (most cases)	Rub only if with pericarditis
Abnormal S_3	Absent unless preexisting	May be present
Abnormal S_4	Absent unless preexisting	Nearly always present
S_4	Intact	Often dull, mushy after first day
Pulmonary congestion	Absent	May be present
Arrhythmia	None (in absence of heart disease)	Frequent
Conduction abnormalities (AV and IV)	None (in absence of heart disease)	Frequent

AV, atrioventricular; IV, interventricular.

    e. distention of the neck veins in which the x and y descent both collapse, departing from a high standing level of pressure.
  2. The echocardiographic diagnosis of constrictive pericarditis is not specific, although certain findings may be helpful in conjunction with the clinical features (Table 29-4).
E. Treatment
  1. Medical management of constrictive pericarditis resembles that of congestive heart failure, because most signs and symptoms are related to systemic congestion.
  2. Diuretics have long been a mainstay to relieve systemic congestion and its symptoms.
  3. The definitive treatment of constrictive pericarditis is always surgical removal of as much of the pericardium as possible.
F. Cardiac compression after cardiac surgery. The rapidly increasing number of patients undergoing cardiac surgery is producing significant increased postsurgical cardiac compression from four major causes: bleeding, pericardial effusion, postpericardiotomy syndrome, and constrictive pericarditis.

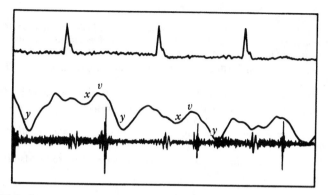

Figure 29-3. Constrictive pericarditis. Jugular venous pulse tracing taken 2.5 months after successful coronary bypass surgery. The patient developed systemic congestion and distention of neck veins with prominent *x* and *y* descents. The *x* trough falls between the first and second heart sounds, and the *y* trough follows the second heart sound on the phonocardiogram.

TABLE 29-4	Echocardiography of Pericardial Scarring and Constriction[a]

A. Pericardial thickening
    1. Condensed parietal pericardial echo
    2. Doubled parietal pericardial echo
B. Adhesions (fibrous or fibrinous)
    1. Adhesive strands seen (2-D) between LVPW and parietal pericardial echo (fluid present)
    2. Parietal pericardium moves with LVPW
        a. Without intervening space
        b. With intervening space = residual pericardial fluid ("halo sign")
C. Constrictive pericarditis
    1. Reduced ventricular size
    2. Atrial dilated
    3. Flat LVPW motion in mid- to late diastole
    4. Usually no posterior "depression" after atrial systole (post-P wave endocardial echo moves <1 mm posteriorly)
    5. Mitral E/F slope sharp
    6. Early atrioventricular valve closure
    7. IVS notchings: sharp posterior, men anterior motion (septal "flip-flop")
        a. During atrial systole
        b. During early diastole
    8. Inspiratory effects
        a. Interatrial and interventricular septa bulge to left
        b. Premature (pre-P wave) pulmonary valve opening (at very high RVDP)
        c. Marked inspiratory post-P wave deepening of pulmonary valve A wave
        d. Mitral and aortic Doppler flow velocities reduced from first inspiratory beat[b]
        e. Tricuspid and pulmonic transvascular velocities increased from first inspiratory beat[b]
D. 2-D only (most of A, B, and C on both M-mode and 2-D)
    1. Pericardium forms immobile single or double "shell"
    2. Ventricular expansion ends abruptly
    3. Atrioventricular valves hyperactive
    4. SVC, IVC, and hepatic veins dilated and lack normal inspiratory narrowing

[a]Most signs are relatively nonspecific.
[b]Distinguish constriction from restrictive cardiomyopathy.
IVC, inferior vena cava; IVS, interventricular spetum; LVPW, left ventricular posterior wall; RVDP, right ventricular diastolic pressure; SVC, superior vena cava; 2-D, two-dimensional.

Selected Readings

Shabetai R, Fowler NO, Fenton JC, et al. Pulsus paradoxus. *J Clin Invest* 1965;44:1882.
The physiology of pulsus paradoxus, an important finding among patients with pericardial effusions with tamponade, is outlined in a landmark study.

Spodick DH. Acute pericardial disease: pericarditis, effusion, and tamponade. *JCE Cardiol* 1979;14:9.
A comprehensive review of pericardial diseases by the world's leading authority.

Spodick DH. Arrhythmias during acute pericarditis: a prospective study of one hundred consecutive cases. *JAMA* 1976;235:39.
Arrhythmias, mostly supraventricular in origin, can occur in patients with acute pericarditis.

Spodick DH. *The pericarditis: a comprehensive textbook.* New York: Marcel Dekker, 1997.

THE ACUTE AORTIC SYNDROMES

Piotr Sobiesczyk, Heather L. Gornik, and Joshua A. Beckman

30

I. OVERVIEW. The acute aortic syndromes are rare yet morbid entities with variable clinical presentation. Mortality due to these disorders increases rapidly with delayed treatment, requiring a high index of suspicion to allow early recognition and management.

II. AORTIC DISSECTION

A. Background

1. Epidemiology of aortic dissection (AD)
   a. Most common acute aortic syndrome
   b. Estimated U.S. annual incidence of 3.5/100,000 may be an underestimate as many patients die before diagnosis is made.
   c. Incidence increases with age.
2. Stanford Classification System
   a. Type A: involves the ascending or proximal aorta
   b. Type B: involves the aorta distal to the origin of the left subclavian artery

B. Pathophysiology

1. Tear in the aortic intima exposes underlying media to blood flow at systemic pressure. The intimal tear propagates, forming a second or "false" lumen.
2. Etiology of AD is variable (Table 30-1). Processes that weaken the aorta's medial layers, such as hypertension, or intrinsic connective tissue disorders, may eventually result in intramural hemorrhage, aortic dissection, or rupture. Iatrogenic causes include previous aortic surgery or catheterization.

C. Prognosis

1. Without intervention, the risk of death approaches 1% per hour in the first 24 hours after AD. For untreated cases, mortality rates are approximately 50% at one week, and upwards of 90% beyond three months.
2. Type A: 30-day mortality with medical management approaches 50%, but 20% with surgical repair.
3. Type B: 30-day mortality rate 10% with medical therapy.

D. Diagnosis

1. Clinical presentation is variable and depends on the aortic segment involved. No pathognomonic physical findings secure the diagnosis. Clinical index of suspicion must be high.
   a. Common symptoms: chest pain (73%), back pain (53%), syncope (10%)
   b. Common sign: hypertension (77% Type B cases, 36% Type A cases).
   c. Less common signs: murmur of aortic insufficiency (31%); hypotension and shock; pericardial tamponade; myocardial ischemia (3%); congestive heart failure (4–7%); malperfusion syndromes (e.g., limb ischemia, neurological impairment or paraplegia, mesenteric ischemia, or renal insufficiency).
2. Diagnostic testing
   a. No reliable blood test at this time for rapid detection of AD.
   b. Chest radiography has limited diagnostic utility.
   c. Electrocardiogram nonspecific (normal in 31% of cases). Ischemic changes may be seen if Type A dissection involves the coronary arteries.
   d. Noninvasive imaging of the aorta establishes the diagnosis. Three available modalities provide similar diagnostic accuracy (Table 30-2). Invasive angiography is rarely required.

TABLE 30-1	Factors Associated with Predisposition to Aortic Dissection

Degeneration of the aortic wall
  Advanced age
  Chronic hypertension
Connective tissue disorders
  Marfan syndrome
  Ehlers-Danlos syndrome
  Familial aortic dissection syndromes
Inflammatory disorders
  Giant cell arteritis
  Takayasu arteritis
Iatrogenic injury
  Catheterization
  Intra-aortic balloon
  Aortic surgery
Congenital disorders
  Bicuspid aortic valve
  Aortic coarctation
  Turner's syndrome
  Noonan's syndrome
Pregnancy
Cocaine use

        (1) Contrast—enhanced computed tomography (CT)
        (2) Transesophageal echo (TEE)
        (3) Magnetic resonance angiography (MRA).
  E. Treatment (Fig. 30-1)
    1. Early surgical consultation is critical. Initial management of hemodynamically stable patient must focus on reducing adrenergic tone and lowering heart rate and dP/dt (Table 30-3).
    2. Type A dissection is a surgical emergency.
    3. Type B dissection is managed medically. Surgery carries high mortality and is reserved for patients with limb or visceral ischemia or contained rupture. Endovascular treatment may play a role in high-risk patients.
    4. Long-term management after initial stabilization requires control of hypertension; β-blocker therapy is central to any strategy to prevent aortic expansion. Periodic imaging of the aorta is essential to detect aneurysm formation, extension of dissection, and impending rupture.

III. INTRAMURAL HEMATOMA
  A. Background
    1. Intramural hematoma (IMH) comprises up to 20% of cases of acute aortic syndromes.
    2. Categorized by Stanford classification system (type A and type B).
  B. Pathophysiology
    1. Variant of AD.
    2. Spontaneous hematoma within the medial layer of the aorta without an identifiable intimal flap. Rupture of the vaso vasorum into the medial layer is most likely mechanism.
  C. Prognosis
    1. Dependent on Stanford classification and similar to that of AD.

TABLE 30-2 Advantages, Disadvantages, and Performance of Aortic Imaging Modalities for Aortic Dissection

Modality	Findings	Advantages	Disadvantages	Sensitivity (%)	Specificity (%)
Transthoracic echocardiography	Diagnostic: - undulating intimal flap in proximal aorta Suggestive: - aortic root dilatation - aortic insufficiency - pericardial effusion	- easy to obtain - performed at bedside - non-invasive	- visualization of aorta limited to aortic root - poor image quality in many patients	70–90 (Type A) 30–40 (Type B)	80
Transesophageal echocardiography	Diagnostic: - undulating intimal flap in aorta - differential flow in true and false lumens Intramural hematoma Suggestive: - aortic root dilatation - aortic insufficiency - pericardial effusion	- quick to perform - performed at bedside - descending aorta can be assessed - valvular and ventricular functional assessment possible	- specially trained personnel needed to perform test - aortic arch may be obscured from overlying bronchus	90–100	70–80
Computed Tomography	Diagnostic: - intimal flap within aorta - presence of dual lumens with differential contrast enhancement Suggestive: - aortic root dilatation - pericardial effusion	- readily available at most centers	- limited visualization of branch vessels - requires intravenous iodinated contrast - unable to assess aortic valve, ventricular function	90–100	80–90
Magnetic Resonance Imaging	Diagnostic: - intimal flap within aorta - presence of dual lumens Suggestive: - aortic root dilatation - pericardial effusion	- excellent sensitivity and specificity - no need for contrast agents - assessment of branch vessels	- not uniformly available - long scanning times - difficult to monitor patients during exam	95–100	95–100
Aortography	Diagnostic: - intimal flap within aorta - presence of dual lumens Suggestive: - aortic root dilation - aortic insufficiency	- excellent branch vessel visualization	- requires assembly of angiography team - requires iodinated contrast agents - invasive - unable to detect IMH - limited sensitivity if dual lumens equally opacified	80–90	90–96

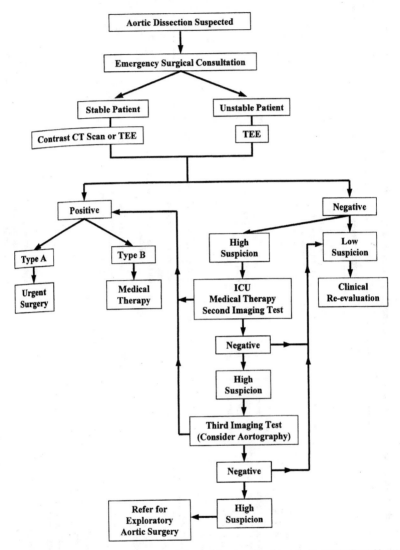

Figure 30-1. Suggested diagnostic and therapeutic algorithm for patients presenting with suspected acute aortic dissection or related entity. CT, computed tomography; ICU, intensive care unit; TEE, transesophageal echocardiogram. (From Shah PB and Beckman JA. Acute aortic syndromes. In: Irwin RS and Rippe JM, eds. *Irwin and Rippe's intensive care medicine*, 5th edition. Philadelphia: Lippincott Williams & Wilkins, 2003, with permission.)

D. Diagnosis

1. Clinical presentation indistinguishable from AD.
2. Pericardial effusion, hemothorax, and hemoperitoneum from rupture of the adventitia herald impending rupture.
3. Diagnosis is made by one of the imaging modalities used to diagnose AD (i.e., CT, TEE, and MRA).

TABLE 30-3	Medical Therapy for Hemodynamically Stable Acute Aortic Dissection		
Therapeutic Goal	**Medication**	**Suggested Dose**	**Desired response**
Pain relief	Morphine sulfate	1–2 mg IV q 3–5 minutes.	Pain relief resulting in reduction of sympathetic tone
Heart rate reduction	Metoprolol	2.5–5.0 mg IV q 2 minutes up to three doses. Follow with 5–10 mg IV q 4–6 hours.	Maintenance of heart rate to between 60 and 70 beats per minute
	Esmolol	500 mcg/kg IV bolus followed by continuous infusion of 50 mcg/kg/min. Titrate up to maximum of 300 mcg/kg/min.	Maintenance of heart rate to between 60 and 70 beats per minute
	Propranolol	1 mg IV q 3–5 minutes (not to exceed 10 mg). Follow with 2–6 mg IV q 4–6 hours.	Maintenance of heart rate to between 60 and 70 beats per minute
Heart rate/blood pressure reduction	Labetalol	20 mg IV over 2 minutes followed by 40 mg to 80 mg IV q 10–15 minutes to a maximum of 300 mg. Start IV infusion at 2 mg/min and titrate to 10mg/min.	Maintenance of heart rate to between 60 and 70 beats per minute; maintenance of systolic blood pressure between 100 and 110 mm Hg
Blood pressure reduction	Sodium nitroprusside	0.25–0.3 mcg/min IV infusion and titrate to 10 mcg/kg/min	Maintenance of systolic blood pressure between 100 and 110 mm Hg
Blood pressure reduction in setting of renal artery involvement	Enalaprilat	0.625–1.25 mg IV q 6 hours	Maintenance of systolic blood pressure between 100 and 110 mm Hg

E. Treatment

1. Initial management identical to that of AD (see Fig. 30-1 and Table 30-3)
2. Surgical repair is recommended for type A IMH (surgical mortality rate of 8% versus 55% with medical therapy).
3. Type B IMH can be managed medically but warrants careful clinical follow-up and serial imaging. Late progression of IMH to dissection, aneurysm, or rupture can be as high as 21%.

IV. PENETRATING ATHEROSCLEROTIC ULCER

A. Background

1. Penetrating atherosclerotic ulcer (PAU) more common in elderly patients with hypertension and severe aortic atherosclerosis.
2. Preferentially involves the descending thoracic and abdominal aorta.

B. Pathophysiology

1. Severe atherosclerotic lesion ulcerates, penetrates through the intimal layer, and results in a discrete ulcer crater.
2. Propagation to dissection can occur but is rare: ulceration can extend through the adventitia resulting in pseudoaneurysm formation or frank aortic rupture. Symptomatic ulcers or ulcers with deep erosion are more likely to rupture. Stable PAU will often progress to aneurysmal dilatation of the aorta.

C. Clinical presentation

1. Occurs in patients with multiple atherosclerotic risk factors and marked systemic atherosclerosis
2. Most patients, if they have symptoms, present with the acute onset of pain in the chest and/or the back and hypertension.
3. Pericardial tamponade, myocardial ischemia, and aortic insufficiency are uncommon because the ascending aorta is a very unusual location for PAU.

D. Diagnosis

1. Diagnosis can be established with contrast CTA, TEE, or MRA.

E. Treatment

1. Optimal treatment strategy of patients with PAU is unknown. Medical therapy is initial choice in absence of false aneurysm formation, frank rupture, or recurrent pain.
2. Blood pressure must be controlled to reduce the shear stress and pulse pressure against the ulcer (Table 30-2).
3. Patients with hemodynamic instability, evidence of aortic rupture, or pseudoaneurysm should undergo immediate surgical therapy.
4. Elective surgical repair indicated in patients with intractable pain, distal embolization from thrombus within the ulcer, or progressive aneurysmal dilatation of the aorta. Endovascular stent grafting is likely to play a future role.
5. Stable patients with PAU must be followed with serial imaging studies.
6. Risk factor modification includes lipid-lowering therapy and smoking cessation.

V. RUPTURED AORTIC ANEURYSM

A. Background

1. Annual incidence of ruptured abdominal aortic aneurysm (AAA) and thoracic aortic aneurysm (TAA) is estimated at 5 to 7 and 3.5 per 100,000 persons, respectively.
2. Due to the progressive risk of rupture with increasing aneurysm diameter, elective repair is recommended when the diameter of the thoracic aorta reaches 6 cm (5 cm in patients with Marfan syndrome) and that of the abdominal aorta reaches 5 to 5.5cm.

B. Prognosis

1. Prognosis of ruptured TAA or AAA is grim. Of patients who develop rupture, 60% will die prior to presentation to medical attention.
2. Operative mortality for patients reaching medical attention is nearly 50%; however, mortality is 100% without surgical intervention.

C. Diagnosis

1. Clinical presentation
   a. Diagnosis should be considered in all patients presenting with acute hemodynamic instability and new onset back, chest, or abdominal pain.
   b. The classic triad of abdominal pain, hypotension, and a pulsatile abdominal mass is present in less than one third of patients and supports the diagnosis of ruptured AAA.

    c. Ruptured TAA can present with acute hemothorax or hemorrhagic pericardial effusion and tamponade. The most common site of rupture is in the descending thoracic aorta.

  2. Diagnostic testing

    a. Imaging studies (CT or abdominal ultrasound) should be obtained only in the stable patient. If there is clinical concern of ruptured TAA or AAA in an unstable patient, immediate surgical exploration should be pursued.

D. Treatment

  1. Ruptured TAA or AAA is a surgical emergency. Immediate surgical consultation is critical for patients with symptomatic or aneurysms with suspected rupture.

Selected Readings

Clouse WD, et al. Acute aortic dissection: population-based incidence compared with degenerative aortic aneurysm rupture. *Mayo Clin Proc* 2004;79(2):176–180.
This study describes the incidence, operative intervention rate, and long-term survival rate of Olmsted County, Minnesota, residents with a clinical diagnosis of acute aortic dissection initially made between 1980 and 1994.

Dake MD, et al. Endovascular stent-graft placement for the treatment of acute aortic dissection. *N Engl J Med* 1999;340(20):1546–1552.
One of the first experiences with stent grafts used for treatment of aortic dissection.

Hagan PG, et al. The International Registry of Acute Aortic Dissection (IRAD): new insights into an old disease. *JAMA* 2000;283(7):897–903.
The IRAD registry describes presentation, management and outcomes of 464 patients with type A and B dissection presenting in the modern era.

Harris JA, et al. Penetrating atherosclerotic ulcers of the aorta. *J Vasc Surg* 1994;19(1):90–98; discussion 98–99.
Discussion of the presentation, natural history, and early experience in of this aortic syndrome.

Hirst AE, Jr, Johns VJ Jr., Kime SW, Jr. Dissecting aneurysm of the aorta: a review of 505 cases. *Medicine (Baltimore)* 1958;37(3):217–279.
A classic paper describing the natural history of aortic dissection.

Hollier LH, Taylor LM, and Ochsner J. Recommended indications for operative treatment of abdominal aortic aneurysms. Report of a subcommittee of the Joint Council of the Society for Vascular Surgery and the North American Chapter of the International Society for Cardiovascular Surgery. *J Vasc Surg* 1992;15(6):1046-1-56.
This consensus statement describes prognosis of patients with catastrophic rupture of aortic aneurysms.

Kaji S, et al. Long-term prognosis of patients with type B aortic intramural hematoma. *Circulation* 2003;108(suppl 1):II307–311.
This report examined 110 patients in Japan with type B aortic dissection or intramural hematoma, focusing on the difference in clinical course between these two entities.

Maraj R, et al. Meta-analysis of 143 reported cases of aortic intramural hematoma. *Am J Cardiol* 2000;86(6):664–668.
This meta-analysis contributed to our understanding of acute intramural hematoma by analyzing the demographic profiles, imaging modalities, pathologic sites, and treatment strategies in relation to outcome in 143 patients with intramural hematoma.

Nienaber CA, Eagle KA. Aortic dissection: new frontiers in diagnosis and management: part I: from etiology to diagnostic strategies. *Circulation* 2003;108(5):628–635.
This review article summarizes current understanding of the pathophysiology of acute aortic syndromes and discusses new developments in their diagnosis.

Sawhney, NS, DeMaria AN, Blanchard DG. Aortic intramural hematoma: an increasingly recognized and potentially fatal entity. *Chest* 2001;120(4):1340–1346.
This review article outlines the pathophysiology, presentation, diagnosis, and management of intramural hematoma.

Shinohara T, et al. Soluble elastin fragments in serum are elevated in acute aortic dissection. *Arterioscler Thromb Vasc Biol* 2003;23(10):1839–1844.
Elastin, an integral component of the aortic wall is released into the bloodstream during aortic wall injury and can serve as a marker of aortic dissection.

Suzuki T, et al. Diagnostic implications of elevated levels of smooth-muscle myosin heavy-chain protein in acute aortic dissection. The smooth muscle myosin heavy chain study. *Ann Intern Med* 2000;133(7):537–541.
Although no biochemical diagnostic assays are currently in clinical use, this study presents initial data on detection of smooth muscle myosin heavy chain in acute aortic dissection and its potential use as a diagnostic tool.

von Kodolitsch Y, et al. Chest radiography for the diagnosis of acute aortic syndrome. *Am J Med* 2004;116(2):73–77.
Chest radiographs on 216 patients presenting with acute aortic syndromes were evaluated to assess their accuracy as a diagnostic tool.

von Kodolitsch Y, et al. Intramural hematoma of the aorta: predictors of progression to dissection and rupture. *Circulation* 2003;107(8):1158–1163.
This multicenter study reports on the natural history of 66 patients presenting with acute intramural hematoma.

I. DEFINITIONS

A. *Hypertensive crisis* is defined as a severe elevation in blood pressure.

   1. *Hypertensive emergencies* and *urgencies* are categories of hypertensive crises that are potentially life-threatening and may occur with chronic essential hypertension, with secondary forms of hypertension, or *de novo* (Table 31-1).

   2. Usually associated with diastolic blood pressures higher than 120 to 130 mm Hg.

B. *Hypertensive emergencies* and *urgencies* are differentiated by the presence or absence of acute and progressive target organ damage (TOD).

   1. In *hypertensive emergencies,* blood pressure elevation is associated with ongoing central nervous system, myocardial, hematologic, or renal TOD.

   2. In *hypertensive urgencies,* the potential for TOD damage is great and likely if blood pressure is not soon controlled.

C. *Accelerated hypertension* and *malignant hypertension* are subcategories of hypertensive crises with exudative retinopathy. They probably represent a continuum of organ damage.

   1. *Accelerated hypertension*: a hypertensive crisis with grade III Keith-Wagener-Barker retinopathy (vasoconstriction and sclerosis [i.e., grades I or II] plus hemorrhages and exudates making this grade III). Exudate is more worrisome than hemorrhage alone.

   2. *Malignant hypertension:* a hypertensive crisis with the presence of Keith-Wagener-Barker grade IV retinopathy plus papilledema.

II. APPROACH TO THE PATIENT

A. In the ICU, therapy must often begin before a comprehensive patient evaluation is completed. A systematic approach offers the opportunity to be both expeditious and inclusive (Table 31-2).

B. A brief history and physical examination should be initiated to assess the degree of TOD and to rule out obvious secondary causes of hypertension.

C. History

   1. History of hypertension or other significant medical disease

   2. Medication use and compliance.

   3. Symptoms attributable to TOD

      a. Neurologic (headache, nausea, and vomiting; visual changes; seizures; focal deficits; mental status changes)

      b. Cardiac (chest pain, shortness of breath)

      c. Renal (hematuria, decreased urine output)

D. Physical examination

   1. Blood pressure readings in both arms. Intraarterial monitoring may be necessary.

   2. Signs of neurologic ischemia, such as altered mental status or focal neurologic deficits

   3. Direct ophthalmologic examination

   4. Auscultation of the lungs and heart

   5. Evaluation of the abdomen and peripheral pulses for bruits, masses, or deficits

E. Ancillary and laboratory evaluation

   1. Electrolytes, blood urea nitrogen and creatinine, complete blood count with differential, assessment of cardiac function, and chest radiography

TABLE 31-1	**Examples of Hypertensive Crises**		

Generalized	Cardiovascular	Neurologic	Renal
Accelerated and malignant hypertension	Acute left ventricular failure	Hypertensive encephalopathy	Acute renal failure
Microangiopathic hemolytic anemia/disseminated intravascular coagulation	Unstable angina pectoris	Subarachnoid hemorrhage	Acute glomerulonephritis
Eclampsia	Myocardial infarction	Intracerebral hemorrhage	Scleroderma crisis
Catecholamine excess (drugs, rebound syndrome, pheochromocytoma	Aortic dissection	Cerebrovascular accident	
Vasculitis	Suture integrity after surgery		

From Vidt DG, Gifford RW. A compendium for the treatment of hypertensive emergencies. *Cleve Clin Q* 1984; 51:421, with permission.

III. TREATMENT

A. The intensity of intervention is determined by the clinical situation.

B. Goal of initial therapy is to terminate ongoing TOD, *not* to return blood pressure to normal levels because cerebral autoregulation determines the initial stop point.

C. Goal is approximately 25% lower than the initial mean arterial pressure or a diastolic blood pressure in the range of 110 to 100 mm Hg.

   1. Patients with acute left ventricular failure, myocardial ischemia, or aortic dissection may require more aggressive treatment

   2. Interventions such as intubation, control of seizures, hemodynamic monitoring, and maintenance of urine output can be as important as prompt control of blood pressure.

TABLE 31-2	**Initial Evaluation of Hypertensive Crisis in the Intensive Care Unit**

Continuous blood pressure monitoring
Direct (intraarterial) preferred
Indirect (cuff)
   Brief initial evaluation—history and physical examination with attention to neurologic, cardiac, pulmonary, renal symptoms
Organ perfusion and function
Blood and urine studies: electrolytes, BUN, creatinine, CBC with differential, urinalysis with sediment; if indicated, serum catecholamines, cardiac enzymes
ECG
Chest radiograph
Initiation of therapy
Further evaluation of etiology once stabilized

BUN, blood urea nitrogen; CBC, complete blood count; ECG, electrocardiogram.
From Vidt DG, Gifford RW. A compendium for the treatment of hypertensive emergencies. *Cleve Clin Q* 1984; 51: 421, with permission.

D. Oral versus parenteral therapy
   1. In the intensive care unit, parenteral therapy with close hemodynamic monitoring is preferred to most quickly and reliably reduce the blood pressure.
   2. Avoid initial reductions in blood pressure more than 20% to 25% because it may exacerbate TOD if evidence of cardiac, cerebrovascular, or renovascular disease is present.

IV. SCENARIOS OF HYPERTENSION
   A. New onset of hypertension
      1. Secondary causes, such as pain, anxiety, new onset of angina, hypercarbia or hypoxia, hypothermia, rigors, excessive arousal after sedation, or fluid mobilization with volume overload, can all lead to short-term elevations in blood pressure.
      2. If antihypertensive agents are necessary, low doses of short-acting agents should be used to avoid sharp drops in blood pressure in this usually self-limited situation.
   B. Perioperative hypertension
      1. Preoperative. Moderate chronic hypertension is not a major risk factor for surgery, "but it is a marker for potential coronary artery disease. β-Blockers have been shown to reduce perioperative cardiovascular complications.
      2. Perioperative. Blood pressure higher than 160/100 mm Hg or an increase of more than 30 mm Hg (systolic or diastolic) above preoperative are worrisome.
      3. Postoperative. Blood pressures can vary widely due to an increase in pressor reflexes and central nervous system activity due to pain, hypothermia with shivering, hypercarbia and hypoxia, or reflex excitement after anesthesia.

V. PHARMACOLOGIC AGENTS (Table 31-3)
   A. Direct vasodilators
      1. Sodium nitroprusside: the most predictable and effective agent for the treatment of severe hypertension. It dilates both arterioles and venules (reducing both afterload and preload) and lowers myocardial oxygen demands.
      2. Nitroglycerin: predominantly dilates the venous system. Useful in patients with cardiac ischemia or congestive heart failure.
      3. Hydralazine: a direct parenteral arterial vasodilator that increases cardiac output and heart rate.
   B. β-Blockers
      1. Parenteral agents include labetalol (nonselective), propranolol (nonselective), metoprolol (selective), and the short-acting esmolol (selective).
   C. Calcium antagonists
      1. Nifedipine: decreases peripheral vascular resistance and increases collateral coronary blood flow in an uncontrolled and unpredictable manner and may result in serious complications
      2. Nicardipine: a rapid-acting systemic and coronary artery vasodilator with minimal effects on cardiac conductivity or inotropy
      3. Nimodipine: recommended only for patients with subarachnoid hemorrhage
      4. Verapamil: an arterial vasodilator that delays atrioventricular conduction and has a negative inotropic effect
      5. Diltiazem: effects intermediate between those of verapamil and of the dihydropyridine group
   D. Angiotensin-converting enzyme inhibitors
      1. Captopril: rapid onset of effect after oral administration (30 minutes) with little change in cardiac output or reflex tachycardia
      2. Enalaprilat: the only parenteral angiotensin-converting enzyme inhibitor
   E. Central agonist:
      1. Clonidine: an oral or transdermal alpha$_2$ central agonist that decreases peripheral vascular resistance. Takes several days to achieve a steady state.
   F. Diuretics: not considered primary agents in managing hypertensive crises because most patients are hypovolemic. In patients who are volume overloaded, loop diuretics, such as furosemide or bumetanide, can help control intravascular volume and maintain urine output.

| TABLE 31-3 | Proper Dosing for Agents to Treat Hypertensive Crisis |

Agent	Administration	Onset	Duration
Direct vasodilators			
Nitroprusside	i.v. infusion: 0.25–10.0 mg/kg/min	Immediate	1–2 min
Nitroglycerin	i.v. bolus: 50–100 mg q10–15 min (total 600 mg); i.v. infusion: 5–200 mg/min	2–5 min	5–10 min
b-Blockers			
Esmolol	250–500 mg/kg/min for 1 min; then 50–100 mg/kg/min/ for 4 min; may repeat	5–10 min	3–5 min
Labetalol	i.v. bolus: 20–80 mg q10 min; i.v. infusion: 2 mg/min	5–10 min	2–4 h
Calcium antagonists			
Nicardipine	i.v. infusion: 5–15 mg/h	5–10 min	1-2 h
Nimodipine	i.v. infusion: 5–10 mg/h ↑ by mg/h, up to 15 mg q30 min, 60 mg q4h × 21 days; repeat	15–30 min	3–6 h
Angiotensin-converting enzyme inhibitors			
Captopril	p.o. 6.25–25 mg, repeat q30 min, if necessary	1 h	1–4 h
Enalaprilat	i.v. bolus: 1.25–5.0 mg (over 5 min) q6h	15–50 min	6–8 h
Central agonists			
Clonidine	p.o. 0.2 mg initially; 0.2 mg/h (total 0.7 mg)		3 h
Miscellaneous			
Fenoldopam	i.v. infusion: 0.1 mg/kg/min; ↑ by 0.05–0.2 mg/kg/h at 20-min intervals	5 min	15–30 min
Hydralazine	i.v. bolus: 10–20 mg	10–20 min	1–4 h
Trimethaphan	i.v. infusion: 0.5–5 mg/min	1–5 min	5–15 min
Phentolamine	i.v. 5–10 mg/min	1–2 min	10–20 min

i.v., intravenous; p.o., oral.

Selected Readings

Breslin DJ, Gifford RW, Fairbairn JF, et al. Prognostic importance of ophthalmoscopic findings in essential hypertension. *JAMA* 1966;195:91.
   The fundoscopic examination, frequently overlooked in daily clinical practice, provides important prognostic information in patients with hypertension.

Calhoun DA, Oparil S. Treatment of hypertensive crisis. *N Engl J Med* 1990;323:1177.
   A review of treatment strategies for use in hypertensive crisis.

Chobanian AV, Bakris GL, Black HR, et al. Seventh report of the Joint National Committee on Prevention, Detection, Evaluation, and Treatment of High Blood Pressure. *Hypertension.* 2003;42:1206–1252.
A complete review of hypertension with specific sections on the treatment of hypertensive emergencies with expert recommendations.

Mangano DT, Layug EL, Wallace A, et al. Effect of atenolol on mortality and cardiovascular morbidity after noncardiac surgery. *N Engl J Med* 1996;335:1713.
β-Blocker therapy has a favorable impact on outcome among patients undergoing noncardiac surgery.

Vaughan CJ, Delanty N. Hypertensive emergencies. *Lancet* 2000;356:411–417.
Focused review of pathophysiology, diagnosis, complications, and management of hypertensive emergencies.

Vidt DG, Gifford RW. A compendium for the treatment of hypertensive emergencies. *Cleve Clin Q* 1984;51:421.
Two of the leaders in hypertension provide an overview of treatment modalities.

32 SYNCOPE
William H. Maisel

I. GENERAL PRINCIPLES
  A. Definition: Sudden/transient loss of consciousness with loss of postural tone.
  B. Accounts for 3% of emergency room visits and 1% to 6% of all hospital admissions.
  C. Cost of diagnosis and treatment approaches $750 million dollars per year.

II. PATHOPHYSIOLOGY
  A. Caused by hypoxia/hypoperfusion of the cerebral cortices and reticular activating system.
  B. Systolic blood pressure less than 70 mm Hg or interruption of cerebral blood flow for 8 to 10 seconds usually results in syncope.
  C. Seizures cause loss of consciousness through global interruption of cerebral electrical activity without necessarily impairing blood flow.

III. DIAGNOSIS
  A. Differential diagnosis
    1. A number of different disease processes can cause syncope (Table 32-1).
    2. Reflex mediated syncope and orthostatic intolerance are most common, whereas neurological, cardiovascular, and psychogenic causes occur with decreasing frequency.
    3. Up to 45% of patients will be labeled as having "syncope of unknown cause" despite a thorough evaluation.
    4. Etiology of syncope has important prognostic significance
    5. In absence of implantable defibrillator, syncope of cardiac etiology has 1-year mortality of 20% to 30% compared with 0% to 12% for patients with noncardiovascular causes of syncope and 6% for those with syncope of unknown etiology.
    6. Younger patients more frequently have syncope due to noncardiovascular cause or syncope of unknown origin and overall have a more favorable prognosis.
    7. Older patients more often have a cardiac etiology or syncope due to polypharmacy.
  B. Initial diagnostic evaluation
    1. Algorithm for the approach to the patient with syncope (Fig. 32-1).
    2. Goal is to differentiate between benign and potentially life-threatening causes.
    3. Presence of cardiovascular disease identifies patients at increased risk of sudden death.
    4. History and physical examination alone allow diagnosis of syncope cause in 45% of patients and suggest a diagnosis in another 40%.
  C. History
    1. Obtain patient's and eyewitnesses' reports of event.
    2. Search for situational or provocative factors, postural or exertional symptoms, and symptoms of cardiac or neurologic origin.
    3. Take a careful medication history.
    4. Past medical history should focus on prior syncopal events, as well as prior cardiac, neurologic, and psychiatric history.
    5. Family history for familial cardiomyopathy, sudden cardiac death, or syncope should also be sought.

TABLE 32-1	Differential Diagnosis of Syncope

Cardiovascular	
Arrhythmia	**Low cardiac output**
Bradyarrhythmia	Obstruction to flow
Sinus node disease	Aortic stenosis
AV node disease	Mitral stenosis
Drug induced	Tricuspid stenosis
Pacemaker malfunction	Hypertrophic cardiomyopathy
	Atrial myxoma
Tachyarrhythmia	Pulmonary stenosis
Ventricular arrhythmias	Pulmonary embolism
Supraventricular arrhythmias	Pulmonary hypertension
	Cardiac tamponade
	Aortic dissection
	Pump failure (cardiomyopathy, MI)

Disorders of autonomic control	
Autonomic insufficiency	
Diabetes mellitus	
Parkinson's disease	
Primary	
Reflex mediated	
Neurocardiogenic (vasovagal/vasodepressor)	
Carotid sinus hypersensitivity	
Situational (cough, defecation, micturition, swallow)	
Neuralgia (trigeminal, glossopharyngeal)	

Neurologic	**Psychiatric**
Cerebrovascular disease (CVA, TIA)	Anxiety disorder/panic disorder
Seizure	Major depression
Hyperventilation	Somatization
Migraine	Münchhausen's
Narcolepsy	Substance abuse
Subclavian steal	

Orthostatic hypotension	**Metabolic**
Volume depletion	Hypoadrenalism
Medication related	Hypoglycemia
	Hypothyroidism
	Hypoxia

AV, atrioventricular; CVA, cerebrovascular accident; MI, myocardial infarction; TIA, transient ischemic attack.

6. Tongue biting, aching muscles, or disorientation following a syncopal episode suggests a seizure, whereas sweating, nausea, vertigo, incontinence, injury, headache, family history of epilepsy, and history of prior concussion are not predictive of seizures.

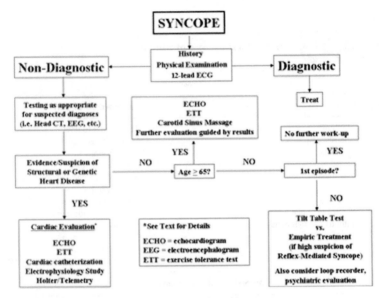

Figure 32-1. Algorithm for the approach to the patient with syncope.

D. Physical examination
1. Should focus on identifying potential clues as to the etiology of the syncopal episode.
2. Orthostatic hypotension as etiology of syncope should be diagnosed only when the history and examination are consistent and other potential etiologies of syncope have been excluded.
3. Murmurs, bruits, signs of heart failure, and so forth might suggest cardiovascular etiology.
4. Neurologic abnormalities such as diplopia, headache, or other focal signs may suggest a neurologic etiology.

E. 12-Lead electrocardiogram (ECG)
1. Half the patients who present with syncope have significant baseline ECG abnormalities.
2. The ECG alone is diagnostic of the cause of syncope in less than 10% of cases.
3. An abnormal ECG suggests the presence of underlying heart disease and warrants further evaluation.
4. The ECG is the only way to diagnose some genetic disorders, including long QT syndrome and Brugada syndrome.

F. Laboratory tests
1. Routine laboratory evaluation not recommended.
2. Blood chemistries and hematologic assessments are appropriate as guided by the history and physical examination.

G. Further cardiac evaluation (Table 32-2)
1. Telemetry/24-hour Holter monitoring
   a. Diagnostic in up to 20% of selected patients (symptoms during monitoring either with or without arrhythmia).
   b. The majority of patients have no symptoms and no arrhythmia during monitoring.
   c. Patient-activated loop recorders, event monitors, and implantable recorders can be used for patients with infrequent but recurrent episodes.

TABLE 32-2	Indications for Cardiac Tests in Patients with Syncope

Test	Indication
Electrocardiogram	All patients at initial presentation
Echocardiogram	Patients with known or suspected cardiac disease (including patients with chest pain, heart murmur, abnormal electrocardiogram, etc.)
Exercise tolerance test	Patients with chest pain, ischemic changes on electrocardiogram, or exercise-induced or postexertional syncope (who do not undergo cardiac catheterization)
Tilt table test	Patients with recurrent syncope or patients with a single episode of syncope accompanied by physical injury, motor vehicle accident, or high-risk setting (pilot, surgeon, window washer, etc.) thought to be vasovagal. Indicated in patients with unexplained syncope after other appropriate workup.
Holter or inpatient ECG telemetry	Patients with symptoms suggestive of arrhythmic syncope (brief loss of consciousness, no prodrome, presence of palpitations), unexplained cause of syncope, underlying heart disease, or an abnormal electrocardiogram
Electrophysiologic studies	Patients with known or suspected structural heart disease and unexplained syncope or patients with no organic heart disease but recurrent syncope and a negative tilt table test

2. Echocardiography
   a. Part of the initial evaluation for patients with known or suspected cardiac disease.
   b. Unselected patients have unanticipated findings 5% to 10% of the time.
3. Exercise testing
   a. Part of the initial evaluation of patients with suspected ischemia or exercise-induced arrhythmias
   b. Rarely reveals the precise cause of syncope (less than 1% have an arrhythmia during exercise testing).
4. Electrophysiology (EP) studies
   a. Well established for detecting ventricular and supraventricular arrhythmias but less sensitive for detecting bradyarrhythmias.
   b. Diagnostic yield is approximately 30% to 50% in patients with syncope.
   c. Low yield in patients without structural heart disease.
   d. Patients with normal hearts and normal ECGs rarely require electrophysiology testing.
   e. A "positive" EP study predicts an increased 3-year sudden death and total mortality rate compared to patients with negative EP studies.
   f. EP studies are insensitive for the detection of arrhythmias in nonischemic cardiomyopathy.
5. Signal average ECG (SAECG) and T wave Alternans
   a. Noninvasive test used to identify higher and lower risk patients.
   b. May be considered as an adjunct to other tests in the evaluation for arrhythmia, but it is not routinely indicated
H. **Evaluation for disorders of autonomic control/reflex-mediated syncope**
   1. A number of syncope syndromes are related to abnormal control of autonomic function (see Table 32-1).

2. More than 50% of patients with syncope of undetermined etiology may have neurally mediated syncope.
3. Tilt table test
   a. May be used to diagnose neurocardiogenic (also known as vasodepressor or vasovagal) syncope.
   b. Among patients with syncope of unknown origin, 25% to 50% will have positive tilt table tests with passive tilt alone, and up to two thirds will have positive tests with the use of isoproterenol.
   c. False-positive (10% to 30%) and false-negative (30% to 35%) test results are common.
4. Carotid sinus massage
   a. Performed by firm massage of the carotid artery for 5 to 10 seconds in an attempt to elicit a baroreflex-mediated vagal response that can cause bradycardia and/or hypotension.
   b. A positive test is: 3 or more seconds of asystole, a 50 mm Hg or greater systolic blood pressure decrease, or a 40 beats per minute or greater decrease in heart rate.
   c. Should not be performed in patients with a carotid bruit, recent myocardial infarction, recent stroke, or history of VT.

I. Neurologic evaluation
1. Patients with focal neurologic signs or symptoms should undergo further evaluation.
2. Additional neurologic testing is rarely indicated in the absence of specific clinical abnormalities or suspicion.
3. Electroencephalography (EEG)
   a. Yields diagnosis of seizure disorder in less than 2% of unselected patients with syncope referred for EEG.
   b. Not recommended as part of the routine evaluation of patients with syncope but should be considered when seizure is strongly suspected.
4. Head computed tomography (CT)
   a. Yields a positive finding in less than 5% of patients with syncope.
   b. Unsuspected central nervous system abnormalities are found in less than 1% of patients without neurologic abnormality on history or physical examination.
   c. Should be reserved for patients with neurologic abnormality and those who have suffered head trauma.

J. Psychiatric evaluation
1. Up to 25% of patients with syncope of unknown etiology have a *Diagnostic and Statistical Manual of Mental Disorders,* fourth edition (DSM-IV) psychiatric diagnosis of panic disorder, generalized anxiety disorder, or major depression.
2. Screening for psychiatric disorders is recommended for patients with recurrent syncope of unclear etiology.

IV. TREATMENT
   A. Hospital admission is suggested for patients with syncope who have:
   1. A history or suspicion of coronary artery disease, chronic heart failure (CHF), or ventricular arrhythmia
   2. Physical signs of significant valve disease, CHF, stroke, or focal neurological disorder
   3. ECG findings of ischemia, arrhythmia, increased QT interval, or bundle branch block
   4. Syncope with injury, rapid heart action, chest pain, or exertion
   5. Frequent episodes
   6. Moderate to severe orthostatic hypotension
   7. Age greater than 70
   B. Intensive care unit (ICU) admission should be strongly considered in syncope patients with sustained ventricular tachycardia (VT), symptomatic nonsustained VT, second- or third-degree heart block, pauses greater than 3 seconds, symptomatic

bradycardia, severe aortic stenosis, severe CHF, evidence of acute ischemia, or ongoing hemodynamic instability.

C. Specific treatment

    1. Arrhythmia. Guidelines for implantation of permanent pacemakers and implantable cardioverter-defibrillators for patients with syncope are summarized in Table 32-3.

    2. Neurally mediated syndromes

        a. Primary treatment is hydration and salt repletion.

        b. β-Adrenergic blockers, selective serotonin-reuptake inhibitors (e.g., fluoxetine), and α-adrenergic agonists (midodrine) have demonstrated efficacy in randomized trials.

        c. Other agents, including volume expanders (e.g., fludrocortisone) and disopyramide, appear useful in some patients.

        d. Patients with recurrent, medically refractory vasovagal syncope associated with marked bradycardia may benefit from implantation of a permanent pacemaker.

        e. Can consider pacemaker implantation in patients with severe bradycardic response to carotid sinus massage after other potential causes of syncope are excluded.

TABLE 32-3	Current ACC/AHA Guidelines for Implantation of Permanent Pacemakers and Implantable Cardioverter-Defibrillators in Patients with Syncope

Device	Indications for implantation[a]
Pacemaker	• Symptomatic sinus pauses or sinus bradycardia (I)
	• Bradycardia and second- or third-degree AV block (I)
	• Recurrent syncope caused by carotid sinus stimulation; minimal carotid sinus pressure induces ventricular asystole of >3 seconds duration in the absence of any medication that depresses sinus node or AV conduction (I)
	• Major abnormalities of sinus node function or AV conduction discovered or provoked at electrophysiology study (IIa)
	• Chronic bifascicular or trifascicular block and syncope not proved to be due to AV block when other likely causes have been excluded, specifically VT (IIa)
	• Recurrent syncope without clear provocative events and with a hypersensitive cardioinhibitory response (IIa)
	• Neurally mediated syncope with significant bradycardia reproduced by a head-up tilt with or without isoproterenol or other provocative maneuvers (IIb)
ICD	• Clinically relevant, hemodynamically significant sustained VT or VF induced at electrophysiology study when drug therapy is ineffective, not tolerated, or not preferred (I)
	• Ventricular dysfunction and inducible ventricular arrhythmias at electrophysiologic study when other causes of syncope have been excluded (IIb)

[a]Indication class in parentheses
Class I: Evidence and/or general agreement that treatment is beneficial
Class IIa: Conflicting evidence and/or divergence of opinion but weight of evidence/opinion is in favor of treatment
Class IIb: Conflicting evidence and/or divergence of opinion with treatment efficacy less well established
ACC, American College of Cardiology; AHA, American Heart Association; AV, atrioventricular; ICD, implantable cardioverter-defibrillator; VT, ventricular tachycardia; VF, ventricular fibrillation

   3. Psychiatric causes. Treatment of the underlying psychiatric disorder abolishes recurrent episodes in most patients.
   D. Special considerations
   1. Patients suspected of having arrhythmic syncope should not drive, pending diagnosis and treatment.
   2. Many states require a 3- to 12-month driving restriction following a syncopal episode.
   3. State laws vary with respect to the patient's and physician's responsibility to report individuals with syncope to their respective department of motor vehicles. Physicians should become familiar with their local requirements.

Selected Readings

Benditt DG, Ferguson DW, Grubb BP, et al. Tilt table testing for assessing syncope. *JACC* 1996;28:263–275.
An excellent review of tilt table testing.

Calkins H. Pharmacologic approaches to therapy for vasovagal syncope. *Am J Cardiol* 1999;84:20Q–25Q.
Excellent review of treatment options for vasovagal syncope.

Gregoratos G, Cheitlin MD, Conill A, et al. ACC/AHA guidelines for implantation of cardiac pacemakers and antiarrhythmia devices: Executive summary. *Circulation* 1998; 97:1325–1335.
Guidelines for which syncope patients should be treated with device therapy.

Grubb BP. Pathophysiology and differential diagnosis of neurocardiogenic syncope. *Am J Cardiol* 1999;84:3Q–9Q.
Comprehensive overview of neurocardiogenic syncope.

Kapoor WN. Evaluation and management of the patient with syncope. *JAMA* 1992; 268:2553–2560.
Classic article on syncope.

Kapoor WN. Syncope. *N Engl J Med* 2000;343:1856–1862.
Classic article on syncope.

Linzer M, Yang EH, Estes III NAM, et al. Diagnosing syncope part 2: unexplained syncope. *Ann Intern Med* 1997;127:76–86.
A review of how to approach the challenge of the patient with unexplained syncope.

Linzer M, Yang EH, Estes III NAM, et al. Diagnosing syncope part 1: value of history, physical examination, and electrocardiography. *Ann Intern Med* 1997;126:989–996.
An excellent review of the diagnostic evaluation of patients with syncope.

Maisel WH, Stevenson WG. Syncope—getting to the heart of the matter. *N Engl J Med* 2002;347:931–933.
A brief review of the approach to the syncope patient.

Soteriades ES, Evans JC, Larson MG, et al. Incidence and prognosis of syncope. *N Engl J Med* 2002;347:878–885.
A comprehensive study on the incidence and prognosis of syncope in the modern era.

Zipes DP, DiMarco JP, Gillette PC, et al. ACC/AHA guidelines for clinical intracardiac electrophysiological and catheter ablation procedures. *Circulation* 1995;92:675–691.
Guidelines to help assist decision making regarding which syncope patients require invasive evaluation.

CARDIAC AND THORACIC-AORTIC TRAUMA

Thomas A. Abbruzzese, Jonathan D. Gates, and John G. Byrne

33

I. PENETRATING CARDIAC INJURY

A. General principles

1. Despite advanced prehospital care, only a minority of patients reach the hospital alive.
2. These injuries are usually the result of violent conflicts involving knives and guns and are less frequently caused by traffic or occupational or recreational accidents.
3. Stab wounds usually lead to single-chamber injury, whereas gunshot wounds frequently lead to multiple-chamber injury, as well as concomitant injuries to other organ systems, resulting in higher mortality.

B. Presentation

1. All penetrating injuries to the chest, neck, and upper abdomen should prompt a thorough evaluation for intrathoracic injury, including cardiac injury.
2. Hypotension is present in almost all patients with penetrating cardiac trauma, but it is not specific and indicates neither the site of injury nor the underlying pathology.
3. Hemopericardium and pericardial tamponade present acutely with a dramatic increase in intrapericardial pressures and impairment of cardiac output. The classic Beck's triad (distant heart sounds, distended jugular veins, and decreased arterial pressure) is not common in hypovolemic patients, making the diagnosis of tamponade difficult.
4. Hemorrhage due to free wall or coronary vessel laceration, or great vessel injury usually manifests as hemothorax and hypovolemia. Chest tubes will exhibit significant drainage, heralding the immediate need for exploration in the emergency room or operating room.

C. Diagnosis

1. Chest radiograph (CXR), although a useful diagnostic tool in trauma, is of little value in penetrating cardiac trauma.
2. Echocardiography is the study of choice, because it can be performed in the trauma resuscitation room and offers accurate, rapid identification of pericardial tamponade or bleeding.
3. The definitive diagnosis of cardiac trauma is established in the operating room.

D. Treatment

1. Emergency department management
   a. All penetrating wounds between the right midclavicular and left midaxillary lines (Fig. 33-1) should be assumed to involve the heart. Impaled objects should be left *in situ*, if possible, until operative exploration.
   b. Treatment begins with the initial survey including airway, breathing, and circulation.
   c. Large-caliber upper extremity intravenous access is established, and volume resuscitation is initiated with crystalloid, colloid, and/or O negative blood.
   d. Hemodynamically stable patients (either initially or after fluid resuscitation) should undergo diagnostic evaluation including thorough physical examination, CXR, and echocardiogram (Figs. 33-2 and 33-3).
   e. Hemodynamically unstable patients (SBP less than 80 to 90 mm Hg or cardiopulmonary arrest) are intubated and a large-bore chest tube is inserted (for absent or decreased breath sounds) to evacuate pneumothorax or hemothorax.

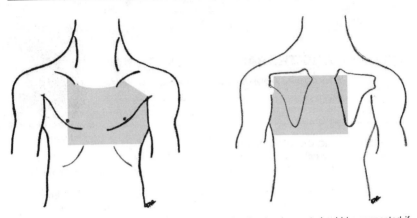

Figure 33-1. Extended anterior and posterior box. Cardiac involvement should be suspected if chest injuries involve the gray zones.

The amount of hemothorax dictates the need for operative exploration (Table 33-1).

    f. Victims of penetrating trauma who have lost signs of life during transfer or on arrival at the hospital should undergo emergent left anterior thoracotomy, opening of the pericardium, clamping of the descending aorta, and control of bleeding in the emergency room. Further repair and closure should be performed in the operating room.

  2. Operative management

    a. Median sternotomy and left anterior thoracotomy are the most common approaches (Fig. 33-4). Other incisions depend on the presumptive diagnosis and should be used only when the diagnostic results dictate such action.

    b. Atrial injuries are controlled with clamps and the defect is repaired with sutures (Table 33-2). Ventricular injuries should be controlled by digital compression, and the defect is repaired with sutures. Larger defects may require cardiopulmonary bypass, aortic cross clamping, and the use of autologous or prosthetic material.

    c. Missiles should be removed surgically because of the risk of embolization, endocarditis, and the erosion of adjacent vessels.

    d. Coronary artery injuries are uncommon but carry a high mortality. Small branches may be ligated, but larger vessels should be either repaired or bypassed.

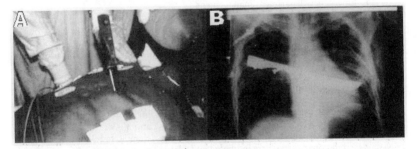

Figure 33-2. *(A)* Stab wound injury in the anterior box. *(B)* Hemodynamic status permitted an anteroposterior chest radiograph prior to operative exploration.

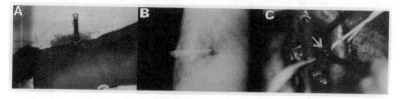

Figure 33-3. *(A)* Stab wound injury in the posterior box. *(B)* Lateral chest radiograph. *(C)* Operative situs through a right thoracotomy. *Thin arrow:* Esophagus. *Interrupted arrow:* Tip of knife. *Dashed arrow:* descending aorta.

    e. Only life-threatening injuries should be repaired at the time of operation; all others should be approached in a future session.

II. PENETRATING THORACIC AORTIC INJURY
A. Background
    1. Injury to the thoracic aorta occurs in 1.4% of gunshot and 0.6% of stab injuries to the chest and carries a mortality rate as high as 93%. Coexistent major injuries are common.
B. Presentation
    1. Most patients arrive at the hospital with minimal or no signs of life, and emergent thoracotomy in the emergency room is the only chance for survival. Patients who arrive hemodynamically stable usually have contained ruptures or fistulous communications with adjacent veins.
C. Diagnosis
    1. Hemodynamically stable patients should undergo CXR, and a chest tube should be placed for absent or diminished breath sounds or for signs of hemothorax.
    2. Hemodynamically unstable patients should undergo emergent left anterior thoracotomy.
    3. Aortography is the gold standard for detecting aortic injury, but it is time-consuming and requires moving the patient to the radiology suite.
    4. Transesophageal echocardiography should be used only if esophagogram has excluded esophageal injury and is not routinely used.
D. Treatment
    1. The operative approach includes primary control of the bleeding during the emergency thoracotomy.
    2. Small lacerations may be repaired through tangential clamping and direct suture. For large defects, replacement of the aorta is performed with a tube graft.

TABLE 33-1	Indications for Urgent Surgical Exploration

1. Hemodynamic instability despite volume resuscitation
2. Excessive chest tube drainage (1.5 to 2.0 L or more total, or >300 mL/h for 3 or more hours)
3. Significant hemothorax on chest radiograph
4. Suspected penetrating cardiac trauma
5. Gunshot wound to the abdomen
6. Penetrating torso trauma, particularly if associated with peritoneal perforation
7. Positive diagnostic peritoneal lavage (particularly with evidence of ongoing hemorrhage)
8. Significant solid-organ or bowel injury

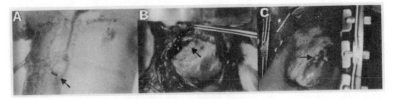

Figure 33-4. *(A)* Stab wound injury in the anterior box. Hemodynamic instability dictated immediate operative exploration *(B)* Operative situs through a median sternotomy. Intraoperative findings revealed left ventricular myocardial laceration and hemopericardium. *(C)* Defect closure by direct sutures with pledgets excluding a diagonal branch of the left anterior descending artery.

III. BLUNT CARDIAC INJURY
A. Background
1. Myocardial contusion can be diagnosed only if suspected. Clinical signs and symptoms are either missing or nonspecific and hemodynamic instability may be due to other causes (Table 33-3).
2. For prognostic and treatment purposes it is helpful to classify patients into two categories: those who are stable or whose hemodynamic instability is not due to their cardiac injury (subacute injury) and those with major life-threatening cardiac injuries who require emergent intervention (life-threatening injury).

B. Presentation
1. Subacute blunt cardiac injury
   a. Many patients are asymptomatic, but common presentations include chest pain, arrhythmias (premature atrial or ventricular contractions, tachycardia, and bradycardia), and pericardial tamponade.
   b. Chest pain is usually an early symptom but may also manifest several hours or even days postinjury and has two forms: an angina-like pain and the usual thoracic pain associated with chest injury.
   c. Mortality in patients with subacute injury is mainly dependent on extracardiac comorbidities.
2. Life-threatening blunt cardiac injury
   a. Present with hemodynamic instability or cardiogenic shock
   b. Myocardial lacerations, rupture (most commonly the right ventricle), or great vessel injury present with hemopericardium and/or hemothorax
   c. Malignant arrhythmias or severe left ventricular dysfunction may also result in cardiogenic shock.
3. Specific presentations
   a. Pericardial tamponade may develop because of hemorrhage after rupture of the myocardium or great vessels, or because of exudation of fluid through the injured pericardium or epicardium.
   b. Chest pain is rather nonspecific.

TABLE 33-2	Cardiac Injuries and Repair Techniques
Myocardial free wall	Primary repair buttressed with felt or pledgets
VSD, papillary muscles	Delayed repair preferred
Coronaries involved	Ligate small or distal vessels
	CABG for proximal vessels, especially LAD

CABG, coronary artery bypass grafting; LAD, left anterior descending; VSD, ventricular septal defect.

TABLE 33-3	Causes of Cardiopulmonary Deterioration Associated with Blunt Trauma

1. Severe central neurologic injury with secondary cardiovascular collapse
2. Hypoxia secondary to respiratory arrest resulting from neurologic injury, airway obstruction, large open pneumothorax, or severe tracheobronchial laceration or crush
3. Direct and severe injury to vital structures, such as the heart, aorta, or pulmonary arteries
4. Underlying medical problems or other conditions that led to the injury, such as sudden ventricular fibrillation in the driver of a motor vehicle or the victim of an electric shock
5. Severely diminished cardiac output from tension pneumothorax or pericardial tamponade
6. Exsanguination leading to hypovolemia and severely diminished oxygen delivery
7. Injuries (e.g., fractured leg) in a cold environment complicated by secondary severe hypothermia

  c. Fatal arrythmias occur, even in cases of blunt trauma with no histological evidence of myocardial contusion.
  d. Injury to the aortic, mitral, and tricuspid valves and the atrioventricular septae occurs and often appears as combined injuries.
  e. Injury to the coronary vessels—including laceration, dissection, thrombosis, or spasm—occurs with low incidence and presents as tamponade, hemorrhage, or ischemia.
C. Diagnosis
 1. The first step in diagnosing blunt myocardial injury is an awareness that such an injury might have occurred.
 2. Evaluation for possible preexisting heart disease is mandatory, so that differentiation between old and new findings can be appreciated.
 3. A 12-lead electrocardiogram (ECG) should be obtained and this, combined with the clinical presentation, will determine whether further diagnostic evaluation or treatment is necessary. However, misinterpretation of preexisting conditions is common (Table 33-4). ECG findings include ST and T-wave abnormalities, conduction abnormalities, atrial or ventricular arrhythmias, or ischemic changes.
 4. Serial measurements of the creatine-kinase-MB/total creatine kinase (CK-MB/CK) ratio should be assessed in conjunction with ECG and troponin I level. Elevations in serum markers—which rapidly return to baseline—indicate only moderate contusions, whereas prolonged elevations are associated with more severe injury.
 5. A CXR is obtained to assess for signs of injury, including mediastinal widening, sternal or rib fractures, tracheal or nasogastric tube displacement, pneumothorax,

TABLE 33-4	Differential Diagnosis of Abnormal ECG Findings After Blunt Cardiac Trauma

Findings preceding the event	Preexisting cardiac disease; old, unrelated finding
	Normal variant
Findings present at the time of the event	First presentation of unrelated cardiac disorder
	Event inducing cardiac disorder
	Alcohol or other extrinsic factors
Findings associated with the event	Catecholamine release
	Hypovolemia
	pH or electrolyte abnormalities
	Cardiac injury secondary to trauma (not force related)

hemothorax, diaphragmatic rupture, and apical capping or indistinct aortic knob. Further evaluation may be performed by computed tomography (CT), according to patient stability and the index of suspicion.

6. Transthoracic echocardiography is performed in the emergency or operating room, while other procedures take place, and should be performed early in patients with hemodynamic instability or ECG changes.

7. Coronary angiography is indicated in patients who present acutely with the suspicion of coronary trauma and require immediate diagnosis and intervention or in patients with persistent symptoms or ECG findings over several days.

D. Treatment

1. ECG and echocardiography have better predictive value and, in the majority of cases, these studies are sufficient to establish diagnosis and guide further management (Fig. 33-5).

2. Hemodynamically stable patients who are less than 55 years of age, have a normal ECG and no history of heart disease, and do not require surgical or neurological observation do not require specific cardiac evaluation and can be discharged from the hospital.

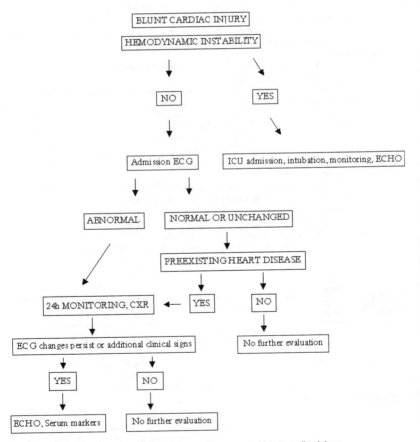

Figure 33-5. Algorithm to approach patients with suspected blunt cardiac injury.

3. An abnormal ECG or history of cardiac disease dictates ECG monitoring and observation for 24 hours. In the absence of arrhythmia, ECG changes, or complications, no further evaluation is needed. If ECG changes progress or persist, then echocardiography should be performed.

4. Hemodynamically unstable patients should undergo cardiac evaluation to identify injury. They are admitted to the ICU, intubated, and undergo ECG monitoring and continuous measurement of arterial and central venous pressures. Echocardiography is performed to estimate the degree of cardiac involvement and identify the specific anatomic injuries.

5. Patients with blunt cardiac injury are treated similarly to those with acute myocardial infarction. Bed rest, oxygen, drug therapy, and electrocardiographic or hemodynamic monitoring are the mainstays of treatment. Analgesics or narcotics should be administered as needed.

6. Drugs that may potentiate arrhythmias should be avoided; however, antiarrhythmic agents may be indicated in rare cases. Digitalis may be used for rate control of atrial fibrillation but should be avoided for sinus tachycardia because it increases electrical instability in contused myocardium. β-Blockers have not been sufficiently studied, but their use appears reasonable for clinically significant myocardial damage or tachyarrhythmias.

7. Diuretics or inotropic agents are indicated if congestive heart failure develops.

8. Anticoagulants should be avoided because they may precipitate intrapericardial or intramyocardial hemorrhage.

9. Volume resuscitation should be done carefully and should be guided by pulmonary wedge pressure, cardiac output, and vascular resistance measurements in patients with major hemodynamic compromise.

10. Valve or septal injuries should be corrected operatively; however, the timing of surgery depends on the hemodynamic stability of the patient. Treatment of all non–life-threatening injuries should be delayed when possible. Occasionally small ventricular septal and most atrial septal defects are treated conservatively but followed up closely.

11. Emergent thoracotomy for patients with blunt cardiac injury who present *in extremis* is almost always futile and should be attempted only if there are no signs of associated brain injury.

IV. BLUNT THORACIC AORTIC INJURY

A. Background

1. The thoracic aorta is particularly susceptible to deceleration injury, the most frequent cause of which is a motor vehicle accident. The incidence in blunt chest trauma victims is 4% among patients who reach the hospital alive and 15% to 17% at autopsy.

2. Aortic injury is often associated other organ injuries that are not limited to the chest.

3. Unlike patients with penetrating injury, most patients with blunt aortic injury are stable enough to undergo diagnostic evaluation.

B. Presentation

1. Clinical presentation varies widely, from hemodynamically stable with radiographic abnormalities to profound hemodynamic instability.

2. The spectrum of aortic injuries includes hemorrhage, dissection, partial or full transection, pseudoaneurysm, and thrombosis. Aortic wall disruption ranges from a small intimal tear to full transection, held together only by the adventitia or the mediastinal reflection of the pleura.

3. Intrapericardial aortic injuries may manifest as acute pericardial tamponade.

C. Diagnosis

1. A CXR is the first diagnostic step. This will typically show a widened mediastinum. Less common findings include indistinct aortic knob, widening of the paratracheal stripe, and pleural effusion.

2. Aortography is required to evaluate the suspected injury and determine the need for operation. However, computed tomography and magnetic resonance imaging are increasingly used.

D. Treatment

1. The first priority is to control aortic wall stress by maintaining systolic blood pressures at or below 100 mm Hg, providing adequate analgesia and sedation and minimizing movement of the thoracic vertebral column.
2. Vasodilators and short-acting β-blockers may be used for blood pressure control, just as would be the case for acute dissection. β-Blockers are particularly suitable because they reduce the blood pressure, the force of arterial upstroke, and the heart rate.
3. Operative correction should be performed as soon as possible. Delay may be acceptable in patients who require operative correction of other, more urgent injuries and sometimes in stable patients with small intimal tears who have major comorbidities that place them in a prohibitive operative risk category. In these cases, aortic repair utilizing endoluminal stent-grafts may represent a better option in the future.
4. Signs of free perforation, such as rapid evolving mediastinal hematoma or pleural effusion, should be indications for emergent operation.
5. Injuries to the aorta distal to the left carotid artery should be approached via a left posterolateral thoracotomy and left heart bypass. If there is no possibility for left heart bypass, a Gott shunt may be used.
6. Defects located between the intrapericardial aorta and aortic arch are best approached via median sternotomy with cardiopulmonary bypass and/or circulatory arrest.
7. Multiple tears may require a combination of these approaches.

Selected Readings

Asensio JA, Berne JD, Demetriades D, et al. One hundred five penetrating cardiac injuries: a 2-year prospective evaluation. *J Trauma* 1998;44:1073–1082.
  This study validated physiologic variables and injury severity scoring systems as predictors of outcome in penetrating cardiac injury.

Bertinchant JP, Polge A, Mohty D, et al. Evaluation of incidence, clinical significance, and prognostic value of circulating cardiac troponin I and T elevation in hemodynamically stable patients with suspected myocardial contusion after blunt chest trauma. *J Trauma* 2000;48:924–931.
  This study demonstrated that elevations of circulating troponin I and T had a low sensitivity in hemodynamically stable patients with suspected blunt cardiac injury and did not correlate with outcome.

Campbell NC, Thomson SR, Muckart DJ, et al. Review of 1198 cases of penetrating cardiac trauma. *Br J Surg* 1997;84:1737–1740.
  Classic description of the prevalence and outcome of traumatic cardiac injuries.

Fabian TC, Richardson JD, Croce MA, et al. Prospective study of blunt aortic injury: Multicenter trial of the American Association for the Surgery of Trauma. *J Trauma* 1997;42:374–380; discussion 380–383.
  Large, multicenter trial of 274 cases of blunt aortic injury that compared the clamp and sew technique with bypass techniques with respect to mortality and paraplegia rates. Mortality was not affected by the type of repair. Clamp and sew as well as bypass times greater than 30 minutes were associated with a higher rate of postoperative paraplegia.

Karalis DG, Victor MF, Davis GA, et al. The role of echocardiography in blunt chest trauma: a transthoracic and transesophageal echocardiographic study. *J Trauma* 1994;36:53–58.
  This comparison study of transthoracic echocardiography (TTE) and transesophageal echocardiography (TEE) demonstrated that of those patients who sustained a myocardial contusion, echocardiography benefited only those who developed a cardiac complication. Additionally, TEE was useful when aortic injury was suspected and the results of TTE were suboptimal.

Minard G, Schurr MJ, Croce MA, et al. A prospective analysis of transesophageal echocardiography in the diagnosis of traumatic disruption of the aorta. *J Trauma* 1996;40:225–230.
  Direct comparison of transesophageal echocardiography (TEE) with aortography in the diagnosis of traumatic aortic disruption. The sensitivity and specificity of TEE were

57% and 91%, respectively, and the sensitivity and specificity of aortography were 89% and 100%, respectively. The authors concluded that aortography remains the gold standard diagnostic method for diagnosing traumatic aortic disruption.

Pasquale M, Nagy K, Clarke J. Practice management guidelines for screening of blunt cardiac injury. In: *EAST: Eastern Association for the Surgery of Trauma* 1998.
Practice guidelines based on meta-analysis for screening patients for suspected blunt cardiac injury by the EAST organization. The guidelines assess the role of ECG, enzyme analysis, echocardiography, radionuclide imaging, and pulmonary arterial monitoring in the diagnosis of blunt cardiac imaging.

Pretre R, Chilcott M. Blunt trauma to the heart and great vessels. N Engl J Med 1997;336: 626–632.
Excellent general review of blunt chest trauma with an emphasis on the heart and great vessels.

Pretre R, LaHarpe R, Cheretakis A, et al. Blunt injury to the ascending aorta: three patterns of presentation. *Surgery* 1996;119:603–610.
Excellent description of the injury patterns observed in blunt aortic injury.

Rozycki GS, Feliciano DV, Ochsner MG, et al. The role of ultrasound in patients with possible penetrating cardiac wounds: a prospective multicenter study. *J Trauma* 1999;46:543–551; discussion 551–552.
Classic study demonstrating the utility of ultrasound in the evaluation of penetrating precordial wounds. The study demonstrated a sensitivity and specificity of 100% and 96.9% of ultrasound in diagnosing acute hemopericardium.

Singh MJ, Rohrer MJ, Ghaleb M, et al. Endoluminal stent-graft repair of a thoracic aortic transection in a trauma patient with multiple injuries: case report. *J Trauma* 2001;51:376–381.
Provocative case report highlighting the potential of endovascular therapies in the trauma setting.

Tyburski JG, Astra L, Wilson RF, et al. Factors affecting prognosis with penetrating wounds of the heart. *J Trauma* 2000;48:587–590; discussion 590–591.
Large retrospective series that demonstrated the physiologic state of the patient at presentation, the mechanism of injury, and the presence of tamponade as the important prognostic factors for penetrating heart injuries.

34 MANAGEMENT OF UNSTABLE ANGINA AND NON–ST-ELEVATION MYOCARDIAL INFARCTION

Eli V. Gelfand and Christopher P. Cannon

I. GENERAL PRINCIPLES
   A. About 1.7 million patients are admitted to the hospital each year in the United States with an acute coronary syndrome (ACS).
   B. Eighty percent of patients do not have ST segment elevations on an initial electrocardiogram (ECG) and are said to have unstable angina and non–ST-segment elevation myocardial infarction (UA/NSTEMI).

II. PATHOPHYSIOLOGY
   A. Caused by rupture of an atherosclerotic plaque and formation of a nonocclusive thrombus.
   B. There is embolization of the thrombus fragments downstream, causing additional myocardial ischemia and necrosis.
   C. The sequence of events in UA/NSTEMI is:
   1. Rupture of a vulnerable atherosclerotic plaque
   2. Platelet activation, aggregation, and adhesion
   3. Secondary activation of plasma coagulation system
   4. Coronary vasoconstriction
   5. Imbalance in myocardial oxygen and demand

III. DIAGNOSIS
   A. Based on new or accelerating symptoms of coronary ischemia, with or without ECG changes
   B. Cardiac biomarker (troponin I or T, or CK-MB) elevation distinguishes NSTEMI from UA
   C. ECG changes in UA/NSTEMI may include:
   1. ST-segment depressions
   2. Transient ST-segment elevations
   3. New T-wave inversions

IV. TREATMENT
   A. Evaluation of patient with possible UA/NSTEMI consists of:
   1. Assessment of the likelihood that the patient's symptoms are indicative of an acute coronary syndrome
   2. Application of risk stratification to identify high versus lower risk patients.
   a. TIMI Risk Score (Table 34-1) provides a rapid way of assessing the patient's risk.
   b. Some therapies have been shown to benefit only high-risk patients, and can thus be targeted to only those patients.
   B. There are three broad aspects of therapy of US/NSTEMI:
   1. Antiischemic therapy: β-blockers, nitrates
   2. Antithrombotic therapy
   a. Antiplatelet therapy: aspirin, clopidogrel, glycoprotein (GP)IIb/IIIa inhibitors
   b. Antithrombin therapy: unfractionated heparin, low-molecular-weight heparins, direct thrombin inhibitors
   3. Overall treatment strategy
   a. Early invasive strategy: cardiac catheterization within 24 to 48 hours with revascularization if feasible
   b. Conservative strategy: medical management with revascularization dictated by recurrent ischemia at rest or on provocative testing.

TABLE 34-1	TIMI Risk Score for UA/NSTEMI
Age ‡65 years	1 pt
Prior coronary stenoses >50%	1 pt
‡3 risk factors for CAD	1 pt
Use of aspirin in the preceding 24 h	1 pt
‡2 anginal events in the preceding 24 h	1 pt
ST segment changes	1 pt
Elevated cardiac biomarkers	1 pt
Total possible score	0–7 points

CAD, coronary artery disease; TIMI, Thrombosis In Myocardial Infarction Study Group.

C. Antiischemic therapy

1. Nitrate therapy is recommended initially, with the use of with sublingual or intravenous nitrates for ongoing ischemic pain.
   a. Nitrates can be safely discontinued on successful revascularization.
2. Beta blockade remains a cornerstone of treatment of ACS.
   a. Intravenous beta blockade followed by oral beta blockade targeted to a heart rate of 50 to 60 beats per minute is recommended for all patients with UA/NSTEMI without major contraindications.

D. Aspirin and clopidogrel

1. **Aspirin**, which reduces events by 50% to 70% as compared with placebo, should be started immediately in all patients.
   a. Initial recommended dose is 162 to 325 mg by mouth
   b. For maintenance therapy, a dose of 75 to 100 mg/day is sufficient
2. **Clopidogrel** should be added to aspirin in all patients with UA/NSTEMI.
   a. Clopidogrel blocks the adenosine diphosphate pathway and decreases platelet activation and aggregation
   b. In the CURE trial, clopidogrel in combination with aspirin and in addition to other standard therapies led to a 20% relative risk reduction in cardiovascular death, myocardial infarction (MI), or stroke compared with aspirin alone.
      (1) Benefit of combination antiplatelet therapy was seen in both low- and high-risk patients with UA/NSTEMI and emerged as early as 24 hours.
      (2) Benefit of pretreatment prior to percutaneous revascularization was also seen with a 31% reduction in cardiac events at 30 days and 1 year.

E. GP IIb/IIIa inhibitors

1. Intravenous GP IIb/IIIa inhibitors have been shown to be beneficial in treating UA/NSTEMI.
   a. For "upstream" management (i.e., initiating therapy when the patient first presents to the hospital), the small molecule inhibitors eptifibatide and tirofiban clearly show benefit
   b. Monoclonal antibody abciximab should be used only in the setting of percutaneous **coronary** intervention.
2. The benefit of GP IIb/IIIa inhibitors is limited to patients at high risk.
   a. In troponin-positive patients there is a 70% reduction in death or MI at 30 days and 6 months, whether or not they underwent revascularization.

F. Heparin and low-molecular-weight heparin

1. Unfractionated heparin (UFH) or low-molecular-weight heparin (LMWH) should be added to the medical regimen for all patients with UA/NSTEMI.
2. Comparative trials of enoxaparin, an LMWH, versus unfractionated heparin have demonstrated its superiority in reducing recurrent cardiac events in patients managed with a conservative strategy, but less so in the setting of an early invasive strategy.

G. Invasive versus conservative strategy

1. Nine randomized trials so far have assessed the merits of an invasive strategy involving routine cardiac catheterization, with revascularization if feasible, versus a conservative strategy in which angiography and revascularization are reserved for patients who have evidence of recurrent ischemia either at rest or on provocative testing.

2. The benefits of the early invasive strategy were seen in intermediate- and high-risk patients and especially in those with ST-segment changes who had a positive troponin, with reductions in recurrent ischemic events.

H. In-hospital management summary

1. Patients with a low likelihood of having UA/NSTEMI should undergo a "diagnostic pathway" evaluation including serial ECGs, cardiac biomarkers, and early stress testing to evaluate for coronary disease. This can be accomplished in an emergency department observation or chest pain unit.

2. Patients with a clinical history suggesting high likelihood of UA/NSTEMI should undergo:

   a. antithrombotic therapy with aspirin, clopidogrel, heparin, or low-molecular-weight heparin

   b. antiischemic therapy with β-blockers and nitrates initially

   c. risk stratification as described earlier

      (1) patients at low risk may undergo conservative strategy, although an invasive strategy is of equal clinical benefit.

      (2) for patients at intermediate and high risk (ST-segment changes, positive troponin, TIMI Risk Score [TRS] of 3 or above), above-mentioned medications plus GP IIb/IIIa inhibition (thus, four antithrombotic agents) are recommended and an early invasive strategy is preferred (Fig. 34-1).

V. LONG-TERM SECONDARY PREVENTION

A. Five classes of drugs receive a strong recommendation from American College of Cardiology/American Heart Association for long-term medical therapy:

1. Aspirin
2. Clopidogrel

Evidence-Based Risk Stratification in UA/NSTEMI

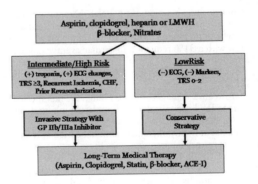

Figure 34-1. Treatment algorithm for non—ST-elevation acute coronary syndrome.

   3. β-blockers
   4. ACE inhibitors
   5. Statins
B. For plaque stabilization, statins and ACE inhibitors are recommended in the long term.
   1. High-dose statins should be used, and a target LDL level should be below 70 mg/dL.
   2. Secondary goal of HDL level higher than 40 mg/dL is reasonable
C. β-Blockers are appropriate antiischemic therapy and may help decrease "triggers" for MI during follow-up.
D. Antiplatelet therapy in the form of aspirin and clopidogrel is continued for at least 12 months and acts by preventing or decreasing the severity of any thrombosis that would occur if a plaque does rupture. After stent implantation, a *mandatory* course of aspirin and clopidogrel is necessary to prevent stent thrombosis as follows:
   1. bare-metal stent: at least 1 month
   2. sirolimus-eluting stent: at least 3 months
   3. paclitaxel-eluting stent: at least 6 months
E. Other goals that should be emphasized prior to discharge include:
   1. Complete smoking cessation
   2. Weight control
   3. Regular exercise
   4. Tight glycemic control in diabetic patients

Selected Readings

Blazing MA, de Lemos JA, White HD, et al. Safety and efficacy of enoxaparin vs unfractionated heparin in patients with non-ST-segment elevation acute coronary syndromes who receive tirofiban and aspirin: a randomized controlled trial. *JAMA* 2004;292:55–64.
One of the studies showing benefit of enoxaparin over unfractionated heparin, but only in patients managed conservatively.

Boersma E, Harrington RA, Moliterno DJ, et al. Platelet glycoprotein IIb/IIIa inhibitors in acute coronary syndromes: a meta-analysis of all major randomised clinical trials. *Lancet* 2002;359:189–198.
The meta-analysis of all trials of GP IIb/IIIa inhibitors for acute coronary syndrome to date.

Braunwald E, Antman EM, Beasley JW, et al. ACC/AHA guideline update for the management of patients with unstable angina and non-ST-segment elevation myocardial infarction-2002: Summary article: A report of the American College of Cardiology/American Heart Association Task Force on Practice Guidelines (Committee on the Management of Patients With Unstable Angina). *Circulation* 2002;106:1893–1900.
The official guideline for management of UA/NSTEMI

Cannon CP, Braunwald E, McCabe CH, et al. Intensive versus moderate lipid lowering with statins after acute coronary syndromes. *N Engl J Med* 2004;350:1495–1504.
The pivotal trial showing that "lower is better" for treatment of LDL cholesterol following acute coronary syndrome.

Cannon CP. Evidence-based risk stratification to target therapies in acute coronary syndromes. *Circulation* 2002;106:1588–1591.
A brief overview of how risk stratification can direct which treatments are used for UA/NSTEMI.

Clopidogrel in Unstable Angina to Prevent Recurrent Events Trial Investigators. Effects of clopidogrel in addition to aspirin in patients with acute coronary syndromes without ST-segment elevation. *N Engl J Med* 2001;345:494–502.
The principal trial demonstrating benefit of clopidogrel in UA/NSTEMI.

Grundy SM, Cleeman JI, Merz CNB, et al. Implications of recent clinical trials for the National Cholesterol Education Program Adult Treatment Panel III Guidelines. *Circulation* 2004;110:227–239.
Definitive guidelines for treatment of LDL cholesterol.

Hamm CW, Heeschen C, Goldmann B, et al. Benefit of abciximab in patients with refractory unstable angina in relation to serum troponin T levels. *N Engl J Med* 1999;340: 1623–1629.
The first study to show that patients with positive troponin should be treated with GP IIb/IIIa inhibitors and that they derive increased benefit over those without positive troponin.

Mehta SR, Yusuf S, Peters RJ, et al. Effects of pretreatment with clopidogrel and aspirin followed by long-term therapy in patients undergoing percutaneous coronary intervention: the PCI-CURE study. *Lancet* 2001;358:527–533.
A trial demonstrating benefit of clopidogrel among patients undergoing percutaneous coronary intervention.

Thomas W. Wallace and James A. de Lemos

I. GENERAL PRINCIPLES

A. Rapid reperfusion of the infarct-related artery (IRA), with either primary percutaneous coronary intervention (PCI) or fibrinolytic therapy is the cornerstone of management for patients with ST-segment elevation myocardial infarction (STEMI).

B. Adjunctive therapy with aspirin, clopidogrel, β-blockers, clopidogrel, ACE inhibitors, and statins further prevents death and major cardiovascular events after reperfusion.

II. PATHOPHYSIOLOGY

A. Rupture of lipid-rich, inflammatory atherosclerotic plaque causes collagen exposure, platelet adhesion, and activation.

B. Fibrinogen binds to platelet glycoprotein IIb/IIIa (GP IIb/IIIa) receptors on adjacent platelets causing platelet aggregation.

C. A fibrin-platelet clot develops as thrombin converts fibrinogen to fibrin.

D. Platelet-fibrin clot completely occludes the IRA causing transmural myocardial injury, manifested by ST-segment elevation on the electrocardiogram (ECG).

III. DIAGNOSIS

A. Differential diagnosis: Rapidly consider/rule out pneumothorax, aortic dissection, pericarditis, tamponade, pulmonary embolism, cholecystitis.

B. History

  1. Angina is classically described as severe, pressure-type pain in midsternum, often with radiation to left neck, arm, or jaw. (Note onset of symptoms.)

  2. Associated symptoms: dyspnea, nausea, vomiting, diaphoresis, weakness.

  3. Silent infarction in 25% of cases, especially in elderly and diabetics.

C. Physical examination

  1. Not helpful in confirming the diagnosis of STEMI.

  2. Examination should focus on eliminating other potential diagnoses and assessing for complications of STEMI (see Table 35-5).

D. ECG

  1. ST elevations (convex) are found in regional distributions with concurrent ST depression in reciprocal leads.

  2. Consider pericarditis with global ST elevations (concave) and PR depressions, early repolarization abnormalities, old left ventricular aneurysm, and Prinzmetal angina.

  3. New left bundle branch block (LBBB) represents large anterior infarction; indication for reperfusion therapy.

E. Cardiac biomarkers

  1. Biomarkers of limited use for diagnosis of STEMI.

  2. Myoglobin is earliest detector of myocardial damage.

  3. B-type natriuretic peptide (BNP) useful in prognostic assessment.

IV. REPERFUSION THERAPY

A. Evolving goals of reperfusion therapy

  1. The goal of reperfusion therapy is rapid and complete restoration of epicardial coronary artery and microvascular blood flow.

  2. Current interventions include pharmacologic, mechanical, and combined reperfusion modalities.

TABLE 35-1	Comparison of Fibrinolytic Therapy and Primary PCI	
	Fibrinolytic therapy	**Primary PCI**
Advantage	Widely accessible Easy to use Rapid administration No subspecialist required	Lower bleeding risk Improved efficacy Less mortality Fewer recurrent MIs Immediate-risk stratification
Disadvantage	More serious bleeding Less efficacy Lower TIMI 3 flow rate Higher mortality Many contraindications	Time delay Limited availability Operator dependent Resource intensive Major commitment needed

PCI, primary coronary angioplasty; MI, myocardial infarction; TIMI, Thrombosis In Myocardial Infarction; TIMI flow, angiographic measure of antegrade coronary flow.

3. Resolution of ST-segment elevation is the best indicator of successful reperfusion (Table 35-1).

B. Time-dependent benefit with reperfusion (mechanical or pharmacologic).
1. If Thrombosis In Myocardial Infarction-3 flow achieved within 1 hour, mortality decreases by 50%.
2. After 12 hours, no mortality benefit with fibrinolytic therapy.

C. Current guidelines for fibrinolytic therapy in non-PCI centers
1. Transfer for primary PCI if patient has access to high-volume PCI center within 90 minutes of onset of symptoms.
2. Transfer to PCI facility if patient has contraindication to fibrinolytic therapy.
3. If (1) and (2) not met, then administer fibrinolytics within 12 hours of onset of symptoms.
4. Less clear guidelines include patients over age of 75, symptoms between 12 and 24 hours, hypertensive and high risk patients.
5. No indication for fibrinolytic therapy if symptoms greater than 24 hours or non-STEMI (Tables 35-2 and 35-3).

D. Limitations to fibrinolytic therapy
1. Intracranial hemorrhage in approximately 1%; higher in elderly, women, low body weight, hypertension.
2. TIMI 3 flow remains 50% to 60%. PCI achieves TIMI-3 in 80% to 90% of cases.

E. Combination therapy with GP IIb/IIIa inhibitors and reduced-dose fibrinolytics
1. Improved microvascular perfusion, decreased recurrent myocardial infarction (MI).
2. No mortality benefit; increases bleed risk; currently not recommended.

F. Rescue PCI after failed fibrinolytic therapy
1. Noninvasive criteria to define successful fibrinolytic therapy include ST-segment resolution greater than 50% to 70%, chest pain resolution, and early peaking of cardiac biomarkers; accuracy of these tools is modest.
2. Persistent ST-segment elevations (even without symptoms) in elderly, diabetics, previous coronary artery disease, or anterior infarction represent high-risk patients who should be considered for rescue PCI.

G. Primary PCI
1. Percutaneous transmural coronary angioplasty (PTCA)
a. Demonstrates mortality benefit when compared with fibrinolytics.
b. Increases TIMI 3 flow, decreases stroke risk, and decreases reocclusion and recurrent MI.
c. Requires skilled technicians in high-volume PCI centers.
2. Intracoronary stenting
a. No survival benefit but decreases reocclusion and restenosis when compared with PTCA.

TABLE 35-2	Comparison of Fibrinolytic Therapies			
	Alteplase	**Reteplase**	**Tenecteplase**	**Streptokinase**
Fibrin-selective	+++	++	++++	—
Half-life	5 min	14 min	17 min	20 min
Dose	15-mg bolus; then 0.75 mg/kg over 30 min; then 0.5 mg/kg over 60 min (max 100-mg total dose)	Two 10-unit bolus doses given 30 min apart	0.53 mg/kg as a single bolus	1.5 million units over 30–60 min
Weight adjusted	Partial	No	Yes	No
Adjunctive heparin	Yes	Yes	Yes	No
Possible allergy	No	No	No	Yes
TIMI 2/3 flow (90 min)	80%	80%	80%	60%
TIMI 3 flow (90 min)	55%–60%	60%	55%–65%	32%
Efficacy vs. tPA	NA	Similar	Equivalent	1% ↑ mortality
Safety	NA	Similar	Similar ICH ↓ non-ICH bleeding	↓ ICH ↓ Overall bleeding
Cost	+++	+++	+++	+

ICH, intracranial hemorrhage; tPA, tissue plasminogen activator (alteplase); TIMI, Thrombosis In Myocardial Infarction; NA, not available; TIMI flow, angiographic measure of epicardial flow.

   3. Adjunctive GP IIb/IIIa inhibitors improve outcomes with primary PCI.
 H. Facilitated PCI
    1. Pharmacologic reperfusion therapy prior to PCI is designed to open the IRA early, followed immediately by definitive therapy with coronary stenting.
    2. Ongoing trials are investigating GP IIb/IIIa inhibitors alone, fibrinolytics alone, and several combinations of fibrinolytics and GP IIb/IIIa inhibitors.

TABLE 35-3	Contraindications to Fibrinolytic Therapy
Absolute contraindications	**Relative contraindications**
Active internal bleeding	Blood pressure consistently >180/110 mm Hg
History of CNS hemorrhage	History of stroke or AVM
Stoke of any kind within the last year	Known bleeding diathesis
Recent head trauma or CNS neoplasm	Active peptic ulcer
Suspected aortic dissection	Proliferative diabetic retinopathy
	Prolonged CPR
	Prior exposure to SK or APSAC (5 days to 2 years) or prior allergic reaction
	Pregnancy
	Major surgery or trauma within 2 weeks
	Anticoagulation use
	Puncture of a noncompressible vessel

CNS, central nervous system; SK, streptokinase; APSAC, anisolylated plasminogen streptokinase activator complex (anistreplase); AVM, arteriovenous malformation; CPR, cardiopulmonary resuscitation.

V. ADJUNCTIVE ANTITHROMBOTIC THERAPY

A. Aspirin and clopidogrel (antiplatelet activity)

   1. Aspirin (ASA) reduces mortality, reocclusion, and reinfarction.

   2. Administer ASA 81 to 325 mg orally at presentation; continue daily.

   3. Clopidogrel is indicated in all patients receiving PCI with intracoronary stent placement. Recent studies also demonstrate decreased rates of death and IM when clopidogrel is administered as an adjunct to fibrinolytic therapy.

B. Unfractionated heparin (UFH) and low-molecular-weight heparin (LWMH)

   1. Adjunctive therapy to tPA-based fibrinolysis.

   2. UFH administered intravenously 60 units/kg bolus, then 12 units/kg/hr. *Data support this dose as optimal in limiting intracranial hemorrhage.*

   3. LMWH may decrease nonfatal ischemic events when combined with full-dose fibrinolysis but may increase life-threatening hemorrhage in the elderly; utility remains under investigation.

C. Warfarin/oral anticoagulation

   1. Warfarin indicated for left ventricular aneurysm, atrial fibrillation.

   2. Direct thrombin inhibitors (with fibrinolytic therapy) have not demonstrated improvements in cardiac outcomes when compared with UFH.

VI. ANTIISCHEMIC THERAPY

A. β-Blockers (BB)

   1. Limits size of infarction, decreases recurrent MI, improves survival.

   2. Prevents arrhythmias and cardiac rupture.

   3. Administer 2.5- to 5-mg IV bolus of metoprolol three times 5 min apart as tolerated, then continue with oral treatment indefinitely.

B. Angiotensin-converting enzyme inhibitors (ACEi)

   1. Prevents congestive heart failure (CHF) and death by halting adverse remodeling of left ventricular chamber.

   2. In 30-day mortality, 7% reduction in 100,000 patients with STEMI.

TABLE 35-4   **Electrical Complications of Acute MI**

Complication	Prognosis	Treatment
Ventricular tachycardia/fibrillation		
Within first 24 to 48 hours	Good	Immediate cardioversion; lidocaine; beta blockers
After 48 hours	Poor	Immediate cardioversion; electrophysiology study/implantable defibrillator; amiodarone
Sinus bradycardia	Excellent	Atropine for hypotension or symptoms
Second-degree heart block		
Mobitz type I (Wenkebach)	Excellent	Atropine for hypotension or symptoms
Mobitz type II	Guarded	Temporary pacemaker
Complete heart block		
Inferior MI	Good	Temporary pacemaker
Anterior MI	Poor	Temporary pacemaker followed by permanent pacemaker
Atrial fibrillation	Good	β-Blocker and/or amiodarone

MI, myocardial infarction.

     3. Decreases recurrent ischemic events through direct vascular effects.

     4. Not necessary in first hours of STEMI, particularly if blood pressure is low.

  C. Nitrates

     1. Decreases myocardial demand by decreasing preload and afterload.

     2. Increases oxygen supply by dilating coronary resistance vessels.

     3. No mortality benefit demonstrated.

     4. Sublingual or intravenous nitrates beneficial for angina, CHF, hypertension.

     5. Contraindicated in right ventricular infarction.

  D. Calcium channel blockers (CCB)

     1. No mortality benefit.

     2. Nifedipine and other dihydropyridines may cause reflex tachycardia and should not be administered without concurrent BB.

     3. Diltiazem and verapamil may be effective in patients with BB contraindications, but they should be avoided in patients with CHF.

VII. COMPLICATIONS. See Tables 35-4 and 35-5.

TABLE 35-5		**Mechanical Complications of Acute Myocardial Infarction**		
		Pathophysiology	**Physical examination**	**Intervention**
VSD	Acute—subacute	Myocardial necrosis of ventricular septum causing left to right flow during systole	Early, soft, high-frequency systolic murmur at mid to LLSB; elevated JVP; RV heave ± thrill; pulmonary congestion	Emergent echo; right heart catheterization: O_2 step-up in RV; IABP; surgery
Acute MR	Early	Myocardial necrosis of papillary muscles that tether mitral valves	CHF symptoms; early systolic, decrescendo, or holosystolic murmur; thrill radiating to apex ± S3.; ECG shows	Emergent echo; right heart catheterization: large v waves. IABP; surgery.
LV aneurysm	Late (weeks to months)	Regional dilatation and dyskinesis of LV. Risk of thrombus formation, arrhythmias, CHF	persistent ST segment elevation. ± pericardial friction rub	Echo; oral anticoagulation
RV MI	Acute	Hypokinesis or akinesis of right ventricle; may involve SA node and/or AV node	Hypotension, bradycardia (Bezold-Jarish reflex); elevated JVP; congested liver; ST elevations in V1, (± V2, V3), V3R, V4R	IV fluids; temporary pacemaker; intubation; emergent catheterization
LV rupture	Acute—Subacute	Myocardial necrosis of LV causing free wall rupture and flow into pericardial chamber	Usually presents as sudden death; hypotension, muffled heart sounds, elevated JVP	Emergent echo; pericardiocentesis[a] emergent surgery

VSD, ventricular septal defect; MR, mitral regurgitation; LV, left ventricle; TTE, transthoracic echocardiogram; TEE, transesophageal echocardiogram; IVF, intravenous fluids. IABP, intra-aortic balloon pump; RV, right ventricle; TR, tricuspid regurgitation; MI, myocardial infarction; SA, sinoatrial; AV, atrioventricular; CHF, congestive heart failure; LLSB, left lower sternal border; JVP, jugular venous pressure; ECG, electrocardiograph.

[a]Pericardiocentesis should be avoided if patient has stable blood pressure, because this may precipitate hemodynamic collapse.

Selected Readings

ACE Inhibitor Myocardial Infarction Collaborative Group. Indications for ACE inhibitors in the early treatment of acute myocardial infarction: systematic overview of individual data from 100,000 patients in randomized trials. *Circulation* 1998;97:2202–2212.
Early administration of ACE inhibitors reduces 30-day mortality by 7%, and most of the benefit is gained in the first week of use. Hypotension and renal dysfunction are significant complications.

Antithrombotic Trialists' Collaboration. Collaborative meta-analysis of randomised trials of antiplatelet therapy for prevention of death, myocardial infarction, and stroke in high risk patients. *BMJ* 2002;324:71–86.
Aspirin, in doses of 75 to 150 mg, is effective in lowering the absolute risks of fatal and nonfatal myocardial infarction or stroke. Brief annotated bibliography.

Antman EM, Anbe DT, Armstrong PW, et al. ACC/AHA Guidelines for the Management of Patients with ST-Elevation Myocardial Infarction. A Report of the American College of Cardiology/American Heart Association Task Force on Practice Guidelines (Committee to Revise the 1999 Guidelines for the Management of Patients with Acute Myocardial Infarction). *J Am Coll Cardiol* 2004;44:671–719.

Antman EM, Ven de Werf F. Pharmacoinvasive therapy: the future of treatment for ST-elevation myocardial infarction. *Circulation* 2004;109:2480–2486.
Excellent historical review of fibrinolytic therapy and recent advances in facilitated PCI.

The Assessment of the Safety and Efficacy of a New Thrombolytic Regimen (ASSENT)-3 Investigators. Efficacy and safety of tenecteplase in combination with enoxaparin, abciximab, or unfractionated heparin: the ASSENT-3 randomised trial in acute myocardial infarction. *Lancet* 2001;358:605–613.
Combinations of tenecteplase with enoxaparin or abciximab show promising reductions in ischemic complications after an acute myocardial infarction, but results are tempered by increased thrombocytopenia, major bleeding complications, and blood transfusions

Cannon CP, Gibson CM, Lambrew CT, et al. Relationship of symptom-onset-to-balloon time and door-to-balloon time with mortality in patients undergoing angioplasty for acute myocardial infarction. *JAMA* 2000;283:2941–2947.
Prospective, observational study of 27,000 patients demonstrates that a door-to-balloon time greater than 120 minutes increases inpatient mortality by 40% to 60%. Furthermore, primary angioplasty at high-volume primary PCI centers has less inpatient mortality than low-volume centers.

Ellis S, da Silva ER, Heyndrickx G, et al. Randomized comparison of rescue angioplasty with conservative management of patients with early failure of thrombolysis for acute anterior myocardial infarction. *Circulation* 1994;90:2280–2284.
A small, randomized trial demonstrating that rescue angioplasty after failed fibrinolytic therapy is beneficial in patients with anterior infarction.

Fibrinolytic Therapy Trialists' (FTT) Collaborative Group. Indications for fibrinolytic therapy in suspected acute myocardial infarction: collaborative overview of early mortality and major morbidity results from all randomised trials of more than 1000 patients. *Lancet* 1994;343:311–322.
Meta-analysis of nine large-scale trials comparing fibrinolytic therapy with control in AMI or unstable angina patients. With 58,000 patients evaluated, mortality at 30 days is reduced by 1.9% with fibrinolytic therapy. Mortality reduction greater in younger patients, ST elevations, new bundle branch block, lower blood pressure, and earlier intervention. Increased mortality observed in ST depressions.

Grines CL, Cox DA, Stone GW, et al. Coronary angioplasty with or without stent implantation for acute myocardial infarction. Stent Primary Angioplasty in Myocardial Infarction Study Group. *N Engl J Med* 1999;341:1949–1956.
In acute MI patients, stent placement demonstrated less need for target-vessel revascularization compared to PTCA. No mortality benefit demonstrated.

The GUSTO Angiographic Investigators. The effects of tissue plasminogen activator, strep-tokinase, or both on coronary-artery patency, ventricular function, and survival after acute myocardial infarction. *N Engl J Med* 1993;329:1615–1622.
A comparison of four fibrinolytic regimens reveals that early and complete reperfusion of the infarct related artery (90 minutes or less) improves mortality and preserves left ventricular function.

The GUSTO V Investigators. Reperfusion therapy for acute myocardial infarction with fibrinolytic therapy or combination reduced fibrinolytic therapy and platelet glycopro-tein IIb/IIIa inhibition: the GUSTO V randomised trial. *Lancet* 2001;357:1905–1914.
No 30-day mortality benefit is achieved when comparing standard-dose reteplase with half-dose reteplase and full-dose abciximab in acute myocardial infarction patients. Combined therapy demonstrated fewer major adverse cardiac events but significantly greater nonintracranial bleeding complications.

Keeley EC, Boura JA, Grines CL. Primary angioplasty versus intravenous thrombolytic therapy for acute myocardial infarction: a quantitative review of 23 randomised trials. *Lancet* 2003;361:13–20.
A thorough review concluding that primary PCI is superior to thrombolytic therapy at high-volume catheterization centers with door-to-balloon times of 90 minutes or less.

de Lemos JA, Braunwald E. ST segment resolution as a tool for assessing the efficacy of reperfusion therapy. *J Am Coll Cardiol* 2001;38:1283–1294.
ST-segment resolution during acute myocardial infarction is a simple, inexpensive, and universally available tool to predict patent IRA, enhanced microvascular flow, morbid-ity, and mortality. This tool should be utilized in clinical trials comparing different reperfusion regimens and as indication for rescue PCI.

Libby P. Current concepts of the pathogenesis of the acute coronary syndrome. *Circulation* 2001;104:365–372.
This article highlights molecular pathways promoting inflammation and resultant en-dothelial dysfunction. Pleiotropic effects of statins, ACE inhibition, diet, and exercise are explored as protective mediators of inflammation.

Montalescot G, Barragan P, Wittenberg O, et al. Platelet glycoprotein IIb/IIIa inhibition with coronary stenting for acute myocardial infarction. *N Engl J Med* 2001;344:1895–1903.
With a combined end point of death, reinfarction, or urgent revascularization of the IRA, abciximab with stent placement is superior to stent placement alone at 30 days and 6 months.

Morrow DA, Antman EM, Charlesworth A, et al. TIMI risk score for ST-elevation myo-cardial infarction: A convenient, bedside, clinical score for risk assessment at presenta-tion. *Circulation* 2000;102:2031–2037.
A simple arithmetic sum of ten baseline variables provides a clinical risk score (30-day mortality from presentation) that is useful in triage and management of fibrinolytic-eligible STEMI patients.

Roe MT, Ohman EM, Maas AC, et al. Shifting the open-artery hypothesis downstream: the quest for optimal reperfusion. *J Am Coll Cardiol* 2001;37:9–18.
Authors explore myocardial blush grade, cardiac marker trends, and ST-segment reso-lution in evaluating microvascular circulation in acute myocardial infarction patients. GP IIb/IIIa inhibitors specifically target restoration of microvascular flow.

Ryan TJ, Antman EM, Brooks NH, et al. 1999 update: ACC/AHA guidelines for the management of patients with acute myocardial infarction. A report of the American College of Cardiology/American Heart Association Task Force on Practice Guidelines (Committee on Management of Acute Myocardial Infarction). *J Am Coll Cardiol* 1999;34:890–911.

Yusuf S, Peto R, Lewis J, et al. Beta-blockade during and after myocardial infarction: an overview of the randomized trials. *Prog Cardiovasc Dis* 1985;27:335–371.
Long-term use of beta-blockade demonstrates overwhelming reductions in mortality and nonfatal reinfarction.

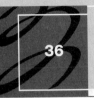

COMPLICATED MYOCARDIAL INFARCTION

36

**Christopher P. Cannon, Leonard I. Ganz,
Peter H. Stone, and Richard C. Becker**

I. BACKGROUND

A. Most complications and the highest mortality occur in the first few months after the acute event (Fig. 36-1); thus, prompt identification and treatment of any established or potential complications are necessary.

II. PATHOPHYSIOLOGY.
It has been well established that the proximate cause of acute myocardial infarction (MI) in most patients is acute coronary occlusion resulting from plaque rupture and platelet initiated thrombosis. The sequelae of coronary occlusion are depicted in Figure 36-2.

III. PROGNOSIS AFTER MYOCARDIAL INFARCTION

A. Factors that play a significant role in determining prognosis after MI:

1. persistent ischemic jeopardy with the potential for recurrent infarction and further loss of myocardial function
2. left ventricular (LV) dysfunction (ejection fraction [EF] <0.40) occurring either in the acute setting or as part of a more insidious process of LV remodeling
3. electrical disturbances that can lead to significant arrhythmias or conduction disorders (Table 36-1)

IV. RECURRENT ISCHEMIA OR INFARCTION.
Recurrent ischemic events after acute MI are a major cause of subsequent mortality.

A. Incidence and clinical consequences. Recurrent infarction may occur in patients whose initial MI was treated with thrombolytic agents and in those whose MI evolved without such therapy. Reinfarction occurs in 4% to 10% of patients after thrombolytic therapy.

B. The consequences of reinfarction with regard to short- and long-term mortality are great. In the Multicenter Investigation of Limitation of Infarct Size (MILIS) study, patients who had infarct extension had an in-hospital mortality more than fourfold higher than patients without extension (30% versus 7%, *p* <.01). In the Thrombosis In Myocardial Infarction (TIMI) trials, patients who had reinfarction had an approximately 2.5 times higher mortality at 1- to 3-year follow-up, compared with those who did not have reinfarction.

C. Prevention

1. Antithrombotic therapy

a. The first component of antithrombotic therapy is aspirin, which has been shown to be of benefit across a wide spectrum of patients with ischemic heart disease. The thienopyridine, clopidogrel, provides further benefit when added to aspirin in patients with acute coronary syndrome (ACS), and in any patient after stent deployment. Glycoprotein (GP) IIB/IIIA receptor antagonists are useful for high-risk patients undergoing percutaneous coronary intervention (PCI).

b. The second component of antithrombotic therapy for prevention of recurrent infarction is heparin. After thrombolytic therapy with tissue-type plasminogen activator (tPA), intravenous unfractionated heparin is necessary to optimize infarct-related artery patency. Low-molecular-weight heparin given subcutaneously has recently been shown to reduce mortality in Acute MI.

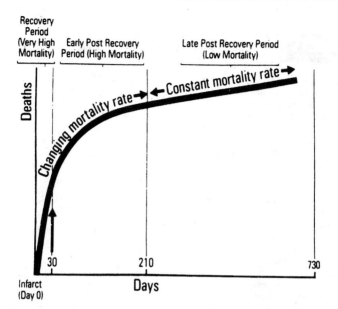

Figure 36-1. Cumulative mortality after an acute myocardial infarction. (From Sherry S. The Anturane Reinfarction Trial. *Circulation* 1980;62[suppl 5]:73, with permission. Copyright 1980, American Heart Association.)

    2. Beta-blockade has been studied extensively and has been found to be benefi-
      cial, especially among patients at highest risk, such as those with heart failure
      or ventricular arrhythmias after MI.
  D. Treatment
    1. An approach to the acute evaluation and treatment of recurrent ischemic events
      is outlined in Figure 36-3.

V. RIGHT VENTRICULAR INFARCTION
  A. Background. Right ventricular infarction occurs clinically in approximately 30%
    of patients with inferior MI (themselves accounting for over half of all MIs) and
    requires special diagnostic evaluation and therapy.
  B. Pathophysiology
    1. Right ventricular infarction is caused by proximal occlusion of the right coronary
      artery. Less often, the left circumflex coronary artery is the infarct-related vessel.

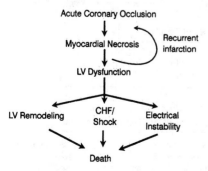

Figure 36-2. Sequelae of acute myocardial infarction. CHF, congestive heart failure; LV, left ventricular.

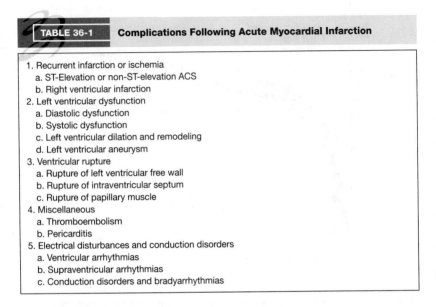

| TABLE 36-1 | Complications Following Acute Myocardial Infarction |

1. Recurrent infarction or ischemia
   a. ST-Elevation or non-ST-elevation ACS
   b. Right ventricular infarction
2. Left ventricular dysfunction
   a. Diastolic dysfunction
   b. Systolic dysfunction
   c. Left ventricular dilation and remodeling
   d. Left ventricular aneurysm
3. Ventricular rupture
   a. Rupture of left ventricular free wall
   b. Rupture of intraventricular septum
   c. Rupture of papillary muscle
4. Miscellaneous
   a. Thromboembolism
   b. Pericarditis
5. Electrical disturbances and conduction disorders
   a. Ventricular arrhythmias
   b. Supraventricular arrhythmias
   c. Conduction disorders and bradyarrhythmias

2. A loss of contractile performance of the right ventricle—a thin-walled chamber—results in reduced left ventricular preload and systemic hypotension. The associated diastolic abnormalities cause RA and systemic venous hypertension.

3. Atrioventricular or sinoatrial nodal block occurs in 10% to 15% of patients with inferior MI but is particularly prevalent in those with right ventricular infarction; nearly 25% of patients with inferior MI with right ventricular infarction exhibit atrioventricular block.

C. Diagnosis

1. The presence of ST-segment elevation in lead V_{4R} has a sensitivity and specificity of 85% to 90% for the diagnosis of right ventricular infarction. Echocardiography is usually definitive.

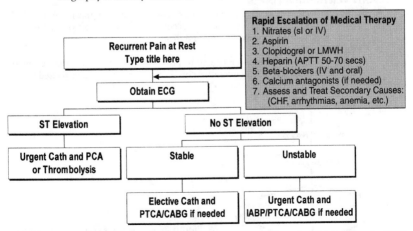

Figure 36-3. Treatment of recurrent ischemic events; SL, sublingually; IV, intravenously; APTT, activated partial thromboplastin time; CHF, congestive heart failure; PTCA, percutaneous transmural coronary angioplasty; IABP, intraaortic balloon pump; CABG, coronary artery bypass grafting.

2. The differential diagnosis for right ventricular infarction includes hypotension resulting from left ventricular (LV) infarction, pericardial tamponade, constrictive pericarditis, and pulmonary embolism.

3. Jugular venous distention and clear lungs distinguish right ventricular infarction from combined right- and left-sided congestion resulting from LV dysfunction.

4. Systemic hypotension is a frequent complication of right ventricular infarction, in which poor right ventricular output leads to decreased LV filling.

D. Treatment

1. Initial treatment of right ventricular infarction involves early reperfusion therapy directed at limiting infarct size.

2. Volume expansion is the mainstay of therapy in patients with hypotension, with the aim of a right atrial or central venous pressure as high as necessary to fill the LV adequately.

3. If volume expansion alone does not restore systemic blood pressure to greater than 90 mm Hg, dobutamine or dopamine should be used to increase right ventricular output.

4. In contrast to left-sided heart failure, in right-sided heart failure venous vasodilators, such as nitrates, should be avoided.

5. If hemodynamically significant sinus bradycardia or atrioventricular block develops, temporary ventricular pacing may be necessary.

VI. LEFT VENTRICULAR DYSFUNCTION (PUMP FAILURE)

A. Background

1. The most important determinant of prognosis after MI is the degree of LV dysfunction (Fig. 36-4).

2. The following factors influence residual ventricular function:
   a. LV function before the acute MI
   b. infarct size
   c. infarct location

B. Pathophysiology

1. The clinical consequence of LV dysfunction is congestive heart failure (CHF).

2. There may be systolic dysfunction, manifested by reduced systemic perfusion and evidence of pulmonary congestion, or diastolic dysfunction, manifested by increases in LV filling pressures and pulmonary congestion, but less evidence of reduced systemic perfusion.

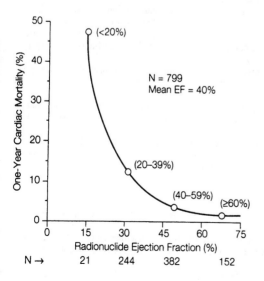

Figure 36-4. Relationship between left ventricular ejection fraction (EF) determined before discharge and 1-year mortality. (From *N Engl J Med* 1983;309:331, with permission.)

3. Diastolic dysfunction occurs almost uniformly in patients with acute MI, although it becomes clinically significant in only one fourth to one third of such patients.

4. It is the most common cause of early mild CHF in the setting of acute MI and can be responsible for acute pulmonary edema.

C. Treatment

1. The treatment goals in patients with diastolic dysfunction include treatment of the pulmonary congestion, which involves diuresis, and treatment of the ischemia.

2. Intravenous nitroglycerin has been used widely because it can be rapidly titrated in response to blood pressure.

3. β-Blockers may be invaluable in patients whose pulmonary congestion is due to isolated diastolic dysfunction.

4. Inotropic agents and mechanical support may also be required in patients with systolic dysfunction.

VII. CARDIOGENIC SHOCK

A. Background

1. The most malignant end of the spectrum of CHF is cardiogenic shock, in which CHF is manifested by frank systemic hypotension and pulmonary congestion.

2. Patients with cardiogenic shock have the highest risk of death after those with MI.

B. Pathophysiology

1. A majority of patients with cardiogenic shock will have large infarctions causing a critical reduction in left ventricular performance.

2. Patients with prior infarctions, multivessel coronary artery disease, or mechanical defects (ventricular septal defect, mitral regurgitation [MR], free wall rupture) should be included in the differential diagnosis

C. Prognosis. Patients with cardiogenic shock following acute MI have an in-hospital mortality rate approaching 70%.

D. Diagnosis. The diagnostic hallmarks of cardiogenic shock are hypotension and hypoperfusion.

E. Treatment

1. The initial goal of treatment for severe CHF is to:

a. ensure adequate oxygenation with supplemental oxygen (and endotracheal intubation, if necessary)

b. maintain systolic blood pressure at 90 mm Hg or greater (MAP >65 mm Hg)

c. provide adequate perfusion of vital organs

2. Diuretics and nitrates diminish pulmonary congestion, but the patient will have no major improvement in cardiac output if preload is compromised.

3. A balanced vasodilator such as nitroprusside reduces both preload and afterload, thereby increasing cardiac output, reducing LV end-diastolic pressure, and alleviating pulmonary congestion.

4. Most effective is administration of both inotropic and vasodilator therapies, with nitroprusside to reduce afterload and dopamine or dobutamine to act as inotropic cardiac stimulants.

5. High-risk patients with cardiogenic shock may require insertion of an intraaortic balloon pump to increase cardiac output as an adjunct in the treatment of severe systolic dysfunction.

6. More important in the treatment of patients with cardiogenic shock is reperfusion of the infarct-related artery. Thus, early angiography and revascularization should be considered, particularly for patients less than 75 years of age.

VIII. VENTRICULAR RUPTURE

A. Background

1. Rupture of the myocardial wall is one of the most serious complications of acute MI.

2. Rupture can occur in the free wall, the interventricular septum (VSD), or the papillary muscle (Table 36-2). Papillary muscle rupture is more common with inferior-posterior MI.

TABLE 36-2	Clinical Profile of Mechanical Complications of Acute Myocardial Infarction		

Variable	Ventricular septal defect	Free wall rupture	Papillary muscle rupture
Age (mean, yr)	63	69	65
Days post-MI	3–5	3–5	3–5
Anterior MI	66%	50%	25%
New murmur	90%	25%	50%
Palpable thrill	Yes	No	Rare
Previous MI	25%	25%	30%
Echocardiographic findings 2-D	Visualize defect may have pericardial effusion		Flail or prolapsing leaflet
Doppler	Detect shunt		Regurgitant jet in LA
PA catheterization	Oxygen step-up in RV	Equalization of diastolic pressures	Prominent V wave in PAO pressure tracing
Incidence	2%–4%	≤10%	1%
Mortality			
Medical	90%	90%	90%
Surgical	50%	Case reports	40%–90%

LA, left atrium; MI, myocardial infarction; PA, pulmonary artery; PAOP, pulmonary artery occlusion pressure, RV, right ventricle; 2-D, two dimensional.
From Pasternak RC, Braunwald E, Sobel BE. Acute myocardial infarction. In: Braunwald E, ed. *Heart disease*, 4th ed. Philadelphia: WB Saunders, 1992, p. 1257; and Labovitz AJ, et al. Mechanical complications of acute myocardial infarction. *Cardiovasc Rev Rep* 1984;5:948, with permission.

3. Free wall rupture occurs in approximately 10% of patients who die of acute MI; those at highest risk are women, hypertensive patients, and those with large infarctions.

4. Rupture usually occurs 3 to 5 days after MI but occurs earlier in patients treated with thrombolytic therapy.

B. Prognosis. Myocardial rupture, particularly of the left ventricular free wall, is associated with a mortality rate exceeding 80%. Prompt surgical repair of myocardial rupture can improve outcome.

C. Diagnosis

1. A high index of suspicion is required for patients with hypotension, severe heart failure or cardiogenic shock, or an unexplained change in clinical states, especially if a new systolic murmur is present.

2. Transthoracic echocardiography is the diagnostic test of choice in patients with suspected ventricular rupture. VSD can be differentiated from MR on the basis of right heart oximetric data with a step up in oxygen saturation between the RA and PA. A new systolic murmur is a clinical feature of VSD and MR.

D. Treatment

1. Pericardiocentesis is potentially lifesaving in patients with free wall rupture but should not delay surgical repair.

2. Supportive measures, intraaortic balloon pump (IABP) placement, and prompt surgical intervention are mainstays of treatment in patients with MR or VSD

IX. THROMBOEMBOLISM

A. Background. Thromboembolism is a recognized complication of acute MI, occurring in 5% to 10% of patients. Both arterial and venous emboli can occur, with LV mural thrombi accounting for most arterial emboli and right ventricular or deep venous thrombi leading to pulmonary embolism.

TABLE 36-3 Arrhythmias During Acute Myocardial Infarction

Category	Arrhythmia	Objective of therapy	Therapeutic options
Ventricular tachyarrhythmias	Ventricular fibrillation	Urgent reversion to sinus rhythm	Defibrillation; lidocaine; amiodarone; bretylium
	Ventricular tachycardia	Restoration of hemodynamic stability	Cardioversion/defibrillation; lidocaine; procainamide; amiodarone
	Accelerated idioventricular rhythm	Observation unless hemodynamic comparomise	Atropine; atrial pacing
	Ventricular premature beats	None	Observation
	Sinus tachycardia	Reduction of heart rate to diminish myocardial work/oxygen demand	Identify and treat underlying cause; beta-blockers
Supraventricular tachyarrhythmias	Atrial fibrillation/flutter	Reduction of ventricular rate; restoration of sinus rhythm	Cardioversion if unstable; beta-blockers, calcium blockers; digoxin; rapid atrial pacing (for flutter); consider anti-arrhythmic therapy
	Paroxysmal supraventricular tachycardia	Reduction of ventricular rate; restoration of sinus rhythm	Vagal maneuvers; adenosine; beta-blockers, calcium blockers; cardioversion if unstable
	Nonparoxysmal junctional tachycardia	Search for precipitating cause (e.g., digitalis toxicity); observation unless hemodynamic compromise	Consider overdrive atrial pacing; consider suppressive antiarrhythmic therapy
Bradyarrhythmias and conduction disturbances	Sinus bradycardia	Increased heart rate only if hemodynamic compromise	Atropine; temporary pacing
	Junctional escape rhythm	Increased heart rate only if hemodynamic compromise	Atropine; temporary pacing
	Atrioventricular block or intra-ventricular conduction block	Increased heart rate; prophylax against progression to high-grade atrioventricular block	Atropine; aminophylline; ventricular pacing

From Ganz LI, Antman EM. Cardiac arrhythmias during acute myocardial infarction. In Antman EM, Rutherford JD, eds. *Coronary care medicine: a practical approach*, 2nd ed. Boston: Martinus Nijhoff, in press. Reprinted with permission by Kluwer Academic Publishers.

TABLE 36-4	Intravenous Antiarrhythmic Drug Dosing During Acute Myocardial Infarction	
Drug	**Bolus**	**Infusion**
Lidocaine	1.0–1.5 mg/kg initially; additional boluses (0.5–0.75 mg/kg every 5–10 min) as necessary to control VT/VF to maximum total load (3.0 mg/kg)	1–4 mg/min
Procainamide	17 mg/kg (maximum 1000 mg) over 15–30 min, monitoring blood pressure	1–4 mg/min
Amiodarone	150 mg over 10 min, monitoring blood pressure	1 mg/min for 6 h, then 0.5 mg/min
Bretylium	5 mg/kg initially; additional boluses (10 mg/kg every 5–10 min) as necessary to control VT/VF to maximum total load (35 mg/kg)	1–2 mg/min

VT/VF, ventricular tachycardia/ventricular fibrillation.

B. Treatment
1. Anticoagulation represents first-line therapy.
2. Fibrinolytic therapy may be considered in patients with cardioembolic stroke but should be undertaken with great caution.

X. PERICARDITIS
A. **Background.** Pericardial irritation occurs in approximately one fourth of patients with acute MI and usually begins 2 to 4 days after MI. It is far more common with ST-elevation MI.
B. **Diagnosis.** Pericarditis may present as an asymptomatic pericardial effusion, early symptomatic pericarditis with or without effusion, or late pericarditis.
C. **Treatment**
1. Aspirin is given to relieve pain and to decrease inflammation; up to 650 mg every 4 hours may be required.
2. Other nonsteroidal antiinflammatory medications relieve pain but may lead to infarct thinning and coronary artery vasoconstriction.
3. Corticosteroids should be avoided.

XI. ELECTRICAL DISTURBANCES
A. **Arrhythmias complicating myocardial infarction**
1. **Background**
   a. Cardiac arrhythmias are an important complication of MI.
   b. In the prehospital phase, ventricular tachycardia and fibrillation probably account for the majority of sudden deaths.
   c. Tachyarrhythmias and bradyarrhythmias are frequently seen in the in-hospital phase of acute MI.
2. **Pathophysiology.** Arrhythmias in the setting of acute MI may be due to reentry, abnormal automaticity, or conduction block; these mechanisms are modulated by ischemia, LV failure, and variations in autonomic tone. Arrhythmias and their treatment are outlined in Tables 36-3 and 36-4.
3. Indications for pacemaker placement during myocardial infarction. (See Chapter 39, "Temporary Cardiac Pacing.")
4. Prophylactic implantation of implantable cardioverter defibrillator (ICD) is recommended in convalescent phase post MR if EF < 30%.

Selected Readings

Becker RC, Gore JM, Lambrew C, et al. A composite view of cardiac rupture in the United States National Registry of Myocardial Infarction. *J Am Coll Cardiol* 1996;27:1321.
Cardiac rupture, although relatively rare, is responsible for 10% to 15% of all deaths after MI. Thrombolytic therapy accelerates the occurrence of rupture, at times within 24 hours of treatment.

Cannon CP. Evidence-based risk stratifications to target therapies in acute coronary syndromes. *Circulation* 2002;106:1588–1591.
A brief overview of the approach to UA/NSTEMS.

Loh E, Sutton MS, Wun CC, et al. Ventricular dysfunction and the risk of stroke after myocardial infarction. *N Engl J Med* 1997;336:251.
The risk of thromboembolism following MI is influenced by ventricular performance. An LV ejection fraction of less than 35% increases the risk of stroke, and therefore long-term anticoagulant therapy should be considered.

Muller JE, Rude RE, Braunwald E, et al. Myocardial infarct extension: occurrence, outcome, and risk factors in the Multi-center Investigation of Limitation of Infarct Size. *Ann Intern Med* 1988;108:1.
MILIS, a landmark study, provided pivotal insights that paved the way for trials of thrombolytic therapy.

TIMI Study Group. Comparison of invasive and conservative strategies after treatment with intravenous tissue plasminogen activator in acute myocardial infarction: results of the Thrombolysis in Myocardial Infarction (TIMI) phase II trial. *N Engl J Med* 1989;320:618.
The rate and clinical relevance of reinfarction after MI was determined in the TIMI phase II trial.

VENTRICULAR TACHYCARDIA
Bruce A. Koplan and William G. Stevenson

37

I. GENERAL PRINCIPLES
A. Definitions
1. **Ventricular tachycardia (VT)**
   a. ≥3 beats at a rate 100 beats per min or greater
   b. QRS width of 0.12 second or greater
   c. Originates from the ventricle
2. **Nonsustained VT (NSVT)**
   a. Terminates spontaneously within 30 seconds without causing severe symptoms
B. Classification (Fig. 37-1)
1. **Monomorphic VT:** Same configuration from beat to beat
   a. Usually due to a circuit through a region of old myocardial infarction (MI) scar.
   b. Idiopathic VT (rare): VT in the absence of an identifiable cause (e.g., structural heart disease, prior MI).
2. **Polymorphic VT:** Continually changing QRS morphology
   a. **Etiologies**
      (1) Active cardiac ischemia (most common)
      (2) Electrolyte disturbance
      (3) Drug toxicity
      (4) Familial
   b. **Torsade de pointes:**
      (1) Unique form of polymorphic VT
      (2) Waxing and waning QRS amplitude during tachycardia associated with prolonged QT interval.
      (3) Secondary to QT-prolonging drugs, electrolyte abnormalities, or familial ion channel disorders (long QT syndrome).
3. **Sinusoidal VT:** Sinusoidal appearance often associated with severe electrolyte disturbance (e.g., hyperkalemia).
4. **Accelerated idioventricular rhythm (AIVR)**
   a. Wide complex, ventricular rhythm at 40 to 100 beats per minute
   b. Usually hemodynamically stable.
   c. Can occur in the first 12 hours after reperfusion of an acute myocardial infarction or during periods of elevated sympathetic tone
   d. Onset is typically preceded by sinus slowing.
   e. Usually resolves without specific therapy
   f. Antiarrhythmic drug treatment is rarely necessary.

II. DIAGNOSIS
A. Differentiating ventricular tachycardia (VT) from supraventricular tachycardia (SVT) in a patient with a wide complex tachycardia (WCT).
1. Differential diagnosis of WCT
   a. VT
   b. SVT with aberrancy (bundle branch block)
   c. SVT conducting of an accessory pathway (Fig. 37-2B)
2. Assume VT until proved otherwise.
3. WCT with a history of MI can be assumed to be VT with better than 95% certainty.

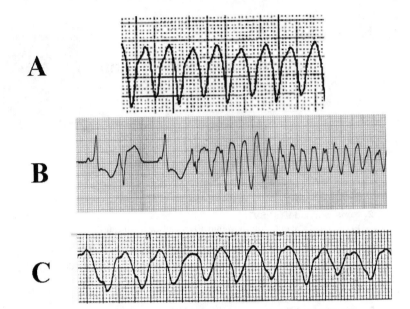

Figure 37-1. Three different wide QRS tachycardias are shown: monomorphic ventricular tachycardia (VT) (*A*) ; polymorphic VT (*B*), and sinusoidal VT due to hyperkalemia (*C*).

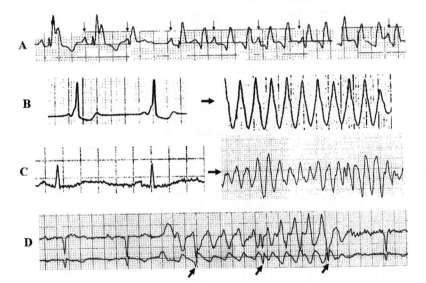

Figure 37-2. Wide complex tachycardias. (*A*) Transition from sinus rhythm to ventricular tachycardia with AV dissociation (P waves identified by small arrows). (*B*) Short PR and delta wave on left, and atrial fibrillation with rapid, wide complex ventricular response in a patient with an accessory pathway. (*C*) Torsade de pointes (*right side*) in a patient with QT prolongation (left side). (*D*) Motion artifact mimicking a wide complex tachycardia. Note that QRS complexes (*large arrows*) are present within the artifact that occurs at the same interval as before and after the onset of the irregular artifactual waveform.

4. If the patient is hemodynamically stable, obtain a 12-lead ECG
5. ECG criteria that favor VT over SVT (Figs. 37-3A and B).
  a. AV dissociation (Fig. 37-2A)
  b. QRS concordance: Absence of an rS or Rs complex in any precordial lead (V_1 through V_6).
  c. rS greater than 100 ms: An interval between the onset of the R and the nadir of the S wave greater than 100 ms in any precordial lead (V_1 through V_6).

VT versus SVT

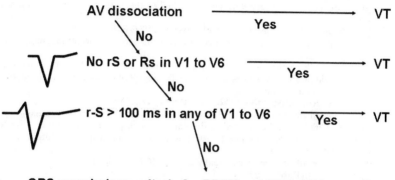

A   QRS morphology criteria for RBBB or LBBB QRS

Wide Complex Tachycardia:
Additional ECG/clinical findings supporting VT vs. SVT

Characteristic	Favors VT	Favors SVT
Capture beats	++	
Fusion beats	+	
Prior known MI or CMP	+	
Irregularly irregular		+
Prior delta wave		+
Onset with a PAC		+
Identical morphology during SR in a patient with IHD		+
QRS >140ms with RBBB or >160ms with LBBB	+	

B

Figure 37-3. (A) Electrocardiographic features to differentiate ventricular tachycardia (VT) versus supraventricular tachycardia (SVT) in patients presenting with wide QRS complex tachycardia. Modified from Brugada et al., *Circulation* 1991. See text for details. (B) Additional clinical and ECG findings to assist with differentiation between VT and SVT in patients with wide complex tachycardia. See text for details. CMP, cardiomyopathy; MI, myocardial infarction; SR, sinus rhythm; IHD, ischemic heart disease.

> **d. Capture beats/fusion beats during tachycardia**
> > **(1)** Occur when a supraventricular beat is able to conduct to the ventricles, depolarizing the ventricle (completely—capture beat, or partially—fusion beat) in advance of the next tachycardia beat.
> > **(2)** Morphologically identical (capture beat) or similar (fusion beat) to the QRS complex seen in sinus rhythm but occur in the midst of a wide QRS complex tachycardia
> **6.** Additional principles
> > **a.** Hemodynamic instability is dependent on the rate and underlying ventricular function and does not differentiate VT from SVT.
> > **b. Electrocardiographic artifacts** can mimic VT/VF (see Fig. 37-2D)

III. TREATMENT. First priority: Determine whether the patient is hemodynamically stable.

> **A. Management of hemodynamically unstable VT/VF** (Fig. 37-4)
> > **1.** Rapid defibrillation (up to three shocks) is the most important measure to improve survival.
> > **2.** If VT/VF persists after defibrillation, epinephri*ne* (1 mg IV every 3 minutes) should be given. Vasopressin (40 units IV, single bolus) is an acceptable alternative to epinephrine.
> > **3. Antiarrhythmic drugs (AAD): see Overview of Drugs**
> > > **a.** Used when cardioversion fails or VT/VF recurs.
> > > **b.** Amiodarone (often used as first-line therapy), procainamide (alternative to amiodarone); lidocaine (most appropriate during suspected acute myocardial ischemia).
> **B. Management of hemodynamically stable WCT** (see Fig. 37-5)
> > **1. Antiarrhythmic** drugs
> > > **a.** Amiodarone
> > > **b.** Procainamide
> > > **c.** Lidocaine

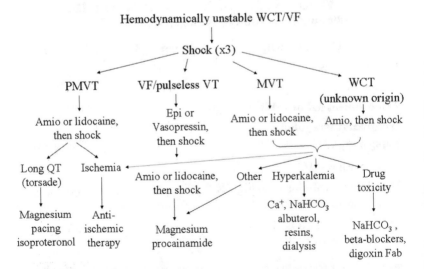

Figure 37-4. Approach to unstable wide complex tachycardia/ventricular fibrillation. This algorithm assumes that cardiopulmonary resuscitation is initiated after the three unsuccessful shocks and maintained until a pulse is achieved. Amio, amiodarone; Epi, epinephrine; MVT, monomorphic ventricular tachycardia; PMVT, polymorphic ventricular tachycardia; VF, ventricular fibrillation; WCT, wide complex tachycardia

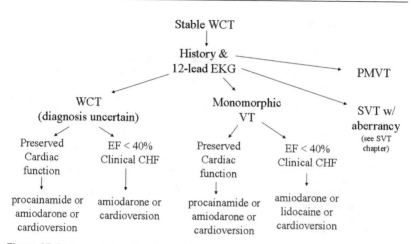

Figure 37-5. Approach to stable wide complex tachycardia. See text for details.

> **2. Electrical cardioversion** is also appropriate initial therapy.
> **3.** If WPW syndrome (see Chapter 38) is suspected (Fig. 37-2B), intravenous procainamide and cardioversion are first-line therapies.

C. Management of polymorphic VT/sinusoidal VT
  1. Correct reversible causes
    a. Cardiac ischemia
    b. Metabolic abnormalities
    c. Drug toxicity including QT-prolonging drugs.
  2. Lidocaine and amiodarone can be considered for recurrent episodes.
  3. Treatment of torsade de pointes
    a. Intravenous magnesium sulfate (1 to 2 g) (can be repeated)
    b. Correction of electrolyte abnormalities
    c. Discontinue QT prolonging medications.
    d. Increasing heart rate with pacing or isoproterenol can be highly effective. Transvenous temporary ventricular pacing is most reliable (target rate of 110 to 120 beats per minute).

D. Implantable cardioverter-defibrillators (ICDs)
  1. May be considered for long-term management of ventricular arrhythmias after acute issues are resolved

E. Management of nonsustained ventricular tachycardia/ventricular ectopy: "First do no harm."
  1. NSVT/PVCs are common in the intensive care unit (ICU).
  2. Treatment
    a. Evaluate for possible aggravating factors (e.g., ischemia, electrolyte disturbance)
    b. β-Blocking agents (if not contraindicated)
    c. In the absence of symptoms, other antiarrhythmic agents should be avoided and may increase mortality.

IV. OVERVIEW OF DRUGS COMMONLY USED FOR MANAGEMENT OF VT/VF IN THE ICU
  A. General principles
    1. Narrow toxic—therapeutic relationship and potential for proarrhythmia necessitate careful monitoring.
    2. Titration to achieve the desired effect is often required.

B. β-Blockers (Class II)
1. Indications
   a. Symptomatic ventricular ectopy
   b. Recurrent sustained ventricular tachyarrhythmias
2. Short-acting agents (e.g., metoprolol tartrate) are preferable in the ICU setting.
   a. Metoprolol
      (1) Can be given orally or as a 5 mg slow intravenous push and repeated every 5 to 10 minutes up to a total of 20 mg IV. Can repeat intravenous boluses every 4 to 6 hours or oral dosing every 4 to 8 hours.
      (2) Esmolol. Useful when there is concern that a β-blocker may be poorly tolerated (short half-life: 2 to 9 min).
         i. 500 mcg/kg IV bolus over 1 minute followed by maintenance dose of 50 mcg/kg per minute titrated for effect up to 300 mcg/kg per minute
3. Adverse effects of β-blockers
   a. Negative inotrope (Avoid with decompensated heart failure)
   b. Bradycardia
   c. Aggravation of bronchospasm

C. Amiodarone
1. Indications
   a. First-line AAD in the recently revised Advanced Cardiac Life Support (ACLS) VF/pulseless VT algorithm.
2. Dosing
   a. 150 to 300 mg IV bolus over 10 minutes, followed by a infusion at 1 mg per minute for 6 hours, then 0.5 mg per minute
   b. Additional 150-mg boluses can be given for breakthrough arrhythmia up to a total load of approximately 2 g per 24 hours and 5 to 8 grams total
   c. Can also be loaded orally (800 to 1600 mg daily for 2 to 3 weeks, with maintenance dose of 400 mg daily for ventricular arrhythmias).
3. Adverse effects
   a. Even though amiodarone causes QT prolongation, torsade de pointes and other proarrhythmias are rare.
   b. Hypotension during IV administration
   c. Bradycardia
   d. Exacerbation of congestive heart failure (negative inotropic effect)
   e. Phlebitis (when administered through a peripheral IV line). Continuous infusions should be administered through a central venous catheter.
   f. Other adverse effects include hepatitis, hyperthyroidism or hypothyroidism, pneumonitis, neuropathy, and tremor.

D. Procainamide
1. First-line agent for WCT (along with amiodarone) for treatment of hemodynamically stable WCT and WCT due to WPW syndrome.
2. Alternative agent for hemodynamically unstable WCT and VF.
3. Dosing: 20 to 30 mg per minute IV infusion loading dose up to a total initial dose of 17 mg/kg followed by a maintenance infusion of 1 to 4 mg per minute
4. Adverse effects
   a. Vasodilatation and negative inotrope.
      (1) Avoid with depressed ventricular function ejection fraction below 40% in favor of amiodarone.
      (2) Blood pressure should be monitored carefully during IV administration.
   b. N-acetyl-procainamide (NAPA), a metabolite of the drug, can increase QTc and cause torsade.
      (1) Monitor serum procainamide and NAPA levels if the drug is continued for greater than 24 hours.
      (2) QTc interval and QRS complex width should be monitored
         i. Discontinue if the QRS widens by more than50% from baseline.
   c. Avoid in patients with significant renal dysfunction.
      (1) NAPA is excreted entirely by the kidney.

E. Lidocaine (IB)

1. Indications
    a. Acute management of life-threatening ventricular arrhythmias, especially when associated with myocardial ischemia. Often ineffective for treatment of sustained VT that is not due to acute myocardial ischemia or infarction; amiodarone, procainamide, and β-blockers are preferable.
2. Dosing: 1 to 1.5 mg/kg IV bolus. Can repeat to a maximum bolus of 3 mg/kg, followed by an infusion of 1 to 4 mg per minute.
3. Adverse effects
    a. Minimal adverse hemodynamic side effects
    b. Neurologic toxicity (seizures, tremors)
4. Class IC AADs (flecainide, propafenone) are rarely used in the ICU for VT/VF and can increase long-term mortality in patients with coronary artery disease and depressed ventricular function.

Selected Readings

Advanced Life Support Working Group of the International Liaison Committee on Resuscitation: ILCOR Advisory Statements: Early defibrillation. *Circulation* 1997;95:2183–2184. *This citation is from the current guidelines on acute management of patients with cardiac arrest.*

Advanced Life Support Working Group of the International Liaison Committee on Resuscitation. International Guidelines 2000 for CPR and ECC. *Circulation* 2000;102:8 (I-1–370). *This citation comes from the current guidelines on cardiopulmonary resuscitation and emergency cardiac care.*

Brugada P, Brugada J, Mont L, et al. A new approach to the differential diagnosis of a regular tachycardia with a wide QRS complex. *Circulation* 1991;83:1649–1659. *This articles describes how to use electrocardiographic criteria to differentiate ventricular tachycardia from supraventricular tachycardia in patients with wide complex tachycardia.*

The Cardiac Arrhythmia Suppression Trial (CAST) investigators. Preliminary report: effect of encainide and flecainide on mortality in a randomized trial of arrhythmia suppression after myocardial infarction. *New Engl J Med* 1989;321(6):406–412. *This study describes the increased mortality risk associated with class IC antiarrhythmic agents used in the patients with coronary artery disease.*

The Cardiac Arrhythmia Suppression Trial II Investigators. Effect of the antiarrhythmic agent moricizine on survival after myocardial infarction. *N Engl J Med* 1992;327:227–233. *This study also demonstrates the increased mortality associated with class IC antiarrhythmic agents when used in patients with coronary artery disease.*

Connoly SJ. Evidenced based analysis of Amiodarone efficacy and safety. *Circulation* 1999; 100:2025–2034. *This article reviews many important studies regarding the efficacy and safety of amiodarone.*

Echt DS, Liebson PR, Mitchell LB, et al. Mortality and morbidity in patients receiving encainide, flecainide or placebo: the Cardiac Arrhythmia Suppression Trial. *N Engl J Med* 1991;324:781–788. *This study demonstrates the increased mortality associated with class IC antiarrhythmic agents when used in patients with coronary artery disease.*

Gorgels et al. Usefulness of AIVR as a marker for myocardial necrosis and reperfusion during thrombolysis in acute MI. *Am J Cardiol* 1988;61:231. *This article describes the association between accelerated idioventricular rhythm and myocardial reperfusion.*

Jawad-Kanber G. Sherrod TR. Effect of loading dose of procaine amide on left ventricular performance in man. *Chest* 1974;66:269–272. *This article describes the hemodynamic and electrophysiologic effects of procainamide.*

MacMahon S, Collins R, Peto R, et al. Effects of prophylactic lidocaine in suspected acute myocardial infarction. An overview of results from the randomized, controlled trials. *JAMA* 1988;260:1910–1916.
This study describes the lack of benefit of prophylactic lidocaine in suspected acute myocardial infarction.

Nalos PC, Ismail Y, Pappas JM, et al. Intravenous amiodarone for short term treatment of refractory ventricular tachycardia or fibrillation. *Am Heart J* 1991;122:1629–1632.
This study demonstrates the usefulness of amiodarone for management of ventricular arrhythmias.

Nasir N Jr, Taylor A, Doyle TK, et al. Evaluation of intravenous lidocaine for the termination of sustained monomorphic ventricular tachycardia in patients with coronary artery disease in patients with or without healed myocardial infarction. *Am J Cardiol* 1994;74:1183–1186.
This study demonstrates the usefulness of lidocaine for management of ventricular arrhythmias in patients with coronary disease.

Tchou P, Young P, Mahmud R, et al. Useful clinical criteria for the diagnosis of ventricular tachycardia. *Am J Med* 1988;84:53–56.
This article describes the ability to use clinical history to assist with the differentiation of ventricular tachycardia from supraventricular tachycardia with aberrancy in patients with wide complex tachycardia.

SUPRAVENTRICULAR TACHYCARDIA

John L. Sapp Jr. and Laurence M. Epstein

38

I. BACKGROUND

A. Definition: Supraventricular tachycardias are those that require involvement of the atrioventricular (AV) node or atria for their perpetuation. They are usually described by mechanism or by their electrocardiographic appearance (Figs. 38-1 and 38-2).

II. MECHANISMS.
There are three main mechanisms underlying supraventricular tachycardias:

A. Abnormal automaticity: inappropriate sinus tachycardia, ectopic atrial tachycardia

B. Abnormal repolarization/triggered activity: atrial premature contractions, multifocal atrial tachycardia

C. Reentry: atrioventricular reentrant tachycardia (AVRT), atrioventricular nodal reentrant tachycardia (AVNRT), atrial flutter

III. RECOGNITION AND DIAGNOSIS (see Figs. 38-1 and 38-2)

A. QRS duration less than 120 msec in *all* surface leads: likely supraventricular SVT may result in a wide complex tachycardia when there is a bundle branch block or intraventricular conduction delay. Wide complex tachycardia in the presence of structura heart disease should be considered ventricular tachycardia until proven otherwise.

B. Irregularly irregular QRS complexes most commonly signify atrial fibrillation (multifocal atrial tachycardia is distinguished by the presence of P waves).

C. Rapid irregularly irregular wide QRS tachycardia may represent atrial fibrillation with preexcitation over an accessory pathway (Wolff-Parkinson-White syndrome).

D. Atrial activity?

1. P wave may be buried in the QRS-T complex. If possible, compare to sinus rhythm tracings.

2. Organized continuous atrial activity faster than 240 beats per minute is classified as atrial flutter. Typical atrial flutter: down-sloping flutter waves in the inferior leads followed by a rapid upstroke, short positive P waves in V1, and an atrial rate of approximately 300 beats per minute. Atypical flutter circuit or ectopic atrial tachycardia may have a different morphology or cycle length.

3. Every P wave is not associated with a QRS (i.e., AV block is present), the tachycardia is unlikely to depend on the AV node. Differential diagnosis: ectopic atrial tachycardia, rarely be seen with AVNRT.

4. A 1:1 relationship between P and QRS deflections? (See Fig. 38-2.) A long RP (RP greater than PR) tachycardia. Differential diagnosis: ectopic atrial tachycardia, less commonly AVRT utilizing a slowly conducting bypass tract or atypical AVNRT. A short RP tachycardia (RP < PR). Differential diagnosis: AVNRT, AVRT, or ectopic atrial tachycardia.

IV. GENERAL MANAGEMENT OF SUPRAVENTRICULAR TACHYCARDIAS.
A general approach to the evaluation and management of supraventricular tachycardias is outlined in Figure 38-3.

A. Assess patient stability

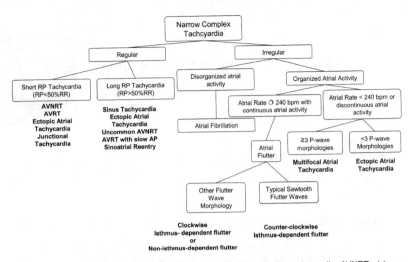

Figure 38-1. Electrocardiographic classification of supraventricular tachycardia; AVNRT, atrioventricular nodal reentrant tachycardia; AVRT, atrioventricular reentrant tachycardia.

B. Identify sinus tachycardia and multifocal atrial tachycardia: treat the underlying causes and control heart rate

C. If unstable: prompt D/C cardioversion

    1. Electrical cardioversion should be **synchronized.** Atrial flutter and other SVTs are usually terminable with a single 50- to 100-joule countershock. Atrial fibrillation often requires 200 to 360 joules.

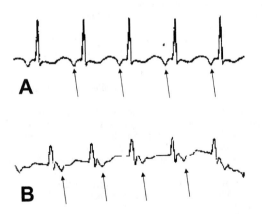

Sinus Tachycardia (Normal P wave morphology)

Atrial Tachycardia (Abnormal P wave morhpology)

Atypical AV Node Reentry Tachycardia

AVRT with slowly conducting Accessory Pathway

AV Node Reentry Tachycardia

Atrioventricular Reentry Tachycardia

Atrial Tachycardia with first degree heart block

Sinus Tachycardia with first degree heart block

Junctional Tachycardia

Figure 38-2. Diagnosis of regular narrow complex tachycardias. *(A)* The RP interval (P waves indicated by *arrows*) is longer than the PR interval. The differential diagnosis is sinus tachycardia (which is associated with a normal or near normal P wave morphology), ectopic atrial tachycardia (which usually has an abnormal P wave morphology), atypical atrioventricular (AV) node reentry tachycardia (in which antegrade propagation is via the "fast pathway" and retrograde activation is via the "slow pathway"), or AV reentry tachycardia utilizing a slowly conducting accessory pathway. *(B)* The RP interval (P waves indicated by *arrows*) is shorter than the PR interval. The differential diagnosis is typical AV nodal reentry tachycardia, atrioventricular reentry tachycardia, ectopic or sinus tachycardia with first-degree heart block (PR prolongation), or junctional tachycardia.

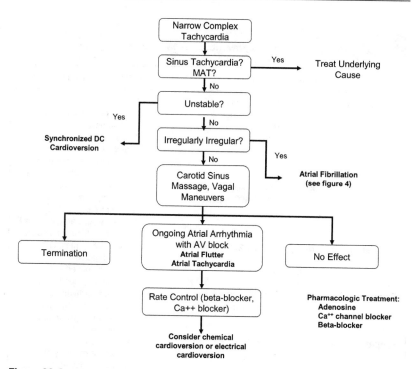

Figure 38-3. Therapeutic approach to narrow complex tachycardia; MAT.

D. Stable patients

1. Vagal maneuvers: carotid sinus massage or a Valsalva maneuver
2. Adenosine: 6 to 12 mg, rapid IV push, followed by saline flush. Carbamazepine and dipyridamole potentiate the actions of adenosine and may prolong its action causing angina or bronchospasm. Methylxanthines (caffeine, theophyllines) antagonize the effects of adenosine and may render it ineffective.
3. IV verapamil, diltiazem or β-blockers may be used (Table 38-1). Vagal maneuvers may be repeated in the presence of drug therapy and may act synergistically.
4. Atrial flutter and atrial fibrillation are unlikely to terminate with these measures, although flutter waves or ectopic P waves may be unmasked, facilitating diagnosis.
5. Type I or type III antiarrhythmic agents may be used for conversion alone or in combination with DC cardioversion.

V. SPECIFIC ARRHYTHMIAS AND THERAPIES

A. Atrial fibrillation
1. Atrial fibrillation is the most common supraventricular tachycardia, and involves chaotic atrial activation. (Fig. 38-4F)
2. Acute treatment (Fig. 38-5.)
   a. Unstable: Synchronized direct current cardioversion is the treatment of choice. Atrial fibrillation may be difficult to convert and require higher energies than other arrhythmias.
   b. Stable: pharmacologic rate control.
      (1) β_1-selective adrenergic receptor antagonists in nonasthmatic patients.
      (2) Non–dihydropyridine calcium channel blockers (e.g., verapamil, diltiazem) may be used in absence of ventricular dysfunction.

TABLE 38-1		Drugs for Supraventricular Tachycardias	
Drug	**Class**	**Dosage**	**Potential adverse effects**
Procainamide	Ia	IV 15 mg/kg not faster than 50 mg/min PO sustained release 250–1,000 mg q6h	Hypotension Lupuslike syndrome, GI symptoms Torsade de pointes, QT prolongation May slow atrial arrhythmia with faster ventricular response
Quinidine	Ia	PO quinidine sulfate 200–400 mg q6 h	Torsade de pointes, QT prolongation GI symptoms May slow atrial arrhythmia with faster ventricular response
Disopyramide	Ia	PO 100–200 mg q6–8 h	Torsade de pointes, QT prolongation Anticholinergic effects Heart failure (negative inotrope)
Flecainide	Ic	PO 200–300 mg load, then 100–200 mg q12 h	Ventricular arrhythmia May slow atrial arrhythmia with faster ventricular response Hypotension
Propafenone	Ic	PO 450–600 mg load, 150–300 mg q8 h maintenance	Hypotension May slow atrial arrhythmia with faster ventricular response
Esmolol	II	IV 0.5 mg/kg over 1–2 minutes, then 0.05–0.2 mg/kg/min maintenance	Bronchoconstriction Bradycardia, heart block, hypotension
Metoprolol	II	IV load 2.5–5 mg q5 min up to 15 mg. May give IV maintenance 2.5–5 mg q6h PO 25–100 mg bid	Bronchoconstriction Bradycardia, heart block, hypotension
Propranolol	II	IV load 0.15 mg/kg PO maintenance 20–80 mg q6h	Bronchoconstriction Bradycardia, heart block, hypotension
Sotalol	II/III	PO maintenance 80–160 mg bid	Bronchoconstriction Bradycardia, heart block, hypotension QT prolongation, torsade de pointes
Amiodarone	III	IV load 5–7 mg/kg over 30–60 minutes, then 1.2–1.8 g per day IV or PO until 10 g administered, then 200–400 daily maintenance PO load 900–1,600 mg/day in 3–4 divided doses until 10 g administered, then 200–400 mg daily maintenance	Hypotension with rapid infusion, phlebitis if given peripherally Pulmonary toxicity, skin photosensitivity and pigmentation

(continued)

TABLE 38-1		continued		

Drug	Class	Dosage		Potential adverse effects
Amiodarone (*continued*)				Hypo/hyperthyroidism, corneal deposits, hepatitis Optic/peripheral neuropathy, bradycardia, Hypotension Interaction with multiple drugs including digoxin and warfarin
Ibutilide	III	IV 1 mg over 10 minutes; repeat once if necessary		QT prolongation, torsade de pointes
Dofetilide	III	PO dose according to creatinine clearance: >60, 500 mcg bid; 40–60, 250 mcg bid; 20–40, 125 mcg bid		QT prolongation, torsade de pointes Contraindicated for creatinine clearance <20 mL/min
Verapamil	IV	IV load 0.075–0.15 mg/kg over 5 minutes		Bradycardia, heart block, hypotension Edema, constipation
Diltiazem	IV	JV load 0.25 mg/kg over 2–5 minutes, then 5–15 mg/hr maintenance PO 60–180 mg bid		Bradycardia, heart block, hypotension Edema, constipation
Digoxin	N/A	IV 0.25 load mg q2–4h up to 1.5 mg PO maintenance 0.125–0.25 mg daily		Bradycardia, heart block, atrial/ventricular tachycardia Interaction with multiple drugs
Adenosine	N/A	IV 6–12 mg bolus followed by saline flush		Transient chest pain, bronchoconstriction, complete heart block Potentiated by dipyridamole, heart transplant and central administration route

(3) Digitalis may be used with relative safety in patients with poor ventricular function but provides only modest control of ventricular rate. It is ineffective in patients with high adrenergic tone or when rapid rate control is required.

(4) Amiodarone effectively controls ventricular rate response during atrial fibrillation when administered intravenously (IV) and is safe for use in patients with low ejection fraction. Intravenous amiodarone should be administered through a central line to avoid phlebitis.

c. Treat underlying causes

(1) Stop offending drugs (e.g., methylxanthine derivatives).

(2) Correct electrolyte abnormalities.

(3) Attend to other cardiac, endocrine (particularly thyroid), and pulmonary disease.

(4) Correct/treat severe metabolic stress, severe noncardiac disease and other hyperadrenergic states.

d. Rate versus rhythm control

(1) Rate control and anticoagulation are a reasonable approach in stable patients with limited symptoms.

(2) Patients in atrial fibrillation less than 48 hours or who have been anti-coagulated (international normalized ratio greater than 2 for at least 3 weeks) are candidates for early cardioversion.

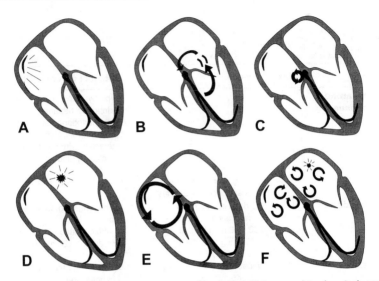

Figure 38-4. Mechanisms of supraventricular tachycardias. *(A)* Inappropriate sinus tachycardia occurs when the sinus node or contiguous areas along the crista terminalis trigger heart rates that are inappropriately fast. *(B)* Atrioventricular (AV) reentry tachycardia uses an accessory pathway for retrograde conduction. Accessory pathways may be manifest (Wolff-Parkinson-White syndrome, pathway can conduct antegrade or retrograde, associated with delta wave on ECG) or concealed (incapable of antegrade conduction). Antegrade propagation via the His-Purkinje system leads to a narrow QRS, and reentry using the accessory pathway as the retrograde limb produces tachycardia. *(C)* AV node reentry tachycardia utilizes two functional pathways within the AV node or approaches to the AV node, most commonly with antegrade conduction along the more slowly conducting pathway and retrograde conduction via the more rapidly conducting pathway. *(D)* Ectopic atrial tachycardia requires the presence of a focus other than the sinus node, which usurps control of the atrial rate. The focus is often located on the crista terminalis, within a venous structure, or near an AV valve. *(E)* Atrial flutter, in its most common (clockwise) form, consists of macroreentry within the right atrium. Activation proceeds up the interatrial septum, across the roof of the right atrium, anterolaterally anterior to the crista terminalis, and inferiorly to the Eustachian isthmus across which it conducts back to the interatrial septum. The atrial rate is usually approximately 300 beats per minute, with conduction to the ventricles limited by the AV node. *(F)* Atrial fibrillation may be initiated by focal ectopy leading to multiple reentrant wavelets within the atria and a high-frequency barrage of impulses activating the AV node. Ventricular activation is limited by the AV node.

(3) Pharmacologic cardioversion: procainamide, flecainide, propafenone, dofetilide, ibutilide, and amiodarone. Class I drugs should always be preceded by rate control.

(4) Unanticoagulated patients in atrial fibrillation for more than 48 hours (or for an uncertain duration) are at elevated risk of thromboembolism. These patients require anticoagulation prior to conversion from atrial fibrillation. An alternative approach is to exclude left atrial thrombus with transesophageal echocardiography, initiate IV anticoagulation, and to proceed to DC cardioversion, followed by oral anticoagulation for at least 4 weeks.

(5) Drug therapy to maintain sinus rhythm includes class Ia, Ic, and III antiarrhythmic agents (see Table 38-1). This approach may be warranted in patients who do not tolerate or are symptomatic in atrial fibrillation. Catheter ablation for atrial fibrillation is a newer approach which may be helpful for selected patients.

(6) Catheter ablation of the AV node with permanent pacemaker implantation may be useful in patients in whom AV nodal blocking medications are not tolerated or in whom rate control is difficult with conventional agents.

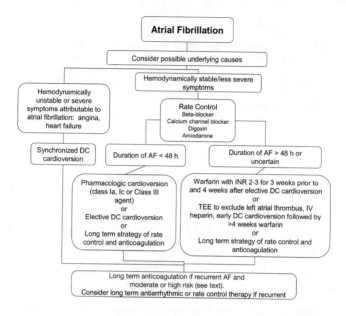

Figure 38-5. Therapeutic approach to atrial fibrillation.

(7) Patients with recurrent atrial fibrillation should be considered for anticoagulation. Low risk patients may be treated with ASA 81–325 mg daily. Moderate risk patients (age 65–75, coronary disease, thyrotoxicosis, diabetes mellitus) may receive either ASA or warfarin. High risk patients (prior stroke/TIA, age >75, history of hypertension, mitral stenosis, ventricular dysfunction, or ≥2 intermediate risk factors) should receive warfarin; target INR 2–3, unless the risk of hemorrhage is excessive.
  e. Atrial fibrillation post–cardiac surgery. Atrial fibrillation is a common sequela to cardiac surgery, occurring in approximately 25% of patients.
   (1) Prophylactic treatment
     i. Beta-blockade administered preoperatively is associated with a 77% reduction in relative risk of atrial fibrillation.
     ii. Amiodarone administered orally preoperatively, or IV postoperatively, has been associated with reductions in the frequency of atrial fibrillation.
     iii. Temporary atrial pacing post–cardiac surgery has also been associated with a decrease in the incidence of postoperative atrial fibrillation.
     iv. In general, all patients undergoing cardiac surgery should receive prophylactic beta-blockade, and those at especially high risk (older age, prior history of atrial fibrillation, mitral valve surgery) may be considered for prophylactic amiodarone therapy.
   (2) Management of atrial fibrillation following cardiac surgery
     i. Unstable patients require urgent cardioversion.
     ii. Stable patients usually require rate control.
     iii. Rate control and anticoagulation are appropriate for most patients; a large proportion of patients will convert spontaneously.
B. Atrial flutter
  1. Usually macroreentry with a single wave-front propagating around the tricuspid annulus, most commonly up the interatrial septum and down the right

atrial free wall, anterior to the crista terminalis, and back across the isthmus between the inferior vena cava and tricuspid annulus (Fig. 38-4E).

2. ECG demonstrates typical flutter wave morphology, a slowly down-sloping initial portion followed by a sharp upward deflection toward the baseline.

3. The clinical presentation and management of atrial flutter are very similar to those of atrial fibrillation. However, rate control can be more difficult to achieve and radiofrequency catheter ablation is more effective for atrial flutter.

4. **Acute treatment**
   a. Rate control, especially prior to attempting chemical cardioversion
   b. Typical atrial flutter is amenable to cure by catheter ablation. The narrow isthmus of atrium between the tricuspid annulus and inferior vena cava can be interrupted by a line of ablation with a high success rate and rare complications
   c. The risk of thromboembolism from atrial flutter is significant. Atrial flutter warrants anticoagulation in the same manner as for atrial fibrillation (see above).

C. AV nodal reentry tachycardia
1. AVNRT is the most common cause of rapid regular supraventricular tachycardia, accounting for up to 60% of cases.
2. Paroxysmal rapid regular narrow complex tachycardia with heart rate often 150 to 250 beats per minute and P waves either buried within the QRS complex or visible at its termination (r' or S wave). A "Short RP" tachycardia.
3. Symptoms: palpitations, pounding in the neck, lightheadedness, shortness of breath, chest pressure, weakness, and fatigue.
4. Presents in third to fifth decade, with a 70% female preponderance
5. Initiated by a critically timed premature complex that blocks in the antegrade "fast" AV nodal pathway, conducts down the "slow" AV nodal pathway, and then reenters retrogradely up the fast pathway (Fig. 38-4C).
6. Atypical AVNRT is caused by reentry antegrade over the fast pathway and retrograde via the slow pathway. A form of long RP tachycardia.
7. **Acute treatment:** see General Management of Supraventricular Tachycardias earlier
8. **Chronic treatment**
   a. Pharmacologic therapy: β-Blockers, calcium blockers, class I and III agents
   b. Catheter ablation is curative with low risk and no need for long-term drug therapy.

D. Atrioventricular reentry tachycardia
1. AVRT is a common form of regular supraventricular tachycardia, accounting for up to 30% of patients.
2. During tachycardia, the QRS usually appears normal, and P waves, if visible, will be seen at the end of the QRS complex, within the ST segment, or within the T wave.
3. The mechanism of tachycardia is reentry; an atrioventricular accessory pathway (AP) is the retrograde limb and the AV node is the antegrade limb (Fig. 38-4B).
4. APs are congenital anomalies of the heart that allow conduction of excitatory impulses across the AV groove, bypassing the AV node.
5. **Acute treatment:** see General Management of Supraventricular Tachycardias earlier
6. **Chronic treatment:** same as for AVNRT

E. Wolff-Parkinson-White syndrome
1. The Wolff-Parkinson-White syndrome (WPW) consists of a short PR interval and ventricular preexcitation (delta wave) due to an accessory pathway, with symptoms of palpitations.
2. The most common arrhythmia associated with WPW is AVRT.
3. The accessory tract may also participate in arrhythmogenesis by allowing rapid ventricular rates during atrial fibrillation. The accessory pathway may permit very rapid ventricular activation during atrial arrhythmias, rarely resulting in ventricular fibrillation.

4. Patients with WPW may be at risk for sudden cardiac death, although the overall risk is rather low, on the order of 0.15% per patient-year.

5. Acute management

   a. Fast preexcited ventricular response to atrial fibrillation (irregular rhythm with varying QRS complexes) should undergo electrical cardioversion.

   b. Stable preexcited atrial fibrillation may be treated with class Ia, Ic, or III drugs. Intravenous ibutilide (1 to 2 mg IV) or procainamide (10 to 15 mg/kg IV) may be effective.

   c. During rapid preexcited atrial fibrillation, AV nodal blocking drugs are contraindicated (digoxin, adenosine, calcium channel blockers, and β-blockers) due to the potential for more rapid ventricular rates.

   d. Treatment of AVRT in patients with WPW: as above.

   e. Chronic therapy

   (1) Patients with symptoms or those in high-risk professions (e.g., airline pilots) should undergo curative catheter ablation.

   (2) Patients with a history of atrial fibrillation with rapid ventricular response or ventricular fibrillation should undergo catheter ablation.

   (3) Patients who are at low risk (intermittent preexcitation or sudden failure of preexcitation during increased atrial rates), yet who experience recurrent AVRT may be treated similarly to patients with concealed accessory pathways or AV node reentry tachycardia. Catheter ablation of the accessory pathway causing WPW offers a high success rate and low complication rate.

F. Ectopic atrial tachycardia

   1. Ectopic atrial tachycardia most likely occurs as a result of abnormal automaticity or triggered activity within the atrium and may be more likely to be associated with structural heart disease than is AVNRT or AVRT.

   2. Narrow complex tachycardia with an RP interval that is usually, but not always, longer than the PR interval, depending on AV nodal conduction properties.

   3. The P wave morphology may or may not be visibly different from sinus.

   4. Ectopic atrial tachycardia may occur in short runs, may be sustained, or even may be incessant.

   5. May be associated with underlying disease (coronary artery disease, myocardial infarction, ethanol ingestion, hypoxia, theophylline toxicity, digitalis toxicity, or electrolyte abnormalities).

   6. Acute treatment

   a. β-blockade

   b. Calcium channel blockade (non-dihydropyridine calcium channel blockers)

   c. Class Ia and Ic antiarrhythmic drugs (with AV nodal blockade), amiodarone.

   7. Chronic treatment

   a. AV nodal blocking agents and antiarrhythmic agents, as above.

   b. Catheter ablation is a viable option for treatment of ectopic atrial tachycardia.

G. Multifocal atrial tachycardia

   1. Multifocal atrial tachycardia is thought to be caused by abnormal automaticity or triggered activity and may be triggered by hypoxia, elevated sympathetic tone, hypokalemia, hypomagnesemia, or theophylline.

   2. It is recognized by a rapid atrial rhythm with at least three P wave morphologies and variable ventricular response.

   3. Acute treatment

   a. Beta-blockade. Caution is required in patients with reactive airways disease.

   b. Calcium channel blockers may be effective and are the treatment of choice in patients with known reactive airways disease.

   c. Underlying triggers must be addressed, including oxygenation, CO_2 clearance, magnesium and potassium repletion, and avoidance of methylxanthine derivatives (e.g., theophylline).

VI. CONCLUSIONS. Supraventricular tachycardias frequently complicate acute medical illness and uncommonly cause severe illness. An organized approach to patients presenting with narrow complex tachycardias facilitates accurate diagnosis and thereby guides therapy. Most SVTs can be medically managed, although DC cardioversion is a highly effective means of restoring sinus rhythm in the unusual circumstance that more conservative measures fail to implement or that time does not permit. Atrial fibrillation is the most common SVT and can usually be managed with a combination of pharmacologic therapy, including anticoagulation and treatment aimed at contributing causes.

Selected Readings

Blomstrom-Lundqvist C, et al. ACC/AHA/ESC Guidelines for the management of patients with supraventricular arrhythmias. *J Am Coll Cardiol* 2003;1493–1531.
Definitive management guidelines for patients with supraventricular tachycardia. Available at cardiosource.com.

Fuster V, et al., ACC/AHA/ESC Guidelines for the management of patients with atrial fibrillation: executive summary: A report of the American College of Cardiology/American Heart Association Task Force on Practice Guidelines and the European Society of Cardiology Committee for Practice Guidelines and Policy Conferences (Committee to Develop Guidelines for the Management of Patients with Atrial Fibrillation). *Circulation* 2001;104(17):2118–2150.
Authoritative reference for the management of patients with atrial fibrillation. Currently in revision. Available at cardiosource.com

Josephson ME. Paroxysmal supraventricular tachycardia: an electrophysiologic approach. *Am J Cardiol* 1978;41:1123–1126.
Review of the presentation and mechanisms of supraventricular arrhythmias.

Kastor J. Multifocal atrial tachycardia. *N Engl J Med* 1990;322(24):1713–1717.
Review of the diagnosis and treatment of multifocal atrial tachycardia.

Maisel WH, Rawn JD, and Stevenson WG. Atrial fibrillation following cardiac surgery. *Ann Intern Med* 2001;135:1061–1073.
Review of the incidence and treatment of atrial fibrillation following cardiac surgery.

Manning WJ, et al. Transesophageal echocardiographically facilitated early cardioversion from atrial fibrillation using short-term anticoagulation: final results of a prospective 4.5-year study. *J Am Coll Cardiol* 1995;25:1354–1361.
Initial, large clinical series looking at the use of transesophageal echocardiography to guide cardioversion for atrial fibrillation.

Morady F, Catheter ablation of supraventricular arrhythmias: state of the art. *PACE* 2004; 27:125–142.
Up-to-date review of the "state of the art" of catheter ablation for the treatment of supraventricular arrhythmias.

I. GENERAL PRINCIPLES
A. Background
1. Pacing options
   a. Transcutaneous
      (1) Primarily used for protection in patients at risk for high-grade atrioventricular (AV) block
      (2) Currently with multifunctional capabilities and can be used for overdrive functions and sensing
      (3) Limitations
         i. Patient discomfort
         ii. Poor capture (particularly with obese patients)
         iii. Large stimulus artifacts
   b. Transvenous
      (1) Supplanted transcutaneous pacing given ease of use and less patient discomfort
2. Algorithm for managing patients with bradycardia (Fig. 39-1)

II. INDICATIONS
A. Overview
1. The indications for temporary pacing in the setting of an acute myocardial infarction (MI) have been well defined and are outlined in a recent consensus guideline from the American Heart Association and the American College of Cardiology (AHA/ACC)
2. No similar guidelines are available for temporary cardiac pacing for other conditions causing bradycardia (i.e., infection, electrolyte abnormalities, drug reactions)
3. Decision to initiate temporary pacing involves three considerations (Tables 39-1 and 39-2)
   a. Is temporary pacing indicated?
   b. Method of pacing (transvenous versus transcutaneous)?
   c. What is the end point? Should permanent pacing be considered?
      (1) Of patients needing temporary pacing, 50% require permanent pacing prior to discharge.
      (2) Transient indications commonly include MI, infection, or overmedication
B. Scope of therapy
1. Bradyarrhythmias
   a. Most common indication is symptomatic bradycardia that is unresponsive to pharmacologic therapy
   b. Classifications
      (1) Sinus node dysfunction
      (2) Conduction block
2. Tachyarrhythmias
   a. Prevention or termination of supraventricular tachycardia (SVT) or ventricular tachycardia (VT)
   b. Rarely used in clinical practice due to efficacy of medications and increased prevalence of implantable cardioverter-defibrillators (ICDs)
   c. Many rhythms are susceptible to pace termination

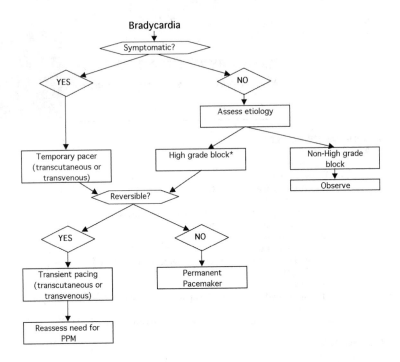

Figure 39-1. Algorithm for management of bradycardia unresponsive to pharmacologic therapy. High grade block includes those listed in Table I-Class I indications (key: PPM-permanent pacemaker)

     (1) SVT reentry (AVNRT, accessory pathway mediated tachycardia)

     (2) VT reentry (scar VT)

  d. No role in management of ventricular fibrillation (VF) or triggered ventricular tachycardia

  e. Prevention of torsade de pointes

     (1) Shortening of QT with pacing to reduce risk of polymorphic VT.

3. MI (Table 39-1)

  a. Ischemia to the conduction system

     (1) Revascularization is primary management, particularly when AV nodal or fascicular blood supply is compromised.

       i. Inferior ischemia (AV nodal blood supply)

       ii. Anterior ischemia (disruption of fascicular blood supply)

     (2) Prognosis

       i. Depends on the extent of underlying ischemia and left ventricular (LV) function

       ii. Death is rare from complete heart block.

  b. Predicting risk of conduction block

     (1) Lamas scoring system based on simple electrocardiographic (ECG) variables

     (2) 1 point each

       i. First-degree AV block

       ii. Second-degree AV block

       iii. Left anterior fascicular block (LAFB) or left posterior fascicular block (LPFB)

| TABLE 39-1 | ACC/AHA Guidelines for Transcutaneous and Transvenous Pacing in Acute Myocardial Infarction |

Placement of Transcutaneous Patches and Active (Demand) Transcutaneous Pacing

Class I	Sinus bradycardia (less than 50 bpm) with systolic BP < 80 mmHg unresponsive to drug therapy
	Mobitz type II second-degree AV block
	Third degree heart block
	Bilateral bundle branch block (alternating right and left bundle branch)
	Newly acquired or age-indeterminate LBBB, RBBB and left anterior fascicular block, or RBBB and left posterior fascicular block
	RBBB or LBBB and first degree AV block
Class II	Stable bradycardia with systolic BP >90 mmHg or hemodynamic compromise responsive to drug therapy
	Newly acquired or age-indeterminate RBBB
Class III	Uncomplicated acute MI without evidence of conduction system disease

Temporary transvenous pacing in setting of acute myocardial infarction

Class I	Asystole
	Symptomatic bradycardia (sinus bradycardia with hypotension, or Type I second-degree AV block with hypotension unresponsive to atropine)
	Bilateral bundle branch block (alternating BBB or RBBB with alternating LAFB/LPFB) any age
	New or indeterminate-age bifascicular block (RBBB with LAFB or LPFB, or LBBB) with first-degree AV block
	Mobitz type II second-degree AV block
Class IIa	RBBB and LAFB or LPFB (new or indeterminate)
	RBBB with first-degree AV block
	LBBB, new or indeterminate
	Incessant VT, for atrial or ventricular overdrive pacing
	Recurrent sinus pauses (>3 seconds) not responsive to atropine
Class IIb	Bifascicular block of indeterminate age
	New or age indeterminate isolated RBBB
Class III	First-degree heart block
	Type I second-degree AV block (Wenkebach) with normal hemodynamics
	Accelerated idioventricular rhythm
	BBB or fascicular block known to exist before acute myocardial infarction

*adapted from 1999 Update of ACC/AHA guidelines for the management of patients with acute myocardial infarction.
Executive Summary and Recommendations JACC 1999;34:890–911

        iv. Right bundle branch block (RBBB)
        v. Left bundle branch block (LBBB)
    (3) Score
        i. 0: Less than 4% risk of developing complete heart block (CHB)
        ii. 1: 12%
        iii. 2: 28%
        iv. 3:45%

III. PROCEDURE
A. Equipment
    1. Transcutaneous
        a. External electrode pads
        b. External pulse generator

TABLE 39-2	Indications for Transvenous Pacing in the Absence of Myocardial Ischemia

Bradyarrhythmias
   Asystole
   Second or third degree AV block with hemodynamic compromise or syncope at rest
   Complete heart block secondary to structural heart disease
   Symptomatic sinus bradycardia
   Prolonged sinus pauses (>3 seconds)
Tachyarrhythmias
   Ventricular tachycardia secondary to bradycardia
   Torsade de pointes associated with structural heart disease, metabolic abnormalities, or drug effects
   Ventricular tachycardia unresponsive to medical therapy
   Supraventricular tachycardia unresponsive to medical therapy
Prophylaxis for procedures or conditions which may promote bradycardia
   General Anesthesia with concomitant conduction block
      Second or third degree AV block
      Intermittent second or third degree AV block
      First degree AV block with bifascicular block
      First degree AV block with LBBB
   Cardiac surgery
      Tricuspid valve surgery
      Ventricular septal defect closure
      Ostium primum repair
   Surgical procedures requiring permanent pacemaker deactivation
   Percutaneous coronary intervention with associated bradycardia
   Right heart catheterization in a patient with associated LBBB
   Cardioversion with sick sinus syndrome
   New Atrioventricular block with endocarditis prior to cardiac surgery
   Lyme carditis with associated conduction block
   Electrophysiology studies

*Not recommended for temporary pacing
Sinus node disease without hemodynamic compromise or syncope at rest

    2. Transvenous
       a. Balloon-tipped electrode catheter
          (1) Platinum or gold tipped catheters
       b. External pulse generator, power source
  B. Technique
    1. Transcutaneous
       a. Electrode placement (anteroposterior or anterolateral)
          (1) Malpositioning may create problems
             i. Excessive skeletal muscle contraction
             ii. Increased output requirements
             iii. Increased patient discomfort
          (2) Output ranges 0 to 140 mA
          (3) Output is increased until a pacer stimulus captures
          (4) Programmed to either primary pacing or demand only
          (5) Threshold is determined (typically 40 to 70 mA)
          (6) Higher outputs improve capture, but associated with pain and skin injury
       b. Pacing rate is determined
          (1) Consideration of rate based on need for protection of symptomatic bradycardia

      c. Length of pacing

        (1) Pacing and sensing should be assessed daily, including measurement of threshold

        (2) Observe for signs of infection

  2. Transvenous

    a. Site (subclavian, internal jugular, brachial, or femoral veins)

    b. Fluoroscopy is helpful in positioning, but not necessary

    c. Electrode catheter placement (Table 39-3)

      (1) Ensure that catheters are functioning appropriately

      (2) Test the balloon integrity by inflating to the recommended volume (3 cc in most balloons)

      (3) Connect the V1 surface lead to the distal electrode to provide continuous intravenous and intracardiac recordings

      (4) Advance the pacing catheter into the sheath (approximately 15 cm)

      (5) Inflate the balloon

      (6) Observe the ECG while advancing the catheter

      (7) Advance to the RV apex

      (8) Deflate the balloon

      (9) Watch for "injury current"

      (10) Determine pacing threshold (Note: threshold can be affected by ischemia, hyperkalemia, hypoxia, and medications.)

TABLE 39-3	**Bedside Positioning of a Temporary Electrode Catheter**

1.) Setup
Sterile preparation (gowns, gloves, masks, drape, hat)
Equipment (pacing electrode catheter, pulse generator, surface electrodes, sheath)
Connections
    V1 surface electrode connects to distal electrode
    Proximal electrode catheter connects to positive pole of pulse generator

2.) Testing components
Inflate balloon to test integrity
Document V1 recordings when inserting electrode catheter into the sheath

3.) Procedure
Carefully advance electrode catheter 15 cm and inflate balloon
Observe V1 transition with advancement of catheter (Figure 4)
    Atrial (p wave) dominant
    Ventricular (QRS) dominant
    Injury current
Stop advancing once injury current is detected

4.) Pacing preparation
Confirm proximal electrode is connected to positive pole of pulse generator
Disconnect distal electrode from V1 surface lead and connect to the negative pole of the
    pulse generator

5.) Pacing
Attempt pacing at 10 milliAmperes (mA) with the highest sensitivity
Observe capture
Determine thresholds and set output 1–2 mA above threshold (generally 3 mA)

6.) Post-procedure
Document distance electrode is within the sheath
Confirm position with a chest radiograph
Routine care of pacemaker and site, including
    Pacing parameters (threshold, rate, sensitivity, output) skin site (observing for infection)

TABLE 39-4	Troubleshooting

Capture
Loss of Capture
    Loose connections
    Electrode catheter malposition
    Increased myocardial stimulation threshold
    Cardiac penetration or perforation
    Lead fracture
    Pulse generator malfunction (including improperly charged)

Sensing
Loss of Sensing
    Inadequate intracardiac signal
    Lead malposition
    Spontaneous complexes falling within refractory period of generator
    Generator malfunction
    Lead fracture
Undersensing intracardiac signals
    Etiology
        Inadequate signal voltage
        Slow rate of change of voltage (slew)
        Prolonged signal duration
    Clinical circumstances
        Acute myocardial infarction and/or ischemia
        Poor electrode position
        Impulse originating in ventricular tissue
        Pacemaker component failure
Oversensing
    P waves
    T waves
    Electromagnetic interference
    Myopotentials
    False signals generated from extension cables

    d. Pacing mode
        (1) Synchronous or asynchronous (fixed)
        (2) VVI most common mode to manage bradycardia
        (3) Determining sensitivity
            i. Lower sensitivity-risk of oversensing ECG artifact and inappropriate suppression of pacing
            ii. Higher sensitivity-risk of inappropriate pacer firing and possibility of pacing on a T wave precipitating polymorphic VT

C. Efficacy
    1. Transcutaneous
        a. Safe and effective
        b. Primary limitation is patient discomfort, which may improve with sedation
        c. Similar achievable hemodynamic response compared with transvenous pacing (both in measured cardiac output and blood pressure augmentation)
    2. Transvenous
        a. High procedural success
        b. Offers a low output with minimal discomfort
            (1) No skeletal muscle capture with pacing

D. Complications
1. Transcutaneous
   a. Local discomfort
      (1) Temporary erythema at the contact site of the electrodes
   b. Skin injury limited due to
      (1) Improved electrode pads
2. Transvenous
   a. Low risk
   b. Complication rate 13% to 18% (includes VT, VF, infection, pericarditis, and cardiac perforation); rare: local thrombus
   c. Component malfunction is rare (Table 39-4)
   d. Benefit of prophylactic antibiotics with permanent pacing systems, but less well established with the temporary systems and only routinely used if sterile technique is broken or suspected infection

E. Contraindications
1. Asystolic arrest victims
   a. No survival benefit from either transcutaneous or transvenous pacing

IV. POSTPROCEDURE CONSIDERATIONS
A. Complications. Low complication rate, generally limited to local discomfort with transcutaneous pacing.
B. Monitoring. The patient needs to be monitored in an intensive care setting while a temporary pacing system is in place.

Selected Readings

Bing OH, McDowell JW, Hantman J, et al. Pacemaker placement by electrocardiographic monitoring. *N Engl J Med* 1972;287(13):651.
Intracardiac electrocardiogram recordings during positioning of a temporary pacing lead.

Donovan KD, Lee KY. Indications for and complications of temporary transvenous cardiac pacing. *Anaesth Intensive Care* 1985;13(1):63–70.
Prospective survey of 153 transvenous pacing lead insertions, with limited complications (7% serious complications, but no deaths), identifying transvenous pacing as a safe and effective treatment for bradyarrhythmias and certain tachyarrhythmias.

Gregoratos G, Cheitlin MD, Conill A, et al. ACC/AHA Guidelines for implantation of cardiac pacemakers and antiarrhythmia devices: executive summary—a report of the American College of Cardiology/American Heart Association Task Force Practice Guidelines (Committee on Pacemaker Implantation). *Circulation* 1998;97(13):1325–1335.
Extensive literature review and guidelines, including ACC/AHA class I, II, and III recommendations for pacing.

Hynes JK, Holmes DR Jr, Harrison CE. Five-year experience with temporary pacemaker therapy in the coronary care unit. *Mayo Clin Proc* 1983;58(2):122–126.
Clinical course of 1,022 patients receiving temporary transvenous pacing with the right internal jugular approach, associated with the lowest complication rate.

Lamas GA, Muller JE, Turi ZG, et al. A simplified method to predict occurrence of complete heart block during acute myocardial infarction. *Am J Cardiol* 1986;57(15):1213–1219.
Report of 698 patients, status-post myocardial infarction, who were analyzed, and predictors for the development of complete heart block were reported, namely referring to first-degree atrioventricular block, Mobitz I and II, atrioventricular block, left anterior fascicular block, left posterior fascicular block, right bundle branch block, and left bundle branch block.

Silver MD, Goldschlager N. Temporary transvenous cardiac pacing in the critical care setting. *Chest* 1988;93(3):607–613.
Description of indications and complications associated with placement of transvenous pacing leads.

40 PERMANENT PACEMAKERS AND ANTIARRHYTHMIC DEVICES

Josh R. Doll and Michael R. Gold

I. PERMANENT PACEMAKERS

A. General principles

1. Most modern pacemakers have a right atrial lead and a right ventricular lead (dual chamber) allowing improved sensing and tracking capabilities and less atrial fibrillation compared with single-chamber devices.
2. Biventricular pacemakers add a left ventricular lead placed via the coronary sinus.
3. Generic pacemaker code to express different pacing modes is shown in Table 40-1.

B. Indications (Table 40-2)

1. Sinus node dysfunction (SND); also known as sick sinus syndrome
2. Atrioventricular (AV) block
3. Bundle branch block: Increased risk of progression to high-degree AV block and sudden death, but not sufficiently high to warrant routine prophylactic pacemaker.
4. Neurocardiogenic syncope and related disorders: Dual-chamber demand pacing can at times decrease episodes of syncope, but is not considered first-line therapy.
5. Orthotopic heart transplantation: Usually for SND.
6. Left ventricular (LV) systolic dysfunction: Cardiac resynchronization therapy (biventricular pacing) has been shown to improve hemodynamics, symptoms, and exercise capacity and reduce hospitalizations among patients with severe heart failure and left bundle branch block.
7. Miscellaneous: Pacing has been utilized but usefulness is not conclusively established.
   a. Long QT syndrome
   b. Hypertrophic cardiomyopathy (no class I or IIa indications).

C. Postprocedure considerations

1. Chest radiography (CXR; two views) routinely obtained after implant to confirm lead placement.
2. Pacemaker parameters routinely interrogated after implantation and at follow-up.
3. Patients are seen 2 to 6 weeks after implantation and every 6 to 12 months thereafter.

C. Complications

1. Battery depletion: Longevity is at least 6 to 8 years and depletion is unusual.
2. Lead dislodgment: May have intermittent contact with endocardium.
   a. Manifest by loss of capture and/or proper sensing.
   b. CXR or fluoroscopy compared to postprocedure film if suspected.
3. Lead insulation break: Results in exposure of conducting wires.
   a. Manifest as oversensing (inappropriate inhibition) and decreased impedance.
   b. Not detectable by CXR (insulation is radiolucent).
4. Pacing wire or electrode fracture: Occurs at points of mechanical stress.
   a. Manifest as loss of capture and high impedance.
   b. May be visible on CXR.
5. Pacemaker infections
   a. May occur early from wound infection or late from generalized sepsis
   b. Usually requires removal of pulse generator and leads
6. Electromagnetic interference

TABLE 40-1	Generic Pacemaker Code

Chamber Paced: 0 = none, A = atrium, V = ventricle, D = dual (atrium and ventricle)
Chamber Sensed: 0 = none, A = atrium, V = ventricle, D = dual (atrium and ventricle)
Response Mode: 0 = none, T = triggered, I = inhibited, D = dual (inhibited and triggered)
Programmability: 0 = none, P = simple (generally rate only), M = multiprogrammable,
  R = rate-responsive
Antitachycardia: 0 = none, P = antitachycardia pacing, S = shock, D = dual (pacing and
  shock)

    a. Electrocautery can cause pacemaker inhibition, so it is prudent to convert the pacemaker to a fixed-rate mode (DOO, VOO) during surgical procedures if patient is pacemaker dependent. (See Table 40-1 for abbreviations.)

    b. This is done with a programmer or by placing a magnet over the generator.

  7. Pacemaker syndrome: Hypotension and palpitations from loss of synchronized atrial systole resulting in atrial contraction against closed AV valves.

    a. Occurs primarily with VVI pacing in patients who are only intermittently paced.

    b. Best treated by upgrading to dual-chamber system.

    c. Alternatively, lower rate limit can be reduced to encourage spontaneous rhythm or increase rate so that patient is 100% paced.

  8. Upper rate limit pacing: Individuals who develop rapid atrial rates may become symptomatic from tracking (sensing and pacing) at the upper rate limit.

    a. Mode-switching feature automatically reverts the pacemaker to a nontracking mode when atrial rate exceeds the programmed rate.

    b. Alternatively, can reprogram to a nontracking mode (e.g., DDI).

  9. Pacemaker-mediated tachycardia (PMT): Ventricular beat produces retrograde P wave, which is sensed by pacemaker and results in ventricular output, which is also sensed, setting up an endless-loop tachycardia.

    a. Can be terminated acutely by application of a magnet (eliminates all sensing).

    b. Most newer pulse generators have algorithms to terminate PMT automatically.

II. IMPLANTABLE CARDIOVERTER DEFIBRILLATORS

  A. General principles

    1. Defibrillation threshold: Minimum amount of energy required for defibrillation.

    2. Sensing: Ability to distinguish between ventricular fibrillation (VF) and ventricular tachycardia (VT) and between supraventricular arrhythmias (including sinus tachycardia) and VF/VT.

    3. After arrhythmia confirmation, there is option of initial low-energy shocks and/ or antitachycardia pacing before delivering full energy shock (tiered therapy).

    4. All current ICDs have pacemaker capabilities (VVI to biventricular).

  B. Indications (Table 40-3)

    1. Secondary prevention: ICDs are superior to antiarrhythmic drugs for the secondary prevention of sudden cardiac death (SCD).

    2. Primary prevention

      a. Ischemic cardiomyopathy: Large, randomized trials have demonstrated efficacy in setting of ischemic heart disease and LV systolic dysfunction.

      b. Dilated (nonischemic) cardiomyopathies: Recent studies demonstrated a reduction of SCD and/or total mortality with ICDs in this population.

  C. Postprocedure considerations. Follow-up as in permanent pacemakers with attention to arrhythmic symptoms (e.g., shocks, palpitations, syncope) and inspection of stored electrograms.

TABLE 40-2 Class I and IIa Indications for Permanent Pacing from the American College of Cardiology/American Heart Association Guidelines for Implantation of Cardiac Pacemakers and Antiarrhythmic Devices

	Class I indications	Class IIa indications
SND	1. Spontaneous symptomatic bradycardia or chronotropic incompetence 2. Symptomatic bradycardia due to necessary pharmacologic therapy	1. SND with heart rate <40 beats/min and symptoms not clearly documented to be related to bradycardia

AV Block	1. Third-degree and advanced second-degree AV block associated with:
	  a. Symptomatic bradycardia.
	  b. Documented periods of asystole or any escape rate <40 beats/min
	  c. Following catheter ablation of the AV junction
	  d. Postoperative block not expected to resolve
	  e. Neuromuscular disease with complete AV block
	2. Second-degree AV block regardless of type with symptomatic bradycardia
		1. Asymptomatic third-degree AV block at any anatomic site with average awake ventricular rate ≥40 beats/min
		2. Asymptomatic type II second-degree AV block
		3. Asymptomatic type I AV block at or below the His bundle found at EPS performed for other indications

BBB	1. Spontaneous high-grade AV block 2. Alternating bundle branch block	1. Syncope not demonstrated to be due to AV block when other causes excluded 2. Incidental finding of HV interval ≥100 ms at EPS without symptoms 3. Incidental finding of pacing induced infra-His block at EPS
Vasovagal Syncope	1. Recurrent syncope due to carotid sinus hypersensitivity.	1. Recurrent syncope without clear provocative event and with a hypersensitive cardioinhibitory response 2. Syncope of unexplained origin when major abnormalities of sinus node function or AV conduction are found or provoked during EPS 3. Significantly symptomatic and recurrent neurocardiogenic syncope associated with bradycardia documented spontaneously or with tilt-table testing
OHT	1. Same as nontransplant	None.
LQTS	1. Sustained pause-dependent VT in which the efficacy of pacing has been clearly documented	1. High-risk individuals with congenital LQTS

SND, sinus node dysfunction; AV, atrioventricular; EPS, electrophysiologic study; BBB, bundle branch block; OHT, orthotopic heart transplant; LQTS, long QT syndrome; VT, ventricular tachycardia.

TABLE 40-3	Class I and IIa Indications for Implantation of ICD from the American College of Cardiology/American Heart Association Guidelines for Implantation of Cardiac Pacemakers and Antiarrhythmic Devices

Class I	Class IIa
1. Cardiac arrest due to VF or VT not due to a transient or reversible cause 2. Spontaneous sustained VT in association with structural heart disease 3. Syncope of undetermined origin with clinically relevant sustained VT or VF induced at time of EPS when drug therapy is ineffective, not tolerated, or not preferred 4. Nonsustained VT in patients with coronary artery disease, prior MI, LV dysfunction, and inducible VF or sustained VT at EPS that is not suppressible by a class I antiarrhythmic drug 5. Spontaneous sustained VT in patients who do not have structural heart disease that is not amenable to other treatments	1. Patients with LV ejection fraction ≤30%, at least 1 month post-MI and 3 months post−coronary artery revascularization surgery

VF, ventricular fibrillation; VT, ventricular tachycardia; LV, left ventricle; MI, myocardial infarction; EPS, electrophysiologic study.

D. Complications
   1. Infection: Pocket infections usually occur early (2 to 12 weeks).
      a. Symptoms include local tenderness, swelling, drainage, erythema, and warmth.
      b. Usually require explantation of entire system.
   2. Pocket hematomas (usually associated with anticoagulation) and seromas usually occur soon after ICD implantation.
   3. Pocket erosions: Occur late in thin individuals at areas of pressure on subcutaneous tissue and require device explantation if skin is broken because infection is presumed.
   4. Oversensing: Suspected if individual receives shocks without precipitating factor and confirmed by the absence of ventricular arrhythmias on stored electrograms.
      a. Possible causes of oversensing and inappropriate sensing are listed in Table 40-4.

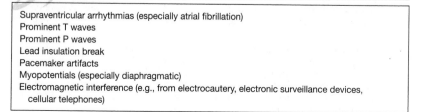

TABLE 40-4	Causes of ICD Oversensing or Inappropriate Sensing

Supraventricular arrhythmias (especially atrial fibrillation)
Prominent T waves
Prominent P waves
Lead insulation break
Pacemaker artifacts
Myopotentials (especially diaphragmatic)
Electromagnetic interference (e.g., from electrocautery, electronic surveillance devices, cellular telephones)

   b. Commonly encountered cause of oversensing in hospital setting is that caused by electrocautery during surgical procedures.

   (1) This interference produces signals within the physiologic range that may be interpreted as QRS complexes by the ICD.

   (2) Defibrillation therapies can be turned off to avoid inappropriate shocks.

   c. Supraventricular arrhythmias (most commonly atrial fibrillation) in the critically ill patient may provoke inappropriate therapy; therefore, the ventricular rate should be controlled with intravenous β-blockers or calcium channel blockers.

5. Increase in defibrillation threshold (DFT)

   a. DFT obtained at implantation and device programmed with large safety margin.

   b. Changes in substrate (e.g., worsening heart failure, ischemia, electrolyte abnormalities) can increase threshold.

   c. Some antiarrhythmic agents can increase threshold (most notably amiodarone).

   d. Device should be retested 4 to 6 weeks after initiation of amiodarone.

Selected Readings

Bristow MR, Saxon LA, Boehmer J, et al. Cardiac-resynchronization therapy with or without an implantable defibrillator in advanced chronic heart failure. *N Engl J Med* 2004;350:2140–2150.
This randomized study showed that cardiac resynchronization therapy reduces heart failure hospitalization and cardiac death, but only when combined with backup implantable cardioverter-defibrillator was total mortality reduced significantly.

Buxton AE, Lee KL, Fisher JD, et al. A randomized study of the prevention of sudden death in patients with coronary artery disease. *N Engl J Med* 1999;341:1882–1890.
This large randomized study showed that antiarrhythmic therapy with implantable cardioverter-defibrillators reduced sudden death and total mortality compared with nonantiarrhythmic medical therapy among patients with coronary artery disease, systolic dysfunction, nonsustained ventricular tachycardia, and inducible ventricular tachycardia.

Cazeau S, Leclercq C, Lavergne T. Effects of multisite biventricular pacing in patients with heart failure and intraventricular conduction defects. *N Engl J Med* 2001;344:873–880.
This was the first controlled study of biventricular pacing demonstrating an improvement of exercise duration and functional status.

Connelly SJ, Kerr CR, Gent M, et al. Effects of physiological pacing versus ventricular pacing on the risk of stroke and death due to cardiovascular causes. *N Engl J Med* 2000;342:1385–1391.
This is the largest randomized study of pacing mode and demonstrated that ventricular pacing does not increase the risk of mortality compared with dual-chamber or atrial pacing.

Connolly SJ, Gent M, Roberts RS, et al. Canadian Implantable Defibrillator Study (CIDS): a randomized trial of the implantable defibrillator against amiodarone. *Circulation* 2000;101:1297–1302.
This study showed a trend toward a reduction in total mortality and a reduction of sudden death with implantable cardioverter-defibrillators versus amiodarone among patients with ventricular tachycardia, ventricular fibrillation, or syncope and inducible ventricular tachycardia.

Connolly SJ, Sheldon R, Thorpe KE, et al. Pacemaker therapy for prevention of syncope in patients with recurrent severe vasovagal syncope: second Vasovagal Pacemaker Study (VPS II): a randomized trial. *JAMA* 2003;289:2224–2229.
This double-blind randomized study showed no significant difference in syncope recurrence with pacing among patients with vasovagal syncope and abnormal tilt-table study. This is contrary to more promising unblinded studies.

Gold MR, Feliciano Z, Gottlieb SS, et al. Dual-chamber pacing with a short AV delay in congestive heart failure: a randomized study. *J Am Coll Cardiol* 1995;26:967–973.
This was the first randomized study of pacing in heart failure and demonstrated that short atrioventricular delay pacing from the right ventricular apex did not improve functional status or ejection fraction.

Gregoratos G, Abrams J, Epstein AE, et al. ACC/AHA/NASPE 2002 Guideline update for implantation of cardiac pacemakers and antiarrhythmia devices: summary article. *Circulation* 2002;106:2145–2161.
These are the current guidelines for pacemaker and implantable cardioverter-defibrillator implantation.

Lamas GA, Lee KL, Sweeney MO, et al. Ventricular pacing or dual-chamber pacing for sinus-node dysfunction. *N Engl J Med* 2002;346:1854–1862.
This study demonstrated that, among patients with sick sinus syndrome, dual-chamber pacing reduces the incidence of atrial fibrillation and pacemaker syndrome.

Maron BJ, Nishimura RA, McKenna WJ, et al. Assessment of permanent dual-chamber pacing as a treatment for drug-refractory symptomatic patients with obstructive hypertrophic cardiomyopathy; a randomized, double-blind, crossover study. *Circulation* 1999;99:2927–2933.
This study showed that dual-chamber pacing did not reduce symptoms among patients with hypertrophic cardiomyopathy despite a reduction of outflow tract gradient.

Moss AJ, Hall J, Cannom DS, et al. Improved survival with an implanted defibrillator in patients with coronary disease at high risk for ventricular arrhythmia. *N Engl J Med* 1996;335:1933–1940.
This primary prevention study showed that implantable cardioverter-defibrillator therapy reduces mortality compared with medical therapy among patients with ischemic cardiomyopathy, nonsustained ventricular tachycardia, and inducible ventricular tachycardia at electrophysiology study.

Moss AJ, Liu JE, Gottlieb S, et al. Efficacy of permanent pacing in the management of high risk patients with the long QT syndrome. *Circulation* 1991;84:1524–1529.
Pacing therapy, particularly in combination with β-blockers can reduce the risk of recurrent syncope and possibly sudden death among patients with long QT syndrome. Today, backup defibrillation is used more commonly with pacemakers for this indication.

Moss AJ, Zareba W, Hall WJ, et al. Prophylactic implantation of a defibrillator in patients with myocardial infarction and reduced ejection fractions. *N Engl J Med* 2002;346: 877–883.
This primary prevention study showed that implantable cardioverter-defibrillators reduce mortality among patients with coronary artery disease and ejection fraction less than 30%.

The Antiarrhythmics versus Implantable Defibrillators (AVID) Investigators. A comparison of antiarrhythmic drug therapy with implantable defibrillators in patients resuscitated from near-fatal ventricular arrhythmias. *N Engl J Med* 1997;337:1576–1583.
This was the first large, randomized study of implantable cardioverter-defibrillators as first-line therapy for secondary prevention of sudden death. Compared with antiarrhythmic therapy (primarily amiodarone), implantable cardioverter-defibrillators were associated with better survival.

41 | EVALUATION OF THE LOW- TO INTERMEDIATE-RISK PATIENT WITH CHEST PAIN: CHEST PAIN CENTERS

Samuel D. Luber, Sean P. Collins, and Alan B. Storrow

I. GENERAL PRINCIPLES
  A. Each year approximately 8 million patients present to U.S. emergency departments (EDs) for chest pain. (Fig. 41-1)
    1. Up to two thirds of these patients are admitted to an inpatient setting; less than half of these patients are discharged with a diagnosis of acute coronary syndrome (ACS).
    2. Of the 3 million patients discharged from the ED without presumed ACS, approximately 40,000 (1% to 2%) ultimately have an acute cardiac event, usually a myocardial infarction.
    3. This ED discharged group represents 20% to 39% of malpractice dollars awarded in the field of emergency medicine.
  B. Classic presentations of unstable angina (UA) and acute myocardial infarction (AMI) do not present diagnostic dilemmas; however, these patients are the minority of ED chest pain presentations.
  C. Many ED patients have atypical symptoms and initial electrocardiograms (ECGs) that are normal or nondiagnostic. Establishing which of these low-risk patients require further evaluation and treatment is often challenging.
  D. Non–ST-segment elevation myocardial infarction (NSTEMI) is two to three times more common than ST-segment elevation myocardial infarction (STEMI). Patients who have NSTEMI have similar long-term prognoses as those with STEMI.
  E. To minimize inappropriate discharge of patients with ACS, many low-risk patients are admitted to an inpatient setting.
    1. This strategy is sensitive for detecting ACS, but the specificity is low.
    2. More than one half of low-risk patients are discharged with a noncardiac diagnosis.
    3. Unnecessary admissions result in a significant cost burden.
  F. The ED-based chest pain center (CPC) concept (Fig. 41-2) was designed to rapidly identify patients in need of reperfusion therapies, reduce unnecessary admissions of low-risk patients, and prevent inappropriate discharge of patients who subsequently have ACS.
  G. Specifically, a CPC provides a mechanism to address four important goals:
    1. earlier diagnosis and treatment of ACS
    2. reduction of inappropriate ED discharges
    3. reduction of inpatient admissions
    4. development of community outreach programs for patients with possible symptoms of acute cardiac ischemia
  H. For ED patients thought to have low or intermediate risk for ACS, CPCs have driven a change from the older concept of inpatient admission to "rule-out" AMI to a period of ED observation to "rule-in" ACS.

II. DIAGNOSIS
  A. History and physical
    1. Classic anginal history is obtained in less than one-half of patients having an AMI, especially in the elderly and in females.
    2. Several risk-factor classification schemes have been developed, but all have limitations for ED use:
      a. Diamond/Forrester likelihood model of coronary artery disease (CAD)
      b. Goldman chest pain protocol for MI diagnosis

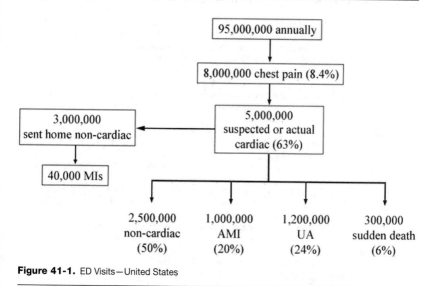

Figure 41-1. ED Visits—United States

    c. Pozen-Selker Acute Cardiac Ischemia Time-Insensitive Predictive Instrument
    d. Agency for Health Care Policy and Research/National Heart, Lung, Blood Institute Unstable Angina guidelines
B. Electrocardiogram
    1. ECG is nondiagnostic in most patients with ACS and provides a specific diagnosis in only 5% of patients.

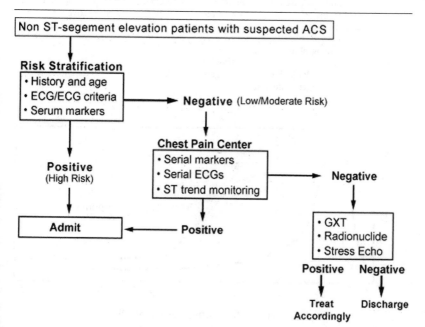

Figure 41-2. Generic Chest Pain Center Flow; ECG, electrocardiographic; GXT, graded exercise testing

2. Patients who present with or develop traditional changes consistent with AMI (ST-elevation or new bundle branch block) are candidates for time sensitive interventions and are excluded from CPC evaluation.

3. Static ECG only captures 10 seconds of the cardiac rhythm. Some CPC protocols employ continuous 12-lead ST-segment monitoring.

C. Cardiac markers (Fig. 41-3)

1. Time-dependent release of serum cardiac biomarkers identifies myocardial necrosis, provides risk stratification, and can drive earlier medical therapy and consideration of invasive reperfusion.

2. Myoglobin is the earliest release marker of myocardial necrosis becoming positive in approximately 2 hours, peaking at 6 to 9 hours, and returning to baseline in 24 to 36 hours.

   a. Many false-positives occur because it is found in skeletal muscle and renal failure; its strength is based on a good negative predictive value.

   b. A 2-hour delta myoglobin has been suggested as useful in excluding the possibility of myocardial necrosis, although its widespread use has been limited by sensitivity issues.

3. Creatine kinase (CK) typically rises 4 to 8 hours after the onset of myocardial necrosis, peaks at 12 hours, and returns to baseline in 48 hours.

   a. It is relatively sensitive for detection of myocardial injury but less specific; it is found in both cardiac and skeletal muscle.

   b. Use of the CK fraction, CK-MB, can greatly improve specificity.

   c. Single determinations are insensitive, but serial levels have been shown to be highly sensitive for AMI within the first 3 to 6 hours.

4. Troponins. Cardiac troponin I (TnI) and T (TnT) have early release kinetics similar to those of CK-MB. However, they remain elevated in the circulation for up to 2 weeks after AMI (Table 41-1).

   a. Useful in delayed ED presentations of AMI.

   b. Highly sensitive and moderately specific markers of myocardial cell damage.

   c. Can be released during brief episodes of ischemia; therefore, troponin elevation may be encountered in situations where CK-MB is negative.

   d. A rise in a cardiac troponin now defines myocardial damage and should be included in all evaluations for ACS, alone or in combination with CK-MB or myoglobin.

D. Point-of-care cardiac marker testing

1. Widely available, highly reliable, and may shorten the time to diagnosis of ACS and subsequent intervention.

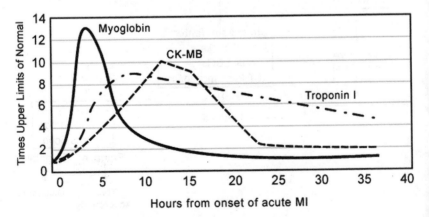

Figure 41-3. Kinetics of Early Serum Markers

TABLE 41-1	Cardiac Troponin Summary

Advantages	Disadvantages
• Risk stratification	• Low sensitivity early (<6 h)
• Sensitivity/specificity > creatine-kinase-MB	• Need for serial sampling
• Detect recent myocardial infarction	• Limited in detection of reinfarction
• Selection of treatment	• Diagnostic "cutoff" confusion
• Detect reperfusion	

   2. Effect on outcome has not been fully studied.

   3. Quicker time to positivity has been associated with worse outcomes.

   4. In the CHECKMATE Study, quantitative, near-patient, multimarker strategies identified more positive patients than single-marker, local laboratory testing and identified them earlier.

E. Rest nuclear imaging

   1. Using technetium-based agents, sestamibi or tetrofosmin, single-photon emission computed tomographic (SPECT) imaging has proved to be safe and effective.

   2. Patients who demonstrate no perfusion defect on resting SPECT imaging while having pain can safely be discharged from the ED and have a low risk for subsequent cardiac events.

   3. Allows a CPC protocol to include patients unable to perform graded exercise testing (GXT), although an elective outpatient stress scan is recommended for those with negative imaging.

   4. Sensitivity is best when injected during pain or within 2 hours of last pain, although the exact relationship between sensitivity loss and time from last pain is not well established.

   5. Cannot differentiate between ischemia and scar; therefore, patient must not have had a prior MI.

F. Provocative testing

   1. If serial serum marker determinations are negative, ST-segment monitoring unrevealing, and chest pain attributes unconvincing, CPC patients may proceed to provocative stress testing.

   2. Graded exercise testing (GXT)

      a. Has been shown to be safe, prognostic, and predictive of underlying CAD.

      b. Positive GXT, generally considered to be horizontal ST-segment depression of 1 mm or greater from baseline, accompanied by ischemic chest pain, results in hospital admission from the CPC.

      c. A normal GXT to an adequate workload after completion of observation and marker testing allows safe discharge.

   3. Stress echocardiography and stress nuclear imaging

      a. Useful in patients unable to physically complete a GXT.

      b. Prognostic for future cardiac events and CAD.

G. Chest pain center protocols

   1. Approximately 2,000 ED-based CPCs in the United States.

   2. Multiple different protocols that focus on evaluating the ACS continuum of acute myocardial necrosis, rest ischemia, and exercise-induced ischemia.

   3. Example protocol (Fig.41-4):

      a. Inclusion criteria: Patients with a clinical presentation consistent with possible ACS and a nondiagnostic ECG. Some institutions have defined levels of risk (see Fig. 41-3).

      b. Exclusion criteria: ST-segment elevation or depression of 1 mm or more, a clinical presentation consistent with unstable angina, or hemodynamic instability.

      c. Serial biomarker testing that includes a cardiac troponin.

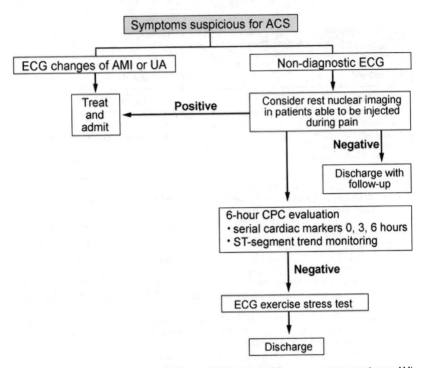

Figure 41-4. University of Cincinnati "Heart ER" Strategy; ACS, acute coronary syndrome; AMI, acute myocardial infarction; UA, unstable angina; ECG, electrocardiograph; CPC, chest pain center

    d. ST-segment trend monitoring (optional, suggested to be of low-yield in the low- to intermediate-risk patient).

    e. After 6 hours without evidence of ACS, provocative testing.

    f. Negative evaluation leads to discharge with appropriate follow-up.

H. Chest pain center cost savings

    1. Multiple retrospective studies have demonstrated significant cost savings by instituting a CPC, commonly crudely defining cost effectiveness as a comparison of hospital charges.

    2. Although not well studied, important issues such as patient satisfaction and identification of other diagnoses of chest pain play an important role.

I. Rapid rule-out protocols

    1. Although not universally accepted, some institutions have shortened their protocols to provide more rapid disposition than a traditional CPC:

        a. Immediate GXT in patients with a nondiagnostic ECG, prior to obtaining results of cardiac enzymes, has been studied and suggested to be safe in low-risk patients.

        b. Others centers have shortened the interval between cardiac marker tests and are dispositioning patients after two sets of negative cardiac enzymes taken as early as 3 hours apart.

Selected Readings

Farkouh ME, Smars PA, Reeder GS, et al. A clinical trial of a chest-pain observation unit for patients with unstable angina. *N Engl J Med* 1998;339:1882–1888.
    A prospective trial of the chest pain center approach analyzing safety and approximating resource use.

Gibler WB, Lewis LM, Erb RE, et al. Early detection of acute myocardial infarction in patients presenting with chest pain and nondiagnostic electrocardiograms: serial CK-MB sampling in the emergency department. *Ann Emerg Med* 1990;19:1359–1366.
The need for serial biomarker testing.

Gibler WB, Runyon JP, Levy RC, et al. A rapid diagnostic and treatment center for patients with chest pain in the emergency department. *Ann Emerg Med* 1988;25:1–8.
A sentinel report of the chest pain center concept.

Goldman L, Cook EF, Brand DA, et al. A computer protocol to predict myocardial infarction in emergency department patients with chest pain. *N Engl J Med* 1988;318:797–803.
One of the most cited aids for emergency department evaluation of potential *acute coronary syndrome.*

Gomez M, Anderson J, Karagounis L, et al. An emergency department-based protocol for rapidly ruling out myocardial ischemia reduces hospital time and expense: results of a randomized study (ROMIO). *J Am Coll Cardiol* 1996;28:25–33.
Important study for establishing a chest pain center.

Graff L, Joseph T, Andelman R, et al. American College of Emergency Physicians information paper: chest pain units in emergency departments–a report from the short-term observation services section. *Am J Cardiol* 1995;76:1036–1039.
Early report on chest pain centers specifically located in emergency departments.

Hamm CW, Goldmann BU, Heeshcen C, et al. Emergency room triage of patients with acute chest pain by means of rapid testing for cardiac troponin T or troponin I. *N Engl J Med* 1997;337:1648–1653.
Prospective emergency department testing for both cardiac troponins.

Hamm CW, Ravkilde J, Gerhardt W, et al. The prognostic value of serum troponin T in unstable angina. *N Engl J Med* 1992;327:146–150.
Establishing the prognostic power of the cardiac troponins.

Kirk JD, Turnipseed S, Lewis WR, et al. Evaluation of chest pain in low risk patients presenting to the emergency department: the role of immediate exercise testing. *Ann Emerg Med* 1998;32:1–7.
Alternative to the traditional chest pain center approach.

Lewis WR, Amsterdam EA. Utility and safety of immediate exercise testing of low risk patients admitted to the hospital for suspected acute myocardial infarction. *Am J Cardiol* 1994;74:987–990.
Alternative to the traditional chest pain center approach.

Lindahl B, Venge P, Wallentin L. Relation between troponin T and the risk of subsequent cardiac events in unstable coronary artery disease. *Circulation* 1996;93:1651–1657.
Establishing the risk-stratification properties of the cardiac tropinins.

McCarthy BD, Beshansky JR, D'Agostino RB, et al. Missed diagnosis of acute myocardial infarction in the emergency department: results from a multicenter study. *Ann Emerg Med* 1994;22:579–582.
Demographics and description of missed myocardial infarction.

Newby LK, Storrow AB, Gibler WB, et al. Bedside multimarker testing for risk stratification in chest pain units–the chest pain evaluation by creatine kinase-MB, myoglobin, and troponin I (CHECKMATE) study. *Circulation* 2001;103:1832–1837.
Prospective point-of-care testing, time to positivity, and a multimarker approach.

Ohman EM, Armstrong PW, Christenson RH, et al. Cardiac troponin T levels for risk stratification in acute myocardial ischemia. *N Engl J Med* 1996;335:1333–1341.
Establishing the risk-stratification properties of the cardiac tropinins.

Pozen MW, Agostino RB, Selker HP, et al. A predictive instrument to improve coronary-care-unit admission practices in acute ischemic heart disease: a prospective multicenter clinical trial. *N Engl J Med* 1984310:1273–1278.
Risk-stratification tool.

Rusnak RA, Stair TO, Hansen K, et al. Litigation against the emergency physician: common features in cases of missed myocardial infarction. *Ann Emerg Med* 1989;18:1029–1032.
Missed myocardial infarction and emergency medicine litigation.

Tatum JL, Jesse RL, Kontos MC, et al. Comprehensive strategy for the evaluation and triage of the chest pain patient. *Ann Emerg Med* 1997;29:116–125.
Sentinel report on rest myocardial perfusion imaging in the emergency department.

Wu A, Apple FS, Gibler WB, et al. National Academy of Clinical Biochemistry Standards of Laboratory Practice: recommendations for the use of cardiac markers in coronary artery diseases. *Clin Chem* 1999;45(7):1104–1121.
Recommendations for biomarker use.

Young GP, Gibler WB, Hedges JR, et al. Serial creatine kinase MB results are a sensitive indicator of acute myocardial infarction in chest pain patients with nondiagnostic electrocardiograms: the second emergency medicine cardiac research group study. *Acad Emerg Med* 1997;4:869–877.
The need for serial biomarker testing.

Pulmonary Problems in the Intensive Care Unit

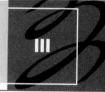

III

A PHYSIOLOGIC APPROACH TO MANAGING RESPIRATORY FAILURE

42

Mark M. Wilson and Richard S. Irwin

I. GENERAL PRINCIPLES

A. Respiratory failure is defined by arterial carbon dioxide tension (P_aCO_2) greater than 50 mm Hg or arterial oxygen tension (P_aO_2) less than 50 to 60 mm Hg.

B. The efficiency of gas exchange is evaluated by measuring the P_aO_2, the P_aCO_2, and the alveolar-arterial (A-a) PO_2 gradient.

1. P_aO_2. The normal value for P_aO_2 depends on the age and body position of the patient:

$$\text{In the upright position, } P_aO_2 = 104.2 - 0.27 \times \text{age (yr)}$$

$$\text{In the supine position, } P_aO_2 = 103.5 - 0.47 \times \text{age (yr)}$$

2. P_aCO_2. The normal P_aCO_2 is 35 to 45 mm Hg and is unaffected by age or body position. Because CO_2 production does not vary widely even in critically ill patients, it can be generally assumed that P_aCO_2 will vary inversely with alveolar ventilation.

3. P_{AO_2}–P_aO_2 gradient. To help interpret a decrease in P_aO_2, one must know the A-a gradient. The alveolar PO_2 (P_{AO_2}) can be calculated from the simplified alveolar air equation:

$$P_{AO_2} = P_{IO_2} - P_aCO_2 / R$$

At sea level and breathing room air the P_{IO_2}, the partial pressure of inspired O_2, can be assumed to be 150 mm Hg. R is the respiratory exchange ratio and is assumed to be 0.8.

The normal A-a gradient is 5 to 10 mm Hg and no more than 20 in an 80 year old, and is a sensitive indicator of intrinsic lung disease. At any age, an A-a gradient exceeding 20 mm Hg should be considered abnormal.

II. PATHOPHYSIOLOGY

A. Hypoxemia

1. Five mechanisms can cause hypoxemia: low P_{IO_2}, hypoventilation, low ventilation-perfusion ($\dot{V}/\dot{Q}$) mismatch, right-to-left shunting, and diffusion impairment.

2. A low P_{IO_2} is generally seen only at high altitude.

3. Diffusion impairment alone is not the major cause of hypoxemia.

4. In the clinical setting, hypoventilation, low $\dot{V}/\dot{Q}$ mismatch, and right-to-left shunting are essentially the only important pathophysiologic causes of hypoxemia.

5. Hypoventilation is a decrease in alveolar ventilation for a given level of CO_2 production resulting from a decrease in minute ventilation from extrapulmonary dysfunction. With no abnormality of gas exchange, the A-a gradient remains normal.

6. In areas of inadequate ventilation for a given level of perfusion (low $\dot{V}/\dot{Q}$ mismatch), pulmonary venous blood has a relative decrease in both PO_2 and percentage of oxyhemoglobin saturation. The result is that P_aO_2 is decreased and the A-a gradient is increased.

7. Right-to-left shunting refers to mixed venous blood going directly into the arterial circulation without having first been exposed to alveolar gas (from cardiac or great vessel, pulmonary vascular, or pulmonary parenchymal conditions). When the shunted blood mixes with the rest of the arterial blood, it lowers the average O_2 content and therefore the average P_aO_2. The A-a gradient is always increased.

B. Hypercapnia

1. Three mechanisms can lead to an elevated P_aCO_2: breathing a gas containing CO_2, hypoventilation, and severe low $\dot{V}/\dot{Q}$ mismatch. Clinically, only the last two are important. Hypoventilation has already been discussed. In patients who cannot augment their alveolar ventilation (e.g., severe chronic obstructive pulmonary disease [COPD] with chronic hypercapnia), hypercapnia can worsen with overfeeding because of an increase in CO_2 production from tissues.

2. The major mechanism causing arterial hypercapnia in patients with severe intrinsic lung disease is severe low $\dot{V}/\dot{Q}$ mismatch. A substantially greater degree of low $\dot{V}/\dot{Q}$ mismatch must be present to cause arterial hypercapnia than to cause hypoxemia.

3. Although not a primary cause of hypercapnia, respiratory muscle overload (from increased work of breathing associated with severe lung derangement) is commonly a contributing factor. Relative hypoventilation, an inability to increase minute ventilation appropriately, also commonly results from respiratory muscle dysfunction or fatigue.

C. Respiratory acid–base disorders

1. Acid–base balance is assessed clinically from the arterial hydrogen ion (H^+) concentration. The ratio of the relative availability of acid versus base determines the H^+ concentration, as shown by the modified Henderson-Hasselbalch equation:

$$H^+ = 24 \times (P_aCO_2 / HCO_3^-)$$

A pH of 7.40 corresponds to a H^+ concentration of 40 nM/L and each change in pH of 0.01 unit corresponds to an opposite deviation in H^+ concentration of 1 nM/L when the pH is 7.28 to 7.45. Outside this range, it is still clinically useful to estimate the H^+ concentration from the pH in this manner because the estimated value will deviate from the true value by no more than 5% to 10%.

2. In primary respiratory acidosis, the P_aCO_2 is elevated because of respiratory system dysfunction. Under normal circumstances, an appropriate compensatory change (i.e., increase) will occur in the HCO_3^- level to help mitigate the effect on H^+ concentration. To determine how long the P_aCO_2 has been elevated, the ratio of $\Delta H^+/\Delta P_aCO_2$ is computed. The kidneys gradually increase the HCO_3^- level to bring H^+ concentration back toward, but not to, normal. The $\Delta H^+/\Delta P_aCO_2$ ratios for acute and chronic respiratory acidosis are 0.8 and 0.3, respectively.

3. The differential diagnosis of respiratory acidosis is the same as that of hypercapnic respiratory failure (Table 42-1). The therapeutic approach is also the same.

4. Primary respiratory alkalosis is defined by a decrease in P_aCO_2 with an accompanying compensatory decrease in HCO_3^-. The duration of respiratory alkalosis involves the same determination of $\Delta H^+/\Delta P_aCO_2$ ratios. The values for acute and chronic respiratory alkalosis are 0.8 and 0.17, respectively. A primary respiratory alkalosis may have a normal or an elevated A-a gradient. The differential diagnosis of respiratory alkalosis with an elevated A-a gradient is the same as that of hypoxemic respiratory failure (e.g., acute asthma, pneumonia, pulmonary embolism, pulmonary edema). The differential diagnosis of respiratory alkalosis with a normal A-a gradient includes central nervous system disorders, pregnancy, high altitude, severe anemia, hyperventilation, and catecholamine, progesterone, or thyroid hormone excess.

III. DIAGNOSIS

A. To determine the cause of hypoxemia one must evaluate the P_aCO_2, the PO_2 (A-a) gradient, and occasionally the patient's response to 100% O_2.

B. During hypoventilation, the P_aCO_2 is always elevated, the A-a gradient is normal (10 mm Hg or less), and the decrease in P_aO_2 is accounted for solely by the low

TABLE 42-1	Causes of Hypercapnia and Their Pathophysiologic Mechanisms[a]	
Site of abnormality	**Disease**	**Mechanism**
Pulmonary disorders of:		Severe ventilation-perfusion mismatch
Lower airways	Chronic obstructive pulmonary disease, asthma, cystic fibrosis	
Lung parenchyma	Environmental/occupational lung disease	
Pulmonary vasculature	Pulmonary embolism (rarely)	
Extrapulmonary disorders of:		Hypoventilation
Central nervous system	Respiratory center depression due to drug overdose, primary alveolar hypoventilation, myxedema	
Peripheral nervous system	Spinal cord disease, amyotrophic lateral sclerosis, Guillain-Barré syndrome	
Respiratory muscles	Myasthenia gravis, polymyositis, hypophosphatemia	
Chest wall	Ankylosing spondylitis, flail chest, thoracoplasty	
Pleura	Restrictive pleuritis	
Upper airways	Tracheal obstruction, epiglottitis, adenoidal and tonsillar hypertrophy, obstructive sleep apnea	

[a]This table is not an exhaustive listing; it includes the more common causes for each involved compartment of the respiratory system.

P_{AO_2}. If the patient is given 100% O_2 to breathe (rarely necessary), there will be a dramatic increase in P_aO_2 (to more than 500 mm Hg).

C. During $\dot{V}/\dot{Q}$ mismatch and right-to-left shunting, the decreased P_aO_2 is typically accompanied by an elevated P_{O_2} (A-a) gradient. During $\dot{V}/\dot{Q}$ mismatch, the P_aCO_2 may or may not be elevated, whereas it is rarely elevated in right-to-left shunt. The P_aO_2 in the patient with $\dot{V}/\dot{Q}$ mismatch shows a dramatic rise in response to 100% O_2 (to more than 500 mm Hg). The patient with right-to-left shunting shows minimal or, in severe cases, no response at all to 100% O_2.

D. Contrast echocardiography or quantitative nuclear medicine perfusion lung scanning can be obtained to differentiate the right-to-left shunt of cardiac, great vessel, or pulmonary vascular origin from a pulmonary parenchymal cause. With cardiac, great vessel, or pulmonary vascular shunting, there will be a too rapid transit of contrast from the venous circulation into the left side of the heart, indicative of a structural/anatomic defect.

E. With hypercapnic respiratory failure (Table 42-1), the A-a gradient or may not be increased. Commonly, a disease process may affect a combination of mechanisms, causing an A-a gradient that is generally only modestly increased (e.g., 15 to 20 mm Hg).

IV. TREATMENT

A. Respiratory failure is managed by combined supportive and specific therapies.

B. In hypoxemic respiratory failure, the major problem is a low P_aO_2. If the mechanism is low $\dot{V}/\dot{Q}$ mismatch, supplemental O_2 will prove effective. If the disease process involves a diffuse pulmonary intraparenchymal shunt, as in the acute respiratory distress syndrome, mechanical ventilation with positive end-expiratory pressure may be required in addition to supplemental O_2. If the problem is a right-to-left cardiac or pulmonary vascular shunt, supplemental O_2 alone will be of limited benefit; emphasis is on specific therapy (i.e., surgical repair of an atrial septal defect, obliteration of a pulmonary arteriovenous fistula).

C. The key initial decision in hypercapnic respiratory failure is whether or not the patient requires intubation and mechanical ventilation. In general, intubation should be strongly considered for patients with acute respiratory acidosis that has not rapidly responded to medical therapy. The patient with a $\Delta H^+/\Delta P_aCO_2$ ratio that signifies chronic respiratory acidosis should be followed closely, but these patients uncommonly need to be intubated. In the acute situation, noninvasive mechanical ventilation or intubation will be needed unless specific therapy can immediately reverse the crisis (e.g., naloxone in heroin overdose). In the acute-on-chronic situation, $(\Delta H^+/\Delta P_aCO_2 = 0.5)$ the trend of the acidosis over time is the crucial factor in deciding on the necessity for intubation.

D. Specific therapy varies greatly by disease, and therefore no broad generalizations can be made. Examples of potential specific therapy include naloxone to offset respiratory center depression from narcotic overdose, inhaled bronchodilators and systemic corticosteroids for asthma and emphysema, or nasal continuous positive airway pressure for obstructive sleep apnea. Details of therapy for the most common of these diseases are presented in subsequent chapters.

Selected Readings

Demers RR, Irwin RS. Management of hypercapnic respiratory failure: a systematic approach. *Respir Care* 1979;24:328.
Provides a systematic approach to the patient with respiratory acidosis and reviews the concept of the Po_2 (A-a gradient).

Murray JF. *The normal lung: the basis for diagnosis and treatment of lung disease.* Philadelphia: WB Saunders, 1976, p.171.
This citation reviews the concept of the A-a gradient and the major mechanisms involved in gas exchange impairment.

Narins RG, Emmett M. Simple and mixed acid-base disorders: a practical approach. *Medicine* (Baltimore) 1980;59:161.
Comprehensive and practical review of acid–base physiology and provides an approach to and differential diagnosis for each of the major acid–base disturbances.

Pratter MR, Irwin RS. Extrapulmonary causes of respiratory failure. *J Intensive Care Med* 1986;1:197.
Reviews how to distinguish extrapulmonary from pulmonary causes of respiratory failure and the mechanisms responsible for arterial hypoxemia and hypercapnia.

Robin ED, Laman PD, Goris ML, et al. A shunt is (not) a shunt is (not) a shunt. *Am Rev Respir Dis* 1977;115:553.
Succinct description of the different right-to-left shunts and how to distinguish them.

West JB. Causes of carbon dioxide retention in lung disease. *N Engl J Med* 1971;284:1232.
Explains how and why $\dot{V}/\dot{Q}$ mismatch is the major cause of hypercapnia in lung disease.

West JB. *Pulmonary pathophysiology: the essentials,* 5th ed. Philadelphia: Williams & Wilkins, 1998:17.
This citation reviews the concept of the A-a gradient and the major mechanisms involved in gas exchange impairment.

I. GENERAL PRINCIPLES

A. Acute respiratory distress syndrome (ARDS) is a state of acute, diffuse alveolar damage characterized by increased capillary permeability, pulmonary edema, and refractory hypoxemia due to right-to-left shunting.

B. A ratio of partial pressure of arterial oxygen (P_aO_2) to fraction of inspired oxygen (F_iO_2) less than 300 indicates an acute lung injury process.

C. ARDS is defined by the following criteria: a P_aO_2 / F_iO_2 ratio less than 200, regardless of the level of positive end-expiratory pressure (PEEP); bilateral pulmonary infiltrates on chest radiograph (CXR); and a pulmonary artery occlusion pressure less than or equal to 18 mm Hg or no clinical evidence of elevated left atrial pressure on the basis of chest radiograph or other clinical data.

II. ETIOLOGY

A. Conditions associated with ARDS include those that cause lung injury directly (gastric aspiration, pneumonia, or other toxic inhalational injury) and those that cause injury indirectly (sepsis, trauma, burns, drug ingestion, pancreatitis). Indirect mechanisms are responsible for most cases of ARDS.

B. Up to one half of all cases of ARDS are associated with the systemic inflammatory response syndrome or sepsis syndrome.

C. The risk of ARDS increases as the number of potential causes (risk factors) increases.

III. PATHOPHYSIOLOGY

A. The initial pathology of ARDS (diffuse alveolar damage) includes interstitial swelling, proteinaceous intraalveolar edema, alveolar hemorrhage, and fibrin deposition. Alveolar flooding characteristically occurs in only some alveoli; others appear to be normal.

B. Degenerative cellular changes occur within 1 to 2 days with deposition of hyaline membranes within the alveoli. The repair from acute lung injury begins quickly after the initial insult.

C. Most of the alveolar edema usually resolves after approximately 1 week. Some patients seem to resolve lung injury with little if any fibrosis, whereas others go on to develop severe parenchymal fibrosis. The reason that outcomes are so variable is unknown.

D. The extensive right-to-left shunt in ARDS (up to 25% to 50% of the cardiac output) results from persistent perfusion of atelectatic and fluid-filled alveoli caused by an ineffective or absent hypoxic pulmonary vasoconstriction response.

E. High airway pressures are almost always required to ventilate patients with ARDS. Respiratory system compliance is dramatically reduced, reflecting the amount of edema and atelectasis that is present and is not a measure of the lung injury as such. If fibrosis develops, the elastic properties of the lung parenchyma can change and then can result in true reductions in lung compliance.

F. The work of breathing in ARDS is increased and may be responsible for 25% to 50% of the body's total oxygen consumption. Mechanical ventilatory support in ARDS reduces the work of breathing so oxygen can be redirected to other vital organs.

G. Given the variety of conditions associated with acute lung injury, it should not be surprising that no characteristic hemodynamic pattern exists. Rather, it is more common for the hemodynamic pattern to reflect the underlying condition itself.

IV. DIAGNOSIS

A. When ARDS presents without preexisting or coexisting conditions, it is easy to recognize.

B. Dyspnea and tachypnea often precede the full development of infiltrates on CXR; however, alveolar infiltrates invariably develop within the next several hours.

C. Dry crackles and scattered rhonchi may be heard throughout the lung fields. Not uncommonly, the chest examination is remarkably normal, despite severe alveolar infiltrates on CXR. The rest of the physical examination is usually normal, unless other organ systems are involved.

D. Because obtaining lung tissue in these critically ill patients is most often impractical, the diagnosis of ARDS is usually made by inference (see foregoing criteria).

V. TREATMENT

A. Specific treatment

1. No specific therapy exists for ARDS. Identified underlying or complicating conditions should be treated with specific therapy on an individual basis.

B. Supportive treatment

1. Mechanical ventilation

a. Noninvasive positive pressure ventilation should be considered first in the setting of progressive respiratory failure from acute lung injury, prior to full-blown ARDS. Should the patient's condition deteriorate further, invasive mechanical ventilation is warranted.

b. Initial ventilator management should include a volume-cycled ventilator in the assist/control mode. Convincing data now favor the use of tidal volumes (V_T) of 6 mL/kg over 12 mL/kg to keep airway plateau pressures no more than 30 to 35 cm H_2O in an attempt to minimize any alveolar overdistension injury. The use of such low V_T can lead to hypercapnia (not necessarily undesirable, see discussions of permissive hypercapnia or controlled hypoventilation strategies) and atelectasis.

c. Attention is being focused on the importance of first recruiting and then maintaining as many alveolar units open as possible. This goal often requires levels of PEEP considerably in excess of those needed simply to lower the F_iO_2 below 0.6 (to minimize additional lung injury from oxygen toxicity).

d. In patients with ARDS whose oxygenation cannot be maintained with more conventional approaches, growing clinical experience with prone positioning and/or the pressure-control mode or even the use of mechanical ventilation in the inverse-ratio mode may be useful strategies for salvaging gas exchange when acceptable P_aO_2 (greater than or equal to 60 to 80 mm Hg) cannot be achieved with PEEP less than 15 cm H_2O or when the use of PEEP is associated with excessive plateau pressures.

e. Clinical experience with other nonconventional modes of ventilatory support (high-frequency ventilation, liquid ventilation, extracorporeal respiratory support, inhaled nitric oxide) is too limited to allow any recommendations on their use.

2. Patient positioning

a. Because of the nonuniform distribution of lung infiltrates in ARDS, repositioning the patient into the prone position can improve oxygenation by relieving atelectasis and by improving the distribution of perfusion relative to ventilation. Improvement occurs in approximately 66% to 75% of patients, usually within minutes. Although gas exchange is likely to improve, studies to date have failed to show an improvement in mortality with prone positioning.

3. Fluid management

a. Patients with ARDS should have fluids restricted and should even undergo diuresis when possible, especially during the first few days after onset of the disorder. The benefits of fluid restriction and diuresis after 3 to 4 days remain unclear. However, hypernatremia and renal hypoperfusion should be avoided.

4. Corticosteroids

a. Several prospective, multicenter, placebo-controlled studies have shown no benefit to the use of high-dose corticosteroids early in the course of ARDS. Corticosteroids also do not appear to be consistently beneficial if they are administered during the fibroproliferative phase of ARDS (7 to 10 days after onset).

5. Exogenous surfactant

a. Because normal surfactant may be dysfunctional in ARDS, the instillation of exogenous surfactant has been proposed as a means to improve airspace stability in ARDS and may add antibacterial and immunologic properties as well. Although the only prospective trial available showed no benefit on 30-day mortality, duration of mechanical ventilation, or physiologic function, the design of the trial and the efficacy of the inhaled drug have been criticized. Interest in exogenous surfactant remains strong, and additional trials with alternative agents in the future are likely.

6. Other pharmacologic therapies

a. No specific medications have been shown to be of benefit in ARDS. Ongoing clinical trials with antioxidants (procysteine), selective pulmonary vasodilators (inhaled nitric oxide, aerosolized prostacyclin), and antiinflammatory agents (eicosanoid inhibitors, selective prostanoids, lisophylline) are currently under way.

VI. COMPLICATIONS

A. The mortality rate for ARDS is approximately 35% to 40%, mostly within the first 2 weeks of the illness.

B. Many patients with ARDS develop a syndrome of multiorgan dysfunction. Recovery depends on adequate support of vital organ systems. Complications of management are common, and include barotrauma, nosocomial pneumonia, deep venous thrombosis, catheter-related infections, and so-called stress-related gastrointestinal bleeding.

C. Outcome for patients is difficult to predict. The number of acquired organ system failures is often the most important prognostic indicator for patients requiring intensive care, including patients with ARDS. The greater the number of failing organs, the worse is the prognosis.

Selected Readings

Albert RK. Prone position in ARDS: what do we know, and what do we need to know? *Crit Care Med* 1999;27:2574.
This editorial summarizes what we have learned regarding prone positioning.

Anzueto A, Baughman RP, Guntupalli KK, et al. Aerosolized surfactant in adults with sepsis-induced respiratory distress syndrome: Exosurf Acute Respiratory Distress Syndrome Sepsis Study Group. *N Engl J Med* 1996;334:1417.
A prospective, multicenter, double-blind, placebo-control study involving 725 patients with ARDS. Continuous aerosolized surfactant had no effect on mortality.

Bernard GR, Artigas A, Grigham KL, et al. The American-European consensus conference on ARDS: definitions, mechanisms, relevant outcomes, and clinical trial coordination. *Am J Respir Crit Care Med* 1994;149:818.
Results of a consensus conference, proposing a standard definition for ARDS and a basic framework for studying and comparing groups of patients with ARDS.

Chatte G, Sab JM, Dubois JM, et al. Prone position in mechanically ventilated patients with severe acute respiratory failure. *Am J Respir Crit Care Med* 1997;155:473.
A descriptive study of 32 patients with ARDS. Significant improvement in arterial oxygenation was documented in prone versus supine positioning.

Knaus WA, Wagner DP, Draper EA, et al. The APACHE III prognostic system: risk prediction of hospital mortality for critically ill hospitalized adults. *Chest* 1991;100:1619.
Refining the APACHE methodology in another large database.

Marini JJ. Lung mechanics in the adult respiratory distress syndrome: recent conceptual advances and implications for management. *Clin Chest Med* 1990;11:673.
An excellent review of the pulmonary pathophysiologic effects of ARDS.

Milberg JA, Davis DR, Steinberg KP, et al. Improved survival of patients with acute respiratory distress syndrome (ARDS): 1983–1993. *JAMA* 1995;273:306.
Describes the temporal trends in ARDS mortality in more than 900 patients seen over a decade at one institution.

Schuster DP. What is acute lung injury? What is ARDS? *Chest* 1995;107:1721.
Raises appropriate questions and concerns regarding the use of the consensus conference definition and criteria for ARDS.

Tomashefski JF Jr. Pulmonary pathology of the adult respiratory distress syndrome. *Clin Chest Med* 1990;11:593.
An excellent review of the pathology of ARDS.

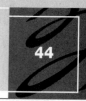

I. GENERAL PRINCIPLES
A. Definitions
1. Asthma is an inflammatory disease of the airways featuring reversible airway obstruction.
2. Status asthmaticus describes a moderate to severe exacerbation of airway obstruction that fails to improve rapidly (usually within 1 hour) with intensive bronchodilator therapy.

II. ETIOLOGY
A. Triggers of asthma exacerbations.
Environmental factors such as viral upper respiratory tract infections, inhaled allergens, pollutants, smoke exposure, and nonsteroidal anti-inflammatory drugs (NSAIDs).
B. Types of asthma exacerbations
1. Slow-onset attacks (>6 hours of deterioration) are most common (~90%).
2. Sudden progression asthma attacks (<6 hours of deterioration) are less common (~10%).

III. PATHOPHYSIOLOGY
A. Pathology
1. Inflammation obstructs the airways by increasing mucus, causing edema and eosinophil infiltration of the airway wall, promoting spasm of smooth muscle, and damaging epithelium.
2. In sudden-progression asthma attacks, neutrophils dominate the inflammation.
B. Physiology
1. Increased airway resistance leads to hypoxemia.
   a. Ventilation-perfusion inequalities mainly account for hypoxemia.
   b. Atelectasis from mucus plugging can cause right-to-left shunt.
2. Persistence of increased airway resistance eventually leads to hypercapnia because of increased work of breathing.

IV. DIAGNOSIS
A. Differential diagnosis
1. Not all wheezing is due to asthma. Obstruction of the airway at any level by any disease process can produce wheezing and dyspnea.
B. Assessment
1. Failure to appreciate the severity of obstruction contributes to mortality.
2. History. High-risk for severe airway obstruction is suggested by prior endotracheal intubation and mechanical ventilation for asthma, aspirin sensitivity, frequent or recent emergency department visits or hospitalizations for asthma, current or recent use of corticosteroids, seizures or syncope during prior exacerbations, poor ongoing medical care, and delay in obtaining medical care.
3. Physical examination
   a. High-risk for severe airway obstruction is suggested by tachycardia (>120 beats/min), tachypnea (>30 breaths/min), diaphoresis, bolt-upright posture in bed, pulsus paradoxus greater than 10 mm Hg, and accessory muscle use.
   b. Cyanosis, respiratory muscle alternans, abdominal paradox, and depressed mental status are late and ominous signs.
   c. Amount of wheezing is a poor way to assess severity of obstruction.

4. Laboratory
   a. Pulmonary function tests (PFTs)
      (1) Obtain an objective measure of maximal expiratory airflow to assess the severity of obstruction whenever possible (PEFR or FEV_1).
      (2) PEFR or FEV_1 less than 50% of baseline is severe obstruction.
   b. Arterial blood gas (ABG) analysis
      (1) Obtain whenever assessment suggests severe obstruction.
      (2) A normal or high pCO_2 is a potentially ominous finding.

V. TREATMENT
A. Bronchodilator therapy
1. β-Adrenergic agonists should be started immediately at presentation.
   a. Short-acting, $β_2$-adrenergic agonists (e.g., albuterol) are the mainstay. One puff of albuterol by metered-dose inhaler (MDI) with spacer device can be given at 1-minute intervals 4 times and repeated every 20 to 30 minutes for up to six doses, if necessary.
   b. Inhaled route of administration is preferable even when severe obstruction is present. When used properly, an MDI with spacer device is as effective as small-volume nebulizer.
2. Cholinergic agonists should be started along with $β_2$-adrenergic agonists.
   a. Muscarinic cholinergic antagonists (e.g., ipratropium) should be used as an adjunct to $β_2$-adrenergic agonists.
   b. Four to eight puffs of ipratropium by MDI with spacer every 6 hours as needed or 0.5 mg by nebulizer every 6 hours as needed.
3. Methylxanthines
   a. Because of toxicity, methylxanthines are mainly reserved for patients not responding to β-adrenergic agonists, cholinergic antagonists, and systemic corticosteroids.

B. Antiinflammatory therapy with corticosteroids
1. Corticosteroids are essential for treating status asthmaticus and should be started at presentation without delay.
2. Oral corticosteroids (e.g., prednisone) are as effective as intravenous therapy (e.g., methylprednisolone). However, many clinicians prefer the intravenous route because gastrointestinal absorption of drugs may be variable in the critically ill.
3. For acute exacerbations of asthma, 60 to 80 mg of methylprednisolone intravenously every 6 to 8 hours is recommended.
4. Once patient shows daily improvement, administer corticosteroids orally. Usually, prednisone is started at 60 mg per day and then gradually tapered over 7 to 14 days. The need for gradual tapering is not well established. The recovering patient should be started on a corticosteroid aerosol.

C. Other therapy
1. Oxygen. Supplemental oxygen therapy should be started immediately. Seemingly paradoxical, inhaled $β_2$-adrenergic agonists may worsen ventilation-perfusion matching and cause hypoxemia unless supplemental oxygen is given.
2. Mechanical ventilation
   a. Decision to intubate is based on repeated clinical assessments of response to therapy, whether hypercapnia is worsening, whether there are signs of muscle fatigue, and whether mental status is deteriorating.
   b. Heliox administration may decrease the need for mechanical ventilation in some acutely ill patients. Do not power nebulizers with heliox given current evidence.
   c. Oral, rather than nasal, route of intubation is preferable. Use an endotracheal tube with internal diameter 8 mm or larger, if possible.
   d. Avoid barotrauma due to dynamic hyperinflation during mechanical ventilation. Controlled hypoventilation is the main strategy that should be used. Physician acceptance of hypercapnia in this setting has been termed permissive hypercapnia. Monitor lung volumes at end inspiration (VEI) to detect, monitor, and manage dynamic hyperinflation.

e. The combination of neuromuscular blocking agents and corticosteroids has been associated with severe myopathy. When paralyzing agents are necessary for ventilating the patient, muscle function always should be allowed to recover partially between repetitive boluses.

D. Additional and unconventional measures. When severe airway obstruction is not responding to conventional therapy and mechanical ventilation, other measures may include helium-oxygen (heliox), general anesthetics (e.g., halothane), magnesium sulfate, bronchoscopy with therapeutic lavage, hypothermia, and extracorporeal life support.

E. Therapies with no established role. There is no established role for fluid administration in excess of euvolemia, mucolytics, or chest physical therapy. Sedatives are contraindicated unless the patient is mechanically ventilated. Antibiotics are used only when there is a strong suspicion of active infection.

Selected Readings

Darioli R, Perret C. Mechanical controlled hypoventilation in status asthmaticus. *Am Rev Respir Dis* 1984;129:385.
Using low respiratory frequency and tidal volume, complications of barotrauma were significantly decreased.

Elshami AA, Tino G. Coexistent asthma and functional upper airway obstruction. *Chest* 1996;110:1358.
Case reports of asthma complicated by functional upper airway obstruction are presented.

Fanta CH, Rossing TH, McFadden ER. Glucocorticosteroids in acute asthma: a critical controlled trial. *Am J Med* 1983;74:845.
Parenteral corticosteroids added to standard bronchodilator therapy caused a significant improvement in lung function at 24 hours compared with standard bronchodilator therapy alone.

Fanta CH, Rossing TH, McFadden ER. Treatment of acute asthma: is combination therapy with sympathomimetics and methylxanthines indicated? *Am J Med* 1986;80:5.
Adding methylxanthines to inhaled β-adrenergic agonists during treatment of acute asthma did not cause significant improvement in lung function compared with β-adrenergic agonists alone.

Feihl F, Perret C. Permissive hypercapnia. *Am J Respir Crit Care Med* 1994;150:1722.
The consequences of hypercapnia and respiratory acidosis are comprehensively reviewed.

Kass JE, Terregino CA. The effect of heliox in acute severe asthma: a randomized controlled trial. *Chest* 1999;116:296.
For patients presenting to the emergency department with acute exacerbations of asthma, heliox (70%/30% helium and oxygen mixture) significantly improved peak expiratory flow rates by 58.4%.

Lanes SF, Garrett JE, Wentworth CE III, et al. The effect of adding ipratropium bromide to salbutamol in the treatment of acute asthma. *Chest* 1998;114:365.
Based on pooled analysis of three clinical trials for acute asthma, addition of inhaled ipratropium bromide to inhaled β-adrenergic agonists caused a small improvement in lung function and modestly decreased need for additional treatment, subsequent exacerbations, and hospitalizations.

McFadden ER. Dosages of corticosteroids in asthma. *Am Rev Respir Dis* 1993;147:1306.
This is an excellent review of corticosteroid use in asthma.

Rizk NW, Kalassian KG, Gilligan T, et al. Obstetric complications in pulmonary and critical care medicine. *Chest* 1996;110:791.
This is a review of obstetric issues in critical care medicine, including a section on the treatment of asthma during pregnancy.

Rodrigo, GJ, Rodrigo C, Hall JB. Acute asthma in adults. *Chest* 2004; 125:1081.
An excellent overview of the assessment and management of status asthmaticus in adults and includes a discussion of noninvasive positive pressure ventilation.

Schwartz SH. Treatment of status asthmaticus with halothane. *JAMA* 1984;251:2688.
One general anesthetic used to treat patients with status asthmaticus refractory to conventional therapy is halothane. Two case reports and the possible risks of halothane are discussed.

Shapiro JM, Condos R, Cole RP. Myopathy in status asthmaticus: relation to neuromuscular blockade and corticosteroid administration. *J Intensive Care Med* 1993;8:144.
Case reports of status asthmaticus complicated by myopathy are described. An association exists between the combination of neuromuscular blocking agents plus corticosteroids and the development of myopathy.

Smith DL, Deshazo RD. Bronchoalveolar lavage in asthma. *Am Rev Respir Dis* 1993;148: 523.
A review of bronchoalveolar lavage in asthma research and as therapy for status asthmaticus.

Tattersfield AE, Knox AJ, Britton JR, et al. Asthma. *Lancet* 2002;360:1313.
An excellent overview of the disease asthma and its management.

Turner, MO, Patel A, Ginsburg S, et al. Bronchodilator delivery in acute airflow obstruction. *Arch Intern Med* 1997;157:1736.
A meta-analysis shows that bronchodilator delivered by metered-dose inhaler or nebulizer is equivalent in the treatment of acute asthma.

U.S. Dept of Health and Human Services, Public Health Service, National Institutes of Health (NIH). *Expert panel report 2: guidelines for the diagnosis and management of asthma.* NIH publication no. 97–4051, 1997.
These are consensus guidelines for the management of asthma.

Williams, TJ, Tuxen, DV, Scheinkestel, CD, et al. Risk factors for morbidity in mechanically ventilated patients with acute severe asthma. *Am Rev Respir Dis* 1992;146:607.
Making ventilator changes to keep volume at end of inspiration by ventilator (VEI) below 20 mL/kg protects against barotrauma in status asthmaticus.

CHRONIC OBSTRUCTIVE PULMONARY DISEASE

Oren P. Schaefer

I. GENERAL PRINCIPLES

A. Definition: Chronic obstructive pulmonary disease (COPD) is a disease state characterized by airflow limitation that is not fully reversible. The airflow limitation is usually both progressive and associated with an abnormal inflammatory response of the lungs to noxious particles or gases.

B. Respiratory failure secondary to COPD leads to 75,000 deaths in the United States annually, is the fourth most common cause of death overall and the second most common cause of permanent disability in people older than 40 years.

C. Deaths from COPD have increased over the last 2 decades.

II. ETIOLOGY

A. Major risk factor is cigarette smoking; correlates with total number of pack-years.

B. Homozygous α_1-antitrypsin deficiency.

C. Other factors that may increase risk include: significant childhood respiratory illnesses, air pollution, increased airway reactivity. Certain occupational exposures may be a risk factor even in the absence of cigarette smoking.

III. PATHOPHYSIOLOGY

A. Expiratory airflow obstruction results from:

  1. Structural airway narrowing, due to inflammatory edema, excessive mucus, and glandular hypertrophy.

  2. Functional airway narrowing, due to destruction of alveolar walls and loss of elastic recoil and radial distending forces. Airway smooth muscle shortening and bronchoconstriction.

  3. Airflow obstruction increases in a dynamic fashion with expiratory effort.

  4. Consequences of severe, chronic airflow obstruction.

    a. Reduced flow rates that limit minute ventilation.

    b. Maldistribution of ventilation.

      (1) Wasted ventilation (high ventilation-perfusion [$\dot{V}/\dot{Q}$] mismatch)

      (2) Impaired gas exchange (low $\dot{V}/\dot{Q}$ mismatch).

    c. Increased airway resistance (and increased work of breathing).

    d. Airtrapping and hyperinflation. Altered geometry places the respiratory muscles at a mechanical disadvantage (reduced maximal force generation).

    e. Blunted respiratory center drive further predisposes to CO_2 retention (select patients).

IV. DIAGNOSIS

A. History

  1. Without a history of cigarette smoking, COPD is unlikely. However, no more than 15% to 20% of smokers develop clinically significant COPD.

  2. Cardinal symptoms are chronic productive cough and dyspnea on exertion.

B. Physical examination

  1. Decreased breath sounds, prolonged expiration, wheezing, hyperinflation, respiratory distress.

  2. Agitation, confusion, or obtundation suggests hypercapnia or hypoxia.

  3. Respiratory muscle fatigue may be heralded by paradoxical respiratory motion.

C. Radiology
1. Findings may include: hyperinflation with flattened diaphragms, increased retrosternal and retrocardiac airspace; vascular attenuation *or* prominence of lung markings; enlarged pulmonary arteries and right ventricular enlargement; regional hyperlucency and bullae.

D. Pulmonary function tests (PFTs)
1. Spirometry demonstrates nonreversible expiratory airflow obstruction and is required to make the diagnosis of COPD.
2. A decreased ratio of forced expiratory volume in 1 second (FEV_1) to forced vital capacity is the hallmark of obstructive airways disease.
3. Global Initiative for Chronic Obstructive Lung Disease (GOLD)
   a. Consensus workshop report with strategy for diagnosis, management, and prevention of COPD.
   b. PFTs used to define the severity of disease (at risk, stage O; mild; stage I; moderate, stage II; severe, stage III; very severe, stage IV).
4. FEV_1 correlates with clinical outcome and mortality.
5. Hypercapnic respiratory failure in COPD not usually seen unless FEV_1 is less than 1 L.
6. PFTs may reveal an increased total lung capacity and residual volume and/or a reduction in carbon monoxide diffusing capacity.
7. Arterial blood gases (ABGs) will diagnose and quantitate the severity of respiratory failure.
8. The relation between the change in P_aCO_2 and the change in hydrogen ion concentration helps determine whether hypercapnia is acute ($\Delta H^+/\Delta PCO_2$ 0.8), acute-on-chronic ($\Delta H^+/\Delta PCO_2$ 0.3–0.8), or chronic ($\Delta H^+/\Delta PCO_2$ 0.3). (See chapter 42.)

E. Exacerbations of COPD
1. Definition: An event in the natural course of the disease (not due to pneumonia, pulmonary embolism, pneumothorax, congestive heart failure) characterized by a change in the patient's baseline dyspnea, cough, and/or sputum beyond day-to-day variability sufficient to warrant a change in management.
2. Acute decompensation most often associated with an acute upper or lower respiratory tract infection. More severe symptoms make bacterial infection more likely.
3. Patient describes increased dyspnea, cough, and sputum production (often with a change in color and character).
4. Airflow obstruction worsens, the work of breathing increases, and mucus production and mucociliary clearance are altered.
5. PFTs and ABGs document worsened expiratory airflow obstruction and gas exchange.

V. TREATMENT
A. Supportive therapy for acute exacerbation
1. Oxygen therapy is required in all hypoxemic patients (PaO_2 <60 mm Hg). with an acute exacerbation. Do not withhold low-flow oxygen for fear that oxygen will aggravate CO_2 retention.
2. Bronchodilator therapy for acute exacerbation
   a. Inhaled β-agonists (albuterol) and ipratropium, in combination
   b. Delivery by small-volume nebulizer or by metered-dose inhaler (MDI) with a spacer is equally effective.
   c. An MDI with an aerosol-holding chamber can deliver bronchodilators to patients receiving mechanical ventilation.
3. Antibiotics for acute exacerbation
   a. Anthonisen type I and type II exacerbations warrant antibiotic therapy. Type I (most severe): Presence of all three cardinal symptoms: increased shortness of breath, increased sputum volume, and sputum purulence. Type II: Presence of two of the three symptoms.
   b. Common organisms include *Haemophilus influenzae*, *Streptococcus pneumoniae*, and *Moraxella catarrhalis*.

4. Corticosteroids for acute exacerbation.
   a. Short-term use of corticosteroids is recommended (10 to 15 days).
   b. Outpatient or emergency department: 30 mg oral prednisolone daily or 40 mg of oral prednisone. Inpatient: 125 mg of intravenous methylprednisolone every 6 hours for 3 days, followed by 60 mg of oral prednisone for 4 days, and then a gradual tapering of the dose to zero.
B. Specific therapy. Institute additional therapy directed at other contributory conditions (e.g., upper respiratory tract infection [antihistamine/decongestants]; aspiration (NPO, speech/swallow therapy).
C. Respiratory failure
   1. Supplemental oxygen to reverse hypoxemia and tissue hypoxia.
      a. Oxygen therapy and a rise in the $PaCO_2$.
         (1) Expect a 10 mm Hg increase in $PaCO_2$. Although CO_2 narcosis may uncommonly occur with excessive oxygen therapy, it is unlikely with low flow-controlled oxygen therapy.
         (2) Results from a change in dead space or shift of the hemoglobin-oxygen binding curve, rather than decreased respiratory drive.
         (3) Should be expected and not specifically treated unless excessive, resulting in acute respiratory acidosis, with central nervous system or cardiovascular effects. Do not discontinue oxygen abruptly, but decrease slowly until the P_aCO_2 returns to an acceptable level.
         (4) Abrupt discontinuation of supplemental oxygen may not result in a quick increase in ventilation and the withdrawal of oxygen further depresses the low alveolar PO_2 and worsens arterial hypoxemia.
   2. Noninvasive positive pressure ventilation (NIPPV)
      a. The favored mode of assisted ventilation if no contraindication exists.
      b. Pressure-support ventilation administered by a tight-fitting face or nasal mask. Improves pulmonary mechanics and gas exchange. May obviate the need for conventional mechanical ventilation.
      c. Contraindications: respiratory arrest, cardiovascular instability, serverely impaired mental status/excessive agitation, recent craniofacial or gastrointestinal surgery, inability to clear secretions or protect airway.
      d. Outcomes: relief of dyspnea, improved pH and ABGs, avoidance of intubation, reduced mortality at 1 year.
   3. Intubation and mechanical ventilation
      a. Indication
         (1) Failure of NIPPV: worsening ABGs and pH in 1 to 2 hours or lack of improvement after 4 hours.
         (2) Severe acidosis (pH <7.2) and hypercapnia ($PaCO_2$ >60 mm Hg).
         (3) Life-threatening hypoxemia (PaO_2/FiO_2 <200 mm Hg).
         (4) Inability to clear secretions and to protect the airway.
         (5) Assessment of the relation between the arterial hydrogen ion concentration and P_aCO_2 helps determine whether intubation may be required urgently (acute acidosis, $\Delta H^+/\Delta PCO_2$ 0.8), be prepared for expectantly (acute-on-chronic, $\Delta H^+/\Delta PCO_2$ 0.3–0.8) or be delayed (chronic, $\Delta H^+/ \Delta PCO_2$ 0.3).
      b. Objectives include support of gas exchange and rest of respiratory muscles.
      c. Regulate ventilatory rate and tidal volume to return pH slowly toward normal.
      d. Hyperventilation of a patient with chronic CO_2 retention can cause marked metabolic alkalosis (i.e., posthypercapnic metabolic alkalosis with risk of seizures or arrhythmias).
      e. "Intrinsic" or "auto" positive end-expiratory pressure (iPEEP or aPEEP).
         (1) Definition: The difference between alveolar pressure and proximal airway pressure measured by the ventilator at end exhalation.
         (2) Results from "airtrapping" from low expiratory flow through obstructed airways.
         (3) Aggravated by rapid respiratory rates, high tidal volumes, low inspiratory flow rates, and ventilation through narrow endotracheal tubes.

TABLE 45-1	Differential Diagnosis of Acute Exacerbation of COPD (Mimics)

Aspiration
Bronchiolitis
Cardiac arrhythmia
Chest wall injury (e.g., rib fracture)
Cystic fibrosis
Lymphangitic carcinomatosis
Metabolic derangements (e.g., hypophosphatemia)
Parasitic infection
Pleural effusion
Pneumonia
Pneumothorax
Pulmonary edema (cardiac vs. noncardiac)
Pulmonary embolism
Sedation (e.g., narcotics, benzodiazepines)
Tracheobronchial infection
Upper respiratory tract infection

(4) Consequences of aPEEP include elevation of inspiratory pressures, hypotension, and increased work for spontaneous or triggered breaths.

(5) Overcome by applying external PEEP equivalent to or slightly less than aPEEP.

(6) Externally applied PEEP reduces inspiratory work; no value in paralyzed patients.

f. Consider mimics of COPD exacerbation that would be treated in different fashion (Table 45-1).

Selected Readings

Anthonisen NR, Monfreda J, Warren CPW, et al. Antibiotic therapy in exacerbations of chronic obstructive pulmonary disease. *Ann Intern Med* 1987;106:196.
Patients with COPD with increased dyspnea, sputum production, and purulence and treated with antibiotics had overall greater treatment success, and fewer relapses, than those given placebo.

Calverley PM. Respiratory failure in chronic obstructive pulmonary disease. *Eur Respir J* 2003;47(suppl):26s–30s.
The physiologic basis of acute respiratory failure in COPD and treatment directed at reducing the mechanical load is reviewed.

Davidson AC. The pulmonary physician in critical care. II: critical care management of respiratory failure resulting from COPD. *Thorax* 2002;57:1079–1084.
The paper describes the physiologic principles behind ventilatory support of patients with COPD to reduce patient–ventilator disharmony and avoid the excessive use of sedation.

Hall CS, Kyprianou A, Fein AM. Acute exacerbations in chronic obstructive pulmonary disease: current strategies with pharmacological therapy. *Drugs* 2003;63:1481–1488.
Review of pharmacologic strategies in the management of acute exacerbations of COPD.

Hill NS. Noninvasive ventilation for chronic obstructive pulmonary disease. *Respir Care* 2004;49:72–87.
Noninvasive positive-pressure ventilation (NIPPV) can reduce the need for intubation and improves outcomes, including lower complication and mortality rates and shortening hospital stay. Patient-selection guidelines and NPPV techniques are reviewed.

Pauwels RA, Buist AS, Calverley PM, Jenkins CR, Hurd SS; GOLD Scientific Committee. Global strategy for the diagnosis, management, and prevention of chronic obstructive pulmonary disease. NHLBI/WHO Global Initiative for Chronic Obstructive Lung Disease (GOLD) Workshop summary. *Am J Respir Crit Care Med* 2001;163:1256–1276.
International GOLD consensus panel guidelines for the assessment and management of stable and exacerbated COPD.

Ranieri VM, Dambrosio M, Brienza N. Intrinsic PEEP and cardiopulmonary interaction in patients with COPD and acute ventilatory failure. *Eur Respir J* 1996;9:1283.
A review of the concepts of intrinsic PEEP in patients with obstructive airway disease and discussion of the use of extrinsic PEEP in ventilatory strategies.

Sethi JM, Siegel MD. Mechanical ventilation in chronic obstructive lung disease. *Clin Chest Med* 2000;21:799–818.
The review covers the pathophysiology of ventilatory failure in acute exacerbations of COPD, including the detection and management of dynamic hyperinflation.

Sethi S. Infectious exacerbations of chronic bronchitis: diagnosis and management. *J Antimicrob Chemother* 1999;43 (suppl A):97.
A review of bacterial acute exacerbations of chronic bronchitis with emphasis on management of the infectious issues.

Snow V, Lascher S, Mottur-Pilson C; Joint Expert Panel on COPD of the American College of Chest Physicians and the American College of Physicians-American Society of Internal Medicine. The evidence base for management of acute exacerbations of COPD: clinical practice guideline, part 1. *Chest* 2001;119(4):1185–1189.
Evidenced-based combined ACCP–ACP practice guideline.

Sutherland ER, Cherniack RM. Management of chronic obstructive pulmonary disease. *N Engl J Med* 2004;350:2689–2697.
An up-to-date review of the subject.

Weinberger SE, Schwartzstein RM, Weiss JW. Hypercapnia. *N Engl J Med* 1989;321:1223.
An excellent discussion of the physiology and therapeutic implications of hypercapnia.

White AJ, Gompertz S, Stockley RA. Chronic obstructive pulmonary disease. 6: The aetiology of exacerbations of chronic obstructive pulmonary disease. *Thorax* 2003;58:73–80.
Exacerbations of COPD are thought to be caused by interactions among host factors, bacteria, viruses, and changes in air quality to produce increased inflammation in the lower airway.

46 EXTRAPULMONARY CAUSES OF RESPIRATORY FAILURE
Mark M. Wilson

I. GENERAL PRINCIPLES
A. The following components make up the extrapulmonary compartment: (a) central nervous system (CNS), (b) peripheral nervous system, (c) respiratory muscles, (d) chest wall, (e) pleura, and (f) upper airway.

B. Impairment of the extrapulmonary compartment produces respiratory failure through the mechanism of hypoventilation; the resultant respiratory failure is always hypercapnic.

C. Extrapulmonary causes can account for up to an estimated 17% of all cases of hypercapnic respiratory failure.

II. ETIOLOGY. See Pathophysiology section.

III. PATHOPHYSIOLOGY
A. Functionally, extrapulmonary disorders lead to hypercapnic respiratory failure because of a decrease in normal force generation (CNS dysfunction, peripheral nervous system abnormalities, or respiratory muscle dysfunction) or an increase in impedance to bulk flow ventilation by chest wall and pleural disorders or upper airway obstruction).

B. Any condition that directly or indirectly impairs respiratory muscle function can result in decreased force generation. If this impairment is severe enough, the level of minute ventilation may be insufficient for the level of production of carbon dioxide.

C. A decrease in central drive to breathe may occur from direct central loss of sensitivity to changes in PCO_2 and pH or as a result of a peripheral chemoreceptor loss of sensitivity to hypoxia, as with CNS depressants (narcotics, barbiturates), metabolic abnormalities (hypothyroidism, starvation, metabolic alkalosis), CNS structural lesions, primary alveolar hypoventilation, and central sleep apnea.

D. Disruption of impulse transmission from the respiratory center in the brainstem to the respiratory muscles may result in respiratory failure. The innervation of the inspiratory respiratory muscles may be involved as part of a generalized process, such as in Guillain-Barré syndrome, myasthenia gravis, amyotrophic lateral sclerosis, neuromuscular junction blockade, or as an isolated abnormality that affects the respiratory system in a variable way that depends on the level of the injury, such as in phrenic nerve palsy and spinal cord trauma.

E. Peripheral nervous system dysfunction severe enough to produce hypercapnic respiratory failure is always associated with a reduced vital capacity (usually less than 50% of predicted value) and markedly decreased maximal inspiratory and expiratory pressures at the mouth (usually less than 30% of predicted).

F. Certain systemic myopathies feature prominent respiratory muscle involvement, such as muscular dystrophies, myotonic disorders, inflammatory and endocrine myopathies, and electrolyte disturbances (hypophosphatemia, hypermagnesemia/hypomagnesemia, hypokalemia, hypercalcemia).

G. Any disorder that causes a decrease in chest wall or pleural compliance (kyphoscoliosis, pleural fibrosis, flail chest, obesity-hypoventilation syndrome, ankylosing spondylitis) or increases airflow resistance from upper airway obstruction (foreign body aspiration, tracheal stenosis, epiglottitis, laryngeal edema, laryngeal/tracheal tumors, obstructive sleep apnea) may culminate in hypercapnic respiratory failure if the resultant respiratory muscle force requirements cannot be sustained.

H. Lateral curvature of the spine (scoliosis) is generally a more important factor in the development of hypercapnic respiratory failure than is dorsal curvature of the spine (kyphosis). Persons with severe deformity (angle of lateral curvature 120 degrees or more) are at the greatest risk of eventual development of respiratory failure.

IV. DIAGNOSIS

A. Arterial hypercapnia in the presence of a normal alveolar-arterial oxygen tension gradient [PO_2(A-a) gradient] on room air is the *sine qua non* of pure extrapulmonary respiratory failure. An A-a gradient less than 20 mm Hg in the presence of an elevated partial pressure of arterial carbon dioxide (P_aCO_2) is, with few exceptions, diagnostic of extrapulmonary respiratory failure.

B. The major differential diagnosis of extrapulmonary respiratory failure is hypercapnic respiratory failure from intrinsic lung disease (chronic obstructive pulmonary disease or asthma).

C. Pulmonary parenchymal disease can exist concomitantly with extrapulmonary respiratory failure and may be suggested by the combination of hypercapnia and mild widening of the A-a gradient to 20 to 30 mm Hg. Even when the A-a gradient exceeds 30 mm Hg, some degree of extrapulmonary dysfunction may be present. When primary pulmonary disease is severe enough to cause hypercapnia, the gradient is generally more than 30 mm Hg.

D. A careful medical history should include an assessment of (but not be limited to): the presence of muscle weakness and any specific muscle groups involved, duration of symptoms, sleep patterns and daytime somnolence, history of trauma or recent viral illness, dietary habits, and drug ingestions or chemical exposures.

E. Measurements of maximal inspiratory pressure (MIP) and maximal expiratory pressure (MEP) at the mouth are easy to perform, noninvasive, and highly predictive of the development of hypercapnic respiratory failure when the problem is decreased respiratory muscle force generation. Although normal predicted values vary (primarily on the basis of age and sex), an MIP not as negative as –30 cm H_2O or reduced to up to 30% of normal is likely to be associated with arterial hypercapnia. MEP is also reduced in this setting and a MEP less than 40 cm H_2O is generally associated with a poor cough and difficulty clearing secretions.

F. Vital capacity measurements may be valuable predictors of the development of arterial hypercapnia and can be performed at the bedside. Although a vital capacity less than or equal to 1 L or less than 15 mL/kg body weight is commonly associated with arterial hypercapnia in patients with neuromuscular weakness, this is a less sensitive predictor than the MIP, particularly in patients with chest wall disorders such as kyphoscoliosis.

G. Significant upper airway obstruction should be considered in the patient who complains of dyspnea in association with stridor (extrathoracic obstruction) or expiratory wheezing (intrathoracic obstruction), particularly if other symptoms suggest an upper airway process (e.g., dysphagia in epiglottitis). Unless the patient is acutely ill, the presence of upper airway obstruction can usually be confirmed in the pulmonary function laboratory with the results of flow-volume loop analysis or by direct visualization.

H. Specific laboratory testing (toxicology screens, thyroid function tests, and levels of magnesium, phosphate, potassium, calcium, and creatinine phosphokinase) and other diagnostic studies (computed tomography, lumbar puncture, electromyography, muscle or nerve biopsy, polysomnogram) should be guided by the patient's presentation and physical examination.

V. TREATMENT

A. The treatment of extrapulmonary respiratory failure can be divided into specific and supportive therapy. A description of specific therapies for each of the numerous potential causes of extrapulmonary respiratory failure is beyond the scope of this chapter.

B. Supportive therapy involves the use of mechanical ventilatory assistance, supplemental oxygen, and techniques of airway hygiene.

C. In the setting of chronic or progressive disease, reversible factors such as pulmonary congestion, infection, retained secretions, and other intercurrent illnesses should be carefully sought and treated.

D. Regardless of the primary cause of respiratory muscle weakness, malnutrition exacerbates muscle weakness and proper nutritional replacement can be beneficial in increasing respiratory muscle strength and function.

Selected Readings

ATS/ERS Statement on Respiratory muscle testing. *Am J Respir Crit Care Med* 2002;166: 518–624.
The latest and definitive word on the topic. Section 10, on pages 610–623 describes how to assess respiratory muscle function in the ICU.

Braun NMT, Arora NS, Rochester DF. Respiratory muscle and pulmonary function in polymyositis and other proximal myopathies. *Thorax* 1983;38:616.
Fifty-three patients with proximal myopathy were extensively studied to determine at what level of muscle weakness hypercapnic respiratory failure is likely and to suggest which tests of pulmonary function or respiratory muscle strength predict this development.

Brooks BR. Natural history of ALS: symptoms, strength, pulmonary function and disability. *Neurology* 1996;47:S71.
Easy-to-read general discussion of the changes that occur and the progression expected in amyotrophic lateral sclerosis.

Defusco DJ, O'Dowd P, Hokama Y, et al. Coma due to ciguatera poisoning in Rhode Island. *Am J Med* 1993;95:240.
An interesting case report on a patient from a nonendemic area for this disease.

Hansen-Flaschen J, Cowen J, Raps EC. Neuromuscular blockade in the intensive care unit: more than we bargained for. *Am Rev Respir Dis* 1993;147:234.
A brief, but important clinical commentary that drew attention to an underappreciated complication of neuromuscular blockade. This article discusses the risk factors and causes of prolonged weakness in this group of patients.

Kelly SM, Rosa A, Field S, et al. Inspiratory muscle strength and body composition in patients receiving total parenteral nutrition therapy. *Am Rev Respir Dis* 1984;130:33.
Small prospective study showing that loss of body mass negatively affects inspiratory muscle strength and contributes to ventilatory failure. Providing nutritional support improves overall nutritional status and inspiratory muscle strength.

Laghi F, Tobin MJ. Disorders of the respiratory muscles. *Am J Respir Crit Care Med* 2003;168:10–48.
Provides a detailed understanding of disease states affecting the respiratory muscles.

NIH Conference. Myositis: immunologic contributions to understanding the cause, pathogenesis and therapy. *Ann Intern Med* 1995;122:715.
A summary of the clinical usefulness of myositis-specific autoantibodies.

Pratter MR, Irwin RS. Extrapulmonary causes of respiratory failure. *J Intensive Care Med* 1986;1:197.
Comprehensive review of the extrapulmonary causes of respiratory failure.

van der Meche FGA, Schmitz PIM, Dutch Guillain-Barré Study Group. A randomized trial comparing intravenous immune globulin and plasma exchange in Guillain-Barré syndrome. *N Engl J Med* 1992;326:1123.
A multicenter trial involving 150 patients treated with either five doses of intravenous immunoglobulin or five plasma exchanges. At 4 weeks from presentation, 53% of the intravenous immunoglobulin group had improved strength versus 34% in the plasma exchange group.

Williams MH Jr, Shim CS. Ventilatory failure. *Am J Med* 1970;48:477.
Good early review of the clinical conditions associated with ventilatory failure and their evaluation.

Zulueta J, Fanburg B. Respiratory dysfunction in myasthenia gravis. *Clin Chest Med* 1994;15: 683.
A general review of the pathophysiology, clinical features, assessment, and manage-

I. GENERAL PRINCIPLES

A. Acute respiratory failure is an important cause of maternal and fetal morbidity and mortality.

B. Thromboembolism, amniotic fluid embolism, and venous air embolism together account for approximately 20% of maternal deaths. Other causes of respiratory failure account for 10% to 15% of maternal deaths.

II. ETIOLOGY

A. Thromboembolic disease

  1. Pulmonary embolism: second leading cause of maternal mortality.

  2. Increases in factors VII, VIII, and X, and fibrinogen; decreased fibrinolytic activity.

  3. Additional risks: venous stasis from uterine pressure on the inferior vena cava, cesarean (C-) section; increased maternal age, multiparity, obesity, and surgery during pregnancy and the early puerperium.

  4. Symptoms, signs, laboratory, radiographic, and ECG findings not specific.

B. Amniotic fluid embolism

  1. Ninety percent occur before or during labor; mortality rate up to 86%.

  2. Predisposing factors: older maternal age, multiparity, amniotomy, C-section, intrauterine fetal monitor, term pregnancy in the presence of an intrauterine device.

  3. Antemortem diagnosis based on clinical setting and exclusion of other causes of respiratory failure.

  4. Finding fetal elements in maternal circulation in blood aspirated from right heart catheters lacks both sensitivity and specificity.

  5. Cardiorespiratory collapse and disseminated intravascular coagulation (DIC) occur simultaneously or in sequence.

  6. Dyspnea, tachypnea, and cyanosis during labor or early puerperium is classic. Shock is first manifestation in 10% to 15%. Excessive bleeding may be the first sign.

  7. Longer survival increases the likelihood of respiratory failure, vascular collapse, and DIC.

C. Venous air embolism

  1. Presentation: sudden, profound hypotension, usually followed by respiratory arrest. Cough, dyspnea, dizziness, tachypnea, tachycardia, and diaphoresis may occur.

  2. Other potential findings: "Mill-wheel" murmur; ECG evidence of ischemia, right heart strain, and arrhythmias; metabolic acidosis.

  3. Obstruction of the pulmonary circulation from air that blocks the apical tract of the right ventricle and fibrin microemboli that obstruct pulmonary arterioles and capillaries. Polymorphonuclear leukocytes may be recruited and activated and lead to tissue damage.

D. Gastric aspiration

  1. Clinical syndromes: Chemical pneumonitis and noncardiogenic pulmonary edema; immediate asphyxia; pneumonia from aspiration of oropharyngeal bacteria

  2. Pathogens are usually oropharyngeal anaerobes.

  3. Risk factors: increased intragastric pressure caused by gravid uterus, progesterone-induced relaxation of the lower esophageal sphincter, delayed gastric emptying during labor, and analgesia-induced decreased mental status.

E. Respiratory infections
1. Community-acquired pneumonia. Organisms to consider: *Streptococcus pneumoniae, Mycoplasma pneumoniae, Haemophilus influenzae,* and respiratory viruses.
2. Primary varicella-zoster infection may progress to pneumonia more commonly than seen in the nonpregnant patient.
3. Coccidioidomycosis associated with an increased risk of dissemination.
4. *Listeria monocytogenes* is rare but has a predilection for pregnant women; commonly results in abortion or neonatal sepsis.

F. Asthma
1. The most common respiratory problem during pregnancy.
2. Assessment includes history, examination, and objective measure of lung function
3. Predictors of hospitalization similar to those of the nonpregnant patient
4. Adequate oxygenation must be ensured.
5. Baseline P_aCO_2 is often already depressed; a P_aCO_2 of 35 mm Hg may represent "pseudonormalization" caused by fatigue and possibly impending respiratory failure.
6. Persistent hypocapnia with respiratory alkalosis (pH >7.48) may result in uterine artery vasoconstriction and decreased fetal perfusion.

G. Tocolytic-induced pulmonary edema
1. β-Adrenergic agonists are used to inhibit preterm labor.
2. β_2-Selective agents (ritodrine, terbutaline) have diminished the frequency of maternal tachycardia, but pulmonary edema remains a serious side effect.
3. Presentation: chest discomfort, dyspnea, tachypnea, rales, and edema on chest radiograph (CXR).
4. May develop after 24 hours; usually after 48 hours of therapy.

H. Pneumomediastinum and pneumothorax
1. Most often seen in the second stage of labor.
2. Presentation: chest or shoulder pain that radiates to neck and arms, mild dyspnea, subcutaneous emphysema.
3. Prolonged, dysfunctional labor is a predisposing factor.

III. DIAGNOSIS
A. Radiology
1. No appreciable increased risk of gross congenital abnormalities or intrauterine growth retardation with exposure to less than 5 to 10 rads. Oncogenic risk also small. Shielding of the abdomen reduces this further.
2. Estimated fetal radiation exposure: CXR, 5 mrad; helical CT, 0.3 to 13 mrad (varies per trimester); pulmonary angiography, <50 mrad; perfusion lung scan, 18 mrad. The average fetal radiation dose with CT is less than that with $\dot{V}/\dot{Q}$ lung scanning during all trimesters.

B. Hemodynamic monitoring
1. Indications for invasive monitoring are similar to those in the nonpregnant patient but also include monitoring the critically ill patient with severe preeclampsia or eclampsia.
2. Cardiac output elevated, central pressures not significantly different in pregnant patient.
3. Monitor fetal heart rate daily or continuously.

IV. TREATMENT
A. Supportive therapy
1. Mechanical ventilation (MV)
   a. Guidelines for intubation and MV same as for nonpregnant patient.
   b. Hyperemia can narrow upper airway; patient at increased risk of upper airway trauma during intubation. Small endotracheal tube may be required.
   c. Decreased functional residual capacity may lower the oxygen reserve. Short period of apnea may result in abrupt decrease in P_aO_2. Prior to intubation, administer 100% oxygen.

    d. Avoid hyperventilation: respiratory alkalosis can decrease uterine blood flow.

    e. Cricoid pressure to decrease gastric inflation and prevent regurgitation.

    f. Adjust minute ventilation for a P_aCO_2 of 30 to 32 mm Hg (normal in pregnancy).

    g. Aim for usual gestational P_aO_2 of more than 95 mm Hg.

    h. Weaning parameters for pregnant patients similar to those for nonpregnant patients. Weaning in the lateral decubitus position may be preferable to avoid compression of the inferior vena cava (IVC).

  2. Reversal of hypotension

    a. Trendelenburg position may further decrease venous return due to IVC compression by the uterus.

    b. Position with right hip elevated 10 to 15 cm (15 degrees) or in the lateral decubitus position.

    c. Hypotension unresponsive to repositioning or fluid resuscitation requires vasopressors.

        (1) α-Adrenergic agents (norepinephrine) improve maternal blood pressure but decrease uterine blood flow (uterine artery vasoconstriction).

        (2) Ephedrine (both α- and β-stimulant) tends to preserve uterine blood flow. Therefore, this is the vasopressor of choice.

  3. Nutrition

    a. Maternal malnutrition may correlate with intrauterine growth retardation and development of preeclampsia. Maternal weight gain correlates with fetal weight gain and a successful outcome.

    b. Enteral route is preferred.

    c. If delivery occurs while mother is receiving total parenteral nutrition, observe the neonate closely for hypoglycemia.

B. Specific therapy

  1. Thromboembolism

    a. Adequate oxygenation; treat hypotension and organ hypoperfusion.

    b. Interrupt clot propagation by anticoagulation with intravenous unfractionated heparin (UFH) or low-molecular-weight heparin (LMWH). UFH and LMWH do not cross the placenta and are not teratogenic. LMWH is the drug of choice because of practical advantages over UFH and because of a lower risk of side effects. Pregnancy and the immediate postpartum period are relative contraindications to thrombolysis.

    c. IVC filter: consider with cardiopulmonary compromise when: no thrombolysis, contraindication to heparin, has recurrent emboli despite anticoagulation.

    d. UFH given for 7 to 10 days; then administer subcutaneously in doses adjusted to prolong the aPTT to 1.5 to 2.5 times control. Continue therapy throughout pregnancy and 4 to 6 weeks postpartum.

    e. LMWH appears safe. May not be associated with osteopenia.

    f. Warfarin, a potent teratogen, is not used.

    g. Pulmonary embolism in late pregnancy or postpartum period, continue anticoagulation at least 3 months.

  2. Amniotic fluid embolism

    a. Treatment is supportive: Adequate ventilation and oxygenation, blood pressure support, and management of bleeding. With active bleeding, transfuse with fresh frozen plasma, cryoprecipitate, and platelets.

    b. Reduce uterine bleeding by manual massage, oxytocin, ± methylergonovine maleate.

    c. With persistent bleeding consider uterine exploration for tears or retained placenta.

  3. Venous air embolism

    a. Left lateral decubitus position may allow air to migrate from RV outflow tract.

    b. Aspiration of air can be attempted with a central venous or pulmonary artery catheter.

    c. Emboli can be decreased in size by providing 100% oxygen.

    d. Anticoagulation, corticosteroids, hyperbaric oxygen suggested but unproved.

4. Gastric aspiration

    a. Prophylactic antibiotics, corticosteroids not beneficial in gastric aspiration.

    b. Antibiotics used when infection complicates chemical pneumonitis.

    c. Antibiotic choice guided by evaluation of respiratory secretions and other cultures.

5. Respiratory infections

    a. Antibiotics similar to those used for nonpregnant patients.

    b. For community-acquired pneumonia: penicillins, cephalosporins, azithromycin, and erythromycin (excluding the estolate), are safe.

    c. Other infections are treated according to usual standards; the safety of drug therapy weighed against the risk of untreated infection.

6. Asthma

    a. Pharmacotherapy similar to that used for the nonpregnant patient.

    b. Prevention or reversal of hypoxemia is paramount. Oxygenation may worsen with bronchodilators; oxygen required in all patients.

    c. High doses of β-agonist carry risk of hypokalemia and pulmonary edema.

    d. High-dose intravenous corticosteroids to help reverse airflow obstruction.

    e. With life-threatening refractory asthma, consider emergency delivery of the fetus by C-section. Decision in part depends on the age and viability of the fetus.

7. Tocolytic-induced pulmonary edema

    a. Discontinuation of tocolytic agent; supplemental oxygen; diuresis; other support as indicated.

8. Pneumomediastinum and pneumothorax (pntx)

    a. Pneumomediastinum almost never requires drainage.

    b. Direct treatment at any underlying cause.

    c. Chest tube drainage: symptomatic patients; mechanical ventilation; enlarging pntx.

    d. Observation: asymptomatic patient with pntx of <20% hemithorax.

Selected Readings

Davies S. Amniotic fluid embolus: a review of the literature. *Can J Anaesth* 2001;48(1): 88–98.
    A review of the literature to determine the natural history, etiology, diagnosis, and potential treatment of amniotic fluid embolus.

Gardner MO, Doyle NM. Asthma in pregnancy. *Obstet Gynecol Clin North Am* 2004; 31:385–413.
    Reviews normal physiology of pregnancy, pathophysiology of asthma in pregnancy, effects of asthma on pregnancy and pregnancy on asthma, goals for the pregnant woman who has asthma, and treatment of chronic and acute episodes of asthma.

Gei AF, Vadhera RB, Hankins GD. Embolism during pregnancy: thrombus, air, and amniotic fluid. *Anesthesiol Clin N Am* 2003;21:165–182.
    Describes clinical characteristics to assist practitioners to distinguish among the different forms of embolism and to institute specific measures of treatment.

Ginsberg JS, Bates SM. Management of venous thromboembolism during pregnancy. *J Thromb Haemost* 2003;1:1435–1442.
    Includes a discussion of the use of low-molecular-weight heparin in the treatment of venous thromboembolism in pregnancy.

Ie S, Rubio ER, Alper B, Szerlip HM. Respiratory complications of pregnancy. *Obstet Gynecol Surv* 2002;57:39–46.
    A review of the common and less common respiratory complications of pregnancy.

Lapinsky SE, Kruczynski, Slutsky AS. Critical care of the pregnant patient. *Am J Respir Crit Care Med* 1995;152:427.
    A review of the critically ill obstetric patient.

Lim WS, Macfarlane JT, Colthorpe CL. Treatment of community-acquired lower respiratory tract infections during pregnancy. *Am J Respir Med* 2003;2:221–233.
Review of lower respiratory tract infection in pregnancy.

Mossman KL, Hill LT. Radiation risks in pregnancy. *Obstet Gynecol* 1982;60:237.
Evaluation of radiation exposures in pregnancy. Procedures to minimize exposure are discussed.

Toglia M, Weg JG. Venous thromboembolism during pregnancy. *N Engl J Med* 1996; 335:108.
An outstanding review of venous thromboembolism in the obstetric patient.

Weinberger SE, Weiss ST, Cohen WR, et al. Pregnancy and the lung. *Am Rev Respir Dis* 1980;121:559.
A comprehensive article on the respiratory physiology of pregnancy.

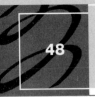

48
VENOUS THROMBOEMBOLISM: PULMONARY EMBOLISM AND DEEP VENOUS THROMBOSIS
Oren P. Schaefer

I. GENERAL PRINCIPLES
   A. Incidence of pulmonary embolism (PE) is greater than 600,000 cases per year in the United States.
   B. Mortality of untreated PE is approximately 30%; with diagnosis, treatment mortality is 2.5%.
   C. Up to 90% of PEs arise from deep venous system of the legs, less commonly in the proximal thigh and iliac veins or inferior vena cava.
   D. Thrombosis and subsequent embolism can occur in upper extremity veins. Risks: central venous catheters, upper extremity exercise, history of congestive heart failure (CHF).

II. PATHOGENESIS
A. Risk factors, acquired
   1. Most common: immobilization, surgery within the last 3 months (especially pelvis and hip).
   2. Others: malignancy, history of venous thromboembolism (VTE), trauma to the lower extremity, CHF, therapeutic estrogen use, postpartum state, and obesity.
B. Risk factors, inherited
   1. Most common: activated protein C (APC) resistance (factor V Leiden mutation). In the United States more than 11 million persons, and 20% to 60% of patients with VTE, have APC resistance.
   2. Others: hyperhomocysteinemia, prothrombin variant 20210, antiphospholipid antibodies.
   3. Rare: deficiencies of antithrombin III, protein C, and protein S; abnormalities in plasminogen or tissue plasminogen activator.

III. DIAGNOSIS
A. Signs and symptoms
   1. Deep venous thrombosis (DVT): most common: leg swelling and tenderness. However:
      a. 95% of patients with symptoms suggestive of DVT have another diagnosis.
      b. 50% to 85% of patients with DVT present without symptoms.
   2. PE: dyspnea, tachypnea, pleuritic chest pain, signs and symptoms of DVT seen in 97%. Findings are nonspecific; symptoms are as likely to be present in those without PE. Syncope is an uncommon presenting symptom. An increased pulmonary second heart sound (P_2) and fourth heart sound more common in patients with PE but found in less than 25%. Consider PE when patients present with three different syndromes:
      a. Acute pneumonia. The most common syndrome mimics acute pneumonia. Accompanied by pleuritic pain and/or hemoptysis
      b. Unexplained dyspnea
      c. Shock
B. Radiographs, electrocardiograms, and arterial blood gases
   1. Chest radiograph is abnormal in more than 80% with PE. Consolidation, atelectasis, pleural effusions, and enlarged central pulmonary arteries with decreased pulmonary vasculature are common. The classic Hampton hump (a pleural-shaped density noted in the costophrenic angle on the posteroanterior projection) is uncommon.

2. ECG is commonly abnormal (in 70%+). Most common findings of sinus tachycardia and ST-segment and T-wave changes are too nonspecific to be of value. The classic S_1-S_2-S_3 and S_1-Q_3-T_3 patterns suggesting cor pulmonale are uncommon.

3. Arterial blood gases are commonly abnormal. Mean P_aO_2 70 ± 16 mm Hg in patients with PE (no different in those without PE). Of patients with proven PE, 15% have a P_aO_2 of ≥85 mm Hg, and 10% to 15% of patients with PE have a normal PAO_2-PaO_2 gradient [(A-a) DO_2].

IV. DIAGNOSIS OF DEEP VENOUS THROMBOSIS
A. Venography
1. The reference standard for the diagnosis of DVT
2. Complications include pain, superficial phlebitis, DVT, and contrast media reactions.
3. Noninvasive tests have supplanted the venogram.

B. Impedance plethysmography (IPG)
1. Overall sensitivity and specificity of 83% and 92%, respectively.
2. False-positive results with tensing of the leg muscles, compression by an extravascular mass, elevated central pressure obstructing venous outflow, or reduced arterial flow.
3. Not sensitive to calf vein thrombosis.
4. Initial negative test in 6% to 26% of symptomatic patients who later develop an abnormal test.

C. Real-time B-mode ultrasonography with color Doppler flow (duplex scan)
1. Permits direct visualization of major vascular channels
2. Doppler signal provides an audible and graphic depiction of blood flow direction and speed.
3. Failure to collapse the vascular lumen completely with gentle probe pressure and the finding of intraluminal echogenic material resulting from clot are diagnostic.
4. Sensitivity for proximal DVT is 97%; specificity is 99%.
   a. False-positive with failure to compress femoral vein due to pregnancy or pelvic tumor
   b. False-negative from missing small clots or misinterpreting total occlusion of the femoral vein because of dilated collateral veins
5. Less sensitive in identifying asymptomatic, isolated calf vein and recurrent thrombosis
6. Predictive value of duplex ultrasound is greater than that of IPG.

V. DIAGNOSIS OF PULMONARY EMBOLISM
A. Ventilation-perfusion lung scan
1. Scans categorized as: normal, near-normal, intermediate, indeterminate, or high probability based on the number and size of the perfusion abnormalities present and whether or not they are matched with abnormalities of ventilation.
2. Positive predictive value (PPV) of a high-probability lung scan is approximately 88%. A prior history of PE decreases the PPV value to 74%.
3. Definition of high-probability lung scan: two or more large (>75% of segment) segmental perfusion defects without corresponding ventilation or radiographic abnormalities or substantially larger than either matching ventilation or chest radiograph abnormalities; two or more moderate segmental (≥25% and ≤75% of segment) perfusion defects without matching ventilation or chest radiograph abnormalities and one large mismatched segmental defect; four or more moderate segmental perfusion defects without ventilation or chest radiograph abnormalities.
4. Normal lung perfusion scan effectively rules out clinically important PE.
5. High-probability (~12%) or normal/near-normal scans (~12%) occur infrequently.
6. Assigning prior clinical probabilities helpful only in concordant situations (infrequent)

   a. High clinical suspicion **AND** high-probability lung scan—PE in 96%.
   b. Low clinical suspicion **AND** low-probability lung scan—PE in only 4%.
   7. With underlying cardiopulmonary disease (chronic obstructive pulmonary disease, congestive heart failure), the frequency of a nondiagnostic scan is higher than in those without underlying disease. Predictive value remains unchanged.
   8. In intensive care unit patients in respiratory failure, the clinical, radiographic, ABG, and V/Q scan findings are unsatisfactory in making a diagnosis.

B. Contrast-enhanced helical (spiral) CT
   1. Sensitivity for central emboli approximately 95% (overall sensitivity 72%); specificity 95%.
   2. Emboli in segmental or small vessels occur in 15% to 30% and may be missed.
   3. However, patients with a negative contrast CT have a rate of subsequent embolism similar to that with a negative $\dot{V}/\dot{Q}$ lung scan and also patients with positive CT and treatment for VTE.
   4. In the high-risk patient, the clinician can consider additional investigation.

C. D-Dimer
   1. Degradation products of cross-linked fibrin. A marker of endogenous fibrinolysis.
   2. D-dimer assays differ in sensitivity, specificity, likelihood ratios, and variability among patients with suspected DVT or PE. Enzyme-link immunosorbent assay (ELISA) and quantitative rapid ELISA D-dimer in general are most clinically useful because they are highly sensitive. The value of the test is in ruling out VTE.
   3. Negative predictive value of greater than 95% for DVT and PE.
   4. Multiple assays available. Less-sensitive assays cannot be used in isolation to rule out VTE.
   5. D-dimer has not been studied extensively in critically ill patients. However, it is of value in ruling out VTE in stable outpatients in the office or emergency department setting.

D. Pulmonary angiography
   1. The gold standard by which to diagnose PE.
   2. Intravascular filling defects and the trailing embolus sign are diagnostic.
   3. Mortality risk 0.1% to 0.5%.
   4. Complications: cardiac perforation, hematoma, contrast media reaction.
   5. A negative angiogram with balloon occlusion excludes the diagnosis of PE.
   6. Diagnostic algorithm. PE in the critically ill. (Fig. 48-1)

VI. TREATMENT
A. Low-molecular-weight heparin
   1. Low-molecular-weight heparin (LMWH) is as effective as or superior to unfractionated heparin (UFH) in the treatment of acute DVT and PE and considered by most to be the drug of choice.
   2. No difference seen in recurrent VTE, bleeding, or mortality.
   3. Dosing is weight based and depends on the particular LMWH
   4. Advantages: subcutaneous administration with fixed dose, once or twice a day, no laboratory monitoring.
   5. LMWH contraindicated in renal failure; dose adjustments required with renal insufficiency.

B. Heparin
   1. UFH is given as a continuous intravenous infusion with an initial loading dose of 60 units/kg (maximum bolus 5,000 units) given on the basis of a strong clinical suspicion unless a high risk or contraindication to anticoagulation exists.
   2. After the loading dose, a continuous infusion is given at 18 units/kg/hour (maximum initial infusion rate 1,800 units/hr). Adjustments are made using a nomogram, to achieve a thrombin clotting time (TCT) of 0.2 to 0.4 heparin U/mL, or an activated partial thromboplastin time (aPTT) 1.5 to 2.5 times mean normal range.
   3. The aPTT is not as accurate as the TCT; use the latter when baseline aPTT is prolonged (e.g., lupus-type inhibitor).
   4. Risk of recurrent VTE increased if adequate anticoagulation not achieved within 24 to 48 hours.

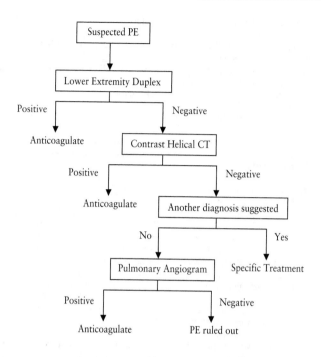

Suspected PE - patients unstable to transport.
- **Lower extremity** (LE) Duplex study. If positive, anticoagulate.
- If no contraindication, anticoagulate with UFH until stability allows transport for CT.
- Consider transthoracic or transesophageal echocardiogram. Right ventricular strain (without other explanation) supports acute PE. RV or PA clot may be visualized.

Figure 48-1. Suggested evaluation algorithm: PE in the stable critically ill patient.

5. Recheck aPTT in 4 to 6 hours after bolus and then every 6 hours for the first 24 to 36 hours or until the therapeutic range has been achieved.
6. If, after the initial loading dose, there is little or no change in the TCT or aPTT, the patient should receive a second loading dose.
7. Complications of UFH
   a. Bleeding occurs in 5% to 20%. A relationship between bleeding and higher levels of anticoagulation exists.
   b. Thrombocytopenia. In most, the platelet count falls modestly. In heparin-induced thrombocytopenia (HIT), due to IgG antibodies, platelet count falls abruptly to less than 100,000 /mm^3. Heparin should be discontinued immediately because of risk of venous and arterial thrombosis. Anticoagulation with nonheparin anticoagulants is required; consider inferior vena cava (IVC) interruption.

C. Warfarin
   1. Initiate warfarin at the time of heparinization.
   2. Leads to depletion of vitamin K–dependent coagulant proteins: factors II, VII, IX, and X; limits carboxylation of anticoagulant proteins C and S.
   3. International normalized ratio (INR) may become therapeutic quickly due to a decrease in factor VII; other coagulant factors may be present in quantity to

generate thrombin. Therefore, warfarin must be overlapped with heparin for 4 or 5 days.

4. After this interval, heparin may be stopped once the INR is in the therapeutic range.

5. Daily dosing is based on the INR, with the goal being 2 to 3.

6. Duration of warfarin therapy. Initial DVT/PE: treat for 6 months; data suggest that the course should possibly be longer. Recurrent VTE: treat for 1 year or longer. Inherited and acquired risk factors and pulmonary hypertension: treatment is indefinite.

7. Complications: Bleeding, most commonly in the gastrointestinal and urinary tracts, in 4.3% to 6%. Risk related to intensity of anticoagulation (14% to 42% when INR is ≥3), concomitant use of aspirin and with comorbid conditions (central nervous system, renal, hepatic, and cardiac disease).

D. Thrombolytic therapy

1. Indication: acute, massive PE with hypotension/hypoxemia despite resuscitation

2. No consensus exists on the use of thrombolytic therapy for acute DVT.

3. Administration of thrombolysis

   a. Discontinue UFH/do not give additional LMWH. Resume this therapy after thrombolysis when the aPTT is less than 1.5 times control value.

   b. Given bleeding risk with thrombolytics consider UFH for 24-hour period following lytic; UFH has short half-life and can be reversed more quickly than LMWH. LMWH has not been studied with thrombolytic therapy.

   c. Agent of choice: t-PA given as 100 mg over 2 hours

   d. Restart heparin when aPTT returns to 1.5 times control or less, followed by warfarin.

4. Contraindications: identical to those for coronary thrombolysis.

E. Inferior vena cava interruption

1. Indications: contraindication to or complication of anticoagulation, documented recurrent VTE despite adequate anticoagulation, chronic recurrent embolism with pulmonary hypertension, and pulmonary embolectomy. May be placed above the renal veins if necessary.

2. Twenty-year efficacy rate of 95% and patency rate of 96%.

3. If possible, anticoagulation should be resumed.

4. Effective in primary prophylaxis in patients with a high risk of bleeding.

5. No benefit to insertion of a filter in patients with free-floating thrombi.

6. Complications: Thrombus at the site of insertion, filter migration, improper filter deployment, proximal clot formation with propagation and embolization, venous insufficiency, and IVC obstruction. Rare: myocardial infarction, vessel perforation, pericardial tamponade, arrhythmia.

F. Pulmonary embolectomy

1. Indications: angiographically documented massive PE with hemodynamic instability and a contraindication to thrombolysis.

2. Mortality rates range from 10% to 75%.

3. Complications: acute respiratory distress syndrome, renal failure, cardiac arrhythmias, mediastinitis, and severe neurologic sequelae.

G. Transvenous catheter extraction of emboli

1. Balloon-tipped catheter guided under fluoroscopy for suction extraction of proximal PE.

2. Indications: Similar to those for embolectomy.

3. Success rates of up to 88% reported with a mortality rate of 27%.

Selected Readings

Arcasoy SM, Vachani A. Local and systemic thrombolytic therapy for acute venous thromboembolism. *Clin Chest Med* 2003;24:73–91.
   This article discusses the role and current areas of controversy for thrombolysis in pulmonary embolism.

Buller HR, Agnelli G, Hull RD, et al. Antithrombotic therapy for venous thromboembolic disease. The Seventh ACCP Conference on Antithrombotic and Thrombolytic Therapy.

Chest. 2004;126(3 suppl):4015–4285.
Recommendations from the expert panel.

Dalen JE. Pulmonary embolism: what have we learned since Virchow? Treatment and prevention. *Chest* 2002;122:1801–1817.
An excellent, comprehensive review of the subject.

Gulsun M, Goodman LR. CT for the diagnosis of venous thromboembolic disease. *Curr Opin Pulm Med* 2003;9:367–373.
Reviews advances in multidetector spiral CT and the combination of CT pulmonary angiography and venography as a one-step evaluation of venous thromboembolic disease.

Holzheimer RG. Low-molecular-weight heparin (LMWH) in the treatment of thrombosis. *Eur J Med Res* 2004;9:225–239.
An up-to-date review on the of LMWH in the treatment of acute venous thrombosis.

Kearon C, Julian JA, Math M, et al. Noninvasive diagnosis of deep venous thrombosis. *Ann Intern Med* 1998;128:663.
An outstanding review. Provides evidence-based recommendations for the diagnosis of deep vein thrombosis in symptomatic, asymptomatic, and pregnant patients.

Kruip MJ, Leclercq MG, van der Heul C, et al. Diagnostic strategies for excluding pulmonary embolism in clinical outcome studies. A systematic review. *Ann Intern Med* 2003; 138:941–951.
Review of strategies to rule out PE incorporating newer technologies such as the D-dimer.

Phillips OP. Venous thromboembolism in the pregnant woman. *J Reprod Med* 2003;48 (suppl):921–929.
The article discusses the management of the pregnant patient with suspected or proven VTE.

Prandoni P, Polistena P, Bernardi E, et al. Upper extremity deep venous thrombosis: risk factors, diagnosis, and complications. *Arch Intern Med* 1997;157:57.
Upper extremity DVT is associated with central venous catheters, thrombophilia, and a previous leg DVT. The diagnostic accuracy of the duplex scan is confirmed. PE is common (36%).

Rashke RA, Reilly BM, Guidry JR, et al. The weight based heparin dosing nomogram compared with a "standard care" nomogram: a randomized controlled trial. *Ann Intern Med* 1993;119:874.
A weight-based nomogram proved superior. More patients reached a therapeutic range sooner, and the risk of recurrent VTE was lower.

Stein PD, Hull RD, Patel KC, et al. D-dimer for the exclusion of acute venous thrombosis and pulmonary embolism: a systematic review. *Ann Intern Med* 2004;140:589–602.
Reviews the studies available on this newer technology, making recommendations for its place in evaluation of VTE, as well as its limitations.

Streiff MB. Vena caval filters: a review for intensive care specialists. *J Intensive Care Med* 2003;18:59–79.
Reviews the literature on indications and complications of vena caval interruption with a filter.

49 MANAGING HEMOPTYSIS
Oren P. Schaefer and Richard S. Irwin

I. GENERAL PRINCIPLES
A. Definitions
1. Hemoptysis: expectoration of blood from the lungs or bronchial tubes
2. Massive hemoptysis: expectoration of 600 mL of blood within 24 to 48 hours
3. Pseudohemoptysis: expectoration of blood from other than the lower respiratory tract

II. ETIOLOGY
A. Nonmassive hemoptysis.
Table 49-1 lists the more common causes of hemoptysis, including bronchitis, bronchiectasis, lung carcinoma, and tuberculosis
B. Massive hemoptysis
1. All causes of hemoptysis may result in massive hemoptysis. Most frequent causes are infection (tuberculosis, mycetoma, bronchiectasis, lung abscess), lung cancer, and diffuse intrapulmonary hemorrhage.
2. Catastrophic, albeit rare causes include rupture of a pulmonary artery from a balloon flotation catheter and tracheoarterial fistula.
C. Idiopathic hemoptysis
1. Despite a systematic diagnostic approach hemoptysis may be idiopathic in 2% to 32%.
2. Most commonly seen in men between ages of 30 and 50 years.
3. Usually presents as nonmassive hemoptysis but can be massive.
4. 10% have recurrence.

III. PATHOGENESIS
A. Bronchial arterial circuit supplies blood to the airways (main stem bronchi to the terminal bronchioles), pleura, intrapulmonary lymphoid tissue, and large branches of the pulmonary vessels and nerves in the hilar regions. The bronchial circulation is responsible for bleeding in approximately 92% of cases.
B. Pulmonary arterial circuit supplies the pulmonary parenchymal tissue, including respiratory bronchioles.

IV. DIAGNOSIS
A. Medical history
1. Consider frequency, timing, duration, anticoagulant use, and travel history (endemic fungi and parasites).
2. Chronic sputum production suggests chronic bronchitis, bronchiectasis, or cystic fibrosis.
3. Orthopnea and paroxysmal nocturnal dyspnea suggests cardiac failure or mitral stenosis.
4. Always consider pulmonary embolism.
5. Consider suction catheter trauma in the intensive care unit.
6. Diffuse intrapulmonary hemorrhage: hemoptysis typical but absence does not rule out.
B. Physical examination
1. Evaluation of the respiratory system
   a. Inspection: evidence of recent or old chest trauma
   b. Auscultation

TABLE 49-1	Common causes of hemoptysis[a]

Tracheobronchial disorders
Acute tracheobronchitis
Bronchiectasis
Bronchogenic carcinoma
Chronic bronchitis
Cystic fibrosis
Gastric acid aspiration
Tracheobronchial trauma
Tracheoarterial fistula

Cardiovascular disorders
Congestive heart failure
Mitral stenosis
Pulmonary arteriovenous fistula
Pulmonary embolism

Hematologic disorders
Anticoagulant therapy
Thrombocytopenia
Disseminated intravascular coagulation

Localized parenchymal disease
Acute and chronic pneumonia
Aspergilloma
Lung abscess
Pulmonary tuberculosis

Diffuse alveolar hemorrhage
Goodpasture's syndrome
Systemic lupus erythematosus
Trimellitic anhydride toxicity
Cocaine inhalation
Viral pneumonitis
Wegener granulomatosis
Bone marrow transplantation
Pulmonary capillaritis

Other
Idiopathic
Iatrogenic (e.g., bronchoscopy, cardiac catheterization)

[a]This list is not meant to be all inclusive. See Hemoptysis chapter in *Intensive Care Medicine*, 5th edition for an expanded list with references.

> **(1)** Unilateral wheeze or rales suggest localized disease.
> **(2)** Diffuse crackles in congestive heart failure and diffuse intrapulmonary hemorrhage.
> **2.** Evaluation of other systems
> > **a.** Skin and mucous membranes
> > > **(1)** Telangiectasias suggest hereditary hemorrhagic telangiectasia.
> > > **(2)** Ecchymoses and petechiae suggest hematologic abnormality.
> > **b.** Neck: with pulsations transmitted to a tracheostomy cannula consider a tracheoarterial fistula or the risk of one.
> > **c.** Cardiovascular: mitral stenosis, pulmonary artery stenosis, or pulmonary hypertension.

C. Laboratory studies
1. Chest radiograph (CXR)
   a. Obtain in every patient (may suggest diagnosis or help localize bleeding site)
      (1) However, do not assume that an abnormality always accurately identifies the site of bleeding.
   b. CXR normal in up to 30%.
2. Complete blood count for evidence of infection, hematologic disorder, or chronic blood loss.
3. Urinalysis may show hematuria or suggest systemic disease associated with diffuse intrapulmonary hemorrhage.
4. Coagulation studies: primary or contributing hematologic disorder.
5. Electrocardiogram
6. High-resolution chest computed tomography (CT) scan may improve yield of bronchoscopy in localizing a bleeding source and point to a diagnosis.

D. Bronchoscopy
1. For diagnosis and localization of the pulmonary hemorrhage.
2. Greatest yield when performed during or within 24 hours of active bleeding.
   a. With active bleeding, localization in up to 91%.
   b. Within 48 hours, localization drops to 51%.
   c. After bleeding stops, localization reduced further.
3. Flexible bronchoscope: ideally used to diagnose lower respiratory tract problems.
4. Rigid bronchoscopy: ideally used for massive hemorrhage.

E. Angiography
1. Can determine the site of bleeding in up to 90%. Not useful in diffuse alveolar hemorrhage syndromes.
2. Can establish a diagnosis not identified by bronchoscopy in only 4%.

V. TREATMENT
A. General considerations
1. Quantify the amount of bleeding; massive hemoptysis is associated with significant mortality.
2. Consider the cause of bleeding.
3. Consider the patient's underlying lung function.

B. Supportive care
1. Bed rest and mild sedation.
2. Cough suppressants should not be used.
3. Supplemental oxygen may be required.
4. Evaluate need for endotracheal intubation (airway protection, assisted mechanical ventilation).
5. If intubation is required, an endotracheal tube with an internal diameter of 8.5 mm will facilitate flexible bronchoscopy.
6. Fluid and blood resuscitation as indicated.
7. Chest physical therapy and postural drainage should be avoided.

C. Definitive care
1. For nonmassive hemoptysis, treatment is directed at the specific cause.
2. Massive hemoptysis is an emergency. The likelihood of death, primarily due to asphyxiation, is directly related to the rate of bleeding.
   a. Treatment aimed at the specific cause
   b. Treatment aimed to stop the bleeding
   c. Lung isolation
      (1) Initial management requires protection of the uninvolved lung from aspiration of blood.
      (2) The bleeding lung should be kept dependent.
      (3) Placement of a double-lumen endotracheal (Carlen) tube can favorably affect bronchial isolation, but these tubes can be difficult to place and may be dislodged easily, and their small diameter may prevent subsequent bronchoscopy.

   d. Rigid bronchoscopy under general anesthesia may be required to clear the airway of aspirated blood.
   e. Therapeutic maneuvers—bronchoscopy
   (1) Fogarty balloon catheter, bronchoscopically positioned, may provide effective tamponade when the bleeding bronchial segment is located.
   (2) Iced saline: lavage of the bronchus leading to the bleeding site may stop hemorrhage.
   (3) Laser coagulation can be used to control bleeding in patients with cancer. Recurrence of bleeding within a few weeks is typical.
   f. Therapeutic maneuvers—angiography
   (1) Embolization can successfully stop bleeding in massive hemoptysis in more than 90% of cases. Rebleeding within 1 to 4 days can occur, and therefore multiple procedures may be necessary. Within 6 months, 20% of patients bleed again.
   (2) Complications that are rare, but serious, include embolization of the spinal arteries and transverse myelitis.
   g. Specific maneuvers for uncommon causes of massive hemoptysis
   (1) Rupture of the pulmonary artery from Swan-Ganz catheter is a rare but serious complication. Deflate balloon, withdraw catheter 5 cm, reinflate balloon with 2 mL of air, allow balloon to float back and occlude vessel. The catheter usually floats to the right pulmonary artery. If not known which artery has ruptured, place patient in the right lateral decubitus position. Once the patient has been stabilized, study the patient angiographically. If a pseudoaneurysm has formed, ablate the feeding vessel with coil.
   (2) Tracheoarterial fistula is a cause of massive hemoptysis. Overinflation of the tracheostomy cuff may stop the hemorrhage as an emergency procedure.
   h. Emergency surgery
   (1) With the exception of immediate intervention to repair a tracheoarterial fistula, the role of emergency surgery remains controversial. Unclear whether emergent surgery for massive hemoptysis provides a survival benefit. Mortality is related to whether the patient is an operable candidate and diagnosis.
   i. Conservative nonsurgical treatment
   (1) Advocated when hemoptysis has an infectious cause.
   (2) In patients with cystic fibrosis, repeated episodes in other areas are likely.
   (3) Severe lung disease (FEV_1 less than 2 L): withhold surgery if assessment suggests a postoperative severe respiratory impairment ($FEV_1 \leq 800$ mL).
D. Approach. Therapy in a given patient depends on etiology, lung function, availability of resources, and local expertise.
   1. Nonsurgical candidates: poor lung function, significant comorbid illness, diffuse lesions. Treat with selective angiography and embolization.
   2. Surgical candidates: resectional surgery should be performed when it will be definitive treatment for the underlying disease.
   3. Diffuse intrapulmonary hemorrhage
   a. Selective arterial embolization and surgery are not options.
   b. For immune-mediated diseases (e.g., Goodpasture's syndrome, SLE) high-dose steroids and cytotoxic agents are recommended.
   c. Post–bone marrow transplantation alveolar hemorrhage requires high-dose steroids.

Selected Readings

Conlan AA. Massive hemoptysis—diagnostic and therapeutic implications. *Surg Annu.* 1985;17:337–354.
   Discusses the value of iced-saline lavage as well as other diagnostic and therapeutic techniques.

Dweik RA, Stoller JK. Role of bronchoscopy in massive hemoptysis. *Clin Chest Med* 1999;20:89–105.
Bronchoscopy plays a central role in the diagnosis and treatment of massive hemoptysis. It allows for localization and acute control of bleeding.

Jean-Baptiste E. Clinical assessment and management of massive hemoptysis. *Crit Care Med* 2000;28:1642–1647.
A complete review of patients with hemoptysis cared for by the intensivist.

Johnston H, Reiza G. Changing spectrum of hemoptysis: underlying causes in 148 patients undergoing diagnostic flexible fiberoptic bronchoscopy. *Arch Intern Med* 1989;149: 1666–1668.
Bronchitis and bronchogenic cancer were found to be more common than bronchiectasis and tuberculosis, a reversal from prior surveys.

Jougon J, Ballester M, Delcambre F, et al. Massive hemoptysis: what place for medical and surgical treatment. *Eur J Cardiothorac Surg* 2002;22:345–351.
The authors aim to define the timing of surgical treatment in management of massive hemoptysis.

Mal H, Rullon I, Mellot F, et al. Immediate and long-term results of bronchial artery embolization for life-threatening hemoptysis. *Chest* 1999;115:996–1001.
Describes embolization in patients with massive hemoptysis. Immediate control of life-threatening hemoptysis was achieved in all but one patient. Long-term control occurred in 45%.

Mullerworth MH, Angelopoulos P, Couyant MA, et al. Recognition and management of catheter-induced pulmonary artery rupture. *Ann Thorac Surg* 1998;66:1242–1245.
Catheter-induced pulmonary artery rupture is uncommon so awareness is essential. Early pulmonary angiography is advocated for accurate diagnosis and treatment by embolization.

Saumench J, Escarrabill J, Padró L, et al. Value of fiberoptic bronchoscopy and angiography for diagnosis of the bleeding site in hemoptysis. *Ann Thorac Surg* 1989; 48: 272–274.
Bronchoscopy had an overall yield of 68% in localizing the site of bleeding. When it was done early, the yield was 91% (vs. 50%). Angiography added little to this.

Tasker AD, Flower CD. Imaging the airways. Hemoptysis, bronchiectasis, and small airways disease. *Clin Chest Med* 1999;20:761–773.
In patients with hemoptysis, CT is now established as a complementary technique to bronchoscopy or as an alternative to bronchoscopy in selected cases.

Yoon W, Kim JK, Kim YH, et al. Bronchial and nonbronchial systemic artery embolization for life-threatening hemoptysis: a comprehensive review. *Radiographics* 2002;22: 1395–1409.
Nonbronchial systemic arteries can be a significant source of massive hemoptysis and a cause of recurrence after bronchial artery embolization. Reviews the techniques, embolic agents, results, and possible complications.

ASPIRATION AND NEAR-DROWNING
Nicholas A. Smyrnios and Richard S. Irwin

I. ASPIRATION
A. General principles
   1. Definitions
   a. Aspiration: taking foreign material into the lungs with the respiratory current. The material may be particulate matter (food particles), irritating fluids, or oropharyngeal secretions containing infectious agents.
B. Pathogenesis
   1. Normal respiratory defenses against aspiration. An aspiration event requires bypassing or overwhelming one or more of these mechanisms.
   a. Aerodynamic filtration—nose, mouth, larynx—particles greater than 10 μm in diameter.
   b. Mucociliary clearance—for particles 2 to 10 μm in diameter
   c. Alveolar detoxification—alveolar macrophage and neutrophil nonspecific killing for particles less than 2 μm in diameter
   d. Cough—provides clearance when mucociliary clearance is inadequate
   e. Immunologic mechanisms—augment the nonimmunologic mechanisms
   f. Swallowing mechanism. Hypopharyngeal muscles move food into the esophagus, the epiglottis covers the larynx, the vocal cords close, and the upper esophageal sphincter relaxes. Pharyngeal swallowing initiates peristaltic waves in the esophagus, which carry the bolus through a relaxed lower esophageal sphincter to the stomach.
   g. For variable periods of time following endotracheal intubation, patients are at risk of aspiration with oral nutrition.
C. Diagnosis
   1. Diagnostic tests available for aspiration are listed in Table 50-1.
D. Treatment
   1. Mendelson syndrome. Aspiration of gastric contents may cause the development of acute respiratory distress syndrome (ARDS). Management of ARDS is described in Chapter 43.
   2. Foreign body aspiration
   a. Particles that do not totally obstruct the trachea removed by bronchoscopy.
   b. Completely obstructing particles removed by subdiaphragmatic thrusts/finger sweeps in unconscious patient or chest thrusts in obese or pregnant patient.
   3. Bacterial pneumonia and lung abscess
   a. Community-acquired most often due to *Streptococcus pneumoniae* and anaerobes.
   b. Nosocomial most often (50% to 74%) due to enteric gram-negative bacilli.
   c. Speech therapy can assess risk of aspiration and often help a patient to develop strategies for swallowing that minimize the risk of further aspiration. Following endotracheal intubation and with tracheostomy tube in place, do not start oral nutrition until patient is cleared.
   4. Exogenous lipoid pneumonia
   a. Caused by animal, vegetable, or mineral oil material aspiration
   b. Exogenous lipoid pneumonias usually resolve on their own.
   c. Surgical repair of achalasia and Zenker's diverticulum
   d. Patients with swallowing problems may require stoppage of oral feedings and initiation of gastrostomy or jejunostomy feedings.

TABLE 50-1	Diagnostic Protocol for Aspiration Syndromes

History

Physical examination
  Baseline examination
  Observation of patient drinking water
Chest radiographs
Lower respiratory studies
  Expectorated samples
  Transtracheal aspiration
  Protected specimen brush with quantitative cultures
  Bronchoalveolar lavage
  Lung biopsy
Upper gastrointestinal studies
  Contrast films
  Endoscopy
  Motility
  Scintiscan
  24-hour esophageal pH monitoring
Speech and swallowing bedside methods for detecting aspiration in tube-fed patients

    e. Patients with tube feedings: elevate head of bed to 45-degree angle.
    f. Gastroesophageal reflux disease treatment: head-of-bed elevation; acid suppression; prokinetic drugs; antireflux diet; nothing to eat for 2 hours before bedtime.
  5. Tracheobronchitis
    a. Intensive care unit patients generally stop aspirating when oral intake is stopped. Do not resume until modified barium swallow confirms swallowing without aspiration.

II. NEAR DROWNING
  A. General principles
    1. Definitions
      a. Drowning: death from suffocation by submersion in water.
      b. Near-drowning: survival, at least temporarily, after suffocation by submersion in water. Requires survival for 24 hours to be called *near-drowning*.
      c. Submersion injury: both drowning and near-drowning taken together.
    2. Statistics
      a. Sixth most common cause of accidental injury death in the United States.
      b. More than 4,400 drownings and an estimated 372,000 near-drownings in the United States annually
      c. Incidence 1.52 per 100,000
      d. Most common in children younger than 5 years, young adults 15 to 29 years, males, Native Americans, African Americans.
      e. States with the highest drowning rates are Alaska and Mississippi.
  B. Etiology
    1. Risk factors
      a. Alcohol. Is #1 risk factor. Thirty-seven to 47% associated with alcohol.
      b. Inadequate adult supervision. Pool, bath tub, large industrial buckets common sites. Fences, sign posting, educational programs, lifeguards minimize risk and improve survival.
      c. Child abuse. 29% to 38% of pediatric submersions related to abuse or neglect.
      d. Seizures. Submersion occurs more frequently in children with epilepsy, perhaps due to poor adherence to anticonvulsant regimen.

    e. Boating. Alcohol and lack of personal flotation devices contribute.

    f. Aquatic sports. Diving, surfing, and water-skiing implicated. Diving and sliding head-first produce most serious injuries. Personal watercraft contribute.

    g. Drugs. Induce sleep, disorientation, impair coordination and swimming.

C. Pathogenesis

  1. Anoxia.

    a. Drowning sequence: panic, breath holding, struggle to surface, gasping, water swallowed, regurgitation and aspiration, break point reached, breath holding overcome by hypercapnia. Involuntary breaths taken with aspiration of water.

    b. Dry near-drowning in 10% to 15% with little fluid aspirated due to laryngospasm.

  2. Hypothermia

    a. Produces both favorable and unfavorable effects.

    b. For survival after long-term submersion, the core body temperature must be reduced quickly and brain metabolic activity slowed rapidly to prevent damage.

    c. Most hypothermic effects are adverse. Causes death three ways:

      (1) vagally mediated asystolic cardiac arrest (immersion syndrome)

      (2) tendency to malignant arrhythmia (separate from immersion syndrome); cardiac arrest from ventricular fibrillation below 25°C and asystole below 18°C.

      (3) loss of consciousness and aspiration as head falls into water

D. Pulmonary effects

  1. Atelectasis due to increased surface tension

  2. Bronchoconstriction

  3. Noncardiogenic pulmonary edema/ARDS

  4. Fresh water inactivates existing surfactant and prevents production for 24 hours.

  5. Hypertonic seawater draws fluid from plasma into the alveoli, causing pulmonary edema. May also damage type II pneumocytes.

  6. Aspiration of gastric contents and particles in fresh and saltwater may lead to ARDS.

  7. Postresuscitation cardiopulmonary resuscitation (CPR) damage, barotrauma, pneumonitis, central apnea, O_2 toxicity. CNS

E. Neurologic effects. Have greatest effect on prognosis. Central nervous system injury due to anoxia.

  1. The time course of anoxia is uncertain. Duration of submersion often unclear and hypothermia may have a protective effect.

  2. Histology: edema, necrosis, mitochondrial swelling in cortex/hippocampus/cerebellum.

  3. Severe anoxic encephalopathy with persistent coma, seizures, delayed language development, spastic quadriplegia, aphasia, and cortical blindness are reported.

  4. Virtually all patients who present with fixed, dilated pupils and coma die.

F. Musculoskeletal effects. Children with anoxic encephalopathy often develop musculoskeletal problems such as contractures, hip subluxation/dislocation, and scoliosis.

G. Serum electrolytes. Minimal impact of electrolyte changes because humans rarely take in enough fluid to cause problems and easily correct small changes that do occur.

H. Hematologic effects. Patients rarely require medical intervention for anemia.

I. Renal effects

  1. Acute tubular necrosis, hemoglobinuria, and albuminuria are all reported.

  2. Diuresis was considered due to hypothermia but is seen in submersion at any temperature.

  3. Metabolic acidosis is frequently present as a result of lactate accumulation.

J. Cardiac effects

  1. Atrial fibrillation and sinus dysrhythmias are common but rarely require therapy.

  2. P–R, QRS, Q–T prolongation and J-point elevation due to hypothermia.

  3. Death due to ventricular fibrillation or asystole.

  4. Transient increase in central venous pressure and wedge pressures and decrease in cardiac output.

K. Infectious complications. Pneumonia is the predominant infection described.

L. DIAGNOSIS

  1. History

   a. Obtain age; history of cardiac, respiratory, neurologic diseases; medications; activities precipitating submersion (i.e., boating, diving, or ingestion of drugs/ alcohol); duration of submersion; temperature and type of water.

2. Physical examination

   a. Tachypnea most common. Tachycardia also common. Use hypothermia thermometer. Standard thermometer underestimates hypothermia and may cause premature stopping of cardiopulmonary resuscitation (CPR).

   b. Examination done to uncover injuries that caused or resulted from submersion.

   c. Neurologic classification

   (1) Category A: alert within 1 hour of presentation. These patients do well.

   (2) Category B: obtunded and stuporous but arousable at evaluation. Eighty-nine to 100 % of these patients survive and permanent neurologic deficits rare.

   (3) Category C: comatose/abnormal respirations/abnormal response to pain. High mortality and survivors have high rate of neurologic dysfunction.

   i. C1: decorticate posturing

   ii. C2: decerebrate posturing

   iii. C3: flaccid

3. Laboratory studies. Obtain hemoglobin, hematocrit, electrolytes, arterial blood gas analysis, blood alcohol level, PT/PTT, serum creatinine, urinalysis, drug screen, cervical spine films, chest radiograph, electrocardiogram.

M. Treatment

1. Initial resuscitation

   a. Mouth-to-mouth resuscitation begun in the water.

   b. Carefully support victim's neck to prevent exacerbation of vertebral injuries.

   c. Full CPR should begin immediately on shore.

   d. Resuscitation must be continued at least until the patient has been rewarmed.

   e. Remove wet clothing and begin external rewarming plus heated O_2 in the field.

   f. Cardiopulmonary bypass should be used in severe cases on arrival at the trauma center.

2. Therapy of underlying cause

   a. Prompt administration of necessary antidotes or other measures

   b. Anticonvulsant levels in known epileptic patients

   c. Neck immobilization until C-spine films cleared for possible head/neck trauma

   d. Correct hypoglycemia and severe electrolyte abnormalities.

3. Treatment of respiratory and other organ failure

   a. Administer oxygen for hypoxemia.

   b. Manage acute respiratory distress syndrome per conventional protocols.

   c. Optimize fluid status and renal blood flow. Severe cases may require dialysis.

   d. Correct cardiac dysrhythmias by rewarming.

4. Neurologic salvage. Maintain adequate oxygenation and cerebral blood flow.

Selected Readings

Colice G, Resolution of laryngeal injury following translaryngeal intubation. *Am Rev Respir Dis* 1992;145:361.
   Describes the effect of prolonged translaryngeal intubation in the upper airway.

Fandel I, Bancalari E. Near-drowning in children: clinical aspects. *Pediatrics* 1976;58:573.
   Review of clinical findings in pediatric victims.

Green GM. Pulmonary clearance of infectious agents. *Annu Rev Med* 1968;19:315.
   Classic article describes pulmonary defense mechanisms against infection.

Logemann JA. Swallowing physiology and pathophysiology. *Otolaryngol Clin North Am* 1988;21:613.
   A comprehensive review of the swallowing mechanisms.

Lorber B, Swenson RM. Bacteriology of aspiration pneumonia: a prospective study of community and hospital acquired cases. *Ann Intern Med* 1974;81:329.
   Epidemiologic findings useful in making treatment decisions.

Modell JH, Conn AW. Current neurological considerations in near-drowning. *Can Anaesth Soc J* 1980;3:197.
Provides commonly used classification system.

National Center for Injury Prevention and Control: *1998 United States unintentional injuries and adverse effects.* Atlanta, Centers for Disease Control and Prevention, 2000.
Provides statistics on near drowning and other injuries.

National Center for Injury Prevention and Control: *Drowning prevention.* Atlanta, Centers for Disease Control and Prevention, 2000.
Effective measures to prevent submersion injuries.

Nelson J, Lesser M. Aspiration-induced pulmonary injury. *J Intensive Care Med* 1997; 12:279.
A review of pulmonary complications of aspiration.

Schwindt WD, Barbee RA, Jones RJ. Lipoid pneumonia. *Arch Surg* 1967;95:652.
Description of the clinical findings of a common syndrome.

Torres A, Serra-Batlles J, Ros E, et al. Pulmonary aspiration of gastric contents in patients receiving mechanical ventilation: the effect of body position. *Ann Intern Med* 1992;116:540.
Elevating the head of the bed is a simple, effective, no-cost measure to prevent aspiration.

51 PULMONARY HYPERTENSION
Oren P. Schaefer

I. GENERAL PRINCIPLES
   A. Definition. A mean pulmonary artery pressure that exceeds 25 mm Hg at rest or 30 mm Hg with exercise.

II. ETIOLOGY
   A. WHO (Evian) Clinical Classification of Pulmonary Hypertension. Categories share similarities in pathophysiologic mechanisms, clinical presentation, and therapeutic options.
   1. Pulmonary arterial hypertension (PAH)
       a. Primary pulmonary hypertension (sporadic, familial)
       b. Related to: collagen vascular disease, congenital systemic-to-pulmonary shunts, portal hypertension, HIV infection, drugs/toxins
   2. Pulmonary venous hypertension
       a. Left-sided atrial or ventricular heart disease
       b. Left-sided valvular hear disease
       c. Extrinsic compression of central pulmonary veins
       d. Pulmonary venoocclusive disease (PVOD)
   3. Pulmonary hypertension associated with disorders of the respiratory system or hypoxemia (Table 51-1)
       a. Chronic obstructive pulmonary disease (COPD)
       b. Interstitial lung disease
       c. Sleep-disordered breathing
       d. Alveolar hypoventilation syndrome
       e. Chronic exposure to high altitude
       f. Neonatal lung disease
       g. Alveolar-capillary dysplasia
   4. Pulmonary hypertension caused by chronic thrombotic or embolic disease
       a. Thromboembolic obstruction of proximal pulmonary arteries
       b. Obstruction of distal pulmonary arteries: pulmonary embolism, *in situ* thrombosis, sickle cell disease
   5. Pulmonary hypertension caused by disorders directly affecting the pulmonary vasculature
       a. Inflammatory (schistosomiasis, sarcoidosis)
       b. Pulmonary capillary hemangiomatosis (PCH)

III. PATHOGENESIS
   A. Three major pathophysiologic categories of pulmonary hypertension (PH).
   1. *Passive*—results from elevated postcapillary pressure
       a. Elevated pulmonary artery balloon occlusion pressure (PAOP) pressure (reflects postpulmonary capillary pressure)
       b. The pulmonary artery end diastolic pressure (P_aED) and PAOP are both elevated; the (P_aED-PAOP) gradient is normal (≤ 5 mm Hg).
       c. Examples are: left ventricular failure, mitral stenosis, obstruction of the major pulmonary veins
   2. *Active*—results from the constriction or obstruction of capillary or precapillary vessels that increases resistance to flow
       a. The PAOP pressure is normal. The (P_aED-PAOP) gradient is elevated (>5 mm Hg).

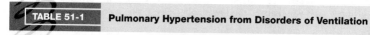

TABLE 51-1	Pulmonary Hypertension from Disorders of Ventilation

Vasoconstriction of precapillary and capillary vascular bed
Structurally normal pulmonary parenchyma and vascular bed
High-altitude pulmonary hypertension (residence at >3,000 m)
Primary central hypoventilation
Obstructive sleep apnea
Obesity-hypoventilation syndrome
Paralytic poliomyelitis
Myasthenia gravis
Pulmonary parenchymal disease
Chronic obstructive pulmonary disease
Cystic fibrosis

Anatomic restriction of the pulmonary capillary bed
Diffuse parenchymal lung disease
Sarcoidosis
Progressive systemic sclerosis
Idiopathic interstitial pulmonary fibrosis
Acute respiratory distress syndrome
Extensive lung resection
Extensive fibrothorax

Vasoconstriction plus anatomic restriction of the vascular bed
Kyphoscoliosis
Chronic fibrotic tuberculosis

    b. Vasoconstrictive stimuli: alveolar hypoxemia, acidemia, hypercarbia.
    c. Includes primary pulmonary artery hypertension.
  3. *Reactive*—PH is initially passive. Upstream pulmonary vasculature responds to chronic passive congestion with an active component superimposed on a passive component.
    a. The PAOP is elevated. The (P_aED-PAOP) gradient is elevated.
    b. Seen in: mitral valve disease (particularly mitral stenosis), pulmonary veno-occlusive disease.

IV. DIAGNOSIS
A. Signs and symptoms
  1. Exertional dyspnea, fatigue, weakness, chest pain, exertional syncope, peripheral edema, abdominal distention. In nonprimary PH symptoms relate to underlying disease.
  2. Examination findings related solely to PH: Large jugular venous A wave, left parasternal (RV) heave, pulmonic ejection click and murmur, enhanced pulmonic component of second heart sound (P_2), RV fourth heart sound, and signs of RV failure. With severe hypertension, one may also find prominent jugular venous V waves, an RV third heart sound, and murmurs of tricuspid or pulmonic regurgitation. With nonprimary PH, signs of the underlying disease are prominent.
B. Chest radiograph
  1. Useful screen for abnormalities of the pulmonary circulation.
  2. Characteristic findings: marked enlargement of the main pulmonary artery segment, dilatation of the central hilar pulmonary artery branches to the origin of the segmental vessels, and constriction of the segmental arteries.

    3. Signs of passive PH (pulmonary venous hypertension): prominence of the upper lobe vessels over the lower lobe vessels; presence of interstitial edema and of alveolar edema.

C. Electrocardiography

    1. Severe PH: right axis deviation in 79%; RV hypertrophy in 87%.

    2. ECG less predictive in COPD due to downward intrathoracic displacement of the heart.

D. Transthoracic Doppler echocardiography

    1. Assess RV and LV function; exclude congenital heart disease, mitral valve disease, and left atrial myxoma. To follow changes after introduction of therapy.

    2. Doppler examination of the regurgitant tricuspid jet allows for estimate of PA systolic pressure (sensitivity 0.79 to 1.00, specificity 0.60 to 0.98).

    3. Consider transesophageal echocardiography in patients with COPD (hyperinflation makes transthoracic echocardiography technically difficult).

E. Pulmonary function tests

    1. To exclude or characterize the contribution of underlying airway or parenchymal disease.

    2. In interstitial fibrosis, vital capacity (VC) less than 50% predicted consider PH at rest; VC between 50% and 80% consider PH with exertion.

    3. In obstructive airway disease, FEV_1 less than 1 L, P_aO_2 less than 50 mm Hg, or P_aCO_2 greater than 45 mm Hg consider PH.

F. Right heart catheterization

    1. Documents elevated PA pressure.

    2. Can classify as active, passive, or reactive based on the (P_aED-PAOP) gradient, or calculation of pulmonary vascular resistance.

G. Other studies

    1. Left heart catheterization: When the origin of PH is not clear; congenital heart disease; acquired obstruction of the main pulmonary veins considered.

    2. Ventilation-perfusion lung scan: With chronic thromboembolic PH, perfusion scans are often high probability; in PAH, previously referred to as primary pulmonary hypertension, normal or low probability.

    3. Pulmonary angiography.

H. Treatment. Treatment rests on proper identification of the underlying condition.

    1. Specific treatment is based on underlying disease.

        a. Pulmonary embolism: anticoagulation, thrombolytics, pulmonary endarterectomy.

        b. Congestive heart failure: diuretics, afterload reduction.

        c. Ventilatory disorders (e.g., COPD): treat with specific intervention.

        d. Alveolar hypoxemia (of any source): supplemental oxygen to achieve SaO_2 greater than 90%.

        e. Obstructive sleep apnea: nasal CPAP; weight loss.

    2. Pulmonary vasoresponsiveness is present in 25% to 30% with PAH (WHO/Evian).

        a. Use short-acting pulmonary vasodilator: prostacyclin, adenosine, nitric oxide.

        b. Requires monitoring with pulmonary artery catheter.

        c. Vasoresponsiveness defined as a 20% decline in pulmonary vascular resistance with an increase in cardiac output, but without any effect on gas exchange or systemic pressure.

    3. Pharmacologic therapy

        a. Calcium channel blockers: diltiazem, nifedipine; use only in those with acute reactivity.

        b. Prostenoids: epoprostenol, treprostinil, inhaled iloprost.

            (1) Continuous intravenous epoprostenol (and calcium channel antagonists) improves symptoms, hemodynamics, and survival.

            (2) Epoprostenol appears to benefit those without vasoresponsiveness as well (vascular wall remodeling and platelet inhibitory effects).

            (3) Common side effects: flushing, headache, jaw pain, diarrhea, nausea, rash, and aches.

    (4) Complications: line-related infection, catheter-associated venous thrombosis, thrombocytopenia.

    (5) Pulmonary edema has resulted when prostanoids given to those with PVOD and PCH.

  c. Endothelin receptor antagonist: Bosentan.

  d. Oxygen to keep SaO_2 greater than 90%.

  e. Warfarin appears to improve survival.

  f. Lung transplantation. Indications: NYHA functional class III/IV despite medical therapy; cardiac index less than 2 L/min/m^2; right atrial pressure greater than 15 mm Hg; mean PAP greater than 55 mm Hg.

  g. Prognosis is variable for patients with pulmonary artery hypertension.

    (1) Mean survival is 3 years from diagnosis. With severe pulmonary hypertension or right heart failure, death usually within 1 year.

    (2) Prognosis clearly improved with NYHA class I or II versus NYHA class III or IV.

    (3) Patients are at risk for progressive right heart failure and sudden cardiac death.

Selected Readings

Barst AJ, Rubin LJ, Long WA, et al. A comparison of continuous intravenous epoprostenol (prostacyclin) with conventional therapy for primary pulmonary hypertension. *N Engl J Med* 1996;334:296.
A randomized trial found therapy with prostacyclin to confer improvements in symptoms, hemodynamics, and survival.

D'Alonzo GE, Bower JS, Dantzker DR. Differentiation in patients with primary and thromboembolic pulmonary hypertension. *Chest* 1984;85:457.
One cannot distinguish the two entities by clinical characteristics. Lung scans in patients with thromboembolic PH were found to be high probability; those with PAH (primary) were normal to low probability.

Dartevelle P, Fadel E, Mussot S, et al. Chronic thromboembolic pulmonary hypertension. *Eur Respir J* 2004;23:637–648.
The diagnosis of chronic thromboembolic pulmonary hypertension (CTEPH) can be difficult; clinically evident acute pulmonary embolism episodes are absent in greater than 50%. CTEPH can be cured surgically. This article reviews this important cause of pulmonary hypertension.

Galie N, Ussia G, Passarelli P, et al. Role of pharmacologic tests in the treatment of primary pulmonary hypertension. *Am J Cardiol* 1995;75:55A.
The article outlines pharmacologic vasodilator testing in the evaluation of primary PAH.

Nazzareno G, Rubin LJ. Pulmonary arterial hypertension. *J Am Coll Cardiol* 2004; 43 (12 suppl 1):S1–S90.
A complete, up-to-date supplement devoted entirely to pulmonary hypertension.

Masuyama T, Kodama K, Kitabatake A, et al. Continuous-wave Doppler echocardiographic detection of pulmonary regurgitation and its application to noninvasive estimation of pulmonary artery pressure. *Circulation* 1986;74:484.
Estimates of pulmonary artery pressure by measuring regurgitant flow velocity in patients with PH. Results correlate with those from right heart catheterization.

McLaughlin VV, Genthner DE, Panella MM, et al. Reduction in pulmonary vascular resistance with long-term epoprostenol (prostacyclin) therapy in primary pulmonary hypertension. *N Engl J Med* 1998;338:273.
Long-term therapy with epoprostenol was found to lower pulmonary vascular resistance beyond that achieved in the short term with intravenous adenosine and had sustained efficacy in the patients who were followed.

Pass SE, Dusing ML. Current and emerging therapy for primary pulmonary hypertension. *Ann Pharmacother* 2002;36:1414–1423.
Reviews epidemiology, pathophysiology, clinical symptoms, and diagnosis of primary pulmonary hypertension. Discusses available current and emerging therapies used to treat this disorder.

Rich S, McLaughlin VV. Lung transplantation for pulmonary hypertension: patient selection and maintenance therapy while awaiting transplantation. *Semin Thorac Cardiovasc Surg* 1998;10:135.
Lung transplantation is considered a definitive treatment of patients with advanced pulmonary vascular disease and PH. With advances in medical management, the guidelines for patient selection for lung transplantation are constantly evolving and are reviewed here.

Runo JR, Loyd JE. Primary pulmonary hypertension. *Lancet* 2003;361:1533–1544.
A timely review with a nice discussion on etiology and pathogenesis.

PLEURAL DISEASE IN THE CRITICALLY ILL PATIENT

Mark M. Wilson

52

I. PLEURAL EFFUSIONS

A. General principles
1. Pleural disease itself is an unusual cause for admission to the intensive care unit (ICU).
2. Exceptions are a large hemothorax for monitoring the rate of bleeding and hemodynamic status, a secondary spontaneous pneumothorax (PTX), and a large unilateral or bilateral pleural effusion causing acute respiratory failure.
3. Pleural disease may be overlooked in the critically ill patient; it is often a subtle finding on clinical examination and chest radiography (CXR).

B. Etiology
1. Pleural effusions are most commonly caused by primary lung disease but may also result from systemic illnesses.
2. Atelectasis is a common cause of small pleural effusions in the ICU.
3. Congestive heart failure (CHF) is the most common cause of all pleural effusions. Most patients have the classic signs and symptoms of cardiomegaly and bilateral small to moderate effusions of similar size on CXR.
4. Hepatic hydrothorax occurs in 6% of patients with liver cirrhosis and clinical ascites.
5. Parapneumonic effusions due to community-acquired and nosocomial pneumonia are common in critically ill patients.
6. If the CXR demonstrates loculation of fluid and pus is aspirated at thoracentesis, then the diagnosis of empyema is established and immediate drainage is needed.
7. Pleural effusions are seen in 3% to 17% of patients with pancreatitis.
8. Pleural effusions occur in 41% to 50% of patients with pulmonary embolism.

C. Pathophysiology
1. Atelectasis causes pleural fluid by decreasing local pleural pressure, thus favoring movement of fluid from the parietal pleural surface into the pleural space. Analysis of the pleural fluid reveals a serous transudate that dissipates once atelectasis resolves.
2. Hepatic hydrothorax results from movement of ascitic fluid through congenital or acquired diaphragmatic defects.
3. Pleural effusions from pancreatitis result from direct contact of the diaphragm with pancreatic enzymes (so-called sympathetic effusion), transfer of ascitic fluid through diaphragmatic defects, a fistulous tract between a pseudocyst and the pleural space, or retroperitoneal movement of fluid into the mediastinum and rupture into the pleural space.
4. Effusions from pulmonary emboli result from increased capillary permeability, imbalance in microvascular and pleural hydrostatic pressures, and pleuropulmonary hemorrhage.
5. Hemothoraces (fluid with a pleural fluid-to-blood hematocrit ratio greater than 50%) result from penetrating or blunt chest trauma; as complications of invasive procedures; with pulmonary infarction, malignancy, or ruptured aortic aneurysm; or as a complication of anticoagulation.

D. Diagnosis
1. Pleural effusions appear on CXR as increased homogeneous densities over the lower lung fields compared with the upper lung fields.

2. Underlying diffuse parenchymal lung disease is common in patients in the ICU and makes the CXR diagnosis of pleural effusion problematic.

3. With hepatic hydrothorax, the CXR usually reveals a normal cardiac silhouette and a right-sided pleural effusion in 70% of patients. The diagnosis is confirmed by demonstrating that pleural and ascitic fluids have similar protein and lactate dehydrogenase concentrations.

4. The CXR in parapneumonic effusions commonly shows a small to large pleural effusion ipsilateral to a new alveolar infiltrate.

5. Effusions from pancreatitis are usually small and left sided (60%) but may be isolated to the right (30%) or bilateral (10%). The fluid is an exudate with glucose values approaching those of the serum and amylase values greater than those of serum.

6. Pulmonary emboli usually produce exudative effusions; however, 20% have transudates as a result of associated atelectasis. Pleural fluid analysis is highly variable and nondiagnostic.

7. A potential life-threatening event, esophageal rupture, requires immediate diagnosis and therapy. The history is usually of severe retching or vomiting or instrumentation of the esophagus. Pleural effusion occurs in 75% and is secondary to mediastinitis. A presumptive diagnosis should be confirmed immediately with lateral decubitus esophagrams. Amylase of salivary origin appears in pleural fluid in high concentration. With seeding of anaerobic organisms from the mouth, the pH falls rapidly and progressively to approach 6.00.

E. Treatment

1. Thoracentesis should be performed if the diagnosis is in question or if the patient's course is other than expected (patient is febrile or has pleuritic pain, unilateral or disparate sized effusions, absence of cardiomegaly, or a partial pressure of arterial oxygen inappropriate for the degree of pulmonary edema).

2. Therapy for effusions due to CHF involves decreasing venous hypertension and improving cardiac output with preload and afterload reduction.

3. Treatment of hepatic hydrothorax is directed at resolution of the ascites with sodium restriction and diuresis. Chemical pleurodesis is uniformly unsuccessful.

4. When the effusion is free-flowing on lateral decubitus CXR and thoracentesis shows a nonpurulent, polymorphonuclear neutrophil–predominant exudate, the patient has a high likelihood of resolution without sequelae over 7 to 14 days using antibiotics alone.

5. Draining the pleural space should be considered in the case of fluid with a positive Gram stain or culture, or when the fluid pH is less than 7.20 (complicated effusion), given the associated increase in morbidity and mortality.

6. No specific therapy is usually necessary for effusions due to pancreatitis; the effusion resolves as the pancreatic inflammation subsides.

7. When sampling of fluid is indicated clinically and the effusion is small, thoracentesis should be performed under ultrasound guidance.

8. Therapeutic thoracenteses are primarily indicated for the relief of dyspnea.

9. The diagnosis of spontaneous esophageal rupture dictates immediate intervention; survival is greater than 90% if primary closure occurs within the first 24 hours.

10. Traumatic hemothorax should be treated with immediate tube thoracostomy.

F. Complications

1. No absolute contraindications exist to thoracentesis; the major relative contraindications are an uncorrectable bleeding diathesis, prior pneumonectomy procedure is formed under ultrasound guidance, and an uncooperative patient.

2. PTX is no more likely to occur in the patient receiving mechanical ventilation than in the patient who is not; however, if a PTX does develop, the patient receiving mechanical ventilation will likely develop a tension PTX (see below).

3. Complications of therapeutic thoracentesis are similar to those for diagnostic thoracentesis, except there appears to be an increased risk of PTX, and three

complications unique to therapeutic thoracentesis may be seen—hypoxemia, unilateral pulmonary edema, and hypovolemia. The reader is referred to Chapter 10 on thoracentesis for further reading.

II. PNEUMOTHORAX

A. General principles. PTX refers to the presence of free air in the confines of the chest cavity (pleural space).

B. Etiology

1. Spontaneous PTX occurs without an obvious cause, either without findings of lung disease (primary spontaneous PTX) or with clinically manifest lung disease (secondary spontaneous PTX) such as chronic obstructive pulmonary disease, status asthmaticus, interstitial lung disease, *Pneumocystis carinii* or necrotizing pneumonias, or cystic fibrosis.

2. Traumatic PTX results from penetrating or blunt chest trauma.

3. Iatrogenic PTX, the most common cause of PTX in the ICU, is a consequence of barotrauma associated with mechanical ventilation or invasive procedures (thoracentesis, central venous catheters).

4. PTX occurs in 1% to 15% of all patients receiving mechanical ventilation.

C. Pathophysiology

1. If the pressure gradient between the airways and pleural space is transiently increased, alveolar rupture may occur; air enters the interstitial tissues of the lung and may then enter the pleural space or decompress to the mediastinum.

2. When PTX occurs, the elasticity of the lung causes it to collapse until the pleural defect seals or the pleural and alveolar pressures equalize.

3. Progressive accumulation of air (and positive pressure) within the pleural space produces a tension PTX. Tension PTX compresses mediastinal structures, impairing venous return to the heart, decreasing cardiac output, and potential fatal cardiovascular collapse. In the setting of mechanical ventilation, 30% to 97% of patients with PTX develop tension.

D. Diagnosis

1. Most iatrogenic PTXs occur at the time of the procedure from direct lung puncture, but delayed (up to 12 to 24 hours later) PTXs have been noted.

2. In the supine patient, PTX gas accumulates in a subpulmonic location and outlines the anterior pleural reflection, the costophrenic sulcus (deep sulcus sign), and the anterolateral border of the mediastinum. The base, lateral chest wall, and juxtacardiac areas should be carefully visualized for evidence of PTX. Up to 30% of PTXs may not be detected initially.

3. PTX in the mechanically ventilated patient usually presents as an acute cardiopulmonary emergency with a mortality rate of 7% if it is rapidly diagnosed clinically, versus a mortality rate of 31% to 77% for delayed diagnoses.

4. The most common CXR signs of a PTX under tension are contralateral mediastinal shift, ipsilateral diaphragmatic depression, and ipsilateral chest wall expansion.

E. Treatment

1. Up to half of spontaneously breathing patients with needle-puncture (iatrogenic) PTX may be managed expectantly without the need for tube drainage.

2. If the patient is receiving mechanical ventilation or if the PTX is large or has caused significant symptoms or gas exchange abnormalities, then tube thoracostomy should be performed as soon as possible. Treatment should not be delayed to obtain CXR confirmation. If a chest tube is not immediately available, placement of a large-bore needle into the anterior second intercostal space on the suspected side will be lifesaving.

Selected Readings

Bartter T, Mayo PD, Pratter MR, et al. Lower risk and higher yield for thoracentesis when performed by experienced operators. *Chest* 1993;103:1873.
   A prospective study of 50 thoracenteses showing the dramatic effect of the level of training in reducing the risk of complications from this procedure.

Collins TR, Sahn SA. Thoracentesis: clinical value, complications, technical problems, and patient experience. *Chest* 1987;91:817.
A prospective study of 129 thoracenteses that highlights the clinical value and limitations of diagnostic thoracentesis.

Rohlfing BM, Webb WR, Schlobohm RM. Ventilator-related extraalveolar air in adults. *Radiology* 1976;121:25.
A descriptive study of the manifestations of extraalveolar air resulting from mechanical ventilation in 38 patients.

Sahn SA. Management of complicated parapneumonic effusions. *Am Rev Respir Dis* 1993;148:813.
A review of the management of complicated parapneumonic effusions that stresses the importance of early diagnosis and treatment to prevent development of this complication.

MECHANICAL VENTILATION: INITIATION
Deborah H. Markowitz and Richard S. Irwin

53

I. GENERAL PRINCIPLES. Mechanisms for respiratory failure and need for mechanical ventilation (MV) include intrinsic lung disease, manifested by hypoxemia and/or pump failure manifested by hypercapnia and hypoxemia. Causes of the latter include central nervous system depression, respiratory muscle fatigue reversible by rest, muscle weakness not reversed by rest, chest wall mechanical defects, and mediators of ongoing disease such as sepsis that affect respiratory muscles. Positive pressure MV is currently the predominant means of providing ventilatory support, as opposed to negative pressure ventilation. MV may be invasive, delivered through an endotracheal tube (ETT) or tracheostomy tube. Noninvasive positive pressure ventilation (NIPPV) interfaces the ventilator with the patient through a full-face or nasal mask.

A. Modes of invasive MV refers to how the ventilator interacts with the patient.

    1. Volume cycled MV delivers a guaranteed preset volume (Vt) with each breath that is specified by the operator. Peak inspiratory pressures (PIP) generated by the ventilator are variable with each breath, depending on the patient's compliance. A "pop-off" pressure can be assigned to prevent excessive peak pressures, which aborts the breath when that pressure limit is reached. All the volume cycled modes can achieve high PIPs if the volume is excessive and/or lung compliance is low. The time that it takes to deliver the Vt (inspiratory time, or Ti) is also controlled by the operator because it is dependent on the volume, inspiratory flow rate ($\dot{V}i$), and wave form characteristics (square or decelerating wave forms), which are all specified by the operator.

        a. Intermittent mandatory ventilation (IMV): At a particular time interval, the machine will deliver the preset volume. None of the breaths are assisted. Spontaneous breaths can be taken by the patient between the mandatory breaths. The time interval between breaths determines the machine-delivered respiratory rate (RR) (e.g., if every 5 seconds a mandatory breath is delivered, the baseline RR is 12 breaths per minute).

            (1) Advantages: assures a minute ventilation ($\dot{V}_E$); can control Ti to maximize passive exhalation in obstructive lung disease states

            (2) Disadvantages: patient asynchrony occurs if different RR or $\dot{V}i$ is desired by the patient.

        b. Assist control (AC): If the patient's intrinsic respiratory rate exceeds the basal rate set by the operator, then all the breaths are assisted. The patient merely initiates a breath and a full inspiratory flow and Vt are delivered with each breath. However, if the patient's intrinsic rate falls below the preset basal rate, then all the breaths delivered are control breaths, spaced at regular time intervals. AC is also a time-triggered mode that delivers a preset volume if the patient does not initiate any spontaneous breaths. During the control and assisted breaths, the Vt and inspiratory flow and characteristics are exactly the same with each breath.

            (1) Advantages: ensures a minimum $\dot{V}_E$; better patient synchrony if higher $\dot{V}_E$ is desired. Can still control Ti to allow for maximum passive exhalation.

            (2) Disadvantages: can potentially induce respiratory alkalosis if high respiratory drive (i.e., liver failure). Patient asynchrony and respiratory muscle fatigue can occur if a different $\dot{V}i$ is required by the patient. I:E ratio can vary because the variable RR can alter the expiratory phase.

        c. Synchronized intermittent mandatory ventilation (SIMV): SIMV is a hybrid between IMV and AC. Three kinds of breaths may be delivered:

spontaneous, assisted, and mandatory breath. If no breaths are initiated within a period of time, a mandatory breath will be delivered. If the machine senses that the patient has taken a spontaneous breath just before the mandatory breath, the machine will recycle and then wait for the next spontaneous breath and assist it.

  i. Advantages: ensures a minimum $\dot{V}_E$

  ii. Disadvantages: It has been shown to be the least beneficial weaning mode. Cannot fully control the I:E ratio given the variability in RR and presence of spontaneous breaths.

2. Pressure-limited MV delivers a flow until a preset pressure limit that is set by the operator is reached. PIP is therefore always the same and is the sum of the preset pressure limit for each breath and the PEEP value (PIP = pressure limit + PEEP). Vt is variable with each breath, according to the patient's compliance.

  a. Pressure support (PS): Every breath is an assisted breath. Each breath is triggered by the patient's respiratory effort. The patient determines the inspiratory flow rate and shape of the wave form as well as the RR. When a preset pressure limit is reached, inspiratory flow slows to less than 0.5 L/min and the machine cycles off.

   (1) Advantages: Better patient synchrony, patient determines $\dot{V}i$ characteristics. Limits PIP. Compliance is easily calculated because PIP closely approximates plateau pressure (Pplt) or end inspiratory hold pressure.

   (2) Disadvantages: If the patient stops breathing then an apnea backup breath is given that is infrequent and less responsive than the backup from AC. Inadequate volumes could be delivered if the ETT is blocked or decreased lung compliance causes present pressure limit to stop inspiratory flow before an adequate Vt is delivered (e.g., pneumothorax).

  b. Pressure control (PC): PC is similar to IMV in that control breaths are delivered at a preset time interval, but with a preset pressure limit rather than a preset volume. Respiratory rate and time to maximal pressure limit are both controlled, and spontaneous breaths can be interspersed between the mandatory breaths.

   (1) Advantages: Can limit PIP and plateau pressure (Pplat) to prevent ventilator-associated lung injury. Can control or extend Ti for inverse ratio ventilation to increase mean airway pressure (MAP) and augment oxygenation. Therefore, given these two advantages, this mode is often used for advanced acute lung injury.

   (2) Disadvantages: Cannot ensure minimal $\dot{V}_E$ with airway obstruction or poor compliance, as in PS mode, because delivered volumes may be low if compliance is high. For normal I:E ratios, PC mode is a standard controlled mode and does not need additional sedation. For inverse ratio ventilation (I:E 4:1), sedation with or without paralysis is necessary because of patient discomfort. Circuit leaks can extend inspiratory time. Exaggeration of inspiratory time can limit time for passive exhalation and induce autoPEEP.

3. Continuous positive airway pressure (CPAP) occurs when the inspiratory and expiratory limbs are pressurized to a preset end expiratory pressure. CPAP functions primarily as an oxygenation and weaning modality.

  a. No inspiratory flow is delivered, so it is not a true positive-pressure MV mode. The patient assumes most of the work of breathing by generating his or her own RR, $\dot{V}i$, Vt, and thus $\dot{V}_E$, closely simulating spontaneous breathing.

  b. Work of breathing (WOB) is reduced compared to complete discontinuation from the MV circuit and delivery of only FiO_2 ("T-piece"). Application of PEEP stents the airways open and allows for better exhaled Vt. CPAP can be used in coordination with flow-by. Flow-by occurs when a stream of gas is delivered across the ventilator circuit, assisting the patient in drawing his or her own Vi and Vt.

   (1) Expiratory positive airway pressure (EPAP): Only the expiratory phase is pressurized. Compared to CPAP, EPAP has a lower mean airway pressure (MAP) and higher WOB.

(2) For those dependent on MV for only oxygenation and not ventilation, CPAP can improve oxygenation without subjecting the patient to the harmful effects of MV.

B. Ventilator settings for invasive positive pressure MV

1. **Fraction of inspired oxygen (FiO_2):** Supplemental oxygen is adjusted to target an oxygen saturation (SaO_2) greater than 90% and/or PaO_2 greater than 60 mm Hg. O_2 should not be withheld for any concern of CO_2 narcosis on MV. O_2 should not be withheld for concern of toxicity, if required. It is believed that clinically significant O_2 toxicity is unlikely to occur with FiO_2 less than 0.6 even with prolonged delivery. Balance between side effects of PEEP, used to lower FiO_2, and O_2 toxicity concern.

2. **Tidal volume (Vt)** is constant in volume-cycled modes and varies with each breath in pressure-limited modes. In patients without lung disease Vt of 8 to 10 mL/kg are used. For obese patients adjustment of the Vt to a value midway between their actual and ideal body weight is reasonable. Lower tidal volumes are recommended for acute lung injury (ALI) of 6 mL/kg. In ARDS, volumes of 6 mL/kg are associated with a lower mortality than 12 mL/kg and targeting a Pplat equal to or less than 30 cm H_2O protects against further lung injury from overdistention and inducing MV related volu-trauma. Vt equal to or less than 8 mL/kg is recommended in patients with obstructive lung disease (asthma, COPD). Limiting Vt decreases expiratory time (Te) and minimizes autoPEEP, where the subsequent breath is started before complete exhalation has occurred.

3. **Inflation pressure limit:** High inflation pressures cause barotrauma. Increased Pplat (end inspiratory hold pressure), rather than PIP, is most injurious, reflecting alveolar overdistention and not airway resistance. No threshold is safe but Pplat equal to or less than 30 cm H_2O is recommended. Permissive hypercapnia by decreasing Vt, RR, or $\dot{V}_E$ allows the operator to achieve a lower Pplat. Use of sedation with or without paralytics can decrease dynamic hyperinflation and allow for lower Pplat. MV pop-off pressure should be set just above the PIP, usually less than 50 cm H_2O.

4. **Sighing:** Periodic increased "sigh" or "yawn" is not currently recommended for routine MV.

5. **Respiratory rate (RR):** RR and Vt determine $\dot{V}_E$. For IMV and PC modes, RR is preset and rates of 12 to 20 beats per minute are reasonable. The AC rate is set below the patient's spontaneous RR to minimize the chance of controlling ventilation with its attendant risk of respiratory muscle atrophy. RR and/or Vt should be adjusted down for autoPEEP.

6. **Sensitivity** relates to the amount of pressure drop in airway pressure that is required before the ventilator senses the patient's effort and assists them during AC and PS. Sensitivities of approximately 0.5 to 1 cm H_2O allow very weak patients to initiate a breath. Higher values make triggering more difficult and are used in conditions with a high respiratory drive (e.g., liver failure) to prevent respiratory alkalosis. The sensitivity is usually set by the respiratory therapist. But one needs to consider whether both the sensitivity value is too high and autoPEEP is present if the patient is making an effort to breathe and the machine is not triggering in assisted modes.

7. **Minute ventilation ($\dot{V}_E$):** $\dot{V}_E$ is not normally specified by operators but is the product of the Vt and RR. Normal individuals maintain normocapnia with a resting $\dot{V}_E$ of approximately 5 L/min. Adjustment of $\dot{V}_E$ is based on $PaCO_2$ as a marker of ventilatory requirements. "Permissive hypercapnia" is employed in ARDS and status asthmaticus to minimize the risk of barotrauma. Do not overventilate patients with chronic CO_2 retention because it can lead to posthypercapnic metabolic alkalosis with its attendant complications. On the other hand, high ventilatory requirements are present in hypermetabolic states (sepsis), or high caloric intake where excess CO_2 production needs to be eliminated. High dead space increases ventilatory requirements for the same CO_2 target.

8. **Inspiratory flow rate ($\dot{V}i$):** Inspiratory flow is usually specified rather than I: E ratio (except in PC mode). The ratio of Vt (liters) to $\dot{V}i$ (L/min) determines

Ti (min). Because RR determines total respiratory cycle time and exhalation is passive, I:E ratio is determined by the above three fixed parameters.

   a. For volume-cycled modes, Ti will be longer and PIP lower for a decelerating wave form and mimics PS mode. Higher $\dot{V}i$ decreases Ti to allow for greater time for passive exhalation and reduce autoPEEP in obstructive lung diseases. Higher $\dot{V}i$ increases PIP but should not affect Pplat. However, there is a theoretical concern that too-rapid lung inflation can cause "deformation injury."

   b. In PS mode, patients determine their own $\dot{V}i$. $\dot{V}i$ is specified for PC ventilation in that one can determine how quickly to achieve the pressure limit.

   c. In asthma and COPD, the expiratory time needs to be lengthened to allow for adequate exhalation of trapped gas. Thus, the I:E ratio needs to be as low as possible, achieved by a short inspiratory time of lower Vt or higher inspiratory flow rates.

 9. Inspiratory hold and inverse ratio ventilation (IRV): No flows are delivered, but passive exhalation is prevented. Ti is regulated in PC mode to precisely control I:E ratio, tantamount to an "inspiratory hold." It is used to recruit collapsed lung units in acute lung injury (ALI) and increase PaO_2, as an alternative to increasing PEEP, which increases Pplat and risks barotrauma. IRV occurs when Ti is greater than Te and is used in severe ARDS to treat hypoxemia.

10. Mean airway pressure (MAP): MAP is the airway pressure averaged over the entire respiratory cycle time, inspiration and exhalation. Attention to MAP is important in ALI in treating hypoxemia, because more time in inspiration, keeping the lung inflated with an inspiratory hold, increases the oxygen driving pressure. An inspiratory hold or IRV, increasing Vt and RR, increases the time spent in inhalation and thus the amount of time in positive pressure. Increasing PEEP and thus exhalation phase pressure increases MAP.

11. Positive end-expiratory pressure (PEEP): PEEP is the maintenance of positive pressure after expiratory flow is completed until the next inspiratory flow is initiated.

   a. Applied PEEP distends airways down to the alveoli to allow for more complete exhalation and CO_2 removal by reducing airtrapping. PEEP improves $\dot{V}/\dot{Q}$ matching, by stenting open alveoli with patent capillaries. It helps distribute alveolar debris and decreases O_2 diffusion distance but does not necessarily drive fluid out of the lung.

   b. Intrinsic PEEP (PEEPi) or autoPEEP is the positive pressure that occurs from incomplete exhalation prior to the initiation of the next breath. Dynamic hyperinflation causes a pressure gradient and a persistent flow. PEEPi is detected on the flow versus time curve when expiratory flow does not return to baseline before the next inhalation. Also, if the end-expiratory occlusion pressure is greater than applied PEEP, then PEEPi is present.

   c. Applied PEEP usually ranges between 0 and 20 cm H_2O and is usually adjusted up or down in 2.5- to 5-cm H_2O increments.

   d. In obstructive diseases, applied PEEP can mitigate the effects of PEEPi in spontaneously breathing patients.

   e. Complications of excessive applied or intrinsic PEEP include overdistention, barotrauma, hypotension from limiting venous return, and decrease in left ventricular diastolic compliance due to lung hyperinflation compressing the lateral cardiac wall.

   f. When applied prospectively, a low PEEP strategy yielded the same outcomes as the high PEEP strategy. Thus, the lowest possible PEEP that promotes adequate oxygenation, in conjunction with other ventilatory strategies, is recommended.

12. Recruitment maneuvers occur when an expiratory hold is applied with high PEEP levels for an extended time to increase PaO_2 by opening collapsed lung units. Levels of 35 to 40 cm H_2O PEEP are held for up to 90 seconds. PEEP equal to or greater than 15 cm H_2O is used after the recruitment maneuver to prevent derecruitment. However, there is no consensus as to the optimal PEEP level, the duration of expiratory hold, or the frequency of repeating the maneuver. There are also no data that show that recruitment maneuvers affect outcomes in ARDS.

C. Noninvasive positive-pressure ventilation (NIPPV) refers to the delivery of ventilatory support without placement of an ETT. Many patient interfaces are available, including mouth pieces and face masks.

1. **Ventilator interfaces:** Oral mouthpieces are subject to excessive air leakage. Masks are more secure and tighter fitting. Nasal masks and pillows are comfortable, allow for talking and even swallowing, but have greater air leaks for that reason. Oronasal or full-face masks are most common in critical care settings to minimize air leaks and ensure quick control over ventilation, but oronasal masks prevent oral secretion evacuation, risk aspiration should emesis occur, risk asphyxiation should the ventilator circuit be interrupted, and cause more nasal bridge skin breakdown.

2. **Ventilators:** Almost any critical care ventilator can be used with the NIPPV interfaces and is sometimes preferable given the higher flow rates that can be delivered and the ability to monitor respiratory rate, Vt and $\dot{V}_E$. However, ICU ventilators may alarm excessively, thus interrupting effective ventilation. More portable ventilators that are primarily available for home usage can be used.

3. **Modes of NIPPV:** Any mode of ventilation can be, including volume-cycled ventilation. Pressure-limited modes are more common with bilevel ventilation. B*i*PAP is the trade name of a ventilator that delivers bilevel positive-pressure ventilation by providing an inspiratory positive airway pressure (IPAP) and expiratory positive airway pressure (EPAP). This is synonymous with PS mode and allows for patient triggering and patient control of $\dot{V}i$ and pattern. The only difference is that of nomenclature. For PS 15 and PEEP 5, the PIP is 20. In BIPAP, for IPAP 15 and EPAP of 5, the PIP is 15, where the pressure gradient for inspiration is the IPAP-EPAP. EPAP should not be confused with CPAP where the inspiratory limb is pressurized to the expiratory limb pressure (IPAP = EPAP). Only when IPAP is greater than EPAP is there a pressure difference during inspiration and thus ventilatory assist. CPAP alone provides airway patency only.

4. **Patient selection:** Patients obviously need to be in respiratory failure and require ventilatory assistance. Ideal candidates for NIPPV are those who are more awake and can protect their airway from aspiration and clear airway secretions by coughing. Less agitated patients are ideal and can tolerate the mask interface without claustrophobia.

5. **Disease states:** The most common uses of NIPPV include COPD exacerbations, cardiogenic pulmonary edema, hypoxic respiratory failure, use in the emergency department for marginal patients to avoid intubation, and for those patients in respiratory distress not desiring intubation for end-of-life considerations. NIPPV can be used as a bridge to hopefully avoid reintubation in a patient who had been extubated. Any condition with copious secretions, such as pneumonia, that requires suctioning is not appropriately treated with NIPPV.

Selected Readings

Brochard L, Mancebo J, Wysocki M, et al. Noninvasive ventilation for acute exacerbations of chronic obstructive pulmonary disease. *N Engl J Med* 1995;333:817.
In-depth discussion of the role of noninvasive mechanical ventilation.

Brochard L. Inspiratory pressure support. *Eur J Anaesth* 1994;11:29.
Good overview of pressure-support ventilation.

Brower RG, Lanken PN, MacIntyre N, et al. Higher versus lower positive end-expiratory pressures in patients with the acute respiratory distress syndrome. *N Engl J Med* 2004;351:327.
Prospective multicenter study indicating that higher levels of PEEP do not lead to better outcomes.

Froese AB, Bryan AC. High frequency ventilation. *Am Rev Respir Dis* 1987;135:1363.
Concise overview of high-frequency ventilation.

Haake R, Schlichtig R, Ulstad DR. Barotrauma pathophysiology, risk factors, and prevention. *Chest* 1987;91:608.
A review of the pathophysiology, risk factors, clinical presentation, and strategies to manage barotrauma.

Hehta S, Hill N. State of the art: noninvasive ventilation. *Am J Respir Crit Care Med* 2001; 163:540–577.
A review of applications and indications for noninvasive ventilation.

Hill NC, ed. *Noninvasive positive pressure ventilation: principles and applications.* Armonk, NY: Futura Publishing Company, 2001.
Applications and indications for noninvasive ventilation.

Marcy TW. Barotrauma: detection, recognition, and management. *Chest* 1993;104:578.
A concise discussion of barotrauma—clinical manifestations and ventilatory strategies.

Marini JJ, Rodriguez RM, Lamb V. The inspiratory work-load of patient-initiated mechanical ventilation. *Am Rev Respir Dis* 1986;134:902.
A look at the patient's component of mechanical workload during MV.

Marini JJ. Evolving concepts in the ventilatory management of acute respiratory distress syndrome. *Clin Chest Med* 1996;17:555.
Offers an update on approaches to management of acute respiratory distress syndrome.

Pepe PE, Marini JJ. Occult positive end-expiratory pressure in mechanically ventilated patients with airflow obstruction. *Am Rev Respir Dis* 1982;126:166.
A discussion of the hemodynamic consequences of $PEEP_i$.

Ranieri VM, Eissa NT, Corbeil C, et al. Effects of positive end-expiratory pressure on alveolar recruitment and gas exchange in patients with the adult respiratory distress syndrome. *Am Rev Respir Dis* 1991;144:544.
Physiologic discussion of PEEP in ARDS.

Slutsky AS. Mechanical ventilation. *Chest* 1993;104:1833.
An excellent review of MV.

MECHANICAL VENTILATION: DISCONTINUATION

54

Deborah H. Markowitz and Richard S. Irwin

I. GENERAL PRINCIPLES

A. Outcome for patients with respiratory failure:
1. Mechanical ventilation (MV) can be discontinued in 80% to 90% of patients within 3 weeks. Of this group 77% can be extubated within 72 hours of the start of MV.
2. Ten to 20% require prolonged MV greater than 21 days. Weaning from MV in this group may take more than 3 months. One-year survival ranges widely between 12% to 93%. Survivor quality of life may be minimally impaired when assessed 2 years later.

B. There are four potentially reversible reasons for prolonged MV.
   a. Inadequate respiratory drive
   b. Inability of the lungs to carry out gas exchange without MV
   c. Inspiratory respiratory muscle fatigue from a variety of causes such as neuromuscular diseases, sepsis, nutritional and metabolic deficiencies, corticosteroids, chronic renal failure. Persistent increased work of breathing (WOB) can be from intrinsic disease or ventilator loads or cardiovascular failure.
   d. Psychological dependency

C. Pump failure from inspiratory respiratory muscle fatigue is probably primarily responsible for failure of discontinuation of MV in most patients on prolonged MV.

D. Cardiovascular failure may prolong MV. Passive pulmonary congestion, leading to increased work of breathing (WOB) during spontaneous breaths. Poor cardiac performance causes inadequate oxygen supply to the respiratory muscles. Some cardiovascular patients cannot be discontinued from MV because the positive intrathoracic pressures during MV paradoxically unload the left ventricle by decreasing transmural pressures. When MV is removed the excess myocardial work resumes.

II. INDICATIONS

A. When to initiate discontinuation trials. Because no objective data exist on when to begin the weaning process, clinical judgment is necessary. A monitored spontaneous breathing (SB) screening trial is recommended when the following criteria are met:
1. Underlying reason for MV has been stabilized and patient is improving
2. Hemodynamically stable and on minimal and unchanging doses of pressors
3. Adequate oxygenation ($PaO_2/FiO_2 > 200$, PEEP < 7.5 cm H_2O, $FiO_2 < 0.5$)

B. Principles of weaning
1. Breathing is a form of continuous muscular exercise and MV discontinuation should reflect principles of muscle training that include stressing respiratory muscles to early fatigue and then resting them. Maintain a structured, progressive program because benefit is transient.
2. Sudden increased WOB with MV discontinuation can cause harmful effects. Monitor closely during the first 5 minutes and return to MV if deterioration.
3. Both physiologic failure and anxiety cause tachycardia, tachypnea, and hypertension, so do not assume anxiety alone is the cause; it may be a consequence thereof.
4. Screening patients daily may reduce ICU stay and time of MV.

C. Predictive indices for successful discontinuation

1. Indices to predict weaning success yield conflicting data. The best results to date are from Yang and Tobin. Their index of rapid shallow breathing (f = respiratory frequency over 1 minute divided by Vt=tidal volume averaged over 1 minute) of 105 (f/Vt in liters) during weaning had the highest positive and negative predictive values. Less than 105 has a positive predictive value of 0.78; 105 or greater has a negative predictive value of and 0.95. Tidal volume equal to or greater than 325 mL was almost as good a predictor. f/Vt should be measured while patients are spontaneously breathing. This index is less accurate when used with pressure support mode because the breaths are assisted and Vt may be augmented.

2. Inability to generate MIP of less than 15 cm H_2O had a negative predictive value of 100%.

3. All markers for weaning had positive predictive values that were lower by at least 0.15 when MV was greater than 8 days as compared to shorter MV duration. Thus, the predictors for successful discontinuation of MV are even less accurate the longer a patient is dependent on MV.

4. Clinical observation of respiratory muscles is not reliable in predicting failure. Both muscle fatigue and any increase in respiratory muscle load, causes a change in rate, depth, and pattern of breathing. Nevertheless, close monitoring is necessary because discontinuation failure is inevitable if these signs are due to fatigue. If these signs never appear, successful discontinuation is likely.

III. PROCEDURE

A. Modes of discontinuation from MV.
The four conventional weaning modes are spontaneous breathing (SB) trials (with or without continuous positive airway pressure [CPAP]), synchronized intermittent mandatory ventilation (SIMV), pressure support (PS), and noninvasive positive pressure ventilation (NPPV). The role of the latter mode is still evolving. Between PS and SB trials, it is possible that successful discontinuation of MV is less determined by the mode than by identification and correction of medical barriers to weaning. However, when compared to other modes, SIMV has nearly consistently performed the worst in clinical trials.

1. **Spontaneous breathing discontinuation trial**
   a. Sudden, complete withdrawal of machine-supported breaths as compared to SIMV and PS, which are gradual-withdrawal modes.
   b. Only one SB trial is recommended in a 24-hour period because no better results are achieved when more frequent discontinuation attempts are tried.
   c. A "T-piece" is attached to the ETT to deliver humidified oxygen for the SB trial. T-tube flow should exceed the patient's inspiratory flow requirement.
   d. A weaning trial should not be attempted until it has been determined that the patient can breathe on his or her own spontaneously.

2. **Continuous positive airway pressure (CPAP):** It is used primarily in conjunction with SB trials. CPAP can minimize the WOB in patients with intrinsic airway obstruction imposed by auto or intrinsic PEEP, augment cardiac function during weaning, and allow monitoring of respiratory rate, $\dot{V}_E$, and Vt during weaning because the ventilator is still attached to the ETT.

3. **Pressure support ventilation discontinuation trial.** There is a gradual decrease of augmented inspired pressure so that the patient gradually assumes the WOB.
   a. Although it is commonly thought that 5 to 7 cm H_2O of PS compensates for ETT and circuit resistance, this has not been shown to be consistently true and there is no simple way of predicting the level of PS that compensates for the resistive loads.
   b. A major adverse effect of PS discontinuation trials is PS-induced central apneas.

4. **SIMV** has been demonstrated by two large randomized prospective trials to be the least effective mode of weaning when compared to SB or PS weaning modes. Therefore, it is not recommended.

5. **NPPV** has been studied in two settings as a weaning mode. In neither has it been shown to be better than PS or SB trials.

  a. The first approach is to extubate directly to NPPV once screening and predictive indices suggest that weaning is close but not likely successful in the short term.

  b. The second uses NPPV as a bridge to avoid reintubation after discontinuation from MV has failed. In this setting, mortality may actually be worse.

B. Recommended SB discontinuation protocol. See full text for details. The salient features are as follows:

  1. Sit the patient in an upright position.

  2. Avoid sedation unless anxiety is overwhelming and a barrier to weaning.

  3. "T-piece" with humidified oxygen at inspiratory flow rates to match inspiratory requirements or keep patient connected to the ventilator and use CPAP mode and 5 cm H_2O.

  4. Continue the trial unless clinical findings, judgment, oxygenation, and cardiac monitoring suggest respiratory muscle fatigue or clinical deterioration with the following parameters:

   a. Clinical criteria of diaphoresis and increased respiratory effort, paradoxical breathing, or use of accessory respiratory muscles is present.

   b. Heart rate greater than 30 beats/min over baseline, profound bradycardia, ventricular ectopy, or supraventricular tachyarrhythmias.

   c. Mean arterial blood pressure equal to or greater than 15 mm Hg or equal to or less than 30 mm Hg from baseline.

   d. Respiratory rate greater than 35 breaths/min for at least 5 minutes, SaO_2 less than 90%, or dyspnea rated by the patient as greater $\geq 5/10$

   e. Although Yang and Tobin outlined arterial blood gas (ABG) criteria for resuming MV at the end of a breathing trial ($PaCO_2 \geq 50$ mmHg or increase >8 mmHg; pHa <7.33 or decrease >0.07; $PaO_2 \leq 60$ mm Hg with FiO_2 of 0.5), routine ABG analysis is not thought necessary in all cases, because blood gas alterations may be a late finding in respiratory muscle fatigue.

  5. When the trial is terminated due to failure, resume the prior MV settings.

C. Duration of discontinuation trials. The optimal duration of a SB trial has not been determined for all patients.

  1. Because reintubation is associated with higher rates of nosocomial pneumonia and mortality, ICU and hospital LOS and transfer to a long-term care rehabilitation facility, the following is recommended:

   a. Patients on short-term MV (<21 days) can be considered for short, well-tolerated SB trials of 30 to 120 minutes that lead to extubation.

   b. Once-a-day SB trials are recommended over other modes.

   c. Longer trials are recommended for prolonged MV (>21 days), those who to have difficulty clearing secretions, or those who have already failed prior extubation attempts. SB trial of at least 24 hours may be appropriate.

IV. POSTPROCEDURE CONSIDERATIONS

A. Considerations regarding extubation

  1. The most common causes of extubation failure are upper airway obstruction (UAO) and inability to protect the airway and clear secretions.

  2. It is not recommended to extubate patients after prolonged MV who continue to have copious secretions that require frequent suctioning ($\geq$ every 2 hours) or who have a weak cough.

  3. Once extubation has taken place, it is cautioned not to feed patients by mouth who have been on prolonged MV until a swallowing evaluation, including a modified barium swallow, assures that there is no aspiration risk. A modified barium swallow is more sensitive in detecting silent aspiration.

B. Managing discontinuation failure

  1. The respiratory muscles are pivotal in the onset and perpetuation of respiratory failure.

  2. Interventions to increase respiratory muscle strength:

   a. Reverse malnutrition.

   b. Correct electrolyte abnormalities (PO_4^-, Mg^{+2}, Ca^{+2}, K^+).
   c. Correct hypoxemia.
   d. Correct chronic hypercapnia during MV.
   e. Reverse hypothyroidism.
   f. Improve cardiovascular function.
   g. Minimize sedation unless anxiety is overwhelming and inhibiting weaning.
   h. Consider the use of progesterone as a respiratory center stimulant.
   i. Consider and evaluate for the possibility of myopathy, polyneuropathy.
   j. Treat sleep deprivation and central fatigue with short-acting sedatives at night.
   k. Improve diaphragmatic function by sitting the patient up during weaning.
   l. Consider using theophylline to stimulate the respiratory center and augment diaphragmatic contraction and suppress its fatigue. Avoid drug interactions with calcium channel blockers that could inhibit the beneficial effects on the diaphragm.
3. Interventions to decrease respiratory muscle demand:
   a. Maximize treatment of systemic disease to decrease metabolic requirements and mitigate cytokine production that can adversely affect muscle function
   b. Prescribe bronchodilators and discontinue β-blockers for increased airway resistance when not needed for comorbid diseases.
   c. Give a course of systemic corticosteroids in exacerbations of chronic obstructive pulmonary disease and asthma.
   d. Prescribe diuretics to reduce pulmonary edema.
   e. Routinely evaluate and treat cardiac dysfunction including myocardial ischemia.
   f. In average size adults, ETT size less than 8 mm internal diameter may increase airway resistance. Therefore, if an ETT size is very small (e.g., 6.5 mm internal diameter), consider replacing the tube with a larger one.
   g. Add CPAP for marginal cardiac function to decrease left ventricular preload.
   h. Determine whether the ventilator is increasing WOB; whether the sensitivity or trigger threshold is appropriate; and whether the inspiratory flow rate or pattern matches patient demand.
   i. Avoid hyperinflation; apply extrinsic PEEP in the presence of inspiratory triggering threshold load from intrinsic PEEP; consider the type of humidification devices because dead space and airway resistance are increased with heat and moisture exchangers rather than heated humidifiers.
   j. Evaluate overfeeding causing increased CO_2 production in chronic hypercapnic patients and the need for increased alveolar ventilation to remove this excess product of metabolism. Overfeeding may precipitate respiratory acidosis or ongoing respiratory muscle fatigue in patients unable to increase alveolar ventilation adequately. Increased total calories, rather than percentage carbohydrates, is the more likely cause of the increased CO_2 production.
4. Potential advantages of tracheostomy tube placement for prolonged failure to wean patients:
   a. Placement of a tracheostomy tube is a more stable means of ventilating and allows for greater flexibility to perform CPAP or SB trails with a trach mask.
   b. The presence of an ETT in the patient's nose or mouth may cause anxiety due to discomfort and frustration from the inability to communicate effectively. Both may interfere with effective discontinuation trials and prolong the duration of MV.
   c. The presence of a tracheostomy tube may alleviate patient frustration by allowing for better communication through mouthing words. Partial cuff deflation may allow vocal cord stimulation and vocalization, even when the patient is still dependent on positive pressure ventilation. During SB trials, vocalization can be attempted with full cuff deflation with gloved finger occlusion of the tube or placement of a one-way valve.
   d. A tracheostomy tube decreases the WOB in some patients by decreasing dead space.

Selected Readings

Brouchard L, Rauss A, Benito S, et al. Comparison of three methods of gradual withdrawal from ventilatory support during weaning from mechanical ventilation. *Am J Respir Crit Care Med* 1994;150:896.
This article is a well-known study comparing methods of weaning.

Cohen IL, Bari N, Strosberg MA, et al. Reduction of duration and cost of mechanical ventilation in an intensive care unit by use of a ventilatory management team. *Crit Care Med* 1991;19:1278.
A team approach to weaning from MV leads to favorable outcomes.

Ely EW, Baker AM, Dunagan DP, et al. Effect of the duration of mechanical ventilation of identifying patients capable of breathing spontaneously. *N Engl J Med* 1996; 335:1864.
Randomized, controlled trial suggesting that an organized team approach used for weaning can influence the duration of MV.

Epstein A, Frutos F, Tobin MJ, et al. Effect of failed extubation on the outcome of mechanical ventilation. *Chest* 1997;112:186.
Risks associated with reintubation.

Esteban A, Frutos F, Tobin MJ, et al. A comparison of four methods of weaning patients from mechanical ventilation. *N Engl J Med* 1995;332:345.
Prospective comparison of three different methods of weaning.

Macklem PT. Respiratory muscles: the vital pump. *Chest* 1980;78:753.
This article provides insight into respiratory muscle fatigue.

Make BJ, Hill NS, Goldberg, et al. Mechanical ventilation beyond the intensive care unit. Report of a consensus conference of the American College of Chest Physicians. *Chest* 1998;133(5 suppl):289S.
Consensus peer group statement of indications and optimal location of caring for acute and long-term mechanically ventilated patients.

Smyrnios NA, Connolly A, Wilson MM, et al. Effects of a multifaceted, multidisciplinary, hospital-wide quality improvement program on weaning from mechanical ventilation. *Crit Care Med* 2002;30:1224.
Evidence that a team approach to weaning from MV leads to a favorable outcome.

Yang KL, Tobin MJ. A prospective study of indexes predicting the outcome of trials of weaning from mechanical ventilation. *N Engl J Med* 1991;324:1445.
An evaluation of several indices proposed to predict weaning success or failure.

RESPIRATORY ADJUNCT THERAPY

55

J. Mark Madison, Cynthia T. French, and Richard S. Irwin

I. AEROSOL THERAPY

A. General principles

1. Inhaled aerosols deliver drugs directly to the airways and lungs, and this decreases doses and side effects and speeds onset of action.

B. Indications

1. Bland aerosols of sterile water or saline theoretically humidify inspired gas, hydrate dry mucosal surfaces, and enhance expectoration. However, routine use to treat respiratory diseases is not established.

2. Mucolytic agents theoretically facilitate expectoration of secretions. Aerosolized N-acetylcysteine (Mucomyst) has low efficacy and may induce bronchospasm. Recombinant human DNAse may be helpful in cystic fibrosis.

3. Aerosolized antimicrobials have no role in treating acute bacterial pneumonia.

a. Inhaled tobramycin for cystic fibrosis if patient is at least 6 years of age, has FEV_1 25% to 75% predicted and is colonized with *Pseudomonas aeruginosa*.

b. Inhaled pentamidine is second-line agent for *P. carinii* pneumonia prophylaxis.

c. Inhaled ribavirin does not have a well-established role in treating respiratory syncytial virus (RSV) infection.

4. Racemic epinephrine (Racepinephrine) decreases laryngeal edema by causing vasoconstriction.

a. Adults: 0.5 mL of 2.25% solution in 3 mL normal saline every 4 to 6 hours.

5. Bronchodilators

a. Inhalation of short-acting β_2-selective adrenergic agonists (e.g., albuterol, pirbuterol) is first-line therapy for asthma and chronic obstructive pulmonary disease (COPD) exacerbations.

b. Long-acting inhaled β_2-selective adrenergic agonists are currently not recommended as treatment for exacerbations of asthma or COPD.

c. Inhaled anticholinergics (e.g., ipratropium bromide) have a role in acute asthma when combined with short-acting β_2-selective adrenergic agonists, are useful in intubated patients to prevent bradycardia during suctioning, and may be useful in select patients with severe bronchorrhea.

6. Inhaled corticosteroids are used to treat stable asthma and COPD and prevent exacerbations.

a. Delivered by metered-dose inhaler (MDI) or dry-powder inhaler

b. No established role during exacerbations of obstructive lung disease

C. Procedure

1. Nebulizers

a. Air-jet nebulizers are a nonpropellant-based option for aerosol delivery. Method is not superior to properly used MDI with spacer/holding chamber.

b. Recommended when patient cannot coordinate use of MDI or drug not available in MDI form.

2. MDIs

a. Pressurized canister that contains drug suspended in propellant

b. Delivery dependent on technique, which requires slow, deep inhalation followed by a breath hold of approximately 10 seconds.

c. Effectiveness improved by spacer and holding chamber

3. Dry-powder aerosols
   a. Available for β-adrenergic agonists and corticosteroids.
D. Postprocedure considerations
   1. Routine use of bland aerosols may cause bronchospasm.
   2. After racemic epinephrine, rebound laryngeal edema may occur. Other complications include cardiac side effects, including tachycardia and angina. Because of these side effects, Heliox (a combination of helium and oxygen) is preferred to decrease airway resistance due to upper airway obstructions (see Administration of Medical Gases).

II. LUNG EXPANSION TECHNIQUES
A. General principles. Techniques used to duplicate a normal sigh maneuver.
B. Indications. To prevent atelectasis and pneumonia by providing periodic hyperinflations.
C. Procedure. Techniques include coached sustained maximal inspiration with cough, incentive spirometry, volume-oriented intermittent positive-pressure breathing, intermittent continuous positive airway pressure (CPAP), or positive expiratory pressure mask therapy.

III. AIRWAY CLEARANCE
A. General principles. Mucociliary clearance and cough are mechanisms for clearing respiratory secretions. Their effectiveness can be augmented therapeutically.
B. Treatment
   1. Mucociliary clearance can be enhanced pharmacologically with inhaled β2-agonists or aminophylline in same doses used for bronchodilation.
   2. Chest physical therapy includes therapeutic positioning, percussion and vibration of the chest wall, and coughing. Indicated in patients with cystic fibrosis and bronchiectasis, and in the unusual patient with COPD who expectorates more than 30 mL of sputum/day, and in patients with lobar atelectasis. Not effective if cough is weak.
   3. Cough effectiveness may be improved by positive mechanical insufflation followed by manual compression of the lower thorax and abdomen in quadriparetic patients, an abdominal push maneuver that assists expiratory efforts in patients with spinal cord injuries, abdominal binding and muscle training of the clavicular portion of pectoralis major in tetraplegic patients, and chest physical therapy. Promising techniques for cystic fibrosis, chronic bronchitis, and bronchiectasis include the flutter valve mucus clearance device, positive expiratory pressure mask therapy, and autogenic drainage. Cough mechanical assist device (insufflator/exsufflator) shows promise in neuromuscular diseases.
   4. Endotracheal suctioning is used when artificial airway present. Preoxygenate with 100% oxygen. Nasotracheal suctioning is rarely, if ever, indicated and has significant complications including death. Nasopharyngeal suctioning is for clearing the upper airway.
C. Postprocedure considerations
   1. Chest physical therapy is infrequently complicated by pulmonary hemorrhage, hypoxemia, rib fractures, increased intracranial pressure, decreased cardiac output, and increased airway obstruction.
   2. Mechanical suctioning may be complicated by tissue trauma, laryngospasm, bronchospasm, hypoxemia, cardiac arrhythmias, respiratory and cardiac arrest, atelectasis, pneumonia, and misdirection of catheter and may result in death.

IV. ADMINISTRATION OF MEDICAL GASES
A. Indications
   1. Oxygen therapy indicated if P_aO_2 less than 60 mm Hg, arterial saturation (S_aO_2) below 90%, and in certain conditions with normal laboratory values or suspicion of tissue hypoxia: acute respiratory failure (hypoxemic or hypercapnic), acute

myocardial infarction, acute asthma, normoxemic hypoxia (e.g., carbon monoxide poisoning), preoperative and postoperative states, and cluster headaches. Administer empirically in cases of cardiac or respiratory arrest, respiratory distress, hypotension, shock, and severe trauma.

2. Helium-oxygen mixtures (Heliox) indicated for postextubation upper-airway obstruction, children with severe croup, laryngeal edema, and in upper airway obstruction due to tracheal tumors or extrinsic compression. Favorable effects in selected patients with acute severe asthma and bronchiolitis who failed conventional therapy.

3. Nitric oxide is a potent pulmonary vasodilator. It is an experimental therapy needing additional study to define appropriate indications.

4. Hyperbaric oxygen therapy (100% oxygen at two to three times atmospheric pressure at sea level) is used to treat decompression sickness, arterial gas embolism, and severe carbon monoxide poisoning. Used as adjunctive therapy in osteoradionecrosis, clostridial myonecrosis, and compromised skin grafts.

B. Procedure

1. Standard dual-prong nasal cannulas deliver oxygen comfortably and allow eating and talking. Flow rates of 0.5 to 1.0 L/min approximate an inspired oxygen fraction (F_IO_2) of 0.24; 2 L/min approximate 0.28.

2. Simple oxygen masks deliver F_IO_2 of 0.35 to 0.50 with flow rates of 5 L/min or greater. Masks can be uncomfortable, need to be removed during eating, and should be used cautiously on sedated, obtunded, or restrained patients. Flows of at least 5 L/min are used to avoid rebreathing CO_2 from mask's reservoir space.

3. Venturi mask delivers oxygen most accurately and up to F_IO_2 of 0.50.

4. Nonrebreathing and partial-rebreathing oxygen masks with reservoir bags can deliver high F_IO_2 (greater than 0.50) when oxygen flows are 8 to 10 L/min.

5. In the hypercapnic, hypoxemic patient, therapy should begin with F_IO_2 of 0.24 or 0.28 by nasal cannula or mask (Venturi is most accurate mask). If the P_aO_2 is still less than 55 mm Hg after 30 minutes, increase oxygen flow incrementally and measure arterial blood gases every 30 minutes for the first 1 to 2 hours or until it is certain that a P_aO_2 of at least 55 mm Hg is being achieved and CO_2 narcosis is not developing. An initial modest increase in P_aCO_2 (5 to 10 mm Hg) is expected in many hypercapnic patients given oxygen and this should not deter delivery of adequate oxygen.

6. Heliox mixtures should contain a minimum of 40% helium to be effective. Higher concentrations of helium can be used as permitted by oxygenation needs.

C. Postprocedure considerations

1. In hypercapnic respiratory failure, there is small risk that supplemental oxygen will worsen alveolar ventilation and lead to CO_2 narcosis.

2. Oxygen therapy should never be abruptly discontinued when hypercapnia has worsened and CO_2 narcosis is a possibility because P_aO_2 may fall lower than it was before any oxygen was given.

3. Complications of oxygen therapy are decreased mucociliary clearance, tracheobronchitis, and pulmonary oxygen toxicity. F_IO_2's greater than 0.50 should be restricted, whenever possible, to less than 48 hours.

V. NASAL CONTINUOUS POSITIVE AIRWAY PRESSURE (Nasal CPAP)

A. General principles

1. Nasal CPAP applies continuous positive airway pressure during the respiratory cycle. Bilevel continuous positive airway pressure (BiPAP) allows independent adjustments of inspiratory and expiratory pressures.

2. CPAP splints the upper airway in obstructive sleep apnea.

B. Indications

1. Nasal CPAP is used to treat obstructive sleep apnea/hypopnea syndrome, chronic left ventricular failure, and Cheyne-Stokes respirations.

2. See Chapter 53 on noninvasive positive pressure ventilation (NIPPV).

C. Procedure

1. Patients usually respond to 3 to 15 cm H_2O of nasal CPAP by tight fitting nasal or full-face mask.

D. Postprocedure considerations

1. Different masks and BiPAP may be tried to improve patient tolerance.

VI. COMMUNICATION ALTERNATIVES

A. General principles. Speech requires air flowing over the vocal cords.

B. Indications. Patients with tracheostomy tubes and need for speech.

C. Procedure

1. Ventilator-dependent with tracheostomy tube:

    a. Partial cuff deflation techniques require close monitoring and ventilator adjustments. Not used routinely.

    b. One-way, positive-closure, no-leak valve (e.g., Passy-Muir valve) should be used only with a fully deflated tracheostomy cuff and extremely close monitoring and adjustments of ventilator. Do not use if cuff is inflated, there is tracheal/laryngeal obstruction, or secretions preventing air from moving around or above the tube, laryngectomy, bilateral vocal cord paralysis, unconsciousness, or unstable medical condition. Not used routinely.

    c. If cuff deflation not tolerated, talking tracheostomy tube (Trach Talk, Portex, Inc.) for whispered speech.

    d. Computer-assisted communication for long-term mechanical ventilation.

2. Non–ventilator-dependent with tracheostomy tube:

    a. Deflation of the tracheostomy cuff (or a cuffless tube) with intermittent gloved finger occlusion.

    b. One-way, positive-closure, no-leak valve (e.g., Passy-Muir valve) attached to tracheostomy tube (cuffless fenestrated and nonfenestrated tubes, metal tubes, and cuffed tubes fully deflated).

    c. Postlaryngectomy consider electronic larynx and Blom-Singer tracheostoma valve for prosthesis-assisted tracheoesophageal speech.

D. Postprocedure considerations

1. Deflating the cuff during mechanical ventilation may decrease gas delivery to the lungs. Close monitoring of tidal volumes and gas exchange are mandatory.

2. Patients with one-way valves should be conscious, able to remove the valve in event of sudden respiratory distress, and able to clear secretions.

Selected Readings

Bach JR. Update and perspective on noninvasive respiratory muscle aids. Part 2. The expiratory aids. *Chest* 1994;105:1538.
An excellent overview of the use of noninvasive respiratory muscle aids. Includes information regarding the cough in-exsufflator device.

Consensus statement: aerosols and delivery devices. *Respir Care* 2000;45:588.
Metered-dose inhalers are underused in the acute care setting.

Dhand R, Tobin, MJ. Inhaled bronchodilator therapy in mechanically ventilated patients. *Am J Respir Crit Care Med* 1997;156:3.
Excellent overview of issues affecting this mode of drug delivery.

Hudgel DW. Treatment of obstructive sleep apnea. *Chest* 1996;109:1346.
Detailed review of treatment options.

Konstan MW, Stern RC, Doershuk CF. Efficacy of the flutter device for airway mucous clearance in patients with cystic fibrosis. *J Pediatr* 1994;124;689.
Good description of and explanation of use of the flutter device.

Newhouse M, Dolovich M. Aerosol therapy: nebulizer vs metered dose inhaler. *Chest* 1987;91:799.
Supporting editorial by experts.

Salathe M, O'Riordan TG, Wanner A. Treatment of mucociliary dysfunction. *Chest* 1996;110:1048.
Excellent review of treatment of mucociliary dysfunction.

Scanlan CL, Thalken R. Medical gas therapy. In: Scanlan CL, Spearman C, Sheldon RL, et al, eds. *Fundamentals of respiratory care*, 6th ed. St. Louis: CV Mosby, 1995:702.
A classic respiratory care text with an excellent description of oxygen masks and other delivery devices.

Turner MO, Patel A, Ginsburg S, et al. Bronchodilator delivery in acute airflow obstruction. *Arch Intern Med* 1997;157:1736.
Meta-analysis, conclusions supporting the use of metered-dose inhaler with spacer.

Vater M, Hurt PG, Aitkenhead AR. Quantitative effects of respired helium and oxygen mixtures on gas flow using conventional oxygen masks. *Anaesthesia* 1983:38:879.
The lower density of helium affects gas flow.

I. GENERAL PRINCIPLES

A. Inhalational injury results in a variety of syndromes with differing pathogenic mechanisms.

B. Agents may cause different syndromes, depending on the intensity and duration of exposure.

C. Workplace exposures and natural disasters may have similar results.

D. Agents may be inhaled as gases, vapors, solid particles, or liquid aerosols. Large particles deposit in the nose and air passages; smaller particles may affect terminal bronchioles and alveoli.

E. Disease is caused by asphyxia, direct toxicity, or systemic reactions.

II. ASPHYXIANTS

A. General principles

1. Simple asphyxiants include carbon dioxide (CO_2), nitrogen (N_2), and methane (CH_4), which are normally present in the atmosphere and can be fatal in increased concentrations.

2. Toxic asphyxiants are present in the atmosphere in minute amounts or are released by manufacturing processes or combustion. They asphyxiate at low concentration and include carbon monoxide (CO), hydrogen cyanide (HCN), hydrogen sulfide (H_2S), and carbon disulfide (CS_2).

3. More than 5,000 deaths are attributed to CO poisoning in the United States each year. Fewer than half are suicides; the rest are accidental. This colorless, odorless, tasteless, nonirritating gas is the most common cause of poisoning and causes 80% of smoke inhalation–related fatalities.

B. Etiology

1. CO_2 accumulates in sealed or poorly ventilated areas.

2. CH_4 is a highly explosive gas released during the breakdown of organic matter. It occurs naturally in the crust of the earth and is also present in mines.

3. Cyanide is encountered as inorganic salts in metallurgy, electroplating, and photoprocessing and in the combustion of natural and synthetic polymers.

4. CO is generated during the combustion of any carbon-containing fuel.

C. Pathophysiology

1. Simple asphyxiants displace oxygen (O_2) from inspired air.

2. Cyanide blocks oxidative phosphorylation and mitochondrial O_2 utilization.

3. The affinity of CO for hemoglobin is 250 times that of O_2. The formation of carboxyhemoglobin (COHb) causes a reduction in the total O_2-carrying capacity of the blood, a left shift of the oxyhemoglobin dissociation curve, and an increased affinity for O_2 at the remaining binding sites. Because of the increased affinity of CO for fetal hemoglobin, infants and fetuses are at greater risk for poisoning.

D. Diagnosis

1. Breathlessness, tachycardia, headache, diaphoresis, syncope, and cardiac arrest may suggest exposure to the simple asphyxiants; severity varies on exposure intensity.

2. Victims of cyanide exposure may give off a distinctive "bitter almond" odor.

3. Clinical features of CO intoxication depend on duration of exposure, concentration involved, and underlying health of the victim. Increasing severity of symptoms correlates with COHb level. Cyanosis is seen more frequently than the "cherry-red" skin color. Signs and prognosis of acute poisoning correlate poorly with COHb levels.

4. In CO poisoning, although arterial O_2 tension (P_aO_2) is normal or near normal, measured O_2 saturation and content are reduced. COHb levels less than 10% are not usually associated with symptoms; levels of 10% to 20% are associated with headaches, tinnitus, dizziness, nausea, and slight behavioral abnormalities; patients with levels of 20% to 40% can present with coma and seizures; levels higher than 40% suggest an increased risk of cardiac arrest.

E. Treatment

1. The basic management for any asphyxiation includes 100% O_2, support of respiratory and circulatory systems, and treating burns and alcohol or drug intoxication.

2. O_2 is the major therapy for CO poisoning. It decreases the half-life of COHb to 40 to 60 minutes or less (vs. 240 minutes breathing room air) by competing with CO for hemoglobin binding sites. Patients with severe poisoning (COHb greater than 40%) or with cardiac or neurologic symptoms are candidates for hyperbaric O_2 therapy.

III. TOXIC GASES

A. General principles

1. Various agents act as toxic irritants to the respiratory tract and cause mucosal edema, impaired mucociliary function, and pulmonary edema with high concentration exposures.

2. Agents in this class include ammonia (NH_3 and ammonium hydroxide in solution), chlorine (Cl_2), phosgene ($COCl_2$, which hydrolyzes to form hydrochloric acid [HCl]), nitrogen dioxide (NO_2), sulfur dioxide (SO_2), formaldehyde, cadmium, mercury, and the metal hydrides.

B. Etiology

1. NH_3 is found in fertilizer production and in chemical, plastic, and dye manufacturing.

2. Cl_2 is used in the production of alkali bleaches and disinfectants and in paper and textile processing. Most exposures result from industrial spills.

3. Firefighters, welders, and paint strippers are exposed to heated chlorinated hydrocarbons, and $COCl_2$ is released in these settings. Because $COCl_2$ is less irritating to the eyes and mucous membranes than Cl_2 or HCl and may be inhaled for prolonged periods without discomfort, the risk of serious injury to the lower respiratory tract is greatly increased.

C. Pathophysiology

1. NH_3, SO_2, and HCl have high water solubility and tend to be highly irritating to conjunctivae, mucous membranes, and upper air passages. Laryngospasm, bronchospasm, and mucous membrane necrosis ensue.

2. Less water-soluble agents (oxides of N_2, $COCl_2$) can penetrate more deeply into the respiratory tree and can cause damage at the alveolar and lower airway levels, resulting in pulmonary edema and bronchospasm. The absence of immediate symptoms with these less water-soluble agents can prolong exposure.

D. Diagnosis

1. These disorders usually occur in the setting of an industrial or transport-related accident.

2. Patients present in acute respiratory distress with evidence of burn injury; skin lesions; intense edema, erythema, and ulceration of the conjunctival and mucous membranes; and possible laryngeal obstruction.

3. Auscultation of the chest may reveal stridor, crackles, and expiratory wheezing.

4. The typical bat-wing distribution of cardiogenic pulmonary edema is less likely on chest radiograph (CXR) than the patchy infiltrates of noncardiogenic pulmonary edema.

E. Treatment

1. Mainstay of management is removal from the site of exposure and immediate administration of O_2.

2. Airway patency should be ensured because of the risk of progressive laryngeal edema over several hours. Bronchospasm is treated with bronchodilators.

3. Intravenous fluids to offset fluid losses from mucosal edema and sloughing from burns.

4. Empiric antibiotics are not indicated, and the early use of corticosteroids is controversial.

IV. HYPERSENSITIVITY PNEUMONITIS

A. General principles. Hypersensitivity pneumonitis (HP) results from an immunologic reaction to inhaled antigens that affects the alveoli and interstitium of the lung but not the airways.

B. Etiology. Exposure to antigens dispersed by contaminated humidification and by climate control systems is most common. Fungal antigens, animal antigens, amebas, insects, and chemicals may also cause HP.

C. Pathophysiology. The unifying features of agents that cause HP are their ability, based on particle size, to penetrate to the distal airways and alveoli, leading to the development of alveolitis.

D. Diagnosis

1. The clinical presentation of HP varies depending on intensity, duration, and recurrence of exposure. Brief, intermittent exposures result in fever, chills, malaise, cough, and dyspnea within 4 to 10 hours of exposure.

2. Patients appear acutely ill, and chest auscultation usually reveals end-inspiratory crackles.

3. A neutrophilic leukocytosis of up to $25,000/mm^3$ with left shift is common.

4. Serum immunoglobulins (IgG, but not IgE) are elevated.

5. The CXR in acute or subacute forms of HP can be normal or show a diffuse nodular or reticulonodular pattern or diffuse patchy infiltrates without any associated adenopathy. In severe cases, the CXR may suggest noncardiogenic pulmonary edema.

6. The lack of response to antibiotics and the recurrent nature of acute HP are helpful in distinguishing this disorder from infectious pneumonia. In chronic HP, CXR findings are pulmonary fibrosis, coarse linear or reticular interstitial infiltrates, and honeycombing.

E. Treatment

1. Acute management of HP includes supplemental O_2 when hypoxemia is evident.

2. Limited courses of corticosteroids may speed resolution in acute and subacute forms but is of limited effect in established fibrosis in the chronic stage. Only leaving the exposure permanently will help prevent disabling pulmonary fibrosis.

V. SMOKE INHALATION

A. General principles

1. Approximately 80% of fire-associated deaths are attributed to smoke inhalational injury.

2. Inhalational injury exerts a synergistic lethal effect when surface burns are present, with a mortality exceeding 50% (vs. a 4% mortality for surface burns only).

B. Pathophysiology

1. Respiratory injuries in fire victims with smoke inhalation can be the result of asphyxia, heat, and exposure to toxic products of incomplete combustion (TPCs). Most deaths are the result of asphyxia.

2. CO and HCN are the two major asphyxiants and frequently occur together. Synergistic toxicity from combinations of TPCs is a definite problem.

3. Direct heat injury is usually limited to the upper respiratory tract. Edema formation and upper airway obstruction occurs in up to 30% of burn patients.

4. Frank pulmonary edema is rare, but it has an associated high mortality (83%).

5. Pulmonary complications can be subdivided based on time of occurrence as early (CO poisoning, upper airway obstruction, tracheobronchial obstruction), delayed for 2 to 5 days (upper airway obstruction, pulmonary edema, pneumonia), and late (pulmonary edema, pneumonia, pulmonary embolism).

C. Diagnosis

1. Classic predictors of smoke inhalation injury include: a consistent exposure history; respiratory signs and symptoms (dyspnea, hoarseness, wheezing, stridor); cervical, facial, and oropharyngeal burns, especially between the nose and mouth; and expectoration of carbonaceous sputum.

2. Initial evaluation should focus on recognition and treatment of CO poisoning and airway obstruction, the major early problems. A delay in symptom onset (hours to days) is not uncommon. Lung examination is inconsistent and may not be abnormal until 24 hours later.

3. High COHb levels are markers of the potential for inhalation of other toxins. Unexplained metabolic acidosis or a lactate concentration greater than 10 mM/L in the presence of normal or mildly elevated COHb levels and normal P_aO_2 suggests cyanide exposure.

D. Treatment

1. Control of the airway is the initial priority. Endotracheal intubation is indicated for stridor, facial burns and smoke inhalation with central nervous system depression, mucous membrane burns, full-thickness burns of the nose and lips, and full-thickness burns of the neck and when signs and symptoms suggest impending obstruction (drooling, hoarseness).

2. Nasotracheal intubation may be preferred over orotracheal intubation in the presence of mouth burns, because the latter may predispose to contractures of the mouth. An endotracheal tube 8 mm or greater in internal diameter is preferable.

3. Corticosteroids have been associated with increased mortality resulting from infection.

Selected Readings

Dolan MC. Carbon monoxide poisoning. *Can Med Assoc J* 1985;133:392.
This article provides an excellent overview of CO poisoning and its management.

Fink J. Hypersensitivity pneumonitis. In: Marchant JA, ed. *Occupational respiratory disease*. Washington, DC: U.S. Department of Health and Human Services, 1986:481.
Provides detailed information on asphyxiants, toxic gases, and hypersensitivity pneumonitis—related acute inhalational injuries.

Frank R. Acute and chronic respiratory effects of exposure to inhaled toxic agents. In: Marchant JA, ed. *Occupational respiratory disease*. Washington, DC: U.S. Department of Health and Human Services, 1986:571.
Provides detailed information on asphyxiants, toxic gases, and hypersensitivity pneumonitis—related acute inhalational injuries.

Goldfrank LR, Bresnitz EA. Toxic inhalants including cyanide. In: Goldfrank LR, Flomenbaum NE, Lewin NA, eds. *Toxicologic emergencies*. Norwalk, CT: Appleton & Lange, 1990:737.
Provides detailed information on asphyxiants, toxic gases, and hypersensitivity pneumonitis–related acute inhalational injuries.

Haponik EF. Smoke inhalation. *Am Rev Respir Dis* 1988;138:1060.
A summary of an American Thoracic Society symposium on the presentation, diagnosis, pathophysiology, and treatment of this complex syndrome.

Olson KR. Carbon monoxide poisoning: mechanisms, presentation, and controversies in management. *J Emerg Med* 1984;1:233.
This article provides an excellent overview of CO poisoning and its management.

DISORDERS OF TEMPERATURE CONTROL: HYPOTHERMIA

57

Mark M. Wilson

I. GENERAL PRINCIPLES

A. Hypothermia occurs when the core temperature is less than 35°C (95°F).

B. On average, 700 people die in the United States each year from accidental hypothermia. The mortality rate for treated hypothermia ranges from 12% to 73%.

C. Heat may be exchanged with the environment by radiation, conduction, convection, or evaporation. *Radiation*, the transfer of thermal energy between objects with no direct contact, accounts for 50% to 70% of heat lost by humans at rest. *Conduction* involves the direct exchange of heat with objects in direct contact with the body. *Convection*, the exchange of heat with the warmer or cooler molecules of air that pass by the skin, may produce rapid heat exchange (the wind chill factor). *Evaporation* of sweat from the skin results in net heat loss. Evaporative heat loss occurs even if a warmer environment surrounds the skin.

D. Impairment of the ability to alter our environment in response to thermal stress (adding or removing clothes, changing level of activity, moving to a different climate) predisposes to an imbalance in heat exchange.

E. Temperature regulation declines with age as a result of deterioration in sensory afferents.

II. ETIOLOGY

A. The most frequent causes of hypothermia are exposure to cold, use of depressant drugs (alcohol, phenothiazines, barbiturates, neuroleptics, paralytics), and hypoglycemia.

B. Other common causes include: hyperglycemia, hypothyroidism, adrenal insufficiency, central nervous system disorders, extensive burns, sepsis, and trauma.

III. PATHOGENESIS

A. The incidence of hypothermia doubles with every 5°C drop in ambient temperature. Wet clothing effectively loses up to 90% of its insulating value. Convective heat loss because of the wind may increase to more than five times baseline values.

B. Alcohol contributes to hypothermia in 14% to 91% of cases. Persons under the influence of alcohol are less likely to perceive danger or to conserve heat by vasoconstriction.

C. Most sedative-hypnotic drugs cause hypothermia by inhibiting shivering and impairing capability for voluntary control of temperature.

D. When the hypothalamus perceives a temperature decrease, it modulates autonomic tone to cause: a decrease in or cessation of sweat production, constriction of the cutaneous vasculature, and involuntary increase in muscle tone so that shivering begins.

E. The shivering phase of hypothermia generally occurs in the range of 35°C to 30°C and is characterized by intense energy production from increased muscle tone and the powerful rhythmic contractions of small and large muscle groups.

F. In the nonshivering phase (less than 30°C), metabolism slows dramatically, at times causing multiple organ failure.

G. Increasing degrees of hypothermia produce malignant dysrhythmias, depressed cardiac function, and hypotension. The electrocardiogram (ECG) in mild hypothermia shows bradycardia with prolongation of the PR interval, QRS complex, and QT interval. At temperatures lower than 30°C, first-degree block is not unusual. At temperatures lower than 33°C, the ECG commonly shows a characteristic J point elevation. Atrial fibrillation is extremely common at temperatures of 34°C to 25°C, and ventricular fibrillation (VF) is frequent below 28°C. Third-degree block and asystole are common when core temperatures drop to less than 20°C.

H. Although blood pressure is initially maintained by an increase in vascular resistance, systemic resistance falls and hypotension is common at temperatures lower than 25°C.

I. Pulmonary mechanics and gas exchange appear to change little with hypothermia. Both tidal volume and respiratory rate decline as core temperature lowers. At temperatures less than 24°C, respiration may cease.

J. As blood pressure decreases during the nonshivering phase, renal blood flow may decrease by 75% to 85%, without a significant change in urine production. This process is termed *cold diuresis* and is due to a defect in tubular reabsorption. The net result is dehydration and a relatively hyperosmolar serum.

K. The brain tolerates hypothermia extremely well; complete neurologic recovery has been described in hypothermic adults after 20 minutes of complete cardiac arrest and after up to 3.5 hours of cardiopulmonary resuscitation.

L. The white blood cell count in mild hypothermia remains normal to slightly elevated; it may drop severely at temperatures lower than 28°C. The hematocrit usually rises in hypothermic patients at a temperature of 30°C (due to dehydration and splenic contraction). Platelet counts drop as temperature decreases (hepatic sequestration), and prolongation of the bleeding time has been noted at 20°C. Platelet levels and function return to normal on rewarming.

M. Hepatic dysfunction is common and involves synthetic and detoxification abnormalities.

N. Hypothermia directly suppresses the release of insulin and increases resistance to insulin's action in the periphery. Elevations in blood glucose, however, are usually mild.

IV. DIAGNOSIS

A. The diagnosis of hypothermia may be suggested by a history of exposure (both intentional, as in an operating room, and unintentional, as in cold water immersion), a high-risk patient profile (elderly, alcoholic, diabetic, quadriplegic, or severely debilitated), clinical examination, and laboratory abnormalities.

B. Cool skin, muscle rigidity, some degree of shivering or muscle tremor, and acrocyanosis are present in most noncomatose patients.

C. Between 35°C and 32°C, the patient may be stuporous or confused; between 32°C and 27°C, the patient may be verbally responsive but incoherent; and at temperatures less than 27°C, most patients are comatose but able to respond purposefully to noxious stimuli. Deep coma is uncommon, but when present it may be difficult to distinguish from death. The criteria for death cannot be applied until core temperature is back near 37°C.

D. Thermometers calibrated to record temperatures lower than 35°C are necessary, and sites that reflect core temperature must be used (bladder, rectal, tympanic, esophageal, or great vessel sites are preferable).

V. TREATMENT

A. Treatment of hypothermia should be aggressive. Wet clothes should be removed and replaced with dry ones if available. The victim should be insulated from cold and wind. Rough handling must be avoided; even minor manipulations can induce VF.

B. Fluid resuscitation, preferably through a central vein, should be attempted in all patients in hypothermic shock. Slightly hypotonic crystalloid fluids should be given after warming to at least room temperature. Pressor agents and procedures (intubation or catheter placement) should not be withheld because of a fear of dysrhythmia.

C. Management of dysrhythmias must be approached in a nontraditional manner because many pharmacologic agents, pacing efforts, and defibrillation attempts do not work in the hypothermic patient. Because atrial dysrhythmias and heart block generally resolve spontaneously on rewarming, therapy is usually unnecessary. Digitalis should be avoided (efficacy is unclear and toxicity increases with rewarming); calcium channel blockers have not been shown to be efficacious. Both procainamide and lidocaine have been of little benefit. Bretylium appears to be the drug of choice and has been shown to both decrease the incidence of VF and increase the likelihood of successful cardioversion. Electrical defibrillation should probably be attempted at least once, but it is unlikely to succeed until the patient's core temperature surpasses 30°C.

D. PCO_2 and pH values uncorrected for temperature may be used to accurately assess these patients. However, because of a decrease in oxygen solubility on warming the arterial blood sample to 37°C, PO_2 values must be corrected for temperature or the presence of hypoxemia may be overlooked. The following formula may be used: decrease the PO_2 measured at 37°C by 7.2% for each degree that body temperature is lower than 37°C.

E. If hypoglycemia is documented, the patient should be given 25 to 50 mg of glucose as a 50% dextrose solution. Because of the ineffective action of insulin and the relatively high serum osmolarity from cold diuresis in hypothermia, treatment with highly concentrated glucose solutions should be delayed until the blood glucose level is measured.

F. Rewarming methods may be divided into three categories: passive external rewarming, active external rewarming, and active central rewarming. Passive external rewarming is the least invasive and slowest rewarming technique. It requires only that the patient be dry, sheltered from wind, and covered with blankets to decrease heat loss, thereby allowing thermogenesis to restore normal temperature. Temperature increase varies inversely with the patient's age; the average rate of temperature increase with this method is only 0.38°C per hour.

G. Active external rewarming by use of warmed air circulated through a plastic blanket surrounding the patient (Bair Hugger) has proved safe and effective in rewarming postoperative patients and appears to work well with other types of hypothermia. This may prove an excellent primary therapy or a useful temporary therapy while interventions for active central rewarming are prepared.

H. Active central rewarming is the fastest and most invasive warming technique available. Safe and effective methods include the following: oxygen that has been humidified and heated to 40°C to 46°C delivered by face mask or endotracheal tube (raises temperature slightly less than 1°C per hour); peritoneal lavage with saline or dialysate fluid heated to 38°C to 43°C and exchanged every 15 to 20 minutes (raises temperature by 2°C to 4°C per hour); and hemodialysis or cardiopulmonary bypass (raises temperature by 1°C to 2°C per hour). The desired rate of rewarming varies according to the patient's cardiopulmonary status and underlying disease. The rewarming methods selected must be appropriate for the individual patient.

Selected Readings

Buckley JJ, Bosch OK, Bacaner MB. Prevention of ventricular fibrillation during hypothermia with bretylium tosylate. *Anesth Analg* 1971;50:587.
A small animal study (31 dogs) that served as the basis for the current choice of bretylium as the first-line antidysrhythmic agent in hypothermia.

Cabanac M. Temperature regulation. *Annu Rev Physiol* 1975;37:415.
This article lays the basic groundwork for discussions of hypothermia.

Herity B, Daly L, Bourke GJ, et al. Hypothermia and mortality and morbidity: an epidemiologic analysis. *J Epidemiol Community Health* 1991;45:19.
The results of a 7-year survey of hospital admissions and deaths in Ireland.

Kurtz KJ. Hypothermia in the elderly: the cold facts. *Geriatrics* 1982;37:85.
This article lays the basic groundwork for discussions of hypothermia.

Raheja R, Puri BK, Schaeffer RC. Shock due to profound hypothermia and alcohol ingestion. *Crit Care Med* 1984;9:644.
A case report highlighting the effects of alcohol-associated hypothermia.

Thompson R, Rich J, Chmelik F, et al. Evolutionary changes in the electrocardiogram of
severe progressive hypothermia. *J Electrocardiol* 1977;10:67.
Another case report focused on the characteristic ECG changes seen in hypothermia.

Wagner JA, Robinson S, Marino RP. Age and temperature regulation of humans in neutral
and cold environments. *J Appl Physiol* 1974;37:562.
This article lays the basic groundwork for discussions of hypothermia.

58

DISORDERS OF TEMPERATURE CONTROL: HYPERTHERMIA
Mark M. Wilson

I. HEAT STROKE
A. General principles
1. Heat stroke is a syndrome of acute thermoregulatory failure in warm environments that is characterized by central nervous system depression, core temperatures usually over 40°C, and typical biochemical and physiologic abnormalities.
2. Mortality may reach 70%. Approximately 4,000 deaths occur annually in the United States.

B. Etiology
1. Causes of heat stroke involve increased heat production and/or impaired heat loss.
2. Exertional heat stroke is typically seen in younger persons who exercise at higher than normal ambient temperatures. Although thermoregulatory mechanisms are typically intact, they are overwhelmed by the thermal challenge of the environment and the great increase in endogenous heat production.
3. Nonexertional ("classic") heat stroke affects predominantly elderly or sick persons and occurs almost exclusively during a heat wave. These patients frequently have some impairment of thermoregulatory control and are more likely to have a compromised cardiovascular response to heat exposure, to have deficient voluntary control and poor acclimatization, and to take drugs that may adversely affect thermoregulation (anticholinergics, diuretics).
4. Impaired voluntary control (schizophrenia, coma, senility) increases the risk of heat stroke when ambient temperatures are high. These patients may fail to perceive a temperature rise or move to a cooler location or change their clothes.
5. Dehydration and impaired cardiovascular status predispose to heat stroke by decreasing skin or muscle blood flow, limiting transfer of heat to the environment.
6. Acclimatization to higher ambient temperatures can greatly increase heat tolerance by increasing cardiac output, decreasing peak heart rate, and lowering the threshold necessary to induce sweating and to increase the volume of sweating.
7. Sweat gland malfunction is *not* inherent to the pathogenesis of this syndrome.

C. Pathophysiology
1. Direct cellular toxicity results from temperatures higher than 42°C; mitochondrial activity ceases, enzymatic reactions become dysfunctional, and cell membrane integrity becomes unstable.
2. Dehydration, metabolic acidosis, and local hypoxia potentiate the damage.
3. Significant muscle enzyme elevation and severe rhabdomyolysis occur commonly in exertional heat stroke but rarely in classic heat stroke.
4. Direct thermal toxicity to the brain and spinal cord rapidly produces cell death, cerebral edema, and local hemorrhage. Stupor or coma is almost a universal feature, and seizures are not uncommon.
5. Hypotension occurs commonly from high output cardiac failure or temperature-induced myocardial hemorrhage and necrosis.
6. Renal damage occurs in nearly all hyperthermic patients; it is potentiated by dehydration, cardiovascular collapse, and rhabdomyolysis. Acute renal failure occurs in 5% of patients with classic heat stroke, and in up to 35% of cases of exertional heat stroke. Urine findings include a characteristic "machine oil" appearance.

7. The liver appears to be particularly sensitive to temperature damage; hepatic necrosis and cholestasis occur in nearly every case and cause death in 5% to 10% of patients.
8. White blood cell counts are typically elevated. Anemia and a bleeding diathesis are frequently present. Disseminated intravascular coagulation is present in most cases of fatal hyperthermia and usually appears on the second or third day after the insult.
9. Potassium levels may be extremely elevated from cell lysis. Hypophosphatemia and hypocalcemia also occur commonly.
10. Direct thermal injury to the pulmonary vascular endothelium may lead to cor pulmonale or acute respiratory distress syndrome. This and the tendency for myocardial dysfunction make pulmonary edema common.

D. Diagnosis
1. Heat stroke should be expected in any patient exercising in ambient temperatures generally greater than 25°C or in susceptible persons during heat waves (ambient peak temperatures exceed 32°C and minimum temperatures do not fall below 27°C).
2. Diagnostic criteria for heat stroke include a core temperature higher than 40°C, severely depressed mental status or coma, elevated serum creatine kinase levels, and a compatible history. Profuse sweating is typical in exertional heat stroke. Lack of sweating is typical in classic heat stroke, but it is not a requirement of diagnosis.
3. Arterial blood gas analysis should be done early in treatment, and values should be corrected for temperature due to altered solubilities of oxygen and carbon dioxide. The net effect is that the patient is more acidotic and less hypoxemic than the uncorrected values imply. For clinical purposes: for each 1°C the patient's temperature exceeds 37°C, one should increase the oxygen tension 7.2%, increase the carbon dioxide tension 4.4%, and lower the pH 0.015 unit.

E. Treatment
1. Primary therapy includes cooling and decreasing thermogenesis. Cooling by either evaporative (placing a nude patient in a cool room, wetting the skin with water, and encouraging evaporation with fans) or direct external methods (immersing the patient in ice water or packing the patient in ice) has proved effective.
2. External methods suffer from inconvenience and the possibility that cold skin may vasoconstrict, thus limiting heat exchange from the core.
3. Dysrhythmias, metabolic acidosis, and cardiogenic failure complicate the early management of hyperthermic crises. Hypotension should be treated initially with normal saline. Dopamine and α-adrenergic agonists should be avoided because of their tendency for peripheral vasoconstriction.
4. Morbidity and mortality are directly related to the peak temperature reached and the time spent at an elevated temperature. Delays in treatment of as little as 2 hours may increase the risk of death up to 70%.

II. MALIGNANT HYPERTHERMIA
A. General principles
1. Malignant hyperthermia is a drug- or stress-induced hypermetabolic syndrome characterized by vigorous muscle contractions, an abrupt increase in temperature, and cardiovascular collapse.
2. Occurs in approximately 1 of every 15,000 patients receiving anesthesia and has a mortality rate between 10% and 30%.

B. Etiology
1. Increased thermogenesis from a defect of calcium metabolism in skeletal muscles causes development of repeated or sustained contractions after specific exposures.
2. The metabolic predisposition to malignant hyperthermia appears to be inherited in an autosomal dominant fashion with variable penetrance and expressivity.

   3. Halothane and succinylcholine are involved in more than 80% of cases.
   4. Other agents have been implicated as well (enflurane, decamethonium, galla-mine, diethyl ether, ketamine, phencyclidine, cyclopropane).
   5. Stress, anoxia, viral infections, and lymphoma have also been reported triggers.
C. Pathophysiology
   1. Direct thermal injury is the predominant cause of toxicity. Pathophysiologic changes parallel those of exertional heat stroke.
   2. Vigorous muscle contractions almost immediately precipitate severe metabolic acidosis; increased carbon dioxide production; and elevations of creatine kinase, aldolase, and lactate dehydrogenase.
   3. Hyperkalemia occurs in minutes to hours and, in combination with tissue hypoxia and acidosis, makes ventricular dysrhythmias more common.
   4. Higher maximal temperatures are usually seen in malignant hyperthermia.
D. Diagnosis
   1. The metabolic predisposition to malignant hyperthermia appears to be inherited in an autosomal dominant fashion with variable penetrance and expressivity.
   2. There is no suitable noninvasive screening test to identify susceptible persons.
   3. Early signs of hyperthermic crisis vary with the agent administered but include muscle rigidity (masseter contractures after succinylcholine), sinus tachycardia, mottling or cyanosis of the skin, supraventricular tachydysrhythmias, and hypertension.
   4. Hyperthermia is typically a late sign in an acute crisis and is rapidly followed by hypotension, acidosis, peaked T waves on the electrocardiogram from hyperkalemia, and malignant ventricular dysrhythmias.
E. Treatment
   1. Direct pharmacologic intervention to decrease thermogenesis is mandatory.
   2. Dantrolene acts by uncoupling the excitation-contraction mechanism in skeletal muscle and by lowering myoplasmic calcium: 1 to 2.5 mg/kg of dantrolene should be given intravenously every 5 to 10 minutes, not to exceed 10 mg/kg. Oral or intravenous dosages of 1 to 2 mg/kg every 6 hours should continue for 24 to 48 hours.
   3. Evaporative cooling, iced saline lavage (gastric, peritoneal), and infusion of chilled solutions may be helpful. Direct external cooling methods are not advised.
   4. Ventricular fibrillation is the most common cause of early death. Procainamide increases uptake of myoplasmic calcium and should be given prophylactically as soon as feasible.
   5. Prophylactic phenobarbital is strongly recommended for seizure prevention.

III. NEUROLEPTIC MALIGNANT SYNDROME (NMS)
A. General principles
   1. NMS results from an imbalance of central neurotransmitters and is characterized by hyperthermia, muscular rigidity, extrapyramidal signs, and recent neuroleptic drug use.
   2. Mental status changes, coma, and catatonia are common.
   3. Incidence rates for NMS range from 0.07% to 2.2% and appear to be declining.
B. Etiology
   1. In all reports of NMS, patients were receiving agents that decrease dopaminergic hypothalamic tone, or the syndrome appeared after withdrawal of dopaminergic agents.
   2. Butyrophenones (haloperidol), phenothiazines, thioxanthenes, and dibenzoxazepines are believed to act as dopamine receptor blocking agents.
   3. Atypical antipsychotic drugs (risperidone, molindone, clozapine, fluoxetine) and metoclopramide and domperidone have also caused NMS.
   4. Drugs acting at the D_2 dopamine binding sites appear to have the greatest potential for causing the syndrome.
C. Pathophysiology
   1. Increased muscular rigidity, akinesia, mutism, and tremor due to hypothalamic dopaminergic imbalance.

2. Motor abnormalities vary but are typically of the parkinsonian type of extrapyramidal reactions. Muscle spasms resolve with the use of centrally acting dopaminergic agents (bromocriptine, amantadine, L-DOPA).
3. Because of the relatively low maximal temperatures in NMS compared with the other hyperthermic syndromes, direct thermal injury occurs less often. Rhabdomyolysis and renal failure are usually mild and may occur in up to one third of patients.
4. Pulmonary complications are the most serious frequent sequelae of NMS, including copious sialorrhea leading to aspiration pneumonia and mechanical ventilation.

D. Diagnosis
1. Onset of symptoms occurs within hours of the initial dose and up to 2 to 4 weeks later.
2. Early symptoms include dysphagia, dysarthria, pseudoparkinsonism, dystonia, and catatonia. Muscle rigidity generally precedes or is concurrent with hyperthermia. Peak temperatures are usually reached within 48 hours of onset of symptoms.

E. Treatment
1. Specific agents (dantrolene, pancuronium, amantadine, bromocriptine, L-DOPA) are used to decrease thermogenesis by reducing muscle contractures.
2. Bromocriptine (2.5 mg three times daily), amantadine (100 to 200 mg twice daily), and carbidopa/L-DOPA (10 to 100 mg three times daily) increase central dopaminergic tone, decreasing the central drive for muscular rigidity and thermogenesis (and directly reduce extrapyramidal side effects). Duration of treatment is usually 1 to 2 weeks.
3. Prophylactic intubation should be strongly considered for patients with excessive sialorrhea, swallowing dysfunction, or coma.
4. Mortality rates less than 10% are possible with appropriate support.

IV. DRUG-INDUCED HYPERTHERMIA. Multiple drugs have been reported to produce hyperthermia. Drug-induced hyperthermia (e.g., serotonin reuptake inhibitors) must be added to the differential diagnosis in any hyperthermic patient.

Selected Readings
Caroff SN, Mann SC. Neuroleptic malignant syndrome. *Med Clin North Am* 1993;77:185.
A well-written general overview of NMS.

Gillman PK. The serotonin syndrome and its treatment. *J Psychopharmacol* 1999;13:100.
A recent, thorough review of what is known of the serotonin syndrome.

Kilbourne EM, Choi K, Jones S, et al. Risk factors for heat stroke: a case-control study. *JAMA* 1982;247:3332.
A case-control study of 156 subjects and 462 matched controls that helped identify important factors associated with heat stroke.

Knochel JP. Heat stroke and related heat disorders. *Dis Mon* 1989;35:306.
A classic review of environmental heat stress illnesses by a foremost authority.

Strazis KP, Fox AW. Malignant hyperthermia: a review of published cases. *Anesth Analg* 1993;77:297.
A compilation and review of the epidemiology, associated various drugs, and mortality rates for the 503 reported cases of malignant hyperthermia reported in the literature to that date.

SEVERE UPPER AIRWAY INFECTIONS

Oren P. Schaefer and Richard S. Irwin

59

I. GENERAL PRINCIPLES

  A. Upper airway anatomy: Nose, mouth, nasopharynx, oropharynx, hypopharynx, paranasal sinuses.

  B. Minor infections in these areas are common; deep neck infections can be fatal.

II. PATHOPHYSIOLOGY

  A. Supraglottitis (epiglottitis). Acute inflammation, usually bacterial, of the supraglottic structures (epiglottis, aryepiglottic folds, arytenoids).

  B. Deep space neck infections. Knowledge of anatomy required to understand manifestations, complications, and treatment.

   1. Submandibular space. Odontogenic infection in up to 90%. Exemplified by Ludwig's angina.

   2. Lateral pharyngeal space (LPS). Two compartments: anterior and posterior.

   4. Retropharyngeal space (RPS). Uncommon; most often are seen in children younger than 6 years.

   5. Descending infections. Any deep neck infection has access to the posterior mediastinum.

   Descending, necrotizing mediastinitis carries a mortality rate of greater than 40%. Develops as soon as 12 hours or as late as 2 weeks from the onset of the primary infection. Mediastinal abscess rupture may result in purulent pleural and pericardial effusions.

  C. Sinusitis. Inflammation/infection of the sinus cavities. Community-acquired versus hospital-acquired.

III. ETIOLOGY

  A. Supraglottitis. *Haemophilus influenzae* type B most common pathogen in both children and adults. Blood cultures in adults are positive in 15%.

  B. Deep space neck infections. Microbiology: Mix of anaerobic and aerobic organisms; the former predominate. *Peptostreptococcus, Fusobacterium,* and *Bacteroides* most frequent. Gram-negative bacilli less common.

  C. Sinusitis. Community-acquired: *H. influenzae, S. pneumoniae,* viruses, and in children, *Moraxella catarrhalis.* Hospital-acquired: greater than 50% of polymicrobial origin. Invasive rhinocerebral mucormycosis in association with diabetes mellitus and acidosis, burns, chronic renal disease, cirrhosis, and immunosuppression. *Aspergillus* in immunocompromised patients.

IV. DIAGNOSIS

  A. Supraglottitis. History and physical examination.

   1. Children: sore throat, dysphagia, followed by stridor. Child leans forward, usually pale and frightened, breathing is slow, and drooling. Presentation and course are usually fulminant. Progression to respiratory arrest may be sudden.

   2. Adults: sore throat, with or without dysphagia; respiratory difficulty less common, muffled voice, drooling, fever, and stridor. Preceding upper respiratory infection common. Duration of symptoms hours to almost a week. Consider supraglottitis when sore throat and dysphagia are out of proportion to visible signs of pharyngitis. Presentation often indolent with higher mortality due to unexpected airway obstruction.

329

3. In children with classic presentation, do not attempt pharyngeal examination. Artificial airway may be needed; the examination can be done in the controlled setting of an operating room. In older patients without distress, initial examination of the pharyngeal structures is recommended.

4. **Radiology.** Lateral soft tissue radiograph of the neck: epiglottic thickening (thumb sign), swelling of the aryepiglottic folds, ballooning of the hypopharynx, narrowing of the vallecula. Perform radiograph only in the stable child.

5. **Other.** Direct visualization required when suspicion high and radiograph normal. Blood cultures are required. Throat culture of no value.

B. **Deep space neck infections.** Important to distinguish the space or spaces involved to prevent potentially devastating complications and to perform early surgical therapy if necessary.

1. Submandibular space. Young, otherwise healthy adults with neck pain and swelling, tooth pain, and dysphagia, dyspnea, tachypnea, stridor, muffled voice, drooling, and tongue swelling. Examination reveals bilateral, woody submandibular swelling, mouth distortion, and fever. Trismus not uncommon and indicates spread to the LPS. Airway obstruction can result from swollen tongue, neck and glottic edema, extension to the epiglottis, and poor control of pharyngeal secretions.

2. Lateral pharyngeal space
   a. Anterior compartment: unilateral trismus (irritation of internal pterygoid muscle), induration, swelling along angle of jaw, high fever, medial bulging of the lateral pharyngeal wall. History of recent upper respiratory infection, pharyngitis, or tonsillitis often present.
   b. Posterior compartment: signs of sepsis, dyspnea. Trismus and tonsillar prolapse are absent. Most patients have no localizing signs.
   c. Complications: Suppurative jugular venous thrombosis; bacteremia; septic emboli; involvement of the carotid artery. Signs of carotid sheath involvement: persistent tonsillar swelling, ipsilateral Horner syndrome, cranial nerve palsies. Impending rupture may be signaled by "herald bleeds" from the nose, mouth, or ears.

3. Retropharyngeal space infections. Children: fever, irritability, refusal to eat, neck often held stiffly (tilted away from the involved side), dyspnea, dysphagia. Respiratory compromise can occur as abscess protrudes anteriorly or ruptures into the airway; aspiration and asphyxiation possible. Adults: fever, sore throat, dysphagia, nasal obstruction, noisy breathing, stiff neck, and dyspnea most common. Pain in or radiating to the posterior neck that increases with swallowing suggests diagnosis. Respiratory distress and chest pain suggest mediastinal extension.

4. Descending infections. Develops 12 hours to 2 weeks from the onset of primary infection.
   Severe dyspnea and pleuritic or retrosternal chest pain are suggestive of mediastinal abscess; rupture may result in purulent pleural and pericardial effusions. Cervical necrotizing fasciitis progresses superficially along neck and chest wall; early in course physical appearance may be deceptively benign. Erythema occurs initially and progresses to dusky skin discoloration, blisters or bullae, skin necrosis. Gas in the tissues can be readily seen on computed tomography (CT) scan.

5. Radiology
   a. Lateral neck radiograph; prevertebral soft tissue swelling and loss or reversal of normal cervical lordosis suggests RPS infection.
   b. CT. Can define neck masses with excellent results and is indicated in all cases.
   c. Ultrasonography. May identify fluid-filled masses and guide needle aspiration for culture and surgical drainage (however, CT is preferable).
   d. Carotid angiography. Recommended if carotid arterial involvement suspected.
   e. Magnetic resonance imaging offers little advantage over CT.

C. **Sinusitis**
1. **History and examination.** Failure of symptom resolution after a typical cold, facial pain, purulent nasal discharge, postnasal drip, nasal obstruction, cough,

and hyposmia. Maxillary toothache, poor response to decongestants, abnormal transillumination, and purulent nasal discharge are independent predictors of sinusitis.

a. Sphenoid sinusitis is uncommon. Delay in diagnosis associated with increased morbidity and mortality. Presentation includes severe headache, often with fever and nasal discharge. Trigeminal hyperesthesia or hypesthesia occurs in 30%.

b. Nosocomial sinusitis occurs in 5% to 8% of intensive care unit (ICU) admissions. Risks: orotracheal and nasotracheal airways, nasogastric tubes, nasal packing. Other factors: corticosteroid use, obtundation, immobility, supine positioning, and blood in the sinuses on admission.

2. Radiology. Sinus radiographs predict culture-positive antral aspirates in 70% to 80% of acute cases. Findings include: air-fluid level, opacification, mucosal thickening of greater than 5 mm in adults. CT scans: to evaluate bony or soft tissue complications.

3. Antral aspirate. Aspiration of the maxillary antrum is the standard technique to diagnose infectious maxillary sinusitis. Aspiration in critically ill patients can help distinguish between infectious and noninfectious sinus involvement as well as direct appropriate antibiotic therapy.

4. Complications: Orbital: cellulitis and abscess, cavernous sinus thrombosis. Intracranial: osteomyelitis, meningitis, epidural abscess, subdural empyema, and brain abscess.

V. TREATMENT

A. Supraglottitis

1. Airway management. In children, early placement of an artificial airway reduces mortality. Intubation for adults is reserved for signs of airway obstruction.

2. ICU observation with equipment and personnel for emergency intubation is required. Humidification and mild sedation can be valuable.

3. Antimicrobial therapy. Active against *H. influenzae.* In adults also cover *Staphylococcus aureus, Streptococcus pneumoniae,* and other streptococcal species. Initial antibiotics given intravenously and continued by mouth for a 10- or 14-day course.

B. Deep space neck infections

1. Airway management. Upper airway obstruction most often complicates submandibular space infections. Endotracheal intubation can be difficult to perform because of trismus and intraoral swelling. Blind intubation is unsafe because of the risk of trauma to the posterior pharyngeal wall or rupture of an LPS or RPS abscess. Intubation with a flexible laryngoscope is recommended.

2. Antimicrobial therapy. Combination of high-dose intravenous (IV) penicillin G and metronidazole recommended. Add agents active against gram-negative bacilli in patients at risk for colonization or if pathogens are identified in culture. With history of penetrating trauma, vertebral disc disease, or IV drug use, include coverage for *S. aureus.*

3. Surgery. Surgical intervention may be necessary despite therapy with antibiotics and needle aspiration. Most important with infection of the RPS and LPS.

4. Lemierre syndrome: acute oropharyngeal infection with invasion into the LPS and secondary septic thrombophlebitis of the internal jugular vein and frequent metastatic infections (in 90% at diagnosis; most commonly to lungs).

a. High clinical suspicion necessary for diagnosis to minimize morbidity and mortality. Seen in wake of infectious mononucleosis.

b. Usual etiologic agent is *Fusobacterium necrophorum.*

c. Swollen and/or tender neck most common sign; red flag with current or recent pharyngitis.

C. Sinusitis

1. Antibiotics

a. Acute: cover *H. influenzae,* Strep species, *M. catarrhalis* in children. Treat 7 to 14 days.

    b. Chronic: additionally consider anaerobes and β-lactamase—producing organisms. Duration of therapy unclear; 3-plus weeks preferred.

    c. Nosocomial: additionally consider facultative gram-negative rods and S. *aureus*.

  2. Topical vasoconstrictors and oral decongestants to facilitate sinus drainage.

  3. Topical/oral steroids to decrease inflammation.

  4. Remove nasopharyngeal tubes.

  5. Surgical drainage for nonresponders or with neurologic signs in sphenoid sinusitis.

Selected Readings

Anon JB, Jacobs MR, Poole MD, et al. Antimicrobial treatment guidelines for acute bacterial rhinosinusitis. *Otolaryngol Head Neck Surg* 2004;130(1 suppl):1–45.
Consensus report on evaluation and treatment of acute sinusitis.

Balcerak RJ, Sisto JM, Bosack RC. Cervicofacial necrotizing fasciitis: report of three cases and literature review. *J Oral Maxillofac Surg* 1988;46:450–459.
The key to successful management of such infections is early diagnosis of the disease process with prompt surgical and medical intervention.

Bansal A, Miskoff J, Lis R. Otolaryngologic critical care. *Crit Care Clin* 2003;19:55–72.
Review of complicated medical conditions that exist in head and neck surgical patients and infectious disorders requiring intensive care unit admission. Intensivists need to be familiar with these procedures and diseases.

Barratt GE, Koopman CF, Coulthard SW. Retropharyngeal abscess: a ten-year experience. *Laryngoscope* 1984;94:455–463.
Discussion of anatomy, bacteriology, radiology, treatment, and complications.

Berger G, Landau T, Berger S, et al. The rising incidence of adult acute epiglottitis and epiglottic abscess. *Am J Otolaryngol.* 2003;24:374–383.
Clinical presentation, diagnostic procedures, treatment, airway management, and complications of 116 consecutive adults with acute epiglottitis are presented. A rise in the incidence of acute epiglottitis and in the number of epiglottic abscesses was established.

Bert F, Lambert-Zechovsky N. Microbiology of nosocomial sinusitis in intensive care unit patients. *J Infect* 1995;31:5–8.
Infections were often polymicrobial and the common pathogens S. aureus, Pseudomonas aeruginosa, Acinetobacter baumannii, *and* Enterobacteriaceae *often drug resistant.*

Blomquist IK, Bayer AS. Life-threatening deep fascial space infections of the head and neck. *Infect Dis Clin North Am* 1988;2:237–264.
A concise review of the three major deep space neck infections.

Dzyak WR, Zide MF. Diagnosis and treatment of lateral pharyngeal space infections. *J Oral Maxillofac Surg* 1984;42:243–249.
Four cases are reviewed with an excellent discussion of anatomy, pathophysiology, therapy, and complications of lateral pharyngeal space infection.

Gidley PW, Ghorayeb BY, Stiernberg CM. Contemporary management of deep neck space infections. *Otolaryngol Head Neck Surg* 1997;116:16–22.
The operative techniques and antibiotics used are discussed. The main complications of jugular vein thrombosis, carotid artery rupture, and mediastinitis are described.

Mayo-Smith MF, Spinale JW, Donskey CJ, et al. Acute epiglottis: an 18-year experience in Rhode Island. *Chest* 1995;108:1640–1647.
A total of 407 cases were identified in children and adults. Epiglottitis now occurs almost exclusively in adults, often with less severe symptoms and a lower incidence of H. influenzae *infection.*

Potter JK, Herford AS, Ellis E 3rd. Tracheotomy versus endotracheal intubation for airway management in deep neck space infections. *J Oral Maxillofac Surg* 2002;60:349–354.
Both methods of airway control have a unique set of complications. Use of tracheotomy allowed earlier movement to a noncritical care unit and was associated with fewer intensive care costs and less overall cost of hospitalization.

Rothrock SG, Pignatiello GA, Howard RM. Radiologic diagnosis of epiglottitis: objective criteria for all ages. *Ann Emerg Med* 1990;19:978–982.
Various measurements on the soft tissue lateral neck radiograph are described in adults and children and are found to have excellent sensitivity for the radiologic diagnosis of epiglottitis.

Solomon P, Weisbrod M, Irish JC, et al. Adult epiglottitis: the Toronto Hospital experience. *J Otolaryngol* 1998;27:332–336.
Soft tissue lateral neck radiographs were abnormal in 88%, but they had a 12% false-negative rate. A rapid clinical course (<12 hours), tachycardia, and positive pharyngeal or blood cultures were factors that selected for a group of patients requiring formal airway intervention.

Talmor M, Li P, Barie PS. Acute paranasal sinusitis in critically ill patients: guidelines for prevention, diagnosis, and treatment. *Clin Infect Dis* 1997;25:1441–1446.
Nosocomial sinusitis is common, is usually caused by gram-negative bacilli or is polymicrobial, and is best evaluated by CT scanning of all paranasal sinuses.

Thadepalli H, Mandal AK. Anatomic basis of head and neck infections. *Infect Dis Clin North Am* 1988;2:21–34.
An excellent review of pertinent anatomy.

Wang LF, Kuo WR, Tsai SM, et al. Characterizations of life-threatening deep cervical space infections: a review of one hundred ninety-six cases. *Am J Otolaryngol* 2003;24:111–117.
A review of 196 patients with an aim to evaluate predisposing factors for complicated deep cervical space infections and prolonged hospitalization.

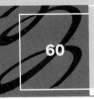

60 ACUTE INFECTIOUS PNEUMONIA
Oren P. Schaefer

I. GENERAL PRINCIPLES
A. Pneumonia in the intensive care unit (ICU)
1. Severe community-acquired pneumonia (CAP)
   a. Mortality rates for patients admitted to the ICU with CAP range from 21% to 54%
   b. There is no uniform definition for severe CAP. Multiple criteria have been published.
   c. Early and effective empiric therapy and ICU admission may improve survival.
   d. Underlying comorbidity and certain medical interventions increase the risk for pneumonia and increase morbidity and mortality (Table 60-1).
2. Nosocomial pneumonia. Definition: pneumonia occurring ≥48 hours or longer after hospital admission and excluding any infection that is incubating at the time of hospital admission.
   a. The infection most likely to contribute to death of hospitalized patients.
   b. Risk factors for nosocomial pneumonia
      (1) Underlying acute illness: predisposes to secondary pneumonia.
      (2) Coexisting medical illness
      (3) Therapies frequently used in the ICU: intubation with mechanical ventilation (increases risk 7- to 21-fold); antibiotic use; colonization with virulent pathogens.
      (4) Malnutrition
      (5) Other risks: general surgery, acute respiratory distress syndrome (ARDS), head injury, advanced age, obesity, cardiopulmonary disease, renal failure, malignancy, diabetes mellitus, endotracheal intubation, and mechanical ventilation (ventilator-associated pneumonia [VAP]), tracheostomy, nasogastric tube, and use of corticosteroids, antibiotics, or H_2 antagonists.

II. PATHOGENESIS.
Understanding normal host defenses (e.g., humoral immunity, cough) and their potential impairments is valuable in assessing those at risk for pneumonia in general and select pathogens in specific (e.g., *Pseudomonas jiroveci* (formerly *carinii*) with impaired cellular immunity).
A. Etiology
1. **Community-acquired pneumonia**
   a. Organism causing pneumonia identified in approximately 50%.
   b. More common organisms: *Streptococcus pneumoniae, Legionella pneumophila, Haemophilus influenzae, Mycoplasma pneumoniae, Chlamydia pneumoniae,* respiratory viruses.
   c. Less common organisms: *Staphylococcus aureus*, anaerobes, enteric gram-negative bacilli.
   d. With severe CAP, *S. pneumoniae* and *Legionella pneumophila* most common.
   e. Frequency of viral infection not known, but likely as high as one third of all cases.
   f. In specific clinical settings, certain pathogens may be more common (e.g., injection drug use, *S. aureus*; neutropenia, *P. aeruginosa*).
2. **Nosocomial pneumonia**
   a. Early-onset (before day 5) consider: methicillin-sensitive *S. aureus, S. pneumoniae,* and *H. influenzae.*

TABLE 60-1	Conditions and Interventions that Increase Risk, Morbidity, and Mortality of Pneumonia[a]
Condition	**Intervention**
Age >65 yr	Antibiotic therapy
Cardiac disease	Gastric acid suppression
Chronic obstructive pulmonary disease	Endotracheal intubation
Diabetes mellitus	Medications
Renal disease	Corticosteroids
Hepatic disease	Immunosuppressants
Malnutrition	Central nervous system depressants
Bronchiectasis	
Malignancy	
Splenic dysfunction	
Immunosuppressive illness	

[a]Underlying comorbidities and certain medical interventions noted in the table not only increase the risk for pneumonia but also increase the morbidity and mortality from it.

    b. Late onset (on or after day 5) consider: enteric gram-negative bacilli (likely drug resistant), *S. aureus* (likely methicillin resistant).

    c. *P. aeruginosa:* more common, especially with steroid use, structural lung disease.

    d. Polymicrobial infections seen in intubated, mechanically ventilated patients.

    e. *S. aureus:* a common pathogen in ICU patients, especially post trauma.

B. Clinical presentation

  1. Community-acquired pneumonia

    a. Signs and symptoms depend on host and bacterial factors. Patients with altered immune function have a more subtle clinical presentation.

    b. Classic symptoms: Fever and chills, pleuritic chest pain, productive cough. Elderly patients may have more indolent presentation (fever without chills, nonproductive cough, headache, myalgias, mental status change).

  2. Nosocomial pneumonia

    a. Clinical diagnosis is poor.

    b. Weighted scoring system using six clinical variables—fever, white blood cell count and differential, presence of pathogens in sputum, purulence of sputum, radiographic changes, and changes in oxygenation—may be helpful.

III. DIAGNOSIS

  A. History. In addition to usual symptoms, consider comorbid illness, medication use, history of immunosuppression, geographic and travel history, and exposure to animals. This information does not help in diagnosis but may suggest specific pathogens.

  B. Physical examination. Not specific for diagnosis of pneumonia. Findings may help predict severity of disease. Consider presence of pleural effusion or metastatic infection. Dermatologic findings may suggest a pathogen (e.g., large crusted lesion in blastomycosis).

  C. Diagnostic testing

    1. Routine laboratory tests. Chest radiograph (CXR), complete blood count, routine chemistry studies, blood cultures, assessment of oxygenation.

    2. Chest radiography. May suggest a specific pathogen but not diagnostic. Multilobar involvement carries worse prognosis. Look for pleural effusion and cavitation.

      a. Limitation of CXR in the ICU must be recognized. Consider noninfectious pneumonia mimics.

    3. Sputum examination. Routine sputum Gram stain and culture remain controversial: approximately 30% do not produce sputum; approximately 25%

may have received prior antibiotics; results often do not affect empiric therapy. Consider sputum evaluation for atypical, opportunistic, or resistant organisms or tuberculosis in proper setting.

4. Culture. Definitive diagnosis only if cultures of blood or pleural or spinal fluid are positive.
   a. Bacteremia is uncommon: 15% or less with CAP, 8% to 15% with nosocomial pneumonia.
   b. Expectorated or suctioned sputum: difficult to interpret (infection vs. colonization)
5. Serology. Routine testing not recommended. Urinary *Legionella* antigen possible value in severe CAP (yield of ~50%); urinary pneumococcal antigen may be of value.
6. Invasive diagnostic culture. Techniques that avoid overgrowth by colonizing rather than pathogenic organisms.
   a. Transtracheal aspiration: limited value and is no longer practiced.
   b. Transthoracic needle aspiration: diagnostic in 50% to 80%; risk of pneumothorax (30%), hemoptysis (10%).
   c. Flexible bronchoscopy
      (1) Protected specimen brush (PSB) with quantitative culture: accurate estimates of the numbers and types of bacteria present when more than 10^3 organisms/mL are isolated before antibiotics are given.
      (2) Bronchoalveolar lavage (BAL): valuable in establishing nonbacterial causes of infection, especially in the immunocompromised patient.
      (3) Bronchoscopy for diagnosis of ventilator-associated pneumonia (VAP) is controversial. Purulent secretions seen surging from distal bronchi during exhalation may be predictive of VAP.
   d. Open lung biopsy: standard for the diagnosis of infection; most often used in the immunocompromised host.
D. Differential diagnosis. In critically ill, diseases that mimic pneumonia such as congestive heart failure, pulmonary embolism, and malignancy may be more common.

IV. TREATMENT
A. Supportive therapy
1. Nutritional therapy. Evaluation and support early in the course
   a. Enteral nutrition preferred; data suggest better preservation of immune function.
   b. Gastric tube is as effective as duodenal/jejunal tube in most.
2. Chest physical therapy (CPT). CPT reserved for patients with pneumonia plus bronchiectasis, cystic fibrosis, and diseases associated with bronchorrhea.
3. Aerosols and humidity. Have little impact. May provoke cough. Mucolytics (e.g., N-acetylcysteine) can precipitate bronchospasm. β_2-Adrenergic bronchodilators can enhance mucociliary clearance, though are best reserved for patients with chronic obstructive pulmonary disease or asthma.

B. Antibiotic therapy. Early, effective antibiotic therapy improves survival in severe CAP.
1. Severe community-acquired pneumonia
   a. Initial therapy: third-generation cephalosporin, plus a macrolide, given intravenously. Alternative is fluoroquinolone plus third-generation cephalosporin.
   b. When *P. aeruginosa* considered: antipseudomonal penicillin or ceftazidime plus aminoglycoside.
   c. With clinically severe pneumonia or in the immunosuppressed host with *L. pneumophila* add rifampin, 600 mg 4 times a day.
2. Nosocomial pneumonia
   a. Treat common pathogens; consider local patterns of infection, resistance, and antibiotic use. Broad initial coverage, narrowed on culture result most effective.
   b. Consider disease severity, risk factors for specific pathogens, time of onset (Table 60-2).
   c. With risk for Pseudomonas or highly resistant gram-negative bacillary pathogen, use combination therapy until cultures demonstrate the absence of such organisms.

TABLE 60-2	Antibiotic Therapy in Nosocomial Pneumonia

Severity of illness	Likely organisms	Therapy[a]
Mild to moderate, no risk factors[b]; severe, early onset, no risk factors	Core organisms[c]	2nd- or 3rd-generation cephalosporin, β-lactam/β-lactamase inhibitor
Mild to moderate, specific risk factors[a]	Core + specific pathogens	Above antibiotics modified for consideration of specific pathogen
Severe, early onset, specific risk factors	Core + *P. aeruginosa*, MRSA, resistant gram-negative bacilli, *Acinetobacter* sp.	Combination antipseudo-monal therapy[d] Consider vancomycin
Severe, late onset, – risk factors	Same	Same

MRSA, methicillin-resistant *Staphylococcus aureus*.
[a]Suggested therapy for hospital-acquired pneumonia based on severity, timing, and risk factors for specific pathogens.
[b]Risk factors for specific pathogens (e.g., anaerobes after recent abdominal surgery).
[c]Core pathogens: *Streptococcus pneumoniae*, methicillin-sensitive *S. aureus*, nonresistant gram-negative bacilli.
[d]Aminoglycoside or ciprofloxacin with an antipseudomonal beta-lactam.

3. Antibiotic resistance. The frequency of resistance among community-acquired organisms and nosocomial pathogens is increasing. An understanding of local resistance patterns is required.
4. Prevention of VAP. Evidence-based strategies include: orotracheal intubation; changes of ventilator circuits only for new patient and if circuits soiled; use of closed endotracheal suction systems; heat and moisture exchangers (with weekly change); semirecumbent positioning. Also consider subglottic secretion drainage and kinetic beds.
5. Drotrecogin alfa (Xigris). Recombinant human activated protein C. Use associated with reduced mortality in patients with septic shock or sepsis-induced ARDS.

Selected Readings

Allen RM, Dunn WF, Limper AH. Diagnosing ventilator-associated pneumonia: the role of bronchoscopy. *Mayo Clin Proc* 1994;69:962.
A discussion of the two diagnostic procedures used most frequently to obtain uncontaminated lower airway secretions during bronchoscopy—protected specimen brush (PSB) and bronchoalveolar lavage (BAL).

Campbell GD, Neiderman MS, Broughton WA, et al. Hospital-acquired pneumonia in adults: diagnosis, assessment of severity, initial antimicrobial therapy, and preventative strategies. *Am J Respir Crit Care Med* 1996;153:1711.
The ATS consensus statement on hospital-acquired pneumonia, including microbiology, diagnostic studies, and therapy, with an excellent discussion on response to therapy and prevention.

Collard HR, Saint S, Matthay MA. Prevention of ventilator-associated pneumonia: an evidence-based systematic review. *Ann Intern Med* 2003;138:494–501.
A literature review and synthesis of evidence-based methods for prevention of ventilator-associated pneumonia.

Heyland DK, Cook DJ, Marshall J, et al. The clinical utility of invasive diagnostic techniques in the setting of ventilator-associated pneumonia: Canadian Critical Care Trials Group. *Chest* 1999;115:1076.

The use of bronchoscopy with PSB and BAL cultures in the mechanically ventilated patient with suspected ventilator-associated pneumonia (VAP) may increase physician confidence in the diagnosis and may allow for greater ability to limit or discontinue antibiotic treatment.

Leroy O, Soubrier S. Hospital-acquired pneumonia: risk factors, clinical features, management, and antibiotic resistance. *Curr Opin Pulm Med* 2004 May;10:171–175.
This review summarizes recent developments regarding risk factors, clinical features, management, antimicrobial resistance, and prevention of hospital-acquired pneumonia.

Mandell LA, Bartlett JG, Dowell SF, et al.; Infectious Diseases Society of America. Update of practice guidelines for the management of community-acquired pneumonia in immunocompetent adults. *Clin Infect Dis* 2003;37:1405–1433.
Updated consensus guidelines from the Infectious Disease Society of America (IDSA). Complements the American Thoracic Society (ATS) statement on community acquired pneumonia (CAP).

Napolitano LM. Hospital-acquired and ventilator-associated pneumonia: what's new in diagnosis and treatment? *Am J Surg* 2003;186:4S–14S.
A comprehensive review of the risk factors, microbiology, diagnosis, treatment, and prevention of hospital associated pneumonia (HAP)/VAP.

Neill AM, Martin IR, Weir R, et al. Community acquired pneumonia: aetiology and usefulness of severity criteria on admission. *Thorax* 1996;51:1010.
The criteria of the British Thoracic Society for severe CAP performed well as a severity indicator at admission (sensitivity 95%, sensitivity 71%). A 36-fold risk of death was found when two of the following were present: respiratory rate greater than 30 per minute, diastolic blood pressure less than 60 mm Hg, blood urea nitrogen greater than 7 mmol/L, and confusion.

Niederman MS, Mandell LA, Anzueto A, et al. American Thoracic Society Guidelines for the management of adults with community-acquired pneumonia. Diagnosis, assessment of severity, antimicrobial therapy, and prevention. *Am J Respir Crit Care Med* 2001;163:1730–1754.
The updated ATS consensus statement on CAP.

Pugin J, Aukenthaler R, Mili N, et al. Diagnosis of ventilator-associated pneumonia by bacteriology analysis of bronchoscopic and nonbronchoscopic "blind" bronchoalveolar lavage fluid. *Am Rev Respir Dis* 1991;143:1121.
"Blind" BAL can be of value in clinical practice; its sensitivity is slightly lower than for bronchoscopic BAL. Clinical scoring criteria for predicting VAP are described.

Rello J, Diaz E. Pneumonia in the intensive care unit. *Crit Care Med.* 2003;31:2544–2551.
A state-of-the-art review on pneumonia in adult patients in the intensive care unit, with special emphasis on new developments in management. A decision tree outlining an approach to the evaluation and management of ventilator-associated pneumonia is provided.

Torres A, González J, Ferrer M. Evaluation of the available invasive and non-invasive techniques for diagnosing nosocomial pneumonia in mechanically ventilated patients. *Intensive Care Med* 1991;17:439.
A complete review of the invasive and noninvasive techniques to diagnose VAP, including bronchoscopic PSB and BAL, as well as percutaneous lung needle aspiration.

Wilkinson M, Woodhead MA. Guidelines for community-acquired pneumonia in the ICU. *Curr Opin Crit Care* 2004;10:59–64.
Severe community-acquired pneumonia requiring intensive care unit admission is a distinct entity with different pathogens, outcomes, and management. The mortality rate in severe community-acquired pneumonia can be more than 50%. Guidelines have been developed to direct clinicians in the management of severe CAP.

Renal Problems in the Intensive Care Unit

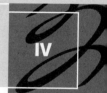

IV

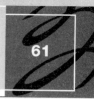

I. NORMAL ACID–BASE PHYSIOLOGY. The pH of extracellular fluid is tightly regulated and normally runs between 7.36 and 7.44. This regulation is made possible largely by the bicarbonate buffer system. Preservation of this buffer reserve depends, in turn, on two renal physiologic processes:

A. Reclamation of filtered bicarbonate, most of which occurs in the proximal tubule; and

B. Disposal of 50 to 100 mEq of metabolically produced hydrogen ion each day. These hydrogen ions are actively secreted by pumps throughout the nephron and buffered either by filtered buffers, such as phosphate anion, or by ammonia.

II. METABOLIC ACIDOSIS

A. Definition: abnormally low plasma pH (also called acidemia) accompanied by a fall in the serum bicarbonate concentration.

B. Classification: normal or expanded anion gap. The anion gap (AG in the following equation) is the difference between the plasma concentrations of the predominant cation (sodium) and anions (chloride and bicarbonate):

$$AG = Na^+ - [Cl^- + HCO_3^-]$$

The normal anion gap is between 6 and 12 mmol/liter.

1. Acidosis with an expanded anion gap

a. Occurs when organic acids accumulate in the plasma. Lactic acidosis is a good example. Each molecule of lactic acid added to the plasma donates a hydrogen ion, which titrates a bicarbonate anion. Each lost bicarbonate anion is replaced by a lactate. Because lactate is an *unmeasured anion,* that is, not appearing in the anion gap calculation, its retention causes an apparent increase in the anion gap. Lactate levels higher than 4.0 mmol/L are considered diagnostic of lactic acidosis.

b. Other forms of metabolic acidosis with expanded anion gap

(1) *Ketoacids,* as occur in diabetic, alcoholic, and starvation-related ketoacidosis

(2) *Renal failure acids,* a heterogeneous group of organic waste acids that accumulate in the uremic state

(3) *Intoxicants,* especially alcohols: methanol, isopropanol, ethylene glycol. An osmolar gap is often present in these cases (see Chapter 62).

2. Acidosis with a normal anion gap (hyperchloremic acidosis)

a. Decrement in plasma bicarbonate concentration is matched by an increase in chloride. See Table 61-1 for causes.

b. Substitution of chloride for bicarbonate can come about as follows:

(1) Exogenous chloride loading (e.g., saline volume expansion; TPN)

(2) Bicarbonate loss, which may occur from either the gastrointestinal tract or the kidney (e.g., diarrhea, type 2, proximal RTA)

(3) Retention of hydrogen ions (e.g., type 1 distal RTA)

C. Clinical presentation

1. Physical examination often reveals Kussmaul respirations (deep, rapid). Hypotension and hypovolemia are often present, particularly in severe acidosis.

2. Hyperkalemia, when present, probably reflects egress of potassium from cells as hydrogen ions enter.

D. Diagnosis

1. This is a simple laboratory diagnosis made on the basis of a low blood pH in association with a reduced plasma bicarbonate concentration.

TABLE 61-1	Causes of Metabolic Acidosis with a Normal Anion Gap

Cause of hyperchloremic acidosis	Cause	Mechanism
Hydrogen chloride overload	Cholestyramine	Intraintestinal exchange of chloride for bicarbonate
	Parenteral alimentation	Exogenous hydrogen chloride loading
Bicarbonate loss	Type 2 renal tubular acidosis	Inadequate proximal tubular bicarbonate reabsorption
	Diarrhea	Bicarbonate loss from gut
H$^+$ retention	Type 1 renal tubular acidosis	Failure of distal nephronal proton pumps
	Type 4 renal tubular acidosis (hypoaldosteronism)	Impaired ammonia production

2. *Respiratory compensation* for metabolic acidosis is caused by chemical stimulation of the brainstem respiratory centers.
   a. To determine whether compensation meets the expected degree, the following formula may be used:

$$\text{Expected } P_{CO_2} \text{ (mm Hg)} = [(1.5 \times HCO_3^-) + 8] - 2$$

   A quicker estimate can be made by comparing the last two digits of the pH (i.e., those to the right of the decimal point) with the carbon dioxide pressure (P_{CO_2}); by mathematical coincidence, these numbers should be approximately equal.
3. The urinary anion gap (UAG in the following equation) is calculated as follows:

$$UAG = (Na^+ + K^+) - Cl^-$$

The urinary anion gap is expected to be negative in patients with metabolic acidosis, because large amounts of ammonium are excreted as a urinary buffer and act as unmeasured cations. A neutral or positive urinary anion gap in an acidotic patient therefore bespeaks a problem in urinary acidification or ammoniagenesis.
E. Multiple acid–base disturbances. Multiple acid–base disturbances are not uncommon.
   1. *Metabolic alkalosis and metabolic acidosis* can occur simultaneously. For example, a patient who has been vomiting copiously may then develop ketoacidosis. Because these two acid–base imbalances tend to offset each other, such a patient may have near-normal blood pH and bicarbonate concentration. The presence of the acidosis is disclosed by the expanded anion gap. The alkalosis, suggested by the history of vomiting, manifests itself as a serum bicarbonate level higher than that expected for the degree of expansion of the anion gap. In other words, the magnitude of the drop in serum bicarbonate (ΔHCO_3) resulting from the acidosis is much less than the magnitude of the expansion of the anion gap ($\Delta A.G.$) Note that the so-called Δ/Δ ratio (the ratio of anion gap increase to bicarbonate decrease) is usually greater than 1.0, even in simple metabolic acidosis. Only when the ratio is greater than 1.6 does a mixed

TABLE 61-2	Recognition of Some Common Complex Acid–Base Disturbances			
Disturbance	**P_{CO_2}**	**HCO_3**	**pH**	**Δ HCO_3 vs. Δ Anion gap**
Metabolic acidosis with metabolic alkalosis	Normal or near normal	Normal or near normal	Normal or near normal	Δ HCO_3 < Δ anion gap
Compound metabolic acidosis	$\downarrow\downarrow$	$\downarrow\downarrow\downarrow$	$\downarrow\downarrow\downarrow$	Δ HCO_3 > Δ anion gap
Mixed respiratory alkalosis with metabolic acidosis	$\downarrow\downarrow\downarrow$	$\downarrow\downarrow$	Normal or near normal	—

disturbance need be invoked. When respiratory alkalosis is superimposed on metabolic acidosis, the P_{CO_2} is lower than would be expected based on simple respiratory compensation alone; the pH is much closer to normal than in compensated metabolic acidosis.

2. *Multiple superimposed metabolic acidoses.* If, for example, a patient with diarrhea develops diabetic ketoacidosis (DKA), the simultaneous presence of hyperchloremic normal-gap acidosis (resulting from the diarrhea) and high-gap acidosis (from the ketoacidosis) is revealed by a drop in bicarbonate far exceeding the extent to which the anion gap has widened. In summary, the recognition of complex acid—base disturbances necessitates attention to anion gap, pH, bicarbonate level, and P_{CO_2} (Table 61-2). An interesting characteristic of ketoacidosis is that, in this particular form of acidosis, the Δ/Δ ratio is usually no greater than 1.0, reflecting the loss of ketoacids, which otherwise could expand the anion gap, in the urine.

F. Treatment

1. Invariably, the best approach to therapy of metabolic acidosis is to treat its underlying cause.

2. Supplementation of bicarbonate should not be considered unless blood pH is less than 7.20 or serum bicarbonate levels are less than 12 mEq/L. Even in these settings, alkali administration is unlikely to help unless the predisposing circumstances are addressed. Bicarbonate deficit may be calculated as follows:

$$HCO_3^- \text{ deficit} = LBM\ (0.5)\ (24 - HCO_3^-_{obs})$$

where LBM is the lean body mass in kilograms, 0.5 is the "bicarbonate space" in liters per kilogram, and $HCO_3^-_{obs}$ is the observed serum bicarbonate. In severe acidosis, or when ongoing bicarbonate losses are severe, the bicarbonate space may increase to more than 0.7.

3. Specific approaches to the therapy of DKA, lactic acidosis, the acidoses associated with toxic ingestions, and the acidosis of renal failure are found elsewhere in this text (Chapters 63, 88, and 107).

III. METABOLIC ALKALOSIS

A. The findings of an elevated plasma pH and bicarbonate concentration establish the diagnosis of metabolic alkalosis.

B. Pathogenesis

1. *Generative phase.* Metabolic alkalosis can be generated in three ways:

a. Loss of hydrogen ion in gastric juice or urine

b. Exogenous bicarbonate loading

c. Loss of fluid with a higher chloride-to-bicarbonate ratio than that of normal extracellular fluid (contraction alkalosis)

   2. *Maintenance phase.* Excess bicarbonate is normally disposed of rapidly. The most common causes of failure to correct a bicarbonate surplus are *hypokalemia* and *hypovolemia.*

C. Classification

   1. Chloride-responsive alkalosis. Chloride-responsive alkalosis, as the name implies, is usually readily treatable with chloride replacement, especially when the triggering problem is corrected. Examples include:

      a. Diuretic use. Loop and thiazide diuretics enhance delivery of sodium to the distalmost segments of the nephron, where sodium–hydrogen ion exchange occurs. Under the presence of aldosterone, stimulated by the diuretic, this exchange is potentiated. The lost hydrogen ion is likely to be excreted with chloride anion. If diuretic therapy is discontinued, the alkalosis resolves readily with replacement of sodium, potassium, and chloride.

      b. Vomiting and nasogastric suction. Gastric juice is rich in hydrogen and chloride ions. Loss of gastric contents, therefore, leads directly to bicarbonate excess. Furthermore, the paucity of hydrogen ion reaching the duodenum lessens the stimulus for pancreatic secretion of bicarbonate into the intestinal lumen.

      c. A transient bicarbonate excess state known as *posthypercapnic alkalosis* occurs after the resolution of compensated respiratory acidosis. Bicarbonate levels rise in a state of sustained hypercapnia; once the hypercapnia resolves, the accumulated bicarbonate is excreted in the urine. Until this bicarbonate "dumping" process is complete, a state of metabolic alkalosis obtains.

   2. Chloride-resistant alkalosis. Chloride-resistant alkalosis is seen in association with obligate losses of hydrogen ion or chloride in the urine. Some examples:

      a. Ongoing diuretic therapy, through the mechanism described earlier.

      b. Mineralocorticoid excess states, such as hyperaldosteronism and Bartter syndrome, are characterized by enhanced distal tubular sodium–hydrogen ion exchange. Patients with Bartter syndrome may also have intrinsic impairment of tubular chloride reabsorption.

D. Clinical presentation. Alkalemia itself is relatively free of adverse clinical effects. Most of the symptoms, such as muscle spasm, paresthesias, and weakness, are more directly attributable to the commonly associated electrolyte imbalances such as hypokalemia, reduced ionized calcium level, and sodium depletion (hypovolemia).

E. Diagnosis

   1. History. Patients should be questioned for vomiting and diuretic use. Bulimic patients and persons who abuse diuretics may not yield this information willingly.

   2. Other clues. The presence of hypertension in a patient with hypokalemic alkalosis should raise suspicion of a mineralocorticoid excess state such as primary hyperaldosteronism. A lifelong history of muscle weakness and of polyuria in a normotensive patient with hypokalemic alkalosis suggests Bartter syndrome.

   3. The *sine qua non* of laboratory diagnosis is the presence of an elevated serum bicarbonate concentration and plasma pH. When a metabolic alkalosis coexists with metabolic acidosis, however, the bicarbonate level may not be raised. The urine chloride concentration may be useful in differentiating among the causes of alkalosis (Table 61-3). Finding less than 15 mEq/L is typical of chloride-responsive alkalosis, greater than 20 mEq/L of chloride-resistant.

F. Treatment

   1. Emergency treatment of metabolic alkalosis is rarely necessary because of the relative paucity of adverse effects associated with this disorder. Only when blood pH is extremely high, such as higher than 7.55, need urgent therapy be contemplated.

   2. *Chloride-responsive alkalosis.* Chloride-containing solutions may be administered, the specific nature of the fluid dictated by the clinical situation.

      a. Because hypovolemia and metabolic alkalosis frequently coexist, it may be necessary to replace much of the chloride deficit as sodium chloride.

      b. Most patients with metabolic alkalosis also have a potassium deficit and are at risk for ongoing potassium wasting, particularly if they are receiving sodium chloride. Potassium chloride may be administered at rates of up to 20 mEq per hour with proper monitoring.

TABLE 61-3	Chloride Concentration in Metabolic Alkalosis

Urine chloride concentration	
<15 mEq/L	**>20 mEq/L**
Vomiting	Mineralocorticoid excess states
Nasogastric suction	Exogenous alkali loading[a]
Recent diuretic use	Ongoing diuretic use
Posthypercapnia	Severe hypokalemia
Exogenous alkali loading[a]	Bartter syndrome and related disorders

[a]The level of chloride excretion in these states depends on whether bicarbonate retention is associated with intrinsic renal tubular damage is present (high urine chloride) or simply hypovolemia (low urine chloride).

    c. For patients with persistent vomiting or those receiving continuous nasogastric suctioning, loss of hydrogen chloride may be attenuated by medications such as H$_2$ blockers that reduce gastric acid output.

    d. *Other options*

       (1) *Acetazolamide* (250 mg intravenously or orally one to four times daily) may be given.

       (2) In severe degrees of alkalemia, it may be useful to give 0.1 N hydrochloric acid. This solution should be administered only through a large vein and at a rate of up to 100 mEq per 6 hours. Ammonium and arginine hydrochloride are alternatives to hydrochloric acid, but they should be avoided in patients with liver or kidney disease, who are at risk of encephalopathy. The dose of hydrogen ion may be calculated using the following equation (which is the mirror image of the "base deficit" equation introduced earlier in the discussion of metabolic acidosis):

$$HCO_3^- \text{ excess} = 0.5 \text{ (body weight) } (HCO_3^-{}_{obs} - HCO_3^-{}_{desired})$$

       (3) Severe alkalosis in patients with renal failure may be treated by dialysis with *chloride-rich dialysis solutions.*

  3. *Chloride-resistant alkalosis.* Therapy of chloride-resistant metabolic alkaloses has two components. Potassium chloride administration is generally necessary. Definitive therapy, however, should be aimed at the cause of the problem. Hypertensive patients should be investigated for primary aldosteronism. If the diagnosis is secured, treatment with *spironolactone,* or, in the case of aldosterone-producing adenoma, *surgery,* may be undertaken. Bartter syndrome is usually approached with nonsteroidal antiinflammatory drugs, amiloride, triamterene, and angiotensin-converting enzyme inhibitors in various combinations.

Selected Readings

Adrogue HJ, Madias NE. Management of life-threatening acid-base disorders (two parts). *N Engl J Med* 1998;338:26 and 107.
   Practical guide for approaching acid–base emergencies.

Battle DC, Hizon M, Cohen E, et al. The use of the urinary anion gap in the diagnosis of hyperchloremic metabolic acidosis. *N Engl J Med* 1988;318:594.
   Shows how to use urinary anion gap in differentiating among forms of renal tubular acidosis as well as nonrenal acidosis.

Black RM. Metabolic acidosis and metabolic alkalosis. In: Irwin RS, Rippe JM, eds. *Irwin and Rippe's intensive care medicine,* 5th ed. Philadelphia: Lippincott Williams & Wilkins, 2003, p.852.
   Source material for this chapter.

Emmett M, Narins RG. Clinical use of the anion gap. *Medicine* 1977;56:38.
Another classic, which provides a conceptual framework for understanding the use of the anion gap, as well as brief descriptions of major clinical anion-gap acidoses.

Friedman BS, Lumb PD. Prevention and management of metabolic alkalosis. *J Intensive Care Med* 1990;5[suppl]:S22.
A practically oriented review.

Kraut JA, Kurtz I. Use of base in the treatment of severe acidemic states. *Am J Kid Dis* 2001;38:703.
The pros and cons of base supplementation in acidemic patients remain a source of great controversy. This review examines the issue in detail.

Madias NE. Lactic acidosis. *Kidney Int* 1986;29:752.
A thorough exploration of the pathophysiology of lactic acidosis and the complex issues surrounding its proper therapy.

Seldin DW, Rector FC. The generation and maintenance of metabolic alkalosis. *Kidney Int* 1972;1:306.
The classic treatise on the pathophysiology of metabolic alkalosis.

Smulders YM, Frissen J, Slaats EH, et al. Renal tubular acidosis: pathophysiology and diagnosis. *Arch Intern Med* 1996;156:1629.
Concise, lucid review of a challenging subject.

DISORDERS OF PLASMA SODIUM AND PLASMA POTASSIUM

David M. Clive and Eric S. Iida

I. DISORDERS OF PLASMA SODIUM

A. Maintenance of normal plasma osmolality depends on (a) water excretory capacity and (b) intact thirst sensation with access to water.

1. Plasma osmolality is estimated as follows:

$$Posm = 2 \times plasma\ Na^+\ concentration + glucose\ /\ 18 + BUN\ /\ 2.8$$

where plasma Na^+ = sodium concentration in mEq/L; glucose = glucose concentration in mg/dL; and BUN is blood urea nitrogen in mg/dL.

2. Sodium concentration is the major determinant of plasma osmolality.

3. Solutes that can raise the measured osmolality but do not result in fluid movements across semipermeable membranes (termed "ineffective" osmoles) include urea, ethanol, ethylene glycol, and methanol.

4. A plasma osmolality increase of 1% to 2% or, more important, a blood pressure or volume decrease of 7% to 10%, stimulates antidiuretic hormone (ADH). A decline in plasma osmolality of 1% to 2% suppresses ADH and results in dilute urine.

B. Hyponatremia

1. **Causes.** Causes of hyponatremia are outlined in Table 62-1.

   a. *The syndrome of inappropriate ADH (SIADH)* is characterized by the following: euvolemia; plasma hypoosmolality; urine osmolality greater than 100 to 150 mOsmol/kg; urinary sodium concentration greater than 20 mEq/L; normal adrenal, renal, and thyroid function; and normal potassium and acid–base balance. Table 62-2 lists major causes of SIADH. Adrenocortical insufficiency and severe hypothyroidism can also cause euvolemic hyponatremia.

   b. *Edematous disorders*, such as congestive heart failure (CHF), liver disease, and nephrotic syndrome, are often characterized by hyponatremia. Patients with these disturbances have a *reduced effective circulating volume*, causing impaired ability to make and excrete free water. By definition, these patients are volume expanded.

   c. *Hypovolemic hyponatremia* is characterized by sodium and water deficits, but with the magnitude of the sodium deficit exceeding that of water. This occurs when patients lose electrolyte-rich fluid, as in vomiting or copious sweating, and replenish only the free water.

2. **Clinical presentation**

   a. Symptoms of hyponatremia include lethargy, confusion, nausea, vomiting, and, in severe cases, seizures and coma. The likelihood of symptoms being present relates to the level of hyponatremia and the rapidity with which it develops.

   b. Physical examination findings: assessment of volume status is essential.

3. **Laboratory diagnosis**

   a. A normal measured plasma osmolality with a low calculated value likely reflects *pseudohyponatremia*, a laboratory artifact caused by severe hyperlipidemia or hyperproteinemia.

   b. *Hyperosmolar hyponatremia* results from an overabundance of osmoles in the extracellular fluid (ECF), drawing water from the cellular space. The influx of water causes the dilution of sodium in the ECF. The most common cause of this syndrome is severe hyperglycemia. Other solutes, such as mannitol, can also induce hyponatremia. When the measured osmolality exceeds the calculated value by more than 10 mOsm/liter, an *osmolar gap* is said to be present. An osmolar gap is a tip-off to the presence of unmeasured osmoles in the ECF.

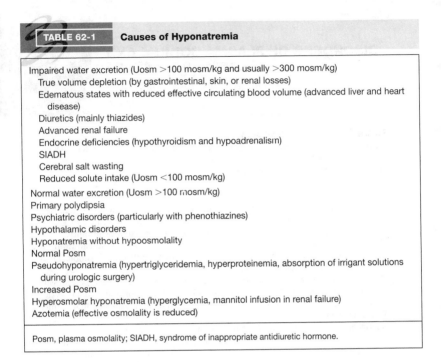

TABLE 62-1 Causes of Hyponatremia

Impaired water excretion (Uosm >100 mosm/kg and usually >300 mosm/kg)
  True volume depletion (by gastrointestinal, skin, or renal losses)
  Edematous states with reduced effective circulating blood volume (advanced liver and heart disease)
  Diuretics (mainly thiazides)
  Advanced renal failure
  Endocrine deficiencies (hypothyroidism and hypoadrenalism)
  SIADH
  Cerebral salt wasting
  Reduced solute intake (Uosm <100 mosm/kg)
Normal water excretion (Uosm >100 mosm/kg)
Primary polydipsia
Psychiatric disorders (particularly with phenothiazines)
Hypothalamic disorders
Hyponatremia without hypoosmolality
Normal Posm
Pseudohyponatremia (hypertriglyceridemia, hyperproteinemia, absorption of irrigant solutions during urologic surgery)
Increased Posm
Hyperosmolar hyponatremia (hyperglycemia, mannitol infusion in renal failure)
Azotemia (effective osmolality is reduced)

Posm, plasma osmolality; SIADH, syndrome of inappropriate antidiuretic hormone.

c. A urine osmolality greater than 100 mOsmol/kg in a hyponatremic patient demonstrates defective urinary dilution. Maximally dilute urine osmolality suggests *primary polydipsia.*

d. Typically, the urine sodium concentration is less than 20 mEq/L with effective volume depletion (patients with reduced true or effective circulating volume) and more than 40 mEq/L with SIADH.

e. Other blood chemistries: the findings of metabolic alkalosis and hypokalemia in cases of hyponatremia should raise the question of thiazide-induced hyponatremia.

TABLE 62-2 Major Causes of the Syndrome of Inappropriate Antidiuretic Hormone Secretion

Pulmonary diseases of any cause
Neurologic diseases affecting the central nervous system
Ectopic production (carcinoma, especially small cell lung)
Drugs (intravenous cyclophosphamide, carbamezapine, chlorpropamide, NSAIDs, cisplatin)
Following major surgery (pain-induced, after mitral commissurotomy for mitral stenosis)
Exogenous antidiuretic hormone or oxytocin
HIV infection (from central nervous system, pulmonary, and malignant causes)
Idiopathic (monitor periodically for underlying disorders)
Cerebral salt wasting

NSAIDs, nonsteroidal antiinflammatory drugs.

Hypouricemia (less than 4 mg/dL) and a low BUN-to-creatinine ratio can be seen in SIADH or *cerebral salt wasting*; in volume depletion, these values are typically normal or elevated.

4. Treatment

  a. *Salt therapy*, usually as isotonic saline, is appropriate in patients with true volume depletion or adrenal insufficiency (along with cortisol replacement). In SIADH, the osmolality of any fluid given must exceed that of the urine or hyponatremia may worsen.

    (1) To estimate the amount of sodium needed to raise the plasma concentration, multiply total body water times the difference between the desired sodium level (a target of about 120 mEq/L is usually adequate) and the current level. Lean body weight times 0.6 for men or 0.5 for women approximates total body water.

    (2) Actual serum sodium concentration should be monitored during the correction phase.

    (3) Take into account any potassium repletion when calculating the amount of sodium to be given because it, too, is osmotically active.

    (4) Patients with sodium levels less than 115 mEq/L or neurologic symptoms may need hypertonic saline given through central access. In asymptomatic patients, one should aim for a rate of rise of plasma sodium not faster than 12 mEq per day (0.5 mEq per hour). With symptomatic patients, one can use an initial rate of correction of 1.5 to 2.0 mEq per hour for the first 3 to 4 hours or longer if the patient remains symptomatic. After initial treatment, one should slow the rate of correction to achieve 12 mEq net over the initial 24 hours.

  b. *Water restriction* is indicated for edematous hyponatremic patients, as well as those with SIADH, primary polydipsia, and advanced renal failure.

  c. Other modalities

    (1) Loop diuretics and demeclocycline (300 to 600 mg twice a day) may help stimulate free water excretion in patients with SIADH.

    (2) Treating the underlying disorder is key for correcting hyponatremia in patients with edematous diseases, for example, angiotensin-converting enzyme inhibition in CHF.

  d. *Osmotic demyelination* (or central pontine myelinolysis) can occur when chronic hyponatremia is corrected too rapidly. Imaging studies may not be positive for up to 4 weeks.

C. Hypernatremia. Table 62-3 lists major causes of hypernatremia.

  1. Clinical presentation

    a. Symptoms of hypernatremia include thirst, lethargy, weakness, irritability, and, with acute elevations in the plasma sodium to more than 158 mEq/L, potentially irreversible twitching, seizures, and coma.

TABLE 62-3   **Major Causes of Hypernatremia**

Unreplaced water loss
Insensible and sweat losses
Gastrointestinal losses
Central or nephrogenic diabetes insipidus
Hypothalamic lesions affecting thirst or osmoreceptor function:
    Primary hypodipsia
    Essential hypernatremia
    Reset osmostat in mineralocorticoid excess
Water loss into cells: severe exercise or seizures
Sodium overload: intake of hypertonic sodium solution

b. Chronic hypernatremia is often asymptomatic; however, if the condition is corrected too aggressively, cerebral edema may ensue.

2. Diagnosis
   a. Clinical
     (1) History may give clues as to causes of water loss (e.g., fever, lack of access to water, perspiration, polyuria).
     (2) Laboratory
   b. Urine osmolality
     (1) In patients with intact hypothalamic and renal function, the urine osmolality will be greater than 700 to 800 mOsmol/kg, reflecting renal water conservation. The urine sodium is low (less than 20 mEq/L) with water loss and volume depletion and high (more than 100 mEq/L) after hypertonic salt ingestion.
     (2) A urine osmolality less than that of the plasma suggests either central (ADH-deficient) or nephrogenic (ADH-resistant) diabetes insipidus.
       (a) *Nephrogenic diabetes insipidus* with polyuria can occur with certain renal diseases, long-term lithium use, hypercalcemia, and severe hypokalemia.
       (b) A historical clue to *central diabetes insipidus* is that the associated polyuria is often abrupt in onset. The water-restriction test can confirm the diagnosis. In this test, the patient discontinues water intake for several hours to stimulate ADH release and to cause the kidney to retain free water, thus leading to a rise in urine osmolality. If no response occurs, one should administer 1-deamino-8-D-arginine vasopressin (DDAVP, a synthetic ADH substitute); if the urine osmolality rises, the patient has central diabetes insipidus. In practice, results may be obscured by incomplete defects, whether central or nephrogenic; direct measurement of the ADH level may be helpful in this situation.

3. Treatment
   a. *Water replacement.* To treat hypernatremia caused by water loss, estimate the water deficit as:

$$CBW[\text{plasma Na} / 140 - 1]$$

where CBW = current (observed) body water = 60% lean body mass.
     This formula applies only to the current free water deficit and not to any simultaneous sodium deficit in hypovolemic patients. The water should be given intravenously in a 5% dextrose solution or orally at a rate of correction not exceeding 0.5 mEq per hour.
   b. For diabetes insipidus
     (1) Central: *DDAVP* by nasal spray (5 to 20 micrograms [mcg] once or twice a day). Potential risks of treatment are water retention and hyponatremia. Other treatment options include chlorpropamide, carbamazepine, and clofibrate.
     (2) Nephrogenic: correct the underlying disorder or remove the offending drug, (although lithium-induced nephrogenic diabetes insipidus may be irreversible). Thiazide diuretics and amiloride diminish polyuria in nephrogenic diabetes insipidus; however, thiazides must be used cautiously in patients on lithium because they may lead to increased tubular lithium reabsorption and toxic levels. Nonsteroidal antiinflammatory drugs may be helpful by promoting the effect of ADH. Restricted dietary sodium and protein lowers solute excretion and thus urine output. Some patients with incomplete nephrogenic diabetes insipidus may be helped by supraphysiologic doses of ADH.

II. DISORDERS OF PLASMA POTASSIUM
   A. Plasma potassium levels reflect the net balance of intake and excretion and shifts between extracellular and intracellular compartments.
     1. Cellular uptake of potassium is mediated by insulin and β-adrenergic stimulation. Conversely, a relative absence of insulin or β-adrenergic stimulation prevents potassium movement into cells. Osmolality also affects transcellular shifts.

TABLE 62-4	Major Causes of Hypokalemia

Decreased intake
Increased entry into cells
   An elevation in extracellular pH
   Increased availability of insulin
   Elevated β-adrenergic activity (e.g., high catecholamine states)
   Hypokalemic periodic paralysis
   Marked increase in blood cell production
   Hypothermia
Increased gastrointestinal losses
Increased urinary losses
   Diuretics
   Primary mineralocorticoid excess
   Loss of gastric secretions
   Nonreabsorbable anions (e.g., HCO_3^- in renal tubular acidosis, β-hydroxybutyrate in diabetic ketoacidosis, hippurate [glue sniffing], penicillin derivatives from high-dose therapy)
   Metabolic acidosis
   Hypomagnesemia
   Amphotericin B
   Salt-wasting nephropathies (e.g., Bartter syndrome, tubulointerstitial disease, hypercalcemia)
   Polyuria
Increased sweat losses
Dialysis

2. Urinary excretion occurs almost exclusively through secretion in the distal tubule and is stimulated by high potassium levels, aldosterone, and a high rate of distal urine flow. Alternate routes of excretion, such as through insensible losses or the gastrointestinal tract, can be significant at times.

B. Hypokalemia. Table 62-4 lists the major causes of hypokalemia.

  1. Clinical presentation

    a. Symptoms and signs

      (1) Muscle weakness, rhabdomyolysis; impaired respiratory muscle function in especially severe hypokalemia

      (2) Cramps and paresthesias occur usually with plasma levels below 2.5 mEq/L

      (3) Reduced smooth muscle tone: ileus, orthostatic hypotension

      (4) Polyuria

    b. Electrocardiogram (ECG) changes include T-wave depression, prominent U waves, and eventually frank arrhythmias.

  2. Diagnosis

    a. Measurement of urinary potassium losses; potassium-depleted healthy persons can reduce potassium excretion to less than 25 to 30 mEq per day.

      (1) Low urinary K^+ excretion rates suggest gastrointestinal loss or prior diuretic use.

        (a) An associated metabolic acidosis generally signifies lower gastrointestinal K^+ losses (i.e., diarrhea or laxative effect).

        (b) Metabolic alkalosis with a low urinary excretion rate suggests surreptitious vomiting or diuretic use. However, severely alkalotic patients may waste potassium in the urine even in these settings.

      (2) High urinary potassium excretion with alkalosis

        (a) Normotensive

          (i) Ongoing diuretic use

          (ii) Bartter syndrome, or other related renal tubular disorder.

(b) Hypertensive
  (i) Renovascular disease
  (ii) Diuretic therapy with underlying hypertension
  (iii) Primary mineralocorticoid excess
(3) High urinary potassium excretion with metabolic acidosis
  (a) Normal anion gap: distal (type 1) renal tubular acidosis.
  (b) Widened anion gap: diabetic ketoacidosis

3. Treatment

a. Mild K^+ depletion

(1) Plasma levels between 3 and 3.5 mEq/L generally produce no symptoms, except in patients with heart disease (especially if taking digitalis) or advanced liver disease.

(2) Diuretic therapy is one of the most common causes of hypokalemia. It can be approached by combining routine agents (i.e., loop diuretics and thiazides) with a potassium-sparing diuretic, or with concurrent potassium supplementation. The latter approach requires careful monitoring and should be avoided if renal insufficiency is present.

(3) Hypomagnesemia can cause renal potassium wasting. Failure to correct underlying magnesium deficiency may make potassium supplementation very difficult.

(4) Forms of supplemental K^+
  (a) Generally, chloride-based preparations correct potassium deficits fastest.
  (b) Use bicarbonate or citrate-based supplements when acidosis is present, as in chronic diarrheal states or renal tubular acidosis.
  (c) Potassium-rich foods are generally less effective.
  (d) Intravenous therapy with a saline solution is preferable to a dextrose-based solution because the latter can stimulate insulin release.

b. Severe K^+ depletion

(1) Oral replacement can transiently raise plasma levels as much as 1 to 1.5 mEq/L after 40 to 60 mEq and by 2.5 to 3.5 mEq/L after 135 to 160 mEq.

(2) Careful monitoring is required; avoid overshoot hyperkalemia while correcting potassium depleted state

(3) More potassium should be given as necessary. A patient with a plasma concentration of 2 mEq/L, for example, may have a potassium deficit of 400 to 800 mEq. Generally, the maximum rate of intravenous administration is 10 to 20 mEq per hour. Higher rates require central access, can disturb cardiac conduction, and should be considered only in extreme circumstances.

(4) In diabetic ketoacidosis, potassium therapy is usually begun once the plasma potassium is 4.5 mEq/L or less (if the patient is making urine) because patients already have a large total-body potassium deficit even if normokalemic, and treatment with fluids and insulin shifts potassium back into cells, leading to severe hypokalemia.

C. Hyperkalemia Table 62-5 lists major causes of hyperkalemia.

1. Clinical presentation

a. Signs and symptoms
  (1) Paresthesias
  (2) Abnormal muscle skeletal and cardiac muscle function including weakness, paralysis, arrhythmias
  (3) Severe symptoms occur when plasma concentrations are greater than 7.5 mEq/L, but substantial interpatient variability exists.

b. ECG Manifestations
  (1) ECG manifestations include symmetric peaking of T waves, reduced P-wave voltage and widening of the QRS complexes, and ultimately a sinusoidal pattern. However, the ECG may not show changes despite higher levels, especially if the rate of rise of potassium has been slow.
  (2) Arrhythmias

TABLE 62-5   **Major Causes of Hyperkalemia**

Increased potassium release from cells
Pseudohyperkalemia
Metabolic acidosis
Insulin deficiency, hyperglycemia, and hyperosmolality
Tissue catabolism and necrosis
β-Adrenergic blockade
Exercise
Other
  Severe digitalis overdose
  Hyperkalemic periodic paralysis
  Succinylcholine
  Arginine hydrochloride
Reduced urinary potassium excretion
  Hypoaldosteronism (see Table 62-6)
  Renal failure and renal tubular disorders
  Effective circulating volume depletion
Drugs
  Dapsone
  Sulfa/trimethoprim
  Nonsteroidal antiinflammatory drugs
  Angiotensin-converting enzyme inhibitors
  Spironolactone and other potassium-sparing diuretics
  Heparin

2. Treatment
    a. Mild hyperkalemia (no ECG changes; plasma potassium level ≤6.5 mEq/L)
        (1) May use cation exchange resin such as sodium polystyrene sulfonate (Kayexalate).
        (2) With a level of less than 6.0 mEq/L, diuretics alone may suffice.
        (3) For maintenance: low-potassium diet and the discontinuation of offending drugs.

TABLE 62-6   **Major Causes of Hypoaldosteronism**

Hyporeninemic hypoaldosteronism
Renal disease, most often diabetic nephropathy
Drugs
  Nonsteroidal antiinflammatory drugs
  Angiotensin-converting enzyme inhibitors
  Cyclosporine
  Spironolactone
HIV infection
Primary adrenal insufficiency
Heparin
Congenital adrenal hyperplasia (21-hydroxylase deficiency is most common)
Isolated impairment in aldosterone synthesis
Pseudohypoaldosteronism (end-organ resistance)
Severe illness

    b. Severe or symptomatic hyperkalemia (>6.5 mEq/L)

        (1) Most rapidly acting therapeutic maneuvers are those that effect K^+ transit into cells.

            (a) *Calcium* (1 ampule of 10% calcium gluconate) stabilizes cell membranes.

            (b) Acts within minutes but is short-lived in effect.

            (c) Should not be given in bicarbonate-containing solutions or precipitates may form.

            (d) Should be prescribed only when absolutely necessary in patients taking digoxin, because hypercalcemia can induce digitalis toxicity.

        (2) *Insulin* (10 U of regular) and glucose (50 mL of 50% solution)

            (a) Can decrease potassium levels by 0.5 to 1.5 mEq/L.

            (b) Effect begins within 15 minutes and lasts for several hours. In a hyperglycemic diabetic patient, use insulin alone.

        (3) *Sodium bicarbonate* (one ampule of a 7.5% sodium bicarbonate solution)

            (a) Works best in patients with metabolic acidosis but is less effective in renal failure.

            (b) Begins to act within 30 to 60 minutes, and the effect lasts for several hours.

        (4) *Albuterol* (20 mg in 4 mL of saline by nasal inhalation or 0.5 mg by intravenous infusion) can lower the plasma potassium concentration by 0.5 to 1.5 mEq/L within 30 to 60 minutes.

        (5) Increasing K^+ excretion (slower but longer-lasting effect)

            (a) *Loop or thiazide diuretics* promote urinary potassium excretion.

            (b) *Cation exchange resins* such as Kayaxelate cause loss of potassium in the stool by exchanging potassium for sodium.

                (i) Can be given orally or by retention enema.

                (ii) Intestinal necrosis and volume overload can potentially complicate treatment.

                (iii) One should consider *dialysis* if the foregoing measures fail, the patient has renal failure, the hyperkalemia is severe, or the patient has marked tissue breakdown with release of large amounts of potassium. Hemodialysis removes potassium many times faster than peritoneal dialysis.

Selected Readings

Black RM. Disorders of plasma sodium and plasma potassium. In: Irwin RS, Rippe JM, eds. *Irwin and Rippe's intensive care medicine*, 5th ed. Philadelphia: Lippincott Williams & Wilkins, 2003, p. 864.
Source material for this chapter.

Gennari FJ. Hypokalemia. *N Engl J Med* 1998;339:451.
A good review.

Lauriat SM, Berl T. The hyponatremic patient: practical focus on therapy. *J Am Soc Nephrol* 1997;8:1599.
Good discussion of risks and issues surrounding treatment, although the approach is more aggressive than presented here.

Miller M, Kalkos T, Moses A, et al. Recognition of partial defects in antidiuretic hormone secretion. *Ann Intern Med* 1970;73:721.
Description of the water-deprivation test and its interpretation.

Scheinman SJ, Guay-Woodford LM, Thakker RV, et al. Genetic disorders of renal electrolyte transport. *N Engl J Med* 1999:340:1177.
Summarizes advances in defining mechanisms of some less common but important disorders that alter potassium and sodium balance, such as Bartter syndrome.

Weiner ID, Wingo CS. Hyperkalemia: a potential silent killer. *J Am Soc Nephrol* 1997;9:1535.
A good review of the subject.

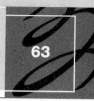

I. OVERVIEW

A. *Acute renal failure* (ARF) means a sudden decline in kidney function.

B. Most important diagnostic features are *azotemia* and *oliguria*.

C. May stem from any of three types of insults:

  1. Impaired renal perfusion, called *prerenal azotemia*

  2. Injury to the renal parenchyma, or *renal* (also called intrinsic or parenchymal) *ARF*

  3. Obstruction of the urinary tract, or *postrenal ARF* (Table 63-1)

II. PRERENAL AZOTEMIA AND AUTOREGULATORY FAILURE

A. Prerenal azotemia arises from a reduction in renal blood flow associated with factors such as hypovolemia, reduced effective circulating volume, selective renal hypoperfusion, and autoregulatory failure (Table 63-2).

B. Correction of causative factors usually restores renal function.

C. Renal response to reduced perfusion, intense conservation of salt and water, provides important diagnostic information. Urinary chemical features include:

  1. Urine sodium concentration (U_{Na}) less than 10 mEq/L

  2. *Fractional excretion of sodium (FE_{Na})* less than 1%. FE_{Na} is the fractional excretion of filtered sodium = 100 × (urine sodium/plasma sodium)/(urine creatinine/plasma creatinine).

  3. Urine osmolality (U_{osm}) greater than 500 mOsmol/kg

  4. BUN-to-creatinine ratio may rise from the normal 10:1 to greater than 20:1; however, this finding is not pathognomonic of prerenal states (Table 63-3).

III. INTRINSIC RENAL DISEASE

A. Glomerular and vascular diseases

  1. Causes of ARF include the following: vasculitis; acute glomerulonephritis; diseases of either the main renal vessels or their branches, such as renal artery or renal vein thrombosis; and microscopic occlusion of smaller vessels, as occurs in a variety of disorders such as atheroembolic renal disease, hemolytic-uremic syndrome, scleroderma, and malignant hypertension.

  2. Diseases of the main renal vessels are discussed in further detail later.

B. Tubulointerstitial diseases

  1. *Acute tubular necrosis (ATN)*

    a. May result from renal ischemia or exposure to nephrotoxins (aminoglycoside antibiotics, radiocontrast agents, heavy metals, myoglobin).

    b. A suggestive history is elicited in 80% of patients with ATN.

    c. Classic urinary findings consist of sloughed renal tubular epithelial cells, epithelial cell casts, and muddy brown granular casts.

    d. In contrast to prerenal azotemia, the FE_{Na} is generally high (more than 1%), a finding suggesting tubular damage with impaired sodium reabsorption. Urinary concentration is also impaired, generally resulting in U_{osm} of approximately 300 mOsmol/kg.

  2. *Acute interstitial nephritis*

    a. Characterized by inflammation of the renal interstitium and tubules.

    b. Often drug induced, with features of allergy: fever, rash, and eosinophilia.

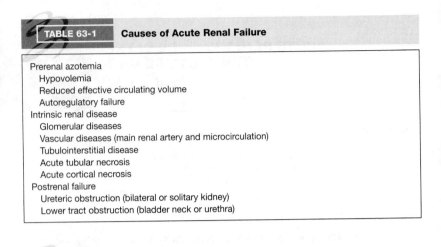

TABLE 63-1   **Causes of Acute Renal Failure**

Prerenal azotemia
  Hypovolemia
  Reduced effective circulating volume
  Autoregulatory failure
Intrinsic renal disease
  Glomerular diseases
  Vascular diseases (main renal artery and microcirculation)
  Tubulointerstitial disease
  Acute tubular necrosis
  Acute cortical necrosis
Postrenal failure
  Ureteric obstruction (bilateral or solitary kidney)
  Lower tract obstruction (bladder neck or urethra)

TABLE 63-2   **Causes of Prerenal Azotemia**

Hypovolemia
Gastrointestinal losses
  Vomiting
  Diarrhea
  Surgical drainage
Renal losses
  Osmotic agents
  Diuretics
  Renal salt wasting disease
  Adrenal insufficiency
Skin losses
  Burns
  Excessive diaphoresis
Hemorrhage
Translocation of fluid ("third-spacing")
  Postoperative
  Pancreatitis
Reduced effective circulating volume
  Hypoalbuminemia
  Hepatic cirrhosis
  Left ventricular cardiac failure
  Peripheral blood pooling (vasodilator therapy, anesthetics, anaphylaxis, sepsis, toxic shock
    syndrome)
  Renal artery stenosis
  Small vessel disease (malignant hypertension, toxemia, scleroderma)
  Renal vasoconstriction (hypercalcemia, hepatorenal syndrome, cyclosporine, pressor agents)
Autoregulatory failure
  NSAIDs (preglomerular vasoconstriction)
  ARBs and CEIs (postglomerular vasodilation)

ARBs, angiotension receptor blockers; CEIs, converting enzyme inhibitors; NSAIDs, nonsteroidal antiinflammatory drugs.

TABLE 63-3	Causes of Blood Urea Nitrogen or Serum Creatinine Elevation Without Reduction of Glomerular Filtration Fate

Increased biosynthesis of urea
  Gastrointestinal bleeding
  Drug administration
    Corticosteroids
    Tetracycline
  Increased protein intake
  Amino acid administration
  Hypercatabolism and febrile illness
Increased biosynthesis of creatinine
  Increased release of creatinine from muscle (rhabdomyolysis)
Drug-interference with tubular creatinine secretion
  Cimetidine
  Trimethoprim
Spuriously elevated creatinine colorimetric assay
  Ketoacids (diabetic ketoacidosis)
  Cephalosporins

IV. POSTRENAL AZOTEMIA

A. May be caused by any lesion impeding urine flow. Common examples:
  1. Prostatic enlargement or tumor
  2. Urolithiasis
  3. Urinary infections
  4. Neoplasms involving the urinary tract
B. For obstruction to cause azotemia, both kidneys must be involved or unilateral obstruction in a patient with only one normally functioning kidney must occur.
C. While cessation of urine flow (anuria) may occur in complete obstruction of the urinary tract, partial obstructions, even high-grade ones, may not be associated with low urine output.
D. Obstruction is usually easily detected by sonography, with hydronephrosis evident.
E. Depending on the site of obstruction, immediate treatment may involve the placement of an indwelling urinary catheter, ureteral stents, or nephrostomy drainage until the underlying cause can be treated.

V. ETIOLOGIES AND PRESENTATIONS OF ARF

A. Two thirds of hospitalized patients with ARF have either ATN or prerenal azotemia.
B. Ischemic ATN results from more profound hypoperfusion than does prerenal azotemia. Ischemia is the most common cause of ARF in the intensive care unit.
C. Often, ARF cases are etiologically multifactorial.
D. Toxin-associated ARF
  1. Myoglobinuric ARF
    a. Occurs as a result of the nephrotoxic effects of the intracellular protein, myoglobin, which is released into plasma during skeletal muscle injury (rhabdomyolysis).
    b. Diagnosis is suggested by serum creatine kinase levels greater than 5,000 µL.
    c. Administration of isotonic bicarbonate-rich fluids (e.g., three ampoules of bicarbonate in 1 L of 5% dextrose in water) and diuretics (e.g., mannitol or loop diuretics) is recommended. Mannitol, however, may cause volume overload if the kidneys are unable to effect diuresis.
    d. Hemoglobinuria is also capable, albeit rarely, of inducing ARF.
  2. Tumor lysis syndrome
    a. Released tumor cell contents, including phosphates, uric acid, and purine metabolites, cause diffuse nephronal microobstruction.

    b. Most commonly occurs during induction of chemotherapy in patients with hematologic and lymphoproliferative malignancies, especially if large tumor burden is present. May occur spontaneously in patients with rapidly growing (high cell turnover) malignancies.

    c. Patients at risk should routinely receive prophylaxis before chemotherapy, including volume expansion, maintenance of diuresis, alkalinization of the urine, and pretreatment with allopurinol.

3. Radiocontrast-induced nephropathy

    a. Follows the administration of intravenous radiocontrast and is associated with rapidly developing, and typically oliguric, ARF.

    b. Serum creatinine generally peaks around 4 days after the procedure, and renal function returns to baseline within 7 to 14 days.

    c. Prevention is key

        (1) Modest hydration before the procedure (0.45% saline, 0.5 to 2.0 mL/kg per hour to start 2 to 6 hours before contrast administration) and to continue 6 hours afterward is advocated.

        (2) Diuretics are to be avoided during this period.

        (3) There may be a benefit to the use of nonionic, low-osmolality radiocontrast media in at-risk patients.

    d. Risk factors include preexisting renal insufficiency, diabetic nephropathy with renal insufficiency, volume depletion, large contrast dose (more than 2 mL/kg), age greater than 60 years, hyperuricemia, hepatic failure, and multiple myeloma.

4. Drug-induced syndromes

    a. *Acute tubular injury.* Drugs exerting direct toxic effects, typically to the proximal tubular epithelium, cause this ATN-type syndrome. Agents include aminoglycoside antibiotics, certain cephalosporins, cisplatin, amphotericin B, and foscarnet. Predisposing risk factors for tubular injury include volume contraction, preexisting renal insufficiency, and liver disease. ARF is usually reversible with drug discontinuation.

    b. *Intratubular microobstruction.* Selected drugs, such as acyclovir, methotrexate, sulfamethoxazole, and low-molecular-weight dextran may precipitate in and obstruct the nephrons. Prevention of tubular obstruction necessitates optimal hydration of the patient and maintenance of high urine flow rate. The syndrome is usually reversible and short-lived.

    c. *Acute interstitial nephritis.* An ever-enlarging list of drugs can cause acute interstitial nephritis (Table 63-4). Among the most common culprits are penicillins, sulfa drugs, thiazide diuretics, and allopurinol. The urine sediment typically shows red and white cells, often including eosinophils. Largely reversible on discontinuation of the drug; protracted cases may benefit from a short course of steroids.

    d. *Autoregulatory failure.* Two patterns of hemodynamically mediated, drug-induced renal failure may occur.

        (1) When the main action of the drug is to permit afferent arteriolar vasoconstriction, such as with nonsteroidal antiinflammatory drugs or vasopressors, failure to autoregulate renal blood flow ensues and prerenal azotemia develops.

        (2) If a drug causing efferent arteriolar vasodilatation, such as a converting enzyme inhibitor, is given to a patient with a fixed impediment to blood flow (e.g., bilateral renal artery stenosis, volume depletion), a sharp reduction in glomerular filtration rate (GFR) may occur.

        (3) Unless severe renal ischemia has occurred, renal failure is promptly reversible after withdrawal of the drug.

5. Renal vascular disease

    a. *Renal artery occlusion.* Generally, ARF is seen only if a thromboembolic event involves both kidneys or a solitary functioning kidney. Renal artery emboli typically occur in the setting of cardiac disease, such as arrhythmia, myocardial infarction, or valvular disease. Clinical hallmarks include acute flank pain, oliguria, and hematuria. Radiologic techniques, including nuclear imaging, computed

TABLE 63-4	Drugs Most Often Implicated in Acute Interstitial Nephritis

Antibiotics
　　Penicillinase-resistant penicillins
　　Cephalosporins
　　Ampicillin
　　Amoxicillin
　　Penicillin G
　　Sulfonamides and sulfa-trimethoprim
　　Rifampin
　　Ethambutol
　　Tetracycline
Diuretics
　　Furosemide
　　Thiazides and related compounds
Nonsteroidal antiinflammatory drugs
　　Ibuprofen
　　Indomethacin
　　Fenoprofen
　　Naproxen
　　Phenylbutazone
　　Mefenamic acid
　　Tolmetin
Miscellaneous drugs
　　Diphenylhydantoin
　　Cimetidine
　　Alpha-methyldopa
　　Allopurinol
　　Captopril

tomography, and arteriography can confirm the diagnosis. Arteriography is the most invasive study and associated with the greatest risks, but it yields the most anatomic information. Therapy is most effective if performed within 24 hours. Options include surgical thrombectomy, supportive care with anticoagulation, and possibly use of fibrinolytic agents.

b. *Renal vein thrombosis.* Situations in which renal vein thrombosis may occur include the nephrotic syndrome, renal cell carcinoma, hematologic disorders characterized by hypercoagulability, sickle cell disease, pregnancy, use of oral contraceptives, and trauma. As in renal artery occlusion, ARF seldom occurs unless both kidneys are simultaneously involved; clinical features are similar as well. Duplex venography and computed tomography can confirm the diagnosis. Treatment involves anticoagulation and possibly fibrinolytic therapy.

c. *Atheroembolic renal disease (cholesterol emboli).* Showers of cholesterol emboli to the kidneys and other organs may occur in patients with severe aortic atherosclerosis, typically after a precipitating event such as aortography, major vascular surgery, or blunt trauma to the abdomen; they may also develop spontaneously or in association with anticoagulant therapy. Blue distal digits, a mottled appearance of the lower extremities (livedo reticularis), and Hollenhorst plaque in the retinal vessels, are suggestive. Laboratory testing may reveal eosinophilia, hypocomplementemia. Urinalysis is generally nonspecific. Patients may suffer minor degrees of azotemia or may progress to irreversible renal failure requiring dialysis.

d. *Renal dysfunction in patients with liver disease.* Although prerenal azotemia is the most common renal syndrome in patients with advanced liver disease, *hepatorenal syndrome (HRS),* or the relentless development of progressive oliguria and azotemia, is the most feared.

(1) HRS is characterized by severe sodium retention unresponsive to volume loading or diuretics.

(2) Although HRS is generally irreversible, barring a recovery of liver function, reports exist of reversal of renal dysfunction with infusions of salt-poor albumin or fresh frozen plasma and peritovenous or portosystemic shunting procedures (including TIPS). Renal function may also improve following successful liver transplantation.

(3) Precise fluid management usually required

    (a) Dietary sodium restriction and diuretics including spironolactone, and paracentesis in hypervolemic patients.

    (b) Colloid infusion should be performed simultaneously with large-volume paracentesis to minimize the risk of hypovolemia and its consequences and may also potentiate the effects of diuretics.

    (c) Recognition of common electrolyte and acid–base disturbances.

        (i) Primary respiratory alkalosis is frequently observed.

        (ii) A mixed acid–base disturbance of respiratory alkalosis and metabolic acidosis often develops in patients who suffer an additional insult, such as sepsis or renal failure.

        (iii) Both potassium depletion and metabolic alkalosis should be avoided because they enhance ammonia synthesis and aggravate hepatic encephalopathy.

VI. DIAGNOSIS

A. History and physical examination

1. History can be helpful because it may establish the chronicity of the problem, reveal underlying previous renal or urinary abnormalities, or identify exposure to nephrotoxic agents or ischemic events.

2. Physical examination may provide diagnostic information. For example, orthostatic hypotension, diminished skin turgor, and dry mucous membranes suggest a diagnosis of prerenal azotemia; bladder distention and prostatic enlargement point to obstructive uropathy.

B. Urine tests

1. Urinalysis

    a. Dipstick test for heme may disclose myoglobinuria or hematuria.

    b. Microscopic analysis of the urine should also be done because formed elements (cells, casts) in the urine can yield information about the nature of the renal failure.

2. Urine chemistries include the FE_{Na}, urinary sodium concentration, and osmolality. Their use was discussed previously.

C. Blood tests.
Serum chemistry studies should be monitored closely to aid in the management of critical acid–base and electrolyte abnormalities. Complete blood count may identify anemia or eosinophilia, pointing to the chronicity of renal failure or the diagnosis of acute interstitial nephritis, respectively. Serologic tests should be ordered only when indicated (e.g., if vasculitis is suspected).

D. Radiography

1. *Renal ultrasound* is safe, quick, and high-yield. It permits the identification and measurement of the kidneys as well as characterization of the parenchyma and collecting systems.

2. *Computed tomography* offers similar benefits, but it should be performed without contrast in the patient with ARF to avoid the added nephrotoxicity of intravenous radiocontrast.

3. *Intravenous pyelography (IVP)* has little role in the evaluation of ARF, because of concerns about radiocontrast-induced nephrotoxicity and because its ability to produce images depends on renal function.

4. *Retrograde pyelography* is reserved for patients in whom there is strong concern for urinary tract obstruction.

5. *Isotopic renal scanning* is a safe and effective method to assess renal perfusion as well as function. It is particularly valuable in the evaluation of suspected renal infarctions or thromboemboli.

E. Renal biopsy. Renal biopsy is reserved for patients who are thought to have parenchymal renal disease. The procedure should be considered when azotemia is of recent onset and unknown cause, when the possibility exists that the patient has a renal disease that may require specialized drug treatment such as steroids or immunosuppressive medication, or when the biopsy may be of prognostic importance.

VII. CONSEQUENCES OF ARF
A. acid–base, fluid and electrolyte disorders
1. Hyperkalemia
   a. This is the most immediately life-threatening electrolyte imbalance encountered in patients with ARF.
   b. Sources of potassium, endogenous or exogenous, need to be identified and regulated if possible. Endogenous sources include tissue breakdown, cell lysis, and hematoma reabsorption. Exogenous sources include diet, intravenous fluids, and medications.
   c. Medications that interfere with potassium regulation, such as nonsteroidal antiinflammatory drugs, heparin, and angiotensin-converting enzyme inhibitors, should be discontinued.
   d. Specific medical interventions besides dietary restriction include diuretics to increase urine flow rate, potassium binding resins, and dialysis if hyperkalemia is severe or refractory to the foregoing interventions (see Chapter 62).
2. Hyponatremia
   a. Acute renal failure markedly limits the kidney's ability to make and excrete free water.
   b. Hypotonic fluids should be avoided or limited to an amount commensurate with the patient's ability to maintain water balance.
3. Metabolic acidosis
   a. Metabolic acidosis that results from reduced tubular hydrogen excretion normally produces hyperchloremic or low anion gap acidosis.
   b. When the GFR is severely impaired, retention of acidic wastes in the extracellular fluid may produce high anion gap acidosis.
   c. Mild metabolic acidosis (serum bicarbonate level no less than 16 mEq/L) does not require therapy.
   d. More marked acidosis requires correction with bicarbonate therapy. Severe acidosis (serum pH less than 7.20) requires therapy with parenteral sodium bicarbonate; however, the patient's extracellular volume status must be monitored carefully because the sodium salt may lead to volume overload, particularly if the patient is oliguric. Acidosis that cannot be treated medically is an indication for dialysis.
4. Volume overload
   a. Despite the reduced tubular reabsorption of sodium that occurs in ATN, the reduction in filtered load of sodium often causes a net state of sodium overload (hypervolemia).
   b. Severely hypervolemic patients (e.g., those with pulmonary vascular congestion) can be managed with aggressive diuretic therapy (i.e., loop diuretics given intravenously in high doses). For patients unable to respond adequately to these agents, dialysis may be indicated.
5. Abnormal calcium and phosphorus metabolism. Phosphate retention in renal failure may lead to perturbation of calcium and phosphorus metabolism. Supplementation of calcium is rarely needed. Dietary phosphate binders may be indicated when hyperphosphatemia is present.
B. Uremia
1. Accumulation of endogenous toxins in the body results in uremia.
2. In general, the syndrome manifests itself when the GFR is reduced to 10 mL per minute or less for at least several days.

3. Uremia may present as vague symptoms such as lethargy, malaise, anorexia, and nausea. Other less subjective manifestations constitute stronger indications for prompt initiation of dialysis, including bleeding diathesis, seizures, coma, and the appearance of a pericardial rub (see Chapter 62).

C. Abnormal drug metabolism
  1. A careful review of all medications is imperative in the care of the patient with ARF. Drugs that are excreted almost entirely by the kidneys will need adjustment in drug dose or dosing intervals.
  2. If dialysis is initiated, adjustments may need to be made to account for clearance with dialysis.

D. Treatment
  1. The *predialysis management* of ARF is outlined in Table 63-5. These simple procedures are applicable to any patient with ARF and may be critical for the patient's survival.
  2. In general, dialysis therapy should be reserved for patients in whom fluid and biochemical parameters cannot be controlled through medical means alone or in patients who develop uremic symptoms. The use of dialysis is discussed in depth in Chapter 64.

E. Prognosis and outcome
  1. Overall, the mortality rate from ARF ranges from 25% to 64%.
  2. Nonoliguria is associated with the best odds of recovery of renal function and approximately half the mortality of oliguric ARF. Recovery of renal function, however, can be expected in most patients who survive ARF, except those who have acute bilateral cortical necrosis or other irreversible forms of parenchymal renal disease.

TABLE 63-5	Predialysis Management of Acute Renal Failure

Fluid balance
  Weigh patient daily
  Monitor input and output
  In volume-depleted patients replace extra cellular fluid with isotonic saline (or bicarbonate)
  In normovolemic or edematous patients, restrict fluid intake (~1,500 mL/d) and sodium intake (<2 g/d)
  Only use diuretics in oliguric patients who are either normovolemic or hypervolemic
Acid/base and electrolyte balance
  Avoid water overload and hyponatremia (restrict free water intake, particularly in oliguric patients)
  Restrict potassium intake (<2 g/d) and treat hyperkalemia
  Supplemental bicarbonate for serum level <15mM
  Use phosphate binders to maintain serum phosphorus <5.0 mg/dL
Drugs
  Avoid nephrotoxins when possible
  Adjust doses of all drugs excreted by the kidneys
  Withhold NSAIDs, ARBs, and CEIs in patients with prerenal azotemia
  Avoid magnesium-containing drugs (antacids, milk of magnesia)
Nutrition
  Restrict protein intake to <0.5 g/kg/d to prevent increased urea synthesis
  Ensure calorie intake to >400 kcal/d to reduce tissue catabolism
Reduction of infectious risks
  Remove indwelling urinary catheter in oliguric, nonobstructed patients
  Strict aseptic technique and rapid removal, when feasible, of
    vascular catheters

ARBs, angiotension receptor blockers; CEIs, converting enzyme inhibitors; NSAIDs, nonsteroidal antiinflammatory drugs.

Selected Readings

Clive DM, Cohen AJ. Acute renal failure in the intensive care unit. In: Irwin RS, Rippe JM, eds. *Irwin and Rippe's intensive care medicine*, 5th ed. Philadelphia: Lippincott Williams & Wilkins, 2003, p. 889.
An extensive review of this subject.

Dubrow A, Flamenbaum W. Acute renal failure associated with myoglobinuria and hemoglobinuria. In: Brenner BM, Lazarus JM, eds. *Acute renal failure*, 2nd ed. New York: Churchill Livingstone, 1988, p. 279.
A good review of pigment-induced ARF.

Eknoyan G. Acute tubulointerstitial nephritis. In: Schrier RW, Gottschalk CW, eds. *Diseases of the kidney*, 6th ed. Boston: Little, Brown, 1997, p. 1249.
A thorough and well-written review of the topic.

Lameire NH, DeVriese AS, Vaholder R. Prevention and nondialytic treatment of acute renal failure. *Curr Opin in Crit Care* 2003;9:481.
An up-to-date review of management of ARF.

Moreau R, Lebrec D. Acute renal failure in patients with cirrhosis: perspectives in the age of MELD. *Hepatology* 2003;37:233.
A current review of a complicated subject.

Murphy SW, Barrett BJ, Parfrey PS. Contrast nephropathy. *J Am Soc Nephrol* 2000;11:177.
A concise overview of the epidemiology, pathophysiology, and prevention of contrast-induced nephrotoxicity.

Murphy SW, Barrett BJ, Parfrey PS. Contrast nephropathy. *J Am Soc Nephrol* 2000;11:177.
A concise overview of the epidemiology, pathophysiology, and prevention of contrast-induced nephrotoxicity.

Nally JV Jr. Acute renal failure in hospitalized patients. *Cleve Clin J Med* 2002;69:569.
Good review with epidemiologic and pathophysiologic overview.

Swan SK, Bennett WM. Nephrotoxic acute renal failure. In: Brenner BM, Lazarus JM, eds. *Acute renal failure*, 3rd ed. New York: Churchill Livingstone, 1993, p. 357.
An in-depth review of various nephrotoxic drugs and the general mechanisms by which they induce ARF.

64 DIALYSIS THERAPY IN THE INTENSIVE CARE SETTING
David M. Clive

I. BACKGROUND
A. Dialysis is used in the treatment of chronic, end-stage renal failure, as well as in acute renal failure (ARF).

B. Most cases of ARF resolve without requiring dialysis. However, intensively ill patients with ARF have a high mortality.

II. HEMODIALYSIS
A. Hemodialysis uses an artificial kidney or dialyzer and a dialysis machine, comprising mechanical blood and dialysate pumps.

    1. Typically, the blood flow rate is ≥ 300 mL/min, and that of dialysate is ≥ 500 mL/min. Dialysate passes through the system once and is discarded, maximizing the gradient favoring transfer of permeant molecules from blood to dialysis.

    2. Membrane composition and surface area also influence clearances, with the newer, higher-porosity membranes achieving high clearances even of solutes with molecular weights exceeding 300 daltons.

    3. Two parameters for determining the "dose" of dialysis given to a patient are as follows:

        a. Kt/V = the volume adjusted fractional clearance of urea, where K is the dialyzer urea clearance, t is time of the dialysis treatment, and V is the volume of distribution of urea.

        b. URR or urea reduction ratio, defined mathematically as [1 $\times$ (post- pre- blood urea nitrogen concentration)] $\times$ 100

        c. These parameters were developed to optimize dialysis prescriptions in patients receiving long-term hemodialysis; their use in ARF is still being defined.

III. HEMOFILTRATION AND HEMODIAFILTRATION
A. Hemofiltration and hemodiafiltration employ extremely high-porosity dialyzers that permit transmembrane filtration of large volumes of plasma ultrafiltrate.

B. They are generally run as continuous procedures and thus collectively are classified as *continuous renal replacement therapy (CRRT)*.

C. Solute movement occurs by convection.

D. In continuous arteriovenous hemofiltration (CAVH), an arteriovenous circuit is used. Blood flow in CAVH is driven entirely by the patient's own hemodynamics, the filtrate being wholly or partially replaced with a physiologic replacement solution.

E. Continuous venovenous hemofiltration is similar to CAVH, but it uses a venovenous circuit in conjunction with a blood pump.

F. Several modifications of hemofiltration are used including:

    1. *Slow continuous ultrafiltration*, in which ultrafiltrate is removed relatively slowly and is not replaced.

    2. *High-volume hemofiltration*, in which a certain portion of the ultrafiltrate is replaced with physiologic crystalloid. High-volume hemofiltration permits substantial convective solute clearance.

    3. *Hemodiafiltration* in which dialysis solution is infused slowly into the CRRT membrane cartridge. This enables solute wastes to be removed both through dialytic and convective transfer and is an extremely effective form of renal replacement therapy in ARF.

IV. PERITONEAL DIALYSIS

A. Peritoneal dialysis, like hemodialysis, affords gradient-driven solute clearance.

B. The gradient may be optimized by using maximal dialysis dwell volumes; 2 to 3 L is typical in an adult patient.

C. Ultrafiltration in peritoneal dialysis is engendered by the osmolality of the dialysate, generally a dextrose-containing solution.

D. Peritoneal dialysis is now rarely used in treating acute renal failure in the intensive care unit.

V. INDICATIONS FOR AND TIMING OF DIALYSIS

A. Absolute indications

1. Serious fluid and electrolyte imbalances, such as hyperkalemia, hypervolemia, and metabolic acidosis, that cannot be managed through more conservative medical means

2. Severe uremic symptoms, namely, uremic pericarditis and severe uremic encephalopathy

3. Life-threatening intoxication with a dialyzable substance

B. Relative indications

1. Minor uremic symptoms, such as nausea and lethargy, bleeding believed to be exacerbated by uremic platelet dysfunction

2. Non–life-threatening chemical imbalances such as moderate hypercalcemia and hypermagnesemia.

VI. TECHNICAL ASPECTS OF HEMODIALYSIS AND HEMOFILTRATION

A. Dialyzers

1. Dialyzers for hemodialysis and hemofiltration are plastic cylinders encasing a bundle of parallel, hollow-fiber capillary tubes through which the blood flows.

2. The dialysate runs countercurrent through the encasing jacket.

3. The two major characteristics to be considered in choosing a dialyzer are, first, the ultrafiltration coefficient (K_{uf}), a function of its aggregate membrane surface area, and, second, permeability. CRRT techniques demand extremely high K_{uf} membranes.

4. *Dialyzer membrane type* is most commonly cellulose acetate or related cellophane-like membranes. The newer polymers, polyacrylonitrile, polymethylmethacrylate, and polysulfone, offer the potential advantage of "biocompatibility," that is, they do not lead to complement activation and cytokine production and are therefore felt by many to improve patient tolerance and outcomes.

B. Dialysates

1. Dialysates are physiologic fluids, that is, their chemical composition is close to that of normal plasma ultrafiltrate.

2. Although there is some variation among solutions, glucose concentrations in dialysates are in the normoglycemic range.

3. Sodium concentration ranges between 135 and 140 mEq/L. In some dialytic protocols, the sodium concentration may be varied as the treatment progresses (sodium "modeling" or "profiling"). This modification helps to control osmolar shift symptoms such as leg cramps, headaches, and dysequilibrium.

4. Potassium content of dialysate solutions is usually prescribed at the time of treatment, particularly in patients receiving short-term dialysis. Potassium removal is an objective of most dialysis treatments. Patients at risk for arrhythmias from hypokalemia, such as those receiving digitalis glycosides, should be dialyzed against a potassium concentration of 3 to 4 mEq/L, unless these patients are floridly hyperkalemic at the outset.

5. The typical concentration of bicarbonate is 30 to 35 mEq/L.

6. The treatment objectives regarding divalent cations in most patients undergoing dialysis are to engender positive calcium balance and modestly negative magnesium balance. Thus, dialysis concentrations of 3.5 and 1.0 mEq/L, respectively, are employed.

7. When dialysis is to be performed in conjunction with CRRT (hemodiafiltration), peritoneal dialysis fluid is generally used. The standard buffer base in peritoneal dialysis stock solutions is lactate; in patients with impaired ability to metabolize lactate, this may pose a problem.

C. Replacement solutions

1. Replacement solutions for CRRT are isotonic, physiologic solutions. Ringer's lactate is popular for this purpose because it contains the full range of major physiologic solutes. Its use is limited in patients with specialized problems such as severe metabolic alkalosis or lactate intolerance. Many centers formulate their own replacement fluids on demand.

D. Anticoagulation

1. Anticoagulation for hemodialysis and CRRT is made necessary by the thrombogenic potential of most dialyzer membranes.

2. Patients who are anticoagulated at baseline or patients with severe bleeding problems may need little or no anticoagulation.

3. Anticoagulation for the typical hemodialysis treatment involves systemic heparinization with a 2,000- to 5,000-U bolus of heparin, followed by an infusion of 1,000 U per hour for the duration of the treatment. The goal is to keep the activated clotting time approximately 50% over baseline.

4. Controlled heparinization protocols must be employed in patients at enhanced risk of bleeding.

    a. "Tight" and "fractional" heparinization protocols target an activated clotting time of 15% and 25% over baseline, respectively.

    b. The safest form of anticoagulation, yet a challenging one to perform, is regional heparinization, in which sodium citrate is infused at low rates into the arterial line of the dialyzer circuit. This technique is used only in the most extreme cases of bleeding risk including:

        (1) Patients with active bleeding or within 14 days of a major operative procedure or intracranial surgery

        (2) Patients within 72 hours of a needle or forceps biopsy of a visceral organ

        (3) Patents with pericarditis

        (4) Patients within 72 hours of a minor surgical procedure.

        (5) Patients anticipated to undergo a major surgical procedure within 8 hours of hemodialysis

5. Anticoagulation in CRRT poses the same basic issues as for hemodialysis, except the anticoagulation, like CRRT, is continuous. The partial thromboplastin time in the arterial line is kept at 50% higher than control. Hemofilters are notoriously prone to thrombosis, probably because of the high protein concentration they develop during the ultrafiltrative process.

E. Angioaccess

1. Angioaccess for acute dialytic procedures in the intensive care unit usually involves the placement of a large-bore, dual-lumen catheter. These are usable as soon as they are inserted, and removable as soon as they are no longer needed, making them ideal for access in most patients with reversible ARF. Catheters may be placed in the femoral, internal jugular, or subclavian location.

2. Femoral venous catheters limit the patient to the supine position and are associated with a high risk of venous thrombosis and infection; they are not recommended for use for more than a few days at a time. Subclavian catheters do not pose the same positional problems as femoral catheters, but they may induce the development of venous stenoses and thromboses. The internal jugular location is preferred for this reason.

3. The basic technique for placing a catheter in any location is to employ sterile technique and local anesthesia. The vessel is cannulated with an introducer needle, and a guide wire is inserted through the needle. The catheter is ultimately passed over the wire (Seldinger technique). Care must be taken to avoid hitting arterial structures. In upper extremity locations, the risk of pneumothorax must be considered. Double-lumen catheters draw from and return into the same vein through different lumina.

4. Vascular access for CRRT is achieved in a similar fashion to that described in the previous paragraph. In CAVH, however, separate arterial and venous catheters are used.

5. In long-term maintenance hemodialysis, fistulas or arteriovenous grafts are the accesses of choice. They cannot be accessed as soon as they are implanted, obviating their use in patients with ARF.

VII. TECHNICAL ASPECTS OF PERITONEAL DIALYSIS

A. Peritoneal dialysates

1. Peritoneal dialysates are less diversified than hemodialysis solutions. The major therapeutic consideration is choosing the dextrose concentration of the dialysate, because this is the method for controlling ultrafiltration.

2. Three strengths are in common use: 1.5%, 2.5%, and 4.25% dextrose. The choice depends on the particular patient's ability to "clear fluid" during peritoneal dialysis; 4.25% dialysate is appropriate for clinically fluid overloaded patients with ARF. Diabetic patients undergoing peritoneal dialysis must have serum glucose concentrations followed closely.

B. Peritoneal access

1. Peritoneal access can be established on an emergency basis using a rigid catheter passed over a stylet. The patient's urinary bladder must be emptied to avoid perforation, because the access site is in the midline between the umbilicus and the symphysis pubis. More electively, soft, Dacron-cuffed catheters (e.g., Tenckhoff catheters) are placed surgically.

VIII. DOSE OF DIALYSIS

A. Adequacy of dialysis appears to affect outcomes in ARF, just as it does in chronic renal failure. Although the specific needs of patients with ARF have not yet been elucidated, it should be assumed they are at least equal to those of patients with chronic renal failure. This means a Kt/V greater than or equal to 1.2 or a URR greater than or equal to 70%.

IX. CONTINUOUS VERSUS INTERMITTENT DIALYSIS THERAPY

A. Nephrologists generally believe that CRRT offers advantages over intermittent hemodialysis in the treatment of ARF.

1. CRRT is better tolerated hemodynamically.

2. CRRT treatments may be modified easily from minute to minute and can be tailored to match a patient's changing daily fluid input.

3. On the down side, CRRT is fairly labor intensive. As already mentioned, it necessitates higher anticoagulation exposure. Further, outcome studies have yet to prove any benefit of CRRT over intermittent treatment.

4. The choice should be made by the physician.

X. DISCONTINUATION OF DIALYSIS

A. Most patients with ARF become dialysis independent within several weeks. Harbingers of renal recovery include:

1. Increase in the urine output in a previously oliguric patient, although the correlation between urine output and glomerular filtration rate is poor.

2. A spontaneously falling serum creatinine level or one that fails to rise between treatments.

B. Discontinuation of dialysis may also be contemplated under less fortunate circumstances, that is, in patients with persistent renal failure who languish or fail despite intensive medical care. Such decisions should reflect close communication between patients (or their representatives) and physicians.

XI. COMPLICATIONS OF DIALYSIS

A. Hemodialysis and CRRT

1. Cardiovascular complications occur more frequently with hemodialysis than with the other blood purification techniques. Hypotension is the most common complication. Its pathophysiology is multifactorial.

2. Hypotension of hemodialysis can be controlled or prevented by cooling of dialysate, which promotes vasoconstriction and improved myocardial contractility and careful volumetric control of ultrafiltration.

3. *Dysequilibrium syndrome* refers to the series of neurologic symptoms, most commonly dizziness and headache, caused by transcerebral fluid movement after dialysis. These fluxes, which result from a transient disparity in solute concentration between the cerebrospinal fluid and the vascular space, can be attenuated by limiting the rate of solute clearance during a patient's first dialyses.

4. Hypoxemia occurs commonly. It is attributed to alveolar hypoventilation and intrapulmonary leukostasis triggered by dialysis membranes. This is rarely a problem, except for patients with significant cardiopulmonary disease.

5. Technical errors such as air embolism and contamination of blood or dialysate lines are unusual when adequate precautions are observed.

6. Bleeding is the most significant problem with CRRT and mandates a cautious approach to anticoagulation, as already noted.

B. Peritoneal dialysis

1. Infections

   a. Peritonitis is the predominant complication of therapy. These infections arise from introduction of pathogens into the dialysis system during dialysate exchanges.

   b. Tunnel infections arise at the catheter exit site and may track subcutaneously into the peritoneum.

   c. The most commonly isolated pathogens are *Staphylococcus aureus* and *S. epidermidis*. Gram-negative bacteria and fungi are occasionally culpable.

   d. When a patient is suspected of having peritonitis associated with peritoneal dialysis, it is recommended to begin therapy with broad-spectrum antimicrobial coverage, to be narrowed once culture reports are available.

Selected Readings

Coladonato JA, Griffith TF, Owen WF Jr. Dialysis therapy in the intensive care setting. In: Irwin RS, Rippe JM, eds. *Irwin and Rippe's intensive care medicine*, 5th ed. Philadelphia: Lippincott Williams & Wilkins, 2003, p.939.
Source material for this chapter.

Daugirdas JT. Dialysis hypotension: a hemodynamic analysis. *Kidney Int* 1991;39:233.
An analysis of the pathophysiology of hemodynamic instability during hemodialysis.

Himmelfarb J, Hakim RM. The use of biocompatible dialysis membranes in acute renal failure. *Adv Ren Replace Ther* 1997;4:72.
Explores the concept of biocompatibility of dialysis membranes and their impact on outcomes in cases of dialysis-dependent ARF.

Kellum JA, Mehta RL, Angus DC, et al. The first international consensus conference on continuous renal replacement therapy. *Kidney Int* 2002;62:1855.
A summary of the current collective experience with CRRT.

Lohr JW, Schwab SJ. Minimizing hemorrhagic complications in dialysis patients. *J Am Soc Nephrol* 1991;2:961.
A thorough discussion of principles of safe anticoagulation in renal replacement therapy.

Pastan S, Bailey J. Dialysis therapy. *N Engl J Med* 1998;338:1428.
A good review of the fundamentals of hemodialysis and peritoneal dialysis.

Ronco C, Bellomo R. Acute renal failure and multiple organ dysfunction in the ICU: from renal replacement therapy (RRT) to multiple organ support therapy (MOST). *Int J Artif Organs* 2002; 25:733.

Tonelli M, Manns B, Feller-Kipman D. Acute renal failure in the intensive care unit: a systematic review of the impact of dialytic modality on mortality and renal recovery. *Am J Kid Dis* 2002;40:875.
The preceding two articles provide excellent overviews of the use of CRRT in the intensive care unit setting.

Infectious Disease Problems in the Intensive Care Unit

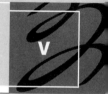

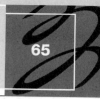

V

APPROACH TO FEVER IN THE INTENSIVE CARE PATIENT

Catherine Yu and Richard H. Glew

65

I. GENERAL PRINCIPLES. Fever is a common problem in the intensive care unit (ICU). Noninfectious and infectious causes of fever and a diagnostic framework for evaluation are discussed.

II. PATHOPHYSIOLOGY OF FEVER
   A. Principal mediator is IL-1. Others such as TNF, IL-6 are similar effectors of fever.
   B. Cytokines interact with receptors in the anterior hypothalamic thermoregulatory area, which releases prostaglandins, resetting the thermoregulatory set point.
   C. Prostaglandins coordinate shivering and peripheral vasoconstriction.

III. MEASUREMENT AND FEVER PATTERNS
   A. Body temperature varies diurnally.
   B. The febrile response may be blunted or even absent in:
      1. Elderly patients
      2. Azotemia
      3. Congestive heart failure
      4. Patients receiving antipyretics or corticosteroids
   C. Fever patterns generally are not helpful in suggesting or establishing specific diagnoses.
      1. Rigors may be seen in bacterial infections but also in viral infections, drug reactions, other inflammatory conditions, and lymphoma.

IV. NONINFECTIOUS CAUSES OF FEVER. Although acute bacterial infections are among the most common and serious causes of fever, fever can be a major symptom with:
   A. Acute vasculitis
   B. Subarachnoid hemorrhage
   C. Dissection of an aortic aneurysm
   D. Mesenteric ischemia
   E. Heat stroke
   F. Hyperthyroidism
   G. Adrenal insufficiency
   H. Malignant hyperpyrexia
   I. Nonanaesthetic agents, such as phenothiazines
   J. Acute alcohol withdrawal
   K. Seizures.
   L. Deep vein thrombosis (DVT) or pulmonary embolism (PE)
   M. Reactions to medications and blood products
   N. Malignant diseases

V. INFECTIOUS CAUSES OF FEVER
   A. The most common sources of bacterial infection include the urinary tract, respiratory tract, and wounds.
   B. Secondary bacteremia can complicate infection in these sites but can also develop as a consequence of vascular invasion.
   C. The gastrointestinal tract can serve as the source for severe infections.
      1. Acute acalculous cholecystitis may occur after surgery and severe trauma.
      2. *Clostridium difficile* colitis
      3. Mesenteric ischemia
      4. Intraabdominal abscess.

371

VI. DIAGNOSIS. Fever in patients in the ICU warrants immediate assessment because the organisms common in nosocomial infections, *Staphylococcus aureus,* gram-negative bacilli, and fungi, may cause necrotizing destruction of tissue and blood infections.

  A. History-taking:
    1. A thorough history should be obtained.
    2. The patient, hospital chart, and caregivers should be reexamined for:
      a. relevant antecedent problems
      b. duration of vascular cannulation
      c. quantity and purulence of sputum or wound drainage
      d. changes in skin condition
      e. apparent abdominal or musculoskeletal pain or tenderness
      f. difficulty in handling respiratory secretions and food
      g. changes in ventilator support requirements
  B. Physical examination should be thorough because it may provide clues to the diagnosis.
    1. Skin examination may demonstrate findings suggestive of:
      a. drug reaction
      b. vasculitis
      c. endocarditis
    2. Intravascular line sites should be inspected.
    3. Spreading erythema, warmth, and tenderness suggests
      a. cellulitis of an extremity
      b. deep venous phlebitis
      c. pyarthrosis
      d. gout
    4. Wound dressings should be removed and examined after the first 24 hours postoperatively.
    5. Fundoscopic lesions may suggest disseminated candidiasis.
    6. Purulent sinusitis can occur in the nasally or orally intubated patient and may have a paucity of symptoms.
    7. Oral lesions may be indicative of recrudescent herpetic stomatitis.
    8. Examination of the lungs can be difficult in the ICU patient.
      a. More sensitive (though nonspecific) indicators of pneumonia:
        i. chest radiography (CXR)
        ii. unexplained deterioration in arterial oxygenation
    9. Unfortunately, pulmonary infiltrates and arterial hypoxemia also can be seen with:
      a. congestive heart failure
      b. acute respiratory distress syndrome
      c. reactions to medications
      d. pulmonary hemorrhage
   10. Cardiac examination
      a. pericardial friction rub resulting from Dressler syndrome
      b. new or changing murmur possibly caused by endocarditis
   11. Abdominal findings
      a. Can be diminished in patients who are elderly, with altered sensorium, or receiving potent analgesics
      b. May be confoundingly positive in the patient with recent surgery
   12. Examination of the genitals and rectum
      a. epididymitits
      b. prostatitis
      c. prostatic abscess
      d. perirectal abscess

VII. LABORATORY STUDIES. Initial laboratory evaluation of fever in the ICU patient should include:
  A. urinalysis and culture
  B. two blood cultures (each obtained from a separate venipuncture or intravascular catheter)

C. CXR
D. sputum Gram stain and culture
   1. Culture of sputum without concomitant Gram stain examination is virtually worthless.
      a. Most ICU patients exhibit pharyngeal colonization with gram-negative bacilli within a few days of hospitalization.
         (1) Culture alone cannot distinguish colonization from infection.
         (2) Other available laboratory evaluations, such as Gram stain, can help to distinguish these two by the absence or presence of polymorphonuclear cells (PMNs) and their abundance. The presence of many PMNs is suggestive of infection or inflammation.
         (3) Clinical features such as changes in ventilatory support, pressor support, leukocyte count, or new fevers also aid in determining whether a culture growth is infection or colonization.
E. All abnormal fluid collections should be sampled for microscopic and chemical analysis and culture.
F. Meningitis is an uncommon nosocomial infection, except in cases of head trauma, neurosurgery, or high-grade bacteremia.
   1. Lumbar puncture should be considered, after soft tissue mass is excluded by noncontrast CT, in
      a. sudden, unexplained change in mental status in the febrile ICU patient
      b. recent neurosurgery or head trauma in a febrile patient
      c. when mental status is difficult to evaluate
G. Symptomatic complaints or physical findings referable to the
   1. liver chemistry studies
   2. serum amylase
   3. abdominal diagnostic imaging

VIII. APPROACH TO INITIAL PRESUMPTIVE ANTIBIOTIC THERAPY. In the acutely ill, unstable patient in the ICU, it may be necessary to begin empiric broad-spectrum antibiotic therapy before an infectious cause is established.
A. Positive cultures
   1. may permit narrowing of the spectrum of antibiotic coverage
   2. additional organisms may need to be covered with added antimicrobial therapy
B. Negative cultures in a patient who has not improved yet is stable on broad-spectrum therapy may indicate that antibiotics could be discontinued and the patient reevaluated.
C. Negative cultures, laboratory findings, and radiologic examinations in a febrile patient who is unimproved or worsened may be a clue to disseminated fungal infection.
D. Patients with intravascular lines and suspected bacteremia should have blood cultures obtained and their lines removed if possible.
E. Empiric antibiotic therapy for the febrile ICU patient should be initiated according to generally accepted principles based on likely pathogens followed by culture-directed therapy.
   1. Such guidelines must be interpreted in light of the types of organisms and patterns of drug resistance prevalent in the specific institution.
   2. Definitive antibiotic therapy is determined by review of the final microbiologic data with identification of the infecting microorganism and its antibiotic susceptibilities.

Selected Readings
Arbo MJ, Fine MJ, Hanusa BH, et al. Fever of nosocomial origin: etiology, risk factors, and outcomes. *Am J Med* 1993;95:505.
   This study looked at 100 patients and found that many had causes of fever other than infection.

Clarke DE, Kimelman J, Raffin TA. The evaluation of fever in the intensive care unit. *Chest* 1991;100:213.
   Review of the fever workup.

Mackowiak PA, Bartlett JG, Bordon EC, et al. Concepts of fever: recent advances and lingering dogma. *Clin Infect Dis* 1997;25:119.

Transcript of a symposium that gives details regarding pathophysiology as well as reviewing causes of fever in selected groups of patients.

Mackowiak PA, LeMaistre CF. Drug fever a critical appraisal of conventional concepts. *Ann Intern Med* 1987;106:728.
Drug fever is common in hospitalized patients, and the diagnosis may be elusive.

Musher DM, Faintein V, Young EJ, et al. Fever patterns: their lack of clinical significance. *Arch Intern Med* 1979;139:1225.
Fever patterns may not be useful in narrowing the differential diagnosis.

Sayer CB, Breder CD. The neurologic basis of fever. *N Engl J Med* 1994;330:1880.
Review of the pathophysiology of fever.

USE OF ANTIMICROBIALS IN THE TREATMENT OF INFECTION IN THE CRITICALLY ILL PATIENT   66

Asimah Quyyum, Richard H. Glew, and Jennifer S. Daly

I. GENERAL PRINCIPLES. This chapter reviews antimicrobial agents used in the treatment of bacterial and fungal infections, outlining important considerations for using each of the agents.

II. β-LACTAM AND RELATED AGENTS

A. Penicillin G and ampicillin
1. Highly active against streptococci, meningococci, and most mouth anaerobes.
2. Both are used with gentamicin for bactericidal killing to treat enterococcal endocarditis (other than cases due to penicillin-resistant isolates of *Enterococcus faecium*).
3. Ampicillin should not be relied on for gram-negative coverage in the intensive care unit (ICU).

B. Penicillinase-resistant semisynthetic penicillins: nafcillin and oxacillin
1. Excellent *in vitro* activity against most isolates of *Staphylococcus aureus*, except methicillin-resistant *S. aureus* (MRSA).
2. Hepatic clearance, no adjustment in dose is necessary in patients with renal insufficiency (Table 66-1)

C. Anti-gram-negative penicillins: piperacillin and mezlocillin
1. Used in combination with an aminoglycoside to treat infection with gram-negative bacteria including *Pseudomonas aeruginosa*.

D. β-Lactam/β-lactamase inhibitor combinations: Ampicillin-sulbactam, ticarcillin-clavulanate, and piperacillin-tazobactam
1. Active against bacteria susceptible to the β-lactam component of the combination and against β-lactamase–producing strains of *S. aureus*, *Bacteroides* sp., *Hemophilus influenzae*, and enteric gram-negative bacilli.
2. These combinations are ineffective against many isolates of *P. aeruginosa*, *Enterobacter cloacae*, *Citrobacter freundii*, and *Serratia marcescens*.

E. First-generation cephalosporin: cefazolin
1. Active against *S. aureus* but not against enterococci, *Listeria monocytogenes*, MRSA, and many coagulase-negative staphylococci.
2. Community-acquired strains of *Escherichia coli*, *Proteus mirabilis*, and *Klebsiella pneumoniae* often are susceptible.
3. Nosocomial isolates of Enterobacteriaceae frequently are resistant.

F. Second-generation cephalosporins: cefotetan and cefoxitin
1. Activity against hospital-acquired gram-negative bacilli is limited. Not recommended for use in the ICU.
2. Moderately good activity *in vitro* against anaerobes, including a majority of *Bacteroides fragilis* isolates.

G. Third-generation cephalosporins: ceftriaxone and cefotaxime
1. Exhibit an expanded spectrum and increased potency against gram-negative organisms compared with older cephalosporins.
2. Should not be used to treat *P. aeruginosa*.

H. Antipseudomonal cephalosporins: ceftazidime and cefepime
1. More potent against *P. aeruginosa* than other cephalosporins
2. Add an aminoglycoside to treat *P. aeruginosa* to avoid development of resistance during therapy

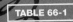

TABLE 66-1	Adjustment of Dosing Required in Patients with Renal Insufficiency

β-Lactam and related agents
Penicillin G
Ampicillin
Piperacillin
Mezlocillin
Ampicillin-Sulbactam
Ticarcillin-Clavulanate
Piperacillin-Tazobactam
Cefazolin
Cefotetan
Cefoxitin
Cefotaxime
Ceftazidime
Cefepime
Imipenem
Ertapenem
Meropenem
Aztreonam

Aminoglycosides
Gentamicin
Tobramycin
Amikacin

Fluoroquinolones
Levofloxacin
Ciprofloxacin

Miscellaneous agents
Trimethoprim-Sulfamethoxazole[a]
Vancomycin
Clarithromycin
Quinupristin/Dalfopristin
Daptomycin

Antifungal agents
Fluconazole
Voriconazole[a]

Antiviral agents
Acylovir
Valacyclovir
Ganciclovir
Valganciclovir

[a]try to avoid in patients with creatinine clearance less than 10 mL/min

3. In ICU patients, the cephalosporins should be employed, at least initially, at maximal doses and frequencies.
I. **Carbapenems: imipenem, ertapenem and meropenem**
   1. Exhibit the broadest spectrum (including anaerobes) of available β-lactams.
   2. Coadministration of an aminoglycoside for treatment of highly resistant gram-negative bacilli is recommended.

J. Monobactam: aztreonam

1. Reserve for treatment of gram-negative infections in penicillin allergic patients.
2. Spectrum and potency against gram-negative bacteria is similar to those of the third-generation cephalosporins
3. Aztreonam has no antibacterial activity against gram-positive or anaerobic bacteria.

III. AMINOGLYCOSIDES, FLUOROQUINOLONES AND TRIMETHOPRIM-SULFAMETHOXAZOLE

A. Aminoglycosides

1. Provide the broadest range of potent bactericidal antibiotic activity against gram-negative bacilli, particularly multiply resistant enteric gram-negative bacilli species.
2. Used in the ICU in combination with an extended spectrum beta-lactam antibiotic for gram negative bacteria
3. Gentamicin is used in combination with ampicillin, penicillin, or vancomycin for treatment of endocarditis caused by enterococci or viridans group streptococci.

B. Fluoroquinolones

1. Broad-spectrum agents highly active against enteric gram-negative bacilli, including enteric pathogens such as *Campylobacter, Salmonella,* and *Shigella* species as well as *H. influenzae.*
2. Indicated in the treatment of complicated urinary tract infections, prostatitis, bacterial diarrhea of diverse causes, invasive (malignant) external otitis, gram-negative bacterial pneumonia, and intraabdominal and intrapelvic infections (in combination with antianaerobic agents).
3. Therapy of gram-negative bacteria such as *P. aeruginosa* and *Acinetobacter* species with fluoroquinolones may induce resistance
4. Streptococci exhibit poor susceptibility in general to quinolones, although levofloxacin and newer compounds have potency against penicillin-resistant *Streptococcus pneumoniae.*
5. Resistance to fluoroquinolones is becoming increasingly common among *S. aureus* isolates, especially MRSA, and among gram-negative bacilli, notably *P. aeruginosa.*

C. Trimethoprim-sulfamethoxazole

1. Trimethoprim-sulfamethoxazole (cotrimoxazole) can be used in the therapy of gram-negative infections including β-lactam–resistant nosocomial bacteria.
2. Cotrimoxazole is the agent of choice in the treatment of *Pneumocystis carinii* pneumonia

IV. ANTI GRAM-POSITIVE AGENTS

A. Vancomycin

1. Used in the therapy of infections due to MRSA and infections due to coagulase-negative staphylococci, especially infection involving prosthetic material and endovascular infections in patients undergoing long-term hemodialysis.
2. Although most enterococci are inhibited by low concentrations of vancomycin, bactericidal killing of these organisms requires the addition of an aminoglycoside (e.g., gentamicin).
3. Resistance to vancomycin is an emerging problem, particularly in strains of *E. faecium* and *S. aureus.*
4. Oral vancomycin (not absorbed from the gastrointestinal tract) is employed to treat only antibiotic-associated colitis caused by *Clostridium difficile.* However, oral metronidazole is preferred for this infection to reduce the selective pressure toward vancomycin-resistant enterococci.

B. Quinupristin/dalfopristin (Synercid)

1. Quinupristin/dalfopristin is a new IV streptogramin antibiotic approved for treatment of infections due to *E. faecium,* including vancomycin-resistant enterococcus (VRE), and complicated skin and soft tissue infections due to *S. aureus.* Use of this drug should be guided by results of laboratory susceptibility testing.
2. A central line for administration is preferred since Quinupristin/dalfopristin may cause local reactions at the infusion site.

C. Oxazolidinones: linezolid

1. Bacteriostatic against MRSA, vancomycin-resistant *S. aureus* (VRSA), VRE and bactericidal against penicillin resistant *S. pneumoniae*.
2. Reserved for treatment of vancomycin or beta-lactam–resistant organisms.
3. Reversible thrombocytopenia may occur if treatment is given longer than 14 days.

D. Cyclic lipopeptide agent: Daptomycin

1. Cyclic lipopeptide agent, concentration-dependent bactericidal activity occurs *in vitro* against a broad spectrum of gram-positive pathogens including MRSA, VRSA, VRE, and penicillin resistant *Streptococcus pneumoniae* (PRSP) causing complicated skin wound, abscesses or infected ulcers, resistant to oxacillin, vancomycin, and linezolid.
2. Dosage approved for use (4 mg/kg) may not be adequate to treat bacteremia or endocarditis.
3. Low frequency of spontaneous development of *in vitro* resistance

V. ANTIANAEROBIC AGENTS

A. Metronidazole

1. Highly active against obligate anaerobes
2. Oral form is completely absorbed, but IV preparation is used in critically ill patients where gastrointestinal absorption may be a limiting factor.
3. Dosages should be reduced in patients with severe hepatic insufficiency.

B. Clindamycin

1. It is active *in vitro* against many gram-positive cocci and anaerobes.
2. It is used to treat bacterial infections of the head, neck, and lungs and pleural space.
3. Use of clindamycin in addition to penicillin in the treatment of necrotizing fasciitis due to β-hemolytic streptococci is recommended, in theory, because of its activity against nondividing organisms present in extremely high inoculum in tissue and by inhibition of protein synthesis decreasing toxin production.

C. Macrolides

1. Azithromycin (or erythromycin) is used to treat pneumonia in the ICU in combination with a cephalosporin or in cases known to be due to nonpyogenic organisms such as *Mycoplasma pneunoniae*, *Chlamydia pneumoniae*, and *Legionella* species.
2. These agents are not usually used as first-line agents for treatment of gram-positive infections in the ICU, although they are used as a substitute for penicillin for oral therapy in β-lactam allergic patients.

VI. ANTI FUNGAL AGENTS

A. Amphotericin B deoxycholate and lipid preparations of amphotericin

1. Amphotericin B in one of its forms is the drug of choice for life-threatening, invasive, or systemic fungal infections.
2. *Candida albicans* generally is susceptible to amphotericin B and to imidazoles. Non-*albicans* species of *Candida* often are less susceptible, and variable activity is evident against species of *Aspergillus* and Zygomycetes species, *Pseudallescheria boydii*, and *Fusarium* species.
3. The combination of amphotericin B plus flucytosine is synergistic against *Candida* species and *Cryptococcus neoformans*.
4. Infections caused by less susceptible fungi (e.g., *Aspergillus*, Zygomycetes species [Mucor], and *Coccidioides immitis*) warrant treatment with higher doses than infections with *Candida* species.
5. Preparations of amphotericin B complexed with cholesteryl sulfate, liposomal vesicles containing phosphatidylcholine distearoylphosphatidylglycerol and cholesterol (AmBisome), a bilayered lipid membrane (Abelcet), and a colloidal dispersion (Amphocil) are more expensive than Ampho B deoxycholate but are advantageous in patients with renal insufficiency that worsens during treatment with amphotericin B (Table 66-2).

B. Fluconazole

1. Available for intravenous and oral use and exhibits good activity *in vitro* against *Candida* species and *Cryptococcus neoformans*.

TABLE 66-2	No Adjustment in Dosing Recommended for Most Patients with Renal Insufficiency
Nafcillin	
Oxacillin	
Ceftriaxone	
Linezolid	
Metronidazole	
Clindamycin	
Moxifloxacin	
Azithromycin	
Erythromycin	
Amphotericin B Deoxycholate	
Lipid preparations of Amphotericin	
Caspofungin	

2. Serum levels are comparable with oral or parenteral administration.
3. Penetrates well into bodily fluids, including cerebrospinal fluid.
4. It inhibits the metabolism and potentiates the effects of warfarin, phenytoin, cyclosporine, tacrolimus, and oral hypoglycemic agents.

C. Voriconazole

1. Drug of choice for invasive aspergillosis infection and refractory infections with *Pseudallesheria/Scedosporium* and *Fusarium species.*
2. Used in fluconazole-resistant species of *C. albicans, C. kruseii,* and strains of *C. glabrata* that are inherently fluconazole resistant.
3. Extensively metabolized by the CYP2C9 and CYP3A4 hepatic enzymes.
4. It is available in IV and PO formulations with excellent tissue penetration.
5. In contrast to Amphotericin B, it is safe in renal failure and has no infusion-related effects.

D. Echinocandins: Caspofungin

1. Used to treat candidemia and other deep infections due to *Candida* species.
2. Has not been studied for initial treatment of *Candida* endocarditis, osteomyelitis, or meningitis
3. Used to treat invasive *Aspergillus fumigatus* infections in patients intolerant or refractory to other antifungals.

VII. ANTIVIRAL AGENTS

A. Acylovir and Valacyclovir

1. Acyclovir is used to treat encephalitis and *Herpes simplex* and *Herpes zoster* (chicken pox) and is available for oral use and as an IV preparation.
2. Valacyclovir, a prodrug for acyclovir, is used orally, is more completely absorbed than acyclovir, and is rapidly hydrolyzed to acyclovir.

B. Ganciclovir and Valganciclovir

1. Ganciclovir is effective in the prophylaxis and treatment of cytomegalovirus (CMV)
2. Valganciclovir is a prodrug for ganciclovir and is the preferred oral form for continuing therapy after IV ganciclovir.

Selected Readings

Balfour HH. Antiviral drugs. *N Engl J Med* 1999;340:1255.
  Use of oral and IV antivirals.

Bisno AL, Steven DL. Streptococcal infections of skin and soft tissues. *N Engl J Med* 1996;334:240.
  Illustrates the use of both clindamycin and a β-lactam to treat necrotizing streptococcal infections

Campbell GDJ, Silberman R. Drug resistant *Streptococcus pneumoniae*. *Clin Infect Dis* 1998;26:1188.
This reference discusses rational for set points for laboratory testing and use on the antibiotics to treat different sites of infection with S. pneumoniae.

Carpenter CF, Chambers HF. Daptomycin: another novel agent for treating infections due to drug-resistant gram-positive pathogens. *Clin Infect Dis* 2004; 38:994.
Review of the newest agent effective against gram-positive organisms.

Denning DW. Echinocandin antifungal drugs. *Lancet* 2003;362:1142.
Update on caspofungin and other echinocandins in development.

Hellinger WC, Brewer NS. Carbapenems and monobactams: imipenem, meropenem, and aztreonam. *Mayo Clin Proc* 1999;74:420.
Good review of the uses and toxicity of these agents.

Marshall FW, Blair JE. The cephalosporins. *Mayo Clin Proc* 1999;74:187.
Overview of these agents.

Patel R. Antifungal agents. Part I. Amphotericin B preparations and flucytosine. *Mayo Clin Proc* 1998;73:1205.
Good review of the amphotericin preparations and their biochemistry and use.

Smith TL, et al. Emergence of vancomyin resistance in *Staphylococcus aureus*. *N Engl J Med* 1999;340:493.
Landmark article on vancomycin-resistant Staphylococci.

BACTERIAL MENINGITIS
Alan L. Rothman

I. GENERAL PRINCIPLES
A. Definition
1. The term *bacterial meningitis* applies to the presence of bacteria in the cerebro-spinal fluid (CSF) with concomitant meningeal inflammation.
   a. Symptoms and signs (see later) are typically related to meningeal irritation.
   b. Altered neurologic function is related to metabolic and circulatory distur-bances more than to direct bacterial invasion of brain tissue.
B. Epidemiology
1. Bacterial meningitis is a rare but serious infection. The overall incidence in the United States is in the range of 2.0 to 2.5 cases per 100,000 population per year but is higher in the very young (<2 years of age) and the elderly.
C. Prognosis
1. Mortality from bacterial meningitis ranges from 10% to 50%, depending on the pathogen; intensive care unit admission is recommended.
2. Independent predictors of outcome: hypotension, alteration in consciousness, and seizures.
   a. Favorable outcome in 91% of patients with none of these present.
   b. Favorable outcome in 43% of patients with two or more present.

II. ETIOLOGY
A. Community-acquired meningitis
1. *Streptococcus pneumoniae* the most common pathogen.
2. *Neisseria meningitidis* is second most common overall, particularly in older children and young adults, and associated with outbreaks.
3. *Haemophilus influenzae* formerly was most common in young children; its incidence has declined more than 90% since introduction of routine infant im-munization.
4. *Listeria monocytogenes* is most often a cause in compromised hosts: infants (age <3 months), older adults (age >50 years), and patients with alcoholism, immunosuppression, or general debility.
B. Nosocomial meningitis. Usually caused by skin or hospital flora (e.g., Staphylo-cocci, aerobic gram-negative bacilli).

III. PATHOGENESIS
A. Bacterial entry via hematogenous route, except after head trauma or neurosurgery.
B. Bacteria that commonly cause meningitis escape host defenses at mucosa and in the blood.
C. Interactions between bacterial components and cells in the brain and meninges lead to infiltration of leukocytes, altered cerebral blood flow, and disruption of cerebral function.

IV. DIAGNOSIS. Clinical evaluation should be compressed to avoid treatment delays. the major objectives are to recognize the diagnosis and define likely pathogen.
A. History
1. Acute onset of fever with headache, photophobia, or stiff neck suggest bacterial meningitis, but consider meningitis in any patient with altered consciousness.

2. Alcohol use, previous head trauma, recent use of antibiotics, ill contacts, and immunosuppression influence the risk for bacterial meningitis, the likely etiology, or the yield of diagnostic tests.

B. Physical examination

1. Nuchal rigidity and altered consciousness suggest meningitis; however, their absence does not exclude the diagnosis.
2. Papilledema or focal neurologic deficits indicate that lumbar puncture should be delayed until a mass lesion is excluded.
3. Petechiae suggest meningococcal meningitis but can be seen in other infections.

C. Laboratory studies

1. Blood
   a. Most tests of limited value for diagnosis of bacterial meningitis but help to identify complications.
   b. Blood cultures are positive in 30% to 80% of patients with community-acquired infection and should be collected before initiation of antibacterial therapy.
2. Cerebrospinal fluid
   a. Lumbar puncture (LP) should be performed promptly except when there is suggestion of a mass lesion. Cerebrospinal fluid (CSF) examination is valuable for diagnosis and management.
   b. CSF white blood cell count typically greater than 1,000 cells/mm^3.
   c. Neutrophils predominate in most cases, often greater than 85% of cells present.
   d. CSF glucose less than 20 mg/dL is strong indication of bacterial infection, but up to 40% of patients have normal values.
   e. CSF protein usually greater than 100 mg/dL.
   f. CSF Gram stain positive in 75% or more of community-acquired infections in the absence of prior antibacterial therapy.
   g. Routine bacterial culture of CSF positive in more than 90% of patients with community-acquired infection.
      (1) Yield is lower when antibacterial drugs given before LP.
      (2) Drug susceptibility should be tested for all CSF isolates.
   h. Stains and cultures for fungi or mycobacteria are of low yield. Reserve for patients with immunosuppression, history suggesting chronic meningitis, or lymphocytic CSF pleocytosis with negative routine culture.

D. Radiologic studies

1. Cranial computed tomography and magnetic resonance imaging normal in 76% of patients with suspected meningitis.
   a. Routine imaging before LP not supported by literature.
   b. Can reserve for patients with focal neurologic deficits or other reason to suspect intracranial mass lesion.

V. TREATMENT

A. Antibacterial therapy

1. General principles
   a. Start empiric therapy as soon as possible after the diagnosis is suspected.
      (1) A brief delay for collection of blood cultures and CSF is acceptable. However, antimicrobial therapy should optimally be started within 30 minutes of the initial evaluation.
      (2) If LP to be delayed further, start therapy as soon as blood cultures obtained.
   b. Continue high-dose therapy for full course (discussed later).
   c. Check on local patterns of antimicrobial resistance.
2. Empiric therapy
   a. Community-acquired meningitis
      (1) Ceftriaxone (usual adult dose, 2 g IV every 12 hours) or cefotaxime (usual adult dose, 2 g IV every 6 hours) the mainstay of empiric therapy.
         i. Active against *S. pneumoniae*, *N. meningitidis*, and *H. influenzae*.
      (2) Add vancomycin (usual adult dose, 1 g IV every 12 hours) if CSF Gram stain shows gram-positive cocci or is negative.
         i. Improved coverage for drug-resistant *S. pneumoniae*.

(3) Add ampicillin (usual adult dose, 2 g IV every 4 hours) for patients younger than 3 months or older than 50 years; those with immunosuppression, alcoholism, or debilitation; or if CSF Gram stain shows gram-positive bacilli.
  i. Coverage for *L. monocytogenes*.
  b. Postneurosurgical meningitis
    i. Vancomycin (usual adult dose, 1 g IV every 12 hours) plus ceftazidime (usual adult dose, 2 g IV every 8 hours)
  c. Patients with drug allergies
    (1) Note: Few good alternatives available; use standard regimen unless documented serious cephalosporin intolerance.
    (2) Vancomycin (for *S. pneumoniae*) plus trimethoprim-sulfamethoxazole (for *L. monocytogenes* and *N. meningitidis*).
  3. Therapy after results of CSF culture
    a. Target therapy based on the identity and susceptibility of the organism.
    b. *S. pneumoniae* infections:
      (1) Fully susceptible strains (ceftriaxone MIC ≤0.5 mg/L): ceftriaxone as a single agent.
      (2) Intermediately resistant strains (ceftriaxone MIC >0.5 and ≤2.0 mg/L): ceftriaxone plus either vancomycin or rifampin.
      (3) Fully resistant strains (ceftriaxone MIC >2.0 mg/L): ceftriaxone plus vancomycin plus rifampin.
        i. Note: optimal therapy is not well defined.
      (4) Repeat LP for infection with intermediately or fully resistant strains; consult an infectious diseases specialist if CSF culture remains positive.
  4. Duration of therapy
    a. *N. meningitidis* or *H. influenzae*: 7 days
    b. *S. pneumoniae*: 10 days; longer for strains not fully susceptible.
    c. *L. monocytogenes*: 14 to 21 days
    d. Gram-negative bacilli (other than *H. influenzae*): 21 days

B. Corticosteroids

  1. Dexamethasone (0.15 mg/kg IV every 6 hours for 2 to 4 days) proven of value in clinical trials.
    a. Reduced neurologic complications of *H. influenzae* meningitis in children.
    b. Reduced mortality of *S. pneumoniae* meningitis in adults.
    c. Early initiation important; greatest efficacy noted when dexamethasone started immediately before first antibiotic dose.

C. Supportive care

  1. Careful fluid management and early recognition and treatment of complications essential.
    a. Potential neurologic complications include seizures and increased intracranial pressure.
    b. Possible systemic complications are hypotension, disseminated intravascular coagulation, metastatic infection.

D. Infection control

  1. Respiratory isolation: 24 hours after start of antibiotic (*N. meningitidis* or *H. influenzae*)
  2. Chemoprophylaxis
    a. *N. meningitidis*: household and daycare contacts, intimately exposed hospital staff (e.g., unprotected intubation); rifampin, ciprofloxacin, or ceftriaxone.
    b. *H. influenzae*: household contacts, if household includes an unvaccinated child younger than 4 years or an immunocompromised child of any age; rifampin.

Selected Readings

Aronin SI, Peduzzi P, Quagliarello VJ. Community-acquired bacterial meningitis: risk stratification for adverse clinical outcome and effect of antibiotic timing. *Ann Intern Med* 1998;129:862.
  A retrospective study of 269 cases of bacterial meningitis that provides a model for the prediction of clinical outcome.

Attia J, Hatala R, Cook DJ, et al. Does this adult patient have acute meningitis? *JAMA* 1999;282:175.
This article provides a review of published data on the sensitivity of the clinical history and physical examination in the diagnosis of meningitis.

Begg N, Cartwright KA, Cohen J, et al. Consensus statement on diagnosis, investigation, treatment and prevention of acute bacterial meningitis in immunocompetent adults. British Infection Society Working Party. *J Infect* 1999;39:1.
This consensus statement lays out detailed recommendations for all aspects of treatment of bacterial meningitis, with an assessment of the strength of the data; however, the statement predates the study by de Gans et al.

Centers for Disease Control. Effect of new susceptibility breakpoints on reporting of resistance in *Streptococcus pneumoniae*—United States, 2003. *MMWR* 2004;53:152.
Susceptibility data from the Active Bacterial Core Surveillance system from 1998 to 2001 showed reduced susceptibility to penicillin and cefotaxime in 30% and 20% of isolates, respectively.

Coant PN, Kornberg AE, Duffy LC, et al. Blood culture results as determinants in the organism identification of bacterial meningitis. *Pediatr Emerg Care* 1992;8:200.
A study of the yield of blood cultures in 169 cases of bacterial meningitis in children.

De Gans J, van de Beek D, European Dexamethasone in Adulthood Bacterial Meningitis Study Investigators. Dexamethasone in adults with bacterial meningitis. *N Engl J Med* 2002;347:1549.
In this randomized, prospective, double-blind placebo-controlled trial, dexamethasone treatment begun before the first dose of antibiotics reduced mortality in adult with bacterial meningitis by 50%.

Durand ML, Calderwood SB, Weber DJ, et al. Acute bacterial meningitis in adults: a review of 493 episodes. *N Engl J Med* 1993;328:21.
The largest review of clinical features and outcome in meningitis in adults, extending over a 27-year period.

Hasbun R, Abrahams J, Jekel J, et al. Computed tomography of the head before lumbar puncture in adults with suspected meningitis. *N Engl J Med* 2001;345:1727.
Abnormal findings on cranial CT scanning among 301 adults with suspected meningitis were associated with increased age, immunocompromise, seizure, abnormal level of consciousness, or focal neurologic findings; the results suggest that routine CT scanning before LP can be avoided in the remaining 40% of subjects.

Jones ME, Draghi DC, Karlowsky JA, et al. Prevalence of antimicrobial resistance in bacteria isolated from central nervous system specimens as reported by U.S. hospital laboratories from 2000 to 2002. *Ann Clin Microbiol Antimicrob* 2004;3:3.
This survey of data from more than 300 U.S. hospitals covering the years 2000 to 2002 found resistance to penicillin and ceftriaxone in 17% and 3.5%, respectively, of CSF isolates of S. pneumoniae.

Odio CM, Faingezicht I, Paris M, et al. The beneficial effects of early dexamethasone administration in infants and children with bacterial meningitis. *N Engl J Med* 1991; 324:1525.
Dexamethasone, begun before the first dose of cefotaxime, reduced the frequency of neurologic sequelae in this clinical trial involving children with predominantly H. influenzae meningitis.

Paris MM, Ramilo O, McCracken GH Jr. Management of meningitis caused by penicillin-resistant *Streptococcus pneumoniae*. *Antimicrob Agents Chemother* 1995;39:2171.
A review of clinical and experimental data on the management of this important problem.

Quagliarello VJ, Scheld WM. Treatment of bacterial meningitis. *N Engl J Med* 1997; 336:708.
An excellent review of all aspects of the treatment of bacterial meningitis, with detailed recommendations.

Scheld WM, Koedel U, Nathan B, et al. Pathophysiology of bacterial meningitis: mechanism(s) of neuronal injury. *J Infect Dis* 2002;186:S225.
An excellent review of the current understanding of the pathogenesis of bacterial meningitis.

Schuchat A, Robinson K, Wenger JD, et al. Bacterial meningitis in the United States in 1995. *N Engl J Med* 1997;337:970.
A picture of the epidemiology of bacterial meningitis in the United States after introduction of the H. influenzae *conjugate vaccines.*

Spanos A, Harrell FE Jr, Durack DT. Differential diagnosis of acute meningitis: an analysis of the predictive value of initial observations. *JAMA* 1989;262:2700.
This analysis of 422 cases derives a model to differentiate bacterial and viral meningitis.

68 INFECTIVE ENDOCARDITIS
Karen C. Carroll and Sarah H. Cheeseman

I. GENERAL PRINCIPLES
A. Definition
1. Infective endocarditis (IE) is a microbial infection of the endothelial lining of the heart, characterized on pathologic study by vegetations.
2. The infected site is usually a valve, but the term *infective endocarditis* encompasses infection of any vascular endothelial surface, usually hemodynamically or structurally abnormal.

B. Classification
1. Two clinical forms of native valve endocarditis have been traditionally delineated.
    a. Acute
    (1) Presents as a fulminant infection, with abrupt onset, high fever, leukocytosis, rapid valve destruction, and systemic toxicity.
    (2) Frequently secondary to *Staphylococcus aureus* and may occur on previously normal valves.
    b. Subacute
    (1) Insidious onset, slow development of the characteristic lesions, and absence of marked toxicity for a long period.
    (2) A high proportion of these cases occur on valves damaged by congenital, rheumatic, or degenerative cardiovascular disease.
    (3) Caused by organisms of relatively low virulence (e.g., viridans streptococci)
2. Prosthetic valve endocarditis

II. ETIOLOGY
A. Most frequently implicated organisms
1. Viridans streptococci most often recovered include *S. sanguis*, *S. mitis*, *S. mutans*, and *S. bovis*. The latter is commonly associated with preexisting colon lesions.
2. Staphylococci, particularly *S. aureus*, have surpassed streptococci in more recent series as the most common cause of IE. Coagulase-negative staphylococci (CNS) are the most common pathogens in early (≤60 days following surgery) prosthetic valve endocarditis (PVE). *Staphylococcus lugdunensis* is associated with valve destruction and usually requires valve replacement.
3. Enterococci are causes of nosocomial bacteremia and less frequently IE.
4. *Haemophilus* not influenzae, *Actinobacillus*, *Cardiobacterium*, *Eikenella* and *Kingella* species (HACEK group) collectively cause 3% to 4% of cases in patients with preexisting valvular disease. *Haemophilus*, *Actinobacillus*, *Cardiobacterium*, *Eikenella*, and *Kingella* species (HACEK group) cause 3% to 4% of cases in patients with preexisting valvular disease.
5. Culture-negative endocarditis is the result of prior antibiotic administration in about 50% of cases. The remainder may be attributed to unusual or noncultivatable organisms such as *Bartonella* sp., *Tropheryma whipplei*, *Brucella* sp., and *Coxiella burnetii*. The microbiology laboratory should be consulted when such diseases are suspected.

III. PATHOGENESIS AND PATHOPHYSIOLOGY
A. Trauma to the valve results in the elaboration of a fibrin-platelet thrombus.

B. Introduced bacteria from transient bacteremia, a distal site of infection, or an indwelling catheter or via injection drug use become trapped in the thrombus.

C. Infection of the fibrin-platelet thrombus results in enlargement of the process into a vegetation and invasion of tissue by the infection with eventual valvular disruption.

D. Specific valve involvement predicts the physiologic consequences:

  1. A vegetation may be so large as to function as a stenotic lesion.

  2. Tissue destruction results in valvular incompetence characterized by a new regurgitant murmur.

  3. Aortic valve disease carries the worst prognosis because of greater potential for spread of infection to the conducting system, emboli to coronary arteries, or propensity to cause heart failure.

E. The vegetations may break off as emboli to the brain, viscera, coronary arteries, and large arteries of the extremities (fungal endocarditis).

IV. DIAGNOSIS

A. IE is diagnosed based on signs and symptoms that reflect the pathology: fever, embolic phenomena, and evidence of valvular dysfunction.

B. Criteria

  1. Histopathologic confirmation of vegetation with infecting organisms on the valve.

  2. Stringent clinical criteria called the Duke Criteria have been devised and revised.

C. History

  1. Most common feature is fever, but this may be minimal or absent among certain patients.

  2. Musculoskeletal complaints such as lower back pain are also common.

  3. Loss of appetite, weight loss, malaise, and night sweats.

  4. Symptoms of complications such as embolism, stroke, congestive heart failure.

D. Physical examination

  1. Mucocutaneous embolic phenomena may be observed.

    a. Petechiae on plantar surfaces of toes and fingers, the conjunctival and buccal mucosa.

    b. Subungual splinter hemorrhages that appear at rest in the hospital.

    c. Osler's nodes and Janeway lesions are uncommon in recent series of endocarditis.

      (1) Osler's nodes are painful, tender, bluish-purple nodular lesions located on the pads of the fingers or toes.

      (2) The Janeway lesion is a painless, pink, nontender macular lesion that is located commonly on the palms or soles.

  2. Any heart murmur is compatible with a diagnosis of endocarditis, but a new regurgitant murmur is of greatest importance.

  3. Splenomegaly is found in nearly half of patients with subacute bacterial endocarditis and in very few of those with acute disease.

  4. Signs of congestive heart failure are not early findings but signal a need to consider cardiac surgical intervention.

E. Laboratory studies

  1. The key to the diagnosis of endocarditis is blood cultures.

    a. Two or three separate blood cultures within a 24-hour interval are recommended.

    b. In adults, 20 to 30 mL of blood per culture is optimal.

    c. In cases that are culture negative, the advice of a clinical microbiologist should be sought regarding the need for special media, such as those for the propagation of *Brucella* sp., *Bartonella* sp., and cell-wall defective forms.

    d. Organisms that are noncultivatable or difficult to cultivate may be detected by serologic studies. Such organisms include *C. burnetii*, the agent of Q-fever endocarditis, *Chlamydia* sp., *Bartonella* sp., and some fungi.

  2. An electrocardiogram is the simplest test for evaluation of perivalvular extension of infection in endocarditis.

    a. Persistent prolongation of the PR interval in the absence of digitalis toxicity; new persistent bundle-branch block, or complete heart block is specific for predicting extension beyond the valve leaflet and the subsequent need for surgery.

3. Echocardiography is a valuable adjunct in the patient with endocarditis. Current roles for echocardiography include:
   a. characterization of underlying valvular disease
   b. clarification of destructive nature of endocarditis
   c. assessment of the persistently febrile patient for evidence of perivalvular extension
   d. assessment of valvular function in prosthetic valve endocarditis
   e. Types of studies:
      (1) Transthoracic two-dimensional (2D) echocardiography (TTE) has an overall sensitivity for vegetation detection of 50%. TTE has very limited ability to detect valve perforations and abscess extension, especially on prosthetic heart valves. Specificity is high at 98% (see Chapter 22).
      (2) Transesophageal echocardiography (TEE) has a sensitivity of 90%, and vegetations as small as 1 mm can be seen. TEE is also superior to TTE for detection of perivalvular abscess, with approximately 87% sensitivity. TEE appears to be the optimal tool to assess prosthetic valve dysfunction (see Chapter 22).

V. TREATMENT
A. Types
   1. Medical: 4 to 6 weeks of intravenous antimicrobial agent(s) bactericidal for pathogen
   2. Approaches for typical pathogens based on American Heart Association Committee on Rheumatic Fever, Endocarditis, and Kawasaki Disease recommendations:
      a. Native valve endocarditis
         (1) Viridans streptococci, *S. bovis* penicillin MIC ≤0.1 µg/mL—Penicillin G (PenG) 12 to 18 mU/d IV continuously or q4h for 4 weeks OR ceftriaxone 2.0 gm/d IV for 4 weeks; Penicillin G at same dose PLUS gentamicin (gent) 1 mg/kg q8h for 2 weeks.
         (2) Viridans streptococci, *S. bovis* MIC >0.1 µg/mL and ≤0.5—Pen G 18 mU/d IV OR cefazolin 2 g q8h PLUS gent 1 mg/kg q8h IV for 2 weeks
         (3) Viridans streptococci, *S. bovis*, nutritionally variant streptococci, susceptible enterococci Pen G 18 to 30 mU/24h IV continuous or q4h OR ampicillin (Amp) 12 g/d continuous or q4h PLUS gent as above for 4 to 6 weeks
         (4) For patients allergic to penicillin or cephalosporins in any scenario above—vancomycin (vanco) 15 mg/kg q12 (max 2 g/day)
         (5) Enterococci resistant to Pen/Amp, vancomycin and HLR to aminoglycosides
            i. Consider infectious diseases consultation
            ii. Potential therapies include quinupristin/dalfopristin (Synercid), linezolid
         (6) Methicillin-susceptible staphylococci (MSSA): tricuspid valve nafcillin OR oxacillin 2 g q4 IV PLUS gent 1 mg/kg q8h IV for 2 weeks
         (7) MSSA left-sided infection: nafcillin OR oxacillin 2 g q4h IV or cefazolin 2 g q8h IV for 4 to 6 weeks PLUS gent 1 mg/kg q8h IV for 3 to 5 days
         (8) Methicillin-resistant *S. aureus* (MRSA): vancomycin 15 mg/kg q12h IV for 4 to 6 weeks; quinupristin/dalfopristin or linezolid for failures or vanco intolerance; daptomycin currently in trials.
         (9) HACEK group bacteria ceftriaxone 2.0 g/d IV for 4 weeks
      b. Prosthetic valve endocarditis
         (1) *Staphylococcus epidermidis*: vancomycin 15 mg/kg q12h IV PLUS rifampin 300 mg PO q8h PLUS gent 1 mg/kg q8h IV for 6 weeks
         (2) MSSA: nafcillin as per native valve PLUS rifampin 300 mg PO q8h for 6 weeks PLUS gent 1 mg/kg q8h for 14 days
         (3) MRSA: Vanco 15 mg/kg q12h PLUS rifampin 300 mg PO q8h for 6 weeks PLUS gent 1 mg/kg q8h IV for 14 days
         (4) Streptococci, enterococci (see Native valve section earlier)
   3. Surgical management
      a. Indications for valve replacement
         (1) Microbiologic failure
         (2) Congestive heart failure requiring more than simple therapy

(3) Other criteria that may warrant early surgery: multiple emboli, certain echocardiographic features, conduction defects, infection with organisms that are difficult to treat, such as *Brucella* sp. *C. burnetii*, *Candida* sp., other fungi.

Selected Readings

Birmingham GD, Rahko PS, Ballantyne F. Improved detection of infective endocarditis with transesophageal echocardiography. *Am Heart J* 1992;123:774.
A careful study of the incremental value of transesophageal over transthoracic echocardiography.

Birmingham MC, Rayner CR, Meagher AK, e al. Linezolid for the treatment of multi-drug resistant, gram positive infections: Experience from a compassionate-use program. *Clin Infect Dis* 2003; 36:159–168.
Included in this large series of patients are clinical and microbiologic outcomes on 40 cases of endocarditis with VRE and MRSA. Important data on complications of therapy is presented.

Brouqui P, Raoult D. Endocarditis due to rare and fastidious bacteria. *Clin Microbiol Rev* 2001;14:177–307.
Comprehensive discussion of the clinical presentation and diagnostic strategies for detecting a broad range of fastidious organisms causing IE, most notably Bartonella *sp., and* T. whipplei.

Carroll KC, Cheeseman SH. Infective endocarditis and infections of intracardiac prosthetic devices. In Irwin RS III and Rippe JM , eds. Irwin and Rippe's intensive care medicine Baltimore: Lippincott Williams and Wilkins, 2003, pp. 1000–1015.
Comprehensive review of all aspects of endocarditis and infection of intracardiac devices.

Chambers HF, Korzeniowski OM, Sande MA, et al. *Staphylococcus aureus* endocarditis: clinical manifestations in addicts and nonaddicts. *Medicine* 1983;62:170.
Classic study defining the differences in staphylococcal endocarditis between injection drug users and all others.

Cheitlin MD, Armstrong WF, Aurigemma GP, et al. ACC/AHA/ASE 2003 guideline update for the clinical application of echocardiography: Summary article. A report of the American College of Cardiology/American Heart Association Task force on practice guidelines (ACC/AHA/ASE Committee to Update the 1997 guidelines for the clinical application of echocardiography.) *J Am Soc Echocardiogr* 2003;16:1091–1110.
Changes to the 1997 guidelines include the addition of the Duke criteria and the value of TEE when TTE is negative in settings of high clinical suspicion and PVE.

DiNubile MJ. Surgery in active endocarditis. *Ann Intern Med* 1982;96:650.
Superb and not-yet-outdated review of indications for cardiac surgery in active endocarditis.

Durack DT, Lukes AS, Bright DK. New criteria for diagnosis of infective endocarditis: utilization of specific echocardiographic findings. *Am J Med* 1994;96:200–209.
Original Duke criteria which incorporated predisposing factors, blood culture information, and echocardiographic findings into probability assessments for predicting likelihood of IE.

Eishi K, Kawazoe K, Kuriyama Y, et al. Surgical management of infective endocarditis associated with cerebral complications: multicenter retrospective study in Japan. *J Thorac Cardiovasc Surg* 1995;110:1745–1755.
A retrospective study of 181 patients with cerebral complications, which concludes that valve replacement surgery may be safely performed 4 weeks or more after the neurologic event.

Li JS, Sexton DJ, Mick N, et al. Proposed modifications to the Duke criteria for the diagnosis of infective endocarditis. *Clin Infect Dis* 2000;30:633–638.
Proposed modified criteria, which have added positive Q-fever serology to major criteria and physical findings and laboratory tests, such as splenomegaly and C-reactive protein, respectively, to the minor criteria.

Moreillon P, Que YA. Infective endocarditis. *Lancet* 2004;363:139–149.
Review article that has an excellent discussion of the pathogenesis and pathophysiology of IE.

Mylonakis E, Calderwood SB. Infective endocarditis in adults. *N Engl J Med* 2001;345:1318–1330.
One of the better-written and more comprehensive recent reviews of endocarditis, complete with color photos of the peripheral stigmata.

Reinhatz O, Hermann M, Redling F, et al. Timing of surgery in patients with acute infective endocarditis. *J Cardiovasc Surg* 1996;37:397–400.
Frequently cited publication on demonstrated improved outcome with surgery when performed prior to deterioration in cardiac performance.

Rosen AB, Fowler VG, Corey GR, et al. Cost effectiveness of transesophageal echocardiography to determine the duration of therapy for intravascular catheter-associated *Staphylococcus aureus* bacteremia. *Ann Intern Med* 1999;130:810.
One of the landmark studies that justifies using transesophageal echocardiography to stratify patients with S. aureus bacteremia to short-duration versus long-duration therapy.

Wilson WR, Karchmer AW, Dajani AS, et al. Antibiotic treatment of adults with infective endocarditis due to streptococci, enterococci, staphylococci and HACEK microorganisms. *JAMA* 1995;274:1706.
Still-current authoritative statement on treatment regimens, with full explanation of the rationale and references.

69

INFECTIONS ASSOCIATED WITH VASCULAR CATHETERS
Suzanne F. Bradley and Carol A. Kauffman

I. GENERAL PRINCIPLES
A. Leading cause of nosocomial bloodstream infections; 250,000 to 300,000 infections each year at a cost of approximately $30,000 per survivor.
B. Highest rates of infectious complications are with short-term central venous, pulmonary artery, and peripheral artery catheters.
C. The longer a peripheral venous or artery catheter or pulmonary artery catheter remains in place, the higher the risk of infection. Change peripheral catheters every 3 days, peripheral artery catheters every 4 days, and pulmonary artery catheters every 5 days.
D. Routine changes of central venous catheters over a guide wire are not recommended. Central venous, first percutaneous intravenous central catheter (PICC), and tunneled semipermanent catheters can remain for weeks to months.
E. Catheter insertion in the lower extremities should be avoided, except in children.
F. Placement of central venous and pulmonary artery catheters always requires maximal sterile barrier precautions (cap, mask, sterile drapes, gowns, gloves).
G. Insertion site disinfection with chlorhexidine appears more effective than povidone-iodine.
H. Use of antimicrobial-impregnated central venous catheters (chlorhexidine-silver sulfadiazine or minocycline-rifampin) may be cost effective for high-risk patients who require catheterization for 1 to 2 weeks but should not be used routinely.

II. ETIOLOGY
A. Coagulase-negative staphylococci (CoNS) are the most common cause of infection.
B. *Staphylococcus aureus* less common but causes many more complications than CoNS.
C. Other gram-positive organisms, such as *Enterococcus* and *Corynebacterium*, can cause central venous catheter-related infections
D. Gram-negative bacilli, such as *Pseudomonas aeruginosa*, less common cause of catheter-related bloodstream infections and usually involve central venous catheters.
E. *Candida* species are an increasing cause of central venous catheter-related bloodstream infections.

III. PATHOGENESIS
A. Initiation of infection
1. A thrombin sheath accumulates on all intravascular catheters.
2. This sheath increases with prolonged catheterization and is less likely to form on subclavian than femoral and internal jugular catheters.
3. Microorganisms adhere to materials, especially fibrin and fibronectin, in the thrombin sheath and form a biofilm that helps protect the organism from antibiotic action.
B. Entry of organisms
1. Microorganisms gain entry at the insertion site and colonize the external catheter surface; most common mode of infection and occurs most often in short-term central and peripheral venous catheters.
2. Contamination of the hub and subsequently the internal catheter lumen occurs more often in tunneled, long-term central venous catheters.
3. Hematogenous seeding from a distant focus (usually gastrointestinal tract) occurs most often in neutropenic patients.

IV. DIAGNOSIS

A. Clinical clues

1. Positive blood cultures with an organism that commonly causes catheter-related bloodstream infection
2. No other source of infection
3. Local inflammation around the catheter entry site

B. Diagnostic methods without removing the catheter

1. Simultaneous cultures drawn from a peripheral vein and the catheter.
2. With catheter infection, the culture from the catheter is positive at least 2 hours earlier than the culture from the peripheral vein.

C. Diagnostic methods requiring catheter removal

1. The catheter is removed, and the tip is cut off with a sterile scissors and sent to the laboratory in a sterile cup.
2. The catheter tip is rolled on an agar plate to determine the number of colonies; 15 or more colonies correlates with infection.

V. TREATMENT

A. General measures

1. For most patients with documented catheter-related infection, the catheter should be removed as soon as possible.
2. If at all possible, another central catheter should not be placed until it is shown that blood cultures are negative.
3. For patients who have limited vascular access and are wholly dependent on a semipermanent catheter for nutrition or medications:
   a. Can attempt to treat with antibiotics alone without catheter removal. Likely to be successful with CoNS infections.
   b. *S. aureus, Candida,* and gram-negative bacillary infections almost always require catheter removal.
   c. Tenderness, swelling, and redness along the insertion site of a semipermanent catheter usually imply a tunnel infection, and the catheter must be removed.

B. Empiric treatment

1. Initial treatment should cover CoNS and *S. aureus.* Empiric treatment for gram-negative bacilli depends on the clinical situation but is generally not needed for most cases.
2. Vancomycin preferred because of activity against methicillin-resistant strains of *S. aureus* and CoNS; a broad-spectrum penicillin or cephalosporin can be added for treatment of gram-negative bacilli, if desired.

C. Coagulase-negative *Staphylococcus*

1. Nafcillin, 2 g q4h, or cefazolin, 2 g q8h, for methicillin-susceptible organisms
2. Vancomycin, 1 g q12h for methicillin-resistant organisms
3. Length of therapy usually 7 to 10 days

D. *S. aureus*

1. Nafcillin, 2 g q4h, or cefazolin, 2 g q8h, for methicillin-susceptible organisms
2. Vancomycin, 1 g q12h for methicillin-resistant organisms
3. Length of therapy
   a. Short-course (2-week) intravenous therapy is appropriate only if the catheter is removed immediately, fever resolves promptly, no metastatic foci are found, and bacteremia resolves as documented by repeatedly negative blood cultures.
   b. Patients with bacteremia or fever persisting more than 3 days after catheter removal and initiation of antibiotics are at high risk for complications, including endocarditis. Transesophageal echocardiography is strongly recommended, and 4 to 6 weeks of therapy is generally needed.
4. Follow closely for relapse or symptoms(e.g., back pain, suggesting metastatic infection).

E. Gram-negative bacilli

1. Third-generation cephalosporin or extended-spectrum penicillin is required; piperacillin-tazobactam, 3.375 g q6h, is reasonable until susceptibility studies return and definitive antibiotic therapy is initiated.
2. Length of therapy: 2 weeks after blood cultures become negative

F. Candida species

1. Candidemia should always be treated with an antifungal agent and clears more quickly if the catheter is removed promptly.
2. Can use fluconazole, 400 mg daily, amphotericin B, 0.5 to 0.7 mg/kg/day, or caspofungin, 50 mg daily until species known.
3. Patients with *C. glabrata* or *C. krusei* fungemia, treat with caspofungin, vericonazole, or amphotericin B; other species, including *C. albicans,* treat with fluconazole.
4. Length of therapy: usually 2 weeks after blood cultures become negative unless other sites involved.

VI. COMPLICATIONS

A. Most common with *S. aureus* and *Candida* infections and with central venous or pulmonary artery catheters.
B. Suppurative thrombophlebitis of the great veins can occur with central venous catheter infection.
C. Metastatic infection, especially of retina and intervertebral disc spaces, can occur with any type of catheter and is most commonly seen with *S. aureus* infections.
D. Endocarditis is increasingly associated with catheter-related bloodstream infections, especially those due to *S. aureus.*

Selected Readings

Chaiyakunapruk N, Veenstra DL, Lipsky BA, et al. Chlorhexidine compared with povidone-iodine solution for catheter-site care: a meta-analysis. *Ann Intern Med* 2002;136:792–801.
Meta-analysis showing reduced risk of catheter-associated bloodstream infections when chlorhexidine, rather than povidone-iodine, was used for insertion site disinfection.

Crnich CJ, Maki DG. The promise of novel technology for the prevention of intravascular device-related bloodstream infection. I. Pathogenesis and short-term devices. *Clin Infect Dis* 2002;34:1232–1242.
Review of methods to prevent infections in short-term indwelling intravascular devices.

Crnich CJ, Maki DG. The promise of novel technology for the prevention of intravascular device-related bloodstream infection. II. Long-term devices. *Clin Infect Dis* 2002;34:1362–1368.
Review of methods to prevent infections in long-term indwelling intravascular devices.

Darouiche RO, Raad II, Heard SO, et al. A comparison of two antimicrobial-impregnated central venous catheters. *N Engl J Med* 1999;340:1.
Controlled randomized trial showing that the use of catheters impregnated with minocycline-rifampin on both internal and external surfaces was superior in preventing bloodstream infections to catheters impregnated only on the external surface with chlorhexidine silver sulfadiazine

McGee DC, Gould MK. Preventing complications of central venous catheterization. *N Engl J Med* 2003;348:1123–1133.
Excellent review of the many complications of central venous catheterization and tips for preventing them.

Mermel LA, Farr BM, Sheretz RJ, et al. Guidelines for the management of intravascular catheter-related infections. *Clin Infect Dis* 2001;32:1249–1272.
Infectious Diseases Society of America guidelines for the diagnosis and treatment of catheter-related infections.

O'Grady NP, Alexander M, Dellinger EP, et al. Guidelines for the prevention of intravascular catheter-related infections. *Clin Infect Dis* 2002;35:1281–1307.
Consensus guidelines from the Centers for Disease Control and many other groups for preventing catheter-related infections.

Raad I, Hanna HA, Alakech B, et al. Differential time to positivity: a useful method for diagnosing catheter-related bloodstream infections. *Ann Intern Med* 2004;140:18–25.
Study shows that if a blood culture taken from a central venous catheter becomes positive at least 2 hours earlier than a simultaneous culture drawn from a peripheral vein, it is likely that the patient has catheter-related bloodstream infection.

Raad II, Hanna HA. Intravascular catheter-related infections. New horizons and recent advances. *Arch Intern Med* 2002;162:871–878.
Excellent overview of pathogenesis, diagnosis, and newer methods to prevent catheter-related bloodstream infections.

Rubinson L, Diette GB. Best practices for insertion of central venous catheters in intensive-care units to prevent catheter-related bloodstream infections. *J Clin Lab Med* 2004;143:5–13.
Practical suggestions for preventing catheter-related infections in intensive care unit patients.

Sheretz RJ, Ely EW, Westbrook DM, et al. Education of physicians-in-training can decrease the risk for vascular catheter infection. *Ann Intern Med* 2000;132:641–648.
Shows that education of house staff in insertion of catheters can reduce nosocomial catheter-related bloodstream infections in the intensive care unit setting.

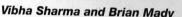

URINARY TRACT INFECTIONS IN THE INTENSIVE CARE UNIT
Vibha Sharma and Brian Mady

70

I. GENERAL PRINCIPLES

A. Urinary tract infection (UTI) remains the most common nosocomially acquired infection in the United States.

B. UTI is a major cause of morbidity in hospitalized patients and, being the most frequently recognized source of gram-negative bacteremia, constitutes a major cause of mortality in critically ill patients.

C. UTIs requiring intensive care management are discussed in this chapter.

D. A separate area of focus is problems associated with catheter-associated UTI (CAUTI).

II. ETIOLOGY AND MICROBIOLOGY

A. The most common cause of UTI is *Escherichia coli*.

B. Other microorganisms frequently associated with UTIs include other Enterobacteriaceae: *Klebsiella, Enterobacter, Proteus,* and *Providencia* species. These are common in hospitalized patients on antibiotics and in patients with anatomic or functional abnormalities in urine flow.

C. In the intensive care unit setting, gram-positive bacterial species occasionally cause UTIs. Enterococci and *Staphylococcus epidermidis* may cause infections in elderly patients or in patients with structural abnormalities.

D. *Staphylococcus aureus* UTI should prompt a search for extrarenal sources of infection, *because* it is frequently seen in patients with bacteremia.

E. *Candida* species and other fungal organisms may complicate urinary catheterization and occasionally lead to fungemia in ascending UTI.

III. PATHOPHYSIOLOGY

A. *E. coli* and other enteric gram-negative aerobic bacteria colonize the human colon and frequently contaminate the lower urinary tract, resulting in ascending infection.

B. Infection in the urinary tract is directly related to the ability of bacteria to adhere to and then colonize the bladder and renal system.

C. Virulence factors for *E. coli* include properties of certain O antigen serotypes, fimbrial adhesions, and production of hemolysin and aerobactin, a siderphore necessary for iron acquisition.

D. Virulence factors for *Proteus mirabilis* include production of hemolysin and IgA protease, flagella, fimbriae, and secretion of urease.

IV. DIAGNOSIS

A. The clinical diagnosis of acute upper UTI is based on the findings of frequency or dysuria with or without fever.

B. Urine analysis is positive for leukocyte esterase and nitrite and white blood cell count greater than 5 per high power field (HPF).

C. Urine cultures should be obtained before the start of antimicrobial therapy.

D. In patients admitted to the intensive care unit (ICU) with a suspicion for pyelonephritis, blood cultures should be obtained in addition to a urine culture.

E. A positive urine culture is classically defined as greater than 10^5 CFU/mL.

F. In some cases, the absence of pyuria and bacteriuria may not exclude the possibility of UTI. Neutropenic patients may not have pyuria, and urine cultures may be negative in acute obstruction.

G. Additional diagnostic methods such as renal ultrasound, computed tomography, magnetic resonance imaging, cystoscopy, or retrograde studies may be necessary to make the diagnosis in complicated cases.

V. TREATMENT

A. Medical management of patients with UTI severe enough to warrant ICU admission consists of stabilization of hemodynamic parameters, supportive measures, and empiric antimicrobial therapy.

B. In patients who are not immunocompromised, coming from the community into the ICU, and have not received prior antibiotic treatment, monotherapy with a third- or fourth-generation cephalosporin or extended-spectrum penicillin or quinolone is recommended.

C. The empiric use of an extended spectrum β-lactamase antibiotic (like a third- or fourth-generation cephalosporin or extended-spectrum penicillin or quinolone) in combination with an aminoglycoside is the standard therapeutic regimen in UTIs associated with gram-negative septic shock and in nosocomial urosepsis.

C. If an enterococcal UTI is suspected, ampicillin with or without an aminoglycoside is initiated. Further definitive therapy with vancomycin (in case of ampicillin-resistant enterococcus or linezolid in case of vancomycin-resistant enterococcus) is based on definitive culture results.

D. Duration of treatment: parenteral therapy is administered until the patient is afebrile; oral therapy should then be continued for about 2 weeks. For pyelonephritis or urosepsis, 2 to 3 weeks of therapy is recommended. Depending on the organism and susceptibility, switching to oral therapy should be considered.

VI. PROGNOSIS

A. Acute pyelonephritis warranting ICU admission can be complicated by septic shock and bacteremia, urinary obstruction, papillary necrosis, or other suppurative complications.

B. Most patients respond to appropriate therapy in 72 hours, which includes targeted antimicrobial therapy and alleviation of mechanical obstruction to urine flow.

C. A search for suppurative complications is necessary if the patient does not respond promptly to conventional therapy.

VII. CATHETER-ASSOCIATED URINARY TRACT INFECTION

A. A major problem in patients in ICUs is determining whether a patient has a catheter-associated UTI versus colonization.

B. The two most common mechanisms of CAUTI are extraluminal infections by direct inoculation at the time of insertion and intraluminal infections by reflux of organisms.

C. Major risk factors for CAUTI are duration of catheterization (≥7 days increases the risk sevenfold), female gender, and age of patient over 60 years.

D. Infection is diagnosed by pyuria, positive urine culture with no more than two microorganisms, and fever.

E. Treatment should include removal of the urinary catheter if possible.

F. If bacteriuria persists after removal of catheter, treatment with a short course of an antimicrobial agent (based on culture results) is adequate.

G. If removal of the catheter is not possible, the catheter should be changed and the patient treated with appropriate antimicrobial agents.

H. Prostatitis, prostatic abscess, or epididymitis may complicate long-term urinary catheters in men.

I. Good hand hygiene, use of clean technique, use of a closed drainage system, ensuring dependent drainage at all times, and, if possible, clean, nonsterile intermittent catheterization are some of the strategies useful for prevention of CAUTI.

VIII. CANDIDURIA

A. Candiduria is frequent in ICU patients taking antimicrobial agents.

B. Quantitative cultures yielding *Candida* species do not have the same diagnostic implications as those yielding a pathogenic bacterium.

C. Removal of the catheter is the best treatment.

D. Persistent fever and candiduria in a patient with no other source for fevers may suggest a Candida UTI.

E. Amphotericin B bladder irrigation is not indicated in this setting.

F. Treatment with short course of Fluconazole 200 mg the first day, followed by 100 mg a day for 4 days is often effective.

G. In patients with prolonged ICU stay and colonization with resistant *Candida* species like *C. krusei* and *C. glabrata*, resistance to Fluconazole is a concern and may warrant use of agents such as amphotericin B or Voriconazole.

Selected Readings

Jacobs LG, Skidmore EA, Freeman K, et al. Oral fluconazole compared with bladder irrigation with amphotericin B for treatment of fungal urinary tract infections in the elderly. *Clin Inf Dis* 1996;22:30.
Comparison of two treatment approaches.

Rosser C, Bare R, et al. Urinary tract infections in the critically ill patient with a urinary catheter. *Am J Surg* 1999;177:287–290.
Notes increase in incidence of urosepsis in patients with increased length of stay in the intensive care unit, increased duration of catheterization, and increase in age.

Rubenstien JN, Schaeffer AJ. Managing complicated urinary tract infections: the urologic review. *Infec Dis Clin North Am* 2003;17{2};333–351.
This article asserts the importance of a combined medical and surgical approach and appropriate imaging in management of complicated urinary tract infections.

Stamm W, Hooton T, Johnson J. Urinary tract infections: from pathogenesis to treatment. *J Infect Dis* 1989; 159(3).
Good article on pathogenesis of urinary tract infection and duration of treatment of pyelonephritis.

Trautner BW, Darouiche RO. Catheter-associated infections: pathogenesis affects prevention. *Arch Intern Med* 2004;164:842–850.
Good review article on approaches to prevent and treat catheter-associated urinary tract infection.

Warren J, Abrutyn E, et al. Guidelines for treatment of uncomplicated acute bacterial cystitis and acute pyelonephritis in women. *Clin Infect Dis* 1999;29:745–758.
Infectious Diseases Society of America (IDSA) guidelines for treatment of women hospitalized with acute pyelonephritis.

71 TOXIC SHOCK SYNDROME, TICK-BORNE ILLNESSES, AND POSTSPLENECTOMY INFECTION
Iva Zivna and Richard T. Ellison III

I. TOXIC SHOCK SYNDROME
A. Background
1. Toxic shock syndrome (TSS) is a toxin-mediated multisystem disease with acute onset of high fever, hypotension, diffuse macular erythroderma, mucous membrane inflammation, severe myalgia, vomiting or diarrhea, and altered consciousness without focal neurologic signs.
2. It arises as a result of infection or colonization with toxin-producing strains of *Staphylococcus aureus* or group A streptococci. Approximately 50% of cases of staphylococcal TSS occur in menstruating women using tampons.

B. Pathogenesis.
S. aureus exotoxins, primarily TSS toxin-1, are superantigens that are able to activate large number of T cells. Activated T cells then release massive amounts of cytokines that mediate the signs and symptoms of TSS.

C. Diagnosis
1. Five clinical features are needed for the diagnosis of staphylococcal TSS: (a) fever, (b) skin and mucous membrane manifestations, (c) desquamation 1 to 2 weeks after the onset of illness, (d) hypotension, and (e) evidence of multiorgan failure.
2. Evidence of *S. aureus* and streptococci on a peripheral blood smear and cultures. Blood cultures are usually negative in *S. aureus* TSS but are positive in streptococcal TSS.

D. Treatment
1. Correct hypovolemic shock rapidly.
2. Surgically treat infected area; remove foreign bodies.
3. Institute therapy with a β-lactamase–resistant antistaphylococcal antimicrobial agent, such as oxacillin, or nafcillin until the bacteriologic diagnosis is confirmed. Alternatives include a first-generation cephalosporin or vancomycin.
4. In streptococcal TSS, also administer clindamycin to block bacterial toxin production.
5. Intravenous immunoglobulin and recombinant human activated protein C (Xygris) should both be considered for severe cases.

II. TICK-BORNE ILLNESSES
A. Rocky Mountain spotted fever
1. Background
   a. Potentially lethal tick-borne disease caused by intracellular parasite *Rickettsia rickettsii*. This disease is characterized by acute onset of fever and rash.
   b. Endemic areas include southeastern part of the United States, primarily North Carolina, and regions of Oklahoma and Arkansas.
2. Pathogenesis. After inoculation and intracellular proliferation, organism attaches to the endothelial cells, causing vasculitis, hemorrhage, edema, and eventually shock.
3. Diagnosis
   1. Clinical manifestation, presence of risk factors, and epidemiologic features.
   2. Evidence of *R. rickettsii* on a skin biopsy or a fourfold rise in specific antibody titers.
   3. Routine laboratory studies are nonspecific.
   4. Treatment. Doxycycline or chloramphenicol.

B. Babesiosis
   1. Background
      a. Babesiosis is a tick-borne disease endemic on the Northeast coast of the United States.
      b. In the United States, babesiosis is caused by protozoa *Babesia microti* that infect red blood cells and result in mild to severe hemolytic anemia. It can occur concurrently in up to 25% of patients with Lyme disease, ehrlichiosis, or anaplasmosis.
   2. Pathogenesis. After inoculation organism multiplies inside the erythrocytes, causing hemolysis. Greater severity and high incidence are seen in asplenic patients.
   3. Diagnosis. Routine laboratory studies are nondiagnostic; diagnosis confirmed by thick and thin peripheral blood smear showing intraerythrocytic parasites.
   4. Treatment
      a. Azithromycin and atovaquone or quinine and clindamycin.
      b. In severe cases transfusion exchange therapy can be effective.
C. Ehrlichiosis and anaplasmosis
   1. Background
      a. Tick-borne diseases caused by intracellular pathogens *Ehrlichia chaffeensis*, *Ehrlichia equi*, and *Anaplasma (Ehrlichia) phagocytophilium*. The most prominent symptoms are high fever, severe headache, and myalgias.
      b. Ehrlichiosis is endemic in the southern part of the United States, especially Arkansas, whereas anaplasmosis is found mainly on the Northeast coast.
      c. Anaplasmosis can occur in up to 25% of patients with Lyme disease or babesiosis.
   2. Pathogenesis
      a. *E. chaffeensis* primarily infect mononuclear leukocytes and form inclusion body "morulae" in the cytoplasma, whereas *E. equi* and *A. phagocytophilium* infect mostly granulocytes.
   3. Diagnosis. Routine laboratory studies are nonspecific; diagnosis confirmed by identification of intraleukocytic morulae, serologic studies, or polymerase chain reaction assays.
   4. Treatment. Doxycycline or chloramphenicol.

III. POSTSPLENECTOMY INFECTION
   A. Background. Postsplenectomy sepsis is a fulminant and frequently fatal illness that occurs in asplenic patients and those with impaired splenic function. The main pathogens are encapsulated bacteria such as *Streptococcus pneumoniae*, *Haemophilus influenzae*, and *Neisseria meningitidis*.
   B. Pathogenesis
      1. Splenectomy impairs three host defenses essential to control of encapsulated bacteria:
         a. production of type-specific antibodies
         b. bacterial phagocytosis by splenic macrophages
         c. activation of the complement pathway
   C. Diagnosis
      1. Signs of sepsis in any splenectomized patient or those with impaired splenic function.
      2. Presence of bacteria on a peripheral blood smear or cultures.
   D. Treatment. Institute broad-spectrum antibiotic therapy with vancomycin and ceftriaxone along with supportive therapy.

Selected Readings
Bakken JS, Dumler JS. Human granulocytic ehrlichiosis. *Clin Infect Dis* 2000;31:554–560.
   This review includes epidemiology, clinical manifestation, laboratory testing, and treatment of human granulocytic ehrlichiosis.

Boustani MR, Gelfand JA. Babesiosis. *Clin Infect Dis* 1996;22:611.
   This informative review provides description of pathogenesis, clinical manifestation, diagnosis, and treatment of babesiosis.

Brigden ML, Pattullo AL. Prevention and management of overwhelming postsplenectomy infection—an update. *Crit Care Med* 1999;27:836.
This detailed review discusses immunology, bacteriology, and management of patients with overwhelming postsplenectomy infection.

Dumler JS, Bakken JS. Ehrlichial disease of humans: emerging thick-borne infections. *Clin Infect Dis* 1995;20:1102.
This is a complete review of epidemiology, pathogenesis, clinical manifestation, diagnosis, and therapy of human ehrlichiosis.

Stevens DL. The toxic shock syndromes. *Infect Dis Clin North Am* 1996;10:727.
This is a review of streptococcal and staphylococcal TSS, including case definitions, pathogenesis, clinical presentation, and treatment.

Thorner AR, Walker DH, Petri WA. Rocky Mountain spotted fever. *Clin Infect Dis* 1998; 27:1353–1360.
This detailed review provides an overview on epidemiology, pathogenesis, clinical manifestations, diagnosis, and treatment of Rocky Mountain spotted fever.

I. GENERAL PRINCIPLES. More aggressive therapies for malignancies and end-stage diseases have resulted in a growing population of persons with defects of the immune system, raising the risk of infectious complications. This chapter focuses on infectious diseases associated with cancer chemotherapy and hematopoietic stem cell transplantation (HSCT) and solid organ transplantation (SOT) resulting primarily in defects of neutrophil function and cell-mediated immunity. Infections associated with HIV disease are discussed in Chapter 73.

II. PATHOGENESIS. Many factors contribute to the risk of infectious complications in the immunocompromised host.

A. The nature and severity of immunosuppression may be affected by the primary disease or its medical and surgical management.

1. Malignancies of neutrophils, T lymphocytes, and antibody production increase the risk of infections from fungal, intracellular, and encapsulated organisms, respectively. Recipients of allogeneic solid organs or hematopoietic stem cells experience a higher rate of infectious complications compared with those receiving autologous tissues.

2. Agents affecting T lymphocyte activity, such as fludarabine and anti-T lymphocyte antibodies, are among the most severe suppressants of cell-mediated immunity.

3. Prevention and treatment of graft-versus-host-disease (GVHD) significantly raises the level of immunodeficiency.

B. Immunocompromised patients may develop infections from endogenous microorganisms or those acquired from an allograft or the environment.

1. Prolonged neutropenia, therapy with broad-spectrum antibiotics or steroids, and total parenteral nutrition predispose patients to fungal infections.

2. Organisms identified in potential donors may be transmitted to and cause infection in the recipient, including herpesviruses, hepatitis viruses, *Toxoplasma gondii*, and *Histoplasma capsulatum*. Similarly, pathogens previously well controlled by the immune system may reactivate, such as herpesviruses cytomegalovirus (CMV), Epstein-Barr virus (EBV), and human herpes virus-6 (HHV-6) and *T. gondii*.

C. Infections often arise from mucosal surfaces and indwelling foreign bodies. Bacteremia and fungemia may occur without an obvious source, although compromised oral or gastrointestinal tract mucosa resulting from chemotherapy, neutropenia, adverse drug reaction, or hypoxemia is the most likely origin of occult bloodstream infection. Solid organ transplantation recipients may also develop infections related to the surgical procedure. Except in patients with impaired cell-mediated immunity and after neurosurgery, central nervous system infections are infrequent in immunocompromised patients.

D. Infections with specific pathogens are most common during predictable time periods following hematopoietic or solid organ transplantation.

1. Typical infections within the first month are similar to those of other hospitalized medical and surgical patients. Reactivation of herpes simplex virus can also occur during this period.

2. Opportunistic infections typically associated with immunosuppression occur most frequently during the second through the sixth months. These pathogens

include herpesviruses, *Pneumocystis jiroveci*, *T. gondii*, *Mycobacterium tuberculosis*, fungi such as *Cryptococcus neoformans*, *Aspergillus*, and endemic species (*Coccidioides immitis* and *Histoplasma capsulatum*), and environmental pathogens such as *Nocardia*, *Listeria*, and *Legionella*.

3. Beyond 6 months, infections common in the general population can also affect immunocompromised patients, including respiratory viruses, community-acquired pneumonia, and urinary tract infections. Adenoviruses, polyoma viruses, and reactivation of varicella-zoster virus (VZV) can occur during this late period. In addition, patients with chronic infections such as CMV and hepatitis viruses, allograft rejection requiring increased immunosuppression, and completed antimicrobial prophylactic drug regimens may develop infections that are more common during earlier periods.

III. DIAGNOSIS

A. Physical examination may be obscured by diminished signs of inflammation, including fever. A thorough history must be taken and a physical examination must be performed initially and repeated daily, with special attention to the oropharynx, sinuses, optic fundi, anorectal region, lungs, skin, recent surgical wounds, and vascular catheter sites.

B. Initial diagnostic tests should include the following: (a) cultures of blood and urine; (b) chest radiograph; (c) culture of sputum in patients with evidence of pulmonary disease; (d) stool culture and *Clostridium difficile* toxin assay in patients with diarrhea; (e) semiquantitative culture of intravenous catheters removed due to fever; (f) swab, aspiration, or biopsy of suspicious skin or mucous membrane lesions for smears, cultures (routine, fungal, and viral), and pathologic examination; (g) other cultures from sites with signs of infection; and (h) studies of liver, biliary tract, pancreas, and renal function if indicated. Diagnosis may require histologic examination and special culture techniques of specimens obtained by tissue biopsy, bronchoalveolar lavage, gastrointestinal endoscopy, surgery, or other invasive procedures.

IV. TREATMENT.

Initial management of immunocompromised patients with suspected infection commonly includes empiric antimicrobial agents. Therapy of a limited number of common clinical syndromes is discussed.

A. Fever and neutropenia without obvious source in adults with cancer.

1. Because of the high risk of life-threatening infections, all febrile patients with an absolute neutrophil count (ANC) of less than 500/mm^3 or a falling ANC of 500 to 1,000/mm^3 should be treated with high doses of intravenous broad-spectrum bactericidal antibiotics promptly after culture specimens are obtained. Recommended empiric antibiotic regimens are listed in the Table 72-1.

TABLE 72-1	Initial Empiric Antibiotic Therapy for Febrile Adult Neutropenic Patients

1. Ceftazidime 2 grams IV every 8 hours plus or minus vancomycin 1 gram IV every 12 hours. Consider discontinuing vancomycin in the absence of a documented pathogen requiring this agent.
2. Alternatives
   - piperacillin/tazobactam 3.375 grams IV every 4 to 6 hours (suspected oral, dental, or other polymicrobial or anaerobic infection)
   - aztreonam 2 grams every 6 hours plus vancomycin 1 gram IV every 12 hours (severe penicillin allergy)
   - imipenem 500 mg IV every 6 hours (suspected extended spectrum β-lactamase–producing organism).
3. Aminoglycosides may be added to β-lactam antibiotics in cases of suspected sepsis with antibiotic-resistant organisms or an abdominal source of infection.

2. Removal of indwelling venous catheters should be considered in cases of (a) bacteremia due to *Staphylococcus aureus*, vancomycin-resistant enterococci, *Pseudomonas* species, *Candida* species, *Corynebacterium jeikeium*, *Bacillus* species, and *Fusarium* species; (b) evidence of tunnel or exit site infection; (c) the presence of septic thrombophlebitis; or (d) persistent or recurrent bacteremia.

3. Patients with fever persisting more than 3 days need to be thoroughly reevaluated. Empiric therapy for *Aspergillus* species and other filamentous fungi with amphotericin B or voriconazole should be considered after 4 to 7 days of fever.

4. Empiric antibiotics may be discontinued when fever and neutropenia have resolved.

B. Fever and pulmonary disease

1. The differential diagnosis includes not only infection (bacteria, fungi, protozoa, viruses, and helminths), but also acute respiratory distress syndrome, bronchiolitis obliterans with organizing pneumonia, malignancy, pulmonary hemorrhage, radiation injury, drug toxicity, and many others.

2. Focal or multifocal infiltrates suggest bacterial or invasive fungal pneumonia. Diffuse interstitial disease is more characteristic of viruses, *P. jiroveci*, or a noninfectious process. Cavitary and nodular disease can be associated with bacteria (e.g., *P. aeruginosa*, *S. aureus*, anaerobes), *Nocardia* species, mycobacteria, *Legionella*, endemic or invasive fungi, and noninfectious processes. Pneumonia due to "atypical" pathogens such as mycoplasma or chlamydia are rare.

3. Patients with fever and pulmonary infiltrates should be started promptly on antibiotics targeting the most likely pathogen(s), such as the combination of a quinolone or a macrolide with a third-generation cephalosporin for common bacteria, trimethoprim-sulfamethoxazole for *P. jiroveci*, or amphotericin B or voriconazole for fungal disease. Bronchoscopy with bronchoalveolar lavage or lung biopsy is indicated in patients with a nondiagnostic evaluation for pulmonary disease or lack of clinical improvement on initial empiric therapy.

Selected Readings

Immunocompromised Host Society consensus conference on epidemiology, prevention, diagnosis, and management of infections in solid organ transplant patients. *Clin Infec Dis* 2001;33(suppl 1):S1–65.
This entire supplement issue is devoted to a variety of topics in transplant infectious diseases.

Nichols WG. Management of infectious complications in the hematopoietic stem cell transplant recipient. *J Intensive Care Med* 2003;18(6):295–312.
A thorough introduction to stem cell transplantation and managing common infectious complications in these patients.

Sullivan KM, et al. Preventing opportunistic infections after hematopoietic stem cell transplantation: the Centers for Disease Control and Prevention, Infectious Diseases Society of America Hematology, and American Society for Blood and Marrow Transplantation Practice Guidelines and beyond. *Hematology* 2001:392–421.
Consensus guidelines for preventing opportunistic infections in hematopoietic stem cell transplant (HSCT) recipients, including chemoprophylaxis, infection control practices, and vaccines.

INTENSIVE CARE OF PATIENTS WITH HIV INFECTION

73

Mark J. Rosen

I. HIV INFECTION AND CRITICAL ILLNESS

A. Background

1. The use of combination therapy directed at human immunodeficiency virus (HIV) ("highly active antiretroviral therapy," or HAART) resulted in a substantial reduction in the incidence of AIDS and its associated mortality.

2. Patients with HIV infection who require treatment in an intensive care unit (ICU) for opportunistic infections are more likely to be those who have not been diagnosed or in whom antiretroviral therapy has not been used or failed.

3. In the last few years, more patients with AIDS have died of non–HIV-associated disorders, especially complications of hepatitis C virus.

B. Pathogenesis

1. HIV infection results in progressive loss of CD4+ lymphocytes and susceptibility to opportunistic infections and neoplasms.

2. When therapy suppresses viral replication, CD4+ cells are restored and immune function improves. This effect has been accompanied by a notable decline in the frequency of opportunistic infections.

C. Diagnosis

1. The CD4+ lymphocyte count is the best surrogate marker of immune function.

2. Measurement of serum viral load (HIV-RNA) is an important guide to antiretroviral treatment.

D. Treatment

1. Nonadherence to antiretroviral therapy and improper regimens lead to poor responses and drug resistance.

2. Admission to an ICU may make administration of HAART difficult because most drugs are administered orally, absorption may depend on when food is given, and drug interactions are numerous and complex.

3. The ICU team should seek a consultant with expertise in antiretroviral therapy when treating HIV-infected patients.

4. Prophylaxis against opportunistic infections should be started or continued in most patients for whom they are indicated.

II. RESPIRATORY FAILURE

A. Background

1. Respiratory failure is the most common reason for ICU admission of HIV-seropositive persons.

2. Pneumocystis jiroveci pneumonia (PCP) is one of the most common causes of admission to ICU, although its incidence is declining.

3. Pneumonia and acute respiratory distress syndrome (ARDS) due to bacterial infection are common causes of respiratory failure.

4. Tuberculosis, fungal infection, and noninfectious HIV-associated pulmonary disorders may also cause respiratory failure.

B. Pathogenesis

1. PCP almost always occurs in patients with CD4+ counts less than 200/μL.

2. The risk of bacterial pneumonia increases as the CD4+ lymphocyte count declines and is higher in injection drug users than in patients in other HIV transmission categories.

3. *Streptococcus pneumoniae* is the most common cause of bacterial pneumonia, but *Pseudomonas aeruginosa* is a significant problem in patients with a history of prior opportunistic infections or CD4+ counts less than 50/μL.

4. Coinfection with HIV and *Mycobacterium tuberculosis* has fueled the resurgence of tuberculosis, including multidrug-resistant tuberculosis.

5. Fungal pneumonia may result from either new acquisition or reactivation of latent disease.

6. Almost all patients with AIDS and cryptococcal pneumonia have CD4+ counts less than 100/μL, and disseminated disease with meningitis is common.

7. Invasive aspergillosis causes necrotizing lung disease in patients with CD4+ counts lower than 30/μL.

8. Fungal diseases in specific endemic areas such as histoplasmosis and coccidioidomycosis may become disseminated in patients with CD4+ counts less than 200.

C. Diagnosis

1. Most patients with HIV and respiratory failure have either bacterial pneumonia or PCP.

2. Bacterial pneumonia usually presents in a similar fashion in patients with and without HIV infection. The diagnostic evaluation is the same in both groups.

3. PCP usually presents with progressive dyspnea and cough, with the chest film showing diffuse granular opacities. Cystic disease with or without spontaneous pneumothorax may also be seen.

4. Definitive diagnosis of PCP requires demonstrating the organism in respiratory specimens. Sputum induction has a high diagnostic yield in many centers.

5. When sputum is negative, flexible bronchoscopy with bronchoalveolar lavage should be considered.

6. Bronchoscopic lung biopsy is usually not performed in patients receiving mechanical ventilation or those with uncorrectable coagulopathy; biopsy may be diagnostic when lavage is negative in PCP, as well as providing rapid diagnosis of other infectious and noninfectious pulmonary diseases.

7. Cavitation, hilar and mediastinal adenopathy, and pleural effusions suggest tuberculosis; in patients with severe immunosuppression, diffuse infiltrates, miliary patterns, or normal chest radiographs are common.

8. Respiratory specimens from HIV-infected patients should always be examined for acid-fast bacilli by smear and culture.

D. Treatment

1. Supportive management (supplemental oxygen, mechanical ventilation, positive end-expiratory pressure) is the same as in patients without HIV infection.

2. Initial therapy for HIV-infected patients with respiratory failure should be directed at *S. pneumoniae*, Haemophilus *influenzae*, and PCP (Table 73-1).

3. Adjunctive corticosteroid therapy given at the start of anti-*Pneumocystis* treatment reduces the likelihood of respiratory failure, deterioration of oxygenation, and death in patients with moderate to severe pneumonia.

4. Response to an empiric regimen does not obviate the need for establishing a specific diagnosis whenever possible. Otherwise, patients are committed to a prolonged course of potentially toxic antimicrobials and corticosteroids for a disorder they might not have.

III. IMMUNE RECONSTITUTION INFLAMMATORY SYNDROME

A. Pathogenesis

1. When HAART inhibits viral replication, there is an increase in the population of memory and naïve T cells, enhancement of lymphoproliferative responses, increased IL-2 receptor expression, and reduced production of some plasma cytokines.

2. These proinflammatory effects underlie immune reconstitution inflammatory syndrome (IRIS).

| TABLE 73-1 | Treatment of Moderate to Severe[a] *Pneumocystis* Pneumonia |

Drug	Dose	Comments
Trimethoprim (TMP)-sulfamethoxazole (SMX)	15–20 mg/kg TMP, 75–100 mg/kg IV SMX IV or PO in three or four divided doses	Drug of choice, but toxicity (rash, fever, nausea, leukopenia) frequent
Pentamidine isoethionate	3–4 mg/kg IV daily	Toxicity: dysglycemia, renal failure, QT interval prolongation, arrhythmias, pancreatitis, hypotension; 50% dextrose must be available
Trimetrexate-leucovorin	45 mg/m² IV daily (plus folinic acid, 20 mg/m² IV or PO q6h)	Not as effective as trimethoprim-sulfamethoxazole but better tolerated
Prednisone	40 mg PO bid, days 1–5; 20 mg PO bid, or 40 mg PO qd, days 6–10; 20 mg PO daily, days 11–21	Recommended as adjunctive therapy along with an anti-*Pneumocystis* agent for all patients with PCP who meet criteria for moderate to severe disease

[a]$P_aO_2 \leq 70$ mm Hg, or $P_{(A-a)}O_2 \geq 35$ to 45 mm Hg breathing room air. *Intensive Care Medicine*, 4th ed. Philadelphia: Lippincott Williams & Wilkins, 1998, Table 91-2, p. 1152.

3. Patients with latent or active mycobacterial infection may develop fever, lymphadenopathy, and opacities on the chest radiograph due to IRIS.
4. Patients recently treated for PCP may also have a paradoxical worsening of pulmonary disease after HAART is introduced.

B. Diagnosis

1. IRIS usually occurs 2 to 8 weeks following immune restoration with HAART.
2. IRIS may not be associated with an increase in circulating T-lymphocytes, because these cells are compartmentalized to areas of inflammation.

C. Treatment

1. The optimal timing of the introduction of HAART in critically ill patients is still unknown.
2. When HAART treatment has been successful, it should usually not be withdrawn.
3. Because IRIS is usually self-limited, treatment should be deferred in patients without life-threatening illness.
4. If necessary, administration of corticosteroids can attenuate the severity of IRIS.

Selected Readings

Hanson DL, Chu SY, Farizo KM, et al. Distribution of CD4+ T lymphocytes at diagnosis of acquired immunodeficiency syndrome-defining and other human immunodeficiency virus-related illnesses. *Arch Intern Med* 1995;155:1537–1542.
Correlates the CD4+ lymphocyte count with the development of specific HIV-associated disorders.

Hirschtick RE, Glassroth J, Jordan MC, et al. Bacterial pneumonia in patients infected with human immunodeficiency virus. *N Engl J Med* 1995;333:845–851.
Describes the etiology and outcomes in a large cohort.

Narasimhan M, Posner AJ, DePalo VA, et al. Intensive care in patients with HIV infection in the era of highly active antiretroviral therapy. *Chest* 2004:125:1800–1804.
Intensive care unit admission rates in HIV-seropositive persons were in the era of HAART than before, and these patients were more likely to be admitted for non-HIV associated disorders.

Narita M, Ashkin D, Hollender ES, et al. Paradoxical worsening of tuberculosis following antiretroviral therapy in patients with AIDS. *Am J Respir Crit Care Med* 1998;158:157–161.

Wislez M, Bergot E, Antoine M, et al. Acute respiratory failure following HAART introduction in patients treated for *Pneumocystis carinii* pneumonia. *Am J Respir Crit Care Med* 2001;164:847–851.
Two case series of respiratory illness due to immune reconstitution inflammatory syndrome.

National Institutes of Health—University of California Expert Panel for Corticosteroid as Adjunctive Therapy for Pneumocystis Pneumonia: consensus statement on the use of corticosteroid as adjunctive therapy for *Pneumocystis pneumonia* in the acquired immunodeficiency syndrome. *N Engl J Med* 1990;323:1500–1504.
Review of studies of adjunctive corticosteroid therapy of PCP, with recommendations for clinical use.

Palella FJ, Delaney KM, Moorman AC, et al. Declining morbidity and mortality among patients with advanced human immunodeficiency virus infection. *N Engl J Med* 1998; 38:853–860.
Documents markedly reduced HIV-associated mortality and morbidity attributable to the use of HAART.

Panel on Clinical Practices for Treatment of HIV Infection. Guidelines for the use of antiretroviral agents in HIV-infected adults and adolescents. Available at http://www.aidsinfo.nih.gov/guidelines/adult/AA. Accessed August 8, 2004
Continually updated information and recommendations by reliable and mainstream experts.

Sundar K, Suarez M, Banogon PE, et al. Zidovudine-induced fatal lactic acidosis and hepatic failure in patients with acquired immunodeficiency syndrome: report of two patients and review of the literature. *Crit Care Med* 1997;25:1425.
Excellent review of this complication of antiretroviral therapy.

2001 USPHS/IDSA guidelines for the prevention of opportunistic infections in persons infected with HIV. Available at http://www.aidsinfo.nih.gov/guidelines/op_infections/OI_112801. Accessed August 8, 2004.
Comprehensive and updated guidelines for the prevention of opportunistic infections in persons with HIV infection.

74 INFECTIOUS COMPLICATIONS OF SUBSTANCE ABUSE
Raul Davaro and Aneetha Thirumalai

I. **GENERAL PRINCIPLES.** Illicit drug use causes more than 25,000 deaths a year and has an economic cost of $100 billion. Infectious complications account for 60% to 80% of hospital admissions and 20% to 30% of deaths in parenteral drug addicts. The current epidemic of HIV infection and hepatitis C is largely related to parenteral drug use.

II. **MANAGEMENT OF THE FEBRILE INJECTION DRUG USER.** Because of a potential life-threatening infection and the lack of discriminating clinical or laboratory features to predict complications, it is recommended that every injection drug user with fever be hospitalized. Risk for clinical withdrawal symptoms and management of this complication is needed to ensure adherence with treatment.

III. **SKIN AND SOFT TISSUE INFECTIONS.** Skin and soft tissue infections are the leading causes of hospitalization in parenteral drug users. The most common skin infections are abscesses and cellulitis. The practice of "skin-popping" is the strongest risk factor for abscess formation. Recent studies showed that the predominant flora are *Staphylococcus aureus, Streptococcus pyogenes, Streptococcus milleri, Fusobacterium* spp, *Veillonella* spp *and Prevotella* spp. Most specimens contain polymicrobial flora. Abscesses should be incised and drained.

Soft tissue infections may be indistinguishable from simple cellulitis in their early stages. The presence of vesicles or bullae, an area of central necrosis within a larger area of erythema, the presence of subcutaneous crepitation, and gas seen in soft tissues on radiographs suggest necrotizing fasciitis. This life-threatening infection requires immediate, aggressive débridement in association with parenteral antibiotics. Empiric therapy should be directed against *S. aureus,* streptococci, anaerobes, and aerobic gram-negative bacilli.

IV. **BACTEREMIA AND ENDOCARDITIS.** Bacteremia is common in the febrile parenteral drug user. Approximately 60% of these bacteremias are due to causes other than endocarditis. Most are caused by skin and soft tissue or vascular infections.

S. aureus is the most common blood culture isolate with increasing rates of methicillin-resistant *S. aureus* (MRSA). Streptococci are the second most frequent and are commonly associated with skin and soft tissue infections.

Polymicrobial bacteremia occurs in about 10% of cases, of which two thirds have *S. aureus* as one of the organisms. Facultative anaerobic organisms, including *Eikenella corrodens,* are associated with saliva-contaminated needles.

Empiric antibiotic therapy should include agents active against MRSA, streptococci, and aerobic gram-negative bacilli.

Infective endocarditis accounts for 6% to 8% of hospital admissions among injection drug users. *S. aureus* sensitive to methicillin is the leading pathogen followed by MRSA, viridans streptococci, *Steptococcus pyogenes, Enterococci, Pseudomonas aeruginosa, Serratia marcescens,* other gram-negative rods and *Candida albicans.* Infections of the right side of the heart often present with fever or pleuropulmonary involvement. A systolic murmur often develops during therapy. On chest radiography, multiple patchy infiltrates indicative of pulmonary emboli strongly suggest the diagnosis. Blood cultures are almost invariably positive. Negative blood cultures in a patient with the appropriate clinical syndrome should raise the possibility that the patient has recently taken antibiotics. Left-sided endocarditis is often complicated by arterial embolization to the renal and cerebral arteries.

Empiric therapy should be directed against staphylococci, streptococci, and aerobic gram-negative bacilli. Right-sided endocarditis typically has a favorable prognosis and responds well to therapy. Limited data suggest that patients without evidence of left-sided involvement, renal failure, extrapulmonary metastatic infections, or MRSA may be treated with a 2-week course of nafcillin or oxacillin, plus an aminoglycoside. In a small study of right-sided *S. aureus* endocarditis, a course of 4 weeks of ciprofloxacin plus rifampin was found to be efficacious. For patients with isolated tricuspid valve involvement and intractable infection, valvulotomy is successful in most cases. Left-sided endocarditis secondary to *P. aeruginosa* has a mortality rate of nearly 70%. A course of 6 weeks of an antipseudomonal β-lactam antibiotic plus an aminoglycoside and early surgical removal of the involved valve is often required. *Candida* endocarditis also has an extremely high mortality rate, even with prompt valve replacement and systemic antifungal therapy.

V. PERIPHERAL VASCULAR INFECTIONS. Septic thrombophlebitis is common and typically presents with fever, bacteremia, and swelling over the involved vein. When the injection site is into the deep tissues of the groin or neck, it may be difficult to distinguish involvement of vascular structures from simple cellulitis, soft tissue abscesses, or fasciitis. If there is a diagnostic dilemma, angiography should be performed to determine whether the vasculature is involved. Septic thrombophlebitis can often be treated with antibiotics alone, although incision, drainage, and removal of the vein are sometimes necessary. Anticoagulation is generally not needed.

Mycotic aneurysm is another frequent vascular complication that results when the user injects a drug directly into the artery. Patients typically present with fever and a tender, pulsatile mass, usually in the groin or the neck.

VI. SKELETAL INFECTIONS. Vertebral osteomyelitis is the most common infection of the axial skeleton. Patients generally present with weeks to months of pain, often without high fevers, and many are afebrile. Typically, tenderness is found over the involved vertebral body, and there is often radiographic evidence of osteomyelitis. Septic arthritis in this group of patients often involves the sacroiliac, sternoarticular, or symphysis pubis joints. Patients usually have weeks to months of pain and tenderness to palpations. Magnetic resonance imaging (MRI) is the imaging study of choice in these patients. Pyogenic bacteria account for almost 90% of bone and joint infections; staphylococci and steptococci cause almost 80% of these infections. *Candida* species may also occur alone or as part of a dissemination syndrome. Biopsy or needle aspiration of the involved bone or joint is imperative to direct therapy, because of the varied microbiology.

VII. HUMAN IMMUNODEFICIENCY VIRUS INFECTION. The spectrum of HIV-related complications among injection drug users differs from that in other HIV-infected populations. Bacterial infections, especially pneumonia, endocarditis, and sepsis, are frequent occurrences. The incidence of bacterial pneumonia in HIV-infected drug users is four times higher than in HIV-negative drug users. Other complications in this patient population include tuberculosis and various opportunistic infections.

VIII. NERVOUS SYSTEM INFECTIONS. Epidural abscess is one of the most frequent central nervous system infections. Pain associated with radicular symptoms is the most common presentation, and symptoms are often indolent. These infections are usually secondary to underlying vertebral osteomyelitis. Computed tomography (CT) and MRI are useful in defining the extent of the infectious process. Staphylococci are the most frequent cause, although other pathogens, including *P. aeruginosa* and *Mycobacterium tuberculosis*, have been recognized. Surgical decompression is often required.

Brain abscesses may occur usually as a result of embolization from either endocarditis or mycotic aneurysm. They are typically multiple and generally are secondary to *S. aureus*. However, a definitive microbiologic diagnosis is imperative.

IX. **SINOPULMONARY INFECTIONS.** Cocaine, heroin, and petroleum distillates are usually snorted, sniffed, or smoked. These forms of abuse lead to cough, bronchospasm, chemical pneumonitis, and pneumomediastinum. "Crack lung" is a syndrome comprising chest pain, hemoptysis, and diffuse pulmonary infiltrates. Complications from injection drug use include pneumonia, empyema, lung abscesses, septic emboli, pulmonary edema, and granulomatosis caused by talc and other contaminants. Bacterial pneumonia may be due to typical community pathogens such as *Streptococcus pneumoniae*, *S. aureus*, *Haemophilus influenzae*, and *Klebsiella pneumoniae*. If there is a recent history of unconsciousness, suggesting aspiration, anaerobes should also be considered. Clinicians must maintain a high index of suspicion for tuberculosis in drug users, particularly if they are infected with HIV. Some studies show that the prevalence of a positive PPD increases with age among individuals actively using intravenous drugs. *Pneumocystis jiroveci* pneumonia and other opportunistic infections must also be considered in patients with HIV infection.

Selected Readings

Asselah T, Vidaud D, et al. Second infection with a different hepatitis C virus genotype in an intravenous drug user during interferon therapy. *Gut* 2003;52:900–902.

Chambers HF, Miller RT, Newman MD. Right-sided *Staphylococcus aureus* endocarditis in intravenous drug abusers: two-week combination therapy. *Ann Intern Med* 1988;109:619.
A small study demonstrating 94% efficacy with 2 weeks of antibiotics.

Dworkin RJ, Lee BL, Sandy MA, et al. Ciprofloxacin with rifampin: a predominately oral regimen for right sided *S. aureus* endocarditis in intravenous drug abusers. *Lancet* 1989;2:1071.
A small study demonstrating efficacy with an oral regimen possibly helpful for patients who refuse intravenous treatment.

Levine DP, Cran LR, Zervos MJ. Bacteremia in narcotic addicts at the Detroit Medical Center. II. Infectious endocarditis: a prospective comparative study. *Rev Infect Dis* 1986;8:374.
A classic two-part series on bacteremia in narcotic addicts.

Marantz PR, Linzer M, Feiner CJ, et al. Inability to predict diagnosis in febrile intravenous drug abusers. *Ann Intern Med* 1987;106:823.
A frequently quoted article showing the need for hospitalization of intravenous drug abusers.

Mathei C, Buntinx F, Van Damme P. Seroprevalence of hepatitis C markers among intravenous drug users in western European countries: a systematic review. *Journal of Viral Hepatitis* 2002;9(3):157–173.

O'Connor PG, Selwyn PA, Schottenfeld RS. Medical care for injection drug users with human immunodeficiency virus infection. *N Engl J Med* 1994;331:450.
A well-written review touching on multiple aspects of caring for the injection drug user with HIV.

Salomon N, Perlman DC, Friedmann P, et al. Prevalence and risk factors for positive tuberculin skin tests among active drug users at a syringe exchange program. *Int J Tuberc Lung Dis* 2000.4:47–54.

TUBERCULOSIS IN THE INTENSIVE CARE UNIT   75
Michael D. Mancenido and Jennifer S. Daly

I. BACKGROUND
A. The changing epidemiologic features of tuberculosis in the United States make this disease more difficult to recognize for all health-care providers, including those in the intensive care setting.

B. Tuberculosis is an acute, subacute, or chronic illness caused by *Mycobacterium tuberculosis*, known for its property as an acid-fast staining bacillus (AFB). *M. tuberculosis* usually affects the lung but may cause disease in other organs of the body.

C. Prompt recognition of tuberculosis and early institution of effective therapy allow successful treatment of the patient and the prevention of transmission.

II. PATHOPHYSIOLOGY
A. The pathogenesis of tuberculosis (TB) involves a complex interaction between bacilli and host.

　1. Primary infection: usually an asymptomatic presentation

　　a. Tubercle bacilli gain entry into the lungs, then become phagocytized by alveolar macrophages. A localized inflammatory process occurs with the development of tubercle granulomas.

　　b. Bacilli multiply and involve adjacent hilar lymph nodes, then disseminate via the bloodstream, infecting the central nervous system, liver, spleen, kidney, and other organ systems.

　　c. Cell-mediated response through the effect of Th1 cytokines brings the infection under control in most normal individuals.

　　d. Tuberculin skin test (TST) usually becomes positive in 2 to 10 weeks.

B. Adaptive host response occurs with manifestations of clinically active or latent TB

　1. Active tuberculosis

　　a. Active TB occurs in about 10% of immunocompetent individuals infected with *M. tuberculosis* over their lifetime. Half of these cases develop within the first 1 to 2 years.

　　b. Associated with classic symptoms of cough, hemoptysis, fevers, night sweats, or weight loss

　2. In patients with defects in cell-mediated immunity:

　　a. The risk of progressive primary or disseminated disease is increased (i.e., the annual risk of developing TB is 5% to 7% among HIV-infected persons)

　　b. These patients have less granulomatous inflammation and more *M. tuberculosis* organisms in tissues.

　3. Latent tuberculosis

　　a. Characterized by a positive tuberculin skin test

　　b. Immunocompetent persons develop a granulomatous inflammatory process and usually control the infection

　　c. Classic symptoms are absent

C. Immune reconstitution inflammatory syndrome

　1. Immune reconstitution inflammatory syndrome (IRIS) is a transient, paradoxical worsening of the patient's condition with fevers, increasing lymphadenopathy, new infiltrates, and acute respiratory distress syndrome (ARDS) after treatment of TB or the underlying immunodeficiency, such as occurs with the initiation of highly active antiretroviral therapy in HIV/AIDS patients.

   2. May occur in patients debilitated by their TB disease. Successful treatment of TB reduces the burden of disease. This facilitates a return of cell-mediated immunity as TB is treated.

   3. In patients with suspected IRIS, the clinician must exclude drug-resistant *M. tuberculosis*, a febrile response to therapy, coinfection with nontuberculous pathogens, or other alternative diagnoses.

III. PROGNOSIS. Worldwide, 2 million people die of TB each year. With medications, most patients with localized disease and adherence to therapy are cured.

IV. DIAGNOSIS

   A. The clinician should have a high suspicion for disease in intensive care unit (ICU) patients with predisposing risks or comorbidities and involvement of particular organ systems

   1. Suspect in high-risk patients
      a. history of positive TST or tuberculous disease
      b. contact with known or suspected TB
      c. presence of fibrotic lung lesions or upper lobe scar
      d. immigration from countries with a high risk for TB
      e. advanced age
      f. alcohol or other drug use
      g. institutional exposure (i.e., congregate living)
      h. immunocompromised host (e.g., with HIV infection, undergoing chemotherapy, or taking steroids or antitumor necrosis factor agents)

   2. Suspect in certain organ or disease states
      a. lungs: respiratory failure from fulminant tuberculous pneumonia, life-threatening (severe) hemoptysis, or ARDS
      b. heart: pericardial tamponade from pericardial tuberculosis
      c. central nervous system: tuberculous meningitis
      d. gastrointestinal: complications of gastrointestinal tract involvement
      e. systemic: disseminated tuberculosis

   B. Chest radiograph: the primary diagnostic and screening test

   1. Immunocompetent patients with pulmonary tuberculosis usually have an abnormal chest radiograph
      a. Primary tuberculosis: lower lobe infiltrate with ipsilateral hilar adenopathy (especially in children)
      b. Reactivation disease: fibrotic and cavitary infiltrates in the apical segment of the upper and superior segment of the lower lobes
      c. Disseminated (miliary) disease: nodules 1 to 3 mm in size
      d. Old disease: upper lobe parenchymal scars or calcified granulomata representing fibrotic foci of healed inactive tuberculosis (Ghon's complex)

   2. Immunocompromised *and immunosuppressed* patients may have a normal-appearing chest radiograph
      a. Patients with dissemination to the lungs may infrequently present as a normal-appearing chest radiograph. Nodules in the size range of 1 to 3 mm can be missed until several days to weeks later with involvement of more lung parenchyma. However, a high-resolution CT scan has a higher sensitivity than chest radiography and may be abnormal.
      b. HIV infected patients with a CD4$^+$ less than 200 may have sputum-culture-confirmed TB with a normal chest radiograph. Other atypical presentations include hilar/mediastinal adenopathy, pleural effusions, diffuse and/or lower lobe opacities.

   C. Detection of *M. tuberculosis*: microscopy (smear) and culture

   1. Sputum microscopy (AFB smear)
      a. Most important diagnostic tool.
      b. Sputum samples positive by auramine-stained smear or Ziehl-Neelsen stain may be examined with direct nucleic acid amplification tests to distinguish *M. tuberculosis* from nontuberculous mycobacteria.

    c. AFB stains and cultures of gastric aspirates, other body fluids, and blood may be diagnostic

  2. Culture

    a. Obtain specimens of sputum as well as infected fluids, blood, bone marrow, lymph nodes, and tissue biopsy (e.g., pleural and pericardial)

    b. Timing: mycobacterial pathogens grow slowly, but liquid media often radiometrically detect *M. tuberculosis* within 2 to 6 days and then identification may be done promptly with genetic probes within 1 to 3 weeks rather than the usual 4 to 8 weeks for growth on routine solid media.

    c. Susceptibility testing: may be available (within 1 to 3 weeks for AFB smear–positive sputum specimens) with direct susceptibility testing. Additional weeks may be needed if the laboratory sends isolates to a reference laboratory after initial isolation.

  3. Pathology: Characteristic histology on biopsy (see earlier pathophysiology section).

V. TREATMENT

  A. Oral therapy: Four drug combination of isoniazid (INH), rifampin, pyrazinamide, and either ethambutol or streptomycin for the initial 8 weeks of therapy.

  B. Intravenous therapy: Rifampin, aminoglycosides (streptomycin or amikacin), and fluoroquinolones may be given intravenously. INH may be given intramuscularly. The use of a fluoroquinolone is needed if resistant *M. tuberculosis* is suspected. INH and rifampin are key components of an ICU treatment regimen.

  C. If IV access cannot be obtained, INH and streptomycin may be given intramuscularly, while rifampin (capsule) and pyrazinamide (tablet) can be delivered via nasogastric tube 4. Referral to an outpatient program with directly administered therapy. Cure rates of over 95% can be achieved with a 6-month regimen among patients with drug-susceptible organisms (isoniazid and rifampin the last 4 months).

  D. Strains resistant to isoniazid and rifampin usually require therapy for 18 or 24 months.

  E. In patients with renal failure, isoniazid and rifampin may be given in standard doses. Ethambutol, pyrazinamide, aminoglycosides, and fluoroquinolones require dose adjustments.

  F. Corticosteroids are used for tuberculous meningitis and tuberculous pericarditis.

VI. INFECTION CONTROL AND RESPIRATORY ISOLATION

  A. Major concern is to prevent nosocomial transmission. Guidelines from the Centers for Disease Control and Prevention and the Occupational Health and Safety Administration form the basis of infection control policy.

  B. Early recognition allows the appropriate use of respiratory isolation and the prompt initiation of treatment. The infectiousness of tuberculosis begins to decrease within days of the initiation of effective therapy. Key components of infection control for TB are the following:

    1. Patients in the ICU should be in single-patient rooms with special ventilation characteristics appropriate for the purposes of isolation. For example, in existing facilities negative-pressure isolation rooms with at least six air changes per hour are appropriate.

    2. Staff should use closed suctioning systems to avoid generation of infectious aerosols as well as submicron filters for air exhausted from ventilated patients.

    3. Health-care workers who will be in contact with the patient need personal protective devices (respirators). These respirators must be able to filter particles 1 micron in size and be fit-tested in health-care workers with a variety of facial characteristics.

    4. Hospital personnel need to have periodic tuberculin skin testing to monitor the effectiveness of infection control measures and allow prompt preventive therapy of staff recently infected with *M. tuberculosis*.

Selected Readings

Centers for Disease Control and Prevention. Prevention and treatment of tuberculosis among patients infected with human immunodeficiency virus: principles of therapy and revised recommendations. *MMWR* 1998;47:1–51.

National guidelines outlining therapy and prophylaxis in HIV-infected patients. The recommendations consider the use of antiretroviral agents and drug interactions with medications used to treat TB disease and TB infection.

Christie JD, Calihan DR. The laboratory diagnosis of mycobacterial diseases. *Clin Lab Med* 1995;15:279–306.
Review of laboratory methods.

Comstock GW. Epidemiology of tuberculosis. *Am Rev Respir Dis* 1982;125:8–15.
Review of traditional studies of epidemiology.

Guidelines for preventing the transmission of *Mycobacterium tuberculosis* in health-care facilities, 1994. *MMWR* 1994; 43:1–143.
This is the standard guideline on which institutional infection control policies are based. The Web site is www.cdc.gov/mmwr/preview/mmwrhtml/00035909.htm

Hill AR, Premkumar S, Brustein S, et al. Disseminated tuberculosis in the acquired immunodeficiency era. *Am Rev Respir Dis* 1991;144:1164–1170.
Tuberculosis may be difficult to diagnose and present in organs other than the lungs in patients with HIV infection.

Horsburgh CR, Feldman S, Ridzon R. Infectious Diseases Society of America. Practice guidelines for the treatment of tuberculosis. *Clin Infect Dis* 2000;31(3):633–639. Epub 2000 Oct 04.
Ten essential practice guidelines for the treatment of active and latent TB infection.

Iseman MD. Treatment of multi-drug resistant tuberculosis. *N Engl J Med* 1993;329:784–791.
Review of therapeutic strategies, medications, and rationale for the treatment of patients with multidrug-resistant TB.

Keiper MD, Beumont M, Elshami A, et al. CD4 T lymphocyte count and the radiographic presentation of pulmonary tuberculosis. A study of the relationship between these factors in patients with human immunodeficiency virus infection. *Chest* 1995:107:74–80.
Review of tuberculosis in HIV-infected patients.

Targeted tuberculin testing and treatment of latent tuberculosis infection. This official statement of the American Thoracic Society was adopted by the ATS Board of Directors, July 1999. This is a Joint Statement of the American Thoracic Society (ATS) and the Centers for Disease Control and Prevention (CDC). This statement was endorsed by the Council of the Infectious Diseases Society of America. (IDSA), September 1999, and the sections of this statement. *Am J Respir Crit Care Med* 2000;161(4 Pt 2):S221–S247.
This is the reference on which today's therapy is based.

Weis SE, Slocum PC, Blais FX, et al. The effect of directly observed therapy on the rates of drug resistance and relapse in tuberculosis. *N Engl J Med* 1994;330:1179–1184.
Review of data supporting the current recommendation for directly observed therapy for patients with TB disease.

I. BOTULISM
A. General principles
1. Botulism is a rare disease that requires prompt diagnosis and treatment to decrease mortality.
2. Disease results from a potent neurotoxin produced by *Clostridium botulinum* and is classified into five types: (a) foodborne botulism, (b) wound botulism, (c) infant botulism, (d) adult infectious botulism as a result of intestinal colonization, and (e) inhalation of aerosolized toxin as a biological weapon.
3. Most of the cases of botulism are foodborne and involve home-canned and - processed foods. Food contaminated with toxin, especially type E, may appear and taste normal. Sometimes, disease associated with toxin types A or B spoils the food and results in gas production.
4. Wound botulism should be considered in parenteral abusers of black tar heroin who present with neurologic symptoms.
5. Pulmonary complications are the principal cause of death.
6. Mortality rate from foodborne botulism is 15%.

B. Etiology
1. The causative agent of botulism is *C. botulinum,* an anaerobic spore-forming gram-positive bacillus that is ubiquitous in nature.
2. Both the vegetative form of the organism and the toxins are heat labile. The spores, however, are highly heat resistant and can survive boiling for hours.

C. Pathogenesis
1. *C. botulinum* toxin (types A, B, E, and rarely F and G) acts at the neuromuscular junctions, where it inhibits the release of acetylcholine at the cholinergic synapses.
2. In adults, intestinal colonization with the organism may occur after intestinal surgery and antibiotic therapy.

D. Diagnosis/clinical presentation
1. The incubation period is usually 18 to 36 hours after the ingestion of the contaminated food.
2. Patients are typically alert and afebrile.
3. Frequent neurologic symptoms include bilateral cranial nerve impairment, dysphagia, diplopia, dysarthria, blurred vision, and upper and lower paralysis or weakness.
4. Ocular findings include extraocular palsies; nystagmus; and dilated, poorly reactive, or fixed pupils.
5. Nausea, vomiting, and abdominal cramps often precede the neurologic manifestations.
6. With wound botulism, fever may be present and the incubation period is from 4 to 14 days.

E. Laboratory studies
1. Botulism can be confirmed by: (a) botulinal toxin detection in the patient's serum, feces, or food; (b) culture; or (c) repetitive nerve stimulation.
2. Complete blood count, electrolytes, serum enzymes, and cerebrospinal fluid are normal unless there are secondary complications.

F. Treatment
1. Therapy must be based on the clinical evidence; laboratory confirmation is often delayed.
2. Remove unabsorbed toxin from the gastrointestinal tract using a nasogastric tube for lavage and a cathartic or a tap water enema.

3. Administer trivalent antitoxin (A, B, E) to neutralize any circulating toxin in the serum. Contact the CDC at 404-639-2206 or 404-639-2888.
4. Meticulous supportive care.
5. Elective intubation should be performed when the vital capacity approaches 30% of the predicted value.
6. Wound botulism is treated with débridement and intravenous penicillin G as well as antitoxin.
7. If the patient is penicillin allergic, use metronidazole.

II. TETANUS

A. General principles
1. Tetanus is a preventable disease.
2. Almost exclusively limited to inadequately immunized persons.
3. The spores of C. *tetani* are found worldwide in soil.
4. Almost any wound may serve as a portal of entry for the organism.
5. Tetanus-prone wounds may be minor and may not appear infected.
6. Cases have also been reported after gastrointestinal surgery, obstetric delivery and abortions, and injections, particularly in drug addicts.

B. Etiology
1. C. *tetani* is a large, spore-forming, anaerobic gram-positive bacillus.
2. The vegetative forms of the organism are easily destroyed by heat and disinfectants. The spores are extremely resistant to physical and chemical disinfection.
3. Tetanus results from the action of tetanospasmin, a potent exotoxin.

C. Pathogenesis
1. After a puncture wound or laceration, spores introduced at the injury site are converted to the vegetative form.
2. The organism proliferates only under anaerobic conditions usually associated with local vascular damage or trauma with tissue necrosis.
3. The organism does not produce tissue injury or evoke an inflammatory reaction.
4. The toxin acts at the motor end plates of the skeletal muscles, the spinal cord, the brain, and the sympathetic nervous system.

D. Diagnosis/clinical presentation
1. Three forms of the disease are described: (a) local, (b) cephalic, and (c) generalized.
2. Local tetanus is present when the muscle spasms are limited to those near the site of injury.
3. In cephalic tetanus, patients have paralysis of the cranial nerves. The incubation period is usually 1 to 2 days and follows an injury to the scalp, face, or neck.
4. The generalized form of the disease is the most common. Incubation is usually 7 days but ranges from 1 to 54 days. Ninety percent begin within 2 weeks.
   b. Patients complain of trismus or lockjaw and have diffuse muscle spasms.
   c. Facial muscles may spasm, resulting in a grinning expression (*risus sardonicus*).
   d. Spasms of the neck and back muscles may result in opisthotonos.
   e. Laryngeal spasms may result in cyanosis and respiratory arrest.
   f. Generalized seizures occur and are often triggered by mild external stimuli.
   g. The sympathetic nervous system stimulation results in profuse perspiration, tachycardia, labile hypertension, and cardiac arrhythmias.
   h. The patient's mental status is usually not impaired.
5. Tetanus is extremely unlikely in a patient with a prior history of tetanus immunization.
6. Sera can be assayed for tetanus antitoxin.
7. Wounds should undergo Gram staining and should be cultured anaerobically for C. *tetani* .
8. Table 76-1 lists certain conditions that may be confused with tetanus.

E. Treatment
1. The mainstay of therapy is meticulous intensive care in a quiet area.
2. A nasotracheal tube or an oral endotracheal tube should be inserted to manage the copious pharyngeal secretions and to prevent airway obstruction. Once the airway is secure, drugs are needed to control the spasms and the seizures.

TABLE 76-1   Causes of Trismus

Local
  Abscesses (alveolar)
  Parotitis
  Fractures
  Infected upper molar teeth
  Cervical lymphadenopathy
  Temporomandibular joint arthritis
Systemic
  Phenothiazines
  Strychnine poisoning
  Trichinosis
Other
  Cerebrovascular accidents
  Acute hysteria

3. The patient should be given human tetanus immunoglobulin. A recent report suggests that administration of the tetanus immunoglobulin by the intrathecal route is preferred over the intramuscular route.

4. The wound should be surgically débrided, and a 10-day course of penicillin administered. Patients who are allergic to penicillin can be given metronidazole or doxycycline.

5. Muscle relaxation can usually be obtained using diazapam. Intrathecal baclofen and intravenous magnesium sulfate may be used to control spasms. Some patients require an agent such as vecuronium or even drug-induced coma. The discontinuation of the sedation is determined by trial and error.

6. Cardiac arrhythmias are common and demand close attention. Hypertension caused by the increased catecholamines often requires treatment with labetalol.

7. The overall case fatality rate is about 11%.

8. Prevention is most important. Patients presenting with an injury with an inadequate tetanus immune status should receive tetanus immunoglobulin (250 U intramuscularly) as well as tetanus toxoid.

Selected Readings

Centers for Disease Control and Prevention (CDC). Botulism in the United States, 1899–1996: handbook for epidemiologists, clinicians, and laboratory workers. Atlanta: CDC 1998. *Review.*

Faust RA, Vicker OR, Cohn I Jr. Tetanus: 2,449 cases in 68 years at Charity Hospital. *J Trauma* 1976;16:704.
Clinical features include muscle spasms and no sensory deficits.

Hughes JM, Blumenthal JR, Merson MH, et al. Clinical features of type A and B foodborne botulism. *Ann Intern Med* 1981;95:442.
Clues to the diagnosis include symmetric neurologic findings, no sensory deficits, and the absence of fever.

Miranda-Filho D, Arraes de Alencar Ximenes R, Alci Barone A, et al. Randomised controlled trial of tetanus treatment with antitetanus immunoglobulin by the intrathecal or intramuscular route. *BMJ* 2004;328:7440–7444.
Intrathecal tetanus immunoglobulin was preferred compared to when the drug was given by the intramuscular route.

Okoromah MDC. Diazepam for treating tetanus. *The Cochrane Database of Systematic Reviews* 2004;2:1–27.
Evidence-based review of diazepam for tetanus.

Pavani K, Crowe C, Reller M, et al. An outbreak of foodborne botulism associated with food sold at a salvage store in Texas. *Clinical Infectious Disease* 2003;37:1490–1495.
Chili from a salvage store was the source.

Santos ML, Mota-Miranda A, Alves-Pereira A, et. al. Intrathecal baclofen for the treatment of tetanus. *Clinical Infectious Diseases* 2004;38:321–328.
Another option to treat spasms.

Shapiro RL, Hatheway C, Swerdlow D. Botulism in the United States: a clinical and epidemiologic review. *Ann Intern Med* 1998;129:221.
This review notes that treatment consists of supportive care and trivalent equine antitoxin.

Weinstein L. Tetanus. *N Engl J Med* 1973:289:1293.
This review describes diagnosis and management.

Gastrointestinal and Hepatobiliary Problems in the Intensive Care Unit

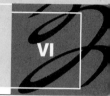

VI

GASTROINTESTINAL BLEEDING: PRINCIPLES OF DIAGNOSIS AND MANAGEMENT

Chandra Prakash

I. GENERAL PRINCIPLES. Acute gastrointestinal (GI) bleeding is a common clinical emergency. Early recognition of clinical and endoscopic prognostic signs helps in the triage to the intensive care unit of patients at risk of rebleeding. Bleeding from the upper GI tract is more common than lower GI bleeding.

    A. Prognosis

        1. The mortality rate from upper GI bleeding remains around 6% to 12%, whereas that from lower GI bleeding typically is less than 5%.

        2. Newer nonsurgical therapies may improve survival.

II. ETIOLOGY

    A. Upper gastrointestinal bleeding

        1. Common causes

            a. Duodenal and gastric ulcers and erosions

            b. Esophageal and gastric varices

            c. Esophagitis

            d. Mallory-Weiss tears

        2. Uncommon causes

            a. Angiodysplasia

            b. Cancer

            c. Dieulafoy's lesions

            d. Portal gastropathy

            e. Other causes, including hemobilia, Cameron's erosions, aortoenteric fistula

    B. Lower gastrointestinal bleeding

        1. Common causes

            a. Diverticulosis

            b. Angiodysplasia

            c. Cancer and polyps, including postpolypectomy bleeding

            d. Colitis, including inflammatory bowel disease, infectious colitis, ischemic colitis

            e. Hemorrhoids

        2. Uncommon causes

            a. Anal fissure, rectal ulcers including stercoral ulcers, solitary rectal ulcer syndrome

            b. Radiation proctopathy and colopathy

            c. Vasculitis

            d. Meckel's diverticulum

            e. Colonic varices

            f. Other, including endometriosis, intussusception, aortoenteric fistula

III. DIAGNOSIS

    A. Clinical presentation

        1. Passage of red or dark red blood in the stool usually indicates lower intestinal bleeding.

        2. Repeated passage of liquid bloody stool indicates ongoing or recurrent bleeding, because fresh blood has laxative properties.

        3. Passage of black, sticky, tarry stool (melena) usually indicates upper GI bleeding.

        4. Melena can persist for several days, and the stool may remain positive for occult blood for up to 2 weeks after GI bleeding has ceased.

        5. Bright or dark red blood in the stool is infrequently seen with an upper GI bleeding source, but, when it occurs, it indicates rapid bleeding; it is usually associated with hemodynamic compromise.

B. Diagnostic tests

1. Nasogastric aspiration

a. Passage of a nasogastric tube may help to detect upper GI bleeding in patients with an obscure bleeding site.

b. However, the nasogastric aspirate may be nonbloody if a tightly closed pylorus prevents reflux of blood from a duodenal bleeding site.

c. Further use of the nasogastric tube for lavage to control bleeding is unsubstantiated, although lavage may help remove clots from the stomach in preparation for endoscopy.

2. Endoscopy

a. Endoscopy is performed when the patient is hemodynamically stable, but resuscitation usually is ongoing at the time of the procedure.

b. When a bleeding site proximal to the jejunum is suspected, esophagogastroduodenoscopy (EGD) is the diagnostic procedure of choice.

c. When a lower GI bleeding source is suspected, sigmoidoscopy or colonoscopy may be helpful after bowel preparation. These procedures may help to detect and treat colonoscopic bleeding sources or to localize fresh blood to a segment of colon and to direct other therapeutic measures.

d. Push enteroscopy evaluates the proximal small bowel when a bleeding site is not found in the upper GI tract or colon with conventional endoscopy.

e. While EGD frequently is performed with therapeutic intent early in the course of bleeding, other endoscopic procedures typically are performed after the bleeding has ceased or in patients with subacute bleeding.

3. Imaging studies

a. A technetium99m-labeled red blood cell scan can detect bleeding rates as low as 0.1 mL per minute and is a reasonable initial imaging test in the patient with signs of active bleeding distal to the upper GI tract.

b. If active bleeding is found, angiography often is indicated for confirmation of the site and administration of intraarterial vasopressin or embolization of the bleeding artery for bleeding control.

c. Patients who continue to bleed despite intraarterial vasopressin may require surgical management.

d. Avoid barium studies in the setting of acute bleeding.

4. Newer techniques

a. Wireless capsule endoscopy may help localize bleeding to the small bowel if no bleeding source is identified on conventional endoscopy.

b. Limitations of this procedure include lack of real-time viewing of images and lack of therapeutic ability.

IV. TREATMENT

A. Initial approach

1. Rapid evaluation

a. Mental confusion, agitation, diaphoresis, mottled skin (livedo reticularis), and cold extremities accompany hypotension with hemorrhagic shock.

b. A quantitative estimate of the amount of bleeding is helpful, because the initial blood count may not reflect the degree of blood loss.

c. Nevertheless, initial blood testing should be performed urgently to obtain baseline hemoglobin/hematocrit values, to measure platelet count and coagulation parameters, and to type and cross-match blood for transfusion.

d. Abdominal pain is not common with GI bleeding and may indicate the presence of hemobilia, intestinal infarction, or perforation.

e. Chest pain may imply a superimposed myocardial infarction or dissecting aneurysm.

f. Previous vascular surgery adds aortoenteric fistula to the differential diagnosis.

2. Resuscitation

a. Resuscitation of the unstable patient takes precedence over other treatments.

b. Recognizing and aggressively treating intravascular volume depletion are of the highest priority and should proceed concurrently with the initial diagnostic evaluation.

    c. Intravenous access with large-bore peripheral catheters or a central venous catheter is needed for aggressive administration of fluids or blood products.

    d. Ongoing massive hematemesis may require endotracheal intubation for airway protection before endoscopy.

    e. Exsanguinating hemorrhage may require immediate surgical management, at times with the assistance of limited endoscopy to help direct the surgical approach.

3. Acid suppression

    a. Rationale for using acid suppression in acute upper GI bleeding is based on the coagulopathy resulting from an acid milieu.

    b. A randomized trial showed that the proton pump inhibitor omeprazole (40 mg orally every 12 hours for 5 days) significantly decreased the incidence of recurrent bleeding and surgery in hospitalized patients with peptic ulcers; the study was restricted to patients who had bleeding peptic ulcers with high likelihood of recurrent bleeding, yet none underwent any commonly performed endoscopic therapies.

    c. Nevertheless, early treatment with oral or intravenous proton pump inhibitors is standard in acute upper GI bleeding.

B. Endoscopy

1. Endoscopic therapy, using thermal devices (heater probe, electrocoagulation, laser), injection therapy (sclerosing solutions, hypertonic saline, epinephrine), or banding devices, offers a convenient and expedient method of treating upper GI bleeding from many causes.

2. These treatments can decrease further bleeding, shorten hospital stay, decrease transfusions, decrease emergency surgery, and lower costs in acute upper GI bleeding.

3. Recurrent bleeding occurs in up to 30% of patients with bleeding ulcers despite successful endoscopic therapy, and continued observation for up to 72 hours is recommended.

4. Endoscopic therapy is of use for some colonic bleeding sites, such as angiodysplasia.

C. Angiographic therapy

1. Intraarterial vasopressin has been used for angiographic management of bleeding from many sites, particularly in the lower GI tract.

2. Vasopressin use is attended by risk of cardiovascular complications.

3. Gelfoam or metal coil embolization of the bleeding artery is an alternative approach that causes localized thrombosis and vessel occlusion; tissue ischemia and perforation are potential complications.

4. In the upper GI tract, angiographic therapy is usually reserved for patients with bleeding peptic ulcer disease in whom endotherapy has failed or who are ineligible for this endotherapy and who have a prohibitive surgical risk.

D. Surgery

1. Surgical consultation should be obtained early in patients with clinical and endoscopic risk factors for high morbidity and mortality.

2. Patients with massive ongoing hemorrhage that overwhelms the resuscitative effort need urgent surgical assessment.

3. Patients who fail to respond to endoscopic or angiographic management also need surgical assessment.

4. Arterial embolization and percutaneous shunts for variceal bleeding are alternatives in high-risk surgical candidates.

Selected Readings

Baradarian R, Ramdhaney S, Chapalamadugu R, et al. Early intensive resuscitation of patients with upper gastrointestinal bleeding decreases mortality. *Am J Gastroenterol* 2004;99:619–622.
Early correction of hemodynamic instability, low blood count, and coagulopathy resulted in a better outcome in patients with upper GI bleeding.

Bini EJ, Cohen J. Endoscopic treatment compared with medical therapy for the prevention of recurrent ulcer hemorrhage in patients with adherent clots. *Gastrointest Endosc* 2003;58:707–714.
Recurrent bleeding, need for transfusions, and hospital stay were reduced after endoscopic therapy compared with medical management alone for peptic ulcer bleeding.

Branicki FJ, Boey J, Fok PJ, et al. Bleeding duodenal ulcer: a prospective evaluation of risk factors for rebleeding and death. *Ann Surg* 1989;211:411.
Recurrent bleeding and mortality were significantly higher with bleeding duodenal ulcers larger than 1 cm in diameter.

Cook DJ, Guyatt GH, Salena BJ, et al. Endoscopic therapy for acute non-variceal hemorrhage: a meta-analysis. *Gastroenterology* 1992;102:139.
A meta-analysis of acute nonvariceal upper GI bleeding showing significant reduction of recurrent bleeding, need for surgical intervention, and mortality after endoscopic hemostatic therapy.

Jensen DM, Machicado GA. Colonoscopy for diagnosis and treatment of severe lower gastrointestinal bleeding: routine outcomes and cost analysis. *Gastroenterol Endosc Clin North Am* 1997;7:477.
Indications, therapeutic potential, and outcomes of urgent colonoscopy in acute lower GI bleeding.

Khuroo MS, Yattoo GN, Javid G, et al. A comparison of omeprazole and placebo for bleeding peptic ulcer. *N Engl J Med* 1997;336:1054.
A significant reduction in recurrent bleeding and need for surgery was noted in omeprazole-treated patients with bleeding peptic ulcers not managed with endoscopic hemostatic techniques.

Longstreth GF. Epidemiology and outcome of patients hospitalized with acute lower gastrointestinal hemorrhage: a population-based study. *Am J Gastroenterol* 1997;92:419.
Diverticulosis is identified as the leading cause of acute lower GI bleeding, and annual incidence rates, recurrence, and mortality are characterized.

Magnano A, Privitera A, Calogero G, et al. The role of capsule endoscopy in the work-up of obscure gastrointestinal bleeding. *Eur J Gastroenterol Hepatol* 2004;16:403–406.
Capsule endoscopy may provide a definitive diagnosis in approximately one half of patients with obscure GI bleeding.

Pennoyer WP, Vignati PV, Cohen JL. Management of angiogram positive lower gastrointestinal hemorrhage: long term follow-up of non-operative treatments. *Int J Colorectal Dis* 1996;11:279.
Angiotherapy with vasopressin infusion or embolization is highly effective in controlling massive lower GI bleeding and has a low recurrence rate.

Peura DA, Lanza FL, Gostout FL, et al. The American College of Gastroenterology bleeding registry: preliminary findings. *Am J Gastroenterol* 1997;92:924.
A wealth of demographic and etiologic information on both upper and lower GI bleeding, including current practice standards.

Reinus JF, Brandt LJ. Vascular ectasias and diverticulosis: common causes of lower intestinal bleeding. *Gastroenterol Clin North Am* 1994;23:1.
An excellent review of the common causes of lower GI bleeding.

Robinson P. The role of nuclear medicine in acute gastrointestinal bleeding. *Nucl Med Commun* 1993;14:849.
Appropriateness of patient selection and timeliness of the study are critical in the use of nuclear medicine studies in the investigation of acute GI bleeding.

Zuckerman GR, Prakash C, Askin MP, et al. AGA technical review on the evaluation and management of occult and obscure gastrointestinal bleeding. *Gastroenterology* 2000;118:201–221.
A comprehensive review and guidelines for management of occult and obscure gastrointestinal bleeding.

Zuckerman GR, Prakash C. Acute lower intestinal bleeding. Part I. Clinical presentation and diagnosis. Part II. Etiology, therapy and outcomes. *Gastrointest Endosc* 1998;48:606–616;1999;49:228–238.
A comprehensive, well-referenced two-part review on current concepts in acute lower GI bleeding.

Zuckerman GR, Trellis DR, Sherman TM, et al. An objective measure of stool color for differentiating upper from lower gastrointestinal bleeding. *Dig Dis Sci* 1995;40:1614.
An objective pocket-sized color card with five stool colors helps to differentiate upper from lower GI bleeding.

STRESS ULCER SYNDROME
Chandra Prakash

I. GENERAL PRINCIPLES
A. Definition
1. Stress ulcers are erosions or ulcers that occur in the upper gastrointestinal (GI) tract with extreme physiologic stress.
2. When associated with clinical bleeding or perforation, the condition is called stress ulcer syndrome (SUS).

B. Description
1. Multiple ulcers or erosions in the proximal stomach, in contrast to distal stomach lesions in peptic ulcer disease.
2. Duodenal ulcers are uncommon in SUS but, when seen, are associated with proximal gastric lesions.
3. As many as 52% to 100% of patients admitted to intensive care units (ICUs) have endoscopic evidence of gastric mucosal injury within the first day but most are asymptomatic.
4. Bleeding from SUS typically occurs within 2 weeks of ICU admission.
5. Abdominal pain is unusual except in the infrequent setting of perforation.

C. Prognosis
1. Mortality rates can be as high as 50% to 80% in patients who bleed, although death usually is attributed to the underlying disease.

II. ETIOLOGY
A. ICU patients with coagulopathy or who require prolonged mechanical ventilation are significantly predisposed to SUS.
B. Renal failure is independently associated with clinically significant bleeding from stress ulcers.
C. Major surgery, hemorrhagic shock, hypotension, major burns, acute intracranial head trauma, and sepsis are other risk factors.
D. The incidence of GI bleeding increases with each risk factor up to two; additional risk factors do not further increase the incidence.
E. Patients with minor burns, chronic brain disease, chronic obstructive pulmonary disease, transient respiratory illness, dialyzed chronic renal failure, myocardial infarction, arrhythmias, and congestive heart failure are presumed not to be at high risk for SUS.

III. PATHOGENESIS
A. Mucosal damage
1. Although gastric acid is essential for stress ulceration, a breakdown of some or all of the following mucosal defense mechanisms also is required:
   a. mucus and mucus-bound bicarbonate, providing an anatomic barrier while buffering intraluminal hydrogen ions;
   b. intact intramucosal blood flow, bringing systemic bicarbonate to buffer intramural pH shifts; and
   c. mucosal cell restitution to rapidly restore of the mucous-cell layer when the epithelium is damaged.
2. Stress results in mucosal ischemia, leading to drops in intramucosal pH from back-diffused hydrogen ions, that is compounded by a deficit of systemic bicarbonate buffer and oxygen.

3. Subsequent reperfusion contributes to the formation of toxic oxygen-derived free radicals and superoxides while decreasing the synthesis of cytoprotective prostaglandins. These effects create a favorable situation for mucosal damage.

4. The role of *Helicobacter pylori* in the pathogenesis remains unknown.

IV. DIAGNOSIS

A. Clinical presentation

1. Stress ulcers come to clinical attention when they bleed.

2. Significant stress ulcer bleeding occurs in 2% to 6% of critically ill patients and presents within 14 days of the onset of physiologic stress or ICU admission as hematemesis, gross blood from the nasogastric tube, or melena.

3. Patients with thermal injury from burns or with acute intracranial disease including head trauma and coma appear to be at increased risk (for Curling ulcers and Cushing ulcers, respectively)

B. Endoscopy

1. The earliest mucosal changes are found in the most proximal part of the stomach and include pallor, mottling, and submucosal petechiae.

2. Superficial linear erosions and ulcers are formed when these lesions coalesce.

3. Eventually diffuse mucosal damage may result, with bleeding and, rarely, perforation.

V. TREATMENT

A. Principles

1. The risk of bleeding and overall prognosis are related to the severity of underlying illness, aggressive management of which should always take precedence.

2. Prophylactic agents enhance mucosal integrity in patients at risk for stress ulceration.

3. Upper GI endoscopy helps establish the diagnosis and determines the need for endoscopic thermal or injection therapy.

4. Acid suppression, preferably with a proton pump inhibitor, is indicated when GI bleeding occurs.

B. Gastrointestinal bleeding

1. Injection of epinephrine or thermal therapy can be attempted during endoscopy.

2. If endoscopic measures fail, angiography can be attempted, using intraarterial vasopressin or embolization if the bleeding site can be demonstrated.

3. If multiple bleeding lesions are present, continuous gastric lavage with 5 to 10 L of ice-cold lactated Ringer's solution over 1 to 2 hours has been advocated.

4. Surgical therapy is reserved for severe, life-threatening hemorrhage that is unresponsive to all other measures.

5. The mortality of total gastrectomy approaches 100% in these critically ill patients, whereas subtotal gastrectomy can be associated with rates of recurrent bleeding approaching 50% from the remnant gastric mucosa.

6. Vagotomy and oversewing of any remaining ulcers during subtotal gastrectomy may decrease the high rate of recurrent bleeding.

C. Prophylaxis. The logic of prophylaxis lies in the assumptions that the formation of stress ulcers can be prevented or that, once these ulcers are formed, the progression from ulcer to bleeding or perforation can be halted.

1. Antacids

    a. Antacids (10 to 80 mL) can be administered through a nasogastric tube every 1 to 2 hours and ideally titrated to keep the gastric pH greater than 4.0, measured 1 hour after administration.

    b. Some antacids may cause diarrhea, may be contraindicated in renal failure, and may affect the bioavailability of oral medications.

    c. Antacid use involves expensive and time-consuming processes of frequent administration and monitoring of gastric pH.

2. Antisecretory drugs

    a. Histamine-2-receptor antagonists are administered intravenously, either as a standard intermittent bolus or by continuous infusion.

(1) Continuous infusion more effectively maintains the desired gastric intra-luminal pH.

(2) Patients with a creatinine clearance of less than 30 mL per minute should receive half the recommended dose, and caution should be exercised in patients with thrombocytopenia.

(3) The optimal gastric pH level is unknown, and the need for 24-hour pH control is not essential for a prophylactic effect.

  b. Although controlled studies are lacking, proton pump inhibitors in usual doses can also be used, including intravenous administration.

3. Sucralfate

  a. Sucralfate coats the early shallow mucosal lesions and protects them from further acid and pepsin damage without altering gastric pH.

  b. It is delivered in the form of a slurry through a nasogastric tube at a dose of 4 to 6 g per day.

  c. Although it is safe for long-term use in critically ill patients, sucralfate should be used with caution in patients with chronic renal insufficiency.

  d. Sucralfate may have a lower incidence of nosocomial pneumonia. It has a low side effect profile and is inexpensive.

4. Other agents

  a. Prostaglandins, free radical scavengers such as dimethylsulfoxide and allopurinol, and the bioflavin meciadanol have also been used for stress ulcer prophylaxis with varying results.

  b. Retrospective studies on burn patients and patients receiving assisted ventilation suggest that upper GI bleeding may be reduced by enteral feeding.

VI. COMPLICATIONS

A. Complications of stress ulcers. Stress ulcers can develop bleeding and, rarely, perforation.

B. Complications of prophylaxis

1. Nosocomial pneumonia as a complication of stress ulcer prophylaxis is a growing concern.

  a. Gastric alkalinization and colonization with gram-negative bacilli are thought to play a causal role, and, consequently, some studies suggest a higher incidence of nosocomial pneumonia in patients who receive antisecretory drugs.

  b. Further studies are needed before one prophylactic agent confidently can be recommended over another because of either higher efficacy or lower complications from treatment.

Selected Readings

Cook D, Guyatt G, Marshall J, et al. A comparison of sucralfate and ranitidine for the prevention of upper gastrointestinal bleeding in patients requiring mechanical ventilation: Canadian Critical Care Trials Group. N Engl J Med 1998;338:791.
A multicenter randomized, blinded, placebo-controlled trial showing a significantly lower rate of gastrointestinal bleeding in mechanically ventilated critically ill patients treated with intravenous bolus ranitidine as compared with nasogastric sucralfate.

Cook DJ, Fuller HD, Guyatt GH, et al. Risk factors for gastrointestinal bleeding in critically ill patients. N Engl J Med 1994;330:377.
This prospective multicenter cohort study identified respiratory failure and coagulopathy as two strong independent risk factors for stress ulcer bleeding.

Cook DJ, Reeve BK, Guyatt GH, et al. Stress ulcer prophylaxis in critically ill patients: resolving discordant meta-analysis. JAMA 1996;275:308.
Histamine-2-receptor antagonists reduce clinically significant stress ulcer bleeding, but data are insufficient to determine the advantage of one medical approach over another.

Cook DJ, Reeve BK, Scholes LC. Histamine-2-receptor antagonists and antacids in the critically ill population: stress ulceration versus nosocomial pneumonia. Infect Control Hosp Epidemiol 1994;15:437.

In critically ill patients, sucralfate results in a lower incidence of nosocomial pneumonia than either antacids or histamine-2-receptor antagonists.

Cook DJ. Stress ulcer prophylaxis: gastrointestinal bleeding and nosocomial pneumonia. Best evidence synthesis. *Scand J Gastroenterol Suppl* 1995;210:48.
This meta-analysis concludes that all stress ulcer prophylactic agents are effective in decreasing the incidence of stress ulcer bleeding, but sucralfate may be associated with a lower risk of nosocomial pneumonia and mortality.

Driks MR, Craven DE, Celli BR, et al. Nosocomial pneumonia in intubated patients given sucralfate as compared with antacids or histamine type 2 blockers. *N Engl J Med* 1987;317:1376.
A randomized trial showing that sucralfate may be preferable to antacids and histamine-2-receptor blockers in mechanically ventilated patients.

Fennerty MB. Pathophysiology of the upper gastrointestinal tract in the critically ill patient: rationale for the therapeutic benefits of acid suppression. *Crit Care Med* 2002;30(suppl):S351–S355.
A discussion of current views regarding the pathophysiology of stress ulcer syndrome.

Jung R, MacLaren R. Proton-pump inhibitors for stress ulcer prophylaxis in critically ill patients. *Ann Pharmacother* 2002;36:1929–1937.
Although effective and safe, the superiority of proton pump inhibitors over other conventional agents has not been established in stress ulcer syndrome.

Langtry HD, Wilde MI. Lansoprazole: an update of its pharmacological properties and clinical efficacy in the management of acid-related disorders. *Drugs* 1997;54:473.
Preliminary studies of lansoprazole show promise in patients at risk for stress ulcers.

Laterre PF, Horsmans Y. Intravenous omeprazole in critically ill patients: a randomized, crossover study comparing 40 with 80 mg plus 8 mg/hour on intragastric pH. *Crit Care Med* 2001;29:1931–1935.
Modest doses of intravenous proton pump inhibitor suppress intragastric pH in critically ill patients.

Levy MJ, Seelig CB, Robinson NJ, et al. Comparison of omeprazole and ranitidine for stress ulcer prophylaxis. *Dig Dis Sci* 1997;42:1255–1259.
A prospective randomized trial concluding that oral omeprazole is safe, effective, and clinically feasible for stress ulcer prophylaxis.

Metz CA, Livingston DH, Smith S, et al. Impact of multiple risk factors and ranitidine prophylaxis on the development of stress related upper gastrointestinal bleeding: a prospective multicenter double-blind randomized trial. *Crit Care Med* 1993;21:1844.
Two concomitant risk factors increased risk for stress ulcer bleeding, but additional risk factors were not detrimental.

Ortiz JE, Sottile FD, Sigel P, et al. Gastric colonization as a consequence of stress ulcer prophylaxis: a prospective randomized trial. *Pharmacotherapy* 1998;18:486.
Bacterial colonization was increasingly likely in patients with a persistently alkaline gastric pH.

Raff T, Germann G, Hartmann B. The value of early enteral nutrition in the prophylaxis of stress ulceration in the severely burned patient. *Burns* 1997;23:313.
Early enteral nutrition prevented stress-related upper gastrointestinal bleeding in burn patients.

Spirt MJ. Stress-related mucosal disease: risk factors and prophylactic therapy. *Clin Ther* 2004;26:197–213.
A review of currently available agents for the prophylaxis of stress ulcer syndrome.

Tryba M, Cook D. Current guidelines on stress ulcer prophylaxis. *Drugs* 1997;54:581.
A review article emphasizing that improvement of oxygenation and microcirculation in the ICU play an important role in preventing stress ulcers.

Yang YX, Lewis JD. Prevention and treatment of stress ulcers in critically ill patients. *Semin Gastrointest Dis* 2003;14:11–19.
A comprehensive review of pathogenesis, risk factors, and management of stress ulcer syndrome.

79

VARICEAL BLEEDING

Chandra Prakash

I. GENERAL PRINCIPLES

A. Acute variceal bleeding occurs in at least 20% of all patients with cirrhosis and varices.

B. The mortality of an acute bleeding episode approaches 30% to 50%.

C. Decompensation from liver disease, aspiration, hepatic encephalopathy, hepatorenal syndrome, septicemia, alcohol withdrawal, and exsanguination all contribute to a poor outcome.

D. Early accurate diagnosis, stabilization of hemodynamics, and immediate hemostasis are critical, as are prevention of recurrent bleeding and prevention and treatment of superimposed complications.

II. PATHOPHYSIOLOGY

A. Portal hypertension

1. The usual cause of portal hypertension is mechanical obstruction to portal venous flow.

2. Other causes include portal vein, hepatic vein thrombosis, and unusual disorders, such as congenital hepatic fibrosis and schistosomiasis.

3. Secondary hemodynamic changes associated with cirrhosis, including peripheral vasodilatation, decreased systemic vascular resistance, increased cardiac output, and splanchnic hyperemia, contribute to increased portal pressure.

B. Development of varices

1. A collateral circulation develops to decompress the portal venous system, the most clinically significant locations being the junctions of squamous and columnar mucosae (gastroesophageal, anal, and peristomal). These collateral vessels progressively enlarge to form varices.

2. Risk factors for variceal rupture include a portosystemic pressure gradient greater than 12 mm Hg, large variceal size, and progressive hepatic dysfunction.

III. DIAGNOSIS

A. Clinical presentation

1. Variceal bleeding typically is brisk, presenting as hematemesis, melena, and varying degrees of hemodynamic instability.

2. Acute bleeding is self-limited in 50% to 60% of cases.

3. Approximately one third of the patients with stigmata of chronic liver disease who present with acute upper gastrointestinal (GI) bleeding have nonvariceal sources of hemorrhage, and endoscopic verification is required.

B. Endoscopy

1. On endoscopy, a fresh fibrin clot may be seen protruding from a varix.

2. Detecting blood pouring from a variceal rent is unlikely.

3. Nonbleeding varices are the most common findings; in such cases, banding or sclerotherapy is warranted because of the high rate of early recurrent bleeding.

IV. TREATMENT

A. Initial resuscitation

1. Appropriate resuscitative efforts should be initiated without delay, even before endoscopic evaluation (see Chapters 77 and 124).

2. Nasogastric aspiration may be necessary when the diagnosis of an upper GI hemorrhage is in doubt; fears of trauma to a varix from the tube largely are unfounded, but good lubrication and careful technique should be exercised.

3. Packed red blood cell transfusion, fresh frozen plasma, and platelet infusion may be necessary before endoscopy, depending on initial laboratory test results.

4. Airway protection with endotracheal intubation is mandatory in the massively bleeding or obtunded patient.

5. Patients with alcoholism should receive thiamine and should be monitored closely for alcohol withdrawal.

B. Pharmacotherapeutic agents

  1. Octreotide is the pharmacotherapeutic agent of choice in acute variceal bleeding.

   a. This synthetic octapeptide shares structural and functional properties with somatostatin in reducing splanchnic blood flow and portal pressure.

   b. Aside from transient nausea and abdominal pain, significant adverse effects are rare.

   c. A bolus of 25 to 100 µg is followed by a continuous infusion of 25 to 50 µg/hour for 48 to 72 hours.

   d. Octreotide is effective in stopping active bleeding from varices and has an important role in the prevention of early recurrent bleeding after initial hemostasis.

  2. Vasopressin, when infused intravenously, is a potent vasoconstrictor that reduces splanchnic blood flow and portal pressure.

   a. Adverse cardiac effects (myocardial ischemia, hypertension) interfere with treatment in nearly 30% of patients and contribute to the limited success rate of this approach.

   b. The starting dose is typically 0.4 U per minute, titrated to a maximum of 1 U per minute if required for bleeding control.

   c. Concurrent intravenous nitroglycerin infusion, titrated to maintain a systolic blood pressure of 100 mm Hg, is recommended. This may prevent side effects from systemic vasoconstriction.

   d. Vasopressin currently is used only when octreotide is not available.

C. Endoscopic therapy

  1. Band ligation is the technique of choice for endoscopic control of bleeding varices.

   a. Small elastic "O" rings are placed endoscopically over the varices.

   b. Subsequent strangulation of the vessel with sloughing and fibrosis of the adjacent esophageal tissues results in the obliteration of the varix.

   c. Active bleeding is controlled in 80% to 90% of patients after one or two treatments.

   d. Band ligation has a lower incidence of esophageal ulceration, stricture formation, perforation, bacteremia, and respiratory failure.

   e. Serial scheduled endoscopic treatment sessions at weekly to monthly intervals ensure obliteration of the varices.

  2. Sclerotherapy

   a. A sclerosant solution is injected into the variceal lumen or into the adjacent submucosa.

   b. This technique is reserved for massive bleeding, wherein visualization of the variceal columns to perform band ligation is impossible, and for gastric variceal bleeding.

  3. Antibiotic prophylaxis is recommended to prevent infection and rebleeding when endoscopic band ligation or sclerotherapy is performed.

D. Transjugular intrahepatic portosystemic stent (TIPS) shunt

  1. TIPS is an iatrogenic fistula between radicals of the hepatic and portal veins, created by interventional radiologists using ultrasonographic and fluoroscopic guidance. An expandable metal stent is left in place, and the portosystemic pressure gradient is reduced to less than 12 mm Hg.

  2. TIPS is recommended if bleeding recurs after two or more endoscopic attempts at prevention, on an emergency basis in active uncontrolled bleeding, or if bleeding has occurred from gastric varices or portal hypertensive gastropathy.

3. The technical success rate in constructing a TIPS is more than 90%, with near-universal success in bleeding control.

4. Some degree of shunt insufficiency is seen in 15% to 60% of patients within 6 months.

5. Doppler ultrasound examination for determining shunt patency is recommended for postprocedure bleeding recurrence. The shunt usually can be revised with little morbidity.

6. After elective shunt placement, 20% to 30% of patients develop transient deterioration of liver function, and up to one fourth of patients may experience new or worsened hepatic encephalopathy.

E. Balloon tamponade

1. Gastric and esophageal balloon devices for direct tamponade of the bleeding varices (Sengstaken-Blakemore, Minnesota, and Linton-Nachlas balloons) may be required for patients with severe or persistent bleeding.

2. Initial success approaches 90%, but rates of recurrent bleeding are high, and definitive plans for portal decompression should be made before deflating the balloon.

3. Complications occur in 15% to 30% of patients; balloon-related deaths occur in up to 6%.

4. Endotracheal intubation should precede balloon placement for airway protection.

F. Other measures

1. Surgical shunts

  a. Surgical shunts are considered in patients with good long-term prognosis who need portal decompression, such as patients with Child A cirrhosis and patients with noncirrhotic portal hypertension.

  b. The utility of surgical shunting in the acutely bleeding patient with cirrhosis is limited by high operative mortality and postprocedure encephalopathy.

2. Nonshunting operations, such as the Sugiura procedure (mucosal transection and devascularization of the esophagus) are infrequently used, because varices reform and bleeding recurs in more than 20% of patients.

3. Embolization of the short gastric veins in gastric variceal bleeding and splenectomy in splenic vein thrombosis are other potential management options.

Selected Readings

Binmoeller KF, Soehendra N. Nonsurgical treatment of variceal bleeding: new modalities. *Am J Gastroenterol* 1995;90:1923.
A clinical review of the nonsurgical modalities available for the therapy of variceal bleeding.

Burroughs AK, Planas R, Svoboda P. Optimizing emergency care of upper gastrointestinal bleeding in cirrhotic patients. *Scand J Gastroenterol Suppl* 1998;226:14.
Of the vasoactive drugs available, somatostatin is the best treatment option, based on meta-analysis of clinical studies.

De Franchis R, Banares R, Silvain C. Emergency endoscopy strategies for improved outcomes. *Scand J Gastroenterol Suppl* 1998;226:25.
This review emphasizes that pharmacotherapy in combination with endoscopic intervention is more effective than endoscopic treatment alone in patients with variceal bleeding.

Haddock G, Garden OJ, McKee RF, et al. Esophageal tamponade in the management of acute variceal hemorrhage. *Dig Dis Sci* 1989;34:913.
Balloon tamponade controlled variceal bleeding in 94%, but 6.4% had fatal complications from the procedure.

Idezuki Y. Transection and devascularization procedures for bleeding from oesophageal varices. *Baillieres Clin Gastroenterol* 1992;6:549.
A review discussing surgery for bleeding esophageal varices and its indications.

Imperiale TF, Teran JC, McCullough AJ. A meta-analysis of somatostatin versus vasopressin in the management of acute esophageal variceal hemorrhage. *Gastroenterology* 1995;109:1289.
Somatostatin is more efficacious with a lower risk of adverse effects when compared with vasopressin.

Patch D, Nikolopoulou V, McCormick A, et al. Factors related to early mortality after transjugular intrahepatic portosystemic shunt for failed endoscopic therapy in acute variceal bleeding. *J Hepatol* 1998;28:454.
Patients with uncontrolled bleeding, advanced liver disease, sepsis, and multiorgan failure have a high mortality rate despite immediate bleeding control by TIPS.

Pohl J, Pollman K, Sauer P, et al. Antibiotic prophylaxis after variceal hemorrhage reduces incidence of early rebleeding. *Hepatogastroenterology* 2004;51:541–546.
Antibiotic prophylaxis reduces incidence of infections as well as early rebleeding after endoscopic treatment of variceal bleeding.

Rossle M, Deibert P, Haag K, et al. Randomized trial of transjugular-intrahepatic-portosystemic shunt versus endoscopy plus propranolol for prevention of variceal rebleeding. *Lancet* 1997;349:1043.
The transjugular shunt was more effective than endoscopic treatment in prevention of recurrent variceal bleeding but resulted in encephalopathy in 36%; there was no survival difference.

Rossle M, Grandt D. TIPS: an update. *Best Pract Res Clin Gastroenterol* 2004;18:99–123.
A review of the indications, technical aspects, complications, and outcome of the TIPS procedure.

Schepke M, Kleber G, Nurnberg D, et al. Ligation versus propranolol for the primary prophylaxis of variceal bleeding in cirrhosis. *Hepatology* 2004;40:65–72.
Variceal band ligation and propranolol are equally effective for the primary prophylaxis of variceal bleeding.

Schoenfeld PS, Butler JA. An evidence-based approach to the treatment of esophageal variceal bleeding. *Crit Care Clin* 1998;14:441.
Evidence from randomized controlled trials indicates that band ligation is more effective than sclerotherapy, that β-blockers and nitrates may prevent the initial episode of bleeding, and that somatostatin may decrease rebleeding rates with or without endoscopic therapy.

Steigmann GV, Goff JS, Michaletz-Onody PA, et al. Endoscopic sclerotherapy as compared with endoscopic ligation for bleeding esophageal varices. *N Engl J Med* 1992;326:1527.
Esophageal band ligation is associated with fewer treatment-related complications and better survival rates when compared with esophageal sclerotherapy for bleeding esophageal varices.

Tripathi D, Helmy A, Macbeth K, et al. Ten years' follow-up of 472 patients following transjugular intrahepatic portosystemic stent-shunt insertion at a single center. *Eur J Gastroenterol Hepatol* 2004;16:1–4.
TIPS is effective in the management of variceal bleeding with a low complication rate.

GASTROINTESTINAL MOTILITY PROBLEMS IN THE CRITICAL CARE SETTING
80
Gregory S. Sayuk and Ray E. Clouse

I. GENERAL PRINCIPLES
   A. Abnormalities of gastrointestinal (GI) motility are common in the intensive care unit (ICU) setting, occurring as a consequence of multiorgan dysfunction, medications, and metabolic derangements.
   B. Up to two thirds of ICU patients are affected, predominantly with disordered gastric and colonic motor function.
   C. Motility disorders manifest as gastric stasis [that can produce gastroesophageal reflux disease (GERD)], colonic dysfunction (abdominal distention, constipation), and diarrhea.
   D. Recognition may be difficult, because typical signs and symptoms are masked in the unresponsive or sedated patient.
   E. GI motility complications prolong ICU stays and nearly double mortality.

II. ETIOLOGY
   A. Causes of gastric stasis (delayed gastric emptying, gastroparesis) include:
   1. Critical illness alone
      a. Burns
      b. Head injury
      c. Pancreatitis
      d. Spinal cord injury
      e. Acute pain
      f. Sepsis
   2. Medications
      a. Anticholinergic medications
      b. Sympathomimetics/pressor agents
      c. Narcotics
      d. Phenothiazines/antipsychotics
   3. Comorbid illnesses
      a. Cirrhosis
      b. Diabetes mellitus
      c. Hypothyroidism (untreated)
      d. Prior gastric surgery and vagotomy
      e. Parkinson disease
      f. Miscellaneous (neuropathy, amyloidosis, scleroderma)
   4. Metabolic derangements
      a. Hypercalcemia
      b. Hypokalemia
      c. Hypomagnesemia
      d. Hyperglycemia
      e. Acidosis/alkalosis
   5. Sympathetic neural stimulation that accompanies many severe medical and surgical illnesses, which results in selective suppression of excitatory motor reflexes and sustained intrinsic inhibitory neural overactivity.
   B. Adverse outcomes from gastric stasis are:
   1. Poor absorption of oral or nasogastric-administered medications
   2. Intolerance to feeding

3. Predisposition to gastroesophageal reflux disease (GERD) and its complications (e.g., GI bleeding); GERD is further exacerbated by supine positioning, use of nasogastric tubes, and mechanical ventilation.
   4. Tracheobronchial aspiration and pulmonary compromise
C. Causes of colonic dysfunction (distention, constipation) include:
   1. Medications and metabolic disturbances that can delay colonic transit (see Causes of gastric stasis earlier).
   2. Medical comorbidities
      a. Burns or trauma
      b. Metabolic or electrolyte imbalances
      c. Hypothyroidism
      d. Organ failure (respiratory failure, acute renal failure)
      e. Infection, either systemic (pneumonia, sepsis) or gastrointestinal (*Clostridium difficile*, cytomegalovirus)
      f. Ischemia (intestinal, cerebrovascular)
      g. Surgical intervention
   3. Autonomic imbalance; this can accompany a host of medical and surgical illnesses and has been incriminated in acute colonic dilatation.
   4. Supine position, because it is not conducive to voluntary elimination.
   5. The withholding or strict limitation of luminal nutrition, a major stimulant of colonic motor function, can act as a contributor.
   6. Combinations of factors are often incriminated in massive colonic dilatation or pseudoobstruction.
D. Causes of diarrhea, a complication seen in at least one third of ICU patients and that interferes with medical management and outcome, include (also see Chapter 84):
   1. Enteral feedings
      a. Of ICU patients receiving enteral nutrition, 40% to 60% develop diarrhea.
      b. Hyperosmolar formulas, higher infusion rates, and colonic fermentation of malabsorbed carbohydrates have been invoked as etiologies.
   2. Infections, including C. *difficile,* and, in immunocompromised patients, cytomegalovirus, Cyclospora, Strongyloides, and Microsporidium
   3. Medications (antacids, antibiotics, lactulose, sorbitol suspensions)
   4. Fecal impaction, with stool overflow around the impaction

III. DIAGNOSIS
A. Gastric stasis (delayed gastric emptying, gastroparesis)
   1. Gastric stasis is suspected with impaired tolerance to gastric feeding, including clinical evidence of oral regurgitation or tracheobronchial aspiration (e.g., airway suctioning of enteral nutrition products).
   2. Gastric residual volumes of 200 mL or greater indicate retention.
   3. More reliable measurements of gastric emptying are accomplished using scintigraphic techniques or the octanoate breath test, but they are rarely performed.
   4. Mechanical obstruction is evaluated by upper endoscopy or radiographic imaging techniques.
   5. GERD, as an outcome of gastric stasis, typically presents with heartburn and regurgitation, though critically ill patients may not relay these symptoms.
      a. Chest pain is an atypical symptom of GERD that requires exclusion of cardiopulmonary explanations.
      b. GERD should be suspected in the setting of unexplained tracheobronchial aspiration, upper GI bleeding, vomiting, or regurgitation.
      c. Endoscopy typically is reserved for evaluation of GERD complications (e.g., GI bleeding) (see Chapters 12 and 77).
B. Acute colonic pseudoobstruction (Ogilvie's syndrome)
   1. Patients typically present with marked abdominal distention, pain, and altered bowel movements.
   2. Progression leads to colonic ischemia and perforation, complications that carry a mortality rate of up to 30%.

3. Colonic distention can be found incidentally on radiographs obtained for other reasons.
4. Plain abdominal films or computed tomography (CT) images demonstrate:
   a. Diffuse dilatation of the colon with normal mucosal markings and haustra.
   b. Absence of small bowel dilatation.
5. A water-soluble contrast enema may be necessary to exclude mechanical obstruction.
6. CT imaging is the most sensitive test for detecting perforation.

C. Diarrhea
1. Diarrhea (see Chapter 84) is defined by change in stool frequency or consistency, but more objectively by a stool weight of greater than 250 g per day.
2. Diarrhea can result in significant nutrient, water, and electrolyte loss, as well as skin breakdown.
3. Review medications for those that may precipitate diarrhea.
4. Maintain high suspicion for antibiotic-associated diarrhea, especially in the setting of unexplained leukocytosis, and diagnose by finding *C. difficile* toxin in the stool.
5. Perform rectal examination to exclude a distal impaction; abdominal radiographs are required to exclude more proximal impaction.
6. Sigmoidoscopy or colonoscopy with biopsy is helpful when diarrhea remains unexplained.

IV. TREATMENT
A. Gastric stasis (delayed gastric emptying, gastroparesis)
1. Initial approach
   a. Eliminate iatrogenic factors and exclude mechanical obstruction.
   b. Minimize or eliminate narcotics and other medications known to slow gastric emptying.
   c. Improve feeding tolerance by positioning the feeding tube ports beyond the pylorus; this maneuver does not eliminate the risk of tracheobronchial aspiration.
2. Pharmacologic treatment
   a. Few prokinetic agents are available.
   b. Metoclopramide is the only clinically approved prokinetic in the United States and is the agent of choice in the ICU.
      (1) The drug accelerates gastric emptying, but does not prevent aspiration pneumonia.
      (2) Significant side effects include confusion, agitation, somnolence, and dystonic reactions.
   c. Intravenous erythromycin, a motilin agonist, accelerates gastric emptying and facilitates post-pyloric tube placement.
      (1) To improve gastric emptying, erythromycin is given at a dose of 1 to 3 mg/kg three to four times daily.
      (2) Side effects include nausea, vomiting, abdominal cramps, and diarrhea.
      (3) Tolerance to the prokinetic effect of erythromycin occurs rapidly with repeated use from downregulation of motilin receptors.
3. Managing GERD as an outcome of gastric stasis
   a. Use conservative measures that may reduce reflux:
      (1) Maintain the head of the bed at a 45-degree elevation.
      (2) Avoid large-bolus tube feedings.
      (3) Consider post-pyloric feeding tube placement.
   b. Pharmacologic treatment also is required:
      (1) Patients with a preceding history of reflux disease should remain on medications at least as effective as their usual acid-suppression regimens.
      (2) Proton pump inhibitors (PPIs) are the most effective acid-suppressant agents.
      (3) PPIs may be given by mouth or by nasogastric tube, using appropriate formulations.
      (4) The intravenous (IV) route may be used when the enteral route is not feasible; pantoprazole and lansoprazole are available in IV preparations.

B. Acute colonic pseudoobstruction (Ogilvie's syndrome)
1. Initial approach
   a. Recognition of potentially reversible precipitants, such as electrolyte imbalances or medications that slow transit, is essential.
   b. Correct electrolyte and metabolic abnormalities
   c. Reduce narcotic medication use.
   d. Give patient nothing by mouth and use low, intermittent nasogastric suction.
   e. Exclude fecal impaction and place a rectal tube.
   f. Follow serial abdominal radiographs every 12 to 24 hours depending on clinical examination.
2. Pharmacologic treatment
   a. Intravenous neostigmine can be used when the patient fails to improve with conservative measures.
   b. Neostigmine 2 mg is given intravenously over 5 minutes in a closely monitored setting.
   c. The medication is contraindicated in face of bradycardia, active bronchospasm, or mechanical bowel obstruction.
3. Colonic decompression
   a. Colonoscopy for decompression is considered when distention worsens or persists and clinical condition of the patient appears compromised.
   b. Overall success of colonoscopic decompression is 88%, though mortality with the procedure in the setting of colonic pseudoobstruction is as high as 2%.
   c. The general value of colonoscopic decompression in colonic pseudoobstruction remains controversial; the procedure should be used selectively.
4. Surgical decompression occasionally is required when physical examination reveals progressive findings of peritoneal irritation or if imaging indicates perforation.

C. Diarrhea
1. Initial approach
   a. Decrease feeding rate in tube-fed patients to improve diarrhea until the gut adapts to the osmotic and volume load.
   b. Identify and correct electrolyte and other relevant metabolic abnormalities.
   c. If possible, discontinue medications potentially responsible for diarrhea, including offending antibiotics in presence of *C. difficile* infection.
2. Pharmacologic treatment
   a. Antidiarrheal agents should be used cautiously in ICU patients; maintain a focus on addressing infectious or other reversible etiologies.
   b. Metronidazole remains the drug of choice for *C. difficile* infection.
      (1) Initiate therapy in the more severely ill ICU patient (i.e., in the setting of fever, leukocytosis, colonic distension) while the toxin assay results are pending, and continue treatment for 14 days in toxin-positive patients.
      (2) The IV administration route is required in patients intolerant of oral metronidazole.
      (3) If broad-spectrum systemic antibiotics cannot be discontinued, maintain metronidazole until their treatment courses are completed.
      (4) Relapse of *C. difficile* infection is common and typically requires retreatment.
      (5) Oral vancomycin is reserved for patients intolerant of or who fail to improve with metronidazole.

Selected Readings

Bosscha K, Nieuwenhuijs VB, Vos A, et al. Gastrointestinal motility and gastric tube feeding in mechanically ventilated patients. *Crit Care Med* 1998;26:1510–1517.
A prospective case series evaluating the fasting and fed gastrointestinal motility characteristics that are possibly responsible for gastric retention in mechanically ventilated patients.

Cerra FB, Benitez MR, Blackburn GL, et al. Applied nutrition in ICU patients. A consensus statement of the American College of Chest Physicians. *Chest* 1997;111:769–778.
The American College of Chest Physicians (ACCP) consensus statement on the general goals and principles of ICU nutrition with comments on emerging therapies and areas of study.

Geller A, Petersen BT, Gostout CJ. Endoscopic decompression for acute colonic pseudo-obstruction. *Gastrointest Endosc* 1996;44:144–150.
A retrospective review of endoscopic decompression for acute colonic pseudoobstruction.

Grundfest-Broniatowski S, Quader M, Alexander F, et al. *Clostridium difficile* colitis in the critically ill. *Dis Colon Rectum* 1996;39:619–623.
A retrospective review of an experience with the management of C. difficile colitis in critically ill patients.

Heyland DK, Tougas G, King D, et al. Impaired gastric emptying in mechanically ventilated, critically ill patients. *Intensive Care Med* 1996;22:1339–1344.
A prospective evaluation of gastric emptying in ICU patients demonstrating delayed gastric emptying compared with healthy controls.

Liolios A, Oropello JM, Benjamin E. Gastrointestinal complications in the intensive care unit. *Clin Chest Med* 1999;20:329–345, viii.
An overview of the GI complications encountered in intensive care medicine.

MacLaren R. Intolerance to intragastric enteral nutrition in critically ill patients: complications and management. *Pharmacotherapy* 2000;20:1486–498.
A summary of the current literature on enteral nutrition complications in the ICU, with recommendations for optimizing patient tolerance.

McClave SA, Snider HL, Lowen CC, et al. Use of residual volume as a marker for enteral feeding intolerance: prospective blinded comparison with physical examination and radiographic findings. JPEN: *J Parenter Enteral Nutr* 1992;16:99–105.
A prospective study assessing gastric residual volumes in an ICU and control population, comparing results to physical examination and radiographic findings.

Ringel AF, Jameson GL, Foster ES. Diarrhea in the intensive care patient. *Crit Care Clin* 1995;11:465–477.
A summary of etiologies of diarrhea in ICU setting and clinical approaches to management.

Ritz MA, Fraser R, Tam W, et al. Impacts and patterns of disturbed gastrointestinal function in critically ill patients. *Am J Gastroenterol* 2000;95:3044–3050.
A review of gastrointestinal motility abnormalities in critically ill patients.

van der Spoel JI, Oudemans-van Straaten HM, Stoutenbeek CP, et al. Neostigmine resolves critical illness-related colonic ileus in intensive care patients with multiple organ failure—a prospective, double-blind, placebo-controlled trial. *Intensive Care Med* 2001; 27:822–827.
A prospective study demonstrating benefit of continuous neostigmine infusion compared with placebo in resolving critical-illness-related colonic ileus.

FULMINANT COLITIS AND TOXIC MEGACOLON

81

Chandra Prakash

I. GENERAL PRINCIPLES
A. Definitions
1. Fulminant colitis
   a. Fulminant colitis implies a serious progression of colonic mucosal inflammation, usually to deeper layers of the colon.
   b. Patients typically manifest severe bloody diarrhea, abdominal tenderness, and systemic toxicity.
2. Toxic megacolon
   a. In the face of fulminant colitis, colonic circular muscle paralysis can precipitate colonic dilatation or toxic megacolon, the term used to describe this entire sequence of events.
   b. Toxic megacolon is most commonly seen as a complication of ulcerative colitis but can occur with both idiopathic and infectious colitis, Crohn disease, amebic colitis, pseudomembranous colitis, and other infections.
   c. Factors associated with increased mortality include age greater than 40 years, the presence of colonic perforation, and delay of surgery.
   d. Early recognition and treatment of toxic megacolon can substantially lower mortality from as high as 50% (with colonic perforation) to less than 15%.

II. DIAGNOSIS
A. Clinical presentation
1. History
   a. Toxic megacolon usually occurs on the background of extensive colitis associated with chronic inflammatory bowel disease.
   b. Toxic megacolon typically occurs early in the course of ulcerative colitis, and 25% to 40% of patients present with the initial attack.
   c. Progressive diarrhea, bloody stool, and crampy abdominal pain are typical symptoms. A paradoxical decrease in stool frequency with passage of bloody "membranes" is an ominous sign.
   d. Manipulation of the inflamed bowel with diagnostic examinations such as barium enema or colonoscopy as well as medications (including vigorous laxatives, antidiarrheals, anticholinergics), electrolyte imbalances, and pH disturbances can contribute to the development of the condition.
   e. Corticosteroids can suppress signs of perforation and peritonitis, but whether these drugs can precipitate toxic megacolon is controversial.
2. Physical examination
   a. Systemic toxicity is heralded by fever and tachycardia and can progress to confusion, agitation, or apathy.
   b. Abdominal pain and distention, with diminished bowel sounds on auscultation, are common.
   c. Peritoneal signs indicate transmural inflammation or perforation, but they may be minimal or absent in elderly patients or in patients receiving corticosteroids.
B. Diagnostic tests
1. Laboratory studies
   a. Leukocytosis is common.
   b. Anemia, hypokalemia, and hypoalbuminemia also can occur.

    c. Laboratory tests should assess the degree of systemic toxicity, fluid and electrolyte deficits, pH disturbances, and the need for blood transfusion.

    d. Stool should be sent for *Clostridium difficile* toxin and other pathogens.

2. Radiologic studies

    a. Plain radiographs of the abdomen reveal loss of haustration and segmental or total colonic dilatation (usually only mild), with mucosal thumbprinting or pneumatosis cystoides coli in severe transmural disease.

    b. Free peritoneal air is an immediate indication for surgery.

    c. Small bowel ileus may accompany toxic megacolon and is a poor prognostic sign for conservative management.

    d. Discrepancies may exist between physical and radiographic findings.

3. Endoscopy

    a. A limited proctoscopic examination may show extensive ulceration with friable, bleeding mucosa, but rarely the examination is normal.

    b. An abdominal radiograph after cautious proctoscopic air insufflation can provide a partial contrast study to define the proximal extent of disease.

    c. More extensive endoscopic examination is contraindicated.

III. TREATMENT

A. General measures

1. Vigorous fluid, electrolyte, and blood replacement must be instituted early in the resuscitative effort, because hemodynamic instability is typical.

2. Total body potassium depletion is common and needs urgent repletion; phosphate, magnesium, and calcium deficiency also should be corrected parenterally.

3. Oral intake is discontinued and nasogastric suction is employed for small bowel ileus.

4. Anticholinergic and narcotic agents should be stopped immediately.

B. Treatment of inflammatory bowel disease

1. When inflammatory bowel disease is diagnosed or suspected, use of parenteral corticosteroids or adrenocorticotropic hormone is essential.

    a. Augmented doses (hydrocortisone, 100 mg every 6 hours, or methylprednisolone, 6 to 15 mg every 6 hours) should be administered.

    b. A continuous infusion may help maintain steady plasma levels. Aminosalicylates (mesalamine, sulfasalazine) have no role in the treatment of fulminant colitis or toxic megacolon and should be withheld until the patient has recovered and has resumed eating.

2. Intravenous cyclosporine (4 mg/kg per 24 hours in a continuous infusion) can be used when severe ulcerative colitis without toxic megacolon fails to improve after 7 to 10 days of intensive intravenous hydrocortisone therapy. The role of cyclosporine in toxic megacolon is controversial.

3. Infliximab infusion may have a role in select causes of severe ulcerative colitis.

C. Antibiotics

1. Broad-spectrum antibiotics are administered intravenously once toxic megacolon or transmural inflammation is suspected and are continued until the patient stabilizes over several days to a week.

2. Broad-spectrum antibiotics should be followed by pathogen-specific therapy in infectious colitis.

3. Metronidazole or vancomycin should be used if *C. difficile* infection is considered likely from the clinical presentation or proctoscopic findings.

D. Surgical indications

1. Surgical exploration

    a. Surgery is indicated if no improvement occurs despite 12 to 24 hours of intensive medical management. Delay of operative therapy may promote higher mortality.

    b. Evidence of colonic perforation is an unequivocal indication for emergency surgery.

    c. Other indications for emergency surgery include signs of septic shock and imminent transverse colon rupture (the most dilated region in most cases of toxic megacolon), especially if the diameter is greater than 12 cm.

d. Hypoalbuminemia, persistently elevated acute-phase reactants, small bowel ileus, and deep colonic ulcers are poor prognostic factors for successful medical therapy.

e. The absence of acute colonic dilatation may permit delay of surgical intervention for 5 to 7 days.

f. The potential for prolonged intensive medical management and complications must be balanced against early surgical intervention to reduce mortality and morbidity.

2. Surgical options

a. The type of operation performed for the treatment of fulminant colitis or toxic megacolon depends on the clinical status of the patient and the experience of the surgeon.

b. Most surgeons prefer a limited abdominal colectomy with ileostomy, leaving the rectosigmoid as a mucous fistula, or oversewing the rectum, using a Hartmann procedure. This allows less operating room time in acutely ill patients, yet leaves the option for a subsequent sphincter-saving ileoanal anastomosis.

c. In less acutely ill patients, a one-stage resection with ileostomy may be appropriate.

Selected Readings

Actis GC, Ottobrelli A, Pera A, et al. Continuously infused cyclosporine at low dose is sufficient to avoid emergency colectomy in acute attacks of ulcerative colitis without the need for high-dose steroids. *J Clin Gastroenterol* 1993;17:10.
Seven of eight patients with acute steroid-resistant ulcerative colitis went into clinical remission with 2 weeks of intravenous cyclosporine infusion.

Caprilli R, Vernia P, Colaneir O, et al. Risk factors in toxic megacolon. *Dig Dis Sci* 1980; 25:817.
The severity of electrolyte imbalance and of metabolic derangement appears to be important in the progression of severe colitis to toxic megacolon.

Caprilli R, Vernia P, Latella G, et al. Early recognition of toxic megacolon. *J Clin Gastroenterol* 1987;9:160.
Persistent small bowel gaseous distention and severe metabolic alkalosis may predict the development of toxic megacolon in severe ulcerative colitis.

Carbonnel F, Lavergne A, Lemann M, et al. Colonoscopy of acute colitis: a safe and reliable tool for assessment of severity. *Dig Dis Sci* 1994;39:1550.
Colonoscopy in acute ulcerative colitis is generally safe and can provide prognostic information in some cases.

Cheung O, Regueiro MD. Inflammatory bowel disease emergencies. *Gastroenterol Clin North Am* 2003;32:1269–1288.
Complications of inflammatory bowel disease, including fulminant colitis and toxic megacolon, are comprehensively reviewed.

Chew CN, Noland DJ, Jewell DP. Small bowel gas in severe ulcerative colitis. *Gut* 1991;32:1535.
Presence of small bowel distention in severe ulcerative colitis predicts poor response to medical therapy.

Gan SI, Beck PL. A new look at toxic megacolon: an update and review of incidence, etiology, pathogenesis, and management. *Am J Gastroenterol* 2003;98:2363–2371.
A discussion of the pathogenesis, diagnosis, investigation, and current management of toxic megacolon.

Gore RM, Ghahremani GG. Radiologic investigation of acute inflammatory and infectious bowel disease. *Gastroenterol Clin North Am* 1995;24:353.
Plain abdominal radiographs, barium studies, and cross-sectional imaging are complementary to endoscopic evaluation in acute enterocolitis.

Imbriaco M, Balthazar EJ. Toxic megacolon: role of CT in evaluation and detection of complications. *Clin Imaging* 2001;25:349–354.
The use of CT scanning in the detection and management of toxic megacolon.

Lichtiger S, Present DH, Kornbluth A, et al. Cyclosporine in severe ulcerative colitis refractory to steroid therapy. *N Engl J Med* 1994;330:1841.

Intravenous cyclosporine is rapidly effective in some patients with severe, corticosteroid-resistant ulcerative colitis.

Meyers S, Janowitz HD. The place of steroids in the therapy of toxic megacolon. *Gastroenterology* 1978;75:729.

The benefit of initiating steroid therapy for toxic megacolon is unclear; when this therapy is initiated, the patient needs to be watched carefully for signs of deterioration.

82

HEPATIC DYSFUNCTION
Kevin M. Korenblat

I. GENERAL PRINCIPLES
   A. Hepatic dysfunction in the intensive care unit (ICU) setting can present as either:
   1. Abnormalities of liver chemistries
   2. Overt manifestations of liver disease (e.g., jaundice, synthetic dysfunction)
   B. Hepatic metabolic processes are frequently disturbed in the setting of critical illness. These processes and their normal physiology include:
   1. Bilirubin metabolism
      a. Bilirubin is the end product of the catabolism of heme, the prosthetic moiety of hemoglobin, myoglobin, and other hemoproteins.
      b. Heme from senescent erythrocytes is the source of 80% of bilirubin.
      c. Unconjugated bilirubin is transported bound to albumin to the liver.
      d. Bilirubin is made water soluble by conjugation with glucuronic acid within the hepatocytes.
      e. Conjugated bilirubin is transported into the bile canaliculus and passed from the bile duct into the intestine.
   2. Drug metabolism
      a. The liver is a major site of first-pass metabolism of medications and other xenobiotics.
      b. The mechanisms of drug metabolism can be categorized as phase I or phase II reactions.
         (1) Oxioreductases and hydrolases catalyze phase I reactions that increase water solubility of substances and potentially generate toxic metabolites.
         (2) The proteins of the cytochrome P-450 family constitute the most important drug-metabolizing enzymes.
         (3) Transferases catalyze phase II reactions that produce biologically less active metabolites.
   3. Hemostasis
      a. The vitamin K–dependent coagulation factors II, VII, IX, and X are produced by the liver.
      b. The liver produces the vitamin K–dependent anticoagulant factors protein C and protein S.

II. ETIOLOGY
   A. Clinical disorders commonly encountered in the critical care setting that result in hepatic dysfunction include:
   1. Ischemic hepatitis
      a. Ischemic hepatitis develops in the setting of reduced liver blood flow, persistent hypotension, or severe hypoxemia.
      b. The causes of ischemic hepatitis are many (Table 82-1).
      c. A clearly documented period of hypotension may not be identifiable.
      d. A variable degree of central vein (zone 3) necrosis and collapse are present on liver histology.
   2. Congestive hepatopathy
      a. Any process that increases hepatic venous pressures (e.g., right heart failure, pericardial disease, pulmonary hypertension) can cause hepatic congestion.
      b. Other diagnoses that may resemble congestive hepatopathy include:
         (1) Budd-Chiari syndrome (hepatic vein thrombosis).

TABLE 82-1	Causes of Ischemic Hepatitis

Hypovolemic shock
  Burns
  Hemorrhage
Cardiogenic shock
Hypoxemia
  Obstructive sleep apnea
Sepsis
Sickle cell crisis
Hepatic artery occlusion post—liver transplantation
Heat stroke

       (2) Sinusoidal obstruction syndrome (venoocclusive disease)
       (3) Inferior vena cava thrombosis at its hepatic portion (obliterative hepato-
          cavopathy).
    c. Long-standing hepatic venous congestion may result in cirrhosis (cardiac
      cirrhosis).
    d. Thick bands of fibrous tissues bridging central to central ("reverse lobula-
      tion") areas is typical of the cirrhosis related to chronic venous congestion.
  3. Total parenteral nutrition (TPN)–related liver injury
    a. Hepatic steatosis and steatohepatitis are the most common hepatic compli-
      cations in adults.
      (1) Asymptomatic elevations in serum chemistries are a common presenta-
          tion of hepatic steatosis and steatohepatitis.
      (2) Deficiencies of essential fatty acids (linoleic acid) or choline may con-
          tribute to the development of steatosis.
    b. TPN-related cholestasis is the predominant clinical finding in infants.
      (1) Conditions associated with the development of cholestasis include large
          doses of lipid emulsion (>1 g/kg per day), short-gut syndrome, and bac-
          terial overgrowth.
      (2) Elevations in serum bilirubin may be mild to severe.
      (3) Cholestasis, particularly in infants, may result in rapid progression to
          cirrhosis and liver failure.
    c. Biliary sludging
      (1) Biliary sludging may develop in more than 50% after 6 weeks of TPN.
      (2) Clinical manifestations of sludging may vary from asymptomatic to cho-
          lecystitis.
  4. Sepsis
    a. Hepatic dysfunction is common in sepsis and is a consequence of:
      (1) Alterations in hepatic blood flow
      (2) Activation of reticuloendothelial cells
      (3) The release of inflammatory cytokines
    b. Elevations in serum aminotransferases two to three times the upper limits of
      the reference range may occur 2 to 3 days after the onset of bacteremia.
    c. Jaundice with serum bilirubin levels five to 10 times the upper limits of the
      reference range may occur.
  5. Drug hepatotoxicity
    a. Myriad patterns are associated with drug-induced liver injury. The pattern
      observed is dependent on the dose and duration of drug exposure and host
      susceptibility factors.
    b. In idiosyncratic drug reactions (e.g., isoniazid, phenytoin), the damage is
      dose independent and unpredictable.
    c. Intrinsic hepatotoxicity is dose dependent, as is seen with acetaminophen
      and methotrexate.

III. DIAGNOSIS

A. History

1. Pertinent historical features include episodes of symptomatic hypotension, a history of right or biventricular heart failure and new medications associated with liver injury.

2. Concurrent symptoms of abdominal or right upper quadrant abdominal pain may suggest mechanical biliary obstruction.

3. The history should be scrutinized for the use of nonprescription medications, including complementary and alternative medicines.

B. Physical examination

1. Physical findings associated with congestive hepatopathy include jaundice, tender hepatomegaly, jugular venous distention, edema, and, in severe cases, ascites.

C. Laboratory studies

1. In ischemic hepatitis, serum aminotransferase tends to rise rapidly to levels 10 to 40 times the upper limits of the reference range. Increases in alkaline phosphatase and bilirubin may rise as transaminase elevations decrease.

2. Hyperbilirubinemia should be further investigated by measuring both direct-reacting (conjugated) bilirubin and indirect-reacting (unconjugated) bilirubin; the latter is calculated by subtracting the direct fraction from the total bilirubin.

   a. Indirect hyperbilirubinemia may result from hemolysis, decreased hepatic clearance due to impairment of bilirubin conjugation, or circumstances in which both processes occur simultaneously.

   (1) Gilbert syndrome and Crigler-Najjar syndrome types I and II are inherited disorders that result in decreased bilirubin conjugation.

   (2) Gilbert syndrome affects 8% of the general population and is characterized by a mild, unconjugated hyperbilirubinemia to levels that rarely exceed 4 mg/dL and normal liver function.

   b. Mixed direct and indirect hyperbilirubinemia or pure direct hyperbilirubinemia can be the result of heritable disorders of bilirubin canalicular excretion, hepatocellular dysfunction, or biliary obstruction.

D. Radiographic studies

1. Sonography of the right upper quadrant with Doppler studies of mesenteric vessels can provide information about liver architecture, diameter of intrahepatic and extrahepatic bile ducts, and flow in hepatic veins, portal vein, and hepatic artery.

2. Combined right heart and transjugular portal pressure measurements can differentiate ascites development from chronic passive congestion caused by hepatic cirrhosis.

IV. TREATMENT

A. Treatment of ischemic hepatitis and congestive hepatopathy is supportive in nature; emphasis should be placed on maintaining organ perfusion and improving venous return.

B. TPN steatosis and steatohepatitis may be amenable to decreasing the carbohydrate load, decreasing total calories (25 to 40 kcal/kg per day), and cycling the infusion schedule.

C. Ursodeoxycholic acid (10 to 45 mg/kg per day) orally has been of variable success in the management of TPN-related cholestasis.

Selected Readings

Berk PD, Wolkoff AW. Bilirubin metabolism and the hyperbilirubinemias. In: Braunwald E, Fauci AS, Kasper DL, et al., eds. *Harrison's principles of internal medicine*, 15th ed. New York: McGraw-Hill, 2001:1715–1720.
A lucid explanation of bilirubin metabolism and approach to the investigation of hyperbilirubinemia.

Buchman AL. Complications of long-term home total parenteral nutrition: their identification, prevention and treatment. *Dig Dis Sci* 2001;46:1–18.
A comprehensive review of all complications of TPN, including those related to the liver and biliary tree.

Faust TW, Reddy KR. Postoperative jaundice. *Clin Liver Dis* 2004;8(1):151–166.
A review of the causes and investigation of hyperbilirubinemia occurring in the setting of surgery.

Kaufmann SS, Gondolesi GE, Fishbein TW. Parenteral nutrition associated liver disease. *Semin Neonatol* 2003;8:375.
Review of TPN-related liver disease with emphasis on effect in infants and the relationship of the underlying cause of gut failure and course of TPN-related liver disease.

Lee WL. Medical progress: drug-induced hepatotoxicity. *N Engl J Med* 2003;349:474–485.
A contemporary review of drug induced liver injury.

Maldonado O, Demasi R, Maldonado Y, et al. Extremely high levels of alkaline phosphatase in hospitalized patients. *J Clin Gastroenterol* 1998;27:342–345.
Sepsis was identified as the cause of serum alkaline phosphatase elevations greater than 1,000 U/l in 10 of 31 patients a single hospital over a 6-month period. Three of the 10 patients with sepsis had acquired immune deficiency syndrome as well.

Seeto RK, Fenn B, Rockey DC. Ischemic hepatitis: clinical presentation and pathogenesis. *Am J Med* 2000;109:109–113.
A case-control study of 31 patients with documented hypotensive episodes and ischemic hepatitis compared with 31 patients with hypotensive episodes from nonhepatic trauma. None of the control group of nonhepatic trauma developed serum transaminase abnormalities consistent with ischemic hepatitis, suggesting that individuals with risk factors for chronic hepatic congestion and superimposed hypotensive episodes are at greater risk for ischemic hepatitis than those with hypotension alone.

I. GENERAL PRINCIPLES

A. Acute liver failure (ALF), also known as fulminant hepatic failure, is an uncommon condition.

B. ALF is defined as the development of encephalopathy within 12 weeks of the onset of jaundice in individuals without preexisting liver disease.

C. ALF can be subdivided into three categories based on the time from jaundice to encephalopathy:

1. Hyperacute liver failure (7 days)

2. Acute liver failure (8 to 28 days)

3. Subacute liver failure (29 to 90 days)

D. Chronic liver failure results from continuous hepatic injury over a prolonged period and typically is characterized by:

1. Cirrhosis of the liver

2. Portal hypertension

II. ACUTE LIVER FAILURE

A. Etiology

1. The causes of ALF are many (Table 83-1). Identification of the cause of ALF is important for several reasons:

a. Specific treatments are available for drug and toxin overdoses.

b. Infectious causes may have implications for public health and be amenable to postexposure prophylaxis.

c. Prognosis varies with cause.

2. A specific cause for ALF may be unidentifiable in as many as 20% of adult cases.

3. Acetaminophen overdose is the most common cause of ALF in the United States.

a. Acetaminophen hepatotoxicity is frequently the consequence of the intentional overdosage at doses greater than 140 mg/kg body weight.

b. Hepatic damage results from the formation of a toxic intermediate, N-acetyl-p-benzoquinone-imine, formed in the process of metabolism of acetaminophen. through the cytochrome P-450 system when cellular glutathione levels are depleted.

c. One third of overdoses may be unintentional and occur in individuals exposed to less than 140 mg/kg body weight. These "therapeutic misadventures" are prone to occur in individuals at risk for either depletion of intracellular glutathione (e.g., chronic alcohol use) or in those with increased cytochrome P-450 2E1 activity (e.g., chronic anticonvulsive exposure).

B. Complications

1. Encephalopathy and cerebral edema

a. By definition, all patients with ALF have encephalopathy, with symptoms ranging from subclinical confusion (grade 1) to coma (grade 4).

b. Cerebral edema occurs in up to 80% of patients with ALF and grade 4 encephalopathy and can result in death from brain herniation.

2. Coagulopathy

a. Prolongation of international normalized ratio (INR) and activated partial thromboplastin time occur as a consequence of reduced hepatic synthesis of vitamin K–dependent coagulation factors.

b. Overt bleeding is uncommon; the combination of severe coagulopathy and platelet dysfunction can result in bleeding from even minor mucosal lesions.

TABLE 83-1	Causes of Acute Liver Failure

Acute viral hepatitis
Hepatitis A
Hepatitis B
Hepatitis C
Delta agent
Hepatitis E
   Cytomegalovirus
   Varicella-zoster virus
   Adenovirus
   Paramyxovirus
Epstein-Barr virus
   Cytomegalovirus
   Herpesvirus
Metabolic disorders
Acute fatty liver of pregnancy
HELLP syndrome
Wilson disease
Reye's syndrome
Cardiovascular disorders
Budd-Chiari syndrome
Sinusoidal obstruction syndrome
Cardiovascular shock
Hyperthermia
Drug and toxins
Acetaminophen
Sodium valproate
Isoniazid
Halothane
Tetracycline
Fialuridine
Amanita phalloides
Cereulide
Hypoglycin

HELLP, a syndrome characterized by *h*emolysis, *e*levated *l*iver enzyme levels, and a *l*ow *p*latelet count.

3. Cardiorespiratory complications
   a. Typical hemodynamic changes in ALF mimic distributive shock: increased cardiac output, decreased peripheral oxygen extraction, and low systemic vascular resistance.
   b. The development of arterial hypertension may herald the development of cerebral edema.
   c. Hypoxemia can result from cardiogenic shock, noncardiogenic pulmonary edema, pneumonia, or alveolar hemorrhage.
4. Renal failure
   a. Renal failure in ALF can result from acute tubular necrosis, prerenal azotemia, or the hepatorenal syndrome.
   b. In acetaminophen overdosage, acute tubular necrosis from the effect of the toxic metabolite on the kidney can be observed in as many as 75% of patients.
5. Metabolic disorders
   a. Lactic acidosis develops as the combined consequence of tissue hypoxia with increased lactate production and impaired hepatic metabolism of lactate. Renal dysfunction also may contribute.

b. Hypoglycemia occurs as a consequence of the loss of hepatic gluconeogenesis and glycogenolysis and signifies severe hepatocellular injury.

6. Infection

a. Patients with ALF are at risk for bacterial and fungal sepsis; impaired neutrophil and Kupffer cell function, decreased bacterial opsonization, bacterial gut translocation, and altered cytokine signaling contribute to immunologic impairment.

b. The most common organisms isolated include Staphylococcus, Streptococcus, gram-negative enteric organisms, and Candida spp.

c. Fungal infections occur late in the course of illness and are associated with high mortality.

d. Signs of infection can be protean; one third of septic subjects may be afebrile and lack leukocytosis.

C. Treatment

1. General measures

a. Early identification of the cause of ALF is critical.

b. Laboratory assessment of hepatic synthetic function, renal function and acid–base status provides useful prognostic information.

c. Invasive hemodynamic monitoring is useful in the management of hemodynamic changes associated with ALF.

2. Sepsis

a. Surveillance cultures of blood, sputum, and urine should be collected with a low threshold for the use of empiric antibacterial or antifungal therapy; the use of prophylactic antibiotics remains controversial.

3. Coagulopathy. The correction of the coagulopathy with fresh frozen plasma (FFP) or platelet transfusion should be reserved for active bleeding or prevention of bleeding during invasive procedures, as excessive blood product transfusion may worsen cerebral and pulmonary edema.

a. Administration of vitamin K is safe but often ineffective.

b. Parenteral administration of recombinant factor VIIa may reverse the coagulopathy and is helpful when there is a need to avoid the large volumes associated with FFP.

4. Encephalopathy and cerebral edema

a. Frequent neurologic examinations, including assessment of level of alertness, papillary response to light, and motor reflexes, are important in the assessment of encephalopathy and intracranial pressure (ICP).

b. Avoidance of excessive oral suctioning and visual and auditory stimuli may prevent sudden increases in ICP; nursing with head of bed at greater than 30-degree elevation may improve cerebral venous drainage.

c. Placement of an ICP monitor is indicated for the identification and treatment of cerebral edema in subjects who are candidates for liver transplantation and progress beyond grade 2 encephalopathy.

    (1) The cerebral perfusion pressure (CPP) is the difference between mean arterial pressure (MAP) and ICP; goals of ICP monitoring are to maintain the CPP above 50 mm Hg and the ICP below 15 mm Hg.

    (2) Risks of ICP monitoring include epidural and intracranial bleeding and infection.

    (3) Treatment options for increased ICP include: permissive hypernatremia, hyperventilation to maintain an arterial carbon dioxide partial pressure of 25 to 30 mm Hg, intravenous mannitol (0.5 to 1 g/kg), and hypothermia to a core body temperature of 32°C.

5. Metabolic disorders

a. Volume resuscitation with colloid is preferable for the treatment of prerenal azotemia.

b. Hemodialysis may be required.

c. Prevention of hypoglycemia is essential for preservation of neurologic function; frequent glucose monitoring and infusions of 10% to 50% dextrose solutions may be required.

TABLE 83-2	Kings College Criteria for Liver Transplantation for ALF

Nonacetaminophen causes of ALF
INR >7.7 (irrespective of grade of encephalopathy)
Or any three of the following:
  Age <10 or >40
  Unfavorable cause
    Non-A, non-B hepatitis
    Drug reaction
    Wilson's disease
  Period of jaundice to encephalopathy >7 days
  INR >3.85
  Serum bilirubin >17 mg/dL
Acetaminophen-related causes of ALF
PH <7.3 (irrespective of grade of encephalopathy)
Or all three of the following:
  Grade III to IV encephalopathy
  INR >7.7
  Serum creatinine >3.4 mg/dL

ALF, acute liver failure; INR, international normalized ratio.

6. Acetaminophen toxicity. The administration of N-acetylcysteine (NAC) is an effective, lifesaving antidote to acetaminophen toxicity.
   a. The decision to use NAC is based on reference to a standardized treatment nomogram and requires knowledge of serum acetaminophen level and time of ingestion.
   b. NAC is most effective when given within the first 24 hours after ingestion; NAC may still be useful even when treatment is delayed more than 24 hours or when signs and symptoms of ALF have developed.
   c. The oral dose of NAC is 140 mg/kg loading dose followed by 17 doses of 70 mg/kg every 4 hours.
   d. Electrolyte imbalances, particularly of hypophosphatemia, are common with acetaminophen-induced liver failure, and correction of electrolyte disorders is essential.
7. Liver transplantation (LT). Patients with ALF without contraindications to LT should be managed at a LT center.
   a. LT with a full-size orthotopic graft, partial graft, or auxiliary graft have all been used in the treatment of ALF.
   b. The Kings College criteria (Table 83-2) can be useful to identify poor prognostic factors that identify individuals who require LT for survival. These criteria are subdivided into acetaminophen and nonacetaminophen causes of ALF.
   c. The admission Acute Physiology and Chronic Health Evaluation (APACHE) II system is comparable to the Kings College criteria in acetaminophen-induced ALF.

III. CHRONIC LIVER FAILURE
A. Etiology
1. Chronic liver failure is the consequence of long-standing hepatic injury from multiple causes (Table 83-3).
B. Pathophysiology
1. Chronic liver injury results in activation of stellate cells within the space of Disse; stellate cell activation leads to the deposition of collagen and, in time, histologic changes of cirrhosis.
2. The time course from injury to cirrhosis is variable and dependent on the nature of the injury, the age at which the injury occurs, environmental factors, and unknown host factors.

TABLE 83-3	Causes of Chronic Liver Failure

Hepatitis B
Hepatitis C
Autoimmune hepatitis
Hereditary hemochromatosis
Alpha$_1$ antitrypsin deficiency
Wilson disease
Nonalcoholic fatty liver disease
Primary biliary cirrhosis
Primary sclerosing cholangitis
Alcohol-related liver disease

3. Cirrhosis also results in endothelial dysfunction and increased resistance to flow within the hepatic sinusoids. Sinusoidal hypertension and endothelial dysfunction produce portal hypertension and its three cardinal features:
   a. Increased resistance to mesenteric vascular flow
   b. Activation of the renal-angiotensin-aldosterone system resulting in sodium and water retention and increased intravascular volume
   c. Increased mesenteric blood flow as a consequence of a hyperdynamic circulation
4. Portal hypertension is responsible for the four main complications of chronic liver disease:
   a. Gastrointestinal bleeding
   b. Ascites
   c. Portosystemic encephalopathy
   d. Hepatorenal syndrome

C. **Diagnosis**
1. History
   a. Common symptoms include fatigue, increased abdominal girth, emotional labiality, day–night sleep reversal, and poor mental concentration.
2. Physical examination
   a. Common physical findings include jaundice, temporal wasting, abdominal ascites, splenomegaly, asterixis, spider angiomata, and male gynecomastia.
3. Blood tests
   a. Varying degrees of thrombocytopenia and leucopenia may be present as a consequence of hypersplenism.
   b. Anemia associated with liver disease is typically macrocytic. In advanced liver disease, a spur cell (acanthocytes) hemolytic anemia may develop.
   c. Elevations in serum transaminases and alkaline phosphatase are variable; hypoalbuminemia and prolongation of INR are common with cirrhosis and indicate synthetic dysfunction.
   d. A mixed direct- and indirect-reacting hyperbilirubinemia is common, particularly in cholestatic liver diseases.
   e. Serum ammonia is a casual marker of encephalopathy and should not supersede physical examination findings in the diagnosis of encephalopathy.
4. Ascites studies
   a. Ascites from portal hypertension is characterized by a difference of greater than 1.1 g/dL between serum albumin and ascites albumin; this difference is known as the serum ascites-albumin gradient (SAAG).
   b. Spontaneous bacterial peritonitis is diagnosed when the neutrophil count in ascites fluid is greater than 250/mm^3 or when bacteria can be cultured from ascites.
   c. The ascites fluid should be inoculated directly into blood culture bottles to increase the potential for identification of bacteria.

| TABLE 83-4 | Child-Pugh-Turcot Scoring System |

Clinical and biochemical measurements	Points scored for increasing abnormality		
	1	2	3
Albumin (g/dL)	>3.5	2.8–3.5	<2.8
Bilirubin (mg/dL)	<4	4–10	>10
International normalized ratio (INR)	<1.7	1.7–2.3	>2.3
Ascites	Absent	Slight	Moderate
Encephalopathy (grade)	None	1 and 2	3 and 4

5. Urine studies
   a. A random urine sodium less than 20 mmol/L is typical but not required for the diagnosis of hepatorenal syndrome.
   b. The severity of chronic liver disease can be graded on the basis of the Child-Turcot-Pugh classification (Table 83-4).

D. Treatment
1. Ascites
   a. Dietary sodium restriction to less than 2 g daily is the first-line treatment of ascites.
   b. The combination of a loop diuretic (20 to 160 mg daily) and spironolactone (50 to 400 mg daily) is effective in the control of ascites in the majority of cases; intravenous diuretics may precipitate renal failure.
   c. Intermittent large-volume paracentesis or transjugular intrahepatic portosystemic shunt (TIPS) is an alternative measures for the control of ascites refractory to diuretics or in those intolerant of diuretics (e.g., hyponatremia, renal insufficiency).
2. Spontaneous bacterial peritonitis (SBP)
   a. The antibiotics of choice in the absence of bacteriologic identification are intravenous third-generation cephalosporins effective against *E. coli*, *Klebsiella* spp., *Streptococcus* spp., and *Staphylococcus* spp.
   b. Intravenous albumin (1.5 g/kg on day 1 and 1 g/kg on day 3) can reduce rates of infection-related renal dysfunction from 30% to 10%.
   c. Repeat paracentesis 48 hours after the initiation of therapy should demonstrate a 50% drop in neutrophil count and sterile cultures.
3. Encephalopathy
   a. Patients should be investigated for precipitants of encephalopathy, including gastrointestinal hemorrhage, infection, and renal failure.
   b. Lactulose orally (15 to 60 mL every 4 to 12 hours) titrated to three to four soft bowel movements per day is effective in most cases of encephalopathy.
   c. Neomycin (500 to 1,000 mg every 8 hours) is also effective in control of encephalopathy.
4. Variceal hemorrhage (see Chapter 79)
5. Hepatorenal (HRS) syndrome
   a. Diuretics should be discontinued.
   b. Volume replacement with intravenous saline 1.5 liters should be given.
   c. Intravenous albumin, 25 to 75 g daily, may be more effective in expanding intravascular volume.
   d. A small series suggests a role for octreotide subcutaneously (100 mcg) every 8 hours, midodrine (7.5 to 12 mg) every 8 hours, and intravenous albumin for treatment of HRS.
6. Liver transplantation
   a. Liver transplantation in appropriately selected subjects can effectively treat all the complications of end-stage liver disease.

b. In the United States, prioritization for liver transplantation is determined by calculation of the Model for End Stage Liver Disease (MELD) score. An online MELD calculator is available at: http://www.unos.org/resources/meldPeldCalculator.asp

Selected Readings

Friedman SL. Liver fibrosis—from bench to bedside. *J Hepatol* 2003;38:S38.
A review of the molecular mechanisms for the development of hepatic fibrosis and strategies to treat and prevent the development of fibrosis.

Gines P, Guevara M, Arroyo V, et al. Hepatorenal syndrome. *Lancet* 2003;362:1819.
A comprehensive and contemporary review of the pathophysiology, diagnosis, and treatment of hepatorenal syndrome.

Gines P, Uriz J, Calahorra B, et al. Transjugular intrahepatic portosystemic shunting versus paracentesis plus albumin for refractory ascites in cirrhosis. *Gastroenterology* 2002;123:1839.
A randomized trial comparing TIPS to paracentesis for management of refractory ascites.

Kamath PS, Wiesner RH, Malinchoc M. A model to predict survival in patients with end-stage liver disease. *Hepatology* 2001;33:464.
A test of the MELD criteria to determine the risk of mortality in patients with chronic liver failure and the applicability of MELD to organ allocation.

Murphy N, Auzinger G, Bernel W, et al. The effect of hypertonic sodium chloride on intracranial pressure in patients with acute liver failure. *Hepatology* 2004;39:299.
A single-center study on the effect of intravenous administration of hypertonic saline to prevent sustained rises in ICP. The methods section includes an excellent description of state-of-the-art approach for the management of ALF.

O'Grady JG, Alexander GJM, Hayallar KM, et al. Early indicators of prognosis in fulminant hepatic failure. *Gastroenterology* 1989;97:439.
The Kings College criteria of prognostic factors that identify individuals who require liver transplantation for survival with ALF.

O'Grady JG, Schalm SW, Williams R. Acute liver failure: redefining the syndromes. *Lancet* 1993;342:273.
A retrospective review of 588 patients with ALF admitted to a single center over a 13-year period before liver transplantation was used for ALF. The report subdivides ALF into its three major forms and reports the rates of survival and cerebral edema for each subgroup.

Ostapowicz G, Fontana RJ, Schiodt FV, et al. Results of a prospective study of acute liver failure at 17 tertiary care centers in the United States. *Ann Intern Med* 2002;137:947.
The three most common causes of ALF at 17 centers participating in the multicenter U.S. Acute Liver Failure Study group were: acetaminophen-induced liver injury (39%), indeterminate (17%), and presumed idiosyncratic drug reaction (13%).

Riordan SM, Williams R. Treatment of hepatic encephalopathy. *N Engl J Med* 1997;337:473.
A comprehensive review of hepatic encephalopathy and its treatment.

Rolando N, Harvey F, Brahm J, et al. Prospective study of bacterial infection in acute liver failure: an analysis of fifty patients. *Hepatology* 1990;11:49.
A prospective study characterizing the high incidence, poor prognosis, and protean nature of bacterial infection in ALF.

Sort P, Navasa M, Arroyo V, et al. Effect of intravenous albumin on renal impairment and mortality in patients with cirrhosis and spontaneous bacterial peritonitis. *N Engl J Med* 1999;341:403.
The landmark study of the effect of intravenous albumin on decreasing rates of renal impairment and in patients with cirrhosis and spontaneous bacterial peritonitis.

Vale JA, Proudfood AT. Paracetamol (acetaminophen) poisoning. *Lancet* 1995;346:547.
A comprehensive review of acetaminophen poisoning and guidelines for use and administration of N-acetylcysteine.

84 DIARRHEA
Chandra Prakash and Ray E. Clouse

I. GENERAL PRINCIPLES
  A. Diarrhea frequently complicates the course of the critically ill patient.
  B. If untreated, it can produce serious fluid and electrolyte imbalance, skin breakdown and local infection, and difficulty with nutritional management.
  C. Diarrhea is the most common nonhemorrhagic gastrointestinal (GI) complication in the intensive care unit (ICU) setting.
  D. The differential diagnosis of diarrhea in patients in the ICU differs considerably from that in the general population; investigation is focused and limited to tests safely performed in the critically ill patient.

II. ETIOLOGY
  A. Iatrogenic causes
   1. Medications
     a. Antibiotics, especially erythromycin, ampicillin, clindamycin, and cephalosporins, may be the most common cause of iatrogenic diarrhea in the ICU.
       (1) Alterations in intestinal flora, breakdown of dietary carbohydrate products, and prokinetic effects (e.g., from erythromycin) are all postulated mechanisms for antibiotic-related diarrhea.
       (2) Additionally, *Clostridium difficile* toxin production can be implicated in 15% to 20% of cases. The toxin produces changes in brush border function, intestinal fluid transport, and GI peristalsis and results in pseudomembranous colitis.
     b. Other medications implicated include magnesium-containing antacids, magnesium and phosphorus supplements, lactulose, colchicine, digitalis, quinidine, theophylline, levothyroxine, aspirin, nonsteroidal antiinflammatory agents, cimetidine, misoprostol, diuretics, β-blocking agents, and chemotherapeutic agents.
   2. Enteral feeding
     a. Diarrhea in enterally fed patients usually is associated with concurrent antibiotic use.
     b. Osmolarity of the enteral solution can play a role in some instances, as can bolus feeding distal to the pylorus.
     c. Enteral formulas high in lactose or fat content may precipitate diarrhea in susceptible patients.
  B. Diarrhea secondary to underlying diseases
   1. Infections and neoplastic disease in immunosuppressed patients, neutropenic enteropathy
   2. Gastrointestinal bleeding, ischemic bowel disease
   3. Postsurgical diarrhea, after cholecystectomy, gastric surgery, pancreatectomy, and in short bowel syndrome
   4. Other causes include fecal impaction and opiate withdrawal.
  C. Diarrhea as a primary manifestation of the disease
   1. Infectious diarrhea
   2. Mucosal inflammation, as in inflammatory bowel disease, graft-versus-host disease (GVHD), celiac sprue
   3. Other causes include sepsis, vasculitis, diabetic diarrhea, renal failure, and adrenal insufficiency

III. DIAGNOSIS

  A. Clinical presentation

    1. History

      a. Attention to historical data (e.g., onset, relation to antibiotic usage or enteral feeding) may lead to prompt diagnosis and management.

      b. *C. difficile*–related diarrhea may occur up to 8 weeks after the offending antibiotic is discontinued.

      c. Abdominal pain suggests ischemia, infection, or inflammatory conditions such as vasculitis or GVHD, depending on the clinical setting.

      d. Bloody diarrhea may indicate overt gastrointestinal bleeding, ischemic colitis, or occasionally pseudomembranous colitis.

      e. Passage of frequent small-volume stools with urgency or tenesmus suggests distal colonic involvement, whereas passage of less frequent, large-volume stools suggests a more proximal process.

    2. Physical examination usually is nonspecific but helpful in assessing severity of volume loss.

      a. Skin rashes or mucosal ulcerations can point toward GVHD, inflammatory bowel disease, or vasculitis; other extraintestinal manifestations of diseases associated with diarrhea should be noted.

      b. An abnormal rectal examination may be the only sign of a partially obstructing fecal impaction.

  B. Laboratory studies

    1. Hyperchloremic metabolic acidosis, hypokalemia, prerenal azotemia, and other serious electrolyte imbalances may occur with severe diarrhea.

    2. Leukocytosis may suggest infection or ischemia.

    3. A falling hematocrit may suggest GI bleeding.

  C. Stool studies

    1. Fresh stool specimens should be sent for *C. difficile* toxin assay and culture for enteric pathogens.

    2. Immunosuppressed patients may need more extensive stool tests, including ova and parasite evaluation and concentration for isolation of *Cryptosporidium, Microsporidium,* or *Isospora belli.*

    3. The stool osmolar gap, which is the difference between expected stool osmolarity $\{[(\text{stool Na}^+) + (\text{stool K}^+)] \times 2\}$ and measured stool osmolarity, may help distinguish between osmotic and secretory causes when diarrhea is severe or protracted and no diagnosis is apparent; an elevated stool osmolar gap (>70 mOsm/L) suggests osmotic causes.

    4. High-volume stool output that persists with fasting supports a secretory origin.

    5. A Sudan stain for fecal fat or stool pH occasionally is helpful (pH is decreased in carbohydrate malabsorption).

  D. Imaging studies

    1. Plain abdominal radiographs can detect partial obstruction, perforation, or changes associated with enteritis or colitis and are recommended in the presence of pain or an abnormal abdominal examination.

    2. Contrast studies including computed tomography and intestinal radiographs may be required in difficult or protracted cases.

  E. Endoscopy

    1. Flexible sigmoidoscopy is useful in diagnosing pseudomembranous colitis, ischemic colitis, cytomegalovirus colitis, herpetic proctocolitis, or GVHD and is usually considered in the presence of bright red rectal bleeding or other indicators of distal colitis.

    2. Mucosal biopsies are helpful on occasion when endoscopic findings are nonspecific or absent.

IV. TREATMENT

  A. General measures

    1. Correction of fluid and electrolyte imbalance needs immediate attention.

    2. Central venous access and monitoring may be necessary in patients with severe fluid loss.

3. Proper patient hygiene and skin care should be maintained, and patient isolation with enteric precautions should be instituted when indicated.
4. Iatrogenic causes of diarrhea are corrected by withdrawal of the offending medications.
5. Enteral feedings suspected of causing diarrhea should be reduced in volume, diluted, given by continuous infusion, or temporarily discontinued.
6. A change in formula to an elemental diet may be indicated in patients with short bowel syndrome, pancreatic insufficiency, radiation enteritis, fistula, or inflammatory bowel disease.
7. In severe cases, total parenteral nutrition may be necessary as a temporary measure.

B. Specific treatment
1. Specific or pathogen-related treatment should be administered whenever possible in both immunocompromised and immunocompetent hosts.
2. *C. difficile* colitis
   a. If *C. difficile*-related diarrhea is suspected, the offending antibiotic should be discontinued when possible; spontaneous improvement often results from this measure alone.
   b. Oral metronidazole (250 to 500 mg three times daily) and oral bacitracin (25,000 units four times daily) are as effective as oral vancomycin (125 to 500 mg four times daily), but they are less expensive.
   c. Vancomycin should typically be reserved for treatment failures and severe cases.
   d. Response is expected within 24 to 48 hours with improvement in diarrhea, pain, fever, and leukocytosis, but treatment should be continued for 7 to 14 days.
   e. As many as 24% of patients have a relapse, and longer retreatment courses are required.
   f. Anion exchange resins such as cholestyramine or colestipol are reportedly useful as adjunctive measures in mild cases or in relapses, but they rarely are required. These agents can bind vancomycin.
   g. Antimotility agents should not be used, because they may lengthen the course of the illness.

C. Symptomatic measures
1. When a cause of diarrhea is not found, palliative treatment lessens fluid losses, patient discomfort, and morbidity.
2. Antimotility agents may decrease the frequency and severity of diarrhea, but monitoring for complications is required (e.g., central nervous system side effects, gut hypomotility).
   a. These drugs include loperamide (4 mg initially, and up to 16 mg per day), diphenoxylate with atropine (20 mg of diphenoxylate four times daily initially, then decrease and titrate to symptoms), and deodorized tincture of opium (6 to 12 gtt two to four times daily).
   b. Octreotide can be used for palliation of diarrhea in patients with acquired immunodeficiency syndrome, GVHD, hormone-producing tumors, and other causes of secretory diarrhea.

Selected Readings

Bartlett JG. Clinical practice. Antibiotic-associated diarrhea. *N Engl J Med* 2002;346:334–339.
A comprehensive discussion of antibiotic-associated diarrhea.

Bartlett JG. Management of *Clostridium difficile* infection and other antibiotic-associated diarrhoeas. *Eur J Gastroenterol Hepatol* 1996;8:1054.
Investigation and therapy of antibiotic-associated diarrhea are outlined in this review.

Brown E, Talbot GH, Axelrod P, et al. Risk factors for *Clostridium difficile* toxin-associated diarrhea. *Infect Control Hosp Epidemiol* 1990;11:283.
Age greater than 65 years, ICU admission, GI procedures, and administration of antibiotics for more 10 days were associated with C. difficile–*associated diarrhea.*

Cataldi-Betcher EL, Seltzer MH, Slocum BA, et al. Complications occurring during enteral nutritional support: a prospective study. *JPEN J Parenter Enteral Nutr* 1983;7:546.

Tube feedings are safely tolerated in most patients, but complications must be recognized and treated promptly.

Cremonini F, Di Caro S, Nista EC, et al. Meta-analysis: the effect of probiotic administration on antibiotic-associated diarrhoea. *Aliment Pharmacol Ther* 2002;16:1461–1467.
Probiotics may benefit patients with antibiotic-associated diarrhea.

Dark DS, Pingleton SK. Nonhemorrhagic gastrointestinal complications in acute respiratory failure. *Crit Care Med* 1989;17:755.
Diarrhea is the most common nonhemorrhagic gastrointestinal complication in the ICU, occurring more frequently in critically ill patients who are administered antacids.

Fekety R. Guidelines for the diagnosis and management of *Clostridium difficile*–associated diarrhea in colitis. *Am J Gastroenterol* 1997;92:739.
Practical guidelines for the management of C. difficile diarrhea.

Guenter PA, Settle RG, Perlmutter S, et al. Tube feeding–related diarrhea in acutely ill patients. *JPEN J Parenter Enteral Nutr* 1991;15:277.
Antibiotic usage was the factor most strongly associated with diarrhea in acutely ill patients administered tube feedings.

Kelly TWJ, Patrick MR, Hillman KM, et al. Study of diarrhea in critically ill patients. *Crit Care Med* 1983;11:7.
Notes the significant incidence of diarrhea in critically ill patients, especially in association with nasogastric feeding.

Sakai L, Keltner R, Kaminski D. Spontaneous and shock-associated ischemic colitis. *Am J Surg* 1980;140:755.
Ischemic colitis carries a high mortality when it is associated with full-thickness necrosis; radiologic findings correlated well with clinical and pathologic evidence of full-thickness necrosis.

Teasley DG, Gerding DN, Olson M, et al. Prospective randomized trial of metronidazole versus vancomycin for *Clostridium difficile*–associated diarrhea and colitis. *Lancet* 1983;2:1043.
Metronidazole and vancomycin have equivalent efficacy and tolerance in treating C. difficile–associated diarrhea, but metronidazole is more economical.

Thielman NM, Guerrant RL. Clinical practice. Acute infectious diarrhea. *N Engl J Med* 2004;350:38–47.
A review of the etiology and management of acute infectious diarrhea.

Yassin SF, Young-Fadok TM, Zein NN, et al. *Clostridium difficile*–associated diarrhea and colitis. *Mayo Clin Proc* 2001;76:725–30.
Clinical presentation, diagnosis, and management of pseudomembranous colitis associated with C. difficile are reviewed.

85 SEVERE AND COMPLICATED BILIARY TRACT DISEASE
Riad Azar

I. GENERAL PRINCIPLES
   A. A wide spectrum of biliary tract diseases are seen in the intensive care unit (ICU).
   B. Presentations range from mildly abnormal blood chemistries to life-threatening septic shock.
   C. Methods used to access the biliary tree for diagnosis and therapy are:
   1. Endoscopic cannulation of the ampulla in the duodenum during endoscopic retrograde cholangiopancreatography (ERCP).
   2. Percutaneous transhepatic cholangiography (PTC) or percutaneous drainage of the gallbladder (cholecystostomy tube).
   3. Operative management through the peritoneal cavity.

II. ETIOLOGY. Several biliary tract disorders are commonly encountered in the critical care setting.
   A. Cholangitis
   1. Typically occurs in patients with bile duct stones or strictures and with recent manipulation of the biliary tree.
   2. The diagnosis should be considered promptly and excluded in ICU patients who are septic; urgent biliary decompression should be achieved.
   3. The clinical manifestations include fever, abdominal pain, and occasionally jaundice; laboratory abnormalities include elevated transaminases, bilirubin, or alkaline phosphatase.
   B. Biliary obstruction
   1. Common causes include gallstone disease, benign stricture, and malignancy; other causes are listed in Table 85-1.
   2. When obstruction presents without cholangitis, the most likely diagnosis is a neoplasm.
   C. Bile leak
   1. Leakage of bile into the peritoneal cavity or pleural space can result from open or laparoscopic cholecystectomy, hepatic resection, liver transplantation or trauma, or percutaneous biliary manipulations.
   2. The resultant bile peritonitis produces dramatic pain, ascites, leukocytosis, and fever.
   D. Acalculous cholecystitis
   1. Typically seen in critically ill patients and can result in significant morbidity and mortality.
   2. The symptoms may be masked by the complicated underlying situation.
   3. This entity warrants a high index of suspicion and aggressive management.
   E. Gallstone pancreatitis
   1. Often results from biliary stone disease; evidence suggests that stone passage or impaction at the ampulla are responsible for gallstone pancreatitis.
   2. Transaminases and bilirubin levels typically are elevated at the onset of the disease.
   3. Abdominal ultrasound can reveal gallstones and possibly a dilated biliary tree.

III. DIAGNOSIS
   ### A. Clinical assessment
   1. Physical examination may reveal icterus, hepatomegaly, ascites, or focal tenderness over the liver or gallbladder; findings range from acute abdomen to nonspecific fever and ileus.
   2. Signs and symptoms of acute cholecystitis often are not readily apparent in the ICU patient.

TABLE 85-1	Causes of Biliary Obstruction

Intrinsic lesions
  Gallstones
  Cholangiocarcinoma
  Benign stricture
Sclerosing cholangitis
  Periarteritis nodosa
  Ampullary stenosis
  Parasites
Extrinsic lesions
Pancreatic carcinoma
Metastatic carcinoma
Pancreatitis
Pancreatic pseudocyst
Visceral artery aneurysm
Lymphadenopathy
Choledochal cyst
Hepatic cyst or cysts
Duodenal diverticulum
Iatrogenic lesions
Postoperative stricture
Hepatic artery infusion chemotherapy

B. Laboratory tests
   1. In acutely ill patients, bilirubin elevation can result from sepsis, drug effects, hemolysis, or other nonbiliary causes.
   2. Alkaline phosphatase can be elevated from other tissues including bone and placenta; concomitant elevation of 5′nucleotidase or γ-glutamyl transferase helps confirm hepatobiliary origin of the enzyme.
   3. Although serum transaminase elevations are the hallmark of hepatocellular injury, elevated levels also can be seen with biliary disease, especially inflammatory and infectious conditions and acute biliary obstruction.
   4. It is important to remember that patients with severe biliary disease can present with normal laboratory values, and abnormal test results may be the first clue to biliary disease in the obtunded or otherwise compromised ICU patient.
C. Plain radiographs
   1. Plain abdominal radiographs usually reveal nonspecific findings (e.g., ileus).
   2. Gallstones are radio-opaque in only 20% of cases.
   3. Air in the biliary tree can result from a prior sphincterotomy, spontaneous biliary–enteric fistula, biliary–enteric surgical anastomosis, and, rarely, infection with gas-producing organisms.
   4. Gas within the gallbladder wall is one sign of acute cholecystitis
D. Ultrasonography
   1. Ultrasonography is extremely useful in the ICU and can be performed at the bedside.
   2. It is sensitive for detecting biliary ductal dilatation and cholelithiasis with an accuracy exceeding 95%.
   3. Ultrasonography does not exclude the presence of stones in the distal common bile duct, because overlying bowel gas obscures the view.
   4. Other diagnoses made readily by ultrasonography are acute cholecystitis, choledocholithiasis, liver lesions, pancreatic masses, abscesses, and ascites.

E. Radionuclide scanning
   1. ^{99m}Tc hepatic iminodiacetic acid (HIDA) scans yield both physiologic and structural information regarding the biliary tract.
   2. Filling of the gallbladder confirms patency of the cystic duct and virtually excludes acute cholecystitis; delayed views and routine pretreatment with cholecystokinin increase the accuracy to more than 90%.
   3. False–positive results can be seen from chronic cholecystitis, prolonged fasting, and long-term parenteral hyperalimentation.
   4. It has a limited role in patients with poor hepatocellular function, complete biliary obstruction, or cholangitis, each of which prevents adequate uptake and excretion of the radiopharmaceutical into the biliary tree.
   5. Significant bile leaks also are identified accurately with HIDA scanning.
F. Computed tomography (CT) and magnetic resonance imaging (MRI).
   1. CT is highly accurate for the detection of the level and cause of biliary obstruction, especially in the pancreatic head region.
   2. In patients with normal renal function, a spiral CT or a dual-phase study (arterial and venous) with thin cuts through the pancreas is better for defining lesions in the pancreas.
   3. MRI techniques that incorporate cholangiopancreatography also provide highly useful images of the liver and entire biliary tree without requiring invasive procedures.
   4. These studies are impractical in many critically ill patients, who often are too sick for transport to the scanners.
G. ERCP and PTC
   1. Both can be performed emergently when necessary, for both diagnosis and therapy of biliary disorders (see below).
   2. Portable fluoroscopy equipment is required for bedside procedures in unstable or moribund patients.

IV. MANAGEMENT
A. Cholangitis and biliary obstruction
   1. If cholangitis is suspected, broad spectrum antibiotics should be started promptly; extended-spectrum penicillins, cephalosporins, and fluoroquinolones are usually recommended.
   2. Aggressive supportive measures should be started with IV fluids and pressors if needed.
   3. Patients should undergo emergent biliary decompression by either ERCP or PTC.
   4. With ERCP a biliary sphincterotomy and stone extraction can be achieved, but placement of a biliary stent can be sufficient for decompression.
   5. If ERCP is not available, PTC is a safe alternative and also provides adequate drainage of the biliary tree.
   6. Definitive therapy for stone disease and palliative therapy for benign or malignant disease can be accomplished during either procedure.
B. Bile leaks
   1. ERCP should be performed as soon as possible once a bile leak is identified.
   2. Most biliary leaks can be managed definitively with biliary decompression and stent placement at ERCP.
   3. Broad-spectrum antibiotics protect against sepsis and abscess formation.
   4. The presence of a large biloma usually requires supplemental percutaneous drainage.
   5. Larger leaks or those associated with ischemia, trauma, or surgical anastomosis, eventually may require surgical repair or bypass.
C. Acute cholecystitis
   1. Percutaneous cholecystostomy under ultrasonographic guidance has become the therapy of choice in patients who are too unstable for operative cholecystectomy when acute cholecystitis does not respond to antibiotics; this can be performed at the bedside in the ICU.

2. The cholecystostomy drainage catheter is left in place until acute symptoms resolve, at which time an elective surgical cholecystectomy can be scheduled.

3. In patients with severe comorbid medical conditions, the tube may simply be removed with or without percutaneous stone extraction.

D. Acute gallstone pancreatitis

1. Most patients with acute gallstone pancreatitis improve with conservative therapy for pancreatitis; early ERCP may be indicated for removal of impacted or retained common bile duct stones, limiting further pancreatic inflammation and preventing cholangitis.

2. Definitive therapy with elective cholecystectomy (or percutaneous cholecystotomy or endoscopic sphincterotomy in nonoperative candidates) is indicated to prevent recurrences.

Selected Readings

Carpenter HA. Bacterial and parasitic cholangitis. *Mayo Clin Proc* 1998;73:473.
The epidemiology, pathogenesis, and clinical manifestations of bacterial and parasitic cholangitis are reviewed comprehensively.

Chang L, Lo SK, Stabile BE. Gallstone pancreatitis: a prospective study on the incidence of cholangitis and clinical predictors of retained common bile duct stones. *Am J Gastroenterol* 1998;93:527.
The best predictor of common bile duct stones in gallstone pancreatitis is serum total bilirubin on hospital day 2; cholangitis is uncommon in this setting.

Elsakr R, Johnson DA, Younes Z, et al. Antimicrobial treatment of intra-abdominal infections. *Dig Dis* 1998;16:47.
New concepts about the treatment of intraabdominal infections, the antibiotics recommended, and the role of invasive procedures are outlined in this well-referenced article.

Fulcher AS, Turner MA, Zfass AM. Magnetic resonance cholangiopancreatography: a new technique for evaluating the biliary tract and pancreatic duct. *Gastroenterologist* 1998;6:82.
Technical refinements allow rapid and comprehensive imaging of the entire biliary tree and pancreatic duct in less than 20 seconds using magnetic resonance cholangiopancreatography.

Hammarstrom LE, Stridbeck H, Ihse I. Effect of endoscopic sphincterotomy and interval cholecystectomy on late outcome after gallstone pancreatitis. *Br J Surg* 1998; 85:333.
Endoscopic sphincterotomy reduced the overall incidence of recurrent pancreatitis after an episode of gallstone pancreatitis.

Kalliafas S, Ziegler DW, Flancbaum L, et al. Acute acalculous cholecystitis: incidence, risk factors, diagnosis and outcome. *Ann Surg* 1998;64:471.
Acute acalculous cholecystitis is a potentially lethal condition in critically ill and postoperative patients that requires a high index of suspicion for accurate diagnosis.

Kavanagh PV, vanSonnenberg E, Wittich GR, et al. Interventional radiology of the biliary tract. *Endoscopy* 1997;29:570.
An excellent review of the techniques available to the interventional radiologist for management of patients with acute biliary tract disorders.

Leung JWL, Ling TKW, Chan RCY, et al. Antibiotics, biliary sepsis and bile duct stones. *Gastrointest Endosc* 1994;40:716.
Imipenem and ciprofloxacin have the highest antimicrobial activity; ciprofloxacin has the highest biliary concentration in patients with duct stones and infected bile.

Ramirez FC, McIntosh AS, Dennert B. Emergency endoscopic retrograde cholangiopancreatography in critically ill patients. *Gastrointest Endosc* 1998;47:368.
Of all ERCPs, 2% are performed on critically ill patients; mechanical ventilation does not compromise technical success.

Ryan ME, Geenen JE, Lehman GA, et al. Endoscopic intervention for biliary leaks after laparoscopic cholecystectomy: a multicenter review. *Gastrointest Endosc* 1998;47(3):261–6.
Endoscopic sphincterotomy, stent placement, or sphincterotomy with stent is effective in healing biliary leaks after laparoscopic cholecystectomy.

Soetikno RM, Carr-Locke DL. Endoscopic management of acute gallstone pancreatitis. *Gastrointest Endosc Clin N Am* 1998;8:1.
A summary of four randomized, controlled trials looking at early endoscopic intervention in acute gallstone pancreatitis.

Sugiyama M, Tokuhara M, Atomi Y. Is percutaneous cholecystotomy the optimal treatment for acute cholecystitis in the very elderly? *World J Surg* 1998;22:459.
Percutaneous cholecystotomy is a safe and effective treatment for acute cholecystitis in the elderly, either as interim treatment or as definitive therapy.

Yusoff IF, Barkun JS, Barkun AN. Diagnosis and management of cholecystitis and cholangitis. *Gastroenterol Clin North Am* 2003;32(4):1145–1168.
An excellent review of the diagnosis and management of biliary diseases and complications.

86

THE BASIC PRINCIPLES OF NUTRITIONAL SUPPORT IN THE INTENSIVE CARE UNIT
Dominic J. Nompleggi

I. GENERAL PRINCIPLES
  A. Severe protein-calorie malnutrition is common in critically ill patients.
  B. In all patients with serious illness, appropriate measures to avoid substrate deficiency and to replenish nutrient deficiency are best recognized promptly and appropriate therapy instituted without delay.

II. PATHOGENESIS
  A. Malnutrition can be present on admission or develop as a result of the metabolic response to injury.
  B. Changes in metabolic response are difficult to assess.
  C. Assessment includes evaluation of clinical, anthropometric, chemical, and immunologic parameters reflecting altered body composition.

III. DIAGNOSIS
A. General assessment
  1. The purpose of nutritional assessment is to identify the type and degree of malnutrition to devise a rational approach to treatment.
  2. Percentage weight loss in the last 6 months, serum albumin level, and total lymphocyte count are commonly used measures to assess nutritional status.
  3. Weight loss of 20% to 30% suggests moderate caloric malnutrition while 30% or greater indicates severe protein-calorie malnutrition; loss of 10% or more over a short period of time also is considered clinically important.
  4. The general appearance of the patient, with emphasis on evidence of temporal, upper body, and upper extremity wasting of skeletal muscle mass, provides a quick, inexpensive, and clinically useful measure of nutritional status.
B. Laboratory assessment
  1. Serum albumin measures visceral protein stores; it is a useful and readily available indicator of kwashiorkor (protein malnutrition).
  2. Serum albumin is not a sensitive indicator of malnutrition in intensive care unit (ICU) patients because it is influenced by numerous factors other than nutritional status (e.g., protein losing states, hepatic function, acute infection or inflammation).
  3. Malnutrition is closely correlated with alterations in immune response as measured by skin test reactivity and total lymphocyte count.
  4. A total lymphocyte count less than 1,000/mm^3 is indicative of altered immune function and is associated with decreased skin test reactivity.
  5. Loss of skin test reactivity is a measure of impaired cellular immunity, which consistently has been found to be associated with malnutrition.
C. Subjective global assessment
  1. Subjective global assessment (SGA) evaluates nutritional status using clinical parameters such as history, physical findings, and symptoms.
  2. The SGA determines whether:
    a. nutritional assimilation has been restricted because of decreased food intake, maldigestion, or malabsorption;
    b. any effects of malnutrition on organ function and body composition have occurred; and
    c. the patient's disease process influences nutrient requirements.

3. In hospitalized patients, SGA has been shown to provide reliable and reproducible results with more than 80% agreement when blinded observers assessed the same patient.

IV. **TREATMENT.** Critical depletion of lean tissue can occur after 14 days of starvation in severely catabolic patients. Nutrition support should be instituted in patients who are not expected to resume oral feeding for 7 to 10 days.

A. **Enteral feeding**

1. Enteral feeding reduces infection and preserves gut integrity, barrier, and immune function.
2. It is the preferred route of nutrient administration.
3. Current recommendations support initiation of enteral nutrition as soon as possible after resuscitation.
4. The only contraindication is a nonfunctioning gut.
5. Enteral feeding technique:
   a. Initiation of enteral feeding distal to the pylorus does not require active bowel sounds or the passage of flatus or stool.
   b. Small-bowel feedings can be given in the presence of mild or resolving pancreatitis and low-output enterocutaneous fistulas (<500 mL/d).
   c. Worsening abdominal distention or diarrhea in excess of 1,000 mL per day, requires a medical evaluation; if distention is present, enteral feedings should be discontinued.
   d. If no infectious cause is found for the diarrhea, antidiarrheals can be administered and feedings continued.
   e. Standard isotonic polymeric formulas can meet most patients' nutritional needs.
   f. Elemental formulas should be reserved for patients with severe small bowel absorptive dysfunction; specialty formulations have a limited clinical role.
   g. Macronutrient goals resemble those for parenteral nutrition (see later): protein requirements should be provided first and dictate the total daily volume needed; remaining macronutrients are in fixed proportions, depending on the formula selected.

B. **Parenteral feeding**

1. Parenteral nutrient administration is recommended when the gastrointestinal tract is nonfunctional or inaccessible or when enteral feeding is insufficient.
2. Parenteral nutrient admixtures are not as nutritionally complete as enteral formulations, but nutritional goals are achieved more often with the former than the latter.
3. Macronutrients
   a. Energy adequate to promote anabolic functions is essential.
   b. Caloric requirements should be based on the usual body weight; a requirement of 25 kcal/kg initially is adequate for most patients.
   c. The protein requirement (1.2 to 1.5 g/kg per day) should be calculated first to ensure protein sparing and maintain lean tissue mass.
   d. Next, approximately 15% to 30% of total calories should be given as fat.
   e. The remaining calories should be given as a carbohydrate.
4. Micronutrients (vitamins, trace minerals) and fluid
   a. Potassium, magnesium, phosphate, and zinc should be provided in amounts necessary to maintain normal serum levels.
   b. Absolute requirements for vitamins, mineral, and trace elements have not yet been determined.
   c. Normal serum and blood levels of vitamins have been established but can vary with the laboratory in which the measurement is obtained.
   d. In general, patients should receive fluid at 25 mL/kg body weight to avoid dehydration.

V. **SUMMARY**

A. Need for nutritional support is determined by the balance between endogenous energy reserves of the body and the severity of stress.

B. Best clinical markers of stress are fever, leukocytosis, hypoalbuminemia, and a negative nitrogen balance.

C. Enteral route should be used to provide nutrients if the gut is functioning.

D. Provision of energy and protein should be tailored to the individual patient.

E. During illness, hypoalbuminemia should be viewed as a marker of injury and not as an indicator of impaired nutrition; normal concentrations are unattainable in many critically ill patients because of large fluid shifts and acute-phase protein synthesis.

F. Goal of short-term nutritional support is to optimize the body's metabolic response to injury by improving immune function, reducing inflammation, maintaining gut barrier function, and minimizing nitrogen deficit.

Selected Readings

Baker JP, Detsky AS, Wesson DE, et al. Nutritional assessment: a comparison of clinical judgment and objective measures. *N Eng J Med* 1982;306:969.
This article validated the accuracy of simple subjective assessment compared with complex objective measurements in nutritional assessment.

Cerra FB, Benitez MR, Blackburn GL, et al. Applied nutrition in ICU patients: a consensus statement of the American College of Chest Physicians. *Chest* 1997;111:769.
The single best reference on ICU nutrition.

Detsky AS, McLaughlin JR, Baker JP, et al. What is subjective global assessment of nutritional status? *JPEN J Parenter Enteral Nutr* 1987;11:8.
This article presents the concept of subjective global assessment as a valid method of nutritional assessment.

Grant JP, Custer PB, Thurlow J. Current techniques of nutritional assessment. *Surg Clin North Am* 1981;61:437.
Excellent review of the methods of nutritional assessment.

Kirby DF, Delegge MH, Fleming CR. American Gastroenterological Association medical position statement: guidelines for the use of enteral nutrition. *Gastroenterology* 1995;108:1282.
Guidelines for the use of enteral nutrition therapy, particularly with reference to the use of specialized formulas.

Klein S, Kinney J, Jeejeebhoy K, et al. Nutrition support in clinical practice: review of published data and recommendations for future research direction. *JPEN J Parenter Enteral Nutr* 1997;21:133.
A state-of-the-art review of the clinical practice of nutrition support, which outlines areas for further research.

Reilly JJ, Gerhardt AL. (Ravitch M, ser. ed.) Modern surgical nutrition. *Curr Probl Surg* 1985;22:1.
Nutrition assessment and therapy for surgical patients.

Endocrine Problems in the Intensive Care Unit

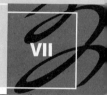

VII

87

I. GENERAL PRINCIPLES. Diabetes mellitus is a common problem in the intensive care unit (ICU). Patients in the ICU with diabetes are particularly vulnerable to the adverse metabolic consequences of stress. Diabetes predisposes to cardiovascular, renal, and infectious complications. Often diabetes itself is the primary problem, as in ketoacidosis and hyperosmolar coma. Adequate control of diabetes minimizes the risk of iatrogenic metabolic complications, cardiovascular complications, poor wound healing, and infection.

II. PATHOPHYSIOLOGY

    A. Normal glycemic control. Blood glucose concentration is tightly regulated, normally ranging only between 60 and 120 mg/dL. Regulation depends in large measure on the presence of appropriate quantities of circulating insulin. Even in the fasting state, insulin continues to regulate the rates of glycogenolysis, gluconeogenesis, lipolysis, and ketogenesis. The key to the ICU management of diabetes is achieving a consistent and appropriate degree of patient "insulinization" at all times.

    B. Diabetes classification system. Diabetes mellitus is not one disease but a group of syndromes sharing the common feature of hyperglycemia. The most common diabetic syndromes are type 1 and type 2. Knowing the diagnosis can assist in the management of diabetes in ICU patients.

        1. Type 1 diabetes. Formerly designated insulin-dependent, ketosis-prone, and juvenile diabetes. Results from autoimmune destruction of pancreatic insulin-producing beta cells. These patients are totally deficient in insulin. They require exogenous insulin for survival. Discontinuation of insulin therapy, even for relatively brief intervals, can lead to serious metabolic complications.

        2. Type 2 diabetes. Formerly designated non–insulin-dependent or adult onset diabetes. The result of relative, rather than absolute, deficiency of insulin. It involves defects in both insulin action and insulin secretion. Some patients with type 2 diabetes can be treated with diet or oral agents, but others need insulin to control hyperglycemia. Infection, metabolic stress, and many medications commonly used in the ICU exacerbate type 2 diabetes and can lead to ketoacidosis, hyperosmolar coma, or lactic acidosis.

        3. Gestational diabetes

        4. Other specific types. Cases of "secondary" diabetes are less common. These can result from genetic defects of beta cell and insulin action and many other factors.

        5. Drug or chemical induced. Thiazide diuretics, HIV protease inhibitors, niacin, calcineurin inhibitors (tacrolimus), isoniazid, pentamidine, zyprexa, hormones (e.g., glucocorticoids, oral contraceptives, α-adrenergic agents, glucagon, growth hormone), Interferon-α, sympathomimetic drugs, antineoplastic agents (e.g., asparaginase, mithramycin, streptozocin).

III. DIAGNOSIS

    A. Diagnostic criteria. All acutely ill patients should be screened for diabetes. Diabetes diagnosed in the ICU may or may not persist after the patient recovers. Criteria for the diagnosis of diabetes include a fasting plasma glucose of 126 mg/dL or greater or a random plasma glucose equal to or greater than 200 mg/dL confirmed by repeat testing on a different day. Impaired glucose tolerance should not be diagnosed in the critically ill because the diagnosis is not valid in patients under stress. ICU patients suspected of having impaired glucose tolerance should be reassessed after recovery.

469

B. **Assessment of severity.** This chapter describes the treatment of diabetes mellitus in the ICU when neither ketoacidosis nor hyperosmolar coma are present. Diabetic ketoacidosis and hyperosmolar coma require urgent treatment (see Chapter 88).

1. Is the patient ketoacidotic? Determined on the basis of history, physical findings, the presence of an anion gap acidosis, and ketonuria or ketonemia. For management, see Chapter 88.

2. Is the patient hyperosmolar? In the presence of extreme hyperglycemia, osmolarity should be measured or calculated. May be associated with severe dehydration, obtundation. For management, see Chapter 88.

3. Is the patient absolutely insulin dependent? Patients with type 1 diabetes and certain individuals with pancreatic diseases require continuous insulin treatment at all times to avoid ketoacidosis.

C. **Evaluation of the ICU patient with preexisting diabetes**

1. Assess cardiac function and peripheral circulation.

2. Occult infections. May include osteomyelitis, cellulitis, cholecystitis, gingivitis, sinusitis, cystitis, and pyelonephritis.

3. Hypertriglyceridemia may cause pancreatitis.

4. Diabetic eye disease. Not a contraindication to anticoagulation, but its severity should be documented before instituting therapy.

5. Assessment of kidney function should include a urinalysis for protein.

6. Autonomic neuropathy. Predisposes to orthostasis, tachyarrhythmias, and intestinal motility disorders; should be suspected in patients with an abnormal pupillary response to light or absence of heart rate response during Valsalva (R-R interval change noted in the electrocardiogram).

7. Poorly controlled diabetes may imply poor nutrition. Patients with uncontrolled diabetes may be thiamine deficient.

D. **Bedside blood glucose monitoring.** Glucose levels are influenced by hematocrit, creatinine concentration, plasma protein concentration, and arterial pO_2. Extremely elevated blood glucose concentrations may be above the range accurately measured by the bedside monitor and should be verified with a serum sample sent to the laboratory. In general, therapy need not be delayed waiting for confirmatory laboratory glucose results.

IV. TREATMENT

A. **Why control diabetes in the ICU?** Maintenance of plasma glucose concentration less than 110 mg/dL with intensive insulin therapy reduces morbidity and mortality in ICU patients. Hyperglycemia is a predictor of mortality after myocardial infarction, and intensive insulin therapy improves long-term prognosis in diabetic patients with acute myocardial infarction and after coronary artery surgery.

Uncontrolled glycemia appears to impair innate immunity, increasing susceptibility of patients with diabetes to infection. Hyperglycemia predisposes to disturbances in sodium, potassium, and phosphate concentrations.

B. **Target blood glucose concentration.** At this writing we recommend that all ICU patients with a plasma glucose concentration greater than 150 mg/dL be treated with a continuous intravenous infusion of regular insulin. Glucose concentration should be maintained above 70 and below 125 mg/dL during treatment with a continuous infusion. Values in this range are not dangerous in a properly staffed ICU and appear to reduce both morbidity and mortality. Whether this recommendation is appropriate for any given ICU patient and ICU environment is a matter of clinical judgment and depends on severity of illness and ICU nursing resources, among other factors. Glucose concentrations greater than 150 mg/dL always require intervention. Blood glucose concentrations less than 70 mg/dL pose the hazard of hypoglycemia.

C. **Misuse of oral agents and sliding scale insulin in the ICU**

1. Oral agents. Oral hypoglycemic agents should not be used in the ICU. Metformin (Glucophage) in particular should be discontinued in critically ill patients because of an increased risk of lactic acidosis.

2. Sliding scale Insulin. Periodic boluses of insulin amplify the risks of hypoglycemia and hyperglycemia and should not be used as primary management of diabetes in the critically ill patient.

D. Intravenous insulin infusion therapy. Recommendations for the institution and management of a continuous insulin infusion in patients with ketoacidosis or hyperosmolar syndrome are given elsewhere. Check glucose concentration hourly until in the target range and every 2 hours thereafter. A patient's sensitivity to insulin and response to therapy cannot be exactly predicted. Concurrent glucose infusions and parenteral or enteral feeding will affect the dose. Use only regular (crystalline) insulin mixed in saline solution. Note that it is entirely appropriate to infuse insulin at low rates (e.g. 0.5 units per hour) and these low rates are often all that is needed to prevent ketoacidosis in a patient with type 1 diabetes. Mixing insulin for infusion at a concentration of 2 U/mL facilitates the infusion of insulin at a low rate.

1. **Insulin adjustment algorithms.** Protocols for management of diabetes in the ICU are developed at the institutional level and require a significant commitment of time and resources to implement. We have found it most practical to construct a series of stepped insulin-adjustment algorithms varying in intensity to account for widely varying insulin requirements in individual patients. Appropriate adjustments in insulin infusion rate must take into consideration the patient's current blood glucose level as well as the rate at which the level has changed from the previous test result. A blood glucose level above the target range may not require an adjustment in the infusion rate if comparison to the prior test result shows the level to be dropping at a sufficient rate. This decision will require the judgment of the individual adjusting the drip. Standard order sets must also account for the management of hypoglycemia and transition from intravenous insulin to subcutaneous or oral therapy as the acute illness resolves. Safe and effective implementation of intensive insulin protocols in the ICU is a team effort, requiring an educated and invested staff at all levels.

2. Factors affecting insulin requirements. Insulin resistance induced by the primary illness and its treatment as well other factors, such as obesity; and the type and amount of nutritional support being given.

   a. Increasing insulin requirements

      (1) An escalating insulin infusion requirement is a sensitive indicator of increasing insulin resistance and requires careful reevaluation of the patient's overall metabolic status.

      (2) Stressors that increase insulin resistance include sepsis, occult infections, heart disease, tissue ischemia, hypoxemia, and medications (most common are glucocorticoids and pressors).

      (3) Instituting or increasing enteral or parenteral nutrition often causes increasing insulin requirements. We recommend that insulin infusion rates not be increased beyond 20 U per hour (480 U/d) without first decreasing any exogenous carbohydrate loads.

   b. Decreasing insulin requirements

      (1) Factors that increase insulin sensitivity in the ICU include improvement in any intercurrent illness, changes in medication, and reductions in enteral or parenteral feeding. Occasionally, hepatic failure, renal failure, or adrenal insufficiency leads to decreased insulin requirements.

      (2) When blood glucose concentrations fall, a common response is to discontinue the insulin drip. For patients with type 1 diabetes, this is always inappropriate because discontinuation of insulin can precipitate hyperglycemia and ketosis within hours. Instead reduce the rate to 1 or even 0.5 U per hour and, if necessary, infuse glucose in a separate intravenous solution. We recommend the same strategy for most other ICU patients as well. Unless their primary disease problem has improved dramatically, they frequently experience recurrent hyperglycemia.

      (3) Patients with diabetes in the ICU should receive continuous intravenous insulin until they demonstrate clear improvement in overall clinical status and stability of glycemic control.

3. Transition to other forms of therapy. When the condition of an ICU patient with diabetes has improved to the point that continuous insulin infusion is no longer needed, subsequent therapy depends on the type of diabetes. Patients with drug-induced (e.g., catecholamine- or steroid-induced) hyperglycemia may

need no further treatment for diabetes. In contrast, all patients with type 1 and many with type 2 diabetes will still require insulin. In these patients, subcutaneous injections of intermediate-acting insulin (e.g., NPH or Lente) should be started before the infusion has been discontinued. It is essential that the intravenous infusion of regular insulin be continued for 2 to 3 hours after the first subcutaneous injection of intermediate-acting insulin. When patients are eating and experience postprandial hyperglycemia, short-acting insulin (e.g., regular or lispro or aspart) can be added. Some stable patients with type 2 diabetes can be managed with oral hypoglycemic agents or diet alone, but that therapeutic decision is best made after discharge from the ICU on a regimen of subcutaneous injections of insulin.

V. COMPLICATIONS

   A. Surgery in the critically ill patient with diabetes. Treatment of hyperglycemia patients who are being prepared for urgent surgery in the emergency department can be initiated with either subcutaneous short-acting insulin or, preferably, a continuous insulin infusion, as described earlier. Critically ill patients with diabetes should be treated with an insulin infusion during surgery. The ICU patient with diabetes who requires surgery should be sent to the operating room or procedure suite with infusions of both insulin and 5% dextrose in half-normal saline. Frequent monitoring of blood glucose is essential. Anesthetic agents may exacerbate hyperglycemia. Regional and local anesthetics are preferable when appropriate.

   B. Special problems

   1. Peritoneal dialysis and diabetes. Critically ill patients with diabetes who are being treated with peritoneal dialysis should in general be maintained on a continuous, low-dose insulin infusion. The use of admixtures of glucose and insulin in the dialysate can lead to unpredictable alterations in glycemia in the presence of intercurrent severe stress.

   2. Hyperalimentation and diabetes. The addition of insulin to parenteral nutrition formulations, although a common practice, is not recommended. There is too much variability among severely ill patients to rely on a fixed ratio of insulin to carbohydrate. Changes in the patient's status can render the fixed ratio inappropriately high or low. If an obese patient receiving hyperalimentation develops severe hyperglycemia and a large insulin requirement, consideration should be given to reducing the amount of carbohydrate administered .

   3. Pearls: key points and pitfalls

   a. Avoid sliding scales! There is no role for variable insulin boluses given only after hyperglycemia has occurred. They do not take into account the rapid changes in status that can occur in the critically ill and lead to fluctuating control. Patients with type 1 diabetes whose insulin is withheld until hyperglycemia occurs can quickly become ketoacidotic.

   b. Regular insulin sensitivity. Patients who have had type 1 diabetes for 15 years or more often develop extreme sensitivity to the effects of regular insulin. The reason is unclear, but such sensitivity frequently contributes to increased "brittleness" in these patients.

   c. The diabetic kidney and radiographic contrast agents. The risk of acute renal failure after angiographic procedures may be reduced by administration of isotonic sodium bicarbonate (at rates of 3 mL/kg per hour for 1 hour before and 1 mL/kg per hour for 6 hours after radiocontrast exposure), minimization of dye loads, and the use of N-acetylcysteine.

Selected Readings

Alberti KG, Zimmet PZ. Definition, diagnosis and classification of diabetes mellitus and its complications. Part 1: diagnosis and classification of diabetes mellitus provisional report of a WHO consultation. *Diabet Med* 1998;15:539–553.
General overview of diabetes by leading international authorities.

Choban PS, Burge JC, Scales D, et al. Hypoenergetic nutrition support in hospitalized obese patients: A simplified method for clinical application. *Am J Clin Nutr* 1997;66:546–550.
Useful guidelines for nutritional management of the obese inpatient.

Ganda OP. Prevalence and incidence of secondary and other types of diabetes, in National Diabetes Data Group, ed. *Diabetes in America.* Bethesda, MD: National Institutes of Health, 1995, pp. 69–84.
Comprehensive review of conditions that can lead to diabetes.

Hirsch IB, McGill JB, Cryer PE, et al. Perioperative management of surgical patients with diabetes mellitus. *Anesthesiology* 1991;74:346–359.
A detailed source of information on the management of diabetes in surgical patients.

Malmberg K. Prospective randomised study of intensive insulin treatment on long term survival after acute myocardial infarction in patients with diabetes mellitus. *Br Med J* 1997;314:1512–1515.
Evidence that glucose control can reduce cardiovascular mortality in both the short and long term.

Merten GJ, Burgess WP, Gray LV, et al. Prevention of contrast-induced nephropathy with sodium bicarbonate: a randomized controlled trial. *JAMA* 2004;291(19):2328–2334.
Contrast nephropathy developed in less than 2% of patients receiving sodium bicarbonate compared with 14% in the group receiving saline.

Queale WS, Seidler AJ, Brancati FL. Glycemic control and sliding scale insulin use in medical inpatients with diabetes mellitus. *Arch Intern Med* 1997;157:545–552.
Evidence that the use of sliding scales leads to excessive hypoglycemia and hyperglycemia in hospitalized patients.

Thompson MJ, Rossini AA, Mordes JP. Management of diabetes in the critically ill patient. In: Rippe J., et al., eds. *Intensive care medicine,* 5th edition. Philadelphia: Lippincott-Williams & Wilkins, 1998, pp. 1251–1258.
The full-length version of this chapter.

Van den Berghe G, Wouters P, Weekers F, et al. Intensive insulin therapy in critically ill patients. *N Engl J Med* 2001;345:1359–1367.
This landmark study has led the way to widespread acceptance of the benefit of tight glycemic control in the ICU setting.

Zerr KJ, Furnary AP, Grunkemeier GL, et al. Glucose control lowers the risk of wound infection in diabetics after open heart operations. *Ann Thorac Surg* 1997;63:356–361.
Evidence that glucose control in the ICU after surgery is important.

DIABETIC COMAS

88 *Michael J. Thompson, John P. Mordes, and Aldo A. Rossini*

I. GENERAL PRINCIPLES
A. The four "diabetic comas"
1. Four causes of stupor and coma are associated with disordered glucose metabolism and often referred to as the "diabetic comas."
   a. Diabetic ketoacidosis (DKA)
   b. Hyperglycemic hyperosmolar syndrome (HHS)
   c. Alcoholic ketoacidosis
   d. Hypoglycemia
2. These four diagnoses should be considered during the evaluation of any patient with altered mental status.

II. DIABETIC KETOACIDOSIS
A. Pathophysiology.
Diabetic ketoacidosis is caused by the total or near-total absence of circulating insulin. Without insulin, glucose no longer enters most types of cells and is neither stored nor metabolized. Glucagon secretion is increased and hepatic glucose production increases without restraint. Stress-responsive hormones accelerate catabolism. Lipolysis accelerates and large quantities of free fatty acids are metabolized to ketone bodies. Most threatening are the accumulation of hydrogen ions, loss of free water, and depletion of electrolytes.

B. Diagnosis
1. **Clinical presentation.** Any person with diabetes can develop ketoacidosis. It most often occurs in patients with type 1 diabetes who have either omitted their insulin or have an intercurrent infection. It occurs in patients with type 2 diabetes who have intercurrent severe infection, trauma, or myocardial infarction. Most patients in DKA are lethargic; about 10% are comatose. Postural hypotension is common, but shock is rare. Patients have rapid, deep (Kussmaul) respiration, and their breath has a sweet fruity odor. Patients in DKA are not febrile unless some other intercurrent disorder is present. The rare cases of hypothermia in DKA are associated with sepsis. Abdominal pain is common and may be accompanied by guarding with diminished bowel sounds. Patients with DKA may be nauseated and vomit guaiac-positive, coffee grounds—like material. Pleuritic chest pain may be present. Hepatic enlargement with fatty infiltration may occur.

2. **Laboratory**
   a. **Plasma glucose.** Plasma glucose concentration in the range of 400 to 800 mg/dL is typical in DKA. Occasionally younger patients maintain blood glucose concentrations less than 300 mg/dL.
   b. **Electrolytes**
      (1) **Sodium.** Serum sodium concentration is variable; decreases occur due to osmotic diuresis and dilution by the osmotic effect of large amounts of extracellular glucose. The "corrected" serum sodium in a patient with a measured concentration of 135 mEq/L and a glucose concentration of 600 mg/dL is $1.6 \times (6 - 1) + 135$, or 143 mEq/L. Hypertriglyceridemia is a common cause of factitiously low sodium concentrations.
      (2) **Potassium.** All patients with DKA are at risk for life-threatening hypokalemia during treatment, despite that the serum potassium concentration is usually elevated at presentation. Total body potassium *loss* (in the range of 200 to 700 mEq) typically occurs. Normal or low concentrations of potassium early in ketoacidosis reflect a very severe potassium deficit.

(3) Phosphorous. Elevated serum phosphate concentrations are common in untreated DKA. After therapy, there is a precipitous decline to subnormal levels.

c. Anion gap acidosis. Arterial blood gas and pH measurements are essential in the management of severe DKA. Uncomplicated DKA presents as an anion gap acidosis. More chronic ketoacidotic states may be associated with hyperchloremic acidosis, probably as a consequence of the loss of neutralized ketone body salts. Rare cases of DKA are complicated by intercurrent metabolic alkalosis, most often from severe vomiting.

d. Plasma ketones. Plasma ketone levels do not necessarily reflect the full extent of ketogenesis because the test measures only acetoacetate (AcAc) and acetone. Beta-hydroxybutyrate (BOHB), a "ketone body" produced from AcAc, is actually an acid alcohol. It is not measured in assays for ketones. Normally, the BOHB:AcAc ratio is 3:1, but acidosis increases the ratio to 6:1 or even 12:1 as pH decreases. Ketone body measurements may initially rise due to conversion of BOHB back to AcAc. Clearance occurs slowly; measurement more often than every 12 hours is generally unnecessary.

e. Mixed anion gap acidosis. A mixed anion gap acidosis may occur in patients with DKA. This can be due, for example, to intercurrent lactic acidosis or salicylate intoxication. To determine whether a nonketone body anion is complicating DKA, multiply the highest positive ketone dilution by 0.1 mM/L to estimate AcAc concentration. Multiply the AcAc concentration by 3 to 6 (depending on the pH) to estimate the BOHB concentration. If the anion gap is greater than the estimated concentrations of AcAc plus BOHB, the presence of an additional unmeasured anion should be considered (e.g., lactate, salicylate, uremic compounds, methanol, ethylene glycol).

f. Other laboratory findings

(1) Renal. The blood urea nitrogen (BUN) of patients with DKA is typically elevated due to prerenal azotemia and increased ureagenesis. AcAc interferes with some creatinine assays.

(2) Hematology. The hematocrit and hemoglobin are usually high. Low values suggest preexisting anemia or acute blood loss. Leukocytoses with a left shift often occur in the absence of intercurrent illness.

(3) Lipids. There is marked elevation of serum triglyceride concentrations; this reverses with insulin therapy.

(4) Other. Serum amylase, lipase, and creatine phosphokinase (CPK) concentrations are sometimes elevated. Uric acid concentrations may be elevated. Ketone bodies interfere with certain transaminase assays.

III. TREATMENT. Treatment of DKA should be directed at four main problems: hypovolemia, electrolyte disturbances, insulin, and identification of the precipitating event.

A. Correction of hypovolemia. Patients in DKA are always hypovolemic. Fluid and electrolyte therapy always takes precedence over insulin therapy, which shifts salt and water from the extracellular (and intravascular) compartments to the intracellular space. The free water deficit generally ranges between 5 and 11 liters, typically about 100 mL/kg. Initial fluid resuscitation should be with an infusion of 0.9% saline. Approximately 2 liters should be given during the first hour to restore blood volume, stabilize blood pressure, and establish urine flow. Another liter of 0.9% saline can typically be given during the next 2 hours. During the first 24 hours, 75% of the estimated total water deficit should be replaced. Urine flow should be maintained at approximately 30 to 60 mL per hour. After the first 2 liters, consider changing to hypotonic 0.45% saline if hypernatremia is present.

B. Electrolytes

1. Sodium, chloride, and potassium. Sodium and chloride are replaced in conjunction with free water as just described. Because serum potassium concentration does not accurately reflect total body potassium, replacement should be initiated early in treatment. Until the serum potassium concentration is known, replacement should be carried out cautiously. The recommended initial repletion rate is 20 mEq per hour as KCl or K3PO4. When the serum value is known, the rate of potassium administration can be adjusted. Typical potassium deficits in DKA are 3 to 5 mEq/kg, but if hypokalemia or normokalemia is present at the time of admission, the deficit may be much higher, up to 10 mEq/kg. If a patient in mild DKA is alert and able to tolerate liquids, potassium should be given orally.

For a variety of reasons, potassium concentration often falls precipitously after starting therapy. Insulin shifts K+ to the intracellular space. As acidemia resolves, buffered intracellular H+ exchanges for extracellular K+. If a nasogastric tube is in place, electrolyte losses resulting from gastric suctioning must also be considered. A sudden reduction in serum potassium concentration can cause flaccid paralysis, respiratory failure, and life-threatening cardiac arrhythmias.

2. **Phosphate.** Initially the concentration of phosphate is elevated, but levels may decrease to less than 1 mM/L within 4 to 6 hours of starting insulin treatment. Persistent severe hypophosphatemia can cause neurologic disturbances, arthralgias, muscle weakness with respiratory failure, rhabdomyolysis, and liver dysfunction. Each vial of potassium phosphate contains 93 mg phosphorus and 4 mEq potassium per milliliter. It is rarely necessary to administer more than one 5-mL ampule of potassium phosphate to a patient in DKA. The hazards of parenteral phosphate administration include hypocalcemia and metastatic calcification. Unless hypophosphatemia is severe (<1.0 mg/dL) and persistent, there is generally no need for treatment.

3. **Bicarbonate.** Most authorities now concur that there is no need for the routine use of bicarbonate therapy in DKA. Fluid and electrolyte replacement alone will ameliorate acidosis, and bicarbonate therapy may produce adverse effects. These include severe acute hypokalemia, late respiratory alkalosis due to paradoxical cerebrospinal fluid acidosis, a shift of the oxygen dissociation curve to the left that results in tissue hypoxia and lactic acidosis, and increased hepatic ketogenesis. In children, bicarbonate therapy may increase the risk of cerebral edema. We recommend bicarbonate therapy (1) when the pH is persistently less than 7.1 after 2 to 3 hours of treatment; (2) in cases complicated by depressed respiratory drive; and (3) when hypotensive shock is unresponsive to rapid fluid replacement. Even in these circumstances, bicarbonate can only "buy time" until metabolic treatment reverses the acidosis. Administer sodium bicarbonate by adding to intravenous fluids, typically two ampules (2×44 mEq, or 2×50 mEq) added to 1 liter of D5W. When the pH is greater than 7.2, treatment should be stopped.

4. **Magnesium.** Hypermagnesemia may occur early in the course of DKA. Mg^{++} concentration generally returns to normal without treatment. In some patients, Mg^{++} stores may be depleted and in rare instances lead to cardiac arrhythmia.

C. **Insulin.** Insulin therapy in DKA should be instituted only after fluid and electrolyte resuscitation is under way. For adults, we recommend a bolus of 10 U of short-acting insulin followed by a continuous intravenous infusion starting at 5 to 10 U per hour. In children, the recommended initial bolus is 0.1 U/kg of body weight and the infusion rate is 0.1U/kg per hour. Insulin should be added to 0.45% saline at a concentration of 0.5 U/mL, and the container swirled before use. Only regular (crystalline) insulin is officially approved for intravenous use. Blood glucose concentration should be measured every 1 to 2 hours after starting the infusion. If the glucose concentration has not decreased by 100 mg/dL, the insulin infusion rate should be doubled. When the glucose concentration has fallen by more than 150 mg/dL, then the infusion rate should be decreased by 50%, but it should never be stopped. The minimum blood glucose concentration during the first 24 hours of treatment should be 200 mg/dL. If it falls below 200 mg/dL, glucose infusion (D5W) should be started, and the insulin infusion rate continued to inhibit ketogenesis. Never stop insulin entirely during the treatment of DKA, even if the infusion rate is reduced to only 0.5 U per hour or less. Serum bicarbonate levels should be near normal before transitioning the patient from intravenous insulin to subcutaneous insulin injections.

D. Identification of the precipitating event. Diabetic ketoacidosis may be the first sign of new-onset type 1 diabetes mellitus. The majority of cases, however, occur in patients known to have diabetes, and it is always necessary to ask why DKA has occurred in this setting. Common underlying causes of DKA include:

1. Omission of insulin therapy

2. Infection

3. Major stressors (e.g., myocardial infarction, trauma)

4. Medication (e.g., high-dose glucocorticoid therapy)

E. Pearls: key points and pitfalls

1. Complications are not infrequent in cases of DKA; some are avoidable.

2. Never stop insulin completely! DKA can recur rapidly, especially in the presence of other intercurrent illnesses. Insulin infusions should always be continued, if only at 0.5 to 1 U per hour, until the patient is well enough to be switched to subcutaneous injections of longer-acting insulin. The infusion can be stopped 2 to 3 hours after the first subcutaneous injection of intermediate-acting insulin is given.

3. Recurrent diabetic ketoacidosis: If ketoacidosis recurs in the ICU despite continued therapy with insulin, severe infection, a severe contrainsulin state (e.g., Cushing's syndrome) or medications (e.g., glucocorticoids) should be suspected.

4. Cerebral edema is a rare complication of DKA in adults, but it occurs occasionally in children. To avoid cerebral edema, the goal of DKA treatment during the first 24 hours is a blood glucose concentration not less than 200 mg/dL.

5. Persistent hypotension should prompt consideration of fluid shifts, bleeding, severe acidosis, arrhythmia, myocardial infarction, cardiac tamponade, sepsis, and adrenal insufficiency.

6. Renal complications include postrenal obstruction, atonic bladder, and acute tubular necrosis secondary to pyelonephritis.

7. Thrombosis of the cerebral vessels and stroke are recognized but uncommon complications of DKA.

IV. HYPERGLYCEMIC HYPEROSMOLAR SYNDROME

A. Pathophysiology. The pathophysiology of HHS involves three interrelated elements:

1. insulin deficiency

2. renal impairment

3. cognitive impairment

Relative lack of insulin is the fundamental defect. Patients have sufficient insulin to inhibit ketone body formation but not enough to prevent glycogenolysis and gluconeogenesis. The resulting hyperglycemia induces an osmotic diuresis, with resultant fluid and electrolyte losses.

Some degree of renal impairment accompanies all cases of HHS. Typical patients with the HHS syndrome are older and have reduced renal blood flow and glomerular filtration rate (GFR). The underlying renal abnormalities in the HHS syndrome may be prerenal, renal, or postrenal. The common result is that affected patients are unable to compensate for the hyperglycemia with an osmotic diuresis.

Invariably, HHS involves acute or chronic impairment of cerebral function. Hyperglycemia leading to an osmotic diuresis and hyperosmolality normally activates a thirst response. A common history for HHS involves an elderly patient with impaired cognitive function due to cerebrovascular disease, dementia, or CNS-depressant medications. Patients with trauma or burns are also susceptible to HHS.

B. Diagnosis

1. Clinical presentation. Patients who develop HHS are typically middle-aged or elderly. They often have a history of mild type 2 diabetes and a prodrome of progressive polyuria and polydipsia lasting days to several weeks. Most patients have underlying diseases; renal and cardiovascular disorders are common. Other intercurrent problems include infection, myocardial infarction, stroke, hemorrhage, and trauma. Additional factors include dialysis, hyperalimentation, and medications (e.g., thiazide diuretics, phenytoin, propranolol, immunosuppressive agents, cimetidine).

Fever is a common finding in HHS even in the absence of infection, but infection must be rigorously excluded in all cases. Patients may have hypotension and tachycardia due to dehydration, and they frequently hyperventilate. Hyperventilation may reflect intercurrent lactic acidosis. Neurological manifestations include tremors and fasciculations. Mental status abnormalities may range from mild disorientation to obtundation and coma. Up to a third of patients with HHS may seize.

2. **Laboratory**
   a. **Blood glucose.** Plasma glucose concentrations in HHS are generally higher than in DKA, usually greater than 600 mg/dL. Values as high as 2,000 mg/dL occur.
   b. **Ketones.** Most patients in HHS are not ketonemic. Serum acetone levels are usually normal or only slightly elevated, seldom exceeding 1:2.
   c. **Arterial pH.** Occasional patients in HHS will develop an intercurrent metabolic acidosis. Most patients in HHS are only mildly acidotic, the average pH being about 7.25 before treatment.
   d. **Osmolality.** Serum osmolality in comatose patients usually exceeds 350 mOsm/kg. Dehydration induces prerenal azotemia.
   e. **Sodium.** The serum sodium concentration in HHS at the time of presentation is variable, ranging between 100 and 180 mEq/L.
   f. **Potassium.** Serum potassium concentration in HHS is also variable, ranging from 2.2 to 7.8 mEq/L.

V. **TREATMENT.** Treatment of HHS should be directed at four main problems: hypovolemia, electrolyte disturbances, insulin, and identification of the precipitating event.
   A. **Correction of hypovolemia.** Patients with HHS are without exception profoundly dehydrated. Within the first 2 hours, 1 to 2 liters of 0.9% saline should be given. Normal saline is recommended, even if hypernatremia is present, to expand the extracellular fluid compartment rapidly. After initial volume expansion and restoration of normotension, subsequent treatment for dehydration in this syndrome emphasizes free water replacement. The average patient requires 6 to 8 liters of fluids during the first 12 hours of treatment.
   B. **Electrolytes.** As soon as adequate urine flow has been established and the degree of hypokalemia estimated, potassium supplementation should be added to the intravenous fluids. A sudden fall in serum potassium concentration frequently accompanies the initial dose of insulin. Serum potassium concentration should be checked frequently and the electrocardiogram monitored for changes. Cardiac arrhythmias induced by hypokalemia may be irreversible, particularly in the elderly.
   C. **Insulin.** Most patients with HHS are more sensitive to insulin than are patients with diabetic ketoacidosis. In addition, blood glucose concentration in HHS can fall precipitously when urine output is reestablished after volume expansion. Treatment with insulin is essential but should be instituted (1) with careful monitoring and (2) only after fluid and electrolyte resuscitation is under way. We do not recommend an initial intravenous insulin bolus. For the infusion, we recommend a starting dose of only 1 to 5 U per hour, depending on individual circumstances. Attempt to maintain blood glucose concentration near 250 mg/dL for the first 24 hours. A rapid fall in blood glucose concentration may cause cerebral edema.
   D. **Identification of the precipitating event.** HHS may be the first sign of newly recognized diabetes mellitus, but the majority of cases occur in patients known to have glucose intolerance. Regardless of the previous glycemic history, it is always necessary to ask why HHS has occurred. Common and easily recognized underlying causes of DKA include infection and major stressors (e.g., myocardial infarction or trauma). Other precipitating events in the elderly can be subtler. These may include drugs that depress the sensorium and inhibit the response to thirst (e.g., anxiolytics and sedatives), drugs that depress renal function (e.g., diuretics leading to prerenal azotemia), and drugs that promote hyperglycemia (e.g., steroids) and other endocrine disturbances (e.g., hypothyroidism or apathetic thyrotoxicosis).

E. Pearls: key points and pitfalls. Patients with HHS may be very sensitive to insulin. Do not be overly aggressive with insulin. Do not give insulin before volume restoration. When insulin is administered to patients with HHS syndrome, glucose shifts from the extracellular to the intracellular compartment. The rapid intracellular movement of free water may precipitate hypotension and shock. Rapid reduction in blood glucose is a major contributor to the development of cerebral edema and a fatal outcome in HHS.

VI. ALCOHOLIC KETOACIDOSIS

A. Pathophysiology. Ethanol metabolism consumes NAD and generates NADH. Sufficient ethanol ingestion can generate an unfavorable NADH:NAD ratio, which in turn impairs gluconeogenesis. Hypoglycemia ensues when glycogen stores are exhausted, explaining the relationship of the disorder to nutritional state. Because of the hypoglycemia, insulin levels are low, which is permissive to the release of free fatty acids from adipose tissue and to the formation of ketone bodies.

B. Diagnosis. The diagnosis depends on the demonstration of hypoglycemia in the setting of ketoacidosis. Definitive demonstration of hypoglycemia has three components: low plasma glucose concentration, neuroglycopenic symptoms (e.g., hunger, headache, confusion, lethargy, slurred speech, seizures, coma) consistent with hypoglycemia, and resolution of those symptoms with administration of glucose.

   1. Clinical presentation. Patients with this disorder may be stuporous or comatose. They are typically chronically alcoholic, but the disorder can occur after binge drinking in adults or accidental ingestion in children. Patients typically have not eaten for days and are prone to nausea, vomiting, and aspiration. Hypothermia and neurologic abnormalities, including trismus, seizures, hemiparesis, and abnormal tendon reflexes, may be observed. Evidence of inebriation is often absent.

   2. Laboratory

      a. Hypoglycemia. Blood glucose concentrations can be as low as 20 mg/dL.

      b. Anion gap acidosis. These patients are usually acidotic, with an arterial pH less than 7.2.

      c. Ketonemia and ketonuria. Both ketoacids and lactate contribute to the unmeasured anion pool in this form of acidosis, but only the former is easily measured and detected.

      d. Other. Liver function tests, amylase, and phosphate are typically normal.

C. Treatment

   1. Fluids and electrolytes. Rehydration with intravenous fluids as appropriate.

   2. Glucose. One ampule of D50W to correct hypoglycemia, being careful to avoid extravasation.

   3. Parenteral thiamine (100 mg) to prevent Wernicke's encephalopathy

   4. Pearls: key points and pitfalls

      a. By the time patients with this disorder are treated, the ethanol has often been metabolized and is no longer detectable.

      b. Administration of sodium bicarbonate is generally not necessary. Treatment with glucose and fluids rapidly reverses the condition by raising the concentration of insulin and thereby inhibiting lipolysis and free fatty acid release.

      c. The presence of urinary ketones in a hypoglycemic patient generally excludes hyperinsulinemia as the cause of the low glucose concentration.

      d. Persons with diabetes treated with insulin or sulfonylurea-class hypoglycemic agents who become intoxicated may develop life-threatening, profound hypoglycemia as a result of the metabolic synergy of ethanol and insulin.

VII. HYPOGLYCEMIC COMA. Hypoglycemia and hypoglycemic coma are discussed in Chapter 92.

Selected Readings

DeFronzo RA, Matsuda M, Barrett EJ. Diabetic ketoacidosis: a combined metabolic-nephrologic approach to therapy. *Diab Rev* 1994;2:209–238.
Comprehensive review that addresses common misconceptions about treatment.

Fulop M. Alcoholic ketoacidosis. *Endocrinol Metab Clin North Am* 1993;22:209–219.
   Detailed review of the causes and treatment of this condition.

Genuth SM. Diabetic ketoacidosis and hyperglycemic hyperosmolar coma. *Curr Ther Endocrinol Metab* 1997;6:438–447.
   Extensive review of these two conditions.

Ishihara K, Szerlip HM. Anion gap acidosis. *Semin Nephrol* 1998;18:83–97.
   Detailed analysis of the diagnosis and analysis of anion gap acidoses.

Okuda Y, Adrogue HJ, Field JB, et al. Counterproductive effects of sodium bicarbonate in diabetic ketoacidosis. *J Clin Endocrinol Metab* 1996;81:314–320.
   Concludes that bicarbonate therapy should be reserved for patients with severely depressed cardiovascular status.

Rossini AA, Thompson MJ, Mordes JP. Diabetic comas. In: Irwin RS, Rippe JM., et al., eds. *Irwin and Rippe's intensive care medicine*, 5th edition. Philadelphia: Lippincott Williams & Wilkins, 2003.
   The full-length version of this chapter.

Wilson HK, Keuer SP, Lea AS, et al. Phosphate therapy in diabetic ketoacidosis. *Arch Intern Med* 1982;142:517–520.
   Concludes that phosphate therapy is usually not essential for DKA management.

I. THYROID STORM

A. General principles

1. Thyroid storm is a rare, life-threatening complication of thyrotoxicosis in which a severe form of the disease is usually precipitated by an intercurrent medical problem.

2. Precipitating factors associated with thyroid storm include infections, stress, trauma, thyroidal or nonthyroidal surgery, diabetic ketoacidosis, labor, heart disease, iodinated contrast studies, thyroid hormone overdose, and radioiodine treatment (especially if there was no pretreatment with antithyroid drugs).

3. Although the cause of the rapid clinical decompensation is unknown, a sudden inhibition of thyroid hormone binding to plasma proteins by the precipitating factor, causing a rise in free hormone concentrations in the already elevated free hormone pool, may play a role in the pathogenesis of thyroid storm.

4. Historically, thyroid storm was frequently associated with surgery for hyperthyroidism but this is rarely seen now.

B. Pathophysiology and Clinical Presentation

1. Symptoms
   a. Thyroid storm is primarily a clinical diagnosis, with features similar to those of thyrotoxicosis but more exaggerated (Table 89-1).
   b. Cardinal features include fever (temperature usually over 38.5°C), tachycardia out of proportion to the fever and mental status changes.
   c. Tachyarrhythmias, especially atrial fibrillation in the elderly, are common, as are nausea, vomiting, diarrhea, agitation, and delirium.
   d. Coma and death may ensue in up to 20% of patients, frequently due to cardiac arrhythmias, congestive heart failure, hyperthermia, or the precipitating illness.

2. Signs
   a. Most patients display the classic signs of Graves disease, including ophthalmopathy and a diffusely enlarged goiter, although thyroid storm has been associated with toxic nodular goiters.
   b. In the elderly, severe myopathy, profound weight loss, apathy, and a minimally enlarged goiter may be observed.
   c. There are no distinct laboratory abnormalities and thyroid hormone levels are similar to those found in uncomplicated thyrotoxicosis; there is little correlation between the degree of elevation of thyroid hormones and the presentation of thyroid storm.

C. Diagnosis

1. The differential diagnosis of thyroid storm includes sepsis, neuroleptic malignant syndrome, malignant hyperthermia, and acute mania with lethal catatonia, all of which can precipitate thyroid storm in the appropriate setting.

2. Clues to the diagnosis of thyroid storm are a history of thyroid disease, history of iodine ingestion, and the presence of a goiter or stigmata of Graves disease.

3. The physician must have a high clinical index of suspicion for thyroid storm, because therapy must be instituted before the return of thyroid function tests in most cases.

D. Treatment

1. Thyroid storm is a major medical emergency that must be treated in an intensive care unit (Table 89-2).

TABLE 89-1	Clinical Features of Thyroid Storm

Fever (as high as 105.8°F)
Tachycardia/tachyarrhythmias
Delirium/agitation
Mental status changes
Congestive heart failure
Tremor
Nausea and vomiting
Diarrhea
Sweating
Vasodilatation
Dehydration
Hepatomegaly
Splenomegaly
Jaundice

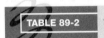

TABLE 89-2	Treatment of Thyroid Storm

Supportive Therapy
Treatment of underlying illnesses
Intravenous fluids
Cooling blanket and/or antipyretics

β-Adrenergic Blocking Drugs
Propranolol: 1 mg IV/min to a total dose of 10 mg then 40 to 80 mg PO q6h, *or*
Esmolol: 500 mg/kg/min IV then 50 to 100 mg/kg/min, *or*
Metoprolol: 100 to 400 mg PO q12h, *or*
Atenolol: 50 to 100 mg PO daily

Antithyroid Drugs
Inhibition of thyroid hormone synthesis
Propylthiouracil: 800 mg PO first does then 200 to 300 mg PO q8h, *or*
Methimazole: 80 mg PO first does then 40 to 80 mg PO q12h

Block release of thyroid hormones from the gland
SSKI: 5 drops PO q8h, *or*
Lugol's solution: 10 drops PO q8h, *or*
Telapaque (iopanoic acid): 1 g PO qd, *or*
Lithium: 800 to 1,200 mg PO qd—achieve serum lithium levels 0.5 to 1.5 mEq/L

Block T_4 to T_3 conversion
Corticosteroids: Dexamethasone 1 to 2 mg PO q6h
Most β-blockers: Propranolol 40 to 80 mg PO q6h
Propylthiouracil
Telepaque (iopanoic acid): no longer available in the United States

Remove thyroid hormones from the circulation
Plasmapheresis, *or*
Peritoneal dialysis, *or*
Cholestyramine: 4g PO q6h, *or*
Colestipol: 20 to 30 mg PO qd

PO, by mouth; SSKI, potassium iodide; T_4, thyroxine; T_3, 3,5,3′-triiodothyronine

2. Treatment includes supportive measures such as intravenous fluids, antipyretics, cooling blankets, and sedation.

3. β-Adrenergic blockers or calcium channel blockers are given to control tachyarrhythmias.

4. Antithyroid drugs are given in large doses, with propylthiouracil (PTU) preferred over methimazole because of its additional advantage of impairing peripheral conversion of thyroxine (T_4) to 3,5,3′-triiodothyronine.

5. PTU and methimazole can be administered by nasogastric tube or rectally if necessary; neither of these preparations is available for parenteral administration.

6. Iodides, orally or intravenously, may be used only after antithyroid drugs have been administered, although the useful radiographic contrast dye iopanoic acid is no longer available in the United States.

7. High-dose dexamethasone is recommended as supportive therapy, as an inhibitor of T4 to T3 conversion, and as management of possible intercurrent adrenal insufficiency.

8. Orally administered ion-exchange resins (colestipol or cholestyramine) can trap hormone in the intestine and prevent recirculation, and plasmapheresis has also been used in severe cases.

9. Treatment of the underlying precipitating illness is essential to survival in thyroid storm.

10. Once stabilized, the antithyroid treatment should be continued until euthyroidism is achieved, at which point a final decision regarding antithyroid drugs, surgery, or ^{131}I therapy can be made.

II. MYXEDEMA COMA

A. General principles

1. Myxedema coma is a rare syndrome that represents the extreme expression of severe, long-standing hypothyroidism.

2. Even with early diagnosis and treatment, the mortality can be as high as 60%.

3. Myxedema coma occurs most often in the elderly and during the winter months; in a recent series, 9 of 11 cases of myxedema coma were admitted in late fall or winter.

4. Other common precipitating factors include pulmonary infections, cerebrovascular accidents, trauma, surgery, congestive heart failure, and the injudicious use of sedatives.

5. The clinical course of lethargy proceeding to stupor and then coma is often hastened by drugs, especially sedatives, narcotics, antidepressants, and tranquilizers, especially in the undiagnosed hypothyroid patient who has been hospitalized for other medical problems.

B. Pathophysiology and Clinical Presentation

1. Symptoms

   a. Cardinal features of myxedema coma are hypothermia, respiratory depression, hypotension, and unconsciousness (Table 89-3).

   b. Most patients have the physical features of severe hypothyroidism, including bradycardia; macroglossia; delayed reflexes; dry, rough skin; and myxedematous facies, which results from the periorbital edema, pallor, hypercarotinemia, and patchy hair loss.

   c. Hypotonia of the gastrointestinal tract is common and often so severe as to suggest an obstructive lesion.

   d. Urinary retention due to a hypotonic bladder is related but less frequent.

2. Signs

   a. Pleural, pericardial, and peritoneal effusions may be present.

   b. The thyroid hormone abnormalities are similar to those in uncomplicated hypothyroidism, with more than 95% of cases resulting from primary hypothyroidism.

   c. Dilutional hyponatremia is common and may be severe.

   d. Elevated creatine kinase concentrations, sometimes markedly so, are encountered frequently, suggesting cardiac ischemia; however, in most cases the MB fraction is normal and an electrocardiogram often shows the low voltage and loss of T waves that is characteristic of severe hypothyroidism.

TABLE 89-3	Clinical Features of Myxedema Coma

Mental obtundation
Hypothermia
Bradycardia
Hypotension
Coarse, dry skin
Myxedema facies
Hypoglycemia
Atonic gastrointestinal tract
Atonic bladder
Pleural, pericardial, and peritoneal effusions

   e. Elevated lactate dehydrogenase concentrations, acidosis, and anemia are common findings.
   f. Lumbar puncture reveals increased opening pressure and high protein content.
C. Diagnosis
   1. The diagnosis of myxedema coma is based on the presence of the characteristic clinical syndrome in a patient with hypothyroidism.
   2. Clues to the diagnosis include symptoms related by family and friends, an outdated container of L-T4 discovered with the patient's belongings, previous treatment with radioactive iodine, or a thyroidectomy scar may be present.
   3. Differential diagnosis includes protein-calorie malnutrition, sepsis, hypoglycemia, exposure to certain drugs and toxins, and cold exposure
   4. What distinguishes myxedema coma from other disorders is the combination of laboratory evidence of hypothyroidism, the characteristic myxedema facies with periorbital puffiness, the skin changes, obtundation, and other physical signs characteristic of severe hypothyroidism.
   5. The physician must have a high clinical index of suspicion for myxedema coma, because therapy must be instituted before the return of thyroid function tests in most cases.
D. Treatment
   1. Myxedema is a medical emergency and must be managed in an ICU setting (Table 89-4).

TABLE 89-4	Treatment of Myxedema Coma

Assisted ventilation for hypoventilation
Hemodynamic support for hypotension
Intravenous glucose for hypoglycemia
Water restriction or hypertonic saline for severe hyponatremia
Passive rewarming for hypothermia
Administer thyroid hormone intravenously
   L-T4: 200–300 µg loading dose, up to 500 µg in the first 24 h[a] and/or
   L-T3: 12.5 µg q 6 h*
Administer hydrocortisone intravenously (100 mg q8h)*
Treat underlying infection and other illnesses, if present
Avoid all sedatives, hypnotics, and narcotics

[a]Note that dosage must be individualized (see text).
L-T4, levothyroxine; L-T3, liothyronine.

2. The mainstays of therapy are supportive care, with ventilatory and hemodynamic support, re-warming, correction of hyponatremia and hypoglycemia and treatment of the precipitating incident, and administration of thyroid hormone.

3. Active heating in myxedema coma should be avoided because it increases oxygen consumption and promotes peripheral vasodilation and circulatory collapse.

   a. An exception is at core temperatures below 28°C, when ventricular fibrillation is a major threat to life; in this case, the rate of rewarming should not exceed 0.5°C per hour until the core temperature is raised to approximately 31°C.

   b. In general, patients should be kept in a warm room and covered with blankets.

4. Sedatives, hypnotics, narcotics, and anesthetics must be minimized or avoided altogether due to their extended duration of action and exacerbation of obtundation in the hypothyroid patient.

5. Because of a 5% to 10% incidence of coexisting adrenal insufficiency in patients with myxedema coma, intravenous steroids are indicated before initiating T4 therapy.

6. Parenteral administration of thyroid hormone is necessary due to uncertain absorption through the gut.

   a. A reasonable approach is an initial intravenous loading dose of 200 to 300 µg L-T4, with another dose of L-T4 given in 6 to 12 hours to bring the total dose during the first 24 hours to 0.5 mg, followed by 50 to 100 µg intravenously every 24 hours until the patient is stabilized.

   b. In the most severe cases, some clinicians recommend using L-T3 at a dosage of 12.5 to 25 µg intravenously every 6 hours until the patient is stable and conscious, followed by a switch to L-T4.

7. Although myxedema coma is associated with a high mortality, many patients can be saved by judicious therapy aimed at correcting the secondary metabolic disturbances and reversing the hypothyroid state in a sustained but gradual fashion, because an effort to correct hypothyroidism too rapidly may completely negate the beneficial effects of the initial treatment.

Selected Readings

Arlot S, Debussche X, Lalau JD, et al. Myxoedema coma: response of thyroid hormones with oral and intravenous high-dose L-thyroxine treatment. *Intensive Care Med* 1991;17:16–18.
This study documents alternatives to the oral route of drug administration.

Brooks MH, Waldstein SS. Free thyroxine concentrations in thyroid storm. *Ann Intern Med* 1980;93:694–697.
In-depth review on the pathophysiology, presentation, and management of myxedema coma and thyroid storm.

Burch HB, Wartofsky L. Life-threatening thyrotoxicosis. Thyroid storm. *Endocrinol Metab Clin North Am* 1993;22:263–277.
In-depth review on the pathophysiology, presentation, and management of myxedema coma and thyroid storm.

Candrina R, DiStefano O, Spandrio S, et al. Treatment of thyrotoxic storm by charcoal plasmaperfusion. *J Endocrinol Invest* 1989;12:133–134.
Adjunctive therapies are important in the management thyroid storm. This study documents several potentially useful therapeutic options.

Hellman R, Kelly KL, Mason WD, et al. Propranolol for thyroid storm. *N Engl J Med* 1977;297:671–672.
Adjunctive therapies are important in the management thyroid storm. This study documents several potentially useful therapeutic options.

Hickman PE, Sylvester W, Musk AA, et al. Cardiac enzyme changes in myxedema coma. *Clin Chem* 1987;33:622–624.
Shows that creatine kinase elevations in myxedema coma are not due to myocardial ischemia.

Holvey DN, Goodner CJ, Nicoloff JT. Treatment of myxedema coma with intravenous thyroxine. *Arch Intern Med* 1964;113:89–96.
This study documents alternatives to the oral route of drug administration.

Hylander B, Rosenquist U. Treatment of myxedema coma—factors associated with fatal outcome. *Acta Endocrinol (Copenh)* 1985;108:65–71.
In-depth review on the pathophysiology, presentation, and management of myxedema coma and thyroid storm.

Jordan RM. Myxedema coma. Pathophysiology, therapy, and factors affecting prognosis. *Med Clin North Am* 1995;79:185–194.
In-depth review on the pathophysiology, presentation, and management of myxedema coma and thyroid storm.

Lazarus JH, Addison AJ, Richards AR, et al. Treatment of thyrotoxicosis with lithium carbonate. *Lancet* 1974;2:1160–1163.
Adjunctive therapies are important in the management thyroid storm. This study documents several potentially useful therapeutic options.

Nee PA, Scane AC, Lavelle PH, et al. Hypothermic myxedema coma erroneously diagnosed as myocardial infarction because of increased creatinine kinase MB. *Clin Chem* 1987;33:1083–1084.
Shows that creatine kinase elevations in myxedema coma are not due to myocardial ischemia.

Pereira VG, Haron ES, Lima-Neto N, et al. Management of myxedema coma: report on three successfully treated cases with nasogastric or intravenous administration of triiodothyronine. *J Endocrinol Invest* 1982;5:331–334.
This study documents alternatives to the oral route of drug administration.

Shakir KM, Michaels RD, Hays JH, et al. The use of bile aced sequestrants to lower serum thyroid hormone concentrations in iatrogenic hyperthyroidism. *Ann Intern Med* 1993;118:112–113.
Adjunctive therapies are important in the management thyroid storm. This study documents several potentially useful therapeutic options.

Yeung SC, Go R, Balasubramanyam A. Rectal administration of iodide and propylthiouracil in the treatment of thyroid storm. *Thyroid* 1995;5:403–405.
These studies document alternatives to the oral route of drug administration.

HYPOADRENAL CRISIS AND THE STRESS MANAGEMENT OF THE PATIENT ON CHRONIC STEROID THERAPY

Christopher Longcope* and Neil Aronin

I. HYPOADRENAL CRISIS

A. General principles. The adrenal glands secrete five types of hormones, but only two of them are critical in the intensive care unit (ICU) setting. Mineralocorticoids (primarily aldosterone) have their major effects on electrolyte balance, and glucocorticoids (primarily cortisol) promote gluconeogenesis but have many other actions. Mineralocorticoids and glucocorticoids are life-maintaining and deficiency of either can result in a hypoadrenal crisis. By contrast, the other three types of adrenal hormones do not play a major role in this disorder.

Hypoadrenal crisis can occur as an acute event in individuals who give little history of previous adrenal problems. A high index of suspicion is necessary because the diagnosis might be easily missed. To establish the diagnosis by biochemical testing requires time. It is wise to perform diagnostic testing procedures before initiating therapy but not to withhold therapy until the results are known.

1. **Etiology.** The most common cause of primary adrenal failure, Addison disease, is autoimmune in nature. Other causes of adrenal failure include hemorrhage secondary to trauma, overwhelming sepsis, circulating anticoagulants or anticoagulant therapy, tuberculosis, fungal disease, amyloidosis, acquired immune deficiency syndrome (AIDS), antiphospholipid syndrome, infarction, irradiation, metastatic disease, and drugs.

   The most common cause of secondary adrenal insufficiency is suppression of corticotropin (ACTH) release by prior glucocorticoid therapy. Pituitary tumors or hypothalamic disease can cause adrenal dysfunction.

2. **Actions of mineralocorticoids and glucocorticoids.** The adrenal cortex secretes aldosterone from the zona glomerulosa and cortisol from the zona reticularis. Aldosterone, which promotes the reabsorption of sodium and the secretion of potassium and hydrogen in the renal tubule, is controlled mainly by the renin–angiotensin system.

   Glucocorticoids promote gluconeogenesis and protein wasting and increase the excretion of free water by the kidney. In large doses, glucocorticoids bind to mineralocorticoid receptors, thereby increasing sodium reabsorption and potassium and hydrogen ion excretion. Glucocorticoids act on numerous tissues, also affecting the sense of well-being, appetite, and mood. They directly inhibit the release of ACTH in the central nervous system. Glucocorticoids have a direct effect on the cardiovascular system and help maintain blood pressure, although the mechanisms are unknown.

   The effects of excess glucocorticoids cause lymphopenia, leukocytosis, and eosinopenia. Excess glucocorticoids can lead to osteoporosis and reduction of hypercalcemia in certain diseases.

   Lack of aldosterone results in sodium wasting, with concomitant loss of water and an increase in renal reabsorption of potassium. A decrease in plasma volume and dehydration occurs, with subsequent increases in blood urea nitrogen (BUN) and plasma renin activity.

   The decrease in circulating levels of cortisol causes a marked increase in circulating levels of ACTH and a corresponding increase in β-lipotropin, from which melanocyte-stimulating hormone activity increases; in long-standing

---

*Deceased

adrenal insufficiency, the skin, especially creases and scars, develops hyperpigmentation. Initially orthostatic, hypotension can progress to frank shock in a crisis. Hypoglycemia and an increase in sensitivity to insulin are commonplace.

B. Diagnosis

1. **Clinical.** Clinical manifestations that suggest adrenal insufficiency can include a nonspecific history of increasing weakness, lassitude, fatigue, anorexia, vomiting, and constipation (with the hypoadrenal crisis, diarrhea can occur). Patients who present with adrenal hypofunction in crisis are hypotensive or in frank shock; they generally have a fever that can be high, show evidence of dehydration, and may be stuporous or comatose. In individuals whose loss of adrenal function occurs as a precipitous event (adrenal hemorrhage during the course of an infection, anticoagulant therapy, trauma, or after surgery), no hyperpigmentation is seen but flank pain is often present. Severely ill patients are often suspected of developing adrenal hypofunction, but the incidence and diagnosis of this entity are controversial.

   In secondary adrenal failure caused by lack of ACTH, the signs and symptoms are essentially those of glucocorticoid deficiency, especially hypoglycemia. ACTH deficiency generally follows deficiency in other anterior pituitary hormones, so that deficits in overall pituitary secretion can lead to signs of other endocrine gland dysfunctions.

   Although clinical signs of adrenal insufficiency raise awareness of its presence, the actual diagnosis of hypoadrenal function requires appropriate laboratory tests.

2. **Adrenal function tests.** In primary adrenal insufficiency, plasma concentrations of cortisol are usually low or in the low to normal range and do not rise after ACTH stimulation. This failure to respond to ACTH is the definitive test for primary adrenal hypofunction and should be carried out on anyone in whom the diagnosis is suspected. Severely ill patients with a serum cortisol less than 20 µg/dL should be suspected of having adrenal insufficiency and should be tested with intravenous (IV) ACTH. The ACTH stimulation is carried out by administering 250 µg of Cortrosyn (synthetic ACTH 1–24) IV, and plasma ACTH and cortisol levels are measured prior to and 30 to 60 minutes after the dose. A normal response is indicated by a stimulated cortisol concentration of more than 20 µg/dL. Although this is the standard test at present, an alternative test has been suggested in which only 1 µg synthetic ACTH is administered IV, with a normal response at 30 minutes of more than 18 µg/dL. With the low-dose ACTH test, patients with secondary adrenal insufficiency show an increase in cortisol, although not to the same degree as those with normal hypothalamic-pituitary adrenal function. Because the analysis of plasma cortisol level cannot be done immediately, in critically ill patients dexamethasone (4 mg IV) can be given before the ACTH test.

   In individuals who develop acute adrenal insufficiency as a result of adrenal hemorrhage, a computed tomography (CT) scan of the adrenal glands can be a very useful diagnostic tool. Individuals with adrenal hypofunction generally show varying degrees of hyponatremia and hyperkalemia and the sodium: potassium ratio is almost always less than 30.

C. Treatment. The management of suspected hypoadrenal crisis depends on the severity of the illness on presentation. The main objective of therapy is immediate administration of a glucocorticoid along with saline and glucose. Because large amounts of hydrocortisone are administered IV in salt-containing solutions, it is not necessary to administer a mineralocorticoid immediately. It is generally believed that individuals in the hypoadrenal state have an approximate 20% deficit of their extracellular fluid volume and should receive at least 3 liters of glucose-containing saline in the first 24 hours.

In critically ill patients, the saline and glucose may have to be given in the first few hours. A bolus of 100 mg of hydrocortisone should be administered IV immediately, and then 100 to 150 mg should be given IV over the next 24 hours. If the patient's condition is deemed sufficiently grave, 4 mg of dexamethasone sodium phosphate can be administered as initial therapy before carrying out the ACTH stimulation. However, because dexamethasone does not have potent salt-retaining activity, hydrocortisone should be used for continuing therapy.

After the initial 24 hours of therapy, the hydrocortisone can be decreased by 50% each day as the situation improves to reach a standard maintenance dose of 20 to 30 mg per day. As the maintenance dose is achieved, a mineralocorticoid (0.1 mg 9α-fluorohydrocortisone acetate) should be added.

In addition to therapy with glucocorticoids, saline, and glucose, any underlying infection should be treated vigorously.

II. GLUCOCORTICOIDS AND STRESS

A. General principles. In normal subjects, the secretion rate of cortisol increases from 10 mg per day to 50 to 150 mg per day during surgical procedures but rarely exceeds 200 mg per day. The degree of response depends, in part, on the extent and duration of surgery.

After the introduction of glucocorticoid therapy, several case reports linked withdrawal of steroids, adrenal suppression, and shock in patients on long-term steroid treatment.

The few studies available suggest that hypotension from inadequate adrenal function is uncommon. Thus, the development of shock in the acutely ill or surgical patient on steroid therapy (or after withdrawal within 1 year) should not be attributed solely to diminished adrenal responsiveness. Adrenal steroids can and should be administered, but other contributing causes of the hypotension should be sought. Suppression of the hypothalamic–anterior pituitary–adrenal axis can occur after only 5 days of glucocorticoid treatment. After long-term administration of corticosteroids, the adrenal axis may respond poorly to appropriate stimuli up to 1 year after steroid withdrawal. Adrenal suppression cannot be predicted based solely on glucocorticoid dosage and duration or a normal basal cortisol.

B. Diagnosis and treatment. Patients on glucocorticoid therapy for at least 4 weeks at either pharmacologic or replacement levels and those who have stopped glucocorticoids within the past year have the highest risk for adrenal suppression. Time permitting, a Cortrosyn test provides information on the adequacy of the adrenal response to stress. An adequate increase in plasma cortisol following corticotropin administration is interpreted to indicate the presence of an intact hypothalamic–anterior pituitary–adrenal axis, and patients who have a subnormal response to Cortrosyn also have a subnormal cortisol response to stress or surgery. For minor surgical procedures, the patient's usual dose of glucocorticoid is probably sufficient, but a single dose of 25 mg hydrocortisone or its equivalent can be given instead. As the extent and duration of surgery increases, the glucocorticoid dose should be increased from 50 to 75 mg per day hydrocortisone, or its equivalent for up to 2 days, to 100 to 150 mg hydrocortisone or its equivalent for up to 3 days.

Hydrocortisone can be rapidly tapered and the patients returned to their usual dose of glucocorticoid if needed.

Selected Readings

Axelrod L. Glucocorticoid therapy. *Medicine* 1976;55:39.
   A review of glucocorticoid action and effects on the hypothalamic-pituitary-adrenal axis; old but still useful.

Barquist E, Kirton O. Adrenal insufficiency in the surgical intensive care unit patient. *J Trauma* 1997;42:27.
   Report on occurrence of acute adrenal insufficiency in the ICU, including diagnostic steps, therapy, and prognosis.

Baxter JD, Tyrrell JB. Evaluation of the hypothalamic-pituitary-adrenal axis: importance in steroid therapy, AIDS, and other stress syndromes. *Advances in Internal Medicine* 1994;39:667.
   Review on evaluating patients for adrenal dysfunction, including tests that are being used and their interpretation.

Henzen C, Suter A, Lerch E, et al. Suppression and recovery of adrenal response after short-term, high-dose glucocorticoid treatment. *Lancet* 2000;335:542–545.
Study emphasizes the high frequency of mild adrenal suppression after glucocorticoid treatment between 5 and 30 days duration. Correspondence (Lancet 2000;335:1458–1459.) raises some uncertainties related to clinical evaluation of the hypothalamic-anterior pituitary-adrenal axis in sick patients.

Kehlet H, Binder C. Adrenocortical function and clinical course during and after surgery in supplemented glucocorticoid-treated patients. *Br J Anaesth* 1973;45:1043.
Evaluation of adrenocortical function and clinical course in glucocorticoid-treated patients during surgery.

Kehlet H, Binder C. Alteration in distribution volume and biological half-life of cortisol during major surgery. *J Clin Endocrinol Metabol* 1973;36:330.
Provides information on the changes in cortisol production and metabolism that occur during stress. One of the few reports giving secretion rates.

Kehlet H, Binder C. Value of an ACTH test in assessing hypothalamic-pituitary-adrenocortical function in glucocorticoid-treated patients. *BMJ* 1973;2:147.
Reports correlating results of prospective ACTH testing and later response to operative stress.

Lamberts SWJ, Bruining HA, de Jong FH. Corticosteroid therapy in severe illness. *N Engl J Med* 1997;337:1285.
Review of the normal adrenal response to stress and the treatment, during stress, of patients with adrenal dysfunction.

Magiakou MA, Chrousos GP. Corticosteroid therapy, nonendocrine disease, and corticosteroid withdrawal. In: Bardin CW, ed. *Current therapy in endocrinology.* St. Louis: CV Mosby, 1997, p. 138.
Reviews adrenal suppression, stress, and therapy.

Masterson GR, Mostafa SM. Editorial II: adrenocortical function in critical illness. *Br J Anaesth* 1998;81:308.
Critical review of studies on adrenocortical dysfunction and critical illness.

Oelkers W. Adrenal insufficiency. *N Engl J Med* 1996;335:1206.
Review of the general topic of adrenal insufficiency, both acute and chronic. Discusses the various tests to be used and treatment.

Salem M, Tainsh RE, Bromberg J, et al. Perioperative glucocorticoid coverage. *Ann Surg* 1994;219:416.
Excellent review of the physiology, diagnosis, and treatment of patients with absent or suppressed adrenocortical function. Recommends lower doses of glucocorticoids than heretofore.

Streeten DHP. Shortcomings in the low-dose (1 μg) ACTH test for the diagnosis of ACTH deficiency states [Editorial]. *J Clin Endocrinol Metab* 1999;84:835.
Discusses the merits and demerits of low-dose ACTH testing. A thoughtful discussion of the article by Thaler and Blevins.

Szalados JE, Vukmir RB. Acute adrenal insufficiency resulting from adrenal hemorrhage as indicated by post-operative hypotension. *Intensive Care Med* 1994;20:216.
Reports on the incidence, diagnosis, and therapy of acute adrenal insufficiency caused by adrenal hemorrhage. This problem is being recognized more frequently than in the past.

Thaler LM, Blevins LS. The low dose (1-μg) adrenocorticotropin stimulation test in the evaluation of patients with suspected central adrenal insufficiency. *J Clin Endocrinol Metab* 1998;83:2726.
An endorsement for the low-dose ACTH test in the diagnosis of adrenocortical dysfunction as proposed by Streeten.

Udelsman R, Ramp J, Gallucci WT, et al. Adaptation during surgical stress: a reevaluation of the role of glucocorticoids. *J Clin Invest* 1986;77:1377.
An argument against supraphysiologic glucocorticoid treatment during stress in adrenal insufficiency. The study was done using cynomolgus monkeys, but is applicable to humans.

I. GENERAL PRINCIPLES

A. Disorders of mineral metabolism (calcium, magnesium, phosphorus) occur frequently in patients admitted to ICUs. They are rarely the primary cause for admission but may exacerbate existing medical situations.

B. Calcium, magnesium, and phosphorus are controlled by interaction of parathyroid hormone (PTH), 1,25-dihydroxyvitamin D (1,25 D), and calcitonin.

II. PATHOPHYSIOLOGY OF CALCIUM DISORDERS

A. In extracellular fluids, calcium is free and bound to albumin or other anions. The free (ionized) form is biologically active. Albumin needs to be measured to interpret total calcium levels.

B. Changes in acid–base balance affect binding of calcium to albumin.

    1. Acidosis decreases binding and increases the free form.

    2. Alkalosis increases binding and decreases the free form.

C. Calcium balance depends on bone resorption and formation, intestinal absorption, and renal excretion.

    a. PTH increases bone resorption and renal calcium reabsorption

    b. 1,25D enhances intestinal calcium absorption

    c. Calcitonin inhibits bone resorption and increases renal calcium excretion

D. Diagnosis of hypercalcemia

    1. Signs and symptoms

        a. Mental manifestations vary from stupor to coma.

        b. Neurologic effects include reduced muscle tone and reflexes.

        c. Intestinal and urologic signs include vomiting, polyuria, polydipsia, and constipation.

        d. Cardiovascular effects include shortening of the QT interval increasing potential for arrhythmias.

    2. Differential diagnosis

        a. Malignancy, especially lung, breast, hematologic (myeloma and lymphoma), head and neck, and renal

        b. Primary hyperparathyroidism

        c. Granulomatous disease

        d. Thyrotoxicosis

        e. Immobilization

        f. Vitamin D intoxication

        g. Addison disease

        h. Familial hypercalciuric hypercalcemia

    3. Depending on the clinical situation, PTH and thyroid-stimulating hormone levels, urine protein electrophoresis, and bone scan can help establish the diagnosis.

E. Treatment of hypercalcemia

    1. Hydration

        a. Pivotal because response is rapid. Aim is to achieve a urine output of 3 to 5L/24h usually requiring 4 to 6L/24h of normal saline

        b. Furosemide (Lasix) 40 to 80 mg intravenously (IV) prevents fluid overload and inhibits renal calcium reabsorption. Electrolyte measurement is mandatory.

    2. Calcitonin

        a. Inhibits bone resorption when a rapid decrease required

  b. Dose is 4 IU/kg body weight subcutaneously or intramuscularly every 12 hours with hydration

  c. Decrease in serum calcium 2 hours after dose and lasts 6 to 8 hours. Average decrease is 9% and lasts 5 to 8 days.

 3. Bisphosphonates

  a. Inhibit bone resorption and provide a more prolonged calcium decrease

  b. Pamidronate disodium (Aredia) (60 mg IV over 4 hours) with hydration

  c. Zolendronic acid (Zometa) (4 mg IV over >15 minutes) with hydration

  d. Calcium normalizes in 70% to 89% of patients with significant decreases within 4 days and duration of response between 17 and 30 days

  e. Renal function needs to be monitored

  f. Retreatment after a minimum of 7 days to allow full response to initial dose. Dose and manner of retreatment identical to initial treatment.

F. Diagnosis of hypocalcemia

 1. Signs and symptoms

  a. Neurologic manifestations include hyperreflexia and tetany

 2. Differential diagnosis

  a. Hypoparathyroidism

  b. Vitamin D deficiency

  c. Hyperphosphatemia

  d. Magnesium deficiency

 3. PTH, 25-hydroxyvitamin D, magnesium, and phosphorus levels usually identify the cause

G. Treatment of hypocalcemia

 1. Depends on severity and chronicity. Symptomatic patients should receive intravenous calcium

 2. Calcium

  a. Calcium gluconate (93 mg of elemental calcium in a 10-mL vial) or calcium chloride (272 mg of elemental calcium in a 10-mL vial) administered in 50 to 100 mL 5% dextrose in water over 10 to 15 minutes

  b. Infusion of 1 to 2 mg calcium/kg per hour continued until ionized calcium is 4.5 mg/dL or the total calcium is 7 mg/dL. Total calcium should be maintained between 8 and 8.5 mg/dL and not higher to avoid hypercalciuria

 3. Vitamin D

  a. Ergocalciferol 50,000 to 100,000 U per day by mouth (PO). Slow onset but wide safety margin

  b. 1,25D (Rocaltrol) 0.25 to 1.0 μg per day PO. More rapid and potent than ergocalciferol but narrower safety margin because of risk of hypercalciuria and hypercalcemia

III. PATHOPHYSIOLOGY OF MAGNESIUM

A. Magnesium circulates in the free form (70%) and bound to albumin (30%).

 1. Albumin needs to be measured to interpret magnesium level.

B. Magnesium levels depend on intestinal absorption and renal excretion.

 1. Decreased renal excretion (e.g., renal failure) increases magnesium levels

 2. Increased renal excretion (e.g., osmotic diuresis or drugs [ethanol, aminoglycosides, cisplatin]) decreases magnesium levels

 3. Decreased intestinal absorption (e.g., accompanying fat malabsorption) decreases magnesium levels

B. Diagnosis of hypermagnesemia

 1. Signs and symptoms

  a. Central nervous system depression (e.g., decreased reflexes, flaccid paralysis, stupor, coma)

 2. Etiology

  a. Most common cause is renal failure, aggravated by use of magnesium-containing antacids.

  b. The hypermagnesemia associated with diabetic ketoacidosis usually reflects dehydration and masks total body magnesium depletion.

C. Treatment of hypermagnesemia
   1. Dialysis for the symptomatic patient when renal function is impaired.
   2. If renal function not impaired, magnesium excretion can be increased by furosemide (Lasix) 40 to 80 mg IV every 1 to 2 hours. Electrolytes must be monitored.
   3. Neuromuscular depressant effects of magnesium in the symptomatic patient can be acutely antagonized by calcium gluconate (93 mg of elemental calcium in a 10-mL vial) administered in 50 to 100 mL 5% dextrose in water over 10 to 15 minutes. Serum calcium levels must be monitored.
D. Diagnosis of hypomagnesemia
   1. Signs and symptoms
      a. Central nervous system excitability which in part may be caused by hypocalcemia. Low magnesium impairs PTH secretion and peripheral responsiveness to PTH, which may result in hypocalcemia.
   2. Etiology
      a. Increased renal excretion due to osmotic diuresis (e.g. hyperglycemia or hypercalcemia) is the most common cause.
      b. Frequently present in patients with malabsorption.
      c. Often encountered in the alcoholic patient due to poor dietary intake
E. Treatment of hypomagnesemia
   1. Symptomatic patient usually has a total body magnesium deficit of 1 to 3 mEq/kg body weight.
   2. Magnesium oxide (Mag-Ox 400) 1 to 2 tabs PO qd 241 mg (19.86 mEq) magnesium/tablet
      a. Monitor serum magnesium and calcium levels.
   3. In the symptomatic patient who cannot take oral medications, magnesium sulfate (97 mg [8 mEq] magnesium per vial) IV. Administer 16 mEq magnesium in 100 mL 5% dextrose in water or 100 mL normal saline over 1 hour. Monitor serum magnesium and calcium levels.

IV. PATHOPHYSIOLOGY OF PHOSPHORUS DISORDERS

A. Most phosphorus is found intracellularly. Because of shifts between intracellular and extracellular compartments, serum phosphorus does not reflect body stores.
   1. Acidosis causes shift of phosphorus from within cells to the extracellular compartment. Serum phosphorus levels may be normal in the acidotic patient despite depletion of total body stores because of this shift.
   2. Low serum phosphorus stimulates renal production of 1,25 D.
B. Diagnosis of hyperphosphatemia
   1. Signs and symptoms. No clinical signs and symptoms of hyperphosphatemia per se. Hyperreflexia and tetany may occur caused by accompanying hypocalcemia.
   2. Differential diagnosis. Most often encountered in patients with renal failure or hypoparathyroidism. In both clinical situations, hyperphosphatemia results from impaired renal excretion
C. Treatment of hyperphosphatemia
   1. Restriction of dietary phosphorus intake
   2. Correction of accompanying hypocalcemia
D. Diagnosis of hypophosphatemia
   1. Signs and symptoms
      a. Muscle weakness, rhabdomyolysis
   2. Differential diagnosis
      a. Impaired intestinal absorption (e.g., malnutrition or use of phosphate-binding antacids)
      b. Increased renal excretion (e.g., hyperparathyroidism, vitamin D deficiency [due to secondary hyperparathyroidism], hyperglycemic states [due to osmotic diuresis], impaired renal handling of phosphorus [vitamin D–resistant rickets])
E. Treatment of hypophosphatemia
   1. Severe hypophosphatemia (<1 mg/dL) may require parenteral therapy

a. Parenteral potassium phosphate (3 mmol phosphate/mL) added to 5% dextrose in 50% normal saline and given over 6 hours. Symptomatic patients may receive 0.16 mmol phosphate/kg body weight. Hypercalcemic patients should receive less (e.g. 0.08 mmol phosphate/kg body weight).

2. Parenteral therapy is contraindicated in patients with renal failure or hypocalcemia.

a. Intravenous phosphate therapy in patient with renal failure may cause hyperphosphatemia and worsen hypocalcemia

3. Mild hypophosphatemia. Potassium phosphate (K-Phos Neutral) 1 to 4 g phosphorus per day PO in divided doses. Diarrhea most common side effect of oral therapy.

Selected Readings

Body JJ, Bartl R, Burckhard T, et al. Current use of bisphosphonates in oncology. *J Clin Oncol* 1998;16:3890.
Discussion of the use of bisphosphonates in cancer patients and their indications for treatment of hypercalcemia of malignancy and metastatic bone pain and for the prevention of the complications of multiple myeloma and metastatic bone disease; 68 references.

Bushinsky DA, Monk RD. Calcium. *Lancet* 1998;352;306.
A review of the mechanisms responsible for abnormalities in calcium homeostasis, the differential diagnosis of hypercalcemia and hypocalcemia, and appropriate therapy; 31 references.

Chan FK, Koberle LM, Thys-Jacobs S, et al. Differential diagnoses, causes, and management of hypercalcemia. *Curr Probl Surg* 1997;34:445.
Extensive discussion of recent advances in molecular biology and genetics that have facilitated the evaluation of patients presenting with hypercalcemia; 253 references.

Li EC, Davis LE. Zolendronic acid: a new parenteral bisphosphonate *Clin Ther* 2003; 25:2669.
A comprehensive review of preclinical and clinical studies of the use of the bisphosphonate in skeletal disorders; 62 references.

Major P, Lortholary A, Hon J, et al. Zolendronic acid is superior to pamidronate in the treatment of hypercalcemia of malignancy; a pooled analysis of two randomized, controlled clinical trials. *J Clin Oncol* 2002;19:558.
Head-to-head studies comparing the effects of the bisphosphonates on hypercalcemia of malignancy; 36 references.

Mundy GR, Guise TA, Hypercalcemia of malignancy. *Am J Med* 1997;103:134.
Clear description of the pathophysiology of hypercalcemia of malignancy; 81 references.

Ross JR, Saunders Y, Edmonds PM, et al. Systematic review of role of bisphosphonates on skeletal morbidity in metastatic cancer. *BMJ* 2003;327:469.
Effects of bisphosphonates on skeletal morbidity in patients with bone metastases; 41 references.

HYPOGLYCEMIA

Michael J. Thompson, John P. Mordes,
and Aldo A. Rossini

92

I. **GENERAL PRINCIPLES.** Hypoglycemia is frequently encountered in emergency departments and must be excluded in every patient with stupor or coma. Cases of refractory, prolonged hypoglycemia of unknown etiology require admission to an intensive care unit (ICU). Severe hypoglycemia can lead to permanent neurologic damage.

No specific blood glucose concentration defines hypoglycemia, although the serum glucose is typically less than 50 mg/dL (2.8 mM). The physiological definition of hypoglycemia is a blood glucose concentration sufficiently low as to cause the release of counterregulatory hormones (e.g., catecholamines) and impair the function of the central nervous system. Specifically, "Whipple's Triad" defines hypoglycemia as: (a) documentation of a low blood glucose concentration, (b) concurrent symptoms of hypoglycemia, (c) resolution of those symptoms after administration of glucose.

II. **PATHOPHYSIOLOGY.** Hypoglycemia can be divided into fasting and nonfasting categories. Nonfasting, postprandial, and reactive hypoglycemic states are not usually life-threatening and are not discussed further here. Fasting hypoglycemia subsumes several subcategories: (a) states of overinsulinization, (b) states of impaired counterregulation, (c) states of inadequate endogenous glucose production, and (d) states in which gluconeogenic substrates are unavailable. Physiologically, most medication-induced hypoglycemia represents fasting hypoglycemia.

A. **Hypoglycemia due to excess insulin**

1. Insulin overdose

   a. Insulin overdose is the most common cause of hypoglycemia. In most cases, the overdose is inadvertent, the consequence of a missed meal or increased intensity of exercise. Patients with long-standing diabetes may be at increased risk of hypoglycemia due to increased sensitivity to regular insulin and defective counterregulatory responses. Intentional overdoses occur in both diabetic and nondiabetic individuals. Self-induced hypoglycemia should be suspected in anyone with access to insulin or oral hypoglycemic agents who experiences unexplained hypoglycemia.

   b. Hypoglycemia is often more severe among patients with long-standing type 1 diabetes because of the presence of a defective counterregulatory response. Impaired glucagon secretory responses are common, and epinephrine responses can also be inadequate. When counterregulation is impaired, adrenergic warning signals such as tremor, diaphoresis, and tachycardia may not occur and neuroglycopenic symptoms (e.g., confusion, combativeness, seizure, coma) can develop rapidly. Inadequate counterregulatory responses can also delay spontaneous recovery from insulin-induced hypoglycemia.

2. Hypoglycemia due to oral agents. Oral agents used to treat type 2 diabetes fall into two classes. Hypoglycemic agents enhance insulin secretion and can cause hyperinsulinemic hypoglycemia. The sulfonylureas and meglitinides belong to this class. Antidiabetic agents promote normoglycemia through other mechanisms. When given as monotherapy they do not cause hypoglycemia, but they can amplify the glucose-lowering activity of insulin and the oral hypoglycemic agents. The thiazolidinediones, biguanides, and α-glucosidase inhibitors belong to this class. Many drugs not used in the treatment of diabetes can also amplify the glucose-lowering activity of oral hypoglycemic agents, and a complete medication history can be critical in the diagnosis of hypoglycemia.

495

a. Hypoglycemic agents
   (1) Sulfonylureas. Sulfonylurea-class oral hypoglycemic agents: This class of drugs enhances insulin secretion by pancreatic beta cells. Sulfonylurea overdose is the leading cause of hypoglycemia in diabetic persons over 60. It typically occurs in the setting of acute or chronic starvation superimposed on mild to moderate liver or kidney failure. Severe hypoglycemia has resulted from inadvertent substitution of an oral hypoglycemic agent for a different medication (e.g., chlorpropamide for chlorpromazine).
   (2) Repaglinide and nateglinide. Repaglinide (Prandin) and nateglinide (Starlix) belong to a new category of oral hypoglycemic agents. Like the sulfonylureas, they increase endogenous insulin secretion, but both repaglinide and nateglinide are rapidly eliminated and have a limited toxicity profile.
b. Antidiabetic agents
   (1) Biguanides. Oral hypoglycemic drugs of the biguanide class induce hypoglycemia much less often than do sulfonylureas. They rarely do so by inhibiting gluconeogenesis during prolonged caloric deprivation.
   (2) Thiazolidinediones. Pioglitazone (Actos) and rosiglitazone (Avandia) are currently the only drugs of the thiazolidinedione class available in the United States. These drugs do not cause hypoglycemia when used as monotherapy but can potentiate hypoglycemia caused by insulin or the sulfonylureas. They act by increasing insulin sensitivity.
   (3) α-Glucosidase inhibitors. Acarbose (Precose) and miglitol (Glyset) are α-glucosidase inhibitors that inhibit the digestion of complex carbohydrates. They have not been reported to cause hypoglycemia when used as monotherapy. Hypoglycemia in patients treated with insulin or sulfonylureas in addition to an α-glucosidase inhibitor may not respond to the oral administration of complex sugars but should respond to monomeric glucose.
3. Hypoglycemia due to other drugs. A number of medications can produce hypoglycemia by increasing circulating insulin concentration. Some of them are listed in Table 92-1.
4. Insulinomas and other tumors. Insulin-secreting pancreatic islet cell tumors are very rare. They classically cause fasting hypoglycemia. Paraneoplastic hypoglycemia may be caused by tumors that secrete insulinlike growth factors. Another unusual cause of hypoglycemia due to insulin in children is nesidioblastosis (nonmalignant islet cell adenomatosis).
5. Autoimmune or antibody-mediated hypoglycemia. A rare condition in which endogenous autoantibodies bind to and activate the insulin receptor.
6. Familial hyperinsulinemic hypoglycemia

B. Hypoglycemia associated with deficiencies in counterregulatory hormones
1. Adrenal disease. Glucocorticoid deficiency commonly causes hypoglycemia in children but not in adults.
2. Pituitary disease. Patients with hypopituitarism may develop hypoglycemia because of deficiencies of growth hormone and/or thyroid hormone.
3. Glucagon. Glucagon deficiency is the rarest cause of hypoglycemia of endocrine origin.

C. Hypoglycemia due to inadequate production of endogenous glucose
1. Liver disease. Hypoglycemia due to abnormal liver function generally does not occur until hepatic injury is severe. Hepatotoxins that can impair gluconeogenesis and cause hypoglycemia include carbon tetrachloride, the *Amanita phalloides* mushroom toxin, and urethane. Hepatic congestion due to severe congestive heart failure rarely causes hypoglycemia.
2. Kidney disease. Symptomatic hypoglycemia occurs in many diabetic patients undergoing dialysis. The cause may involve increased glucose-stimulated insulin release due to the high glucose concentration in the dialysate and impaired clearance of insulin due to the underlying renal disease. Spontaneous fasting hypoglycemia has been reported to occur in nondiabetic patients with end-stage renal disease.

TABLE 92-1	Drugs and Toxins Associated with Hypoglycemia

Drugs that increase circulating insulin concentrations	Drugs that impair gluconeogenesis	Unknown mechanism of action
Direct Stimulants of Insulin Secretion	*Hepatotoxins (Amanitatoxin)*	Acetazolamide—Diamox
Acetohexamide (Dymelor)	Acetaminophen	Acetylsalicylic acid (Aspirin)
Chloroquine (Aralen)	(Tylenol, Tempra)	Aluminum hydroxide
Chlorpropamide (Diabinese)	Propoxyphene (Darvon)	(Dialume)
Disopyramide (Norpace)	*Agents that Decrease Activity*	Captopril (Capoten)
Glimepiride (Amaryl)	*of Gluconeogenic Enzymes*	Chlorpromazine (Thorazine)
Glipizide (Glucotrol)	Metoprolol (Lopressor)	Cimetidine (Tagamet)
Glyburide (Micronase,	Nadolol (Corgard)	Diphenhydramine (Benadryl)
Diabeta, Glynase)	Phenformin	Doxepin (Sinequan, Adapin)
Glibenclamide	Metformin (Glucophage)	Enalapril (Vasotec)
Pentamidine (Pentam)	Pindolol (Visken)	Ethylenediaminetetraacetic
Quinidine	Propranolol (Inderal)	acid (EDTA, Versene)
Quinine	*Hypoglycin*	Haloperidol (Haldol)
Ritodrine (Yutopar)	*Ethanol*	Isoxsuprine
Terbutaline (Brethine,		Lidocaine (Xylocaine)
Bricanyl)		Lithium (Eskalith)
Tolazamide (Tolinase)		Oxytetracycline (Terramycin)
Tolbutamide (Orinase)		Para-aminobenzoic acid
Trimethoprim/		(PABA)
Sulfamethoxazole		Para-aminosalicylic acid
(Bactrim, Septra)		(PASA)
Agents that Enhance the		Phenytoin (Dilantin)
Action of Sulfonylureas		Ranitidine (Zantac)
Bishydroxycoumarin		Sulfadiazine
(Dicoumarol)		Sulfisoxazole (Gantrisin)
Imipramine (Tofranil)		Warfarin (Coumadin)
Phenylbutazone (Butazolidin)		

Adapted from Seltzer HS. Drug-induced hypoglycemia: A review of 1418 Cases. *Endocrinol Metab Clin North Am* 1989;18:163–183. A sampling of common trade names is shown in parenthesis; the enumeration of trade names is not exhaustive. Data for some listed agents may be very limited.

3. **Ethanol-induced hypoglycemia (alcoholic ketoacidosis).** Ethanol inhibits gluconeogenesis and the hepatic uptake of gluconeogenic precursors. Hypoglycemia can occur more than a day after the ingestion of ethanol. Ketonuria and ketonemia are usually present. Children and chronic alcohol abusers are most susceptible. The condition most commonly occurs in the setting of poor food intake and depleted glycogen stores. More information can be found in Chapter 88.

4. **Drugs.** Some of the many drugs and poisons that do not increase circulating insulin but nonetheless cause hypoglycemia are listed in Table 92-1. β-Blockers prevent the normal glycogenolytic and gluconeogenic response to hypoglycemia and may mask adrenergic symptoms. Salicylate intoxication causes hypoglycemia commonly in children but only very rarely in adults. Hypoglycemia associated with angiotensin-converting enzyme inhibitors have been reported in patients with diabetes.

5. **Sepsis.** Sepsis has occasionally been implicated as a cause of hypoglycemia. Septic hypoglycemic patients are often acidotic, and the fatality rate is high.

6. Congenital enzymatic deficiencies. Typically produce hypoglycemia in the context of glycogen storage disease or impaired hepatic gluconeogenesis. These uncommon conditions usually present in infancy.

D. Fasting hypoglycemia due to the unavailability of gluconeogenic substrate. The prototypic disease in which substrate deficiency leads to hypoglycemia is nonketotic hypoglycemia of childhood. The hallmark of the disease is a low basal blood concentration of the gluconeogenic precursor alanine.

III. DIAGNOSIS
A. Clinical presentation
1. Adrenergic signs and symptoms. Caused by counterregulatory hormones (catecholamines) released in response to hypoglycemia. The most prominent symptoms and signs are weakness, palpitations, anxiety, diaphoresis, tachycardia, peripheral vasoconstriction, and widening of the pulse pressure. These findings may be absent in patients taking sympatholytic drugs (e.g., prazosin, clonidine, and β-blockers) and in patients with long-standing diabetes (see later).
2. Neurological signs and symptoms. Signs of neuroglycopenia include hunger, headache, confusion, slurred speech, and other nonspecific behavioral changes. These can progress to lethargy, obtundation, seizures, and coma.
3. Cardiac manifestations. In the ICU setting, hypoglycemia and the sympathoadrenal response to it can be associated with supraventricular and ventricular tachycardias, atrial fibrillation, and junctional dysrhythmias. Electrocardiographic abnormalities include T-wave flattening, increased Q-T interval, ST segment depression, and repolarization abnormalities. Bradycardias have also been attributed to hypoglycemia but only rarely.
4. Prolonged hypoglycemia. Can be associated with hypothermia, hypokalemia, hypophosphatemia, and respiratory failure.

B. Laboratory. Obtain blood and urine samples from comatose hypoglycemic patients when they are first seen. This will allow appropriate assays for sulfonylureas or insulin to be performed later, if indicated.
1. Blood glucose concentration. The normal plasma glucose concentration is 60 to 120 mg/dL (3.3 to 6.7 mM). Whole blood glucose and capillary fingerstick glucose levels are 15% to 20% lower. Fingerstick blood glucose determinations can be less accurate at the lower end of their scale. Symptoms of hypoglycemia generally occur when the glucose concentration is less than 50 mg/dL (2.8 mM) in plasma or less than 40 mg/dL (2.2 mM) in whole blood. After about 48 hours of starvation, however, many individuals, particularly women, have a plasma glucose concentration less than 50 mg/dL (2.8 mM). After 72 hours of fasting the plasma glucose concentration may approach 40 mg/dL (2.2 mM) in asymptomatic individuals. Comparably "low" plasma glucose concentrations also occur in pregnancy, during which the normal fasting plasma glucose concentration is 60 mg/dL or less (3.3 mM). Factitious hypoglycemia may occur as a result of storing blood samples at room temperature before testing. Glucose concentration in the test tube may decline at a rate of about 7% per hour. The effect is enhanced if large numbers of white blood cells are present as the result of severe leukocytosis or leukemia.
2. Ketonuria. Low plasma glucose concentrations are associated with low circulating insulin levels that in turn promote lipolysis and ketogenesis. Hypoglycemia associated with ketonuria is unlikely to be due to overinsulinization.
3. Detection of drugs and toxins. If oral agent abuse is suspected, serum and urine should be screened for sulfonylurea compounds. Not readily available as part of toxic screens, testing for sulfonylurea drugs must be requested specifically.
4. Detection of surreptitiously injected insulin. When abusive insulin self-administration is suspected, obtain simultaneous insulin and C-peptide blood concentrations during a hypoglycemic episode. Insulin and C-peptide are normally cosecreted by the pancreas in equimolar quantities, but the latter is not present in commercial insulin. Insulinomas are often small and difficult to visualize radiographically. In patients with suspected

insulinoma, a fasting immunoreactive insulin (IRI, measured in µU/mL) and glucose (mg/dL) should be obtained. If the IRI/glucose ratio is greater than 0.3, the insulin concentration may be inappropriately high. Another useful test is the serum concentration of proinsulin, which is typically elevated to more than 30% of the insulin concentration in cases of insulinoma.

5. Other. Additional tests should be ordered as appropriate. In general, these should always include studies of hepatic and renal function. A cosyntropin test may be performed if adrenal insufficiency is suspected.

IV. TREATMENT
A. Specific therapies

1. Glucose. Treat presumed or documented hypoglycemia in the patient with stupor or coma with an intravenous injection of 50 mL of D50W over 3 to 5 minutes. The treatment is lifesaving in the presence of hypoglycemic coma and harmless when given to patients with coma due to other causes. Avoid subcutaneous extravasation; the solution is hypertonic and can cause local tissue damage and pain. Treatment with D50W usually leads to improved mental status within minutes, but patients who are elderly or who have had very prolonged hypoglycemia may respond slowly. Most cases of hypoglycemia in the ICU can be treated with glucose alone.

If a patient is sufficiently alert and cooperative, oral carbohydrates (e.g., sucrose in orange juice, glucose tablets) may be given. Hypoglycemia in patients taking α-glucosidase inhibitors should be treated with monomeric glucose or fructose (e.g., fruit juice) because these drugs delay absorption of complex sugars including sucrose.

The most common error in management is inadequate treatment leading to recurrence of symptoms. After the first bolus of D50W is given, an infusion of D5W or D10W glucose should be started in any patient whose hypoglycemic episode is not due to exogenous short- or intermediate-acting insulin. Severe cases of unexplained hypoglycemia require intensive care monitoring. Blood glucose should be monitored every 1 to 3 hours and the serum glucose concentration maintained at a target level of at least 100 mg/dL.

To determine whether parenteral glucose is no longer needed, the infusion should be discontinued and blood glucose concentration measured every 15 minutes. If a patient is unable to maintain a blood glucose concentration greater than 50 mg/dL or if the patient becomes symptomatic, reinstitution of glucose therapy is necessary.

When the cause of hypoglycemia is sulfonylurea ingestion, the patient should usually be admitted to the hospital because continuous intravenous glucose is mandatory. The half-life of many drugs in this class is more than 24 hours. Meals should be provided if the patient can eat. It is particularly important that glucose infusions be continued while patients recovering from a sulfonylurea overdose are asleep. Patients with this condition may require 2 to 3 days of intravenous glucose therapy. The somatostatin analogue octreotide, which inhibits insulin secretion, may be used as an adjunct to the treatment of severe oral agent overdosage.

2. Glucagon. Glucagon is a useful drug, particularly in out-of-hospital treatment of hypoglycemia. It is useful in the emergency department or ICU if hypoglycemic coma occurs in a patient without intravenous access. It is most effective in patients with ample liver glycogen stores.

3. Agents that block insulin secretion. When refractory hypoglycemia is due to an insulinoma or nesidioblastosis, it may rarely be necessary to supplement glucose infusion therapy with drugs that inhibit insulin secretion. These include diazoxide and the somatostatin analogue octreotide.

4. Consider efforts to prevent drug absorption and increase elimination. Activated charcoal adsorbs sulfonylureas, and urinary alkalinization may enhance excretion of drugs in this class. Charcoal hemoperfusion is probably not indicated except in the setting of renal failure and massive overdose.

5. Steroids. When the etiology of severe, refractory hypoglycemia is obscure, adrenocortical steroids may be given to increase gluconeogenic substrates and inhibit insulin action in the periphery.

B. Pearls: key points and pitfalls

1. Manage the precipitating factor. Glucose corrects hypoglycemia but not its cause. The commonest cause of hypoglycemia is inadvertent insulin overdosage due to changes in diet, increases in exercise, or injection of the wrong kind of insulin. Other causes of hypoglycemia include drugs and intercurrent illnesses including renal or hepatic failure. A patient should not be discharged until one of these processes, outlined in the section on pathophysiology, is identified or an appropriate follow-up plan is formulated.

2. Think about drugs. Many drugs cause hypoglycemia. In particular, persons with diabetes who become intoxicated may develop life-threatening, profound hypoglycemia because of the metabolic synergy of ethanol and insulin.

3. Measure urinary ketones. The presence of urinary ketones in a hypoglycemic patient generally excludes hyperinsulinemia as the cause of the low glucose concentration.

4. Beware of recurrent hypoglycemia. Many sulfonylurea-class oral hypoglycemic agents have a very long duration of action. Prolonged treatment is often required in cases of sulfonylurea overdose.

5. Be alert for "hypoglycemia unawareness." Patients with diabetes may fail to perceive the symptoms of hypoglycemia, especially when it occurs precipitously. Hypoglycemia unawareness can be due to frequent hypoglycemic episodes and to medicines that interfere with recovery from hypoglycemia (e.g., β-blockers). Patients who have had diabetes for many years experience blunting of the normal counterregulatory response to hypoglycemia and may also become exquisitely sensitive to regular insulin (and therefore become hypoglycemic rapidly).

Selected Readings

Cryer PE. Diverse causes of hypoglycemia-associated autonomic failure in diabetes. *N Engl J Med* 2004;350(22):2272–2279.
A review of hypoglycemia in diabetes by a leading authority.

Klonoff DC, Barrett BJ, Nolte MS, et al. Hypoglycemia following inadvertent and factitious sulfonylurea overdosages. *Diab Care* 1995;18:563–567.
Excellent review of this common cause of hypoglycemia.

Mordes JP, Thompson MJ, Rossini AA. Hypoglycemia. In Irwin RS Rippe J., et al., eds. *Irwin and Rippe's intensive care medicine*, 5th edition. Philadelphia: Lippincott Williams & Wilkins, 2003.

Whipple AO. The surgical therapy of hyperinsulinism. *J Int Chirurgie* 1938; :237–276.
The source article for the classic definition of hypoglycemia.

I. GENERAL PRINCIPLES

A. Critical illness causes multiple nonspecific alterations in thyroid hormone concentrations in patients who have no previously diagnosed intrinsic thyroid disease that relates to the severity of the illness.

B. Despite abnormalities in serum thyroid hormone parameters, there is little evidence that critically ill patients have clinically significant thyroid dysfunction.

C. Although a wide variety of illnesses tend to result in the same changes in serum thyroid hormones, these changes are rarely isolated and often are associated with alterations in other endocrine systems, such as reductions in serum gonadotropin and sex hormone concentrations and increases in serum adrenocorticotropic hormone (ACTH) and cortisol.

D. The sick euthyroid syndrome should not be viewed as an isolated pathologic event but as part of a coordinated systemic reaction to illness that involves both the immune and endocrine systems.

II. PATHOGENESIS

A. Although the cause of the alterations in thyroid hormone economy in critical illness is largely unknown, cytokines, such as tumor necrosis factor α, interleukin-1, and interleukin-6, have been shown to reproduce many of the features of the sick euthyroid syndrome in both animal and human studies when administered in pharmacologic doses.

B. Whether the sick euthyroid syndrome results from activation of the cytokine network or simply represents an endocrine response to systemic illness resulting from the same mediators that trigger the cytokine cascade remains to be determined.

III. PATHOPHYSIOLOGY

A. Alterations in peripheral metabolic pathways

1. The major pathway of metabolism of T_4 is by sequential monodeiodination by type 1 deiodinase (D1) to generate T_3 (activating pathway) or type 3 deiodinase (D3) to generate rT_3 (inactivating pathway).

2. One of the first alterations in thyroid hormone metabolism in acute illness is inhibition of D1 in peripheral tissues, which is affected by a wide variety of factors (Table 93-1) and subsequent impairment in T_4 to T_3 conversion.

3. Since more than 80% of T_3 is derived from deiodination of T_4 in peripheral tissues, T_3 levels fall soon after the onset of acute illness.

4. In contrast, D3 is unaffected by acute illness, so inner ring deiodination of T_4 to produce rT_3 is unchanged; however, because D1 also deiodinates rT_3, degradation is impaired and levels of this inactive hormone rise in proportion to the fall in T_3 levels.

B. Alterations in the pituitary–thyroid axis

1. Synthesis and secretion of thyroid hormone are under the control of the anterior pituitary hormone thyrotropin (TSH) in a classic negative feedback system.

2. Although serum TSH levels are usually normal early in acute illness, levels often fall as the illness progresses due to the effects of a variety of inhibitory factors that are common in the treatment of the critically ill patient (Table 93-2).

3. The use of dopamine; increased levels of glucocorticoids, either endogenous or exogenous; and inhibitory signals from higher cortical centers also may play a

TABLE 93-1	Factors Inhibit T$_4$ to T$_3$ Conversion in Peripheral Tissues

Acute and chronic illness
Caloric deprivation
Malnutrition
Glucocorticoids
β-Adrenergic blocking drugs (e.g., propranalol)
Oral cholecytographic agents (e.g., iopanoic acid, sodium ipodate)
Amiodarone
Propylthiouracil
Fatty acids
Fetal/neonatal period

T$_4$, thyroxine; T$_3$, thyronine

role in decreasing TSH secretion, as well as certain thyroid hormone metabolites that are increased in nonthyroidal illness.

C. Alterations in serum binding proteins
1. Both T$_4$ (99.97% bound) and T$_3$ (99.7% bound) circulate in the serum bound primarily to thyronine-binding protein (TBG), and the binding of thyroid hormones to TBG is affected by a variety of factors in acute illness (Table 93-3).
2. Because only the unbound hormone has any metabolic activity (free hormone concept), changes in either the concentrations of, or binding to, TBG would have major effects on the total serum hormone levels; however, minimal changes in the free hormone concentrations, and thus overall thyroid function, are actually seen.

TABLE 93-2	Factors that Alter TSH Secretion

Increase	Decrease
Chlorpromazine	Acute and chronic illness
Cimetidine	Adrenergic agonists
Domperidone	Caloric restriction
Dopamine antagonists	Carbamazepine
Haloperidol	Clofibrate
Iodide	Cyproheptadine
Lithium	Dopamine and dopamine agonists
Metoclopramiide	Endogenous depression
Sulphapyridine	Glucocorticoids
X-ray contrast agents	IGF-1
	Metergoline
	Methylsergide
	Opiates
	Phenytoin
	Phentolamine
	Pimozide
	Somatostatin
	Serotonin
	Surgical stress
	Thyroid hormone metabolites

TSH, thyroid-stimulating hormone.

TABLE 93-3	Factors That Alter Binding of T4 to TBG

Increase binding	Decrease binding
Drugs	
Estrogens	Glucocorticoids
Methadone	Androgens
Clofibrate	L-Asparaginase
5-Fluorouracil	Salicylates
Heroin	Furosemide
Tamoxifen	Antiseizure medications (e.g., phenytoin, tegretol)
Systemic factors	
Liver disease	Inherited
Porphyria	Acute Illness
HIV infection	
Inherited	

T_4, thryoxine ; TBG, thyronine-binding globulin.

D. Stages of the sick euthyroid syndrome

1. Low T_3 state

a. Common to all the abnormalities in thyroid hormone concentrations seen in critically ill patients is a substantial depression of serum T_3 levels, which can occur as early as 24 hours after the onset of illness and affects over half of patients admitted to the medical service.

b. The decrease in serum T_3 levels can be explained solely by inhibition of D1 and subsequent impairment of peripheral T_4 to T_3 conversion.

c. Clinically, these patients appear euthyroid, although mild prolongation in Achilles reflex time is found in some patients.

2. High T_4 state

a. Serum T_4 levels may be elevated early in acute illness due to either the acute inhibition of T_4 to T_3 conversion or increased TBG levels.

b. Increased serum T_4 levels are seen most often in the elderly and in patients with psychiatric disorders.

c. As the duration of illness increases, nondeiodinative pathways of T_4 degradation increase and return serum T_4 levels to the normal range.

3. Low T_4 state

a. As the severity and the duration of the illness increases, serum total T_4 levels may decrease into the subnormal range as a result of a decrease in the binding of T_4 to TBG; a decrease in serum TSH levels, leading to decreased production of T_4; and an increase in nondeiodinative pathways of T_4 metabolism.

b. The decline in serum T_4 levels correlates with prognosis in the intensive care unit (ICU), with mortality increasing as serum T_4 levels drop below 4 μg/dL and approaching 80% in patients with serum T_4 levels less than 2 μg/dL.

c. Despite marked decreases in serum total T_4 and T_3 levels to the hypothyroid range, the free hormone levels are often normal; thus, the low T_4 state is more likely a marker of multisystem failure in these critically ill patients than a true hormone-deficient state.

4. Recovery state

a. The alterations in thyroid hormone concentrations resolve as the illness resolves.

b. This stage may be prolonged and is characterized by modest increases in serum TSH levels.

c. Full recovery, with restoration of thyroid hormone levels to the normal range, may take up to several months after the patient is discharged from the hospital.

IV. DIAGNOSIS

   A. The routine screening of an ICU population for the presence of thyroid dysfunction is not recommended because of the high prevalence of abnormal thyroid function tests and the low prevalence of true thyroid dysfunction.

   B. Whenever possible, it is best to defer evaluation of the thyroid–pituitary axis until the patient has recovered from acute illness.

   C. When thyroid function tests are ordered in a hospitalized patient, it should be with a high clinical index of suspicion for the presence of thyroid dysfunction.

   D. Because every test of thyroid hormone function can be altered in the critically ill patient, no single test can definitively rule in or rule out the presence of intrinsic thyroid dysfunction (Table 93-4).

   E. Thyroid function tests
   1. TSH assays
      a. Although the sensitive TSH assay is currently the best screening test for thyroid dysfunction in the healthy, ambulatory patient, this does not hold true for the ill patient.

TABLE 93-4	Tests of Thyroid Function in the ICU		
Tests	**Typical normal range**	**Use**	**Limitation in acute illness**
TSH	0.4–5.0 mU/L	Best initial test to determine thyroid status in healthy patients	Loss of specificity, abnormal in up to 20% of hospitalized patients
Total T_4	4–12 mg/dL	Measures bound and free hormone in serum	Affected by alterations in serum binding proteins
T_4- or T_3-resin uptake	25%–35%	Estimate of the serum protein binding sites	Affected by alterations in serum binding proteins
Thyroid hormone binding ratio (THBR)	0.8–1.15	Estimate of the serum-protein binding sites	Affected by alterations in serum binding proteins
Free T_4 Index (FTI)	1–4 with resin uptake 4–12 with THBR	Estimate of free T_4 concentrations	Affected by alterations in serum binding proteins
Free T_4, analog method	0.7–2.1 ng/dL	Direct measurement of free T_4 concentrations	May not be any more reliable than FTI
Free T_4, equilibrium dialysis method	0.7–2.1 ng/dL	Gold standard for measurement of free T_4 concentrations	Expensive, time-consuming to perform, not readily available
Total T_3	75–180 ng/dL	Measures bound and free hormone in serum	Levels fall in all hospitalized patients, never a first-line test
Free T_3	200–400 pg/dL	Direct measurement of free T_3 concentrations	No advantage over total T_3
Thyroid autoantibodies (anti-Tg, anti-TPO)	Negative	Determines presence of autoimmune thyroid disease	Second-line test, may help predict presence of thyroid dysfunction

b. Abnormal TSH values have been reported in up to 20% of hospitalized patients, more than 80% of whom have no intrinsic thyroid dysfunction on follow-up testing when healthy.

c. Abnormal TSH values require additional biochemical and clinical evaluation before a diagnosis of thyroid dysfunction can be made.

2. Free T_4 concentrations

a. Total T_4 measurements alone are of little use in the acutely ill patient because abnormalities in binding to serum proteins are commonplace.

b. Measurement of true serum free T_4 concentrations is time-consuming and expensive; thus, estimates of the free T_4 concentrations are obtained by either the free T_4 index (FTI) or the free T_4 by analogue measurement.

3. Total T_3

a. There is no indication for the routine measurement of serum T_3 levels in the initial evaluation of thyroid function in the critically ill patient, because serum T_3 concentrations are affected to the greatest degree by the alterations in thyroid hormone economy resulting from acute illness.

b. The only setting in which serum T_3 levels may be helpful is in the presence of a suppressed sensitive TSH value when an elevated serum T_3 concentration will differentiate between thyrotoxicosis and the sick euthyroid syndrome.

4. Thyroid autoantibodies

a. The presence of thyroid autoantibodies (antithyroglobulin and antithyroid peroxidase) determines the presence of autoimmune thyroid disease but does not necessarily indicate thyroid dysfunction.

b. Thyroid autoantibodies do add to the specificity of abnormal TSH and FTI values in diagnosing intrinsic thyroid disease.

F. Diagnostic approach

1. A reasonable initial approach is to obtain both FTI and TSH measurements in patients with a high clinical suspicion for intrinsic thyroid dysfunction.

2. Assessment of these values in the context of the duration, severity, and stage of illness of the patient will allow the correct diagnosis in most patients.

3. If the diagnosis is still unclear, measurement of thyroid antibodies may be helpful as a marker of intrinsic thyroid disease.

4. Only in the case of a suppressed TSH and a midnormal to high FTI is measurement of serum T_3 levels indicated.

V. TREATMENT

A. General ICU patients

1. The question of whether the sick euthyroid syndrome in critically ill patients represents an adaptive or a pathologic response to illness remains unclear.

2. Supplemental thyroid hormone therapy, in the form of either L-T_4 or L-T_3, has not been shown to have any effect on morbidity or mortality and, thus, is not indicated in the routine ICU patient with the sick euthyroid syndrome.

B. Specialized patients

1. Cardiac bypass patients. Although there is a theoretical basis for the use of T_3 to correct the acute drop in serum T_3 levels during cardiac bypass, the clearly demonstrable benefit of T_3 repletion in animals has not been translated into similar benefit in humans undergoing coronary artery bypass in controlled clinical trials.

2. Brain-dead cardiac donors. T_3 has been used to "resuscitate" cardiac function in potential heart donors with preexisting cardiac dysfunction, suggesting that T_3 may be beneficial to stabilize or improve cardiac function before cardiac transplantation. However, these studies have yet to be confirmed.

3. Premature infants. Some degree of transient hypothyroxinemia is present because of the immaturity of thyroid function; however, studies have shown no beneficial effect on developmental outcome at 24 months.

This chapter is based on Farwell AP. The sick euthyroid syndrome in the intensive care unit. In Irwin RS, Cerra FB, Rippe JM, eds. *Irwin and Rippe's intensive care medicine,* 5th edition. Philadelphia: Lippincott Williams & Wilkins, 2003, pp. 1205–1216.

Selected Readings

Baloch Z, et al. Laboratory medicine practice guidelines. Laboratory support for the diagnosis and monitoring of thyroid disease. *Thyroid* 2003;13:3–126.
Guidelines published by the largest professional society of physicians and scientists dedicated to research and treatment of thyroid disease in the United States.

Braverman LE, Utiger RD, eds. The thyroid, 9th ed. Philadelphia: Lippincott Williams & Wilkins, 2005.
The most current and thorough text on clinical thyroidology.

Brent GA, Hershman JM. Thyroxine therapy in patients with severe nonthyroidal illnesses and low thyroxine concentration. *J Clin Endocrinol Metab* 1986;63:1–8.
Initial article demonstrating that L-T_4 replacement therapy in the sick euthyroid syndrome is of no benefit and may be harmful. Classic article on the use of thyroid hormone indices as predictors of mortality in the critically ill patient.

Farwell AP. Sick euthyroid syndrome. *J Intensive Care Med* 1997;12:249–260; Farwell AP. Thyroid gland disorders. In: Fink M, Abraham E, Vincent J-L, eds. *Textbook of critical care*, 5th ed. Philadelphia: WB Saunders/Harcourt Press, 2005.
Recent reviews with details of the points discussed in this chapter with extensive references.

Hashimoto H, Igarashi N, Yachie A, et al. The relationship between serum levels of interleukin-6 and thyroid hormone in children with acute respiratory infection. *J Clin Endocrinol Metab* 1994;78:288–291.
Representative article on the attempts to link the development of the sick euthyroid syndrome to cytokine production during illness.

Kaptein EM, Weiner JM, Robinson WJ, et al. Relationship of altered thyroid hormone indices to survival in nonthyroidal illness. *Clin Endocrinol (Oxf)* 1982;16:565–574.
Classic article on the use of thyroid hormone indices as predictors of mortality in the critically ill patient.

Klemperer JD, Klein I, Gomez M, et al. Thyroid hormone treatment after coronary artery bypass surgery. *N Engl J Med* 1995;333:1522–1527.
This article examines the role of thyroid hormone replacement therapy in the sick euthyroid syndrome in three specialized conditions.

Novitzky D. Novel actions of thyroid hormone: the role of triiodothyronine in cardiac transplantation. *Thyroid* 1996;6:531–536.
This article examines the role of thyroid hormone replacement therapy in the sick euthyroid syndrome in three specialized conditions.

Slag MF, Morley JE, Elson MK, et al. Hypothyroxinemia in critically ill patients as a predictor of high mortality. *JAMA* 1981;245:43–45.

Spencer C, Elgen A, Shen D, et al. Specificity of sensitive assays of thyrotropin (TSH) used to screen for thyroid disease in hospitalized patients. *Clin Chem* 1987;33:1391–1396.
Classic article documents the development and use of sensitive TSH assays by the investigators who developed these assays.

Spencer CA. Clinical utility and cost-effectiveness of sensitive thyrotropin assays in ambulatory and hospitalized patients. *Mayo Clin Proc* 1988;63:1214–1222.
Classic article documents the development and use of sensitive TSH assays by the investigators who developed these assays.

Van den Berghe G, de Zegher F, Lauwers P. Dopamine and the sick euthyroid syndrome in critical illness. *Clin Endocrinol (Oxf)* 1994;41:731–737.
Documents the effects of dopamine on TSH secretion, a major mediator of abnormal thyroid function tests in the ICU.

van Wassenaer AG, Kok JH, de Vijlder JJM, et al. Effects of thyroxine supplementation on neurologic development in infants born at less than 30 weeks gestation. *N Engl J Med* 1997;336:21–26.
This article examines the role of thyroid hormone replacement therapy in the sick euthyroid syndrome in three specialized conditions.

Hematologic Problems in the Intensive Care Unit

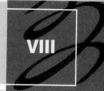

VIII

I. INTRODUCTION

A. Coagulation pathways

1. *In vivo* the extrinsic pathway is the trigger (freshly exposed subendothelial tissue factor [TF] activates factor VII). The intrinsic pathway is the amplifier, beginning with factor XI activation by thrombin (generated by the extrinsic pathway) and factor IX activation by the TF/factor VIIa complex. Factor XII, which initiates the intrinsic pathway *in vitro*, does not regulate coagulation reactions *in vivo*.

2. The coagulation reactions require calcium and phospholipid (provided by platelets and other cells) for assembling the complex of catalytic proteins and their substrates and cofactors (factor V and factor VIII). The most important assemblies are the "tenase" complex, which cleaves and activates factor X (the extrinsic tenase includes TF/factor VIIa/calcium/phospholipid/factor X and the intrinsic tenase includes factor IXa/calcium/phospholipid/cofactor VIIIa/factor X); and the "prothrombinase" complex, which cleaves prothrombin to thrombin (and includes factor Xa/calcium/phospholipid/cofactor Va/prothrombin).

3. The coagulation reactions are terminated by proteins C and S (which are activated by thrombin and then bind and inhibit cofactors VIIIa and Va) and by the protease inhibitors antithrombin III (which binds to and inhibits thrombin and factor Xa) and tissue factor pathway inhibitor (TFPI, which binds to and inhibits the TF/factor VIIa/calcium/phospholipid/factor Xa complex).

4. The fibrin clot is gradually eliminated by dissolution mediated by plasmin, which is formed when tissue or urokinase plasminogen activator (secreted and bound by endothelium) cleaves plasminogen. Coagulation activation is directly coupled to the inhibition of fibrinolysis by thrombin-activatable fibrinolysis inhibitor (TAFI), which inhibits the activation of plasminogen by tPA.

B. Diagnostic studies

1. Blood for the prothrombin time (PT), activated thromboplastin time (aPTT), and thrombin time (TT) are drawn in blue-top (citrate anticoagulated) tubes. The blood is recalcified and coagulation is stimulated by brain tissue factor, kaolin or thrombin, respectively (Fig. 94-1).

2. Several tiers of diagnostic testing are presented (Table 94-1).

3. An elevated aPTT can be worked up by using the flow chart in Figure 94-2.

C. Therapeutic options

1. Blood products: typed and cross-matched packed red cells; random-donor or pheresis platelets; fresh-frozen plasma (FFP); cryoprecipitate (use very rarely for fibrinogen deficiency or dysfunction); purified or recombinant factors (use only for specific factor deficiencies).

2. Use judiciously: to avoid transfusion-associated infections, volume overload, and graft-versus-host disease (use irradiated blood products in patients after solid organ or bone marrow transplant or in patients with lymphomas, Hodgkin disease, and acute lymphoblastic lymphoma).

3. In the intensive care unit, red cell transfusions should be used strictly for hemodynamic stabilization; one study showed that using an arbitrary hemoglobin (Hgb) target of 10 g/dL worsened outcome at 30 days.

4. In the critical care unit (CCU), however, outcome may be improved by maintaining the Hgb at 10 to 11 g/dL among elderly patients with acute myocardial infarction.

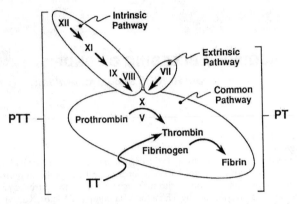

Figure 94-1. The "cascade" or "waterfall" model of blood coagulation forms the basis of routine coagulation testing. The activated partial thromboplastin time (aPTT) is the time it takes for recalcified blood to clot after added kaolin activates factor XII. The prothrombin time (PT) is the time it takes for recalcified blood to clot after added tissue factor complexes with FVII and to activate FX. The thrombin time (TT) is the time it takes recalcified blood to clot after added thrombin cleaves fibrinogen and fibrin polymers form.

    5. Hemostatics are shown in Table 94-2. Except for DDAVP to prevent or treat mild von Willebrand disease or platelet function defects, they are rarely used in the ICU.

II. THE SURGICAL PATIENT
  A. General principles
    1. Establish rank order of structural (i.e., surgical) versus functional (i.e., coagulopathy) defect.
    2. Venous thromboembolism (VTE) prophylaxis is essential; low-molecular-weight heparin and fondaparinux are best treatments in most cases, except in patients receiving spinal anesthesia (where infusional unfractionated heparin may be best) and in patients with brain or spinal cord trauma (where prophylaxis with intermittent pneumatic compression is usually best).
  B. Etiology and pathophysiology
    1. Iatrogenic: extracorporeal circulation diminishes coagulation factors and platelets, and causes a transient platelet function defect.
    2. Neurosurgical trauma: releases tissue factor and causes disseminated intravascular coagulation (DIC).

TABLE 94-1	**Tiers of Diagnostic Testing**			
	First tier	**Second tier**	**Third tier**	**Fourth tier**
Coagulation factor disorder	PT aPTT Thrombin time	Mixing studies D-dimer (or FDPs)	vWF antigen Ristocetin cofactor Factor levels	Lysis by urea vWF multimers α2 Antiplasmin
Platelet disorder	Platelet count	Bleeding time Platelet aggregation	[14C] Serotonin release Electron microscopy	

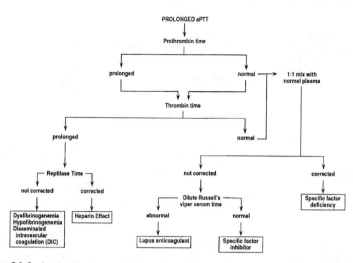

Figure 94-2. An algorithm for evaluating an elevated aPTT.

3. Multiple trauma: large vessel bleeding with massive blood loss leads to dilutional coagulopathy and thrombocytopenia.

4. Large bone fracture results in risk for fat embolism and resulting DIC.

C. Diagnosis: In addition to vital sign monitoring, serial platelet counts and the PT/aPTT, it is important to look for signs of bleeding, including looking with CT scans or other noninvasive means. Reoperation with exploration for fixable structural lesions is often needed.

D. Treatment

1. Blood product support, including red cells, platelets, and FFP.

2. In a patient with VTE or on long-term warfarin therapy, it is important to know how to provide adequate anticoagulation while minimizing perioperative bleeding (Table 94-3).

3. How to dose FFP (Table 94-4).

E. Complications: Watch out for dilutional coagulopathy and thrombocytopenia in patients with hypovolemic shock from massive hemorrhage.

TABLE 94-2	Hemostatic Drugs			
Drug	**Indication**	**Dose**	**Onset**	**Duration**
Desmopressin	Acute bleeding before biopsy or emergency surgery	0.3 µg/kg (IV, SC) 300 µg (intranasally) q 12–24 h 4–5 doses	30–60 min 60–90 min	6–12 hours 6–12 hours
Conjugated estrogens	Chronic, recurrent bleeding	0.6 mg/kg IV infusion q day × 5–7 days	7 days	2 weeks
	Before elective surgery	50 mg po q day × 5–7 days		
IV, intravenously; SC, subcutaneously; po, by mouth.				

TABLE 94-3	Perioperative Management of Anticoagulation

Clinical setting	Preoperatively	Postoperatively
Acute venous thromboembolism (VTE)		
Within 2 weeks	IVC filter	IVC filter
Within 2–4 weeks	IV heparin stopped 6 h preop	IV heparin (1,000 U/h) started 12 h postop
After 4 weeks	Stop warfarin for 3–4 days (INR <1.5)	IV heparin (1,000 U/h) started 12 h postop
Recurrent VTE	Stop warfarin for 3–4 days (INR <1.5)	Low-molecular-weight heparin (e.g., enoxaparin 30 mg bid or 40 mg q day) Started 12 h postop
Acute arterial thrombosis within 1 month	IV heparin stopped 6 h preop	IV heparin (1,000 U/h) started 12 h postop
Mechanical heart valve	Stop warfarin for 3–4 days (INR <1.5)	Low-molecular-weight heparin started 12 h postop
Chronic atrial fibrillation	Stop warfarin for 3–4 days (INR <1.5)	Low-molecular-weight heparin started 12 h postop

TABLE 94-4	How to Dose Fresh Frozen Plasma

Step 1: Establish target INR			Step 2: Convert INR to % activity of prothrombin complex		Step 3: Calculate dose of FFP (or prothrombin complex)
Bleeding risk	Thrombosis risk	Target INR	Initial INR	Prothrombin activity	
High	High	1.5–2.0			Target % prothrombin activity: Initial% prothrombin activity × body weight in kg = mL of FFP or IU of prothrombin complex
	Moderate	1.5		5%	
	Low	1.0	>5	10%	
			4.0–4.9	12%	
Moderate	High	2.0	3.3–3.9	15%	
	Moderate	1.5	2.6–3.2	20%	
	Low	1.0	2.2–2.5	25%	
			1.9–2.1	30%	
Low	High	2.0	1.7–1.8	40%	
	Moderate	2.0	1.4–1.6	100%	
	Low	1.5	1.0		

III. THE HEART DISEASE PATIENT (coronary artery disease, native and prosthetic valve disease)

A. General principles
   1. The CCU patient with an acute coronary syndrome (ACS) is often rendered hemostatically "paralyzed" by anticoagulant, fibrinolytic, and antiplatelet drugs.
   2. The coronary surgery patient who undergoes extracorporeal circulation will suffer transient (<24 hours) platelet dysfunction and somewhat longer (1 to 2 days) thrombocytopenia and hyperfibrinolysis.
   3. The patient with a prosthetic valve typically presents on warfarin anticoagulation with an iatrogenic hemostatic defect that may need to be reversed and then reinstituted rapidly.

B. Etiology and pathophysiology
   1. The cause of the hemostatic defect in ACS and with prosthetic valves is the drugs used to minimize thrombotic risk. In ACS this could include the antiplatelet agents aspirin, clopidogrel, and platelet glycoprotein (Gp) IIb-IIIa inhibitors *and* heparin (*but* usually not GpIIb-IIIa inhibitors plus fibrinolytics). With a prosthetic valve, warfarin, or warfarin plus aspirin is the usual treatment.
   2. The cause of the hemostatic defect in patients undergoing extracorporeal circulation is the artificial membranes that compose the heart-lung pump. These membranes activate the intrinsic coagulation pathway and complement. Such activations lead to enhanced fibrinolysis (probably because of tPA release from the vascular endothelium) and platelet activation, leading to both consumption (and therefore thrombocytopenia) and the circulation of platelets that have released most of their proaggregatory granules ("spent" platelets).

C. Diagnosis
   1. The diagnosis of a hemostatic defect is mainly clinical: increased bleeding during treatment for ACS. It can be confirmed by routine testing (see Table 94-1). The challenge is to maintain vigilance about dangerous bleeding, such as hemopericardium, coronary artery dissection, and even large femoral hematomas following arterial puncture.

D. Treatment
   1. Stop drugs.
   2. Reverse drugs (for example, reverse heparin with protamine 1 mg/100 U of circulating heparin).
   3. Blood product support (for example, use 6 to 10 units random donor platelets within 24 hours of extracorporeal circulation even when the count is greater than $100,000/\mu L$ so as to treat the acquired platelet function defect).
   4. Pharmacologic interventions are rarely used, although the protease inhibitor aprotinin is approved for use by the FDA to minimize perioperative blood loss in patients undergoing coronary bypass grafting, and it has been used outside the United States to treat severe postoperative bleeding in the SICU. It may work because it inhibits the excessive activity of plasmin.

E. Complications
   1. The major complication to avoid when treating bleeding due to defective hemostasis in heart disease patients is thrombosis. Life-threatening progression of coronary artery occlusion or prosthetic valve dysfunction is an ever-present possibility, and one must never injudiciously optimize hemostasis without vigilantly monitoring its effect on the heart. The therapeutic index of interventions must be followed frequently.

IV. THE INFECTED PATIENT

A. General principles. Overwhelming bacteremia resulting in sepsis can be accompanied by thrombocytopenia or DIC. The ICU is also a place where iatrogenic events are common, such as bleeding from vitamin K deficiency or catheter thrombosis extending into the deep venous system of the arm.

B. Etiology and pathophysiology
   1. Gram-negative or -positive bacteremia has many effects on the coagulation system. In general, however, circulating endotoxin or exotoxin triggers systemic coagulation,

leading to fibrin deposition and platelet activation and consumption. This leads to DIC in as many as 30% to 50% of all patients with bacteremia.

2. In patients without DIC, bacteremia is typically accompanied by some degree of thrombocytopenia, including severe thrombocytopenia that is gradually reversible after the bacteremia is cleared.

3. Vitamin K deficiency develops in patients who are suboptimally nourished and receiving intravenous antibiotics for at least 1 week. The combination of poor vitamin K intake and decreased bacterial vitamin K production leads to acquired deficiency. It is so common that vitamin K is usually added to total parenteral nutrition when it is used in the ICU setting.

4. Catheter thrombosis is due to a device disturbing all three elements of Virchow's triad: the blood, blood flow, and the vessel. There is no evidence that catheter thrombosis is a harbinger of either hypercoagulability or bacterial colonization of the device.

C. Diagnosis

1. The diagnosis of DIC encompasses a quadrad of findings: thrombocytopenia, elevated PT/aPTT, elevated D-dimers (D-dimers are the products of plasmin-digested cross-linked fibrin), and microangiopathic hemolytic anemia. These findings alone are not completely specific for DIC (e.g., they can also be found in liver disease, hypertensive crisis, and renal allograft rejection), but when they represent DIC it is usually self-evident because of their clinical context.

2. The diagnosis of bacteremia-associated thrombocytopenia rests solely on establishing a temporal relationship between the two phenomena; no diagnostic studies, other than those that rule out DIC, are useful.

3. Vitamin K deficiency is easy to diagnose: the PT rises during ICU admission, the elevated PT corrects with mixing, the vitamin K–dependent coagulation factors are decreased (factors II, VII, IX, and X) and all other coagulopathies are excluded.

4. Catheter thrombosis can sometimes be heralded by blood or infusate leaking from the subclavian or intrajugular vein. It is suspected when a line stops functioning and the ipsilateral arm swells. Like a lower extremity venous thrombosis, an upper extremity occlusion can be reliably diagnosed by an ultrasound/Doppler study.

D. Treatment

1. DIC is treated by treating the bacteremia. If dangerous bleeding (more common) or thrombosis (uncommon) is associated with bacteremia and DIC, they are addressed by additional specific interventions. In both cases, coagulation factor replacement with FFP and platelet transfusions must be given as intensively as required to reverse the measurable clinical and laboratory abnormalities. Fibrinogen repletion with cryoprecipitate is rarely required during infection-associated DIC because fibrinogen levels are rarely depleted very greatly. In the patient with peripheral ischemia or infarction (e.g., nose and earlobes; or fingers and toes in patients with peripheral arterial insufficiency), a heparin infusion (500 to 1,000 U per hour) without bolus is sometimes started after hemostasis is restored as fully as possible.

2. Vitamin K deficiency is always treated with parenteral vitamin K. In a patient with the coagulopathy of vitamin K deficiency who is exsanguinating, FFP (dosed according to Table 94-4) will rapidly restore hemostasis, whereas the parenteral vitamin K gradually reverses the problem (over 48 to 96 hours).

E. Complications. ICU patients with sepsis (without or with DIC) who are very sick (APACHE II score of >24) for less than 24 hours may receive activated protein C (drotrecogin). Activated protein C cleaves and inactivates the coagulation cofactors V and VIII and might be expected to cause bleeding. In fact, it is associated with bleeding in about 10% of those who receive it (no more than placebo), including 3.5% major bleeding (2.5% more than placebo). In uncontrolled settings (outside of clinical trials) there were 8 intracranial bleeds of 520 patients (1.5% incidence). In a patient with life-threatening bleeding, the first step is to stop the infusion. FFP should then be given to correct an elevated PT and aPTT and, because activated protein C will impair hemostasis for some time after its infusion is finished, the FFP should be continued for at least 1 day after the infusion is stopped. Other than protein C activity (which is not a routinely rapidly available measurement), there are no ways to monitor the specific effects of recombinant activated protein C on hemostasis within an ICU setting.

V. THE TRANSPLANT PATIENT

A. General principles

  1. The dangerous situation faced by transplant patients is multiorgan failure. This is uncommon in renal transplants and common in heart-lung and bone marrow transplantation. The coagulopathy that accompanies multiorgan failure is complex but usually involves DIC and decreased coagulation factor synthesis by the liver.

  2. Bone marrow or stem cell transplant (BMT) patients suffer from hemorrhagic cystitis, diffuse alveolar hemorrhage (DAH), and gastrointestinal (GI) bleeding.

  3. Liver transplant patients are at risk for acquired coagulation factor deficiencies, dysfibrinogenemia, and thrombocytopenia.

B. Etiology and pathophysiology

  1. Multiorgan failure is multifactorial and related to operative issues, restoration of organ function, infection, and graft rejection. It can occur anytime after transplant, but the period of greatest risk is in the immediate posttransplant period.

  2. Hemorrhagic cystitis develops within a few weeks in up to 50% of those who receive high-dose cyclophosphamide or ifosfamide as pre-BMT conditioning. These agents are directly toxic to the bladder mucosa. Acute DAH affects about 5% of all BMT recipients. It usually occurs within 4 weeks of the procedure (often after granulocyte recovery) and is considered to represent an inflammatory insult converging from many different causes. GI bleeding is related to BMT-associated gut epithelial toxicity and thrombocytopenia related to bone marrow underproduction.

  3. Liver transplant patients are at risk for poor hemostasis related to the predictable coagulation factor deficiencies, as well as a unique underproduction thrombocytopenia due to thrombopoietin (TPO) underproduction, because the liver is the principal site of TPO synthesis.

C. Diagnosis

  1. In all cases, the diagnosis rests on clinical issues that are rarely subtle.

  2. In many cases of DAH, bronchoscopy with lavage is used to establish DAH as the cause of an acute respiratory distress syndrome-type clinical picture in a patient who is rapidly deteriorating post-BMT.

D. Treatment

  1. Multiorgan failure is treated by supportive measures, including blood support.

  2. Treatment of bleeding in patients after BMT begins with platelet transfusions. They are used for everyone whose count falls below 10,000 to 20,000/µL and, in patients with overt hemorrhage, they are used to try to maintain a count close to 50,000/µL. Hemorrhagic cystitis may require bladder lavage and the instillation of a sclerotic agent such as alum; failing this, radical cystectomy is then performed. Patients with DAH are usually treated with corticosteroids (up to 2 g/day solumedrol); recombinant activated factor VII has recently been reported to be an effective treatment for DAH.

  3. Disordered hemostasis among liver transplant patients is often most dangerous in the perioperative setting and massive surgical blood loss is not uncommon. An elevated PT and aPTT requires the administration of FFP (or prothrombin complex—see Table 94-4). When the TT is elevated and the fibrinogen level is very low, fibrinogen repletion with cryoprecipitate is indicated. When the platelets are low from underproduction, rather than hypersplenism secondary to portal hypertension, administration of TPO is theoretically beneficial; because it is not yet FDA approved, it can be used only with IRB approval for compassionate use in a single patient, and therefore platelet transfusions (irradiated random donor platelets) are usually used. Recombinant activated factor VII has been used successfully as a hemostatic during liver transplant surgery, but the experience is too small to be able to predict that it generally possesses a favorable therapeutic index.

E. Complications

1. The preservation of transplant function is top priority and toward that end, one often accepts some degree of collateral damage. The converse is that treating collateral damage (for example, stopping sirolamus in a patient with DAH) can place the patient at risk for graft rejection. Vigilant monitoring and assessing the risk-benefit of all interventions is to be expected.

2. The prognosis of DAH is reputedly poor, with mortality approaching 50% (greater in allogeneic than autologous BMT). Because corticosteroids may not alter the natural history of the disease, the utility of recombinant activated factor VII (NovoSeven) has been investigated. Thus far too few patients have been studied to establish its general risks or benefits, although one must be concerned about both expense and the theoretical possibility of causing systemic hypercoagulability.

VI. THE OBSTETRICAL PATIENT

A. General principles

1. The central issue in managing a pregnant woman who is bleeding or at risk is to establish how the problem will affect both the fetus and the mother.

2. The central issue in managing a woman who is bleeding postdelivery is to make the diagnosis and begin treatment rapidly.

3. A pregnant woman is most likely to develop petechiae or bruising from thrombocytopenia, which is rarely very dangerous to the mother or fetus. In contrast, vaginal bleeding is an obstetrical emergency and a postpartum woman who develops bleeding must be considered a potential catastrophe and be managed accordingly.

B. Etiology and pathophysiology

1. The most commonly encountered problem is thrombocytopenia: the platelet count falls to below 150,000/μL in approximately 7% of pregnant women (of whom 75% are incidental, 21% are related to a hypertensive disorder, and 4% are from ITP). Other causes are the fairly benign preeclampsia-associated *HELLP* (*h*emolytic anemia with *e*levated *l*iver enzymes and *l*ow *p*latelets) and the potentially devastating thrombotic thrombocytopenic purpura (TTP; see below).

2. Vaginal bleeding may represent abruptio placentae or intrauterine fetal demise (IUD). Both will also cause DIC.

3. Life-threatening bleeding and systemic collapse often result from amniotic fluid embolism, which occurs in approximately 1/40,000 deliveries.

C. Diagnosis

1. Pregnancy-associated ITP usually causes a platelet count to fall below 50,000/μL. ITP, HELLP, and TTP are distinguished by clinical severity. There are no diagnostic studies for ITP, but HELLP and TTP are accompanied by distinct laboratory abnormality profiles.

2. Abruptio placentae and IUD are diagnosed by examination, sonography, and fetal heart sound measurement.

3. Amniotic fluid embolism usually causes cardiopulmonary collapse with refractory oxygenation and DIC accompanied by very low fibrinogen levels.

D. Treatment

1. ITP is treated whenever there is bleeding. In the absence of bleeding, ITP is treated when the platelet count falls below 20,000/μL, 30,000/μL, and 50,000/μL during the first trimester, second/third trimester, and delivery, respectively. Treatment is with intravenous immunoglobulin (IVIG) or steroids, both of which are safe during pregnancy.

2. Preeclampsia, eclampsia, and HELLP are treated with antihypertensive agents and often corticosteroids. In preeclampsia, magnesium sulfate decreases the risk of seizures and progression to eclampsia. These are temporizing measures only. The only definitive treatment for these thrombocytopenic disorders, as well as for abruptio placentae and IUD, is fetal or infant delivery.

3. TTP is treated as described later.

    4. Amniotic fluid embolism is treated with supportive care, including fibrinogen repletion with cryoprecipitate when the fibrinogen is very low and bleeding continues despite FFP and platelets.

E. Complications

    1. Pregnancy-associated thrombocytopenia and ITP are expected to have excellent maternal and fetal outcomes.

    2. Thrombocytopenia from preeclampsia, eclampsia, and HELLP develops before term in about 80% of all patients affected. Treatment as previously described will permit fetal maturation and a relatively healthy delivery in almost all cases. The major complication is a 3% to 5% risk of maternal seizures.

    3. The mortality from untreated TTP and all cases of amniotic fluid embolism as at least 80%. When pregnancy-associated TTP is recognized and treated, maternal mortality is less than 20%. The impact on the fetus or neonate is not known.

VII. THE PATIENT WITH AN ACQUIRED COAGULATION FACTOR INHIBITOR

A. General principles

    1. The most common acquired inhibitor is a factor VIII inhibitor.

    2. Major bleeding occurs in 80% of these patients, and the inhibitor is lethal in about 20%.

B. Etiology and pathophysiology

    1. The inhibitor is usually an IgG molecule that binds to factor VIII and inhibits its capacity to modulate the intrinsic tenase complex (see earlier).

    2. It usually arises without any prodrome or antecedent diagnosis, but it can also be found associated with cancer, lupus, pregnancy, and lymphoproliferative disorders.

C. Diagnosis

    1. An elevated aPTT that doesn't correct with mixing.

    2. A lupus inhibitor is ruled out.

    3. Factor VIII activity is decreased or absent.

    4. An inhibitor can be quantified using the Bethesda unit (BU = the reciprocal of the dilution of the affected person's plasma that causes a 50% reduction in factor VIII activity when mixed with normal plasma).

D. Treatment

    1. A treatment approach is presented later.

    2. Some patients improve with high-dose IVIG or plasma exchange.

    3. All patients (Table 94-5).

E. Complications

    1. One third of inhibitors disappear, but the rate of resolution is unpredictably slow.

    2. Almost all postpartum inhibitors disappear within 30 months and tend not to recur with subsequent pregnancies.

    3. An inhibitor secondary to an underlying disease sometimes responds to disease treatment.

VIII. THE PATIENT WITH THROMBOCYTOPENIA

A. General principles

    1. Severe thrombocytopenia due to underproduction (from disease or cancer treatments) is almost always associated with bleeding, including life-threatening bleeding.

    2. Severe thrombocytopenia from immune thrombocytopenia can be relatively benign. Less than 5% of patients with ITP die from bleeding; when they die, it is from intracranial hemorrhage.

    3. TTP is an emergency requiring rapid diagnosis and treatment to prevent death.

B. Etiology and pathophysiology

    1. Cancer-associated thrombocytopenia is from decreased marrow megakaryocytopoiesis. It is part of the natural history of all leukemia patients and is commonly encountered in all cancer patients receiving intensive chemotherapy, including hematopoietic stem cell transplantation.

    2. ITP is due to splenic macrophage-mediated destruction of IgG-coated platelets. The antibody may be an autoimmune event, it may be part of another disease process (such as lupus or chronic lymphocytic leukemia), or it may be drug induced.

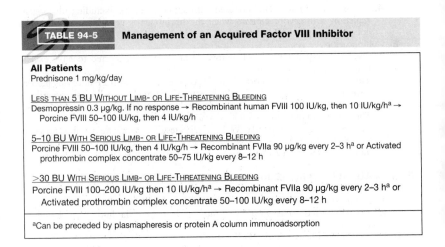

TABLE 94-5	Management of an Acquired Factor VIII Inhibitor

All Patients
Prednisone 1 mg/kg/day

LESS THAN 5 BU WITHOUT LIMB- OR LIFE-THREATENING BLEEDING
Desmopressin 0.3 μg/kg. If no response → Recombinant human FVIII 100 IU/kg, then 10 IU/kg/h[a] → Porcine FVIII 50–100 IU/kg, then 4 IU/kg/h

5–10 BU WITH SERIOUS LIMB- OR LIFE-THREATENING BLEEDING
Porcine FVIII 50–100 IU/kg, then 4 IU/kg/h → Recombinant FVIIa 90 μg/kg every 2–3 h[a] or Activated prothrombin complex concentrate 50–75 IU/kg every 8–12 h

>30 BU WITH SERIOUS LIMB- OR LIFE-THREATENING BLEEDING
Porcine FVIII 100–200 IU/kg then 10 IU/kg/h[a] → Recombinant FVIIa 90 μg/kg every 2–3 h[a] or Activated prothrombin complex concentrate 50–100 IU/kg every 8–12 h

[a]Can be preceded by plasmapheresis or protein A column immunoadsorption

3. TTP is often due to an acquired antibody to the ADAMTS-13 protease that breaks down super-sticky plasma large von Willebrand factor (vWF) multimers. The presence of the large vWF multimers in circulation leads to platelet attachment, activation, and aggregation thereby clogging up the arteriolar circuit of many organs, including the heart, brain, lungs, gut, and kidneys.

C. Diagnosis
   1. Underproduction thrombocytopenia is a clinical diagnosis that rarely requires a bone marrow examination to prove that megakaryocytopoiesis is poor or absent.
   2. ITP is also a clinical diagnosis. Everyone requires HIV testing, and patients over the age of 60 require a bone marrow examination to evaluate for occult underproduction thrombocytopenia, typically from myelodysplasia.
   3. TTP is considered to be diagnosed by a clinicopathologic pentad: fever, thrombocytopenia, microangiopathic hemolytic anemia, neurologic signs, and renal insufficiency. ADAMTS13 can be measured and is low in the majority of "*de novo*" TTP cases. The PT, aPTT, and D-dimer levels are usually normal.

D. Treatment
   1. Bleeding from underproduction thrombocytopenia is treated with platelet transfusions. One unit of platelets should raise the blood platelet count by 5,000 to 10,000/μL unless the patient is alloimmunized or has ongoing destruction (ITP, TTP) or sequestration (hypersplenism). Recombinant interleukin 11 is FDA approved for the treatment of thrombocytopenia resulting from chemotherapy in patients with solid tumors. Its small and gradual effect limits its utility, and it probably shouldn't be used for ICU patients with thrombocytopenia and bleeding.
   2. All ICU patients bleeding from ITP requires high-dose IVIG (e.g., 1 μg/kg per day for 2 days) plus oral prednisone 2 mg/kg per day. If an ITP patient is exsanguinating, massive platelet transfusions are given (e.g., 20 units) to adsorb out the antiplatelet antibody and ultimately permit a reasonably good increase in the blood platelet count. The target platelet count in someone with severe bleeding or intracranial bleeding is at least 50,000/μL and probably should be greater than 100,000/μL.
   3. TTP is treated with high-volume plasma exchange. Corticosteroids (e.g., solumedrol 200 mg divided into four doses) may also be useful.

E. Complications
   1. The main complication of platelet transfusions is alloimmunization. This limits their effectiveness because alloantibody-coated transfused platelets are cleared very rapidly by splenic macrophages. The risk of leukemia patients becoming

alloimmunized is driven below 5% when they are given leukodepleted or UVB-irradiated random donor platelets or by using single-donor platelets.

2. At least one third of all ITP responses are transitory, so that relapse of associated bleeding is a predictable outcome. Such relapses are treated with either IVIG or an increase in daily prednisone dosage, and they are often cured by splenectomy.

3. TTP patients who don't respond to plasma exchange with FFP are sometimes exchanged with cryoprecipitate-poor plasma, which has very little vWF. Failing this, splenectomy has been shown to effect excellent clinical response and cures. Among the 90% of TTP patients who recover, perhaps 20% will relapse. The relapses are treated much the same as the first episode. Splenectomy often stops relapses in those with frequent, chronic, relapsing TTP.

Selected Readings

Hebert PC, Wells G, Blachman MA, et al. A multicenter, randomized, controlled trial of transfusion requirements in critical care. *N Engl J Med* 1999;340:409–417.
The authors conclude that, except for patients with acute MI or unstable angina, a restrictive strategy for red cell transfusions is best.

Kroll MH. *Manual of coagulation disorders.* Malden, MA: Blackwell, 2001, p. 241.
A broad overview by one of the authors of this chapter provides more depth, details, and references framed within a narrative text.

Levi M, Ten Cate H. Disseminated intravascular coagulation. *N Engl J Med* 1999;341:586–592.
This review presents an outline of the subject, focusing on etiology and pathogenesis. The management section addresses in some detail those interventions beyond the famously fundamental maxim "treat the underlying illness."

Moake JL. Thrombotic microangiopathies. *N Engl J Med* 2002;347:589–600.
This is a classic review that is as beautifully illustrated as it is informative.

Nevo S, Vogelsang GB. Acute bleeding complications in patients after bone marrow transplantation. *Curr Opin Hematol* 2001;8:319–325.
This article reviews bleeding problems after hematopoietic stem cell transplantation and emphasizes the importance of treating thrombocytopenia with platelet transfusions.

Schulman S. Care of patients receiving long-term anticoagulation. *N Engl J Med* 2003;349:675–683.
This is a terrific review of the many practical issues involved in optimizing the therapeutic index of warfarin and treating bleeding due to overanticoagulation.

Siegel JP. Assessing the use of activated protein C in the treatment of severe sepsis. *N Engl J Med* 2002;347:1030–1034.
Breaks the subject down into the many details that must be considered when using activated protein C in the ICU. As important as the details are, the tone of the paper emphasizes the point that no one should ever receive activated protein C injudiciously.

Warren HS, Suffredini AF, Eichacker PQ, et al. Risks and benefits of activated protein C treatment of severe sepsis. *N Engl J Med* 2002;347:1027–1030.
Breaks the subject down into the many details that must be considered when using activated protein C in the ICU. As important as the details are, the tone of the paper emphasizes the point that no one should ever receive activated protein C injudiciously.

95

CONGENITAL COAGULOPATHIES
Renée Killian, Michael A. Coyne,
and Arthur R. Thompson

I. GENERAL PRINCIPLE. Congenital bleeding tendencies are most often due to deficient activity of clotting factors VIII or IX (hemophilia) or to loss of functional von Willebrand factor activity in von Willebrand disease. Other deficiency states are rare but should be considered if these common disorders have been excluded and there is a strong clinical suspicion.

II. HEMOPHILIAS
   A. Hemophilias are due to a genetic mutation resulting in a deficiency or absence of specific clotting protein activities, namely factor VIII (hemophilia A) or factor IX (hemophilia B).
      1. X-linked, recessive disorder, primarily manifested in males; 10% to 15% of female carriers may have levels sufficiently low to be symptomatic, usually mild.
      2. Of affected males, 30% to 50% are severe; others have moderately severe or mild bleeding tendencies.
      3. Estimates between 30% and 50% of new cases occur spontaneously, with no family history.

III. DESCRIPTION
   A. Prevents formation of a stable fibrin clot; may form soft, useless "liver clot."
   B. Bleeding may be internal or external, spontaneous (especially with severe hemophilia), or posttrauma.
   C. Results in prolonged oozing and poor wound healing.
   D. Clinical presentations of hemophilia A and hemophilia B are essentially identical.

IV. CLASSIFICATION
   A. Normal plasma range of clotting activity for factors VIII and IX is 50% to 150%.
   B. Clinical presentation generally correlates with baseline, intrinsic levels.
      1. Severe: less than 1% normal activity, characterized by frequent bleeding episodes with or without (spontaneous) trauma.
      2. Moderate: 1% to 5%, characterized by generally less frequent bleeding episodes, infrequent spontaneous bleeds, abnormal bleeding with trauma expected.
      3. Mild: 6% to 35%, bleeding expected to follow trauma or surgery. Female symptomatic carriers (~10% of carriers) may present as mild hemophilia.

V. EPIDEMIOLOGY
   A. Estimated to occur in 1 of 5,000 live male births.
   B. Factor VIII deficiency accounts for approximately 80% of all hemophilia.

VI. CLINICAL COMPLICATIONS
   A. Hemophilic inhibitors (alloimmune responses)
      1. Alloantibodies develop in up to 30% of those with severe hemophilia A and only about 1% to 3% in severe hemophilia B. Can occur in mild hemophilia A, especially following a period of intensive treatment.
      2. Acquired hemophilia
         a. Autoantibodies that neutralize factor VIII clotting activity (acquired hemophilia A) occur in approximately 0.1% of the general population; most common in the seventh and eighth decades of life but can affect all ages.

      b. Comorbid conditions include rheumatoid arthritis, peripartum period, malignancy, systemic lupus erythematosus (SLE), drug reactions, other autoimmune disorders, dermatologic conditions, multitransfusion among others; the majority have no comorbid condition.

VII. PROGNOSIS
    A. Early, consistent treatment and prevention of bleeding offers best outcome with the least incidence of disability, morbidity, or mortality.
    B. Life span is comparable to unaffected individual, with the exception of an unrecognized, untreated intracranial hemorrhage or development of an inhibitor.

VIII. DIAGNOSIS
    A. Presentation
      1. Family history of bleeding disorder.
      2. In absence of family history, diagnosis tends to be earlier in life with increased severity of disease and often because of abnormal bruising.
      3. Typical diagnostic presentations
        a. Circumcision (prolonged oozing).
        b. Mouth, mucous membrane bleed (e.g., tongue, torn frenulum).
        c. Easy, "lumpy" bruising. (Consider a bleeding disorder in children with easy bruisability when abuse is suspected.)
          (1) Hemarthrosis (if spontaneous, likely severe).
          (2) Prolonged oozing after minor surgery or tooth exfoliation or extraction (if mild severity of hemophilia and first clinically significant bleeding episode).
          (3) Routine preoperative screen with prolonged APTT.

IX. DIFFERENTIAL DIAGNOSIS
    A. Unusual bleeding elicits detailed personal and family bleeding history, including any treatment and response to treatment as well as complications.
    B. Normal complete blood count (CBC), prothrombin time (PT) (INR) bleeding time test, platelet count, and fibrinogen.
    C. Prolonged activated thromboplastin time (aPTT), which corrects on 1:1 mix, suggests factor deficiency (XII, XI, IX, VIII); partial correction, suspect inhibitor development.
    D. Sudden onset of first bleeding episode in an adult, no personal or family history, low factor VIII or IX, suspect autoantibody inhibitor development.
    E. If only PT prolonged, consider FVII deficiency.
    F. If both PT and PTT prolonged, consider FX, FV (or vitamin K deficiency, liver disease, warfarin, disseminated intravascular coagulation [DIC]).

X. HISTORY
    A. Easy bruisability, especially "lumpy" bruises.
    B. Prolonged or delayed bleeding after dental extractions or surgery.
    C. Unusual muscle injuries, history of compartment syndrome, persistent "sprain" injury.
    D. Delayed wound healing after surgery, trauma, childbirth, menorrhagia.
    E. Anyone in family with bleeding problems.
    F. History of transfusion due to excessive bleeding.
    G. Joint hemarthrosis.
    H. CNS hemorrhage.

XI. MANIFESTATIONS
    A. Serious sites of bleeding require immediate assessment and intervention. (See Treatment section and Table 95-1.)
      1. Intracranial (may be spontaneous and may present as irritability and vomiting in infants/children).
      2. Spinal cord.
      3. Throat or anterior neck.

TABLE 95-1	Factor Replacement Doses (All antihemophilic factors are administered intravenously)
Hemophilia A or factor VIII deficiency	**Hemophilia B or factor IX deficiency**
Routine dose = 25–30 units/kg Examples: early joint or muscle bleed, epistaxis, hematuria Major dose = 40–50 units/kg Examples: head, GI, prior to invasive procedure (e.g., LP), large joint or muscle bleeds, mouth bleeds, and sutures	Recombinant factor IX Routine dose = 50–70 units/kg Examples: early joint or muscle bleeds, epistaxis, hematuria Major dose = 120–150 units/kg Examples: head, GI, prior to invasive procedure (e.g., LP), large joint or muscle bleeds (e.g., iliopsoas), mouth bleeds, and sutures

Special note: For patients with factor VIII or IX inhibitors, it is imperative to coordinate treatment with a Hemophilia Care Center or a physician knowledgeable in managing such patients.
GI, gastrointestinal; LP, lumbar puncture.

   4. Intraabdominal.
   5. Limb compartments.
   6. Ocular.
 B. Hemarthrosis, bleeding into a joint.
   1. Pain, heat, erythema, decreased range of motion, bubbling or tingling sensation (early symptoms), swelling (late).
   2. Hematoma, bleeding into a muscle, either skeletal or "visceral."
      a. Early, pain, tenseness, rigidity, swelling.
      b. Late, altered posture, guarding, severe pain and loss of motion, bruising with gravitational discoloration (subcutaneous hematoma often delayed).
   3. Iliopsoas (spontaneous flexion of hip and leg on affected side) may not exhibit swelling but can result in significant blood loss requiring immediate treatment with factor and emergency hematology consult. These patients may present with "abdominal" pain.
      a. Majority of muscle bleeding episodes respond to factor replacement without fasciotomy.
      b. Complications of untreated muscle bleeds with nerve and blood vessel compression include foot drop, wrist contracture or loss of limb, pseudotumors.
   4. Superficial, nonexpanding subcutaneous hematomas that do not threaten mobility or function and are not associated with deeper muscle hematomas are generally not treated.

XII. OTHER SITES OF BLEEDING
 A. Gastrointestinal: hemoptysis (Mallory-Weiss tear, varices, upper gastrointestinal ulceration); melena (gastritis, gastroenteritis, varices); miscellaneous (hemorrhoids, intussusception, Meckel's diverticulum), angiodysplasia.
 B. Hematuria usually benign: force fluids, no antifibrinolytics, may require routine factor dose; may or may not be related to kidney stones.
 C. Mucous membrane bleeding or epistaxis: if unable to control bleed himself, may require routine dose of factor or antifibrinolytic therapy with epsilon aminocaproic acid (Amicar).
 D. Oral cavity: same as C.
 E. Retropharyngeal: give major dose of factor, airway precautions, then take any tests, observe, admit.
 F. Menorrhagia in symptomatic carriers may require factor or DDAVP (if factor VIII deficient), Amicar, or gynecologic consult.

XIII. PHYSICAL EXAMINATION

A. May be unremarkable during early onset of a bleeding episode.

B. Later presentations may be dramatic for swelling, heat, muscle rigidity, immobility, acute pain, pallor, signs or symptoms of increasing intracranial pressure, loss of consciousness, airway obstruction.

C. Unexpected oozing from central line puncture site, unexplained muscle bleeding, unexplained blood loss (i.e., dropping hematocrit).

XIV. TREATMENT

A. Dosing guidelines
   1. In previously diagnosed individuals, treatment should be guided by suspicion of bleeding-related problem, not confirmation.
   2. Factor replacement needs to be given following a head injury regardless of physical findings or Geneva coma score.
   3. Repeat dosing is often required due to short half-life of infused factor.
   4. Treatment of choice for either hemophilia A or B is recombinant factor concentrate; some patients elect to treat with a plasma-derived concentrate. Cryoprecipitate is no longer recommended for hemophilia A. Persons with mild hemophilia A and non–life- or limb-threatening bleeding episodes may respond to arginine desmopressin (DDAVP)[1] if previously shown to respond. See Table 95-1.

B. Indications for treatment
   1. Any new or unusual headache, particularly one following trauma.
   2. Any significant injury to head, neck, mouth, or eyes or evidence of bleeding in those areas.
   3. History of accident or trauma that might result in internal bleeding.
   4. Necessity of a surgical or invasive procedure, including biopsy, aspiration, or intramuscular injection or blood gases.
   5. Heavy or persistent bleeding from any site.
   6. Severe pain or swelling at any site.
   7. Suspected bleeding into a joint or muscle.
   8. All open wounds requiring surgical closure, wound adhesive, or steri-strips.
   9. Gastrointestinal bleeding.
   10. Acute fractures, dislocations, and sprains.

C. Monitoring treatment
   1. Clinical response is critical to evaluate.
   2. Factor activity assays can help document recovery and survival, especially in dosing for major surgery where hemostatic levels must be maintained for 10 to 14 days until sufficient wound healing has occurred to prevent rebleeding.
   3. aPTT may be used as a rough guide if specific factor assays are not available.

D. Supportive care
   1. Appropriate analgesia for acute pain related to bleeding episode. No aspirin (ASA) at any time and no nonsteroidal antiinflammatory drugs (NSAIDs) during an acute bleed.
   2. May require additional bolus of factor just prior to surgery or invasive procedure.
   3. RICE (rest, ice, compression, elevation).
   4. Extended factor replacement as needed for wound healing and relief of symptoms; consult with a hematologist.

XV. COMPLICATIONS

A. Hemophilic arthropathies (synovitis, progressive arthritis). Older patients may have severe joint arthropathies, multiple joint replacements, or disability.

B. Septic arthritis occasionally occurs and may be "spontaneous" or follow joint replacement.

C. Viral/infectious: patients born and treated before 1985 may have been exposed to HIV and hepatitis B and C.

D. Of patients with clinically significant or high titer inhibitors, necessitating the use of "bypass" agents for bleeding episodes, immunosuppression can be achieved in

---

[1]DDAVP dosing: 0.3 µg/kg diluted in 50 mL normal saline and infused intravenously over 20 to 30 minutes.

up to two thirds but requires daily factor VIII infusions (immune tolerance induction protocols) usually for several months.

E. Possibility of thrombotic event especially with older, intermediate purity or activated factor IX concentrates.

XVI. VON WILLEBRAND DISEASE. Autosomally inherited; most common hereditary bleeding disorder with three main subtypes.

A. Diagnosis

1. von Willebrand antigen measures amount of protein.

2. Ristocetin cofactor (RCo) assay measures activity.

3. Factor VIII may be decreased (types 1 or 3).

4. Prolonged bleeding time, or PFA closure times (not specific).

5. Platelet aggregation studies usually show decreased agglutination to ristocetin (RIPA).

6. High-molecular-weight multimers decreased in types 2A and 2B.

B. Presentation/symptoms

1. Abnormal mucosal bleeding, especially epistaxis

2. Menorrhagia

3. Easy bruisability

4. Prolonged oozing or delayed wound healing similar to that in hemophilias

C. Treatment

1. Most useful to know precise diagnosis to guide treatment.

a. DDAVP useful in most patients with mild type 1, some with type 2A but contraindicated in type 2B, and not effective in patients with type 3.

b. For patients unresponsive to DDAVP, or where it is contraindicated or where response is unknown in the face of serious or potentially life-threatening bleeding, factor replacement with plasma-derived concentrate containing functional von Willebrand factor (usually with factor VIII) is recommended. The two currently licensed in the United States are Humate-P and AlphanateSD/HT. Both have undergone procedures that inactivate lipid-enveloped viruses including (HIV, HBV, and HCV).

c. Treatment dose varies with severity of disease and clinical situation with 50 to 60 RCo units/kg as an average starting dose (range is 40 to 80 U/kg) for bleeding or just prior to invasive procedure.

d. In emergency when factor is not available, cryoprecipitate may be used and usually as a pool of bags from 15 to 20 donors, although potencies vary and there is no viral inactivation.

Selected Readings

Bolton-Maggs PHB, Pasi KJ. Haemophilias A and B. *Lancet* 2003;361:1801–1809.
Pathophysiology, molecular genetics, diagnosis, complications, management, research, and global organizations.

Ludlam C, Keeling D, Barrowcliffe T, et al. Guidelines on the selection and use of therapeutic products to treat haemophilia and other hereditary bleeding disorders; United Kingdom Haemophilia Centre Doctors' Organisation. *Haemophilia* 2003; 9:1–23.
Evidence-based guidelines on selection and use of therapeutic products to treat hemophilia.

Mannucci PM. Treatment of von Willebrand's disease. *N Engl J Med* 2004; 351:683–694.
Description of classification, diagnosis, treatment, and future areas for research.

Thompson AR. Other bleeding disorders. In Young N, Gerson S, High KA, eds. *Clinical hematology.* Philadelphia: Elsevier, 2006.
Diagnostic and therapeutic considerations for rare deficiencies of other coagulation factors (fibrinogen, prothrombin, and factors V, VII, X, XI, and XIII).

I. DEFINITION
A. Less than 150,000/μL, generally not significant until less than 100,000/μL

B. Relative; acute drop from a higher platelet count may be pathologic.

II. PATHOPHYSIOLOGY
A. Decreased production

B. Increased destruction, consumption

C. Increased sequestration in enlarged spleen

D. Dilutional. Effect of massive transfusion and fluid resuscitation less than predicted on the basis of volume replacement alone.

E. States with multiple causes of thrombocytopenia: cirrhosis with portal hypertension, hepatitis, HIV, other viral illnesses, patients with multiple medical problems on multiple drugs.

III. DIAGNOSIS
A. Complete blood count with peripheral smear examination. Rule out pseudothrombocytopenia due to platelet clumping.

B. Coagulation testing. Identify associated coagulation abnormalities.

C. Additional blood tests
   1. Viral titers and antibody
   2. Immune disorders: antibody testing
   3. Other: see specific disorders

D. Radiologic
   1. Abdominal ultrasound: evaluation of spleen size
   2. CT scanning: evaluation for lymphoproliferative disease

E. Bone marrow examination indications
   1. Unclear pathophysiology
   2. Multiple cytopenias
   3. Suspected infiltrative process

IV. THERAPY
A. Transfusion therapy indications
   1. Bleeding or necessary invasive procedures
   2. Prophylactic: very severe (<10,000/μL) thrombocytopenia
   3. Other blood components as indicated to correct coagulation abnormalities
   4. Platelet transfusion relatively contraindicated:
      a. Thrombotic thrombocytopenic purpura (TTP) unless bleeding present; worsened thrombotic tendency reported.
      b. Immune thrombocytopenia unless bleeding present; poor or short-lived response.
      c. Heparin induced thrombocytopenia (HIT) without bleeding, unknown.

B. Nonspecific therapy for bleeding
   1. Antifibrinolytic agents: epsilon aminocaproic acid (Amicar)
   2. Recombinant factor VIIa (Novo Seven®): controversial; may be indicated in acute intracranial or other life-threatening bleeding in patients without response to platelet transfusion.

C. Secondary thrombocytopenias: direct therapy at underlying cause(s).

D. Primary thrombocytopenia: depends on specific disorder (see later).

V. DECREASED PLATELET PRODUCTION
- **A.** Platelet specific
  1. Drugs, ethyl alcohol (ETOH), viral (e.g., HIV, hepatitis C virus)
  2. Decreased thrombopoietin: liver disease
  3. Amegakaryocytic thrombocytopenia
  4. Congenital thrombocytopenia
- **B.** Multiple cytopenias
  1. Marrow toxins: drugs, alcohol, radiation
  2. Nutritional (e.g., B_{12}, folate)
  3. Metabolic (e.g., thyroid disorders)
  4. Primary marrow disorders: stem cell disorders, marrow infiltration
  5. Hemophagocytic syndrome
- **C.** Diagnosis
  1. Peripheral blood smear
     - **a.** Abnormal morphology: Congenital, myelodysplasia, myeloproliferative
     - **b.** Red blood cell abnormalities
       - **(1)** Teardrops, nucleated red blood cells: marrow infiltrative diseases
       - **(2)** Macrocytosis: B_{12} or folate deficiency, myelodysplasia
     - **c.** White blood cell abnormalities
       - **(1)** Immature forms: leukemia
       - **(2)** Multilobed neutrophils, bizarre forms: B_{12} or folate deficiency, myelodysplasia
- **D.** Therapy: direct at underlying or associated disorder

VI. INCREASED SPLENIC SEQUESTRATION
- **A.** Etiology
  1. Portal hypertension
  2. Myeloproliferative disease
  3. Lymphoma
  4. Storage and infiltrative diseases of spleen
  5. Chronic hemolysis
  6. Granulomatoses: tuberculosis, sarcoidosis
- **B.** Diagnosis
  1. Imaging: abdominal ultrasound, CT
  2. Biopsy of apparently pathologic tissue, bone marrow
- **C.** Treatment: direct at underlying cause

VII. DISORDERS OF INCREASED PLATELET DESTRUCTION
- **A.** Platelet lifespan less than normal 10 days
- **B.** Immune: autoimmune or alloimmune
- **C.** Nonimmune: isolated or combined platelet consumption

VIII. AUTOIMMUNE THROMBOCYTOPENIAS
- **A.** Etiology
  1. Idiopathic (idiopathic thrombocytopenic purpurpa, or ITP)
  2. Drugs
  3. Associated with other autoimmune disease (e.g., systemic lupus)
  4. Associated with malignancy (e.g., lymphoproliferative disease)

IX. ITP
- **A. General principles**
  1. Acute ITP may present with severe thrombocytopenia ($<5,000/\mu L$)
  2. Initial presentation typically abrupt in onset
  3. Petechiae, bruising, mucosal bleeding most common manifestations
- **B.** Epidemiology
  1. Adults: 90% chronic relapsing disorder
  2. Children: 90% acute, self-resolving disorder
  3. Most common in young females (female:male ratio = 3:2).

C. Etiology
   1. Idiopathic, may present following acute viral illness
   2. May be initial presentation of connective tissue disease, lymphoproliferative malignancy, HIV infection
   3. May be associated with antiphospholipid antibody syndrome
D. Pathophysiology
   1. Antibody against glycoproteins on platelet membrane
   2. Reticuloendothelial, especially splenic, platelet clearance
E. Diagnosis
   1. Clinical: presentation, therapeutic response.
   2. Laboratory testing
      a. Other peripheral blood and hemostatic measurements normal unless the patient has been bleeding.
      b. Rule out associated disorders when indicated by history or clinical presentation.
      c. Antiplatelet antibodies generally not helpful in diagnosis.
      d. Bone marrow examination not required unless diagnosis uncertain. Normal to increased numbers of megakaryocytes without other abnormalities.
F. Treatment
   1. Acute
      a. Immunoglobulin therapy: rapid response
         (1) Rh-positive patients who have not undergone splenectomy: anti-RhD immunoglobulin (WinRho) 50 to 75 μg/kg IV. Complications: fever, chills, acute hemolysis. *Or,*
         (2) Immunoglobulin 2 g/kg IV administered over 2 to 5 days. Complications: severe headache, renal failure, aseptic meningitis.
      b. Corticosteroids
         (1) Usual prednisone dose 1 to 2 mg/kg
         (2) Acute emergency: up to 1 g methylprednisolone IV
         (3) Platelet transfusion. Markedly decreased transfused platelet survival. Transfuse only the patient with significant bleeding.
      c. Antifibrinolytic agents. Epsilon aminocaproic acid (Amicar) starting dose 1 g by mouth or IV every 6 hours. Increase as needed to 20 g total daily dose. Contraindication: urinary tract bleeding
   2. Chronic. Options for patients who relapse after immunoglobulin therapy or prednisone taper include splenectomy, pulse corticosteroids, alkylating agents, monoclonal antibody (pituximab), immunosuppressive agents, others.
G. Complications
   1. Therapeutic complications may interfere more with quality of life and be more severe than bleeding risk in mild or moderately thrombocytopenic patients (30,000 to 100,000/μL).
   2. Chronic steroid therapy and immunosuppression: severe osteoporosis, infections, and other complications
H. Prognosis. Severe refractory ITP: 10% to 25% risk of significant bleed during disease course

X. DRUG-ASSOCIATED AUTOIMMUNE THROMBOCYTOPENIA
A. General principles
   1. Multiple drugs implicated
   2. Most common offenders: quinine and derivatives, antibiotics, thiazide diuretics
   3. Heparin a special case (see later).
B. Diagnosis
   1. History of drug exposure
   2. Laboratory testing
      a. Drug-dependent platelet autoantibody
      b. No other blood or hemostatic abnormalities identified
   3. Contraindicated: rechallenge with suspect drug for diagnosis
C. Therapy
   1. Discontinue suspected offending agent(s)

2. Intravenous gamma globulin therapy: administer as for ITP
3. Plasma exchange in severe refractory cases

XI. HEPARIN-INDUCED THROMBOCYTOPENIA
  A. General principles
  1. Immune reaction to heparin may be associated with life-threatening prothrombotic state: heparin-associated thrombocytopenia with thrombosis syndrome (HATT).
  2. Discontinue all heparin therapy while considering the diagnosis.
  B. Pathophysiology
  1. Heparin binds to platelet factor 4 (PF4), creates antigenic complex.
  2. Antibody bound to PF4 in presence of heparin causes platelet activation, aggregation, thrombin generation.
  3. Thrombin generation further activates platelets.
  4. Large and small venous and arterial vessel thrombosis may occur.
  C. Diagnosis
  1. Clinical
    a. Any type of heparin exposure
    b. More than 50% fall in platelet count to less than 100,000/μL
    c. Onset commonly 3 to 7 days after initial heparin exposure
  2. Laboratory
    a. PF4 enzyme-link immunosorbent assay (ELISA) (sensitive, may be nonspecific)
    b. Serotonin release assay: specific, specialized laboratories only
    c. Heparin: platelet aggregation studies, specialized laboratories only
  D. Treatment
  1. Discontinue all heparin exposure
  2. Rule out thrombosis: Doppler studies
  3. Anticoagulation with direct thrombin inhibitors (DTIs)
    a. Hirudin: renal clearance
    b. Argatroban: hepatic clearance
    c. Bivalirudin: patients with renal or hepatic failure or both
    d. DTIs have no antidote
  E. Prognosis: HATT associated with up to 50% serious morbidity and mortality without direct thrombin inhibitor therapy

XII. ALLOIMMUNE THROMBOCYTOPENIAS. Antibodies against foreign platelet antigens encountered through transfusion or pregnancy cause posttransfusion purpura (see next section), HLA alloimmunization and refractoriness to transfused platelets, and neonatal alloimmune thrombocytopenia (NATP).

XIII. POSTTRANSFUSION PURPURA (PTP)
  A. General principles. Severe thrombocytopenia occurs 5 to 10 days posttransfusion of cellular blood components. Most common in multiparous women.
  B. Pathophysiology
  1. Alloimmunization occurs through pregnancy or transfusion to common platelet antigen. Allogeneic platelet destruction with recall of antibody.
  2. Mechanism of associated autologous platelet destruction poorly understood.
  C. Diagnosis. Laboratory: strong serum antibody, IgG or IgM class, most commonly against platelet antigen PLA-1
  D. Treatment
  1. Immunoglobulin 2 g/kg administered IV over 2 to 5 days
  2. Plasma exchange in refractory cases
  3. Poor responses to platelet transfusion

XIV. NONIMMUNE THROMBOCYTOPENIA
  A. Combined consumption
  1. Associated with fibrinogen deposition and consumption (e.g., disseminated intravascular coagulation [DIC])
  2. Sepsis, malignancy, obstetric complications, massive tissue injury, snake bite

  B. Diagnosis
     1. Peripheral blood smear
        a. Bands, toxic granulations, Dohle bodies: sepsis
     2. Abnormal coagulation tests
        a. Increased prothrombin time (PT), partial thromboplastin time (PTT), thrombin time
        b. Falling fibrinogen level
        c. Increased D-dimers
  C. Treatment
     1. Direct at underlying cause
     2. Support with transfusion therapy for bleeding
  D. Isolated platelet consumption
     1. Vascular injury, high shear flow: vasculitis, intravascular prosthetic devices
     2. Microangiopathic hemolysis (e.g., thrombotic thrombocytopenic purpura [TTP], hemolytic uremic syndrome [HUS])

XV. MICROANGIOPATHIC HEMOLYTIC ANEMIAS

  A. General principles. Isolated platelet consumption associated with intravascular hemolysis. Patients present with end-organ signs and symptoms resulting from microvascular thrombosis.
  B. Etiology
     1. TTP
     2. HUS
     3. Associated with *Escherichia coli* O157:H7 or Shigella species infection
     4. Malignant arterial hypertension
     5. Drug-induced: cyclosporine, mitomycin C, pentostatin, others
     6. Pregnancy: may be associated with elevated liver enzymes
     7. HIV
  C. Diagnosis
     1. Peripheral blood smear: red cell fragmentation (schistocytes)
     2. Elevated parameters of intravascular hemolysis (LDH, bilirubin)
     3. Normal coagulation tests
  D. Treatment
     1. Discontinue offending agents.
     2. Treat underlying disorder.
     3. HUS, TTP: see next.

XVI. THROMBOTIC THROMBOCYTOPENIC PURPURA

  A. General principles
     1. Acute presentation of severe to moderate thrombocytopenia
     2. Usually presents with fever, neurologic signs or symptoms, or renal abnormalities
  B. Etiology
     1. Autoimmune
     2. Congenital
     3. Drug related
     4. HIV
  C. Pathophysiology
     1. Deficiency of von Willebrand factor cleaving enzyme (ADAMTS-13) results in persistence of large multimeric forms and increased platelet adhesion.
     2. Formation of platelet thrombi in microvasculature leads to end-organ disease.
     3. Intravascular hemolysis by increased shearing forces.
  D. Diagnosis
     1. Laboratory
        a. Red cell fragments on peripheral blood film
        b. Elevated LDH; indirect bilirubin may be elevated
        c. Hemostasis parameters otherwise normal
        d. Creatinine may be increased; hematuria may be present
        e. Usefulness of ADAMTS-13 level and antibody controversial

   E. Treatment
      1. Medical emergency: plasma exchange lifesaving; replacement fluid must be plasma
      2. Infuse fresh frozen plasma (4 to 6 units in an adult) if plasma exchange delayed
      3. Corticosteroids: role unclear
      4. Refractory: splenectomy, vincristine, immunosuppression
      5. Drug related or HIV; plasma exchange not generally helpful; remove offending agent
   F. Prognosis: 90% mortality rate without rapid institution of therapy

XVII. HEMOLYTIC UREMIC SYNDROME
   A. Pathophysiology
      1. Deposition of platelet thrombi in small and medium-size vessels
      2. No deficiency of ADAMTS-13
   B. Treatment
      1. Primarily supportive (e.g., dialysis)
      2. Plasma exchange of value in some patients
      3. Majority of cases resolve with supportive care

Selected Readings

Dempfle CE. Coagulopathy of sepsis. *Thromb Haemost* 2004;91(2):213–224.
   Review of the pathogenetic mechanisms and treatment of DIC associated with infection.

George JN, Raskob GE, Shah SR, et al. Drug-induced thrombocytopenia: a systematic review of published case reports. *Ann Intern Med* 1998;129(11):886–890.
   Review of drug-related thrombocytopenias and approach to their management.

George NJ, Woolf SH, Raskob GE, et al. Idiopathic thrombocytopenic purpura. A practice guideline developed by explicit methods for the American Society of Hematology. *Blood* 1996;88:3.
   Immune thrombocytopenic purpura diagnosis and management guidelines by a panel of experts.

Portielje JEA, Westendorp RGJ, Kluin-Nelemans HC, et al. Morbidity and mortality in adults with idiopathic thrombocytopenic purpura. *Blood* 2001;97:2549–2554.
   Follow-up study of clinical outcome in patients with ITP.

Tsai HM, Lian EC. Antibodies to von Willebrand factor-cleaving protease in acute thrombotic thrombocytopenic purpura. *N Engl J Med* 1998;339:1585–1594.
   The classic paper describing the relationship of ADAMTS-13 and TTP.

Vesely SK, George JN, Lammle B, et al. ADAMTS13 activity in thrombotic thrombocytopenic purpura-hemolytic uremic syndrome: relation to presenting features and clinical outcomes in a prospective cohort of 142 patients. *Blood* 2003;102:60–88.
   Large observational study of TTP and HUS.

Warkentin TE, Greinacher A. Heparin-induced thrombocytopenia: recognition, treatment, and prevention: the Seventh ACCP Conference on Antithrombotic and Thrombolytic Therapy. *Chest* 2004;126:311S–337S.
   Excellent review of the clinical presentation, pathogenesis, diagnosis, and management of HIT.

Warkentin TE, Smith JW. The alloimmune thrombocytopenia syndromes. *Transfu Med Rev* 1997;11:296–307.
   Review of platelet alloantigen systems and related immune thrombocytopenias.

I. ANTIPLATELET AGENTS

A. Aspirin

  1. General principles

   a. A salicylic acid derivative (acetylsalicylic acid)

   b. Generally is well absorbed from the gastrointestinal tract, but the rate of absorption is dependent on the gastric acidity and presence of food and is erratic with the enteric-coated forms

  2. Indications

   a. Prevention of myocardial infarction (MI) and sudden death in patients with chronic stable angina pectoris

   b. Prevention of death and MI in patients with prior MI or unstable angina pectoris

   c. Treatment of acute MI

   d. Prevention of death and stroke in patients with prior ischemic stroke or transient ischemic attack (TIA)

  3. Pathophysiology

   a. Mechanism of action

    (1) Irreversibly inactivated by acetylation cyclooxygenase-1 (COX-1).

    (2) COX-1 is a key enzyme in the synthesis of the platelet thromboxane A_2 (TXA_2), a proaggregatory and vasoconstricting molecule.

    (3) The inactivation persists for the life span of platelets (7 to 10 days).

   b. Administration and monitoring of anticoagulation

    (1) Dose of 75 to 81 mg per day for prevention of MI and stroke is effective.

    (2) For treatment of acute MI, dose of 160 mg per day is recommended.

    (3) After cardiac revascularization procedures, recommended dose is 325 mg per day.

    (4) Aspirin administration results in the prolongation of the bleeding time, but it rarely rises above the upper limit of normal and is not used for patient monitoring.

   c. Reversal of anticoagulation: platelet transfusions for clinically significant bleeding

  4. Complications

   a. Bleeding

    (1) Risk of minor bleeding is 5%, and of major bleeding 1%.

    (2) The risk of hemorrhagic stroke was not significantly different in one large study.

   b. Bronchospasm, angioedema, or urticaria in sensitive patients

   c. Reye's syndrome: acute hepatic failure in children with certain viral infections

II. CLOPIDOGREL

A. General principles

  1. A thienopyridine derivative

  2. Well absorbed after oral administration, and the absorption rate is not significantly affected by food.

B. Indications

  1. Recent MI, recent stroke, or established peripheral arterial disease

  2. Acute coronary syndrome (ACS)

C. Pathophysiology
1. **Mechanism of action**
   a. Irreversibly inhibits platelet aggregation
   b. Inhibits binding of adenosine diphosphate (ADP) to platelet purinergic P2Y$_{12}$ receptor and subsequent ADP-mediated activation of the glycoprotein IIb/IIIa complex
   c. Dose-dependent inhibition of platelet aggregation seen after 2 hours of single dose, with steady-state reached between days 3 and 7 with daily administration
2. **Administration and monitoring of anticoagulation**
   a. Dose of 75 mg orally daily
   b. In ACS start with loading dose of 300 mg, then 75 mg daily, concurrent with aspirin
3. **Reversal of anticoagulation**
   a. Platelet transfusions for clinically significant bleeding
D. Complications
1. **Bleeding**
   a. Incidence of bleeding 2% versus 2.7% on aspirin
   b. Incidence on clopidogrel and aspirin: 3.7% major and 5% minor bleeding
2. Low risk of neutropenia
3. Low risk of thrombotic thrombocytopenic purpura

III. GLYCOPROTEIN IIB/IIIA INHIBITORS
A. General principles
1. Abciximab is the Fab fragment of a chimeric human-murine monoclonal antibody that binds to and blocks the glycoprotein (GP) IIb/IIIa receptor of human platelets.
2. Tirofiban is a nonpeptide antagonist of the GP IIb/IIIa receptor.
3. Eptifibatide is a cyclic heptapeptide antagonist of the GP IIb/IIIa receptor.
B. Indications
1. ACS
2. Adjunct in patient undergoing percutaneous coronary intervention (PCI)
C. Pathophysiology
1. **Mechanism of action**
   a. Target final common pathway of platelet aggregation
2. **Administration and monitoring of anticoagulation**
   a. Abciximab
      (1) Patients with unstable angina who are planned to undergo PCI within 24 hours: bolus of 0.25 mg/kg followed by 18- to 24-hour IV infusion of 10 mcg/min, concluding 1 hour after PCI
      (2) Patients undergoing PCI: bolus 0.25 mg/kg given 10 to 60 minutes before the PCI, followed by IV infusion of 0.125 mcg/kg/min (maximum 10 mcg/min) for 12 hours
   b. Tirofiban: IV infusion of 0.4 mcg/kg/min for 30 minutes, then 0.1 mcg/kg/min; reduce by half in severe renal insufficiency
   c. Eptifibatide
      (1) ACS: IV bolus of 180 mcg/kg then continuous infusion at 2 mcg/kg/min for up to 72 hours, reduce infusion rate (but not bolus) by 50% if creatinine clearance less than 50 mL/min
      (2) PCI: bolus 180 mcg/kg immediately before PCI, followed by infusion at 2 mcg/kg/min and second bolus 10 minutes after the first one; continue infusion for 12 to 24 hours
   d. All three agents usually administered with concurrent aspirin and heparin
3. **Reversal of anticoagulation**
   a. Tirofiban and eptifibatide can be removed by hemodialysis
      (1) Complications
         (a) Bleeding
            ■ Vascular access site bleeding is the most common
            ■ Intracranial bleeding risk not significantly higher than in controls

    (ii) Thrombocytopenia: platelet count less than 50,000 noted in about 1% of patients

IV. ANTICOAGULANTS
A. Heparin
  1. General principles
    a. Naturally occurring glycosaminoglycan
    b. Extracted from porcine intestinal mucosa or bovine lung
    c. Mixture of fragments with a molecular weight of 5,000 to 30,000
    d. Has an immediate onset of action when given IV, and an onset within 20 to 60 minutes when given subcutaneously (SC)
    e. Cleared primarily by the reticuloendothelial system
    f. The half-life of IV heparin is 60 to 90 minutes; prolonged in patients with liver and renal disease
  2. Indications
    a. Acute venous thromboembolism (VTE)
    b. ACS and arterial embolism
    c. Prevention of arterial embolism (atrial fibrillation)
    d. Prevention of VTE in critically ill or surgical patients
    e. Maintenance of IV catheters
    f. Prevention and treatment of deep vein thrombosis (DVT) in pregnancy (coumadin contraindicated because of its teratogenicity)
  3. Pathophysiology
    a. Mechanism of action
      (1) Forms complexes with antithrombin (AT)
        (i) Binding of heparin to AT induces a conformational change in AT
        (ii) Increases activity of AT 1,000- to 4,000-fold
        (iii) AT inactivates thrombin (factor IIa), factor Xa, to lesser degree factors XIIa, XIa, and IXa
        (iv) Does not inactivate clot-bound thrombin (AT binding site is masked by fibrin)
        (v) Less important is direct binding to platelets and to heparin cofactor II
      (2) Activity expressed in prolongation of the activated partial thromboplastin time (aPTT), thrombin time (TT), and in higher doses prothrombin time (PT)
    b. Administration and monitoring of anticoagulation
      (1) Full-dose IV anticoagulation
        (i) Intravenous dose of 80 units/kg IV bolus then 18 units/kg/hr for most indications, adjusted to aPTT of 1.5 to 2.5 times control
        (ii) Activity monitored by aPTT, 4 to 6 hours after infusion started, then at least once daily
        (iii) "Heparin protocols" more effective in achieving therapeutic anticoagulation than ad hoc approach
      (2) Full-dose SC administration (e.g., pregnant woman)
        (i) 7,500 to 15,000 units SC every 12 hours
        (ii) Dose adjusted base on "mid-dose" (6 hours postinjection) aPTT to 1.5 to 2 times control
      (3) Prophylactic SC administration
        (i) Fixed dose of 5,000 units SC every 12 hours
    c. Reversal of anticoagulation
      (1) Stop IV heparin 4 hours prior to a procedure (short half-life) in noncirrhotic or renal failure patients
      (2) Urgent reversal
        (i) Protamine sulfate by slow IV infusion (20 mg/min and no more than 50 mg over any 10-minute period)
        (ii) Dose of 1 mg of protamine/100 units of heparin remaining in the circulation, for continuous IV infusion, approximately half of the preceding hourly dose of heparin

(iii) Small, repeated doses may be required for SC heparin reversal

(iv) Small (1%) risk of anaphylactic reaction to protamine

4. Complications

   a. Bleeding

   (1) In 5% to 10% of fully anticoagulated patients

   (2) More correlated with patient's risk status than level of anticoagulation

   b. Thrombocytopenia

   (1) HIT type 2

   (i) Immune mediated, by antibodies to heparin-platelet factor 4 complex, resulting in platelet activation

   (ii) Frequency of 1% to 3% of patients on full-dose heparin but can occur with any heparin exposure (flushes, heparin-coated catheters)

   (iii) Decrease in platelet count to below 150,000 or 50% of pretreatment number

   (iv) Window of onset is 5 to 10 days from heparin exposure

   (v) May occur sooner with prior heparin sensitization, or, rarely, cases of delayed HIT have been reported

   (vi) Associated with high risk of venous and arterial thrombosis: 30% to 80% over a 30-day period

   (vii) Frequently diagnosed *after* a thrombotic event

   (viii) When suspected, stopping of all heparins and initiation of alternative anticoagulation with a direct thrombin inhibitor (DTI) while awaiting confirmatory serologic tests is recommended

   (ix) Usually does not result in bleeding, and platelet transfusions should be avoided

   (x) Defer coumadinization until platelets recover above 100,000 and patient is fully anticoagulated with a DTI to avoid exacerbation of the thrombotic tendency from transient protein C deficiency

   (2) Type 1

   (i) Nonimmune platelet aggregation and sequestration

   (ii) Frequency estimated at 10% to 20%

   (iii) Decrease in platelet count within 1 to 4 days of starting heparin

   (iv) Platelet count usually stays above 100,000/μL

   (v) Not associated with thrombotic events

   (vi) No change in management necessary

   c. Osteoporosis

   (1) In a long-term, high-dose heparin administration, pregnant patients at higher risk for osteoporosis (17% in one study, 2% to 3% incidence of vertebral fractures)

   (2) Resolves within 1 year in most cases

V. LOW-MOLECULAR-WEIGHT HEPARINS (LMWHs)

   A. General principles

   1. Derived from unfractionated heparin (UFH) by chemical or enzymatic means

   2. Molecules about one third the size of UFH

   3. Better bioavailability and more reliable dose response than UFH

   4. Onset of action of 20 to 60 minutes after SC administration

   5. Cleared largely by renal excretion

   6. Have half-live of 3 to 6 hours after SC administration

   B. Indications

   1. VTE

   2. ACS and arterial embolism

   3. Prevention of arterial embolism (atrial fibrillation)

   4. Prevention of VTE in critically ill or surgical patients

   C. Pathophysiology

   1. Mechanism of action

   a. Form complexes with antithrombin (AT)

   (1) LMWH/AT complexes have less thrombin-inhibiting activity than UFH/AT

(2) The result is higher anti-factor Xa to antithrombin activity ratio (3:1 vs. 1:1)

(3) Do not inactivate clot-bound thrombin (AT binding site is masked by fibrin)

2. Administration and monitoring of anticoagulation

    a. Given SC for both full anticoagulation and prophylaxis

      (1) Enoxaparin

        (i) Acute VTE: 1 mg/kg SC every 12 hours, 1.5 mg/kg SC once a day has comparable efficacy

        (ii) Prophylaxis of VTE in medical patients with severely restricted mobility: 40 mg SC once a day

        (iii) Prophylaxis of VTE after hip or knee replacement surgery: 30 mg SC every 12 hours, or 40 mg SC once a day

        (iv) Unstable angina or non–Q-wave myocardial infarction: 1 mg/kg SC every 12 hours

      (2) Dalteparin

        (i) Unstable angina or non–Q-wave myocardial infarction: 120 IU SC every 12 hours

        (ii) Prophylaxis of VTE after hip replacement surgery: 5,000 IU SC once a day

        (iii) Prophylaxis of VTE after abdominal surgery: 5,000 IU SC once a day

    b. No predictable effect on aPTT when given in therapeutic doses

    c. Clinical efficacy correlates with anti-factor Xa activity, but measuring that is rarely indicated

    d. Avoid LMWHs in patients with renal failure

3. Reversal of anticoagulation

    a. Stop LMWH 12 to 24 hours prior to a procedure

    b. Urgent reversal

      (1) Protamine sulfate 1 mg/100 anti-Xa units of LMWH

      (2) Neutralization of the anti-factor Xa is less than complete due to lack of binding to the very-low-molecular weight heparin chains

D. Complications

    1. Bleeding

      a. Incidence under 5% on the prophylactic dose and treatment for VTE, higher (17%) in patients with ACS

      b. Injection site hematoma incidence up to 5%, may be higher with prolonged administration, rarely serious

      c. Hematoma after spinal anesthesia: incidence higher with concurrent use antiplatelet agents, NSAIDs, other anticoagulants

    2. Thrombocytopenia

      a. HIT

        (1) Incidence lower than with UFH (between 0 and 0.5%)

        (2) Pathogenesis and management as discussed previously for heparin

        (3) LMWHs should not be administered to patients suspected of or diagnosed with HIT

VI. FONDAPARINUX

A. General principles

    1. Synthetic pentasaccharide

    2. Rapidly and completely absorbed after SC injection

    3. Excreted unchanged in urine

    4. The elimination half-life is 17 to 21 hours in normal renal function

    5. Clearance decreased in patients with renal impairment (by 25% to 55%), elderly, and patients weighing less than 50 kg

    6. Contraindicated in patients with severe renal impairment (creatinine clearance <30 mL/min) and with body weight less than 50 kg

    7. Do not use in patients receiving spinal anesthesia

B. Indications. Prevention of DVT in patients undergoing: hip fracture surgery, hip replacement surgery, or knee replacement surgery

C. Pathophysiology

    1. Mechanism of action

    a. Binds selectively to antithrombin
    b. Potentiates neutralization of factor Xa by antithrombin
    c. Does not inactivate thrombin
    d. Does not affect fibrinolytic activity or bleeding time at the recommended dose

  2. Administration and monitoring of anticoagulation
    a. Fixed dose of 2.5 mg given SC once daily
      (1) Adjust dose for renal impairment, and use with caution in elderly patients
      (2) Initial dose should be given 6 to 8 hours after surgery and continued for 5 to 9 days after hip or knee replacement: longer course (24 days) recommended for hip fracture surgery
    b. Routine monitoring of anti-factor Xa activity not necessary, and the anti-Xa assay has to be calibrated by fondaparinux (the standard used for LMWHs is not appropriate for that purpose)

  3. Reversal of anticoagulation
    a. No specific antidote is available
    b. Partially cleared by hemodialysis

D. Complications
  1. Bleeding
    a. Incidence comparable to that with enoxaparin
    b. Risk higher with increasing age
    c. Most episodes during the first 4 days of therapy
  2. Thrombocytopenia in 3% of patients
  3. Elevation of serum aminotransferases

VII. DIRECT THROMBIN INHIBITORS

A. General principles
  1. Novel agents, not requiring antithrombin as a cofactor
    a. Argatroban
      (1) A synthetic molecule, derived from L-arginine
      (2) Has rapid onset of action, and steady-state levels are attained within 1 to 3 hours
      (3) Metabolized in the liver
      (4) The half-life is 40 to 50 minutes; prolonged in liver disease
    b. Lepirudin
      (1) A recombinant hirudin analogue
      (2) Acts rapidly
      (3) Cleared by kidneys
      (4) The half-life is 1.3 hours; markedly prolonged in renal failure
    c. Bivalirudin
      (1) A synthetic analogue of recombinant hirudin
      (2) Acts within 2 minutes given IV, and peak plasma bivalirudin levels occur within 2 hours of SC doses
      (3) Elimination of bivalirudin is predominantly via metabolic clearance; approximately 20% of a dose is excreted unchanged in the urine
      (4) The plasma half-life of IV bivalirudin is 25 minutes
    d. Ximelagatran
      (1) An oral prodrug of melagatran
      (2) Melagatran is a dipeptide and structurally resembles the sequence N-terminal to the thrombin cleavage site on the fibrinogen alpha chain
      (3) After oral intake and absorption, ximelagatran is rapidly and extensively metabolized to melagatran through hydrolysis and reduction
      (4) Half-life of melagatran is 2.5 to 4.3 hours
      (5) Melagatran is primarily excreted unchanged in urine

B. Indications
  1. Bivalirudin is approved for prevention of ischemic complications during coronary angioplasty
  2. Lepirudin and argatroban are indicated for anticoagulation in patients with HIT to prevent thromboembolic complications

3. Argatroban has additional indications of treatment of thrombosis associated with HIT and use in patients undergoing PCI who are at risk for or have HIT

4. Ximelagatran has no FDA-approved indication at the time of this writing; has been studied in VTE prophylaxis and stroke prevention in atrial fibrillation

C. Pathophysiology

   1. Mechanism of action
      a. Bind directly to the thrombin active site
      b. Inhibit thrombin-catalyzed activation of coagulation factors
      c. Inactivate both free and clot-bound thrombin
   2. Administration and monitoring of anticoagulation
      a. Argatroban
         (1) HIT
            (a) Continuous IV infusion initiated at 2 mcg/kg/min
            (b) Anticoagulation is monitored by aPTT 2 hours after initiation of therapy or dose change; the target is 1.5 to 3 times baseline, not to exceed 100 seconds
            (c) Reduce dose by 75% in hepatic insufficiency
            (d) Because argatroban prolongs INR, recommended transition when used with warfarin:
               (i) At doses up to 2 mcg/kg/min: stop argatroban when INR is above 4, repeat INR in 4 to 6 hours, and if INR is below the desired range, restart argatroban and repeat the procedure daily until therapeutic INR achieved
               (ii) At doses above 2 mcg/kg/min reduce argatroban dose temporarily to 2 mcg/kg/min, repeat INR in 4 to 6 hours and if over 4, follow the procedure above
         (2) PCI
            (a) Bolus of 350 mcg/kg/min and infusion at 25 mcg/kg/min
            (b) Monitored by ACT 5 to 10 minutes after the bolus and every 20 to 30 minutes
            (c) Additional boluses and infusion rate adjustments may be needed to achieve target ACT of 300 to 450 seconds
   3. Lepirudin
      a. Dose with a bolus of 0.4 mg/kg (up to 110 kg), followed by a continuous infusion at 0.15 mg/kg
      b. Anticoagulation is monitored by aPTT 4 hours after initiation of infusion or change of infusion rate, and at least daily thereafter; the target is aPTT-to-control ratio of 1.5 to 2.5
      c. Any aPTT ratio out of range should be confirmed by repeating, before dose adjustment, unless urgent reasons to react
      d. For aPTT ratio above the target range, stop the infusion for 2 hours and restart at rate reduced by 50% without a bolus
      e. For aPTT ratio below the target, increase the infusion by 20%
      f. The infusion rate of 0.21 mg/kg should not, in general, be exceeded
      g. The dose needs to be reduced in patients with renal insufficiency
      h. Between 40% and 70% of patients treated for more than 5 days develop nonneutralizing antilepirudin antibodies that decrease renal clearance of the drug and result in a lower dose requirement
   4. Bivalirudin
      a. Bolus of 1 mg/kg followed by a continuous infusion of 2.5 mg/kg per hour for 4 hours, and if needed, an additional IV infusion of bivalirudin 0.2 mg/kg per hour for up to 20 hours
      b. Subcutaneous doses of 1 mg/kg every 8 hours have been given for DVT prophylaxis in orthopedic surgery patients (not an approved indication)
   5. Reversal of anticoagulation
      a. No specific antidote to either agent is available
      b. Discontinuation of the drug and supportive measures are recommended

D. Complications
  1. Bleeding
      a. Appears not to be higher than in a control HIT group (5% to 15%)
      b. Intracranial hemorrhage incidence when used with thrombolytics was 0.6% to 1%, compared to 0% with DTIs used alone

VIII. WARFARIN

A. General principles
  1. A chemically synthesized racemic mixture of two optically active enantiomers, S-warfarin is five times more potent than R-warfarin
  2. Rapidly absorbed from the gastrointestinal tract, and circulates 99% bound to plasma albumin
  3. Prolongation of PT usually occurs within 48 hours, but effective anticoagulation not until several days later
  4. Metabolized in the liver
  5. Has a half-life of 36 to 42 hours
B. Indications
  1. Atrial fibrillation
  2. VTE
  3. Cardiac valve replacement
  4. After MI
C. Pathophysiology
  1. Mechanism of action
      a. Inhibits the postribosomal γ-carboxylation of the glutamic acid in the vitamin K–dependent factors (II, VII, IX, X, protein C and S)
      b. The reflection of the depletion of factor VII is prolongation of the PT
  2. Administration and monitoring of anticoagulation
      a. Loading dose usually not recommended
      b. Maintenance dose depending on metabolism, diet, concurrent medications
      c. The INR is used for anticoagulation monitoring (standardizes different thromboplastin preparations used for PT measurement)
      d. INR of 2 to 3 is therapeutic for most indications
         (1) Artificial valves require INR of 2.5 to 3.5
         (2) High-intensity anticoagulation (INR 3 to 4) for antiphospholipid antibody syndrome not better than moderate intensity (INR 2 to 3)
      e. Duration of anticoagulation
         (1) For thrombosis provoked by a major reversible risk factor such as surgery, venous catheter: 3 months
         (2) For unprovoked, "idiopathic" VTE or associated with a nonreversible risk factor such as active cancer: 6 months or indefinite anticoagulant therapy is indicated
            (i) Continuing anticoagulation beyond 6 months resulted in a 95% reduction in the risk of recurrent venous thromboembolism, at a cost of 4% rate of bleeding per patient-year
            (ii) Conventional-intensity warfarin therapy is more effective than low-intensity warfarin therapy for the long-term prevention of recurrent VTE. The low-intensity warfarin regimen INR (1.5 to 1.9) does not reduce the risk of clinically important bleeding
  3. Reversal of anticoagulation
      a. Warfarin withdrawal
         (1) INR will decrease from therapeutic to completely reversed after 3 to 5 days
         (2) The best option for the majority of nonbleeding patients with INR in 4.5 to 6.9 range, considering the balance of risks of bleeding versus thrombosis
         (3) The risk of bleeding rises exponentially when INR is above 6.9, and warfarin withdrawal alone is not appropriate in such situations
      b. Vitamin K

(1) Oral vitamin K is more effective than SC. The dose of 1 to 3 mg will decrease INR to at least therapeutic range within 24 hours in the majority of patients.

(2) IV administration results in a rapid correction of anticoagulation, with effect on PT within 4 to 6 hours and provides 70% of its INR correction within 8 hours

    (a) The dose of 0.5 to 1 mg is used to bring INR to the therapeutic range

    (b) In bleeding patients, dose of 5 mg is cited to be the most useful by some authors, but 10 mg is frequently used

  c. Coagulation factors replacement

    (1) Fresh frozen plasma (FFP)

      (a) For urgent anticoagulation reversal, recommended dose is provided in **Chapter 94**

      (b) Repeat every 6 hours (the half-life of factor VII), or administer concurrent vitamin K IV

      (c) Large volume is required; may cause fluid overload

    (2) Prothrombin complex concentrates (PCC)

      (a) Different commercial preparations have wide variation of the coagulation factors content (II, VII, IX, X)

      (b) The advantage over FFP is less volume required

      (c) May predispose to thrombosis

    (3) Recombinant human factor VIIa concentrate

      (a) Off-label use, supported by recent literature, should be directed by a hematologist

      (b) Doses of 15 to 20 mcg/kg (versus 90 mcg/kg for hemophilia) have been effective

      (c) May be administered very rapidly (over 3 to 5 minutes)

      (d) Clinical efficacy does not correlate with prothrombin time

D. Complications

  1. Bleeding

    a. The annual risk is 0.6% for fatal bleeding, 3% for major hemorrhage, and 10% for minor events

    b. The incidence of bleeding is directly proportional to the intensity of anticoagulation and time spent at a high INR

  2. Warfarin-induced skin necrosis

    a. Results from an imbalance of vitamin K–dependent procoagulants (prothrombin complex) and anticoagulant proteins (protein C and S)

    b. Associated with heterozygous protein C deficiency (only in one third of cases), acquired functional protein C deficiency, protein S deficiency, factor V Leiden mutation, antiphospholipid antibodies

    c. The incidence related to high (>10 mg) loading doses of warfarin

    d. Occurs during first few days of the warfarin therapy

    e. Cutaneous vessels become occluded by fibrin thrombi

    f. Erythematous macules appear over breasts, trunk, extremities, penis, and marginate, and become edematous over period of hours and eventually become necrotic

    g. Treated with administration of a protein C–containing product

IX. THROMBOLYTIC THERAPY

A. General principles

  1. Urokinase

    a. An enzyme obtained from human neonatal kidney cells grown in tissue culture

    b. Rapidly cleared by the liver, with elimination half-life of 12 minutes

    c. Activates both fibrin-bound and circulating fibrinogen, resulting in systemic fibrinolysis (is not fibrin specific)

  2. Alteplase

    a. A human tissue plasminogen activator (tPA)

    b. Produced by recombinant DNA technology from genetically modified Chinese hamster ovary cells

    c. Has a half-life in plasma of 5 minutes, but because of fibrin binding the effect can persist for up to 1 hour

    d. Is fibrin–specific; binds to fibrin in a thrombus, producing local thrombolysis, with relatively little systemic effect

  3. Reteplase

    a. A genetically engineered nonglycosylated mutant of tPA, containing only the second kringle and catalytic domains

    b. Produced by recombinant DNA technology in *E. coli*

    c. Has a half-life of 13 to 16 minutes

    d. Is fibrin specific, but less so than alteplase

  4. Tenecteplase

    a. A modified human tPA

    b. Produced by recombinant DNA technology from genetically modified Chinese hamster ovary cells

    c. Has a terminal phase half-life of 90 to 130 minutes

    d. Is more fibrin specific than alteplase

B. Indications

  1. Urokinase

    a. Is approved for the lysis of massive (lobar or multiple segments) pulmonary emboli (PE), and PE with hemodynamic instability; no longer approved for acute MI or central venous access device (CVAD) clearance

    b. Off-label use for CVAD occlusions

  2. Alteplase is approved for:

    a. Acute MI

    b. Acute ischemic stroke within 3 hours of the onset of symptoms

    c. Massive PE (lobar or multiple segments), with or without hemodynamic instability

    d. Clearance of occluded CVAD

  3. Reteplase

    a. Approved for acute MI

    b. Off-label use for pulmonary embolism

  4. Tenecteplase is approved for acute MI

C. Pathophysiology

  1. Mechanism of action

    a. Thrombolytics catalyze cleavage of endogenous plasminogen to generate plasmin, except for streptokinase, which activates plasminogen via an intermediate step.

    b. Plasmin degrades the fibrin matrix of the thrombus.

  2. Administration and monitoring of anticoagulation

    a. Urokinase

      (1) Pulmonary embolism: loading dose, 4,400 IU/kg IV over 10 minutes, followed by continuous infusion, 4,400 IU/kg/hr IV for 12 hours

      (2) Occluded catheter: 5,000 IU instilled into occluded catheter, up to two doses may be used

      (3) Coagulation tests and measures of fibrinolytic activity do not reliably predict either efficacy or risk of bleeding in patients receiving urokinase.

        (i) Obtain aPTT, PT, hematocrit, and platelet count before starting thrombolytic therapy.

        (ii) If heparin has been given it should be discontinued and the aPTT should be less than twice the normal control value before thrombolytic therapy is started.

        (iii) After urokinase administration, anticoagulation treatment (if indicated) should be started after the aPTT has decreased to two times the normal control value.

    b. Alteplase

      (1) Acute myocardial infarction: Accelerated infusion: patients over 67 kg, total dose 100 mg IV, give 15 mg IV bolus, 50 mg over 30 minutes, then 35 mg over 60 minutes

(2) Acute myocardial infarction: Accelerated infusion: patients 67 kg or less, 15 mg IV bolus, then 0.75 mg/kg over 30 minutes, then 0.50 mg/kg over 60 minutes

(3) Acute myocardial infarction: 3-hour infusion: weight 65 kg or more, 60 mg IV in the first hour (6 to 10 mg of which to be given as bolus), 20 mg over the second hour, and 20 mg over the third hour

(4) Acute myocardial infarction: 3-hour infusion: weight less than 65 kg, 1.25 mg/kg IV administered over 3 hours, give 60% in the first hour (10% of which to be given as bolus), give remaining 40% over the next 2 hours

(5) Acute ischemic stroke: 0.9 mg/kg IV (*not* to exceed 90 mg), infused over 60 minutes with 10% of the dose given as an initial bolus over 1 minute

(6) Pulmonary embolism: 100 mg IV infused over 2 hours; heparin should be instituted near the end of or immediately following the infusion when the PTT or thrombin time returns to twice normal or less

(7) Central venous catheter occlusion: in patients 10 kg to 29 kg, 1 mg/mL, dose equal to 110% of catheter lumen volume, maximum of 2 mL; in patients 30 kg or greater: 2 mg/2 mL instilled into occluded catheter, up to two doses may be used

(8) When used for acute MI and pulmonary embolism, alteplase is given concurrently with heparin (unlike urokinase or streptokinase); activated clotting time (ACT) may be used to guide heparin dosing

c. Reteplase
   (1) Acute myocardial infarction: 10 unit IV bolus, two doses given 30 minutes apart
   (2) Pulmonary embolism: 10 unit IV bolus, two doses given 30 minutes apart

d. Tenecteplase. Acute myocardial infarction: single IV bolus over 5 seconds; less than 60 kg, 30 mg; 60 to 69 kg, 35 mg; 70 to 79 kg, 40 mg; 80 to 89 kg, 45 mg; 90 kg or above, 50 mg

3. Reversal of anticoagulation
   a. No specific antidote is available.
   b. Plasmin inhibitors (tranexamic acid or epsilon-aminocaproic acid) may be considered for major bleeding.
   c. If heparin was administered concurrently, protamine reversal may be considered.
   d. Cryoprecipitate may be used if fibrinogen levels are less than 100 mg/dL.

D. Complications
   1. Bleeding
      a. Incidence varies depending on the indication, concomitant therapy, and procedures.
      b. Contraindications and precautions should be strictly observed (published elsewhere).
      c. The incidence of hemorrhagic stroke in MI patients was 0.7% for alteplase, 0.8% for reteplase, and 0.9% for tenecteplase.
      d. In patients treated with alteplase for ischemic stroke, the incidence of hemorrhagic stroke was 15.4% versus 6.4% for placebo.
   2. Cholesterol embolization (rare)
   3. Allergic reactions: in 1% to 4% of patients receiving streptokinase; under 1% for other agents
   4. Hypotension: not secondary to bleeding or anaphylaxis

Selected Readings

Alving BM. How I treat heparin-induced thrombocytopenia and thrombosis. *Blood* 2003;101: 31–37.
   A review article about managing HIT.

Crowther MA, Ginsberg JS, Julian J, et al. A comparison of two intensities of warfarin for the prevention of recurrent thrombosis in patients with the antiphospholipid antibody syndrome. *N Engl J Med* 2003;349:1133–1138.
   A prospective study, suggesting that moderate-intensity warfarin (INR 2 to 3) is appropriate for patients with the antiphospholipid antibody syndrome and venous thrombosis.

Deveras RA, Kessler CM. Reversal of warfarin-induced excessive anticoagulation with recombinant human factor VIIa concentrate. *Ann Intern Med* 2002;137:884–888.
An article describing clinical experience of managing bleeding, overanticoagulated patients with recombinant factor VIIa.

Geerts WH, Heit JA, Clagett GP, et al. Prevention of venous thromboembolism. *Chest* 2001;119:132S–175S.
Review of the literature related to the risks and prevention of VTE.

Hamm CW. Anti-integrin therapy. *Ann Rev Med* 2003;54:425–435.
A broad review of the three available platelet glycoprotein IIb-IIIa inhibitors, including their therapeutic utility and limitations and their toxicity (bleeding and thrombocytopenia). Fine-tuning the heparin therapy appears to be the best way to decrease bleeding while maintaining efficacy.

Kearon C, Ginsberg JS, Kovacs MJ, et al. Comparison of low-intensity warfarin therapy with conventional-intensity warfarin therapy for long-term prevention of recurrent venous thrombo-embolism. *N Engl J Med* 2003;349:631–639.
Conventional-intensity warfarin therapy (INR 2 to 3) is more effective than low-intensity warfarin therapy (INR 1.5 to 1.9) for the long-term prevention of recurrent venous thrombo-embolism. The low-intensity warfarin regimen does not reduce the risk of clinically important bleeding.

Konstantinides S. Should thrombolytic therapy be used in patients with pulmonary embolism? *Am J Cardiovasc Drugs* 2004;4:69–74.
Review of recent data on the use of thrombolysis in pulmonary embolism.

Levine GN, Ali MN, Schafer AI. Antithrombotic therapy in patients with acute coronary syndromes. *Arch Intern Med* 2001;161:937–948.
A summary review of clinical trial data.

Makris M, Watson HG. The management of coumarin-induced over-anticoagulation. *Br J Haematol* 2001;114:271–280.
A comprehensive review of the topic.

Ridker PM, Goldhaber SZ, Danielson E, et al. Long-term, low-intensity warfarin therapy for the prevention of recurrent venous thromboembolism. *N Engl J Med* 2003;348:1425–1434.
Long-term, low-intensity warfarin (INR 1.5 to 2.0) was associated with a 48% reduction in the composite end point of recurrent venous thromboembolism, major hemorrhage, or death.

I. GENERAL PRINCIPLES

A. Hypercoagulable states, also referred to as thrombophilia, are hereditary or acquired disorders that significantly increase the risk of thrombosis by altering the normal hemostatic balance toward inappropriate clot formation.

B. Secondary hypercoagulable states include a variety of acquired or situational conditions that are associated with thromboembolic complications.

C. Venous thromboembolism (VTE), including deep venous thrombosis (DVT) and pulmonary embolism (PE), affects roughly 2 million people in the United States annually, with incidence rates ranging from 1 per 10,000 in young adulthood to greater than 1 per 1,000 in the seventh decade of life.

D. Many, if not most, venous thrombotic events occur in the setting of multiple prothrombotic stimuli that may include a well-defined clinical risk factor in addition to a primary or secondary hypercoagulable state.

E. Clinical risk factors for VTE include:

  1. Strong risk factors (odds ratio >10)

    a. Major general surgery

    b. Hip or knee replacement

    c. Fracture of the lower extremity

    d. Major trauma

    e. Spinal cord injury

  2. Moderate risk factors (odds ratio 2 to 9)

    a. Central venous catheter

    b. Arthroscopic knee surgery

    c. Congestive heart failure or respiratory failure

    d. Paralytic stroke

    e. Previous VTE

  3. Weak risk factors (odds ratio <2)

    a. Bed rest longer than 3 days

    b. Immobility due to sitting (e.g., prolonged air or car travel)

    c. Increasing age

    d. Obesity

    e. Laparoscopic surgery

    f. Varicose veins

F. Arterial thrombotic events most commonly occur in the setting of underlying atherosclerotic disease and acute platelet activation (e.g., diseased coronary or internal carotid arteries leading to myocardial infarction or ischemic stroke, respectively), peripheral vascular disease and cardiac sources of thromboemboli.

II. ETIOLOGY

A. Inherited primary hypercoagulable states include a number of disorders that range from common genetic polymorphisms (among Caucasians) associated with low relative risks of thrombosis to more rare mutations with high risks.

B. Most genetic conditions are autosomal dominant, such that heterozygous carriers are susceptible to complications. Exceptions include hyperhomocysteinemia, in which homocysteine levels are affected by oral intake of folate, B_6, and B_{12}, and persistent elevation of factor VIII coagulant activity, for which the underlying genetic cause is undefined.

1. Weakly thrombogenic disorders, relative risk (RR) of VTE and prevalence in Caucasians:
   a. Factor II (prothrombin) G20210A mutation; threefold RR; 3% prevalence
   b. Factor V G1691A mutation (factor V Leiden; associated with activated protein C [APC] resistance); threefold to sixfold RR; 3% to 5% prevalence
   c. Hyperhomocysteinemia; twofold to threefold RR; prevalence unknown
   d. Persistent, unexplained elevation of factor VIII coagulant activity; threefold to sixfold RR; prevalence unknown
2. Rare and/or strongly thrombogenic disorders, RR of VTE and prevalence:
   a. Protein C deficiency; sevenfold RR; 0.3% prevalence
   b. Protein S deficiency; up to 12-fold RR; 0.02% prevalence
   c. Antithrombin III (AT III) deficiency; up to 20-fold RR; 0.02% prevalence
   d. Dysfibrinogenemia; unknown relative risk; rare cases/families reported
3. Disorders of unclear clinical significance (data currently inconclusive):
   a. Elevated levels of factor IX, factor XI, fibrinogen, lipoprotein (a) or thrombin activatable fibrinolysis inhibitor (TAFI)
   b. Decreased levels of free tissue factor pathway inhibitor or plasminogen
   c. Genetic polymorphisms affecting factor VII, factor XIII, fibrinolytic mediators or platelet membrane glycoproteins

C. Antiphospholipid antibody (APLA) syndrome is an important acquired primary hypercoagulable state, occurring sporadically or with rheumatologic disorders.
   1. APLA syndrome refers to venous and/or arterial thrombosis associated with antibodies against phospholipid-binding proteins and/or antibodies that exhibit lupus anticoagulant (inhibitor) activity. Additional features may include thrombocytopenia, recurrent fetal loss, and livedo reticularis.
   2. APLAs include anticardiolipin antibodies (ACLAs; IgG, IgM, or IgA), anti-beta-2-glycoprotein I (anti-β2GPI), antiprothrombin, and others.
   3. Although APLAs usually occur in association with lupus anticoagulant activity, these antibodies are not identical and may occur separately.
   4. Nonspecific ACLAs are detectable in 5% to 10% of healthy adults. IgM, IgA, and low-titer IgG may be transiently induced by infections or drugs, and such cases are not associated with thrombotic risk.
   5. APLAs and/or lupus anticoagulant occur in 12% to 30% of patients with systemic lupus erythematosus, and carry a 50% to 70% risk of thrombosis.
   6. Thrombosis risk in patients with APLAs but without rheumatic disease is undefined and unpredictable, but clinical events are usually associated with high-titer IgG ACLA, anti-β2GPI, and/or lupus anticoagulant activity.
   7. APLA syndrome is implicated in 10% of unexplained VTE cases.
   8. Arterial events associated with APLA syndrome include stroke, myocardial infarction, and peripheral arterial thromboemboli.
   9. Catastrophic APLA syndrome refers to rapidly progressive, fulminant, multisystem vascular occlusion associated with high-titer APLAs.

D. Secondary hypercoagulable states include:
   1. Pregnancy/puerperium
   2. Female sex hormones (contraceptives, hormone replacement)
   3. Cancer (especially gastrointestinal adenocarcinomas and brain tumors)
   4. Chemotherapy or hormonal therapy for cancer
   5. Myeloproliferative disorders with elevated red cell mass (i.e., polycythemia vera) and/or elevated abnormal platelets (i.e., essential thrombocythemia)
   6. Paroxysmal nocturnal hemoglobinuria (PNH)
   7. Inflammatory bowel disease
   8. Nephrotic syndrome
   9. Disseminated intravascular coagulation (DIC) and sepsis
   10. Heparin-induced thrombocytopenia (HIT) with thrombosis (HITT)

E. Initial VTE events with weakly thrombogenic inherited disorders often occur in the setting of an additional acquired or situational prothrombotic risk factor (e.g., during pregnancy in a woman with heterozygous factor V Leiden).

F. Combined disorders impart a high risk of VTE and recurrence, and include:
   1. Homozygous alleles for factor V Leiden or for the factor II mutation
   2. Multiple inherited disorders (e.g., factor V Leiden and protein C deficiency)
   3. APLA syndrome in a patient with an inherited disorder
   4. A secondary hypercoagulable state plus a primary hypercoagulable state
   5. Central venous catheter–associated thrombosis related to factor V Leiden or factor II mutation.

III. PATHOPHYSIOLOGY

A. Normal hemostasis is controlled by endothelial cell products, platelets, circulating and clot-bound procoagulants, natural anticoagulants (including the APC complex and AT III), and fibrinolytic mediators.

B. Primary hypercoagulable states affect single or multiple steps in hemostasis:
   1. Factor II mutation leads to elevated factor II level and procoagulant activity.
   2. Factor V Leiden (APC resistance) is associated with reduced site-specific cleavage and inactivation of activated factor V (Va) by APC.
   3. Hyperhomocysteinemia causes endothelial cell and vascular dysfunction.
   4. Persistent factor VIII elevation putatively leads to factor VIII overactivity.
   5. Protein C deficiency impairs the anticoagulant activity of the APC complex.
   6. Protein S deficiency impairs the anticoagulant activity of the APC complex.
   7. AT III deficiency impairs the anticoagulant activity of AT III.
   8. Dysfibrinogenemia leads to the formation of fibrin clot that is structurally abnormal and less susceptible to fibrinolysis.
   9. APLAs induce prothrombotic effects on platelets and endothelial cells and appear to impair certain natural anticoagulants and fibrinolytic mediators.

C. Secondary hypercoagulable states and clinical VTE risk factors may cause:
   1. Slow blood flow and enhanced coagulation (CHF, immobilization, tumor)
   2. A prothrombotic imbalance of procoagulants and natural anticoagulants (female sex hormones, pregnancy, cancer, nephrotic syndrome)
   3. Activation of procoagulants and platelets (cancer, sepsis and DIC, inflammatory bowel disease, HITT, trauma, surgery)
   4. Hyperviscosity and/or platelet activation (myeloproliferative disorders)

IV. DIAGNOSIS

A. Clinical presentation

1. Venous system thrombotic complications predominantly occur in patients with inherited and acquired primary hypercoagulable states.
   a. DVT and/or PE
   b. Thrombosis in unusual anatomic locations:
      (1) Hepatic vein (Budd-Chiari syndrome)
      (2) Portal, splenic, and/or mesenteric veins
      (3) Axillary vein (in the presence or absence of a central venous catheter)
      (4) Cerebral veins
   c. Recurrent superficial thrombosis (always consider occult cancer)
   d. Initial VTE is often associated with an additional acquired/situational risk factor (e.g., oral contraceptives, pregnancy, postsurgical immobilization)
2. Multiple (≥ 3) spontaneous early trimester abortions or a single late abortion
3. Arterial thromboembolic events are not commonly associated with primary or secondary hypercoagulable states. Exceptions include:
   a. APLA syndrome and catastrophic APLA syndrome
   b. Moderate-severe hyperhomocysteinemia (or homocysteinuria)
   c. Occasional patients with protein S deficiency or dysfibrinogenemia
   d. Cancer (including emboli secondary to marantic endocarditis)
   e. Myeloproliferative disorders and PNH
   f. HITT and DIC
4. Suspect HITT or DIC in a critically ill or postsurgical patient with thrombocytopenia and new or progressive VTE or arterial thrombosis.

B. Laboratory studies

1. Standard diagnostic algorithms that utilize pretest and posttest probabilities, imaging modalities and D-dimer levels are useful to evaluate for suspected VTE in patients with hypercoagulable states. Additional considerations:

   a. Some D-dimer assays have low specificity for cancer-associated VTE.

   b. Tumor-related compression/infiltration may obscure vascular imaging studies.

   c. Paradoxical emboli, through a patent foramen ovale, should be evaluated in patients with cerebral arterial events and a history of prior DVT or PE.

2. Thorough physical examination and general laboratory screening are required to rule out disorders associated with secondary hypercoagulable states.

   a. Urinalysis to assess for nephrotic syndrome

   b. Complete blood counts to assess for myeloproliferative disorders

   c. Age-appropriate physical examination (including rectal, prostate, pelvic, and breast examinations), chest radiography, and general chemistries to assess for occult malignancy

   d. Extensive screening for occult cancer is not indicated, except with specific signs or symptoms (e.g., unexplained weight loss, hemoptysis, melena).

3. The laboratory assessment for a suspected primary hypercoagulable state is based on a risk-stratification schema (Fig. 98-1).

   a. Higher-risk patients should undergo a full evaluation for both common and rare genetic and acquired disorders. These disorders often present as spontaneous (unprovoked) events at a younger age.

   b. Lower-risk patients should be evaluated for the common and weakly thrombogenic hereditary disorders and for APLA syndrome.

4. Although some of the laboratory assays can be obtained and reliably interpreted at the time of the acute event, a number of limitations and confounding factors must be considered during the evaluation (Table 98-1).

   a. Assays for factor VIII coagulant activity and free protein S antigen activity should be delayed for many weeks after the acute event. Acute inflammation can secondarily increase factor VIII levels (as an acute-phase response) and may decrease free protein S (because free protein S is complexed with C4b-binding protein, an acute phase protein).

   b. C-reactive protein (CRP) level should always be obtained with the factor VIII assay, as an internal control for inflammation. An unexplained elevation of factor VIII coagulant activity (i.e., >150%) should be reevaluated (with CRP) to confirm a positive result.

   c. Warfarin decreases the activity levels of protein S and protein C (both are vitamin K–dependent factors), whereas AT III activity is lowered by heparins.

   d. Other confounding factors are listed in Table 98-1.

5. APLAs found in patients with thrombosis should be confirmed as positive, persistent, and likely causally associated by repeating the assays in 6 weeks.

6. Laboratory screening of asymptomatic adult relatives of a patient with a confirmed hereditary disorder is indicated to identify carriers at risk and their need for aggressive prophylaxis and monitoring during prothrombotic situations.

7. Screening of children at risk of inheriting a genetic disorder can be deferred until after age 14, because of the very low risk of a VTE in an affected child.

V. TREATMENT

A. Initial therapy of thrombotic event

1. Initial therapy of patients with hypercoagulable states and an acute VTE or arterial event is similar to the treatment for general medical-surgical patients with thrombosis.

   a. Intravenous infusion of unfractionated heparin (UFH), to maintain the activated partial thromboplastin time (aPTT) at 1.5 to 2 times control, or therapeutic doses of low-molecular-weight heparin (LMWH)

   (1) Patients with AT III deficiency often require very high doses of UFH to maintain the aPTT in the therapeutic range. Antithrombin concentrate is available and indicated for patients who are resistant to UFH and/or

Higher-Risk Patients

- Unprovoked VTE at <45 y.o.

- Multiple VTE events

- Strong family history of VTE

- Poor obstetric history (≥3 early abortions or single late trimester abortion)

- Single life-threatening event or thrombosis in an unusual anatomic site

- History of rheumatologic or autoimmune disease (suspect APLA syndrome)

⬇

- APC resistance (APCR) assay (clotting assay)

- DNA test for factor V Leiden (as an alternative to the APCR test or to confirm the genotype in a patient with an abnormal APCR result)

- DNA test for factor II G20210A mutation

- Plasma homocysteine level

- Factor VIII coagulant activity (chromogenic assay) with C-reactive protein assay (as a control for inflammation-induced factor VIII elevation)

- APLA serology panel (including anti-β2GPI) and lupus anticoagulant (clotting assay)

- Protein C activity assay

- Protein S activity assay and/or free protein S antigen level

- AT III activity assay

- Fibrinogen functional assay (thrombin time or kinetic fibrinogen assay)

Lower-Risk Patients

- Unprovoked VTE at ≥45 y. o.

- VTE at <45 y.o. during pregnancy or on oral contraceptives

- A predisposed event at < 45 y. o. with a prior history of VTE or strong family history

⬇

  - APC resistance (APCR) assay (clotting assay)

  - DNA test for factor V Leiden (as an alternative to the APCR test or to confirm the genotype in a patient with an abnormal APCR result)

  - DNA test for factor II G20210A mutation

  - Plasma homocysteine level

  - Factor VIII coagulant activity (chromogenic assay) with C-reactive protein assay (as a control for inflammation-induced factor VIII elevation)

  - APLA serology panel (including anti-β2GPI) and lupus anticoagulant (clotting assay)

Figure 98-1. Risk-stratified laboratory evaluations of patients with suspected primary hypercoagulable states. VTE, venous thromboembolism; y.o., years old.

TABLE 98-1	Clinical and Pharmacological Factors that can Affect the Results and Interpretation of Hypercoagulable Laboratory Evaluations
Confounding factor	**Affected laboratory test**
Heparin	AT III activity (↓)
Warfarin	Protein C activity (↓), protein S activity (↓)
Liver disease	AT III (↓), protein C (↓), protein S (↓)
Nephrotic syndrome	AT III (↓), ±protein S (↓)
Inflammation, AIDS	Factor VIII coagulant (↑), protein S (↓)
DIC	AT III (↓), protein C (↓), ±protein S (↓)
Estrogens	APC resistance assay (↑), factor VIII (↑), protein S (↓)

DIC, disseminated intravascular coagulopathy.

have recurrent thrombosis, severe thrombosis, and for those requiring prophylaxis when heparin is contraindicated.

(2) In patients with APLA syndrome and lupus anticoagulant activity that affects the baseline aPTT, the aPTT values during UFH therapy are unreliable because of the confounding effect of the lupus anticoagulant. Therefore, monitoring of UFH therapy must be accomplished by either assaying plasma heparin levels (therapeutic range corresponds to anti-factor Xa activity levels of 0.3 to 0.7 IU/mL) or by using a lupus-insensitive aPTT reagent. An alternative approach is to use therapeutic doses of LMWH rather than UFH.

(3) UFH and LMWH are safe and the agents of choice in pregnant women with acute thrombosis. Warfarin is teratogenic and therefore avoided.

(4) LMWH therapy should be monitored in patients with renal disease, pregnancy, and morbid obesity (conditions that could affect levels) and the dose adjusted to maintain the anti-Xa level at 0.6 to 1 IU/mL at 4 hours after a twice-daily dose or 1 to 2 IU/mL after a once-daily dose.

(5) The platelet count should be monitored while on UFH and LMWH, and HIT suspected when the platelet count falls to <100,000/mL or less than 50% below baseline within 5 to 10 days (in the absence of other etiology) and/or with progressive or new thrombosis on therapeutic heparin.

b. Warfarin should be introduced early (at initial presentation, if low risk of bleeding) and the dose adjusted to achieve a stable international normalized ratio (INR) of 2 to 3 for 48 hours prior to discontinuing heparin.

(1) Warfarin is teratogenic and, therefore, contraindicated in the first trimester of pregnancy.

(2) Warfarin should be started at a low dose (e.g., 2 mg/day) and slowly increased in patients with protein C deficiency or protein S deficiency, to avoid the complication of warfarin-induced skin necrosis.

(3) Arterial thromboemboli associated with APLA syndrome may require higher-intensity warfarin (e.g., an INR at 2.5 to 3.5) to prevent recurrence (this is controversial).

2. Thrombolytic therapy (catheter directed) should be considered for limb-threatening DVT or PE associated with hemodynamic compromise and right ventricular (RV) dysfunction. Thrombolysis cannot otherwise be routinely recommended because of the high risk of hemorrhage and lack of data showing superiority over heparin therapy in preventing postthrombotic syndrome (PTS) or PE after DVT.

3. Central venous catheter–associated superior vena caval thrombosis requires catheter removal, heparin therapy, and, in some cases, thrombolysis. Nonocclusive thrombosis of the subclavian, innominate, or peripheral veins can often be treated successfully with heparin while retaining the catheter.

B. Contraindications to anticoagulation

1. Absolute contraindications:
   a. Active bleeding
   b. Severe bleeding diathesis or coagulopathy
   c. Platelet count equal to or less than $20,000/\mu L$ and unsupportable with platelet transfusions
   d. Recent (within 10 days) neurosurgery, ocular surgery, or intracranial bleed

2. Relative contraindications:
   a. Mild to moderate bleeding diathesis or thrombocytopenia
   b. Recent major trauma or abdominal surgery (within 2 days)
   c. Recent gastrointestinal or genitourinary bleeding (within 14 days)
   d. Multiple brain metastases
   e. Severe hypertension (systolic >200 mm Hg or diastolic >120 mm Hg)

3. Alternative management includes placement of an inferior vena cava (IVC) filter to prevent PE with acute lower extremity DVT. IVC filter is also indicated with recurrent PE despite optimal anticoagulation for lower extremity DVT.

C. Ongoing therapy

1. Warfarin is dose adjusted to maintain the INR at 2 to 3. Although lower-intensity warfarin, to maintain the INR at 1.5 to 2, is superior to placebo for secondary prophylaxis at greater than 3 months after VTE, this level of anticoagulation is inferior to an INR of 2 to 3 when extended for more than 6 months after VTE.

2. Therapeutic-dose LMWH may be given safely throughout pregnancy and is the agent of choice for women with pregnancy-associated VTE.

3. Therapeutic-dose LMWH may be given chronically to patients who are either intolerant of warfarin or who have recurrent events on warfarin (e.g., with cancer-associated VTE). Bone mineral density studies should be obtained periodically (e.g., annually) to assess for heparin-induced osteoporosis.

4. Compression stockings may reduce the incidence of chronic PTS after lower extremity DVT; they are also helpful for PTS symptom management.

D. Duration of anticoagulation

1. The decision to stop or continue therapeutic anticoagulation is based on the relative risks of bleeding weighed against the risks of recurrence.

2. The risk of recurrence after VTE relates to the presence of additional prothrombotic factors at the time of the initial event, the number of previous events, the specific hypercoagulable state(s) and their associated recurrence risks, and the presence of residual PTS.

3. In patients without a strongly thrombogenic hypercoagulable state, VTE recurs in roughly 31% of men and 9% of women within 5 years after a first event. Multiple factors affect the risk and decision to continue anticoagulation in these patients.
   a. A first uncomplicated VTE (i.e., without PTS) provoked by a major transient risk factor (e.g., major surgery, major medical illness, leg casting) has a low risk of recurrence; thus, 3 months of conventional anticoagulant therapy is adequate for secondary prophylaxis.
   b. A first idiopathic event or one provoked by a minor transient risk (e.g., oral contraceptives) requires at least 6 to 12 months of full anticoagulation. Longer duration of treatment (≥ 2 years) is recommended with persistent D-dimer elevation, PTS, or venous insufficiency on follow-up duplex study.
   c. Patients with multiple idiopathic VTEs or persistent significant risk (e.g., severe PTS) should receive therapeutic anticoagulation indefinitely.
   d. Patients with heterozygous factor V Leiden, heterozygous factor II mutation, hyperhomocysteinemia, or a reversible secondary hypercoagulable state (e.g., treated cancer or pregnancy) have a low risk of recurrence after a single uncomplicated event (without PTS); therefore, 6 to 12 months of full anticoagulation may be adequate. Longer duration treatment should be considered with persistent venous or D-dimer abnormalities and/or after an unprovoked VTE event.

4. A higher risk of recurrence after a first event is associated with persistent factor VIII elevation, protein C deficiency, protein S deficiency, or residual venous insufficiency; thus, extended anticoagulation ($\geq$12 to 18 months) should be considered.

5. The risk of recurrent VTE is very high after a single event in patients with AT III deficiency, dysfibrinogenemia, multiple hypercoagulable states, or APLA syndrome; thus, anticoagulation should be continued indefinitely.

6. The risk of recurrence is also very high after two or more spontaneous events in patients with any hypercoagulable disorder; thus, anticoagulation should be continued indefinitely.

7. Indefinite anticoagulation is indicated after a single life-threatening event or thrombosis in an unusual site (e.g., mesenteric or cerebral vein).

E. Prophylactic anticoagulation

1. LMWH or UFH should be given in high-risk situations (e.g., during surgery or prolonged immobilization) in an asymptomatic carrier (without prior VTE history) or in a patient with a prior VTE but currently off anticoagulation.

2. LMWH should be given during pregnancy and 6 weeks postpartum to a woman with recurrent fetal wastage or late miscarriage and either APLAs (combined with daily low-dose aspirin) or a genetic hypercoagulable state.

3. LMWH should be given during pregnancy and 6 weeks postpartum to women with a known hypercoagulable state and prior history of VTE (and currently off anticoagulation) or in asymptomatic women with known high-risk due to AT III deficiency or combined hereditary disorders.

VI. COMPLICATIONS

A. Pregnancy-associated complications of the APLA syndrome and many of the hereditary hypercoagulable states include:

1. Increased risk of VTE
2. Spontaneous early abortions and late-trimester miscarriages
3. Intrauterine growth retardation, placental abruption, and severe preeclampsia

B. Symptomatic PTS occurs in up to 20% of patients with DVT.

C. PE is estimated to contribute to 200,000 VTE-related deaths annually.

D. Treatment-related complications of VTE include anticoagulant-induced bleeding and HIT with or without thrombosis.

1. Bleeding occurs in 2% to 7% of patients during initial therapy with UFH.
2. Major bleeding occurs in roughly 1% during initial therapy with LMWH.
   (3) Major bleeding occurs in 1% of patients per year on standard warfarin.
3. HIT occurs in roughly 3% of patients receiving UFH and at a lower frequency among patients receiving LMWH.
   a. New or progressive venous or arterial thrombosis occurs in 10% to 40% of patients with HIT; therefore, continued anticoagulation is indicated.
   b. LMWH is not a suitable alternative anticoagulant for HIT because of cross-reactivity with antiheparin antibodies.
   c. Lepirudin, argatroban, and danaproid sodium are acceptable alternative anticoagulants for HIT in nonpregnant patients. Bivalirudin and fondaparinux are used off-label.
   d. For critically ill patients, argatroban or lepirudin offers the advantage of short half-life, if bleeding occurs. Argatroban (or danaproid) is preferred in patients with renal insufficiency (lepirudin is excreted by the kidneys), whereas lepirudin is preferred with liver dysfunction.
   e. The anticoagulant of choice in pregnant patients with HIT is undefined, but lepirudin and fondaparinux have been used anecdotally.

E. Chronic indwelling IVC filters placed for contraindications to anticoagulation are associated with a significant incidence of occlusion, PE, and recurrent DVT if anticoagulation cannot be reinstituted while the filter is in place.

Selected Readings

Alving BM. How I treat heparin-induced thrombocytopenia and thrombosis. *Blood* 2003; 101:31–37.
A concise summary of alternative anticoagulants and management approaches for heparin-induced thrombocytopenia in medical and surgical patients, including considerations for critically ill patients in the intensive care unit and patients undergoing dialysis, coronary artery bypass, or coronary interventional procedures.

Anderson FA Jr, Spencer FA. Risk factors for venous thromboembolism. *Circulation* 2003;107(23 suppl 1):I-9–I-16.
A comprehensive general review of clinical, situational, hereditary, and acquired pro-thrombotic risk factors.

Ansell JE, Weitz JI, Comerota AJ. Advances in therapy and the management of antithrombotic drugs for venous thromboembolism. *Hematology (Am Soc Hematol Educ Program)* 2000;266–284.
Contains a review of thrombolytic therapy for VTE that emphasizes the positive outcomes related to surrogate end points of radiographic improvement and quality-of-life symptomatic relief.

Bates SM, Ginsberg JS. Treatment of deep-vein thrombosis. *N Engl J Med* 2004;351:268–277.
An excellent overview of diagnostic and management strategies with clinical practice guidelines for patients with DVT and possible hypercoagulable states.

Bauer KA. Management of thrombophilia. *J Thromb Haemost* 2003;1:1429–1434.
An overview and management recommendations for acute VTE associated with hyper-coagulable states with an emphasis on special considerations, including antithrombin III deficiency, protein C deficiency, pregnancy, and duration of therapy.

Bauer KA. The thrombophilias: well-defined risk factors with uncertain therapeutic implications. *Ann Intern Med* 2001;135:367–373.
A general overview of diagnostic approaches and management considerations in patients with primary hypercoagulable states.

Büller HR, Agnelli G, Hull RD, et al. Antithrombotic therapy for venous disease. The Seventh ACCP Conference on Antithrombotic and Thrombolytic Therapy. *Chest* 2004; 126 (suppl): 401S–428S.
Evidence-based treatment guidelines for initial therapy and secondary prophylaxis.

Crowther MA, Ginsberg JS, Julian J, et al. A comparison of two intensities of warfarin for the prevention of recurrent thrombosis in patients with the antiphospholipid antibody syndrome. *N Engl J Med* 2003;349:1133–1138.
This randomized, double-blind trial found no differences in the rates of recurrent thrombosis among 114 patients with antiphospholipid antibody syndrome treated with conventional-intensity warfarin (to an INR of 2 to 3) compared to high-intensity warfarin (to an INR of 3.1 to 4). Of note, however, only 27 patients had arterial thrombosis, and previous studies have suggested that higher-intensity warfarin may be more important for those patients.

Crowther MA, Kelton JG. Congenital thrombophilic states associated with venous thrombosis: a qualitative overview and proposed classification system. *Ann Intern Med* 2003;138: 128–134.
A review of hereditary hypercoagulable states based on the proposed pathophysiologic mechanisms, including factor VIII elevation and other less well understood abnormalities.

de Groot PG, Derksen RHWM. Antiphospholipid antibodies: update on detection, pathophysiology, and treatment. *Curr Opin Hematol* 2004;11:165–169.
A concise review of pathophysiologic antiphospholipid antibodies, with an emphasis on anti-beta-2-glycoprotein I.

Ginsberg JS, Bates SM. Management of venous thromboembolism during pregnancy. *J Thromb Haemost* 2003; vol. 1435–1442.

A comprehensive overview of diagnostic considerations and treatment recommendations for pregnant women with acute VTE or an increased risk of thrombosis related to a prior history of VTE and/or associated primary hypercoagulable states.

Hassell K. The management of patients with heparin-induced thrombocytopenia who require anticoagulation therapy. *Chest* 2005;127(suppl);1S–8S.
Recent review of HIT management strategies.

Hendler MF, Meschengieser SS, Blanco AN, et al. Primary upper-extremity deep vein thrombosis: high prevalence of thrombophilic defects. *Am J Hematol* 2004;76:330–337.
This retrospective, single-center study detected a primary hypercoagulable state (including antiphospholipid antibodies, hyperhomocysteinemia, factor V Leiden, factor II G20210A mutation, or protein S deficiency) in 75% of the 24 patients with effort-related or spontaneous upper extremity DVT, similar to other studies (but not all) of upper extremity DVT in patients without anatomic abnormalities.

Kearon C, Ginsberg JS, Kovacs MJ, et al. Extended Low-Intensity Anticoagulation for Thrombo-Embolism Investigators. Comparison of low-intensity warfarin therapy with conventional-intensity warfarin therapy for long-term prevention of recurrent venous thromboembolism. *N Engl J Med* 2003;349:631–639.
This randomized, double-blind study of 738 patients with an unprovoked VTE (two thirds of whom had a history of multiple VTEs) found that prolonged warfarin (for a mean duration of 2.4 years) at an INR of 2 to 3 was superior to warfarin at an INR of 1.5 to 2 (hazard ratio of 2.8 for recurrent VTE). Bleeding complications were not different; therefore, prolonged conventional-intensity warfarin may be appropriate after an unprovoked DVT in patients with a low risk of bleeding.

Kovalevsky G, Gracia CR, Berlin JA, et al. Evaluation of the association between hereditary thrombophilias and recurrent pregnancy loss: a meta-analysis. *Arch Intern Med* 2004;164:558–563.
This systematic review and meta-analysis of the published literature revealed that heterozygosity for factor V Leiden or for the factor II G20210A mutation doubles the risk of experiencing two or more miscarriages in the first or second trimester. Screening for these abnormalities is therefore recommended in women with recurrent pregnancy loss.

Kupferminc MJ. Thrombophilia and pregnancy. *Reprod Biol Endocrinol* 2003;1:111.
An overview of the published data and evidence linking many of the primary hypercoagulable states with severe preeclampsia, intrauterine growth retardation, abruptio placenta, and stillbirth.

Kyrle PA, Minar E, Bialonczyk C, et al. The risk of recurrent venous thromboembolism in men and women. *N Engl J Med* 2004;350:2558–2563.
In this prospective follow-up study, men had a 3.5-fold higher risk of recurrent VTE compared to women, and this difference was not due to fewer subsequent events among women who had an initial estrogen-induced VTE. These observations may help determine the risk versus benefit of prolonged secondary thromboprophylaxis in women after a first event.

Levine JS, Branch DW, Rauch J. The antiphospholipid syndrome. *N Engl J Med* 2002;346:752–763.
An excellent review of epidemiologic, diagnostic, clinical, and treatment considerations of antiphospholipid antibody syndrome.

Martinelli I, Taioli E, Battaglioli T, et al. Risk of venous thromboembolism after air travel: interaction with thrombophilia and oral contraceptives. *Arch Intern Med* 2003;163:2771–2774.
This case-controlled study of 210 patients with VTE found a 16-fold increased risk of VTE when recent air travel was combined with a hypercoagulable state (predominantly factor V Leiden or the factor II G20210A mutation) compared to the roughly twofold odds ratio of an event with recent air travel alone.

Nambi V, Gomes M, Deitcher S. Goal-oriented thrombolytic therapy for venous thromboembolic disease. *Clinical Advances in Hematology & Oncology* 2004;2:169–172.

An overview of risks, benefits, and limitations of systemic and catheter-directed thrombolytic therapy for DVT and PE.

Prandoni P, Lensing AW, Prins MH, et al. Below-knee elastic compression stockings to prevent the post-thrombotic syndrome: a randomized, controlled trial. *Ann Intern Med* 2004;141:249–256.

This randomized trial of 180 patients found that routine use of knee-length compression stockings for 2 years following a symptomatic lower extremity DVT decreased the incidence of clinical postthrombotic syndrome by 50% (i.e., 25% versus 49%), as determined by a standardized clinical scoring system.

Proven A, Bartlett RP, Moder KG, et al. Clinical importance of positive test results for lupus anticoagulant and anticardiolipin antibodies. *Mayo Clin Proc* 2004;79(4):467–475.

This retrospective laboratory-based study found no significant predictive value of IgM or IgG anticardiolipin antibodies and/or lupus anticoagulant activity for thrombotic complications among 137 patients with systemic lupus erythematosus, other autoimmune diseases, or cancer or patients without those diseases, suggesting that other antibodies, such as anti-beta-2-glycoprotein I (which was not studied in this cohort), are likely more predictive of risk.

Tormene D, Simioni P, Prandoni P, et al. The incidence of venous thromboembolism in thrombophilic children: a prospective cohort study. *Blood* 2002;100(7):2403–2405.

This prospective cohort study observed no thrombotic events over a mean observation period of 5 years (range 1–8 years) among 81 affected children (ages 1 to 14 years) from families with hereditary hypercoagulable states. Thus, screening a susceptible child for possible inheritance of a hypercoagulable state can be safely delayed until after the age of 14 years.

Van Rooden CJ, Rosendaal FR, Meinders AE, et al. The contribution of factor V Leiden and prothrombin G20210A mutation to the risk of central venous catheter-related thrombosis. *Haematologica* 2004;89:201–206.

This prospective study of 252 consecutive patients, using weekly blinded Doppler ultrasound examinations, found that factor V Leiden or the factor II G20210A mutation imparts a 2.7-fold relative risk for catheter-related thrombosis. These data may justify the use of prophylactic anticoagulation in patients with known hypercoagulability and central venous catheters.

99 THE HEMOLYTIC ANEMIAS
Pamela S. Becker

I. GENERAL PRINCIPLES

A. Hemolytic anemias can be of profound severity in the intensive care unit setting, due to causes such as severe autoimmune hemolytic anemia, overwhelming disseminated intravascular anticoagulation, or sepsis with an organism that carries a hemolytic toxin, among others.

B. One should suspect hemolytic anemia in the critically ill patient if the hematocrit fails to rise despite transfusion, if there is an unexplained high lactate dehydrogenase (LDH) or bilirubin, or hemoglobinuria without red cells on microscopic urinalysis.

C. One confounding difficulty in the diagnosis is that the reticulocyte count may not be elevated in severely compromised patients because of bone marrow suppression.

II. PATHOPHYSIOLOGY

A. Patients with chronic hemolytic anemia rely on increased erythroid production to compensate for the red blood cell destruction demonstrated by an elevated reticulocyte count.

B. This level of increased production renders a susceptibility to three different types of crises:
1. Aplastic
2. Hemolytic
3. Megaloblastic

C. Parvovirus B19 is a classic cause of the aplastic crisis, and bacterial infections can cause hemolytic crises.

D. Megaloblastoid crises arise because of relative folate deficiency, which can occur during adolescence (with growth spurts) or during pregnancy.

E. Chronic hemolytic anemia is associated with pigment gallstones at an early age because of the chronic elevation of bilirubin in the bile (increased concentration leading to more precipitation) and iron overload from chronic increased absorption and/or chronic transfusions.

III. DIAGNOSIS

A. The signs and symptoms of hemolytic anemia as well as the laboratory features (Table 99-1) are a result of both the increased red cell destruction and compensatory red cell production.

B. On physical examination, patients with hemolytic anemia may exhibit pallor and jaundice.

C. There may be splenomegaly in patients with ongoing active hemolytic anemia.

D. Individuals with chronic hemolytic conditions may have overexpanded marrow due to erythroid hyperplasia, resulting in "chipmunk" facies (broad cheekbones, protruding maxillary bones), and extramedullary erythropoiesis, resulting in hepatosplenomegaly.

E. If there is rapid intravascular hemolysis, there can be hemoglobinemia (pink-colored plasma), hemoglobinuria (red-colored urine), and hemosiderinuria.

F. Haptoglobin binds free intravascular hemoglobin and is cleared through the liver, resulting in a low serum haptoglobin level.

G. With both intravascular and extravascular hemolysis, there can be elevation in serum bilirubin, with the majority being indirect (unconjugated) bilirubin because the reticuloendothelial cells convert the hemoglobin released from destroyed red cells to bilirubin, and an elevation in serum LDH because this enzyme is released from the destroyed red cells.

TABLE 99-1 **Laboratory Evaluation in Hemolytic Anemia**

Test	Intravascular	Extravascular	Comment
Bilirubin, indirect	Yes	Yes	Elevated
Lactate dehydrogenase	Yes	Yes	Elevated
Reticulocyte count	Yes	Yes	Elevated
Plasma hemoglobin	Yes		Brisk intravascular
Osmotic fragility	Not prominent	Yes	Hereditary spherocytosis
Coombs' test	Yes, esp. in cold AIHA	Yes	Immune causes
Ham's test	Yes	–	PNH
Sucrose hemolysis	Yes	–	PNH
Urine hemosiderin	Yes	–	PNH, PCH
DIC screen	Yes	Yes	Positive in DIC
Blood smear			Abnormal forms
Hgb electrophoresis	Yes	Yes	S or C hgbs and others
Haptoglobin	Yes	Possibly	Low

AIHA, autoimmune hemolytic anemia; PNH, paroxysmal nocturnal hemoglobulinuria; PCH, paroxysmal cold hemoglobulinuria; DIC, disseminated intravascular coagulation.

H. The chronic elevation of serum bilirubin can result in pigment gallstones and cholecystitis.

I. An increased reticulocyte count reflects the compensatory overproduction of red cells.

J. More specific tests can document or support the cause of the hemolytic anemia. For example, there is increased osmotic fragility in conditions leading to spherocytosis, such as hereditary spherocytosis or autoimmune hemolytic anemia.

K. Autoimmune hemolytic anemia (AIHA) can be diagnosed by the direct Coombs' test, also known as the DAT (direct antiglobulin test), which demonstrates the presence of immunoglobulin and/or complement present on the red cell, or by the indirect test, which demonstrates antibody detected in the serum.

L. The disseminated intravascular coagulation (DIC) screen (FDP, D dimer, and antithrombin III) is positive in DIC.

M. Historically, the diagnosis of paroxysmal nocturnal hemoglobinuria (PNH) was by acid hemolysin (Ham's test) or sucrose hemolysis (sugar water) test, both of which demonstrate the sensitivity to complement-mediated lysis.

N. The current method of diagnosis of PNH is by flow cytometry analysis demonstrating lack of proteins bound via the PI membrane anchor, such as CD59.

IV. ETIOLOGY

A. Hemolytic anemias arise from destruction of red blood cells caused by intrinsic defects (usually inherited) or extrinsic conditions. This destruction can occur in the blood vessels, leading to intravascular hemolysis, or in the extravascular compartment, primarily in the spleen and liver, with the participation of the reticuloendothelial system.

B. Intrinsic disorders

  1. Hemoglobinopathies

   a. Sickle cell disease. Sickle cell disease arises from a point mutation in beta hemoglobin, leading to sickle hemoglobin (Hb S), which is predisposed to polymerization when deoxygenated. Homozygous individuals with SS disease are affected. Several complications of sickle cell syndromes can be life-threatening, due to sickling and infarction in major organs. About 10% of patients experience cerebrovascular accidents, usually in childhood. Acute chest syndrome occurs in 40% of patients, a result of thrombosis in the pulmonary vessels leading to local hypoxia, then increased sickling and eventually to hypoxemia in a progressive downward spiral. It can be difficult to distinguish pulmonary infarct from infection. Pulmonary hypertension is an independent risk factor for death in patients with sickle cell disease. Splenic sequestration crisis, also more common in children, can cause a profound drop in hematocrit and an exacerbation of hemolysis, and can be associated with splenic infarct or rupture. Patients also are susceptible to sepsis due to encapsulated organisms such as *Streptococcus pneumoniae* and *Escherichia coli*, due to absent splenic function due to recurrent infarction by 1 to 2 years of age. Other complications of sickle cell disease include delayed growth and development; chronic hemolytic anemia with hematocrit in the range of 18 to 30; pain crises (especially abdomen, chest, joints) requiring narcotic administration with predisposing factors of dehydration, vasospasm, and infection; systolic ejection murmur due to hyperdynamic state; eventual right heart failure due to recurrent pulmonary infarction and pulmonary hypertension; inability to concentrate urine due to microinfarcts of the renal medulla; renal papillary infarcts resulting in hematuria; renal failure; recurrent joint effusions; osteomyelitis most likely due to Staphylococcus, although Salmonella may be an etiology in these patients; recurrent bony infarcts leading to vertebral deformities; aseptic necrosis of femoral head; dactylitis (hand-foot syndrome); hepatic infarct; retinal infarcts; proliferative retinopathy; and chronic ankle ulcers. There are compound sickle syndromes, such as sickle-hemoglobin C and sickle-beta thalassemia, both of which are associated with chronic sickling but milder anemia, and certain complications including splenomegaly, retinopathy, and avascular necrosis of the femoral head.

   b. Thalassemia. Thalassemia arises from insufficient synthesis of alpha or beta globin. It can range in severity from the silent carrier state in alpha thalassemia with deletion of a single alpha globin gene, to thalassemia major in patients who completely lack production of beta globin. Patients with thalassemia major develop massive hepatosplenomegaly and chipmunk facies due to extramedullary erythropoiesis, complete transfusion dependence, with consequent development of transfusional iron overload leading to congestive heart failure and cirrhosis. Thalassemia minor is milder and generally does not require transfusion support.

2. Membrane defects. Several inherited defects of red cell membrane proteins lead to hereditary hemolytic anemia. The most frequent types are hereditary spherocytosis and hereditary elliptocytosis. The majority of cases are mild, but there are severe forms resulting in transfusion-dependent anemia despite splenectomy. There can also be inherited defects of lipid synthesis such as abetalipoproteinemia, which leads to acanthocytosis (cells have irregular projections), and the absent low density lipoprotein (LDL) leads to vitamin E deficiency, oxidant sensitivity, and hemolysis.

3. Metabolic defects. These defects arise because of enzyme deficiencies critical to the Embden-Meyerhof or glycolytic pathway and the hexose monophosphate (HMP) shunt necessary for ATP production or maintenance of the reduced state of the heme iron. Examples of these enzyme deficiencies include G6PD deficiency, which leads to hemolysis with infections or certain oxidant drugs such as primaquine, nitrofurantoin, sulfamethoxazole, chloramphenicol, phenacetin, dapsone, methylene blue, vitamin K; glutathione synthetase deficiency; pyruvate kinase (PK) deficiency; glucose phosphate isomerase (GPI) deficiency; triose phosphate isomerase (TPI) deficiency; and phosphofructokinase (PFK) deficiency.

4. Paroxysmal nocturnal hemoglobinuria (PNH). PNH is an acquired clonal stem cell disorder resulting from a defect in synthesis of the phosphatidyl-inositol (PI) membrane anchor for a number of proteins, including decay accelerating factor (DAF; an inhibitor of C3 convertase). Because of the decreased binding of DAF, there is increased sensitivity to complement leading to intravascular hemolysis, resulting in variable hemoglobinuria, classically worse at night, and significant iron deficiency through urinary loss (+ urine hemosiderin test). Patients also suffer from episodic abdominal pain attributed to venous thromboses (hepatic, portal, splenic, mesenteric veins) due to a defect in platelets. The disorder can evolve into or from aplastic anemia.

C. Extrinsic disorders

1. Autoimmune hemolytic anemia (AIHA). About half of patients with warm AIHA exhibit both IgG and C'3 on the red blood cell and one third only IgG, and this type is often associated with other autoimmune disorders or malignancies and extravascular hemolysis. Cold agglutinin disease (cold AIHA) is characterized by antibodies that bind better at 4°C, usually due to an IgM antibody, and hemolysis is also primarily extravascular but can be intravascular due to complement fixation. It is associated with infections such as *Mycoplasma pneumoniae* and infectious mononucleosis or malignancies. Drug-induced AIHA can arise by three mechanisms: Hapten (antibodies directed to the drug bound to the RBC membrane), for example, penicillin with positive DAT for IgG, indirect neg. in absence of drug; Immune complex–"innocent bystander" (circulating complexes of antibody-drug bound to serum protein), for example, quinidine, where there is an antibody directed to the drug-protein complex which settles on RBCs, fixing complement, leading to a positive DAT for C'3; and Drug-induced autoantibody, for example, procainamide, usually with anti-Rh specificity, leading to a positive DAT for IgG, and possibly, a positive indirect Coombs' test as well.

2. Microangiopathic hemolytic anemia

   a. Disseminated intravascular coagulation (DIC). The blood vessels become partially occluded by fibrin deposition, and the red cells become caught on fibrin strands, leading to fragmentation and hemolysis. There is also consumption of platelets and coagulation factors, leading to thrombocytopenia and prolongation of the prothrombin time (PT) and partial thromboplastin time (PTT). The DIC screen demonstrates high fibrin degradation products, increased level of D-dimer, and low levels of antithrombin III.

   b. Thrombotic thrombocytopenic purpura (TTP). There are five clinical features in the presentation of TTP: fever, renal dysfunction, neurologic sequelae including seizure, hemolytic anemia, and thrombocytopenia. The hemolytic anemia is manifested by elevation in the reticulocyte count, LDH, and schistocytes present on the peripheral blood smear. The etiology is related to an accumulation of high-molecular-weight von Willebrand factor (VWF) multimers, due to absence of the VWF cleaving protease ADAMTS-13. There are hereditary forms with deficiency of this protease and acquired forms due to autoantibody formation.

   c. Hemolytic uremic syndrome (HUS). Hemolysis and renal dysfunction are the most prominent features, although there can also be mild thrombocytopenia. Fragmented cells are also seen on the peripheral blood smear. This entity can be difficult to distinguish from TTP, but a recent study has found that there is a different pattern of von Willebrand factor multimers.

   d. Other vascular abnormalities. Hemangiomas are focal proliferations of small blood vessels that can cause localized intravascular coagulation. With carcinomatosis metastatic deposits of cancer cells lodge in blood vessels. Renal vascular disorders such as malignant hypertension can lead to vessel narrowing or abnormal vessels in glomerulonephritis. Inflammation of small vessels can occur in polyarteritis nodosum or systemic lupus. All of these abnormalities of vessels can lead to shearing of red cells and hemolysis.

3. Mechanical damage. Red cells rupture under high shear stresses due to mechanical damage. This damage is reflected by abnormal shapes, including schistocytes, helmet cells, and fragments. The damaged cells are removed by the spleen.

   a. "Waring blender" syndrome. This syndrome occurs due to damage from prosthetic heart valves or stenotic, calcified heart valves, especially the aortic valve.

   b. March hemoglobinuria. The stomping of feet or hand surfaces over long distances causes red cell damage.

c. Toxins. Certain toxins and venoms result in profound hemolysis. Classical examples include *Clostridium welchii* sepsis, in which a phospholipase damages RBC phospholipid, leading to rapidly progressive and often fatal intravascular hemolysis, and snake or brown spider venoms.

d. Chemical injury. The RBC membrane can be injured by arsenic, copper, and high O_2 tension such as hyperbaric oxygen, presumed to be due to membrane oxidation.

e. Burn injury. Thermal burns cause direct damage to RBC membrane, resulting in spherocyte and schistocyte formation, especially when third-degree burns are sustained over greater than 20% of the body surface area.

f. Malaria, babesiosis. Malaria parasites directly invade red cells resulting in "knobs" formed on the membranes. These knobs lead to increased ion permeability, increased lipid fluidity, reduced deformability, increased oxidant production, and, ultimately, hemolysis.

g. Liver disease. Severe liver disease results in spur cell anemia, characterized by acanthocytosis due to the accumulation of unesterified cholesterol in the red cell membrane and hemolytic anemia with extravascular hemolysis. It is a late complication of liver dysfunction and augurs for a high mortality rate.

h. Hypersplenism. Splenomegaly from any cause can result in sequestration of blood cells and lead to a decline in any or all of the blood counts.

V. TREATMENT

A. One general supportive measure that should be instituted for all patients with hemolytic anemia is folic acid supplementation, 1 mg daily for chronic hemolytic anemia, 5 mg daily during acute hemolytic crises.

B. Patients with intravascular hemolysis may lose iron through hemoglobinuria, become iron deficient, and require supplementation.

C. During times of exacerbations and hemodynamic compromise, patients may require transfusion support with red blood cells.

D. The threshold for transfusion support is usually a hemoglobin in the range of 7 to 8, as the oxygen-carrying capacity falls below a hemoglobin of about 7.

E. Patients with a hemoglobin exceeding 10 are unlikely to benefit from red cell transfusion.

F. Splenectomy can ameliorate the hemolytic anemia related to many of the etiologies (see later).

VI. SPECIFIC THERAPY

A. Sickle cell disease

1. Treatments include penicillin prophylaxis in children; pneumococcal vaccine; folic acid supplementation (1 mg daily); hydration with hypotonic fluid, oxygen, analgesics, evaluation for infection and organ damage for sickle pain crisis; deferroxamine for iron overload; hydroxyurea to increase Hgb F production and decrease frequency of crises.

2. Empiric antibiotic coverage in febrile patients should include medications that cover encapsulated organisms, such as cephalosporins.

3. Patients with aplastic crisis related to parvovirus B19 infection require red cell transfusion support until the reticulocyte count rises.

4. Patients with acute central nervous system symptoms, acute chest syndrome with hypoxia, undergoing eye surgery or surgery under general anesthesia, or angiography, priapism, cardiac symptoms, or for a period of a few years after stroke should be considered for exchange transfusion.

5. Exchange transfusion is performed by phlebotomy of one unit at a time of whole blood, with replacement with packed red cell transfusions.

6. The exchange should be down to the range of about 30% Hb S.

7. Patients with extensive alloimmunization can have severe hemolytic transfusion reactions; red cell transfusion should be conservatively applied in these patients, and leukocyte-depleted, phenotypically matched red cells should be administered.

8. Allogeneic stem cell transplantation offers a potentially curative option for those with poor prognosis.

B. Thalassemia. The strategy is to transfuse to a hemoglobin of 9 to 10.5 g/dL to prevent marrow expansion and splenomegaly; administer folate; perform splenectomy; administer deferroxamine for iron overload, and allogeneic stem cell transplantation offers a potential curative option in selected cases where the transplant can be performed prior to advanced liver disease.

C. Membrane defects. For chronic hemolysis leading to moderate to severe anemia, transfusion dependence, and/or chronic jaundice, patients can be referred for splenectomy.

D. Metabolic defects. G6PD deficiency can be managed by avoidance of oxidant drugs or ingestion of chemicals such as moth balls or foods such as fava beans; pyruvate kinase deficiency generally requires splenectomy.

E. PNH. The therapy includes judicious use of iron supplements when needed for iron deficiency and anticoagulation as needed for development of abdominal thromboses. Patients may require red cell transfusions during times of stress and excessive hemolysis. Androgen therapy may improve blood counts, and allogeneic stem cell transplant can be curative. The latest approach is a monoclonal antibody, eculizumab, directed against a complement protein, currently in clinical trial.

F. AIHA. The treatments for autoimmune hemolytic anemia include withdrawal of drug for the drug-induced variety, folate supplementation, and immunosuppression for the spontaneous warm and cold autoimmune hemolytic anemias or drug-induced autoantibody type. The immunosuppressive agents include steroids, cyclophosphamide, and azathioprine. In addition, danacrine and IV immune globulin can be effective. In cases of relapse after withdrawal of immunosuppressive medication, or in severe hemolysis, splenectomy should be performed. Rituximab (anti-CD20 antibody) may be highly effective.

G. DIC. The management is largely supportive, with replenishment of red cells, platelets, fresh frozen plasma, and cryoprecipitate and treatment of the underlying cause (e.g., sepsis, tissue necrosis) until resolution.

H. TTP. The treatment of TTP is plasmapheresis and infusion of cryoprecipitate-poor plasma. Chronic, relapsing TTP has been treated with splenectomy, and more recently, rituximab.

Selected Readings

Dhaliwal G, Cornett PA, Tierney LM Jr. Hemolytic anemia. *Am Fam Physician* 2004;69:2599–2606.
General review of hemolytic anemia.

Engelfriet CP, Overbeeke MAM, von dem Borne AEG. Autoimmune hemolytic anemia. *Semin Hematol* 1992; 29:3–12.
Reviews all of the different types of autoimmune hemolytic anemias with their occurrence in conjunction with systemic disease.

Gallagher PG, Forget BG. Spectrin genes in health disease. *Semin Hematol* 1993;30:4–20.
An overview of some inherited hemolytic anemias due to membrane defects.

Kazazian HH. The thalassemia syndromes: molecular basis and prenatal diagnosis in 1990. *Semin Hematol* 1990;27:209–228.
Reviews the details of the thalassemias.

Moake JL. von Willebrand factor, ADAMTS-13, and thrombotic thrombocytopenic purpura. *Semin Hematol* 2004;41:4–14.
Review of the pathogenesis of thrombotic thrombocytopenic purpura.

Nathan DG, Stranahan RA, Orkin SH, et al. *Nathan and Oski's hematology of infancy and childhood*, 6th ed., 2003.
Provides a thorough discussion of all aspects of inherited and childhood anemias.

Peters LL, Lux SE. Ankyrins: structure and function in normal cells and hereditary spherocytes. *Semin Hematol* 1993;30:85–118.
Reviews the molecular basis of hereditary spherocytosis.

Salama A, Mueller-Eckhardt C. Immune-mediated blood cell dyscrasias related to drugs. *Semin Hematol* 1992;29:54–63.

Reviews the mechanisms of drug-induced immune hemolytic anemias as well as other immune cytopenias.

Shinar E, Rachmilewitz EA. Oxidative denaturation of red cells in thalassemia. *Semin Hematol* 1990;27:70–82.
Covers all the oxidative hemolytic anemias.

Steinberg MH. Management of sickle cell disease. *N Engl J Med* 1999;340:1021–1030.
Describes the detailed clinical features and treatment of sickle cell disease.

Steinberg MH, Forget BG, Higgs DR, et al. eds. *Disorders of hemoglobin: genetics, pathophysiology, and clinical management;* Cambridge: Cambridge University Press, 2001.
Provides a thorough discussion of all hemoglobin defects.

I. GENERAL PRINCIPLES

A. Indications

    1. Support of oxygen delivery

    2. Correction of hemostatic abnormalities

        a. Bleeding patient

        b. Preprocedure

    3. Support of the patient with massive hemorrhage

II. RED BLOOD CELLS (RBCs). Unit total volume. 300 to 350 mL. Approximately 200 mL red blood cells, 50 mL plasma or less, preservative approximately 50 mL. No platelet activity.

A. Indications

    1. Anemia signs/symptoms requiring rapid reversal

    2. Chronic hypoproliferative anemia

    3. Hematocrit (Hct) less than 30% in patient with cardiovascular disease or older than 65 years; thresholds for younger patients not established

B. Therapeutic effect. 1 mL/kg increases Hct 0.5% to 0.7% in a stable patient

C. Emergency uncross-matched blood

    1. To maintain cardiopulmonary stability during massive hemorrhage

    2. O or type specific if known

        a. Avoid Rh-positive in females of childbearing age, children. Anti RhD (Rhogam) within 48 hours if Rh exposure occurs to Rh-negative patient.

        b. Risk increases in previously transfused/multiparous patient.

III. WHOLE BLOOD (where available)

A. Plasma not removed from donor unit or added to RBC.

B. Most coagulation factors at stable levels. Decreased factors V, VIII.

C. Indications: massive transfusion, coagulopathic bleeding patient

IV. PLATELETS

A. Platelet concentrates

    1. 60 mL plasma each

    2. Single units from 1 unit donor blood in pools of 4 to 8 for transfusion

B. Apheresis

    1. 200 to 400 mL, $\cong$ 4 to 6 pooled platelet concentrates

    2. Can collect from designated, matched donors for the refractory patient

V. INDICATIONS

A. Thrombocytopenia

    1. Prophylactic transfusion: platelet counts 5,000 to 10,000/μL.

    2. Bleeding patient: 50,000/μL to 100,000/μL. Consider bleeding site: higher for intracranial, pulmonary, and so forth.

    3. Preprocedure: 30,000 to 100,000/μL. Consider site, accessibility.

B. Platelet dysfunction

    1. Congenital, medications, sepsis, obstetrical, extracorporeal circuits, uremia

    2. Transfusion threshold depends on defect. Greater than 100,000/μL for bleeding.

VI. CONTRAINDICATIONS. Relatively contraindicated: Thrombotic thrombocytopenic purpura (TTP), idiopathic thrombocytopenic purpura (ITP) unless bleeding. See section on thrombocytopenia.

VII. THERAPEUTIC EFFECT
  A. 1 platelet concentrate (1 unit) raises count 5,000 to 10,000/mL in 70-kg adult with normal size spleen.
  B. Decreased platelet increments and survival with increased spleen size.
  C. Transfused platelets survive 3 to 5 days. Decreased survival with conditions of increased destruction, fever, sepsis.
  D. Will correct platelet dysfunction only if states toxic to platelet do not persist (e.g., uremia, antiplatelet agents).

VIII. PLASMA
  A. 200 to 250 mL from 1 unit of blood.
  B. Fresh frozen plasma (FFP): frozen within 8 hours of collection; transfuse within 24 hours of thawing.
  C. Thawed plasma: can be held up to 5 days after thawing. Slight decreased levels of factors V and VIII.
  D. Must be ABO compatible. Rh not important. Universal type AB for emergency.
  E. Indications
    1. Documented coagulation factor deficiency(ies). Usually prothrombin time greater than 1.5 times normal.
      a. Bleeding patient
      b. Preparation for invasive procedure
      c. No available recombinant or factor concentrate. Use recombinants or concentrates for hemophilia, von Willebrand disease.
    2. Massive transfusion with coagulopathy
    3. Liver disease
      a. Multifactorial hemostatic defect
      b. Large volumes of plasma may not correct abnormal coagulation tests
    4. Warfarin reversal
      a. May require recurrent transfusion to maintain normal levels
      b. Vitamin K for reversal if time allows
    5. TTP
      a. Plasma exchange
      b. Plasma infusion when exchange delayed
  F. Dosage. Therapeutic effect: increase in factor levels of greater than 10% required for significant hemostatic improvement. See Table 100-1 for general guidelines.

TABLE 100-1	**Fresh Frozen Plasma–Dosage for Transfusion**

Volume of 1 U FFP: 200 to 250 mL
1 mL plasma contains 1 U coagulation factors.
1 U FFP contains 220 U coagulation factors.
Factor recovery with transfusion ≅ 40%
1 U FFP provides ~80 U coagulation factors.
70 kg × 0.05 = plasma volume of 35 dL (3.5 L)
80 U = 2.3 U/dL = 2.3% (of normal 100 U/dL)
In a 70-kg patient:
1 U FFP increases most factors ~2.5%
4 U FFP increase most factors ~10%

From Gernsheimer T. *Blood component therapy 2004.* Published by the Puget Sound Blood Center, Seattle, WA, 2004.
FFP, fresh frozen plasma

IX. CRYOPRECIPITATE

A. Each bag (5 to 15 mL) provides a frozen precipitate of 1 unit plasma.

B. Provides high concentration of fibrinogen.

C. Provides von Willebrand factor, factors VIII, XIII (emergent use only, see later).

D. Indications

    1. Bleeding or prior to procedure in patients with fibrinogen less than 100 mg/dL.

        a. DIC

        b. Massive transfusion

        c. Obstetrical emergencies

        d. Severe liver disease

    2. Uremic platelet dysfunction uncorrected by desmopressin (DDAVP)

E. Dosage

    1. Each bag provides 75 to 100 mg fibrinogen

    2. Multiple bags pooled for infusion

    3. Emergent replacement factor VIII or von Willebrand factor *only* when recombinant or factor concentrate unavailable. 150 U/bag.

X. TRANSFUSION RISKS

A. Infectious risk/unit

    1. HIV, less than 1:1,900,000

    2. Hepatitis C, less than 1:1,900,000

    3. Hepatitis B, 1:1,000,000

    4. HTLV I and II, 1:641,000

    5. West Nile virus, extremely low, screened by polymerase chain reaction (PCR)

    6. Cytomegalovirus (CMV), risk varies by region, depends on patient diagnosis. See Table 100-2 for indications.

    7. Bacterial contamination, platelets tested for contamination. RBC less than 1:30,000.

B. Transfusion reactions

    1. Acute hemolytic transfusion reaction

        a. Signs and symptoms: fever, flushing, chills, back/flank pain, anxiety, hypotension, DIC, hematuria, anuria, renal failure.

        b. ABO incompatibility with RBC most common, less commonly minor antigen mismatch.

        c. Diagnosis: check all patient and blood identifiers; patient sample and blood bag to blood bank for hemolysis workup and retype and cross-match.

        d. Therapy: hydration, treat DIC with blood components as indicated.

    2. Delayed hemolytic transfusion reaction

        a. Recall of antibody formed by prior transfusion or pregnancy 5 to 10 days posttransfusion.

        b. Hemolysis of transfused units results in falling hematocrit, increased bilirubin, LDH

        c. Transfuse with antigen matched RBCs as indicated for anemia.

    3. Febrile transfusion reactions

        a. Due to white blood cells and cytokines in plasma of unit. Common in recurrently transfused.

        b. Rule out bacterial contamination for high fevers, severe rigors, hypotension, DIC, by Gram stain and culture of blood bag, patient blood.

        c. Prevent future reactions with acetaminophen pretransfusion, leukoreduced blood components.

    4. Allergic reaction

        a. Usually due to sensitization to foreign plasma proteins, including IgA in deficient individuals.

        b. Urticaria: Treat with diphenhydramine. Prevent future reactions with antihistamine, volume reduction of platelets if severe.

        c. Treat severe life-threatening reactions with epinephrine. Prevent future reactions with steroids, washing of cellular components to remove plasma.

    5. Transfusion-related acute lung injury (TRALI)

        a. Rapidly worsening dyspnea, bilateral lung infiltrates onset 15 minutes to 6 hours after beginning transfusion. All component types implicated.

| TABLE 100-2 | Indications for Blood Component Modification | | |

	CMV NEG.[a,b]	Irradiation[c]	Leukocyte reduced
BM/stem cell transplant candidate	X	[d]	[e]
Organ transplant candidate	X		Candidates for heart and kidney transplant
Chemo Rx only		[f]	[g]
AIDS/HIV+	X		
Febrile RXN's[h]			X
Neonate	X	X	
Any lymphopro-liferative malignancy		X	

[a]For patients with negative or unknown CMV serology.
[b]Leukocyte depletion may be used if CMV negative blood components are not available.
[c]All components for stem cell transplant patients require irradiation. All directed donations from family members or HLA-matched donors require gamma irradiation.
[d]Gamma irradiation is required pretransplant for patients who may receive nonmyeloablative ("mini") transplants.
[e]Required to prevent alloimmunization pretransplant only.
[f]Irradiation may be indicated in severely immunosuppressive chemotherapy, such as is used to treat patients with acute leukemia.
[g]Leukocyte-reduced blood is recommended for patients who will undergo multiple cycles of chemotherapy that will require platelet transfusion support.
[h]If uncontrolled by leukocyte depletion, volume depletion of platelets prior to transfusion may decrease febrile reactions.
From Gernsheimer T. *Blood component therapy 2004.* Published by the Puget Sound Blood Center, Seattle, WA, 2004.
BM, bone marrow; Rx, prescription; RXNs, reactions

     b. Etiology: patient or donor human leukocyte antigens (HLA) or white blood cell (WBC) antibodies.

     c. Therapy: supportive. Spontaneous improvement 72 to 96 hours after onset.

XI. BLOOD COMPONENT MODIFICATIONS

  A. Indications. See Table 100-2 for indications in specific disorders.

    1. Irradiation: prevention of transfusion-associated graft versus host disease. Prevents donor lymphocyte replication and engraftment following antigenic stimulation.

    2. Leukocyte reduction

      a. Cellular components filtered to remove WBCs

      b. Prevent febrile reactions, cytomegalovirus (CMV) transmission, and alloimmunization to HLA antigens

    3. CMV seronegative

      a. Prevention of CMV transmission in a CMV-negative, immunosuppressed patient.

      b. Leukocyte reduction probably equivalent to use of CMV seronegative components.

4. Volume reduction (platelets only)
  a. Limit transfused plasma to patient with volume overload or plasma protein allergies.
  b. Platelets may be lost or damaged by centrifugation.
5. Washed
  a. Patients with severe, life-threatening plasma protein allergies
  b. Removes all plasma from cellular blood components.
  c. Large platelet loss and damage. RBC must be transfused in 24 hours or wasted.

Selected Readings

Bowden RA, Slichter SJ, Sayers M, et al. A comparison of filtered leukocyte-reduced and cytomegalovirus (CMV) seronegative blood products for the prevention of transfusion-associated CMV infection after marrow transplant. *Blood* 1995;86:3598–3603.
Demonstrates the equivalence of leukocyte reduction and use of CMV seronegative blood to prevent CMV infection.

Corwin HL, Gettinger A, Pearl RG, et al. Epo Critical Care Trials Group. Efficacy of recombinant human erythropoietin in critically ill patients: a randomized controlled trial. *JAMA* 2002;288:2827–2835.
Randomized trial of the usefulness of erythropoietin in the critical care patient to avoid transfusion.

Cosgriff N, Moore EE, Sauaia A, et al. Predicting life-threatening coagulopathy in the massively transfused trauma patient: hypothermia and acidosis revisited. *J Trauma* 1997;42:857–862.
An evaluation of factors that are associated with coagulopathy in the patient with massive hemorrhage.

DeLoughery TG, Liebler JM, Simonds V, et al. Invasive line placement in critically ill patients: do hemostatic defects matter? *Transfusion* 1996;36:827–831.
This study evaluates the importance of hemostatic abnormalities in the complication rate of line placement.

Hébert PC, Wells G, Blajchman MA, et al. A multicenter, randomized, controlled clinical trial of transfusion requirements in critical care. *N Engl J Med* 1999;340:409–417.
Large, multicenter randomized trial comparing liberal and restrictive transfusion strategies and outcomes in critical care patients.

Heddle NM, Klama L, Singer J, et al. The role of the plasma from platelet concentrates in transfusion reactions. *N Engl J Med* 1994;331:625–628.
Large randomized trial comparing leukocyte reduction with volume reduction to prevent transfusion reactions.

Kleinman S, Caulfield T, Chan P, et al. Toward an understanding of transfusion-related acute lung injury: statement of a consensus panel. *Transfusion* 2004;44:1774–1789.
Consensus statement of an increasingly recognized and poorly understood complication of transfusion.

Kuriyan M, Carson JL. Blood transfusion risks in the intensive care unit. *Crit Care Clin* 2004;20:237–253, ix.
General review of transfusion issues in the critical care patient.

Practice guidelines for blood component therapy—a report by the American Society of Anesthesiology Task Force on Blood Component Therapy. *Anesthesiology* 1996;84:732–747.
Many hospital guidelines for transfusion of blood components for hemostatic defects are based on these recommendations by the American Society of Anesthesiology.

Rebulla P, Finazzi G, Marangoni F, et al. The threshold for prophylactic platelet transfusions in adults with acute myeloid leukemia. *N Engl J Med* 1997;337(26):1870–1875.
Randomized trial comparing bleeding risks at 10,000 versus 20,000 platelets/mL thresholds for platelet transfusions in patients undergoing therapy for acute leukemia.

Stramer SL, Glynn SA, Kleinman SH, et al. Detection of HIV-1 and HCV infections among antibody-negative blood donors by nucleic acid-amplification testing. *N Engl J Med* 2004;351:760–768.
Residual risk of HIV and HCV infection from transfusion with current methods of detection.

The Trial to Reduce Alloimmunization to Platelets Study Group. Leukocyte reduction and ultraviolet B irradiation of platelets to prevent alloimmunization and refractoriness to platelet transfusions. *N Engl J Med* 1997;337:1861–1869.
Classic study of leukocyte reduction for prevention of alloimmunization to HLA antigens with leukocyte reduction in patients with acute leukemia.

Wu WC, Rathore SS, Wang Y, et al. Blood transfusion in elderly patients with acute myocardial infarction. *N Engl J Med* 2001;345:1230–1236.
This study examines the effect of hematocrit and transfusion on morbidity and mortality in the setting of acute myocardial infarction in the older patient.

I. GENERAL PRINCIPLES

A. Definition and description. Granulocytopenia (also known as neutropenia) refers to an absolute decrease in the circulating level of granulocytes or neutrophils. Classically, neutropenia is defined as an absolute neutrophil count (ANC) less than 500 cells/mm^3 or less than 1,000 cells/mm^3 with a predicted nadir of less than 500 cells/mm^3 [ANC = total white blood cells × (% neutrophils + % bands)]. Agranulocytosis refers to a profound decrease in granulocytes and is most commonly used when the condition is drug induced.

B. Classification. The severity of granulocytopenia is often graded according to the neutrophil nadir; severe (grade 4) neutropenia is associated with a profound increase in the risk for opportunistic infections. The National Cancer Institute uses the following grading scale (ANC/mm^3):

$$\text{Grade 1} = \text{ANC} \geq 1{,}500 \text{ to} < 2{,}000$$

$$\text{Grade 2} = \text{ANC} \geq 1{,}000 \text{ to} < 1{,}500$$

$$\text{Grade 3} = \text{ANC} \geq 500 \text{ to} < 1{,}000$$

$$\text{Grade 4} = \text{ANC} < 500$$

C. Epidemiology. Before the availability of potent antiretroviral therapy, the frequency of leukopenia among patients with acquired immune deficiency syndrome (AIDS) was as high as 70%; etiology was commonly multifactorial (though drug toxicities predominated). Neutropenia, however, is most commonly associated with cancer chemotherapy. Risk factors for neutropenia among patients undergoing treatment for malignancy include:

1. Cancer type (hematologic malignancy > solid tumor)
2. Malignant infiltration of bone marrow
3. Older patient age
4. Decreased performance status or level of nutrition, or both
5. Profound sepsis
6. Chemotherapy correlates:
    a. Degree of regimen-related myelotoxicity
    b. Dose of therapy (induction > maintenance)
    c. Degree of neutropenia with previous chemotherapy cycles

D. Clinical syndromes and prognosis. The primary concern for the neutropenic patient is the risk for opportunistic infection, which is highly correlated with the severity and duration of neutropenia. Neutropenia after chemotherapy is associated with a higher risk of infection than neutropenia due to other causes as a result of the commonly present damage of mucosal surfaces (mucositis) that allows bacterial and fungal translocation into the bloodstream. Though fever is often the first sign of infection, infections may be present without fever.

1. Febrile neutropenia
    a. Bacteremia present in only 20%
    b. Microbiologic diagnosis achieved in only 50%
    c. Noninfectious causes of fever: underlying malignancy (e.g., B-symptoms of lymphoma or Sweet's syndrome), tumor lysis syndrome, drug fever, hyperacute graft-versus-host disease (after allogeneic hematopoietic cell transplantation)
    d. Mortality 70% if antibiotics delayed

2. Neutropenia without fever

   a. Occult infection may manifest as hypothermia or hypotension, or both.

   b. Elderly patients or those receiving corticosteroids may not develop fever.

   c. Prophylactic antibacterial agents are generally not indicated without signs/symptoms of infection.

II. ETIOLOGY. Commonly classified according to mechanism (Table 101-1) or extrinsic/intrinsic causes:

A. Extrinsic causes

   1. Drugs

   2. Sepsis

   3. Alcohol

   4. Nutritional deficiencies

   5. Autoimmune neutropenia (associated with antineutrophil antibodies)

   6. Other immune destruction

   a. Collagen vascular disease (e.g., systemic lupus erythematosus)

   b. Felty syndrome (rheumatoid arthritis, splenomegaly, low white cell count)

   7. Hemodialysis

   8. Splenic sequestration (e.g., with severe cirrhosis)

   9. Viral infections

   a. Cytomegalovirus (CMV)-associated neutropenia in organ and hematopoietic cell transplant recipients.

   b. Parvovirus B19 infections occasionally cause pure red cell aplasia and, in a few cases, neutropenia.

   10. Bone marrow infiltration by malignancy or other infections (i.e., histoplasmosis, tuberculosis)

TABLE 101-1	Mechanisms of Neutropenia

Decreased Production

Drug induced: chemotherapeutic agents, antiinfectives (β-lactams, sulfonamides, metronidazole, vancomycin, isoniazid, ciprofloxacin, nitrofurantoin, zidovudine, ganciclovir, acyclovir), antithyroid agents (propylthiouracil, methimazole), anticonvulsants (phenytoin, carbamazepine), cardiovascular agents (captopril, procainamide, quinidine, calcium channel blockers, hydrochlorothiazide), antiinflammatory agents (gold salts, nonsteroidal antiinflammatory agents, penicillamine), psychiatric agents (phenothiazines, meprobamate, imipramine/desipramine, selective serotonin reuptake inhibitors), gastrointestinal drugs (azulfidine, cimetidine/ranitidine, metoclopramide)

Viral infections: infectious mononucleosis, hepatitis, cytomegalovirus, measles, rubella, varicella

Congenital disorders: Kostmann syndrome (severe congenital neutropenia), cyclic neutropenia, myelokathexis, glycogen storage disease type 1b, other congenital immunodeficiency syndromes

Alcohol

Radiation

Nutritional deficiencies: B_{12}, folate deficiencies

Replacement of marrow by tumor or leukemia

Aplastic anemia

Increased Destruction

Drug induced: penicillin, quinidine, procainamide

Immune mediated: autoimmune neutropenia, Felty syndrome, systemic lupus erythematosus

Miscellaneous: hypersplenism, hemodialysis, paroxysmal nocturnal hemoglobinuria

11. Though neutropenic patients are at risk for a variety of infections (see Management section), infections per se are rarely the cause of isolated neutropenia.

B. Intrinsic causes

   1. Severe congenital neutropenia

   2. Cyclic neutropenia

   3. Shwachman-Diamond syndrome

   4. Glycogen storage disease

   5. Other congenital immunodeficiencies (e.g., X-linked agammaglobulinemia, common variable immunodeficiency)

   6. Functional neutropenic defects (e.g., chronic granulomatous disease)

III. PATHOPHYSIOLOGY

A. Granulocytopenia may be due to:

   1. Decreased or ineffective marrow production

   2. Increased destruction secondary to immune or nonimmune causes

   3. Redistribution from the circulating to the marginal pool (see Table 101-1)

B. Mechanism

   1. Chemotherapeutic agents

      a. Granulocyte or neutrophil nadir usually occurs between 10 and 14 days after therapy.

      b. Melphalan, carmustine, and busulfan cause later neutrophil nadirs (at 30 to 36 days); neutrophils may not recover for 6 weeks.

   2. Hematopoietic cell transplantation

      a. Recipients of autologous bone marrow transplants have severe neutropenia that lasts approximately 12 days, compared to more than 25 days among recipients of matched, unrelated allogeneic bone marrow.

      b. For myeloablative hematopoietic cell transplantation, duration of neutropenia depends on the stem cell source:

         (1) Use of peripheral blood stem cells significantly shortens the duration of neutropenia.

         (2) Use of unrelated cord blood lengthens neutropenia to a month or more.

   3. Radiation: Radiation of marrow proliferative areas such as pelvis, skull, ribs, spine, and sternum can also directly damage marrow stem cells and result in pancytopenia.

   4. Drugs

      a. Alcohol can cause clinically significant neutropenia (when taken in large doses); other factors (e.g., folate deficiency and congestive splenomegaly) often play a role.

      b. A variety of other drugs can damage marrow stem cell production through idiosyncratic reactions. A partial list is shown in Table 101-1.

   5. Systemic processes

      a. Renal failure: Transient granulocytopenia caused by peripheral consumption has been observed in patients with renal failure on hemodialysis; this resolves within 1 to 2 hours after dialysis is stopped.

      b. Anaphylaxis: Anaphylactic reactions to endotoxin or foreign proteins may stimulate complement activation, leading to transient neutropenia.

      c. Marrow infiltration: Diseases that replace the marrow such as acute leukemia can present as an isolated neutropenia, though most patients are pancytopenic.

   6. Chronic and congenital neutropenia (for more detailed review, see Selected Readings)

      a. Cyclic neutropenia results from mutation in neutrophil elastase gene, leading to oscillations of neutrophils and monocytes with 21-day periodicity.

      b. Glycogen storage disease results from deficiency in glucose-6-phosphate translocase enzyme.

      c. Functional defects in neutrophil oxidative burst (e.g., Chediak-Higashi syndrome) or chemotaxis (e.g., leukocyte adhesion deficiency).

IV. DIAGNOSIS

A. Clinical presentation and manifestations

1. Chemotherapy-induced neutropenia: fever, stomatitis, gingivitis, perirectal inflammation, or cellulitis may be presenting signs.
2. Neutropenia unrelated to chemotherapy: signs and symptoms may be variable.
   a. Cyclic neutropenia may present as repetitive episodes of fever, mouth ulcers, pharyngitis, and lymphadenopathy in a child.
   b. Shwachman-Diamond syndrome may present with exocrine pancreatic insufficiency signs, short stature, and bone marrow dysfunction.

B. Differential diagnosis (see Table 101-1)

C. History.
A review of the history and the clinical setting should identify obvious precipitating factors, such as recent chemotherapy or suspect drugs; if not, the patient should be evaluated for occult infections including viral diseases.

1. **Physical examination.** A detailed, daily physical examination should focus on the following sites:
   a. Skin: lesions such as ulcers, ecthyma gangrenosum, erythema multiforme, and Sweet's syndrome may be a manifestation of an underlying systemic infection or condition.
   b. Sinuses
   c. Fundi
   d. Oropharynx
   e. Lung
   f. Abdomen and perirectal area: though the perianal area should be examined for tenderness or fluctuance suggestive of a perirectal abscess, a digital rectal examination should not be performed in the neutropenic patient.
   g. Surgical sites, including bone marrow aspirate sites
   h. Intravenous line sites, including sites of former catheterization

2. **Laboratory studies**
   a. Previous blood counts should be obtained to determine chronicity.
   b. Peripheral blood smear should be examined to rule out a primary hematologic disorder.
   c. Bone marrow aspirate and biopsy should be obtained if diagnosis is in question, to demonstrate the presence of a marrow infiltrative process.
      (1) Chromosomal abnormalities may be diagnostic in patients with acute leukemia.
      (2) Vacuolated bone marrow cells suggest a drug-induced idiosyncratic effect.
   d. Patients with a history of poor nutrition (or those in the intensive care unit for prolonged periods without folate supplementation) should have serum and erythrocyte folate levels measured.
   e. Antinuclear antibodies or latex fixation studies may implicate collagen vascular diseases.
   f. Although assays for antineutrophil antibodies are relatively nonspecific, a positive test and characteristic bone marrow may suggest an autoimmune process.

3. **Radiologic studies.** If pulmonary symptoms are present, chest radiograph or high-resolution chest computed tomography (CT), or both, should be ordered. Altered mental status or neurologic deficits may warrant head CT or magnetic resonance imaging (MRI), or both. As clinically indicated, other sites may be investigated (e.g., sinus and abdomen CT).

V. TREATMENT.
Therapy depends on the cause and the degree of the neutropenia and whether associated infection with or without fever is present.

A. Drug-induced neutropenia

1. Suspected drug should be withdrawn if possible.
2. Most patients with drug-induced granulocytopenia recover spontaneously and uneventfully after 10 to 14 days.
3. Anecdotal reports have suggested that drug-induced agranulocytosis responds to granulocyte-macrophage colony-stimulating factor (GM-CSF).

B. Chemotherapy-induced neutropenia: **Colony-stimulating factors**. Though granulocyte colony stimulating factor (G-CSF) and granulocyte-macrophage (GM)-CSF can shorten the duration of neutropenia following myeloablative chemotherapy, there is little evidence that this translates into measurable benefit in terms of infectious complications or survival. Nevertheless, use of G-CSF or GM-CSF is a reasonable therapeutic maneuver in a patient who is profoundly and persistently neutropenic and at high risk for mortality resulting from documented infections.

C. HIV-induced neutropenia: In neutropenic HIV-positive patients, the use of GM-CSF and G-CSF increases neutrophil and CD4+ lymphocyte counts and augments neutrophil function; these changes are not sustained once growth factor is withdrawn.

D. Intrinsic neutropenia: colony-stimulating factors may also be useful in the setting of neutropenia from intrinsic causes such as cyclic neutropenia.

V. COMPLICATIONS. Infections with a wide variety of pathogens are the primary complications attributable to neutropenia, with risk highest among those with severe (ANC <100) and prolonged neutropenia.

A. Febrile neutropenia: Defined as a single oral temperature of more than 38.3°C (37.8°C axillary) or persistent oral temperature of 38.0°C (100.4°F) or greater for 1 hour or more.

1. Risk of infection is higher in patients with neutropenia after chemotherapy due to:

a. concurrent chemotactic and phagocytic defects in remaining neutrophils

b. concurrent disruption of skin and mucosal defenses

c. use of long-term indwelling catheters that serve as a portal of entry

d. obstruction of lymphatics, biliary tract, gastrointestinal, or urinary systems by tumors

e. immune defects associated with underlying malignancy (e.g., abnormal antibody production with multiple myeloma or T-cell defects with Hodgkin disease).

2. Management

a. Search for cause using:

(1) physical examination and review of symptoms as above

(2) blood cultures from central lines and periphery

(3) other cultures as clinically indicated (wounds, urine if symptoms present)

(4) chest radiography

b. Institute empiric broad-spectrum antibacterial therapy (Figs. 101-1 and 101-2 and Table 101-2).

(1) Monotherapy with an antipseudomonal cephalosporin, penicillin, or carbapenem (i.e., ceftazidime, cefepime, piperacillin/tazobactam, imipenem, or meropenem) is equivalent to combination of these agents with aminoglycosides, yet is associated with lower costs and renal toxicity.

(2) In patients who are allergic to penicillin or cephalosporins, reasonable choices are aztreonam and ciprofloxacin. Note that antimicrobial resistance is becoming problematic for quinolones, and quinolone therapy is not appropriate for patients on quinolone prophylaxis.

(3) Broader or dual coverage may be considered for:

(a) Hemodynamically unstable patients (for whom an aminoglycoside, given on a daily dosing schedule, may also be added empirically)

(b) Patients with presumed anaerobic infection (such as typhlitis or perineal infection, for whom metronidazole may be added or a carbapenem selected) (Fig. 101-1).

(c) Patients with obvious catheter tunnel infections, known colonization with methicillin-resistant *Staphylococcus aureus*, or severe mucositis, in whom vancomycin could be added empirically

■ The use of vancomycin for empiric coverage is discouraged for most patients because of an absence of trials documenting clear benefit and the risk for selecting resistant organisms.

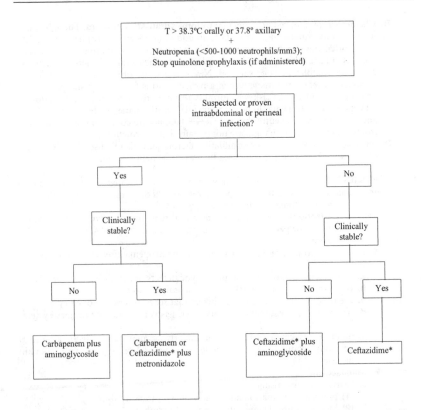

Figure 101-1. Suggested empirical antibacterial therapy for patients with febrile neutropenia. Vancomycin may be added empirically to the above regimens for those at high risk for infection with gram-positive bacteria (see text).

- If vancomycin is used empirically, blood cultures remain negative, and there is no clinical response to its administration after 48 to 72 hours, vancomycin should be discontinued.

  c. Criteria for discontinuation of antibiotic therapy (Fig. 101-2)
  d. Persistent febrile neutropenia
  - **(1)** Definition: fever that persists after 5 to 7 days of broad-spectrum antibacterial therapy without an identified focus
  - **(2)** Raises concern for invasive fungal infection
  - **(3)** Management
    - **(a)** Search for cause
      - Focused examination and review of systems
      - Repeat blood cultures
      - Directed CT scans: lungs (to look for early signs of mould infection); sinus/head/abdomen if symptoms present
    - **(b)** Treatment
      - Patients who have lower risks for mold infections may be treated successfully with fewer toxicities using fluconazole or itraconazole (*Candida* species are the primary infectious agents of concern).
      - Agents that have excellent documented activity against molds should be provided to patients who have high risks or develop

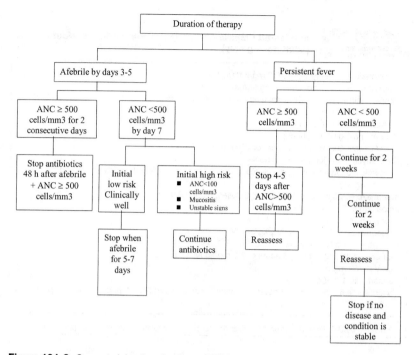

Figure 101-2. Suggested duration of antibacterial therapy for neutropenic fever of unknown origin (Infectious Disease Society of America [IDSA] guidelines).

persistent fever in the setting of azole prophylaxis (i.e., lipid formulations of amphotericin B, caspofungin, and perhaps voriconazole [see Selected Readings]).

■ No single trial using empiric antimold therapy for persistent febrile neutropenia has shown convincingly a benefit in outcomes in those already receiving anti-*Candida* prophylaxis.

■ Early diagnostics with markers such as serum galactomannan and CT scans may allow for a more targeted or preemptive approach rather than current standard empirical therapy.

B. Sepsis

    1. Usually indicates bacteremia or candidemia in neutropenic host (with or without fever)

    2. Management

        a. Search for cause:

            (1) Culture blood, urine, and respiratory secretions; stool, cerebrospinal fluid (CSF), and/or other specimens from clinically or radiographically abnormal sites should be cultured and stained for bacteria, viruses, and fungi.

            (2) Biopsies may also be helpful for culture and histopathology (particularly of new focal skin lesions).

            (3) Other appropriate diagnostic tests as indicated (e.g., stool for *Clostridium difficile* toxin or CSF for cryptococcal antigen)

        b. Institute empiric broad-spectrum antibiotic therapy.

            (1) Combination broad-spectrum antipseudomonal β-lactam (as above) *plus* an aminoglycoside may improve responses.

            (2) Check for vancomycin indications (as stated earlier) and apply if present.

TABLE 101-2	Suggested Empiric Antibiotic Dosage for Febrile Neutropenia (adult dosing only)

Amphotericin B deoxycholate 0.8 mg/kg/day IV[a]
Amphotericin B lipid complex 5 mg/kg/day IV
Caspofungin 70 mg IV × 1 dose, then 50 mg IV q 24 hours
Cefepime 2 g IV q 8 hours
Ceftazidime 2 g IV q 8 hours
Ceftriaxone 2 g IV q 24 hours
Ciprofloxacin 400 mg IV q 8 hours or 750 mg PO q 8 hours
Clindamycin 600–900 mg IV q 8 hours
Gentamicin 5 mg/kg/day IV; check blood level 10 hours after first dose (should not be >4.5 mg/dL)
Itraconazole 200 mg IV q 12 hours × 2 doses, then 200 mg qd or 2.5 mg/kg po q 12 hours[a]
Imipenem 500 mg IV q 6 hours
Levofloxacin 750 mg po or IV q 24 hours
Liposomal amphotericin B 3 mg/kg/day IV[a]
Meropenem 1 g IV q 8 hours
Metronidazole 500 mg IV q 6 hours or 7.5 mg/kg IV q 6 hours
Pen V K 750 mg po q 12 hours
Vancomycin 1 g IV q 12 hours
Voriconazole 6 mg/kg IV q 12 hours × 2 doses, then 4 mg/kg IV q 12 hours or 200 mg po q 12 hours

[a] indicated by U.S. Food and Drug Administration for persistent febrile neutropenia despite broad-

    c. Remove indwelling catheters if:
       (1) persistent sepsis syndrome with positive blood cultures
       (2) obvious catheter tunnel infection
       (3) signs of embolic disease (e.g., multiple pulmonary nodules with positive blood cultures)
       (4) any blood culture positive for difficult-to-eradicate organisms (e.g., nontuberculous mycobacteria, *Bacillus* spp., *Corynebacterium JK*, and *Candida* spp.)
    d. Standard supportive care
       (1) goal-directed volume resuscitation
       (2) tight glycemic control
       (3) glucocorticoid supplementation if documented inadequate adrenal reserve
C. Pulmonary infiltrates
    1. Differential diagnosis
       a. Noninfectious causes
       b. Infectious causes
    2. Management
       a. Empiric antimicrobial therapy as workup proceeds
          (1) antibacterial therapy with antipseudomonal agents for lobar or diffuse consolidation, or both
          (2) mold-active azole or amphotericin product if aspergillosis suspected
       b. Pursue diagnosis:
          (1) Sputum/endotracheal suction specimens (though contamination with upper airway flora may complicate interpretation).
          (2) Strongly consider early bronchoalveolar lavage (BAL) to direct therapy.
             (a) Process for Gram stain, quantitative bacterial culture, fungal prep, and culture

(b) In the appropriate epidemiologic setting and clinical picture (e.g., radiograph suggests an atypical pathogen), further tests including cytologic examination and special stains for bacteria, *Pneumocystis*, *Legionella*, immunofluorescent antibody stains for respiratory viruses and CMV, and cultures for viruses (including respiratory viruses and the human herpesviruses) should be considered as well.

(3) Directed noninvasive tests may be useful in certain scenarios.

(a) Blood antigen detection (e.g., galactomannan for *Aspergillus* and *Legionella* urinary antigen)

(b) Nasopharyngeal wash specimens for viral antigen detection and culture (RSV, parainfluenza, influenza) sputum and tracheobronchial aspirate cultures

(4) If these tests are nondiagnostic and the patient fails to respond to empiric antibacterial therapy, video-assisted or open lung biopsies may be useful to establish a diagnosis.

Selected Readings

Coyle TE. Hematologic complications of human immunodeficiency virus infection and the acquired immunodeficiency syndrome. *Med Clin North Am* 1997;81:449.
Hematologic abnormalities are among the most common manifestations of advanced HIV infection. This excellent review is detailed and well written, with an extensive background reference list.

Crawford J, Dale DC, Lyman GH. Chemotherapy-induced neutropenia. Risks, consequences, and new directions for its management. *Cancer* 2004;100:228–237.
This paper represents a review of management of patients with cancer and treatment-induced neutropenia.

Dale DC. Severe chronic neutropenia. *Semin Hematol* 2002;39(2):73–140.
This is a compilation of articles on the mechanisms, diagnosis, and treatment of severe chronic neutropenia.

The EORTC International Antimicrobial Therapy Cooperative Group. Ceftazidime combined with a short or long course of amikacin for empirical therapy of gram-negative bacteremia in cancer patients with granulocytopenia. *N Engl J Med* 1987;317:1692–1698.
This important trial was the first (and only) study to demonstrate a significant clinical benefit associated with the use of long-course combination therapy with an aminoglycoside among patients with neutropenia and gram-negative bacteremia.

Hughes WT, Armstrong D, Bodey GP, et al. 2002 guidelines for the use of antimicrobial agents in neutropenic patients with cancer. *Clin Infect Dis* 2002;34:730–751.
This is a series of practice guidelines commissioned by the Infectious Disease Society of America that provides evidence-based guidelines for diagnosis and management of neutropenic patients with unexplained fever.

Maher DW, Lieschke GJ, Green NM, et al. Filgrastim in patients with chemotherapy induced febrile neutropenia, a double-blind, placebo controlled trial. *Ann Intern Med* 1994;121:492.
This study randomized 218 patients with cancer and febrile neutropenia to receive granulocyte colony-stimulating factor (G-CSF) or placebo. Neutrophil recovery was accelerated with G-CSF treatment and the duration of febrile neutropenia was shortened, resulting in a decreased risk for prolonged hospitalization.

Marr KA. Empirical antifungal therapy—new options, new tradeoffs. *N Engl J Med* 2002; 346(4):278–280.
This editorial briefly reviews the randomized studies comparing treatment with antifungal agents for fever during neutropenia and issues in study design.

Marr KA. Fungal infections in hematopoietic stem cell transplant recipients. *Current Treatment Options in Infectious Diseases* 2001;3:533–541.
This article reviews the current antifungal management strategies (and drugs) for patients with persistent febrile neutropenia.

Peckham D, Elliott MW. Pulmonary infiltrates in the immunocompromised: diagnosis and management. *Thorax* 2002;57(suppl II):ii3–ii7.
This prospective study of 200 episodes of pulmonary infiltrates among non-HIV immunocompromised hosts illustrates that invasive bronchoscopic techniques have the highest diagnostic yield and impact on therapeutic decisions compared with noninvasive techniques.

Rubin M, Hathorn JW, Marshall D, et al. Gram positive infections and the use of vancomycin in 350 episodes of fever and neutropenia. *Ann Intern Med* 1988;108:30.
The use of vancomycin for empiric coverage of febrile neutropenic patients is a controversial area. This article provides support for withholding vancomycin in routine empiric therapy but adding it when clinical or microbiologic data suggest the need for it.

Schiel X, Hebart H, Kern WV, et al. Sepsis in neutropenia. Guidelines of the Infectious Diseases Working Party (AGIHO) of the German Society of Hematology and Oncology (DGHO). *Ann Hematol* 2003;82(suppl 2):S158–S166.
This article focuses on the pathophysiology, diagnosis, and treatment of sepsis in the neutropenic setting.

Vellenga E, Uyl-de Groot CA, de Wit R, et al. Randomized placebo-controlled trial of granulocyte-macrophage colony-stimulating factor in patients with chemotherapy-related febrile neutropenia. *J Clin Oncol* 1996;14:619.
This is a randomized, placebo-controlled trial of granulocyte-macrophage colony-stimulating factor (GM-CSF) versus placebo in 134 patients with chemotherapy-related febrile neutropenia. This trial demonstrated that GM-CSF shortened the period of neutrophil recovery but did not affect the number of days for resolution of fever or the duration of hospitalization.

I. GENERAL PRINCIPLES

A. Leukemias are curable with chemotherapy.

B. Approximately 30% of adults with acute leukemia can be cured of disease.

C. High-dose chemotherapy followed by either autologous or allogeneic stem cell transplantation is now used as a curative therapy for high-risk patients with acute and chronic leukemia.

D. Four types of leukemia

  1. Acute lymphoblastic leukemia

  2. Acute myelogeneous leukemia

  3. Chronic lymphocytic leukemia

  4. Chronic myelogeneous leukemia

II. ETIOLOGY

A. Most cases idiopathic

B. Acute myelogeneous leukemia may arise as result of prior chemotherapy or radiotherapy

C. Acute myelogeneous leukemia may arise from a myelodysplastic syndrome

D. Not usually familial in origin, no lifestyle risk factors known

III. PATHOPHYSIOLOGY

A. Acute lymphoblastic leukemia (ALL) occurs primarily in children, but also in adults.

  1. Leukemia involvement in bone marrow

  2. May also have mediastinal mass, leukemic meningitis, and testicular involvement

B. Acute myelogeneous leukemia (AML) more common in adults

  1. Monocytic variants can have skin, gum, and central nervous system (CNS) infiltration

  2. Acute promyelocytic leukemia can have disseminated intravascular coagulation (DIC) and bleeding

C. Chronic lymphocytic leukemia. Often indolent disease of elderly

D. Chronic myelogeneous leukemia. Can progress to acute leukemia (myeloid or lymphoid blast crisis)

IV. DIAGNOSIS

A. History: fatigue, shortness of breath, infection, and bleeding

B. Exam: pallor, petechiae, sometimes splenomegaly

C. Laboratory: anemia, thrombocytopenia, white blood count may be normal, high, or low

D. Peripheral smear: increased immature cells

E. Definitive diagnosis: bone marrow aspirate and biopsy with flow cytometry, histochemical stains, and cytogenetics

F. Acute leukemia defined as >20% blasts in the marrow

V. TREATMENT

A. Acute lymphoblastic leukemia

  1. Induction chemotherapy with four to five chemotherapy drugs, such as asparaginase, prednisone, vincristine, adriamycin, and cyclophosphamide

    2. CNS prophylaxis with intrathecal chemotherapy

    3. Intensification and maintenance chemotherapy over 18 to 24 months (outpatient)

  B. Acute myelogeneous leukemia

    1. Induction chemotherapy with idarubicin and cytosine arabinoside

    2. Consolidation chemotherapy with high dose cytosine arabinoside

    3. Stem cell transplantation for patients at high risk of relapse, often based on cytogenetics

    4. Acute promyelocytic leukemia treated with chemotherapy plus retinoic acid

  C. Chronic lymphocytic leukemia

    1. Observation until disease progression

    2. Fludarabine therapy, then antibody therapy with Rituxan or Campath, or both

  D. Chronic myelogeneous leukemia

    1. Tyrosine kinase inhibitor, Gleevec (outpatient)

    2. Allogeneic stem cell transplantation for disease progression

VI. COMPLICATIONS

  A. Leukostasis

    1. Occurs when the white blood cell (WBC) count, predominantly blasts, greater than $100,000/mm^3$

    2. More common in AML than ALL, because blasts larger

    3. Pulmonary infiltrates, hypoxia, visual changes, mental status changes, CNS bleeding

    4. Treatment for leukostasis

      a. Intravenous fluids

      b. Prompt initiation of chemotherapy

      c. Hydroxyurea to lower WBC

      d. Leukopheresis

      e. Avoid red blood cell (RBC) transfusions, which can increase viscosity

  B. Bleeding

    1. Occurs as result of thrombocytopenia or disseminated intravascular coagulation (DIC)

    2. Increased risk of spontaneous bleeding with platelet count below $10,000/mm^3$

    3. Treatment for bleeding

      a. Platelet transfusion when platelet count less than 10,000 or evidence of bleeding

      b. Irradiated, filtered blood products only

      c. Patients who are alloimmunized to platelets may benefit from human leukocyte antigen (HLA)-matched platelets (nonfamily member if patient a candidate for stem cell transplant)

      d. DIC (seen with acute promyelocytic leukemia) treated with fresh frozen plasma, platelets, and chemotherapy to treat leukemia

  C. Infection

    1. WBC high, but abnormal WBC function—patient functionally neutropenic

    2. Chemotherapy also suppresses immune system

    3. Bacterial infections

      a. Gram-positive infections—staphylococcal, streptococcal—related to indwelling catheters

      b. Gram-negative infections—*Escherichia coli*, pseudomonas—related to damaged intestinal tract

    4. Fungal infections

      a. Increased with low counts, antibiotics, indwelling catheter, parenteral nutrition

      b. Candida—skin, lung, liver

      c. Aspergillus—lung, sinuses

    5. Other infections

      a. *Pneumocystis jiroveci* pneumonia—particularly in patients with ALL who are receiving steroids

      b. Herpes simplex virus, herpes zoster

TABLE 102-1   Side Effects from Chemotherapy Agents

Drug	Alopecia	Nausea/ vomiting	Bone marrow suppression	Other
Cytosine arabinoside (ARA-C)	+	+	++	Fever, renal failure, cerebellar toxicity
Idarubicin, daunorubicin	++	++	++	Cardiac, mucositis, vesicant
Etoposide	+	+	+	Hypotension
All trans retinoic acid (ATRA)				Increased white blood cells Lung infiltrates
Cyclophosphamide (Cytoxan)	+	++	++	Hemorrhagic cystitis
Prednisone				Muscle weakness, edema, glucose intolerance
Vincristine		+		Neuropathy
Asparginase				Pancreatitis, coagulopathy
Gleevec			+	Elevated liver tests, rash
Fludarabine		+		Increased risk late infection

6. Treatment for infections

   a. Treat fever immediately as presumptive infection.

   b. Fever workup includes history and physical examination, blood and fungal cultures, urine culture, and chest radiography.

   c. Treat first with gram-negative coverage to include pseudomonas—such as a third-generation cephalosporin.

   d. If fever persists for more than 2 days, add gram-positive coverage, such as vancomycin.

   e. If fever persists for more than 5 to 7 days, add empiric antifungal coverage with amphotericin or voriconazole.

   f. Preventive regimens should include gram-negative coverage such as levaquin, antifungal coverage such as fluconazole, and (for patients with ALL) Bactrim or equivalent.

D. Tumor lysis syndrome

   1. Rapid destruction of tumor cells

   2. High uric acid, low calcium, high potassium

   3. Can progress to acute renal failure

   4. Treatment of tumor lysis syndrome

   a. Start prevention before chemotherapy

   b. Hydration

   c. Alkalinization of urine

   d. Allopurinol or (for patients at very high risk) intravenous uricolytics

E. Chemotherapy toxicity—summarized in Table 102-1

Selected Readings

Anderson JE, Kopecky KJ, Willman CL, et al. Outcome after induction chemotherapy for older patients with acute myeloid leukemia is not improved with mitoxantrone and etoposide compared to cytarabine and daunorubicin: a Southwest Oncology Group study. *Blood* 2002;100:3869–3876.

Comparison of two chemotherapy regimens for older patients with AML, with results favoring the standard approach of anthracycline and cytarabine

Anttila V, Elonen E, Nordling S, et al. Hepatosplenic candidiasis in patients with acute leukemia: incidence and prognostic implications. *Clin Infect Dis* 1997;24:375.

Review of 562 patients with acute leukemia, describing the incidence of serious Candida infections.

Chanock SJ, Pizzo PA. Infectious complications of patients undergoing therapy for acute leukemia: current status and future prospects. *Semin Oncol* 1997;24:132.
Comprehensive update of infectious complications in leukemic patients.

Cripe LD. Adult acute leukemia. *Curr Probl Cancer* 1997;21:1.
Excellent review of pathogenesis, diagnosis, and treatment strategies of acute leukemia.

Dutcher JP, Schiffer CA, Wiernik PH. Hyperleukocytosis in adult acute nonlymphocytic leukemia: impact on remission rate, duration, and survival. *J Clin Oncol* 1987;5:1364.
Description of the negative correlation between leukostasis and survival.

Heckman KD, Weiner GJ, Davis CS, et al. Randomized study of prophylactic platelet transfusion threshold during induction therapy for adult acute leukemia: 10,000/μL versus 20,000/μL. *J Clin Oncol* 1997;15:1143.
No difference seen in bleeding episodes whether 10,000 or 20,000 platelets used as a threshold for transfusion.

Hughes TP, Kaeda J, Branford S, et al. Frequency of major molecular responses to imatinib or interferon alpha plus cytarabine in newly diagnosed chronic myeloid leukemia. *N Engl J Med* 2003;349:1423–1432.
Landmark study revealing the superiority of Gleevec as upfront therapy in CML.

Keating MJ, Flinn I, Jain V, et al. Therapeutic role of alemtuzumab (Campath-1H) in patients who have failed fludarabine: results of a large international study. *Blood* 2002;99:3554–3561.
Multicenter study outlining the utility of Campath as second-line therapy in CLL.

Linker C, Damon L, Ries C, Nararro W. Intensified and shortened cyclical chemotherapy for adult acute lymphoblastic leukemia. *J Clin Oncol* 2002;20:2464–2471.
Description of popular treatment regimen for ALL.

Tallman MS, Nabhan C, Feusner JH, et al. Acute promyelocytic leukemia: evolving therapeutic strategies. *Blood* 2002;99:759–767.
Reviews the use of retinoic acid for induction therapy and arsenic for salvage therapy.

Thomas ED, Clift RA, Feiffer F, et al. Marrow transplantation for the treatment of chronic myelogenous leukemia. *Ann Intern Med* 1986;104:155.
The classic reference describing one of the first diseases to be cured by bone marrow transplantation.

I. SUPERIOR VENA CAVA SYNDROME

A. General principles

1. Due to obstruction of blood flow in the superior vena cava (SVC).
2. Etiology includes intrinsic obstruction by thrombosis, direct tumor invasion, or extrinsic tumor compression.

B. Etiology

1. Most cases due to lung and breast cancer and lymphoma.
2. Other causes are mediastinal or radiation fibrosis and thrombosis (e.g., indwelling central venous line).

C. Diagnosis

1. SVC syndrome is a clinical diagnosis.
2. Symptoms and signs (Table 103-1) are related to poor venous return, increased intravenous pressure, and collateral vessel engorgement.
3. Radiographic studies are usually diagnostic.
   a. Chest radiograph (CXR) is abnormal in more than 80%.
   b. Contrast chest computed tomography (CT) may localize the mass and suggest impending complications (e.g., vertebral spread).
   c. Magnetic resonance imaging (MRI) may be useful if venous access cannot be obtained for contrast-enhanced CT.
   d. Superior vena cavagram is rarely necessary to confirm the diagnosis.
4. Specific tissue diagnosis is often needed, because approximately 60% of patients present without a known diagnosis of cancer.
   a. Tissue diagnosis should be accomplished using the simplest, least invasive method, beginning with thoracentesis, bronchoscopy, mediastinoscopy, and proceeding to thoracoscopy and finally to limited thoracotomy if necessary.
   b. Routine diagnostic procedures carry little excess risk in patients with elevated venous pressures. However, patients with tracheal compression or stridor represent a true medical emergency and should be treated emergently.

D. Treatment

1. Nonspecific methods to decrease venous pressures
   a. Bed rest in reverse Trendelenburg position
   b. Diuretics (maintaining adequate intravascular volume), decreased salt intake, and oxygen
2. Steroids, although commonly prescribed, are of limited benefit.
3. Anticoagulation and thrombolysis may benefit patients with intravascular thrombosis in the setting of an indwelling central venous catheter, if the clot is 5 days old or less.
4. Histology and tumor stage generally dictate initial treatment.
   a. Radiation therapy (RT) is the treatment of choice for most patients and may be lifesaving for tracheal compression.
   b. Patients with Hodgkin's lymphoma, germ cell tumors, or limited stage small cell lung cancer have a poor long-term outcome with RT alone, and initial chemotherapy is preferred.
   c. If extrinsic tumor compression is present, the placement of intraluminal metal stents within the SVC provides more rapid relief of symptoms in a higher proportion of patients than either RT or chemotherapy.

TABLE 103-1	Common Symptoms and Signs of Superior Vena Cava Syndrome	
Symptom or sign		**Incidence (%)**
Facial swelling		43
Trunk and/or extremity swelling		40
Dyspnea		20
Chest pain		20
Cough		20
Dysphagia		20
Dizziness		10
Syncope		10
Visual disturbance		10
Thoracic vein distention		67
Neck vein distention		59
Facial edema		56
Tachypnea		40
Plethora of face		19
Cyanosis		15
Upper extremity edema		9
Paralyzed true vocal cord		3
Horner's syndrome		2

II. EPIDURAL SPINAL CORD COMPRESSION

A. General principles. Epidural spinal cord compression (ESCC) is a common complication of cancer, causing pain and sometimes irreversible loss of neurologic function.

B. Etiology and pathophysiology

1. Increasing intradural pressure or direct invasion from enlarging vertebral body metastases, retroperitoneal lymphadenopathy extending through the paravertebral neural foramina, a pathologic vertebral collapse, or intradural metastases.

2. Vascular compromise leads to spinal cord infarction and rapid, irreversible loss of function.

3. The most common tumors are lung, breast, prostate and kidney cancer; lymphoma; and myeloma.

C. Diagnosis

1. **Clinical presentation**

   a. Back pain is the initial symptom in more than 90% of patients.

   b. Motor weakness, varying from minimal to paralysis, occasionally progresses to paraplegia within hours.

   c. Sensory deficits are rare initially but usually develop at some point.

   d. Loss of bowel or bladder control is a late and poor prognostic sign.

2. **Importance of early diagnosis**

   a. Early diagnosis of ESCC is essential to prevent paralysis.

   b. Patients who begin treatment when paraplegic almost never regain ambulation.

   c. ESCC must be considered in any patient with a known diagnosis of cancer (or whose symptoms suggest the presence of undiagnosed malignant disease) who presents with unexplained back pain.

3. **Diagnostic evaluation**

   a. Thorough neurologic examination and plain spine radiographs (looking for pedicle loss, vertebral compression fractures, and osteoblastic or osteolytic bone lesions).

(1) In one study, plain spine radiographs accurately predicted the presence or absence of spinal epidural metastases in 83% of cases, with a sensitivity of 81% and a specificity of 86%.

(2) If either physical examination or radiographic study is abnormal, further spine imaging, such as with MRI or myelography, is necessary to exclude ESCC.

b. Contrast-enhanced MRI is preferred for diagnosing location and extent of ESCC.

c. CT myelography may be necessary if timely MRI is unavailable or if the patient cannot lie still.

(1) Contrast medium is introduced through the lumbar spine until obstruction is encountered. The anatomy above the obstruction is then defined by a cisterna magna or cervical spinal tap.

(2) Rarely, myelography can result in further neurologic deterioration when cerebrospinal fluid (CSF) pressure below a complete block is reduced by the lumbar puncture.

D. Treatment

1. Corticosteroids (e.g., dexamethasone 10 to 24 mg IV bolus followed by 16 to 24 mg) should be started as soon as ESCC is suspected. Higher initial doses (e.g., dexamethasone 100 mg) may enhance analgesia but do not improve neurologic outcome.

2. Laminectomy

a. Laminectomy was previously considered only in patients with symptomatic progression during or after RT, rapidly progressing neurologic deficits, or the need for spinal stabilization.

b. More recent data suggest that all patients with ESCC (except those with lymphoma or intraspinal tumors) should be considered for initial aggressive radical resection.

(1) The superiority of initial tumor debulking was shown in a landmark study that randomly assigned 101 patients with ESCC (excluding those with lymphoma) to radical resection followed by RT or RT alone.

(2) Patients undergoing resection were three times more likely to regain ambulation and maintain ambulation for the duration of their remaining life span, whereas those undergoing RT alone spent two thirds of their remaining life span unable to walk.

(3) The postoperative complication rate is much lower when surgery is undertaken initially rather than as a salvage procedure after failing RT.

3. Radiation therapy is necessary following laminectomy and is the treatment of choice for patients who are not candidates for aggressive radical resection.

4. Chemotherapy may be considered in patients with chemoresponsive malignancies (e.g., small cell lung cancer, lymphoma).

III. HYPERCALCEMIA OF MALIGNANCY

A. General principles

1. Hypercalcemia is the major metabolic abnormality recognized in patients with cancer, occurring in approximately 10% of all patients.

2. It is most common in patients with breast and lung cancer and multiple myeloma.

B. Etiology and pathophysiology. Three mechanisms cause hypercalcemia in cancer patients:

1. Osteolytic metastases

2. Hypercalcemia in the absence of bone metastases, which most frequently occurs with lung (squamous cell), kidney, and pancreas cancer, is caused by ectopic tumor production of parathyroid hormone-related protein (PTHrP).

3. Hypercalcemia associated with hematologic malignancies (e.g., multiple myeloma) can be caused by direct bone invasion, or local production of humoral factors (e.g., osteoclast activating factor).

4. The final common pathway is increased osteoclast activation.

C. Diagnosis

1. **Clinical manifestations** depend on the degree of elevation of ionized serum calcium and the rate of rise. Symptoms and signs are less apparent when the rate of calcium rise is prolonged.

   a. Change in mental status (e.g., lethargy or depression) can be subtle, but in the extreme, may include psychotic behavior, obtundation, or coma.

   b. The most characteristic ECG changes are prolonged PR interval, occasionally producing high-grade AV block, and shortened QT interval. The spectrum of digitalis-toxic arrhythmias develops more easily in hypercalcemic patients.

   c. The earliest renal consequence is a decrease in concentrating ability with polyuria; dehydration and prerenal azotemia follow. Tubular damage from nephrocalcinosis can result in acidosis, glycosuria, hypomagnesemia, and aminoaciduria.

   d. Gastrointestinal symptoms include anorexia, nausea, vomiting, constipation, and abdominal pain.

2. **Laboratory studies.** Most laboratories report total serum calcium level rather than the biologically active ionized calcium level.

   a. Mild hypercalcemia is defined as a corrected serum calcium between 11 and 12 mg/dL (2.8 to 3 mmol/liter); moderate, 12 to 14 mg/dL (3 to 3.5 mmol/L); severe, greater than 14 mg/dL (>3.5 mmol/L).

   b. Approximately 40% of total serum calcium is bound to protein, primarily albumin. Because 1 g of albumin binds 0.8 mg of calcium, a corrected serum calcium value can be calculated by adding 0.8 mg/dL to the measured serum calcium for each 1 g/dL decrease in serum albumin below 4.0 g/dL.

   c. In multiple myeloma, total serum calcium may be spuriously elevated because hyperglobulinemia leads to increased binding of calcium; in such cases, ionized calcium should be measured.

3. **Differential diagnosis.** Once the presence of hypercalcemia is established, many potential causes can be eliminated by the patient's history (Table 103-2).

TABLE 103-2	Differential Diagnosis of Hypercalcemia

Cancer
  With bone metastasis (solid tumor)
  Without bone metastasis (solid tumor)
  Hematologic (multiple myeloma, leukemia, lymphoma with bone involvement)
Primary hyperparathyroidism
Toxic
  Thiazides
  Milk-alkali syndrome
  Vitamin D or A toxicity
Endocrine
  Thyrotoxicosis
  Adrenal insufficiency
  Pheochromocytoma (usually in association with primary hyperparathyroidism)
Granulomatous disease
  Tuberculosis
  Sarcoidosis
Immobilization (especially with underlying bone disease)
Artifactual
  Hyperalbuminemia or hypergammaglobulinemia
  Venous stasis (prolonged tourniquet application)

D. Treatment

1. The best treatment is specific and effective treatment of the underlying malignancy.
2. Avoid thiazide diuretics because they promote renal tubular calcium resorption.
3. Hypercalcemic patients are usually volume depleted, and initial therapy is fluid replacement with normal saline at 150 to 300 mL per hour. Benefit is usually temporary and insufficient to normalize the calcium level in the majority of patients.
4. In the euvolemic patient, furosemide can be used to maintain urine output and enhance calciuresis. Further volume depletion must be avoided. Total intake and output, weight, serum electrolytes, and urine electrolytes (at least within the first 12 hours) should be closely monitored.
5. The treatment of choice is parenteral bisphosphonates, such as zoledronic acid (4 mg over 15 minutes) or pamidronate (60 to 90 mg over 2 hours). The onset of action is within 24 hours.
6. If a decrease in serum calcium is required urgently (e.g., obtunded patient or ECG changes), calcitonin (4 IU/kg) has an onset of action of 4 to 6 hours.
   a. Tachyphylaxis limits efficacy to the first 48 hours, even with repeated doses.
   b. Calcitonin is a relatively weak agent, lowering serum calcium by a maximum of 1 to 2 mg/dL (0.3 to 0.5 mmol/L).
   c. Concurrent steroids can delay development of tachyphylaxis, but do not enhance the hypocalcemic effect.
7. Intravenous phosphate therapy can lower markedly elevated calcium levels within several hours but is reserved for acute situations if other measures fail or the patient is severely hypophosphatemic.
   a. Phosphates should not be given to patients who have elevated phosphate levels or significantly impaired renal function.
   b. Doses should be given slowly over 6 to 8 hours; rapid IV infusions may cause severe hypotension and hypocalcemia.
8. Dialysis is a treatment of last resort for severe hypercalcemia but may be needed in patients with renal failure.
9. Corticosteroids may be useful for patients with hematologic malignancies or breast cancer.
10. Gallium nitrate (200 mg/m^2 intravenously daily for 5 days) may be considered for refractory patients.
11. In the absence of effective antineoplastic treatment, hypercalcemia typically recurs, and retreatment is required every 3 to 4 weeks.

IV. MALIGNANT PERICARDIAL DISEASE

A. Etiology and pathogenesis

1. Malignant cells gain access to the pericardial space by direct invasion or hematogenous or lymphatic spread, most commonly from breast and lung cancer.
2. Tumor cells block subepicardial lymphatic drainage, leading to fluid buildup in the pericardial space. Increasing intrapericardial pressure compresses all cardiac chambers, leading to cardiac tamponade.
3. The same pathophysiology may result from restrictive or effusive pericardial disease that develops from direct pericardial tumor growth or radiation fibrosis.

B. Clinical manifestations

1. Symptoms of cardiac tamponade include facial swelling, dyspnea, cough, orthopnea, and ill-defined chest discomfort.
2. Physical examination may show signs of low cardiac output (diaphoresis, cool extremities), tachycardia, pulsus paradoxus, jugular venous distention, distant heart sounds, narrowed pulse pressure, a pericardial friction rub, venous hypotension, and, if severe, cardiogenic shock.
3. Electrocardiographic abnormalities include electrical alternans (rare) or, more commonly, tachycardia, diffuse S-T wave abnormalities, loss of voltage, T-wave inversions, or atrial arrhythmias.
4. CXR often shows enlargement of the cardiac silhouette.

C. Diagnosis

1. Echocardiography is the procedure of choice for the diagnosis of pericardial effusions and should be performed emergently if tamponade is suspected.
2. Chest CT may show pericardial thickening and reveal tumor extent and location.
3. Cardiac catheterization is seldom needed to confirm the diagnosis.

D. Treatment. Cardiac tamponade requires prompt treatment.

1. Supportive measures (IV volume expansion and supplemental oxygen) should be provided while preparing for definitive therapy.
2. Because of decreased diastolic filling, medications that lower blood pressure, reduce preload, or decrease heart rate (e.g., diuretics or β-blockers) should be avoided or used with extreme caution.
3. Pericardiocentesis is the initial diagnostic procedure of choice in the workup of pericardial effusion of possible malignant origin and may be lifesaving for patients with tamponade.
   a. A 16- to 22-gauge needle is attached to a syringe and inserted at roughly a 45-degree angle below the xiphoid process cephalad toward the tip of the scapula. Advancement into the myocardium usually reveals an injury pattern on the ECG.
   b. Removal of as little as 50 cc may be sufficient to improve hemodynamics.
   c. The most common complications are right ventricular puncture, hemopericardium, and ventricular ectopy.
4. Prolonged catheter drainage is often accomplished by threading a pigtail catheter into the pericardial space utilizing the Seldinger catheter over a guide wire technique.
   a. Intrapericardial instillation of sclerosing agents (e.g., bleomycin 30–60 U) through the intrapericardial catheter, particularly if used in conjunction with systemic therapy, may prevent further symptomatic recurrence.
   b. Three available surgical approaches—subxiphoid pericardial window placement, limited thoracotomy with pleuropericardial window placement, and thoracotomy with pericardiectomy—provide alternative modes of treatment in a patient with an expected reasonable survival.

E. Prognosis. Prognosis is usually poor. Systemic antitumor treatment can be considered for chemotherapy-responsive cancers (breast, lymphoma). Radiation therapy may be useful in selected cases.

Selected Readings

Ahman FR. A reassessment of the clinical implications of the superior vena cava syndrome. *J Clin Oncol* 1984:2:961.
This large series of 1,986 cases of superior vena cava syndrome are reviewed, with particular emphasis on the safety of diagnostic procedures and the benefit of proceeding with a diagnostic study before embarking on treatment.

Byrne TN. Spinal cord compression from epidural metastasis. *N Engl J Med* 1992; 327:614.
This is an excellent recent summary of pathophysiology, presentation, and diagnostic approach to epidural spinal cord compression.

Liu G, Crump M, Goss PE, et al. Prospective comparison of the sclerosing agents doxycycline and bleomycin for the primary management of malignant pericardial effusion and cardiac tamponade. *J Clin Oncol* 1996;14:3141.
In this study, 27 patients were randomly assigned to intrapericardial instillation of bleomycin or doxycycline for the management of pericardial effusion after placement of a draining catheter. Although both were equally effective, bleomycin resulted in significantly less morbidity.

Major P, Lortholary A, Hon J, et al. Zoledronic acid is superior to pamidronate in the treatment of hypercalcemia of malignancy: a pooled analysis of two randomized, controlled clinical trials. *J Clin Oncol* 2001;19:558.
In a randomized study directly comparing pamidronate and zoledronic acid for the treatment of hypercalcemia of malignancy, a single dose of zolendronate (4 mg) normalized

the corrected serum calcium level in 87% to 88% of patients, compared with only 70% of those receiving pamidronate (90 mg). Moreover, the median duration of calcium control was longer for those receiving zolendronate (32 to 43 days versus 18 days).

Patchell R, Tibbs PA, Regine WF, et al. A randomized trial of direct decompressive surgical resection in the treatment of spinal cord compression caused by metastasis (abstract). *Proc Am Soc Clin Oncol* 2003;22:1.

This preliminary report of a randomized trial demonstrated the superiority of initial aggressive surgical resection and postoperative radiation therapy compared to radiation therapy and salvage surgery, in patients initially presenting with epidural spinal cord compression that was not due to lymphoma or an intraspinal tumor.

Rodichok LD, Harper GR, Ruckdeschel JC, et al. Early diagnosis of spinal epidural metastases. *Am J Med* 1981;70:1181.

This is a classic article describing a study of 87 patients with back pain and a diagnosis of cancer. The use of the neurologic examination and plain radiographs of the spine to predict the risk for epidural cord compression is described.

Spodick DH. Acute cardiac tamponade *N Engl J Med* 2003;349:684.

A contemporary review of the pathophysiology underlying cardiac tamponade, and management of this condition.

Wilkes JD, Fidias P, Baikus L, et al. Malignancy-related pericardial effusion. *Cancer* 1995;76:1377.

This article reviews 127 cases of malignant pericardial effusion from the Roswell Park Cancer Institute, demonstrating that subxyphoid pericardiotomy is a safe intervention that effectively relieves pericardial effusion in 99% of cases with less than 10% recurrence and reoperation rates. An excellent review of surgical approaches to the management of pericardial effusion is provided.

Pharmacology, Overdoses and Poisonings

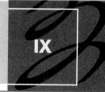

IX

I. GENERAL PRINCIPLES

A. Applied pharmacokinetics is the process of using measured drug concentrations, pharmacokinetic principles, and pharmacodynamic information to optimize drug therapy for individual patients.

B. The change in drug concentration over time is related to the rate and amount of drug absorption and administration, volume of distribution, and rate of drug distribution and elimination.

C. Alteration in drug disposition can be affected by many physiologic changes resulting from underlying disease, sepsis, or injury and alter the response to pharmacotherapy.

D. Many pharmacokinetic and pharmacodynamic alterations can be anticipated by knowing the patient's physiologic status.

E. Failing to appreciate the influence of physiologic status, which is dynamic and may change substantially during the hospital course, leads to a higher risk of treatment failure or serious drug-induced toxicity.

II. DRUG ABSORPTION

A. The rate of drug absorption or administration influences or determines the time required to achieve therapeutic serum concentrations.

B. Serum concentrations are assumed to have reached steady-state conditions after a drug has been administered for a period at least five times its half-life.

C. Bioavailability after ingestion is influenced by the fraction of active drug in its formulation, the rate of product dissolution, chemical properties of the dissolved drug, gastrointestinal (GI) motility, blood flow to the GI tract, blood pH, and surface area available for absorption, all of which can be altered by certain disease states, drugs, and surgery.

D. First-pass effect or metabolism refers to the phenomenon whereby a proportion of an oral dose of a drug is metabolized by the liver or gut before it reaches the systemic circulation. In certain overdose situations, the first-pass metabolism can become saturated, with a resultant increase in the bioavailability of drugs such as cyclic antidepressants, phenothiazines, opioids, and β-blockers.

III. DRUG DISTRIBUTION

A. The rate and extent of drug distribution depend on its chemical properties (protein and tissue binding, lipid solubility) and physiologic status of the patient.

B. The volume of distribution (V_d) represents the theoretical volume into which a substance distributes in the body at equilibrium. It can be used to estimate the plasma drug concentration when a known amount of the drug has been ingested or given: $V_d = dose/Cp$, where Cp is the plasma drug concentration.

   1. The larger the volume of distribution, the lower the serum drug's concentration relative to a dose and vice versa.

   2. Drugs with low V_d (<1 L/kg) are distributed primarily in the extracellular fluid and include aminoglycosides, phenobarbital, salicylates, and lithium.

   3. Drugs with large volumes of distribution (>1 L/kg) have extensive tissue distribution and include digoxin, cyclic antidepressants, and phenytoin.

C. The distribution of most drugs follows first-order kinetics (i.e., the plasma or serum drug level declines at a rate equal to a constant fraction of the level per unit of time) and can be characterized by a half-life (the initial α phase half-life), the time required for the drug level to decline by 50%.

IV. PROTEIN BINDING

A. The plasma proteins albumin and α-acid glycoprotein (AAG) are responsible for 95% of all drug binding. Anionic drugs and weak acids (e.g., phenytoin, warfarin, salicylates) tend to bind to albumin, whereas cationic drugs and weak bases (e.g., quinidine, propranolol, lidocaine) usually bind to AAG.

B. Only the unbound or free fraction of the drug is pharmacologically active.

C. Decreased protein binding occurs when protein levels are decreased or saturated (e.g., in overdoses) and increases drug effects.

  1. Malnutrition, sepsis, burns, renal disease, and liver disease can all decrease albumin concentration and increase the percentage of free drug.

  2. Traumatic injuries, surgery, burns, psychiatric conditions, acute inflammation, and myocardial infarction are associated with large increases in AAG and, consequently, decrease circulating concentrations of free drug.

V. DRUG ELIMINATION

A. The elimination of most drugs follows first-order kinetics. The elimination half-life, $t_{1/2}$, equals $0.693/K_e$, where K_e is the elimination rate constant.

B. Zero-order elimination occurs when a constant quantity of drug is eliminated per unit of time, of which ethanol, at intoxicating levels, is an example.

C. Michaelis-Menten kinetics is a combination of first-order elimination kinetics at low drug concentrations and zero-order elimination at higher concentrations. It characterizes drugs that are eliminated by capacity-limited or saturable enzyme systems (e.g., aspirin, phenytoin, theophylline).

D. Total body clearance, a measurement of the body's ability to eliminate a substance from blood or plasma over time, is equal to the sum of all clearance processes—renal, hepatic, gastrointestinal, pulmonary, and artificial. It can be calculated by multiplying the rate constant of elimination by the volume of distribution ($Cl = K_e \times V_d$).

  1. If renal clearance accounts for 50% or more of total clearance, dosing regimens must be adjusted in patients with renal dysfunction to maintain appropriate serum drug concentrations.

   a. When a drug is freely filtered and neither secreted nor reabsorbed, renal clearance is equivalent to glomerular filtration rate (GFR).

   b. When renal function is stable, creatinine clearance (CrCl) and serum creatinine (SCr) are highly correlated and SCr can be used to estimate CrCl and, thus, GFR: CrCl (mL/min) = $(140 - \text{age}) \times$ lean body weight/$72 \times$ SCr (multiply by 0.85 for women).

   c. Many disease states are associated with altered creatinine production, leading to poor correlation between SCr and GFR. In some instances, the actual CrCl should be measured using an 8-hour urine collection.

  2. Hepatic clearance depends on blood flow to the liver, the intrinsic activity of hepatic enzymes, and the fraction of drug that is unbound and free to interact with these enzymes.

   a. Alterations in hepatic blood flow caused by drugs, surgical procedures, or disease states such as shock or heart failure cause significant changes in the rate of elimination of drugs such as aminoglycosides, lidocaine, meperidine, and ranitidine.

   b. Cytochrome mixed-function oxidase enzyme systems can be induced by specific drugs (phenobarbital, rifampin) and, thus, affect the metabolism of other drugs (acetaminophen, theophylline).

   c. Liver disease decreases the clearance of many drugs.

VI. DOSING CONSIDERATIONS

A. End-organ responses to illness or injury (e.g., oxygen clearance, cardiac output, serum proteins, vascular volume, extracellular fluid volume, metabolic rate, urinary urea nitrogen,

TABLE 104-1	Flow-Limited Agents Frequently Used in the Intensive Care Unit		
Gentamicin	Ranitidine	Netilmicin
Tobramycin	Ampicillin	Vancomycin
Amikacin	Ceftazidime	Meperidine
Cefazolin	Lidocaine	Imipenem
Piperacillin	Aztreonam	

urinary catecholamines, regional shunting in blood flow, amino acid utilization, organ blood flow) can result in changes in drug disposition.

B. Variation in dosage requirements is not readily predictable by common organ function tests, such as serum creatinine or liver function profiles.

C. Three physiologic variables that the clinician can use to make qualitative assessments and inferences regarding a drug's disposition characteristics are cardiac output, organ function, and serum protein concentration.

D. The disposition of many drugs is dependent on organ blood flow for clearance.

   1. The clearance of drugs with high intrinsic hepatic elimination rates and those eliminated primarily by glomerular filtration can be characterized as flow limited (Table 104-1). For such agents, quantitative approaches using serum drug measurements can be used to calculate dosages necessary to attain desired serum concentrations, improve survival, and decrease the length of intensive care unit (ICU) stay.

   2. Drugs with low intrinsic hepatic and renal elimination are categorized as capacity limited (Table 104-2), meaning clearance is primarily dependent on hepatic enzyme activity rather than on blood flow. The effect of disease states on dosage is complex and less predictable than the flow-limited agents.

E. The qualitative pharmacokinetic effect on many agents used in the ICU can be anticipated by knowing the patient's response to underlying diseases, fluid balance, injury, sepsis, and the drug's physiologic clearance properties.

   1. Classifying the physiological state as hypermetabolic or hypometabolic is useful to anticipate decreased or increased dosage requirements.

     a. Increased cardiac output, oxygen clearance, energy requirements, metabolic rate, and blood flow to the kidney and liver characterize the hypermetabolic state, which is usually secondary to burns, traumatic injury, and sepsis.

      (1) As blood flow to the organ increases, drug clearance and dosage requirements can increase, particularly with agents that have flow-limited characteristics.

      (2) Drug clearance generally increases in parallel with blood flow as long as the intrinsic function of the organ is not altered by medical complications, altered renal function, altered hepatic function, or drugs.

TABLE 104-2	Capacity-Limited Agents Frequently Used in the Intensive Care Unit		
Drug	**Binding sensitive**	**Binding insensitive**	**Unknown**
Phenytoin	Yes		
Clindamycin	Yes		
Lorazepam			Yes
Theophylline		Yes	
Midazolam	Yes		
Cimetidine		Yes	
Diazepam			Yes

   b. A hypometabolic state is characteristic of congestive heart failure, shock, and multiple-system organ failure.

   (1) The functional (drug elimination) capacity of the kidney and liver decreases markedly with the onset of changes in blood chemistry and clinical indicators of organ failure.

   (2) Changes in drug disposition can occur before the change in blood chemistry or other physiologic markers are evident.

2. Fluid shifts between physiologic spaces can affect the distribution of drugs to tissue compartments for many agents.

   a. Intravascular and extracellular fluid volumes are increased in patients with traumatic injury, congestive heart failure, and renal failure.

   b. They are decreased with dehydration and acute blood loss.

3. Changes in the concentration and total amount of serum proteins secondary to disease or injury can affect the amount of free drug and patient response.

   a. Drugs with capacity-limited clearance may be sensitive or insensitive to serum protein levels, depending on whether their binding is high ($>50\%$) or low, respectively (Table 104-2).

   b. With decreased albumin levels, as may occur with burns, malnutrition, sepsis, and renal and liver disease, the free fraction and effect of anionic drugs that are highly bound to albumin (see Chapter 90) is greater for the same total serum drug concentration.

   c. With increased α_1-acid glycoprotein, an acute-phase reactant synthesized by the liver in response to acute inflammation, injury, myocardial infarction, and psychiatric and surgical stress, cationic drugs that are highly bound to this protein have lower free fractions and less drug available for the pharmacologic activity.

Selected Readings

Abraham E. Host defense abnormalities after hemorrhage, trauma, and burns. *Crit Care Med* 1989;17:934.
Review article that provides an overview of the abnormalities of the immune system after significant stress (e.g., hemorrhage, trauma, burns).

Bodenham A, Shelley MP, Park GR. The altered pharmacokinetics and pharmacodynamics of drugs commonly used in critically ill patients. *Clin Pharmacokinet* 1988;14:347.
A review article on the altered pharmacokinetics and pharmacodynamics of common drugs used in the ICU. Limited data show delayed drug clearance, altered volumes of distribution, and prolonged elimination half-lives, which can affect the ICU course.

Boucher BA, Rodman JH, Jaresko GS, et al. Phenytoin pharmacokinetics in critically ill trauma patients. *Clin Pharmacol Ther* 1988;44:675.
This study of phenytoin pharmacokinetics of 12 patients to trauma intensive care showed a substantial clinically significant fall in serum concentrations. Possible mechanism may include changes in protein binding or induction of phenytoin metabolism.

Cloyd J. Pharmacokinetic pitfalls of present antiepileptic medications. *Epilepsia* 1991;32:S53.
A helpful review of the factors that cause fluctuations in antiepileptic drugs.

Cockcroft DW, Gault MH. Prediction of creatinine clearance from serum creatinine. *Nephron* 1976;16:31.
Describes the formula used to predict creatinine clearance from serum creatinine, including its derivation and factors to correct for age and body weight.

Durbin CG. Neuromuscular blocking agents and sedative drugs: clinical uses and toxic effects in the critical care unit. *Crit Care Clin* 1991;7:489.
A review article on the indications, contraindications, and toxicity of neuromuscular blocking agents, with a brief discussion of conditions that can affect dosing in the ICU.

Evans W, Schentag J, Jusko W, eds. *Applied pharmacokinetics: principles of therapeutic drug monitoring.* Vancouver, WA: Applied Therapeutics, 1990.
Extensive discussion on general aspects of pharmacokinetics and in-depth discussions on the pharmacokinetics and dose-response data of various commonly monitored drugs.

Farina ML, Bonati M, Lapichino G, et al. Clinical pharmacological and therapeutic considerations in general intensive care: a review. *Drugs* 1987;34:662.
An extensive review of the clinical pharmacology in intensive care settings with a focus on a problem-oriented approach rather than a drug-focus review.

Griebel ML, Kearns GL, Fiser DH, et al. Phenytoin protein binding in pediatric patients with acute traumatic injury. *Crit Care Med* 1990;18:385.
A study of pediatric patients with acute head injury that demonstrated significant elevations in phenytoin-free fractions and recommended monitoring both free and total serum phenytoin to prevent toxicity.

Hickling KG, Begg EJ, Perry RE, et al. Serum aminoglycoside clearance is predicted as poorly by renal aminoglycoside clearance as by creatinine clearance in critically ill patients. *Crit Care Med* 1991;19:1041.
A prospective study of 18 critically ill patients treated with gentamicin or tobramycin, which demonstrated that individualized pharmacokinetic dosing is the only effective method of achieving target serum concentrations.

Klotz U. Pathophysiological and disease-induced changes in drug distribution volume: pharmacokinetic implications. *Clin Pharmacokinet* 1976;1:204.
Reviews the effect of various disease states on a drug's volume of distribution and the clinical implications of these effects.

Mann HJ, Fuhs DW, Cerra FB. Pharmacokinetics and pharmacodynamics in critically ill patients. *World J Surg* 1987;11:210.
A review article on the pharmacokinetic effects of cardiac, renal, and hepatic failure, with recommendations for the dosing of commonly used medications in the intensive care setting.

McLean AJ, Morgan DJ. Clinical pharmacokinetics in patients with liver disease. *Clin Pharmacokinet* 1991;21:42.
A review article on the pathology of liver disease and its effect on metabolism, with suggestions regarding modification of drug dosages.

Murray M. P450 enzymes: inhibition mechanisms, genetic regulation, and effects of liver disease. *Clin Pharmacokinet* 1992;23:132.
An overview of the importance of hepatic P450 enzymes and the effect of drug interaction and hepatic disease on their level of function.

Pond SM, Tozer TN. First-pass elimination: basic concepts and clinical consequences. *Pharmacokinetics* 1984;9:1.
Detailed discussion of first-pass elimination, its effect on bioavailability of drugs, and implications on clinical and therapeutic effects.

Reed R, Wu A, Miller-Crotchett P, et al. Pharmacokinetic monitoring of nephrotoxic antibiotics in surgical intensive care patients. *J Trauma* 1989;29:1462.
A study demonstrating the importance of pharmacokinetic analysis of nephrotoxic antibiotics to maintain therapeutic levels in surgical intensive care patients.

Rosenberg J, Benowitz NL, Pond S. Pharmacokinetics of drug overdose. *Clin Pharmacokinet* 1981;6:161.
Detailed discussion of the pharmacokinetic differences that occur when drugs are taken in overdose. Several specific drugs are reviewed in this context.

Shelly MP, Mendel L, Park GR. Failure of critically ill patients to metabolize midazolam. *Anaesthesia* 1987;42:619.
Impaired ability of critically ill patients to metabolize midazolam was demonstrated in six patients with septic shock.

Shoemaker WC. Circulatory mechanisms of shock and their mediators. *Crit Care Med* 1987;15:787.
Discussion of the limitations of the traditional approach to circulatory physiology that presents an approach founded on a model based on survival pattern.

Sue YJ, Shannon M. Pharmacokinetics of drugs in overdose. *Clin Pharmacokinet* 1992;23:93.

A review of the altered patterns of absorption, distribution, and metabolism or elimination that occur during drug overdose and a discussion of the clinical implications.

Tillement J, Lhoste F, Giudicelli JF. Diseases and drug protein binding. *Clin Pharmacokinet* 1978;3:144.
Discussion of diseases that decrease protein binding of drugs as a result of hypoalbuminemia and whether this reduction has clinically significant modifications on pharmacologic effects of drugs.

Whipple J, Ausman R, Franson T, et al. Effect of individualized pharmacokinetic dosing on patient outcome. *Crit Care Med* 1991;19:1480.
Prospective, randomized clinical study showing that individualized pharmacokinetic and aminoglycoside dosing may improve the clinical outcome of ICU patients.

Winter ME, Koda-Kimble MA, Young LY, eds. *Basic clinical pharmacokinetics*, 2nd ed. Vancouver, WA: Applied Therapeutics, 1988.
Simplified explanations of pharmacokinetic concepts and chapters on the calculation of doses for commonly monitored drugs, with multiple examples.

I. GENERAL PRINCIPLES. Goals and priorities in the evaluation and treatment of the patient with a chemical exposure and potential poisoning include:
- **A.** Recognition (diagnosis) of poisoning
- **B.** Identification of the offending agents
- **C.** Prediction of potential toxicity
- **D.** Assessment of severity
- **E.** Provision of supportive care
- **F.** Prevention of chemical absorption
- **G.** Prevention or reversal of poisoning by the use of antidotes
- **H.** Enhancement of chemical elimination
- **I.** Safe disposition
- **J.** Prevention of reexposure

II. EVALUATION
- **A.** Recognition of poisoning
  1. Diagnosis is often made on the basis of a history of chemical exposure, a clinical course consistent with poisoning, and exclusion of other causes.
  2. Poisoning should always be considered in patients with metabolic abnormalities (especially acid–base disturbances), gastroenteritis, or changes in mental status of unclear cause.
  3. Signs and symptoms of poisoning typically develop within minutes to an hour of an acute exposure, progress to a maximum within several hours, and gradually resolve over a period of hours to a few days.
- **B.** Identification of the offending agent
  1. Poison Centers, Poisindex, Material Safety Data Sheets (MSDS), and Internet search engines can be used to identify the contents of unknown pills and products.
  2. Plants; mushrooms; and venomous insects, reptiles, and other animals can be identified by experts from local specialty societies, colleges, botanical gardens, and zoos.
  3. The mental status and vital signs provide the most useful information for identifying the cause of poisoning by an unknown agent. Using these parameters, the physiologic state can usually be characterized into one of four categories, and a differential diagnosis can then be formulated (Table 105-1).
     - **a.** Common causes of seizures are tricyclic antidepressants, cocaine, amphetamines, antihistamines, theophylline, and isoniazid (INH).
       - **(1)** Seizures are usually generalized, but carbon monoxide, hypoglycemic agents, and theophylline can cause focal seizures.
       - **(2)** Central nervous system (CNS) hemorrhage is a complication of poisoning, and a computed tomography (CT) scan of the brain should be obtained if focal signs and symptoms are present.
     - **b.** Laboratory studies
       - **(1)** Anion and osmolar gaps and serum ketone and lactate levels can provide important diagnostic clues (Fig. 105-1).
         - **(a)** The anion gap, calculated by subtracting the serum chloride and bicarbonate concentrations from the serum sodium concentration, is normally 13 ± 4 mEq/L.
         - **(b)** The serum osmolality is normally 290 ± 10 mOsm/kg of H_2O, and the normal osmolar gap—the difference between the serum osmolality

TABLE 105-1 Differential Diagnosis of Poisoning Based on Physiologic Abnormalities, Underlying Mechanisms, and Specific Causes

	Physiologic state		
Excited (CNS stimulation with increased vital signs)	Depressed (CNS depression with decreased vital signs)	Discordant (mixed CNS and vital sign abnormalities)	Normal
Sympathomimetics Amphetamines Bronchodilators (β agonists) Catecholamine analogues Cocaine Decongestants Ergot alkaloids Methylxanthines Monoamine oxidase inhibitors Thyroid hormones **Anticholinergics** Antihistamines Atropine and other belladonna alkaloids Cyclic antidepressants Cyclobenzaprine Muscle relaxants Mydriatics (topical) Nonprescription sleep aids Parkinsonian therapeutics Phenothiazines Plants/mushrooms **Hallucinogens** LSD and tryptamine derivatives	**Sympatholytics** α-Adrenergic antagonists Angiotensin-converting enzyme inhibitors β-Adrenergic blockers Calcium-channel blockers Clonidine gestants Cyclic antidepressants Decongestants (imidazolones) Digitalis Neuroleptics **Cholinergics** Bethanechol Carbamate insecticides Echothiophate Myasthenia gravis therapeutics Nicotine Organophosphate insecticides Physostigmine Pilocarpine Urecholine **Opioids** Analgesics Antidiarrheal drugs Fentanyl and derivatives	**Asphyxiants** Carbon monoxide Cyanide Hydrogen sulfide Inert (simple) gases Irritant gases Methemoglobinemia Oxidative phosphorylation inhibitors Herbicides (nitrophenols) **Membrane active agents** Amantadine Antiarrhythmics Beta-blockers Cyclic antidepressants Fluoride Heavy metals Lithium Local anesthetics Meperidine/propoxyphene Neuroleptics Quinine (antimalarials) **AGMA[a] inducers** Alcoholic ketoacidosis Ethylene glycol Methanol (formaldehyde)	**Nontoxic exposure** **Psychogenic illness** **Toxic time bombs** Acetaminophen Agents that form concretions *Amanita phalloides* and related mushrooms Anticholinergics Cancer therapeutics Carbamazepine Chloramphenicol Chlorinated hydrocarbons Digitalis preparations Dilantin kapseals Disulfiram Enteric-coated pills Ethylene glycol Heavy metals Immunosuppressive agents Lithium Lomotil (atrophine and diphenoxylate) Methanol Methemoglobin inducers (some)

Marijuana	Heroin	Paraldehyde	Monoamine oxidase inhibitors
Mescaline and amphetamine derivatives	Opium	Metformin (biguanide hypoglycemics)	Paraquat
Psilocybin mushrooms	**Sedative-hypnotics**	Salicylate	Opioids
Phencyclidine	Alcohols	Toluene	Organophosphate insecticides (some)
Withdrawal syndromes	Anticonvulsants	Valproic acid	Podophyllin
β-Adrenergic blockers	Barbiturates	**CNS syndromes**	Salicylates
Clonidine	Benzodiazepines	Disulfiram	Sustained-release formulations
Cyclic antidepressants	Bromide	Extrapyramidal reactions	Thyroid hormone synthesis inhibitors
Ethanol	Ethchlorvynol	Isoniazid (GABA lytic)	Viral antimicrobials
Opioids	Gamma hydroxybutyrate	Neuroleptic malignant syndrome	
Sedative-hypnotics	Glutethimide	Serotonin syndrome	
	Methyprylon	Solvent (hydrocarbon)	
	Muscle relaxants	Strychnine (glycinergic)	

From Irwin RS, Rippe JM. *Irwin and Rippe's intensive care medicine*, 5th ed. Philadelphia: Lippincott Williams & Wilkins, 2003, p. 1328.
[a]Low-lactate increased anion gap metabolic acidosis.

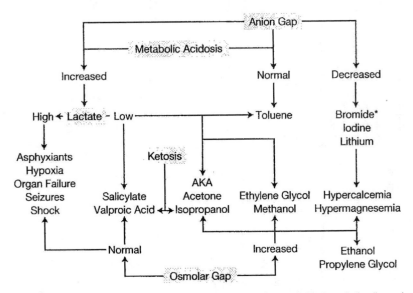

Figure 105-1. Use of the anion gap, osmolar gap, and serum lactate and ketones in the diagnosis of poisoning. Asterisk, see text for other (rare) causes; AKA, alcoholic ketoacidosis.

(measured by freezing point depression) and the calculated serum osmolality—is 5 ± 7 mOsm/kg.

■ The serum osmolality is calculated by doubling the serum sodium concentration and adding the result to the serum glucose and blood urea nitrogen (BUN) concentrations (assuming that all concentrations are measured in millimoles per liter).

■ If glucose and BUN are measured in milligrams per deciliter, dividing these values by 18 and 3, respectively, will give their approximate concentrations in millimoles per liter.

■ The approximate concentration of low-molecular-weight solutes that increase the serum osmolality by 1 mOsm/kg of H_2O, calculated on the basis of their molecular weights, is shown in Table 105-2.

■ Toxic solute concentrations can be estimated by multiplying concentration listed in the table by the excess osmolar gap.

(2) Pregnancy testing is recommended in women of childbearing age.

(3) Hypokalemia can be caused by barium salts, β-agonists, diuretics, methylxanthines, and toluene.

(4) Hyperkalemia can be caused by α-agonists, β-blockers, cardiac glycosides, and fluoride.

(5) Potential hepatotoxins include acetaminophen, ethanol, halogenated hydrocarbons (e.g., carbon tetrachloride), heavy metals, and mushrooms (e.g., *Amanita* species).

(6) Renal dysfunction can be caused by ethylene glycol, agents causing rhabdomyolysis or hemolysis, nonsteroidal antiinflammatory drugs, and toluene.

c. Electrocardiographic (ECG) findings

(1) Ventricular tachydysrhythmias can result from myocardial irritation (enhanced automaticity) or reentry mechanisms (due to delayed cardiac conduction).

(a) Myocardial irritants include sympathomimetics, cardiac glycosides, and halogenated hydrocarbons.

TABLE 105-2	Effects of Some Solutes on Serum Osmolality

Solute	Approximate concentration required to increase serum osmolality by 1 mOsm/kg
Alcohols, glycols, and ketones	
Acetone	5.8 mg/dL
Ethanol	4.6 mg/dL
Ethylene glycol	5.2 mg/dL
Isopropanol	6.0 mg/dL
Methanol	2.6 mg/dL
Propylene glycol	7.6 mg/dL
Electrolytes	
Calcium	4.0 mg/dL (1 mEq/L)
Magnesium	2.4 mg/dL (1 mEq/L)
Sugars	
Mannitol	18 mg/dL
Sorbitol	18 mg/dL

Source: Irwin RS, Rippe JM. *Irwin and Rippe's intensive care medicine*, 5th ed. Philadelphia: Lippincott Williams & Wilkins, 2003, p. 1330.

(b) Delayed cardiac repolarization and depolarization are manifested by an increased QRS duration and prolonged QTc interval, respectively. Causes include amantadine, types I and III antidysrhythmic agents, β-blockers, fluoride, heavy metals (e.g., arsenic, thallium), magnesium, normeperidine, organophosphate insecticides, potassium, cyclic antidepressants, antipsychotics, quinine, and related antimalarial drugs.

(2) Atrioventricular block and bradydysrhythmias can be caused by β-blockers, calcium channel blockers, cardiac glycosides, organophosphate insecticides, and phenylpropanolamine.

d. Radiographic findings

(1) Radiopaque agents are identified by the mnemonic CHIPE (chlorinated hydrocarbons, calcium salts, heavy metals, iron salts, iodinated compounds, phenothiazines, packets of drugs, and enteric-coated tablets).

(2) The chest radiograph may demonstrate infiltrates following inhalation of irritant gases (e.g., chlorine, noncardiogenic pulmonary edema), fumes (e.g., metal oxides), vapors (e.g., isocyanates), and some ingestions (e.g., paraquat, salicylates).

e. Toxicology testing

(1) Comprehensive toxicology screens are often neither clinically useful nor cost-effective. They are not immediately available, can detect only a small fraction of all chemicals, and are not always reliable.

(a) A false-negative result can occur when the toxin is not included in the assay panel, or the concentration of the toxin is below the level of detection by the assay.

(b) The physician should speak directly with the laboratory technician to determine whether the assay is appropriate for the toxin being considered.

(2) Quantitative acetaminophen and salicylate concentrations should be obtained in all patients suspected of overdose.

C. Prediction of potential toxicity

1. Depends on dose and time since exposure as well as identity of the exposure agent.

2. Assume a worst-case scenario (maximal possible dose, maximum toxicity from estimated dose)

   3. Criteria for a nontoxic exposure
      a. Patient is asymptomatic by both history and physical examination.
      b. Amount and identity of all chemicals and time of exposure are known with high degree of certainty.
      c. Exposure dose is less than the smallest dose known or predicted to cause toxicity.
      d. Time elapsed since exposure is greater than the longest known or predicted interval between exposure and peak toxicity.
   4. Beware of agents causing delayed toxicity (toxic time-bombs; see Table 105-1).
 D. Assessment of severity
   1. The severity of poisoning is primarily determined by findings on physical examination (Table 105-3).
   2. The number and type of ancillary tests required to assess metabolic or organ function is determined by clinical severity and by the nature of the exposure.
      a. Patients who are symptomatic or suicidal should have serum electrolytes, BUN, creatinine, and glucose measurements; urinalysis; and 12-lead ECG.
      b. Patients with grade 2 or greater stimulant or depressant poisoning (see Table 105-3) should also have a complete blood count, coagulation studies, serum amylase, calcium, magnesium, creatine phosphokinase, hepatic enzyme levels, and a chest radiograph.
      c. Agents for which quantitative measurements are necessary or desirable for optimal patient management include acetaminophen, acetone, alcohols, antiarrhythmic agents, antiepileptic drugs, barbiturates, carbon monoxide, digoxin, electrolytes (including calcium and magnesium), ethylene glycol, heavy metals, lithium, salicylate, and theophylline.

III. TREATMENT
 A. Provision of supportive care
   1. Supportive care includes monitoring (e.g., behavioral, cardiac rhythm, pulse oximetry, urine output, vital signs) and is the primary therapy for most poisoned patients.

TABLE 105-3   **Physiologic Grading of the Severity of Poisoning**

Severity	Signs and symptoms	
	Stimulant poisoning	Depressant poisoning
Grade 1	Agitation, anxiety, diaphoresis, hyperreflexia, mydriasis, tremors	Ataxia, confusion, lethargy, weakness, verbal, able to follow commands
Grade 2	Confusion, fever, hyperactivity, hypertension, tachycardia, tachypnea	Mild coma (nonverbal but responsive to pain); brainstem and deep tendon reflexes intact
Grade 3	Delirium, hallucinations, hyperpyrexia, tachyarrhythmias	Moderate coma (respiratory depression, unresponsive to pain); some but not all reflexes absent
Grade 4	Coma, cardiovascular collapse, seizures	Deep coma (apnea, cardiovascular depression); all reflexes absent

From Irwin RS, Rippe JM. *Irwin and Rippe's intensive care medicine*, 5th ed. Philadelphia: Lippincott Williams & Wilkins 2003, p. 1328.

2. Respiratory care

   a. Prophylactic intubation may be required for patients with central nervous system (CNS) depression to prevent aspiration of gastric contents and is recommended for those who cannot respond to and by voice or who are unable to sit upright and drink fluids without assistance.

   b. Using the gag reflex to assess the need for intubation should be abandoned. Many normal individuals have an absent gag reflex and many comatose patients will gag if sufficiently stimulated and yet be unable to protect their airway. In addition, attempting to elicit a gag reflex may itself induce vomiting and cause aspiration in a patient with an altered mental state.

   c. Prophylactic or therapeutic intubation may also be required for patients with extreme behavioral or physiologic stimulation who require aggressive pharmacologic therapy with sedative, antipsychotic, anticonvulsant, or paralyzing agents.

   d. Even in comatose patients, pretreatment with a sedative and a neuromuscular blocking agent can facilitate intubation.

   e. Extracorporeal membrane oxygenation and CO_2 removal (ECMO and ECCOR), cardiopulmonary bypass, partial liquid fluorocarbon ventilation, hyperbaric oxygen, nitric oxide, and synthetic surfactants should be considered in patients with reversible poisoning who cannot otherwise be adequately oxygenated or ventilated.

3. Cardiovascular therapy

   a. Maintenance or restoration of a normal blood pressure, pulse, and sinus rhythm are the goals of therapy.

   b. Invasive hemodynamic (e.g., arterial, central venous, pulmonary artery pressure) monitoring may be necessary for optimal treatment.

   c. Hypotension (in the absence of an extremely fast or slow heart rate) should initially be treated with intravenous normal saline. A direct-acting vasopressor with inotropic activity (e.g., norepinephrine, epinephrine, high-dose dopamine) should be infused for refractory hypotension.

   d. Hypertension often responds to nonspecific sedation with a benzodiazepine. If severe or if chest pain, ECG evidence of ischemia, headache, papilledema, or encephalopathy are present, specific therapy is indicated. A nonselective sympatholytic (e.g., labetalol) or the combination of an α-blocker and a peripheral vasodilator (e.g., esmolol with nitroprusside) is preferred in patients with sympathomimetic poisoning. A vasodilator alone can be used if hypertension is associated with a normal heart rate or reflex bradycardia.

   e. The treatment of ventricular tachydysrhythmias includes correction of electrolyte and metabolic abnormalities. Lidocaine is generally safe.

   (1) Sodium bicarbonate, hypertonic saline, or hyperventilation may be effective for wide-complex tachycardias caused by antiarrhythmic agents, cyclic antidepressants, and possibly other membrane-active agents.

   (2) Procainamide and other IA and IC antiarrhythmic agents are contraindicated in patients with prolonged QRS and QT intervals.

   f. Symptomatic bradycardia should be treated with atropine and dopamine or epinephrine. When due to β-blocker and calcium channel blocker poisoning, treatment includes intravenous calcium, glucagons, and glucose-insulin-potassium infusion.

   g. External or internal electrical cardiac pacing and intraaortic balloon pump counterpulsation or cardiopulmonary bypass should be considered in patients who are unresponsive to routine therapy.

4. Neuromuscular therapy. Treatment of neuromuscular hyperactivity is necessary to prevent or limit rhabdomyolysis and thermogenesis (hyperthermia). Hyperactivity from sympathomimetic or hallucinogen poisoning and drug withdrawal should initially be treated with sedation using benzodiazepines. Benzodiazepines are preferred to neuroleptic agents (e.g., chlorpromazine, haloperidol) because the latter are more likely to cause hypotension.

   a. Seizures are treated with benzodiazepines and barbiturates.

   b. Administration of pyridoxine is necessary to stop seizures caused by INH.

    c. Paralyzing (neuromuscular blocking) agents should be given to patients who fail to respond to sedatives and anticonvulsants. During such therapy, seizures should continue to be monitored (by electroencephalograph) and treated to prevent permanent neurologic damage.

B. Prevention of chemical absorption

1. Decontamination is recommended in all patients who present within an hour or two of exposure, unless the exposure is clearly nontoxic.

2. Body surfaces exposed to acids or alkali should be immediately irrigated until the pH is between 5 and 8.

3. Oral activated charcoal is the recommended method of decontamination for most ingestions. The optimal dose is at least 10 times the weight of the ingested toxin or a maximum of 1 to 2 g/kg of body weight. Activated charcoal is not recommended for ingestions of alkali, acids, and hydrocarbons with low systemic toxicity. It does not effectively bind inorganic salts (e.g., iron, lithium).

4. The routine use of gastric lavage or syrup of ipecac is not supported by current data.

5. Whole bowel irrigation (WBI), the oral administration of large volumes (0.5 L per hour in children aged 6 to 12 years and 2 L per hour for older patients) of a balanced electrolyte solution (e.g., Golytely) until the rectal effluent is clear may be useful for ingestions of enteric-coated or sustained-release formulations, potentially toxic foreign bodies, and agents that are poorly adsorbed by activated charcoal.

6. Endoscopy can be used to remove foreign bodies or break up drug masses in the stomach. It should be reserved for patients with severe or potentially lethal poisoning, such as those with large amounts of heavy metal visible in the stomach on radiography and those who deteriorate or have rising drug levels despite attempts at gut decontamination by other methods.

7. Cathartics have not been shown to prevent absorption and are recommended as an adjunct to charcoal to prevent constipation from charcoal. Cathartics are contraindicated in patients with caustic ingestions, not recommended in patients with renal insufficiency, and unnecessary in patients with diarrhea.

C. Prevention or reversal of poisoning by the use of antidotes

1. Selective antidotes (Table 105-4) act by competing with chemicals for target sites or metabolic activation pathways, by neutralizing them as a result of antibody-antigen reactions or by binding them (i.e., chelation), by promoting their metabolic detoxification, and by antagonizing their autonomic effects via activation or inhibition of opposing neuronal pathways.

2. Nonselective antidotal therapy includes correcting metabolic derangements and enhancing nonmetabolic chemical elimination.

3. The safe use of selective antidotes requires knowledge of the specific indications, contraindications, dosing, and potential complications (see subsequent chapters for details).

D. Enhancement of chemical elimination

1. The elimination of some toxins by nonmetabolic routes can be enhanced by diuresis, alkalization of the urine, multiple-dose activated charcoal (MDAC), WBI, and extracorporeal techniques.

2. The choice of the technique is dependent on the actual or predicted severity of poisoning and its reversibility, the function of intrinsic detoxification mechanisms, and the potential risks of the intervention and its efficacy in removing the toxin.

3. Urinary alkalinization (urine pH above 7.5) can enhance the renal excretion of acidic chemicals (chlorphenoxyacetic acid herbicide 2,4-D,chlorpropamide, difluinisal, fluoride, phenobarbital, sulfonamides, and salicylates) by ion trapping.

    a. An alkalinizing solution for infusion can be created by adding 134 mEq (3 ampules) of sodium bicarbonate to a liter of D5W.

    b. It is administered at the same rate as the desired urine output.

    c. Acid–base and electrolyte parameters (particularly potassium and magnesium) and respiratory function must be carefully monitored.

4. MDAC can enhance the elimination of previously absorbed chemicals by binding them within the gastrointestinal tract as they are excreted in the bile,

TABLE 105-4	Chemicals and Toxic Syndromes with Specific Antidotes

Agent/condition	Antidotes
Acetaminophen	N-Acetylcysteine
Anticholinergic poisoning	Physostigmine
Anticoagulants	Phytonadione (vitamin K), protamine
Benzodiazepines	Flumazenil
β-Adrenergic antagonists	Glucagon, calcium salts
Calcium channel blockers	Calcium salts, glucagon
Carbon monoxide	Oxygen, hyperbaric oxygen
Cholinergic syndrome	Atropine, pralidoxime
Cyanide	Nitrites, thiosulfate, hydroxycobal
Digoxin (digitalis)	Fab antibody fragments, magnesium
Dystonic reactions	Benztropine, diphenhydramine
Ethylene glycol	Ethanol, 4-methylpyrazole; pyridoxine, thiamine
Envenomations (arthropod, snake)	Antivenins
Fluoride	Calcium and magnesium salts
Heavy metals (arsenic, mercury, lead)	British anti-lewisite (dimercaprol), dimercaptosuccinic acid, D-penicillamine, calcium disodium, ethylenediaminetetraacetic acid
Hydrogen sulfide	Oxygen, nitrites
Iron	Deferoxamine
Isoniazid (hydrazines)	γ-Aminobutyric acid agonists, pyridoxine
Methanol	Ethanol, 4-methylpyrazole; folate
Methemoglobinemia	Methylene blue
Opioids	Naloxone, nalmefene, naltrexone
Sympathomimetics	Adrenergic blockers
Vacor (N-3-pyridylmethyl-N'-p-nitrophenylurea)	Nicotinamide (niacinamide)

From Irwin RS, Rippe JM. *Irwin and Rippe's intensive care medicine*, 5th ed. Philadelphia: Lippincott Williams & Wilkins, 2003, p. 1332.

secreted by the stomach or intestine, or passively diffuse back into the gut lumen. MDAC can also enhance the elimination of agents administered parenterally. The recommended dose of activated charcoal is 0.5 to 1 g/kg every 2 to 4 hours. Cathartics can cause water and electrolyte imbalance and are recommended only with the initial dose of charcoal.

5. Extracorporeal methods include hemodialysis, hemoperfusion, hemofiltration, plasmapheresis, peritoneal dialysis, and exchange transfusion. Hemodialysis can effectively remove barbiturates, bromide, chloral hydrate, ethanol, ethylene glycol, isopropyl alcohol, lithium, methanol, procainamide, theophylline, salicylates, and possibly heavy metals. Patients should be monitored for a rebound (increase) in blood levels and clinical toxicity after the termination of extracorporeal therapies.

E. Safe disposition

1. Intensive care unit admission is recommended for patients with coma (grade 2 or greater), hypotension (systolic pressure <90 mm Hg), respiratory depression (Pco_2 >45 mm Hg or intubated), a nonsinus cardiac rhythm (including second- or third-degree atrioventricular block), seizures, extremes of temperature,

severe hypertension, agitation, hallucinations, or metabolic abnormalities and those who require antidotal or enhanced elimination therapy.

   2. Patients who are less ill, stable, or asymptomatic and who need close or continuous visual observation (e.g., one-to-one suicide precautions) and close or continuous monitoring of cardiac rhythm and vital signs can be admitted to an intermediate care unit, telemetry unit, or emergency department observation unit.

   3. Suicidal patients require psychiatric evaluation, disposition, and follow-up.

F. Prevention of reexposure

   1. The environment of children should be poison proofed.

   2. Substance abusers (recreational users and addicts) should be counseled regarding attendant medical risks and given the opportunity for rehabilitation through referral for behavior modification, supervised withdrawal, and abstinence or maintenance therapy.

   3. Adults with accidental poisoning should be educated regarding the safe use of drugs and other chemicals.

   4. Workplace exposures should be reported to the appropriate governmental agency (e.g., Occupational Safety and Health Administration and/or local health department), and workers should be warned to avoid reexposure.

Selected Readings

Bond GR. Home syrup of ipecac use does not reduce emergency department use or improve outcome. *Pediatrics* 2003;112:1061–1064.
This study suggests that there is no reduction in resource utilization or improvement in patient outcome from the use of syrup of ipecac at home.

Goldfrank LR, Flomenbaum NE, Lewin NA, et al. Vital signs and toxic syndromes. In: Goldfrank KR, Flomenbaum NE, Lewin NA, et al., eds. *Toxicologic emergencies*, 7th ed. New York: McGraw-Hill, 2002.
A discussion of the classic clinical manifestations of a variety of toxicologic exposures.

Krenzelok E, Vale A. Position statements: gut decontamination. American Academy of Clinical Toxicology, European Association of Poisons Centres and Clinical Toxicologists. *J Toxicol Clin Toxicol* 1997;35:695–786.
This review discusses the role of various gut decontamination therapies in poisoned patients.

Nice A, Leikin JB, Maturen A, et al. Toxidrome recognition to improve efficiency of emergency urine drug screens. *Ann Emerg Med* 1988;17:676–680.
The application of classic clinical manifestations correctly identified the drug or class causing intoxication in overdosed patients.

Olkkola K. Effect of charcoal-drug ratio on antidotal efficacy of oral activated charcoal in man. *Br J Clin Pharmacol* 1985;19:767–773.
This in vitro study demonstrated the effective drug-to-charcoal ratio to be 1:10 by weight.

Pond SM, Lewis-Driver DJ, Williams G, et al. Gastric emptying in acute overdose: a prospective randomized controlled trial. *Med J Aust* 1995;163:345–349.
This study failed to demonstrate clinical benefit from gastric emptying in all overdosed patients. However, when severity of illness was controlled for, patients with gastric emptying benefited.

Smilkstein MJ, Steedle D, Kulig KW, et al. Magnesium levels after magnesium containing cathartics. *J Toxicol Clin Toxicol* 1988;26:51–65.
This study demonstrated increased serum magnesium concentrations in human volunteers with normal renal function who were administered magnesium cathartics in repeated fashion.

Tenenbein M, Cohen S, Sitar DS. Whole bowel irrigation as a decontamination procedure after acute drug overdose. *Arch Intern Med* 1987;147:905–907.
This human volunteer study demonstrated the effectiveness of whole bowel irrigation in decreasing drug absorption.

I. BACKGROUND

A. Acetaminophen (APAP) is the most common drug involved in intentional and unintentional overdoses in the United States.

B. It is an active ingredient in hundreds of products, including combinations with opioid analgesics, antihistamines, and decongestants.

II. PATHOPHYSIOLOGY

A. In therapeutic doses, approximately 90% of APAP is metabolized by hepatic conjugation with sulfate or glucuronide to form inactive metabolites. A small portion is excreted unchanged in the urine.

B. The remaining fraction undergoes oxidation by the cytochrome P-450 mixed function oxidases (CYP2E1) to yield the toxic intermediate NAPQI (*N*-acetyl-para-benzoquinoneimine), which then reacts with reduced glutathione (GSH) to form inactive products that are excreted in the urine.

C. NAPQI is a highly reactive electrophile that destroys both hepatocytes (centrilobular necrosis) and renal tubular cells. After overdose, the conjugation pathway becomes saturated, increasing the amount of APAP metabolized by the P-450 enzymes. GSH can then become depleted, allowing NAPQI to produce hepatotoxicity.

D. Single ingestions of more than 7.5 g in an adult and more than 150 mg/kg in children should be considered potentially toxic. Toxicity can also occur after repeated ingestions of therapeutic or slightly greater doses of APAP, especially in persons who have conditions associated with increased cytochrome P-450 activity (chronic alcoholics) or glutathione depletion (malnutrition or acute illness).

III. DIAGNOSIS

A. Acute APAP toxicity can be divided into four phases based on the time after ingestion.

1. Stage 1 (0.5 to 24 hours). Patients may be asymptomatic or may be experiencing nausea, vomiting, and malaise.

2. Stage 2 (24 to 48 hours).

   a. Patients have symptoms of hepatitis, including right upper quadrant abdominal pain, nausea, fatigue, and malaise.

   b. Elevation of aminotransferase levels usually occurs between 24 and 36 hours after ingestion, but in severe cases can occur by 16 hours.

   c. Complications during stage 2 are related to the degree of liver and renal injury.

3. Stage 3 (72 to 96 hours).

   a. Liver injury becomes most pronounced, resulting in prolonged prothrombin time, elevated bilirubin, marked elevation of aminotransferases (>1,000 IU/L), metabolic acidosis, and hypoglycemia.

   b. Clinical symptoms reflect the degree of hepatic failure and encephalopathy. Oliguric or anuric renal failure can result from renal tubular necrosis. Pancreatitis and myocardial necrosis have also been reported.

   c. Most patients go on to full recovery, even those with markedly elevated aminotransferase levels. Death can occur 3 to 7 days after ingestion as a result of intractable metabolic disturbances, cerebral edema, or coagulopathy.

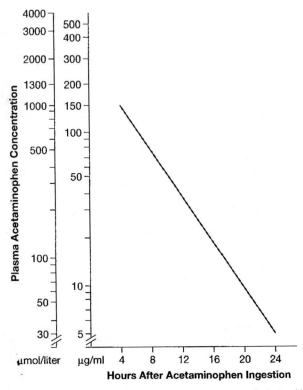

Figure 106-1. Rumack-Matthew acetaminophen treatment nomogram. Patients with acetaminophen concentrations on or above the line require treatment with *N*-acetylcysteine.

    4. Stage 4 (4 days to 2 weeks).
        a. Patients who survive even with severe liver toxicity regain normal liver function. Recovery is often complete in 5 to 7 days in patients with minimal toxicity but can take 2 weeks or more in patients with more serious toxicity.
        b. No known cases have been seen of chronic or persistent liver abnormalities from APAP poisoning.
  B. Laboratory studies. Obtain a serum APAP concentration between 4 and 24 hours after an acute single ingestion.
    1. If it falls on or above the treatment line on the Rumack–Matthew nomogram, the patient should be considered at risk for hepatotoxicity (Fig. 106-1).
    2. A single APAP concentration within 4 to 24 hours after ingestion should be sufficient to plan appropriate therapy, except in selected situations:
        a. if the time of ingestion is unknown and continued APAP absorption is a concern, or
        b. an extended-release formulation is suspected. In this case, a second APAP concentration should be obtained 4 to 6 hours after the initial one.
    3. If a patient is found to be at risk for toxicity, a complete blood count, electrolytes, blood urea nitrogen (BUN), creatinine, glucose, prothrombin and international normalized ratio (INR) time, aminotransferase levels, and bilirubin level should be obtained at admission and repeated every 24 hours until toxicity has resolved or been excluded.

IV. TREATMENT

A. Gastrointestinal (GI) decontamination.

   1. Activated charcoal (see Chapter 105) should be administered for recent acute overdoses.

   2. Although charcoal can decrease the enteral absorption of the antidote N-acetylcysteine (NAC), this effect is clinically insignificant.

B. Antidotal therapy

   1. The specific antidote for APAP toxicity is NAC. Although several mechanisms explain its benefit in preventing APAP-induced liver and renal injury, it primarily acts as a glutathione precursor and substitute.

   2. Begin NAC therapy after an acute overdose if the serum APAP concentration is in the toxic range on the nomogram, if the ingested amount is potentially toxic and more than 8 hours has elapsed since ingestion, or if serum aminotransferases are elevated and the patient has a history of APAP ingestion. In the latter two instances, NAC can be continued or discontinued when the APAP concentration becomes available.

   3. The 72-hour oral treatment regimen consists of NAC (Mucomyst) given as a 140 mg/kg loading dose followed by 17 doses of 70 mg/kg, one dose every 4 hours. The 20% NAC solution should be diluted at least 3:1 with a carbonated or fruit beverage to improve palatability.

   4. Aggressive antiemetic therapy may be needed to treat APAP- or NAC-induced vomiting. Metoclopramide, droperidol, or ondansetron can be effective. NAC can also be given by a slow, continuous infusion through a gastric or duodenal tube. If vomiting occurs within 1 hour of any dose, that dose should be repeated.

   5. A 20-hour intravenous NAC (Acetadote) treatment protocol was recently approved for use in the United States.

C. Special considerations

   1. Late NAC administration (>24 hours after overdose) has shown clinical benefit in patients with APAP-induced fulminant liver failure.

   2. Pregnant women should be treated according to standard guidelines, regardless of gestational age of the fetus.

   3. The nomogram has no validity in chronic APAP overdose. Patients with elevated APAP levels and no hepatotoxicity can be treated with NAC until the APAP is negligible. Patients who develop hepatotoxicity should be given a full course of NAC.

D. Liver transplantation

   1. Liver transplantation can be lifesaving in patients with severe liver failure.

   2. Clinical criteria that predict mortality, and hence the need for liver transplantation, include:

      a. pH less than 7.30 after fluid resuscitation

      b. Serum creatinine greater than 3.4

      c. Prothrombin time greater than 100 seconds (INR >6.5)

      d. Grade III/IV encephalopathy

V. COMPLICATIONS.
If the patient survives, complete recovery of hepatic function can be expected.

Selected Readings

Cetaruk EW, Dart RC, Hurlbut KM, et al. Tylenol Extended Relief overdose. *Ann Emerg Med* 1997;30:104–108.
   Case series of patients with overdoses of extended-release preparations of acetaminophen (APAP) that demonstrated peak levels after 4 hours, suggesting the need for another APAP concentration measurement 4 to 6 hours after the first.

Harrison PM, Wendon JA, Gimson AE, et al. Improvement by acetylcysteine of hemodynamics and oxygen transport in fulminant hepatic failure. *N Eng J Med* 1991;324:1852–1857.
   Study of patients with acetaminophen-induced fulminant hepatic failure that demonstrated increases in oxygen delivery and consumption in response to acetylcysteine, perhaps accounting for its beneficial effect on survival in these patients.

Kao LW, Kirk MA, Furbee RB, et al. What is the rate of adverse events after oral N-acetylcysteine administered by the intravenous route to patients with suspected acetaminophen poisoning? *Ann Emerg Med* 2003; 6:741–750.
Recommended procedure and case series reporting the indications and adverse events associated with administration of the oral N-acetylcysteine preparation by the intravenous route.

Keays R, Harrison PM, Wendon JA, et al. Intravenous acetylcysteine in paracetamol induced fulminant hepatic failure: a prospective controlled trial. *BMJ* 1991;303:1026–1029.
A controlled trial of patients with paracetamol-induced fulminant hepatic failure demonstrating decreased cerebral edema and increased survival in patients receiving intravenous N-acetylcysteine therapy compared with those who did not.

Mitchell JR, Thorgeirsson SS, Potter WZ, et al. Acetaminophen-induced hepatic injury: protective role of glutathione in man and rationale for therapy. *Clin Pharmacol Ther* 1974;16:676–684.
An animal study demonstrating that glutathione-like nucleophiles protect hepatocytes from injury caused by the reactive acetaminophen metabolite.

Renzi FP, Donovan JW, Martin TG, et al. Concomitant use of activated charcoal and N-acetylcysteine. *Ann Emerg Med* 1985;14:568–572.
A human volunteer study showing no difference in N-acetylcysteine levels after oral consumption between subjects who received charcoal and those who did not.

Rumack BH, Matthew H. Acetaminophen poisoning and toxicity. *Pediatrics* 1975;55:871–876.
One of the first reviews to describe the toxicology of acetaminophen and proposals for treatment.

Rumack BH, Peterson RC, Koch GG, et al. Acetaminophen overdose: 662 cases with evaluation of oral acetylcysteine treatment. *Arch Intern Med* 1981;141:380–385.
One of the first and largest patient series to demonstrate the effectiveness of oral N-acetylcysteine treatment and the use of a nomogram to predict toxicity.

Smilkstein MJ, Knapp GL, Kulig KW, et al. Efficacy of oral N-acetylcysteine in the treatment of acetaminophen overdose: analysis of the National Multicenter Study (1976–1985). *N Engl J Med* 1988;319:1557–1562.
Outcome study of more than 2,000 patients with acetaminophen poisoning treated with oral N-acetylcysteine demonstrating a time-dependent relationship for its maximal efficacy.

Whitcomb DC, Block GD. Association of acetaminophen hepatotoxicity with fasting and ethanol use. *JAMA* 1994;272:1845–1850.
A retrospective case series of patients suggesting that acetaminophen hepatotoxicity appears to be enhanced by fasting and alcohol ingestion.

ALCOHOLS AND GLYCOLS
Steven B. Bird

I. BACKGROUND
A. Ethanol (grain or beverage alcohol), methanol (wood alcohol), isopropanol (isopropyl or rubbing alcohol), and ethylene glycol are central nervous system (CNS) depressants.

B. CNS depressant potency increases as the carbon atom chain length increases.

II. PATHOPHYSIOLOGY
A. Ketoacidosis and hypoglycemia are caused by the hormonal, nutritional, metabolic, and intravascular volume changes caused by the consumption of ethanol and other alcohols.

B. The formation of toxic metabolites by hepatic alcohol dehydrogenase (ADH) is responsible for the renal toxicity of ethylene glycol, the ocular toxicity of methanol, and the increased anion gap metabolic acidosis (AGMA) caused by both.

C. The most common sources of methanol and ethylene glycol are automotive windshield washer fluid, gasoline antifreeze, and radiator antifreeze.

III. DIAGNOSIS
A. Clinical presentation
  1. Ethanol
    a. Patients with acute ethanol intoxication can present with varying degrees of altered consciousness, including agitation, slurred speech, ataxia, stupor, and coma.
    b. Death from respiratory depression, aspiration, or cardiovascular collapse can occur in severe poisoning.
  2. Isopropyl alcohol
    a. Isopropanol produces an ethanol-like intoxication.
    b. Symptoms of gastritis (e.g., abdominal pain, nausea, vomiting, possibly hematemesis) may also be present.
    c. Its acetone metabolite causes a spurious increase in serum creatinine. Therefore, an elevated creatinine level with normal blood urea nitrogen (BUN) can be a clue to the diagnosis.
  3. Alcoholic ketoacidosis and hypoglycemia
    a. Patients with alcoholic ketoacidosis usually present with a recent history of binge drinking, poor nutritional intake, vomiting, and little or no measurable ethanol in their blood.
    b. Laboratory findings include mild to moderate AGMA and mild ketonemia. Dehydration is invariably present.
    c. Signs and symptoms of ethanol withdrawal may be present.
    d. Hypoglycemia causes an altered mental status ranging from agitation to confusion and coma.
    e. Symptoms of increased sympathetic activity caused by catecholamine release (e.g., diaphoresis, tachycardia) may also be present.
  4. Ethylene glycol and methanol
    a. Because of their low molecular weight, high levels of an alcohol or ethylene glycol increase the serum osmolality. Hence, an elevated serum osmolality or osmolal gap is a clue to their presence.

    b. Ethylene glycol and methanol poisoning should be suspected in all patients with a history of ingesting alcohol substitutes or in those who have an unexplained AGMA.

    c. Initially, an ethanol-like intoxication along with nausea, vomiting, and occasionally seizures dominates the clinical picture.

    d. Renal failure is a common sequelae of ethylene glycol poisoning. Calcium oxalate crystalluria may be present. Cardiopulmonary effects (e.g., tachypnea, cyanosis, cardiogenic or noncardiogenic pulmonary edema) can occur in severe cases.

    e. In methanol toxicity, neurologic, ophthalmologic, and gastrointestinal symptoms predominate. Patients are frequently alert on admission and complain of headache and dizziness.

       (1) Visual symptoms are usually experienced acutely when the serum pH drops below 7.2.

       (2) Blurred vision, photophobia, scotomata, eye pain, partial or complete loss of vision, and visual hallucinations (e.g., bright lights, "snowstorm") have been reported.

       (3) Methanol can produce hemorrhagic gastritis and pancreatitis, resulting in abdominal pain, nausea, vomiting, and diarrhea.

B. Evaluation

  1. Patients with a history of ethanol ingestion and mild to moderate intoxication need only a serum ethanol level and a fingerstick blood sugar evaluation. Those with severe intoxication or an unreliable history should have electrolytes, BUN, creatinine, glucose, complete blood count, arterial blood gas, ethanol level, magnesium, calcium, phosphorus, liver function tests, prothrombin time, electrocardiogram, chest radiograph, and urinalysis.

  2. Evaluation of known or suspected isopropanol poisoning should also include serum isopropanol and acetone serum levels.

  3. Evaluation of known or suspected ethylene glycol and methanol poisoning should include quantitative serum levels of these compounds.

  4. Microscopic examination of the urine for crystals should also be performed.

IV. TREATMENT

A. General measures

  1. Initial treatment includes supportive measures such as airway management, intravenous (IV) fluids, and cardiac monitoring.

  2. Gastric aspiration via a nasogastric tube should be considered in patients with severe poisoning and within a few hours of isopropanol, ethylene glycol, or methanol ingestion.

  3. Activated charcoal (see Chapter 105) should be considered when coingestants are suspected.

  4. Intravenous naloxone (2 mg) and thiamine hydrochloride (100 mg) should also be considered.

  5. If bedside glucose testing reveals hypoglycemia, IV dextrose (25 to 50 g) should be administered.

B. Alcoholic ketoacidosis and hypoglycemia

  1. IV fluids, glucose, and thiamine should be given for dehydration and to reverse the ketogenic process.

  2. Prolonged hospitalization and refeeding of malnourished patients may be required.

  3. The IV bolus of dextrose should be followed by a high carbohydrate meal or an infusion of 10% dextrose in patients with hypoglycemia.

C. Ethylene glycol and methanol

  1. Large doses of sodium bicarbonate may be required to treat metabolic acidosis.

  2. Primary antidotal therapy is 4-methylpyrazole (fomepizole, Antizole)

    a. Prevents formation of toxic metabolites by competitively inhibiting the enzyme ADH.

   b. Induces its own metabolism. Therefore the dose changes over time.
   c. Consult package insert for dosing during concomitant hemodialysis.
3. If 4-methylpyrazole is not readily available, a continuous ethanol infusion (to a goal of a serum concentration of 100 to 150 mg/dL) may be used temporarily. Methanol and ethylene glycol are then eliminated slowly via pulmonary and renal excretion.
4. Indications for antidotal therapy include:
   a. An ethylene glycol or methanol level greater than 20 mg/dL
   b. Unexplained AGMA and a low lactate level
   c. Visual disturbances
   d. Calcium oxalate crystalluria
   e. Unexplained coma with a high osmolar gap and low ethanol level
5. Patients poisoned by ethylene glycol should receive pyridoxine (100 mg) and thiamine (100 mg) IV daily until ethylene glycol levels are unmeasurable and acidemia has cleared.
6. Patients with methanol poisoning should be given IV leucovorin (1 mg/kg, maximal dose 50 mg) every 4 hours for a total of six doses.
D. Hemodialysis
   1. Effectively removes ethanol, isopropanol, ethylene glycol, and methanol, as well as their toxic metabolites, and can correct metabolic abnormalities.
   2. Should be considered in patients with severe poisoning who are unresponsive to other measures and in patients with ethylene glycol or methanol levels greater than 100 mg/dL (particularly those treated with ethanol).

V. COMPLICATIONS

   A. Renal failure from ethylene glycol poisoning usually resolves after several weeks to several months but can be permanent.
   B. Blindness due to methanol may be irreversible.

Selected Readings

Adams SL, Mathews JJ, Flatherty JJ. Alcoholic ketoacidosis. *Ann Emerg Med* 1987;16:90–97.
   Case presentation and review of the clinical and laboratory features of alcoholic keto-acidosis.

Baud FJ, Galliot M, Astier A, et al. Treatment of ethylene glycol poisoning with intrave-nous 4-methylpyrazole. *N Engl J Med* 1988;319:97–100.
   Case report of the clinical and kinetic data of ethylene glycol treated with intravenous 4-methylpyrazole.

Brent J, McMartin K, Phillips S, et al. Fomepizole for the treatment of methanol poisoning. *N Engl J Med* 2001;344:424–429.
   Case series of the effective treatment of methanol toxicity with the alcohol dehydroge-nase inhibitor 4-methylpyrazole.

Charness ME, Simon RP, Greenberg DA. Ethanol and the nervous system. *N Engl J Med* 89;321:442–454.
   An important review of the neurologic complications associated with ethanol abuse, intoxication, withdrawal, Wernicke encephalopathy, dementia, cerebellar degeneration, and central pontine myelinolysis.

Dethlefs R, Naraqi S. Ocular manifestations and complications of acute methyl alcohol intoxication. *Med J Aust* 1978;2:483–485.
   Clinical series of 24 men with methanol toxicity, showing that the incidence of perma-nent ocular abnormalities correlated with metabolic acidosis.

Hoffman RS, Smilkstein MJ, Howland MA, et al. Osmol gaps revisited: normal values and limitations. *J Toxicol Clin Toxicol* 1993;31:81–93.
   A study of 321 adults that evaluated the limitation of the osmol gaps in adults and con-cluded that small osmol gaps should not be used to eliminate a toxic alcohol ingestion.

Hoffman RS, Goldfrank LR. Ethanol-associated metabolic disorders. *Emerg Med Clin North Am* 1989;7:943–961.
An excellent review and discussion of the fluid, electrolytes, acid–base, glucose, and nutritional complications caused by elevated ethanol levels.

Jacobsen D, Hewlett TP, Webb R, et al. Ethylene glycol intoxication: evaluation of kinetics and crystalluria. *Am J Med* 1988;84:145–152.
A review of the two types of calcium oxalate crystals that are formed in the metabolism of ethylene glycol.

Jacobsen D, McMartin KE. Methanol and ethylene glycol poisonings: mechanism of toxicity, clinical course, diagnosis and treatment. *Med Toxicol* 1986;1:309–334.
A review article on methanol and ethylene glycol toxicity with excellent discussion of the similar clinical and biochemical characteristics that both compounds share.

Kruse JA, Cadnapaphorochni P. The serum osmol gap. *J Crit Care* 1994;9:185–197.
An in-depth review article on the different clinical indications for the use of osmol gap. Includes a helpful discussion regarding the limitations of its use.

LaCouture PG, Wason S, Abrams A, et al. Acute isopropyl alcohol intoxication: diagnosis and management. *Am J Med* 1983;75:680–686.
A review article focusing on the clinical presentation and management of isopropyl toxicity. Includes a helpful discussion of the differences between common toxic alcohols.

Martensson E, Olofsson U, Heath A. Clinical and metabolic features of ethanol-methanol poisoning in chronic alcoholics. *Lancet* 1988;1:327–328.
A study of 84 chronic alcoholic patients who ingested an ethanol-methanol, suggesting that treatment should be based on the clinical presentation and acidosis and not solely on methanol blood concentrations.

I. BACKGROUND

A. Antidepressants include a variety of drugs that have a cyclic component to their structure, including tricyclic antidepressants (TCAs), monoamine oxidase inhibitors (MAOIs), and selective serotonin reuptake inhibitors (SSRIs) (Table 108-1).

B. Toxic effects include central nervous system (CNS) and cardiovascular depression, arrhythmias, and seizures as well as monoamine oxidase inhibitor (MAOI) drug and food interactions and the serotonin syndrome.

II. PATHOPHYSIOLOGY

A. Pharmacology

1. Tricyclic antidepressants (TCAs) inhibit the reuptake of norepinephrine (NE), dopamine (DA), and serotonin (5-HT) in the CNS. Other effects include post-synaptic blockade of histamine, dopamine (DA), acetylcholine (Ach), 5-HT, and NE as well as GABA receptors. Peripheral α-receptor blockade contributes to hypotension. Class IA antiarrhythmic effects (i.e., Na$^+$ channel blockade) largely mediate the cardiac and neurologic toxicity.

2. Other cyclic agents inhibit the reuptake of 5-HT and have varying degrees of NE reuptake inhibition. Bupropion is unique in that its structure resembles amphetamine, which partly explains its propensity for causing seizures.

3. Selective serotonin reuptake inhibitors (SSRIs) inhibit the reuptake of 5-HT but have minimal effects on other neurotransmitters.

4. MAOIs inhibit MAO enzymes that degrade biogenic amines (E, NE, 5-HT, DA) in nerve terminals and the gut wall. This leads to increased catecholamine stores in nerve terminals, which are released by indirect-acting sympathomimetics such as amphetamines, ephedrine, and tyramine. It also increases the bioavailability of ingested amines (sympathomimetic drugs and tyramine/tryptophan in food).

5. The serotonin syndrome (SS) results from excessive CNS serotonergic activity due to increased 5-HT production (e.g., from ingested tryptophan), increased presynaptic release (e.g., by sympathomimetics), reuptake inhibition (e.g., by cyclic and SSRI antidepressants), receptor agonism (e.g., by bromocriptine, L-dopa, lithium, and tryptans), and inhibited metabolism (e.g., by MAOIs).

B. Pharmacokinetics

1. Cyclic antidepressants are well absorbed orally with peak serum concentrations occurring 2 to 6 hours after ingestion. Volume of distribution is large; protein binding is extensive. Metabolism is predominately hepatic. Many have active metabolites. Elimination half-life is variable and ranges from 8 to 30 hours. Absorption and elimination may be prolonged after overdose. Bupropion is available in a sustained-release formulation and can display significantly delayed peak serum concentrations, causing delayed toxicity.

2. Although readily absorbed, maximal MAO inhibition may not occur until 2 to 3 weeks after beginning MAOI therapy. Maximal effects are also delayed after acute overdose. Because most MAOIs are irreversible inhibitors of MAO, inhibition of MAO activity may persist for 2 to 3 weeks after overdose or cessation of therapy (until new enzyme can be synthesized).

TABLE 108-1	Antidepressants

Monocyclic
Bupropion

Bicyclic
Venlafaxine

Tricyclic
Amitriptyline
Imipramine
Doxepin
Trimipramine
Clomipramine
Desipramine
Protriptyline
Nortriptyline

Tetracyclic
Maprotiline
Mirtazapine

"Atypical" tetracyclic
Trazadone
Nefazodone

Heterocyclic
Loxapine
Amoxapine

MAOI
Moclobemide
Pargyline
Phenelzine
Tranylcypromine
Isocarboxazid

SSRI
Fluoxetine
Paroxetine
Sertraline

MAOI, monoamine oxydase inhibitor; SSRI, selective serotonin reuptake inhibitor.

III. DIAGNOSIS
A. Clinical manifestations
1. Monocyclic and heterocyclic antidepressants
   a. Can cause seizures as well as CNS depression.
      (1) Seizures due to bupropion are usually brief, may occur with therapeutic dosing and without any prodrome, and can be delayed up to 24 hours after overdose with sustained-release preparations.
      (2) Seizures due to amoxapine can be recurrent and prolonged, leading to rhabdomyolysis.
   b. Cardiotoxicity appears limited, although reports of conduction delay exist.
2. Bicyclic antidepressants
   a. Generally cause only mild sedation and tachycardia.
   b. Venlafaxine can cause seizures, QRS and QT widening, and ventricular dysrhythmias.
3. Tricyclic antidepressants

    a. Onset and progression of toxicity following TCA overdose is rapid, beginning within 30 minutes and peaking within 2 to 6 hours.

    b. Early manifestations include tachycardia, mild hypertension, and other anticholinergic effects.

    c. Coma, seizures, hypotension, and dysrhythmias may ensue.

    d. ECG findings include intraventricular conduction delays, repolarization abnormalities, ventricular tachydysrhythmias, bradycardia, atrioventricular (AV) block, and asystole.

        (1) Sinus tachycardia is the earliest finding.

        (2) With increasing toxicity, slowing of conduction through the right bundle shifts the overall QRS axis rightward, causing a terminal 40-msec axis of 130 to 270 degrees in the frontal plane. This is recognized as a widened S wave in leads I and aVL and an R wave in aVR.

        (3) The QRS, QT, and JT intervals also become prolonged.

        (4) Sinus tachycardia with aberrant conduction is often mistaken for ventricular tachycardia.

        (5) An R wave greater than 3 mm or greater than the S wave amplitude in AVR and a QRS greater than 0.16 second are associated with severe clinical toxicity.

        (6) JT (and hence QT) prolongation can occur with therapeutic doses.

    e. Anticholinergic effects may also become prominent during emergence from coma.

4. Tetracyclic antidepressants

    a. CNS and cardiovascular toxicity due to maprotiline is similar to that from TCAs.

    b. Less pronounced effects are seen with mirtazapine overdose.

5. "Atypical" tetracyclic antidepressants

    a. Overdose commonly causes tachycardia and CNS depression.

    b. QT prolongation and torsade de pointes (TdP) can occur.

6. MAOIs

    a. Acute overdose

        (1) Toxicity may not develop until 6 to 24 hours after ingestion and can last for several days.

        (2) Initial manifestations are due to sympathetic hyperactivity and include agitation, confusion, tremor, and hyperreflexia increased vital signs (BP, HR, RR, and T).

        (3) This may be followed by cardiovascular collapse as excitatory neurotransmitter stores become depleted.

        (4) Complications include rhabdomyolysis, electrolyte abnormalities, lactic acidosis, and multisystem organ failure.

    b. Drug and food interactions

        (1) Patients taking MAOIs who ingest indirect-acting sympathomimetics (amphetamines, ephedrine, phenylephrine) or food high in tyramine (aged cheese, smoked and pickled meats, red wine, pasteurized light and pale beers) can rapidly (30 to 60 min) develop a "hypertensive crisis" with agitation, tachycardia, hyperthermia, and seizures.

        (2) The duration of effect of all sympathomimetics may be prolonged, regardless of the route of administration.

7. Selective serotonin reuptake inhibitors

    a. Overdose in isolation generally results in mild CNS depression and tachycardia.

    b. Citalopram (and possibly escitalopram) can cause seizures, QT prolongation, and wide-complex tachycardia with doses greater than 600 mg.

8. Serotonin syndrome

    a. Can be caused by all antidepressants, alone or in combination, in therapeutic doses and overdose, or when combined with other serotonergic agents. It is most common during chronic therapy, when the dose is increased or another serotonergic agent is added.

TABLE 108-2	The Hunter Serotonin Toxicity Criteria: Decision Rules[*]

In the presence of a serotonergic agent:
1. IF (spontaneous clonus = yes) THEN serotonin toxicity = YES
2. ELSE IF (inducible clonus = yes) AND [(agitation = yes) OR (diaphoresis = yes)] THEN serotonin toxicity = YES
3. ELSE IF (ocular clonus = yes) AND [(agitation = yes) OR (diaphoresis = yes)] THEN serotonin toxicity = YES
4. ELSE IF (tremor = yes) AND (hyperreflexia = yes) THEN serotonin toxicity = YES
5. ELSE IF (hypertonic = yes) AND (temperature >38°C) AND [(ocular clonus = yes) OR (inducible clonus = yes)] then serotonin toxicity = YES
6. ELSE serotonin toxicity = NO

[*]Dunkley EJ, Isbister GK, Sibbritt D, et al. The Hunter Serotonin Toxicity Criteria: simple and accurate diagnostic decision rules for serotonin toxicity. *Q J Med* 2003;96:635–642.

    b. Manifestations include altered mental status, increased muscle activity (hyperreflexia, clonus), and autonomic findings (hypertension/hypotension, tachycardia, hyperthermia).
    c. The diagnosis is based on the history of drug exposure and examination findings (Table 108-2.)
B. Evaluation
    1. All patients with antidepressant poisoning should have an electrocardiogram (ECG), serum electrolytes, BUN, creatinine, and glucose.
    2. Those with an abnormal ECG should also have serum Mg^{2+} and Ca^{2+} levels.
    3. Those with significant CNS depression or seizures should have a chest radiograph and creatine phosphokinase (CPK).
    4. Frequent clinical and ECG reevaluations should be performed.
    5. Drug concentrations are not readily available and have no utility in the management of overdose.
    6. False-positive urine immunoassay results for TCAs may be caused by carbamazepine, cyclobenzaprine, cyproheptadine, diphenhydramine, prochlorperazine, perphenazine, quetiapine, and thioridazine.

IV. TREATMENT
    A. General measures
        1. All patients with potential poisoning should have cardiac monitoring and intravenous access.
        2. Advanced life support measures should be instituted as necessary. Supportive measures should include treatment of underlying hypoxia, acidosis, hypokalemia, or hypomagnesemia.
        3. Hypotension should initially be treated with intravenous saline. If no response after 2 L, administer vasopressors (see Chapter 105). Intraaortic balloon pump (IABP) and partial cardiac bypass could be used for the treatment of refractory hypotension.
        4. Seizures should be treated with benzodiazepines.
        5. Activated charcoal (see Chapter 105) should be considered for recent acute overdose. For bupropion SR ingestion, whole bowel irrigation (see Chapter 105) should also be considered.
    B. Cyclic antidepressant overdose
        1. Patients with cyclic antidepressant overdose who remain or become asymptomatic and have a normal ECG may be discharged after 6 hours of observation.
        2. Overdose with sustained-release bupropion is an exception and necessitates admission for 24 hours due to potential for delayed seizures.

3. Patients who are symptomatic or have ECG changes should have cardiac monitoring and be observed until normal.
4. Patients with coma, seizures, hypotension, or arrhythmias should be admitted to an ICU.
5. Administer intravenous sodium bicarbonate to patients with TCA overdose and QRS greater than 100 msec) or VT.
6. Avoid class IA or IC antiarrhythmic agents for TCA-induced ventricular tachycardia (VT). Lidocaine (class IB) may be considered because it does not depress conduction; however, it is often ineffective. Electrical cardioversion may be necessary for VT with cardiovascular instability.
7. Administer intravenous magnesium sulfate for prolonged QT and TdP. Overdrive pacing, electrical cardioversion, or isoproterenol infusion can also be used.
8. Physostigmine can be given for anticholinergic agitation and delirium but is contraindicated if TCA effects are noted on ECG or if a period of observation has not excluded worsening toxicity.
9. Patients with tachycardia and hypertension following bupropion overdose should be treated with benzodiazepines for seizure prophylaxis.

C. MAOI overdose and drug and food interactions
1. Treat behavioral hyperactivity with benzodiazepines. Intubation and neuromuscular paralysis (along with cooling measures) may be necessary in patients with hyperthermia.
2. Treat hypertension and tachycardia only if severe. Use easily titratable and reversible agents such as intravenous nitroprusside and esmolol.
3. Treat hypotension with direct-acting vasopressors such as epinephrine and norepinephrine (avoid dopamine).
4. MAOI overdose requires admission to the ICU for at least 24 hours, even in the absence of symptoms, because toxicity can be delayed.

D. Serotonin syndrome
1. Generally responds to withdrawal of the causative agent(s) and supportive care.
2. Administer benzodiazepines to reduce motor activity and control hyperthermia. As with MAOIs, neuromuscular paralysis and intubation may become necessary.
3. Cyproheptadine, a selective 5-HT_{2A} antagonist, may be beneficial. Administer an initial dose of 8 mg (orally or by gastric tube). Repeat dose if symptoms do not improve after 2 hours or if symptoms recur. The maximum dose is 24 mg per day.
4. Symptoms usually resolve in 24 to 48 hours.

V. COMPLICATIONS
A. Pulmonary aspiration, pneumonia, rhabdomyolysis, and sepsis are common in patients with coma and seizures.
B. Shock or anoxia can result in multiple-organ dysfunction.
C. Hypertensive crisis from MAOI interactions can result in intracranial hemorrhage.

Selected Readings
Boehnert M, Lovejoy FH. Value of the QRS duration versus the serum drug level in predicting seizures and ventricular arrhythmias after an acute overdose of tricyclic antidepressants. *N Engl J Med* 1985;313:474.
This paper correlates the degree of QRS prolongation to the risk of subsequent seizures or cardiac dysrhythmia. This study provides the rationale for alkalinization of serum with a QRS duration greater than 100 msec.

Linden CH, Rumack BH, Strehlke C. Monoamine oxidase inhibitor overdose. *Ann Emerg Med* 1984;13(12):1137.
This review provides an overview of the pathophysiology, presentation of, and treatment for MAOI toxicity.

Sternbach H. The serotonin syndrome. *Am J Psychiatry* 1991;148:705–713.
   This is a landmark review of 38 cases of serotonin syndrome from which a set of diagnostic criteria, known as the Sternbach criteria, was developed.

Tokarski GF, Young MJ. Criteria for admitting patients with tricyclic antidepressant overdose. *J Emerg Med* 1998;6:121.
   Provides a review of TCA toxicity and rationale for determining patient disposition.

I. BACKGROUND

A. Illicit forms of cocaine include the hydrochloride salt and its alkalinization products, freebase and crack.

B. Cocaine hydrochloride is water soluble, is readily absorbed from any mucosal surface, and can be administered intravenously (IV).

C. Freebase and crack are insoluble in water but can be smoked.

D. Oral overdose can occur in "body packers" (people who attempt to smuggle cocaine by ingesting wrapped and sealed packets of drug) and "body stuffers" (those who swallow or conceal loosely wrapped packets in body cavities when encountered by law enforcement agents) when packets rupture or leak.

II. PATHOGENESIS

A. Cocaine promotes the release of neurotransmitters (e.g., dopamine, norepinephrine) while also blocking their reuptake in the central and sympathetic nervous system.

B. Cocaine is also a local anesthetic that blocks initiation and conduction of nerve impulse by decreasing axonal membrane permeability to sodium ions; at high doses, this class 1 antiarrhythmic effect contributes to cardiotoxicity.

C. Cocaine is rapidly metabolized by liver esterases and plasma cholinesterase and by nonenzymatic hydrolysis. Only small amounts are eliminated as unchanged drug in urine. Patients with pseudocholinesterase deficiency can be at greater risk of toxicity because of their reduced capacity for metabolism through the pseudocholinesterase pathway.

D. After IV injection or inhalation, a subjective euphoric response occurs in 3 to 5 minutes, with a cardiovascular response peaking in 8 to 12 minutes and lasting approximately 30 minutes. After nasal insufflation (snorting), a euphoric effect occurs within 15 to 20 minutes after exposure; cardiovascular changes and plasma levels peak within 20 to 60 minutes; and effects last several hours. Time to onset, time to peak effect, and duration of effect are somewhat longer following ingestion. Effects can be markedly delayed and prolonged following packet ingestion.

III. CLINICAL PRESENTATION

A. Signs and symptoms of acute poisoning include elevated pulse, blood pressure, respirations, and temperature, the magnitude of which is roughly proportional to the degree of toxicity.

1. Patients with mild poisoning can have normal or nearly normal vital signs. Other manifestations include anxiety, agitation, euphoria, headache, tremors, twitching, nausea, vomiting, diaphoresis, mydriasis, and pallor.

2. Patients with moderate poisoning can manifest mild to moderately increased vital signs, confusion, hallucinations, hyperactivity, clonus, increased muscle tone, abdominal cramps, and brief tonic-clonic seizures. Tea-colored urine should alert the physician to the possibility of rhabdomyolysis and potential renal failure.

3. Patients with severe poisoning have markedly abnormal vital signs with malignant hyperthermia, tachydysrhythmias, and status epilepticus or coma with flaccid paralysis. Other manifestations include apnea, cyanosis, and Cheyne-Stokes respirations. Cardiovascular collapse, bradycardia, and hypotension are preterminal events.

4. Laboratory abnormalities include leukocytosis, hypokalemia, and hyperglycemia.

B. Chronic nasal use can result in rhinitis, epistaxis, and septal perforation. Systemic manifestations of chronic use include anorexia, weight loss, insomnia, formication, impotence, depression, paranoia, and psychosis.

C. Evaluation should focus on the cardiac, pulmonary, and neurologic systems. Continuous electrocardiographic (ECG) monitoring and frequent monitoring of vital signs, including core body temperature, are essential.

1. Patients with moderate to severe toxicity should have the following: an electrocardiogram and chest radiographic study; analysis of complete blood count, electrolytes, glucose, blood urea nitrogen, creatinine, arterial blood gas, urinalysis, creatine, and phosphokinase; and qualitative toxicologic analysis of blood and urine.

2. Finding cocaine and metabolites in the urine supports the diagnosis. However, because urine screening can detect cocaine metabolites for as long as 3 days after exposure, a positive screen does not equate with clinical toxicity.

3. Standard protocols for ruling out myocardial infarction and ischemia should be followed in patients with chest pain of potential cardiac origin.

4. Patients with a persistent or severe headache, abnormal neurologic examination, or prolonged seizures require computed tomography scan and lumbar puncture to rule out subarachnoid hemorrhage.

5. Occult infections (e.g., endocarditis, hepatitis, pneumonia, epidural abscess) should be excluded in those with hyperthermia, particularly injection drug users.

IV. TREATMENT

A. Advanced life support measures should be instituted as necessary.

B. All patients should have close observation with IV access, and continuous ECG monitoring is necessary.

C. Supplemental oxygen, dextrose (25 g IV), and thiamine (100 mg IV) should be administered to patients with altered mental status, seizures, or coma.

D. Agitation, anxiety, and seizures can be treated with benzodiazepines (BZD), such as midazolam (2 to 5 mg IV), diazepam (2 to 10 mg IV), or lorazepam (1 to 4 mg IV).

E. Status epilepticus should be treated aggressively with IV BZD.

1. Early paralysis and short-acting barbiturates (amobarbital, thiopental, pentobarbital) should be employed in refractory cases. Rocuronium (0.6 mg/kg) or vecuronium (0.08 to 0.1 mg/kg) is the preferred paralytic agent.

F. Paralysis, along with aggressive cooling measures, is also indicated in patients with severe hyperthermia.

G. Moderate hypertension and tachycardia usually respond to BZD sedation.

1. Severe hypertension, particularly if associated with chest pain, is best treated with titratable IV agents, such as phentolamine (1 to 2 mg per dose), nitroglycerin, and nitroprusside.

2. Phentolamine can be effective in reducing myocardial oxygen demand and improving coronary blood flow.

3. β-Adrenergic blocking agents (labetalol, esmolol, propranolol) are relatively contraindicated because they may worsen coronary vasospasm.

4. Myocardial ischemia should otherwise be treated as usual. Adjunctive therapy with BZD is recommended.

H. Dysrhythmias should be treated according to standard advanced cardiac life support (ACLS) protocols. Treatment of ventricular dysrhythmias should also include sodium bicarbonate.

I. Hypotension requires active fluid resuscitation. If vasopressor therapy is indicated, a direct-acting drug (e.g., norepinephrine) is preferred because cocaine depletes neurotransmitters and prevents their reuptake.

J. Gastrointestinal decontamination should include activated charcoal for recent ingestions (see Chapter 105).

K. Body packers or stuffers should be treated with multiple-dose charcoal plus laxatives or whole-bowel irrigation (see Chapter 105).

1. Endoscopic removal of intact packets must be performed with caution because packet rupture can occur.

2. If signs or symptoms of cocaine toxicity are present or if intestinal obstruction occurs, immediate surgical intervention is indicated.

V. COMPLICATIONS

A. Complications can be acute or occur hours to days after actual cocaine use.

B. Cerebrovascular complications include cerebrovascular accidents, subarachnoid or intracerebral hemorrhage, and cerebral vasculitis.

C. Cardiovascular complications include myocardial, bowel, and kidney ischemia; infarction; skin necrosis; and aortic dissection.

D. Cerebral and renal vasculitis and cardiomyopathy have been reported.

E. Pulmonary infarcts, barotrauma, eosinophilia with granuloma formation, and noncardiogenic pulmonary edema can occur.

F. Inhalational exposure can result in cough, hemoptysis, reactive airway disease, pneumonitis ("crack lung"), and barotrauma (e.g., pneumothorax, pneumomediastinum).

Selected Readings

Gay GR, Inaba DS, Sheppard CW, et al. Cocaine history, epidemiology, human pharmacology and treatment. A perspective on a new debut for an old girl. *J Toxicol Clin Toxicol* 1975;8:149.
Excellent discussion about historical usage of cocaine.

Hollander JE. The management of cocaine-associated myocardial ischemia. *N Engl J Med* 1995;333:1267.
An excellent review article on the management of cocaine-associated chest pain.

Hollander JE, Hoffman US. Cocaine induced myocardial infarction: an analysis and review of the literature. *J Emerg Med* 1992;10:169.
Identification of a group of young individuals at risk for myocardial infarction.

Isner JM, Estes M, Thompson PD, et al. Acute cardiac events temporally related to cocaine abuse. *N Engl J Med* 1986;315:1438.
A report of seven patients with cardiac toxicity associated with nonintravenous use of cocaine.

Lange HA, Cigarroa RG, Flores ED, et al. Potentiation of cocaine-induced coronary vasoconstriction by beta-adrenergic blockade. *Ann Intern Med* 1990;112:897.
Randomized, double-blind, placebo trial in cardiac catheterization laboratory showing effects of β-adrenergic blockade.

McCarron MM, Wood JD. The cocaine body packer syndrome. *JAMA* 1983;250:1417.
A prospective study of 75 body packers.

Mouhaffel AH, Madu EC, Satmary WA, et al. Cardiovascular complication of cocaine. *Chest* 1995;107:1426.
A concise review of the cardiovascular complication of cocaine.

Pollack CV, Biggers DW, Carlton FB, et al. Two crack cocaine body stuffers. *Ann Emerg Med* 1992;21:1370.
A discussion about the controversies regarding the management of cocaine body stuffers.

Roth D, Alarcon FJ, Fernandez JA, et al. Acute rhabdomyolysis associated with cocaine intoxication. *N Engl J Med* 1988;319:673.
A description of a group of cocaine-intoxicated patients with rhabdomyolysis and renal failure.

Spivey WH, Euerle B. Neurologic complication of cocaine abuse. *Ann Emerg Med* 1990; 19:1422.
A concise review of the neurologic complication of cocaine abuse.

110 NONSTEROIDAL ANTIINFLAMMATORY DRUGS
Ivan E. Liang

I. GENERAL PRINCIPLES
  A. Nonsteroidal antiinflammatory drugs (NSAIDs) include aspirin, other salicylates, and a variety of other aspirinlike drugs. NSAIDs have analgesic, antipyretic, and antiinflammatory activity.

  B. Therapeutic effects and gastrointestinal and renal side effects are caused by inhibition of cyclooxygenase and prostaglandin synthesis.

  C. Aspirin is the only NSAID with significant antiplatelet activity.

II. PATHOPHYSIOLOGY
  A. Salicylates
    1. Absorption can continue for 24 hours after an acute overdose because of delayed dissolution of tablets or formation of gastric concretions.

    2. Following single therapeutic doses, salicylate is metabolized in the liver to the inactive metabolites. The remaining 10% of the dose is excreted unchanged in the urine.

    3. When serum concentrations exceed 20 mg/dL, the metabolism becomes saturated and elimination changes from first-order to zero-order kinetics and the half-life increases from about 2.5 hours to as long as 40 hours. Renal excretion of salicylate then becomes the most important route of elimination.

    4. Following overdose, direct stimulation of the respiratory center in the medulla by toxic salicylate concentrations results in a respiratory alkalosis.

    5. The accumulation of salicylate in cells causes uncoupling of mitochondrial oxidative phosphorylation, which leads to the characteristic increased anion gap metabolic acidosis.

  B. NSAIDs
    1. Nonsalicylate NSAIDs are rapidly absorbed following ingestion; they have small volumes of distribution and are highly protein bound.

    2. In contrast to salicylates, the metabolism of most nonsalicylate NSAIDs is not saturable and elimination follows first-order kinetics.

III. CLINICAL PRESENTATION
  A. Salicylates
    1. Salicylate poisoning can occur with acute as well as chronic overdose.

    2. Severity should be assessed by direct evaluation of acid—base status (Table 110-1) and clinical manifestations, rather than by the serum salicylate level or the Done nomogram.

      a. Mild poisoning is defined by the presence of alkalemia (serum pH >7.4) and alkaluria (urine pH <6). Signs and symptoms include nausea, vomiting, abdominal pain, diaphoresis, headache, tinnitus, and tachypnea.

      b. Moderate poisoning is defined by a normal or alkaline serum pH and aciduria (urine pH <6). Gastrointestinal tract and neurologic symptoms are more pronounced. Arterial blood gas and electrolyte analysis reveals combined respiratory alkalosis and metabolic acidosis with an increased anion gap.

      c. Severe poisoning is defined by the presence of acidemia and aciduria. Signs and symptoms include coma, seizures, respiratory depression, shock, or noncardiogenic pulmonary edema. Because of gastrointestinal, renal, and insensible fluid losses, dehydration is invariably present and often underestimated.

TABLE 110-1	Severity of Salicylate Poisoning		
Grade	Plasma pH	Urine pH	Underlying metabolic abnormality
Mild	>7.4	>6.0	Respiratory alkalosis
Moderate	=7.4	<6.0	Combined respiratory alkalosis and metabolic acidosis
Severe	<7.4	<6.0	Metabolic acidosis with or without respiratory acidosis

From Irwin RS, Rippe JM, eds. *Irwin and Rippe's intensive care medicine*, 5th ed. Philadelphia: Lippincott Williams & Wilkins, 2003, p. 1553.

B. Other NSAIDs

1. Metabolic acidosis, coma, seizures, hepatic dysfunction, hypotension, and cardiovascular collapse are relatively common after phenylbutazone overdose.
2. Other nonsalicylate NSAIDs rarely cause severe poisoning. Typical findings include nausea, vomiting, abdominal pain, headache, confusion, tinnitus, drowsiness, and hyperventilation. Symptoms usually last several hours.
3. Tonic-clonic seizures and muscle twitching have been reported after mefenamic acid overdose.

IV. EVALUATION

A. Salicylates

1. Initial laboratory evaluation should include arterial blood gases, electrolytes, glucose, blood urea nitrogen, and creatinine level and urinalysis.
2. In patients with moderate to severe poisoning, further evaluation should include determinations of serum calcium, magnesium, and ketones; liver function tests; complete blood cell count; coagulation studies; and an electrocardiogram and chest radiograph.
3. Because patients often confuse aspirin and acetaminophen, toxicology testing should be done for both substances.
4. Serial salicylate levels should be performed to assess for continued drug absorption and the efficacy of decontamination and elimination therapies.

B. Other NSAIDs

1. The diagnostic evaluation of patients with acute NSAID overdose is the same as for salicylates.
2. Evaluation of acid—base, electrolyte, and renal parameters is particularly important.
3. Additional ancillary testing is dictated by clinical severity.

V. MANAGEMENT

A. Salicylates

1. Resuscitative measures should be instituted as necessary. If endotracheal intubation and mechanical ventilation are instituted, hyperventilation is essential to prevent acidemia and the resultant increased tissue penetration of salicylic acid into the central nervous system (CNS).
2. Noncardiac pulmonary edema should be treated with intubation and positive end-expiratory pressure (PEEP) rather than diuretics.
3. Because CNS hypoglycemia can occur despite a normal serum glucose, obtain a finger stick blood sugar or empirically treat with D50W in patients with altered mental status.
4. Gastrointestinal tract decontamination should be performed in all patients with intentional overdoses and in those with accidental ingestions of greater than

150 mg/kg. It may be effective for as long as 24 hours following overdose and in patients with spontaneous vomiting, because of delayed absorption and concretion formation.

   a. Activated charcoal without cathartic is the preferred therapy that should be given to all patients.

   b. Gastric lavage and endoscopy may have a role in patients with large ingestions and rising drug levels despite charcoal therapy.

5. The administration of multiple-dose charcoal may enhance salicylate elimination and should also be considered but the clinical efficacy of this therapy is debatable.

6. Initial fluid therapy should be intravenous 5% dextrose in normal saline or 5% dextrose in one half normal saline with one ampoule (50 mEq) of sodium bicarbonate and potassium (10 to 20 mEq/L), with 1 to 3 L given over the first 1 to 2 hours.

7. Electrolyte abnormalities should be corrected.

8. Salicylate elimination can be enhanced by urinary alkalinization and diuresis and extracorporeal removal.

   a. Indications for urinary alkalinization include systemic symptoms, acid—base abnormalities, or salicylate levels greater than 30 mg/dL after an acute overdose.

     (1) The goal is to achieve a urine pH of 7.5 or greater and a urine output of 2 to 4 mL/kg per hour (Table 110-2).

     (2) Additional boluses of bicarbonate should be given to correct acidemia.

     (3) Acetazolamide should not be used to alkalinize the urine, because it can cause a concomitant systemic acidosis, which may promote tissue distribution of salicylate and result in clinical deterioration.

     (4) Alkali therapy should be withheld if the serum pH is greater than 7.55.

   d. Hemodialysis is indicated in patients with severe poisoning and in those with moderate poisoning who fail to respond to alkaline diuresis.

     (1) It is generally necessary for patients with serum levels greater than 1,000 mg/L (100 mg/dL) after an acute intoxication and 600 mg/L (60 mg/dL) after chronic intoxication, but severe or progressive clinical toxicity is the most important indication.

     (2) It is essential for a successful outcome in those with coma, seizures, cerebral or pulmonary edema, or renal failure.

B. Other NSAIDs

1. The treatment of nonsalicylate NSAID poisoning is supportive and symptomatic.

2. Advanced life support measures and invasive monitoring may be required in severe cases.

3. Renal function should be monitored carefully in patients with abnormal urinalysis, underlying renal disease, or advanced age.

4. Gastrointestinal tract decontamination with activated charcoal is recommended for patients who present soon after ingestion (see Chapter 105).

TABLE 110-2   **Alkaline Diuresis Therapy of Salicylate Poisoning: Fluid and Electrolyte Therapy**[a]

Grade	Intravenous solution	NaHCO$_3$ (amp/L)	Potassium (mEq/L)
Mild	D$_5$NS	1	20
Moderate	D$_5$½NS	2	40
Severe	D$_5$W	3	60

From Irwin RS, Rippe JM, eds. *Irwin and Rippe's intensive care medicine*, 5th ed. Philadelphia: Lippincott Williams & Wilkins, 2003, p. 1557.
D$_5$NS, 5% dextrose in normal saline; D$_5$½NS, 5% dextrose in one-half normal saline; D$_5$W, 5% dextrose in water; NaHCO$_3$, 50 mEq sodium bicarbonate/50 mL ampule (8.4%).
[a]Initial treatment should include hydration with 1-3 L of a saline solution containing dextrose (see text).

Selected Readings

Balali-Mood M, Critchley JA, Proudfoot AT, et al. Mefenamic acid overdose. *Lancet* 1981; 1354.
  A case series of mefenamic acid overdose that showed a high number of patients with neurologic toxicity such as seizures and muscle twitching.

Brenner BE, Simon RR. Management of salicylate intoxication. *Drugs* 1987;24:335.
  A review article on salicylate toxicity with a discussion of the different bedside tests for salicylates.

Duffens KR, Smilkstein MJ, Bessen HA, et al. Falsely elevated salicylate levels due to diflunisal overdose. *J Emerg Med* 1987;5:499.
  A case report and discussion of the cross-reactivity of diflunisal with the immunoassay and colorimetric assay for salicylates.

Dugandzic RM, Tiemey MG, Dickinson GE, et al. Evaluation of the validity of the Done nomogram in the management of acute salicylate intoxication. *Ann Emerg Med* 1989; 18:1186.
  A retrospective study of 55 acute salicylate intoxications, which demonstrated that management decisions should be based on the clinical presentation and serum salicylates level.

Gabow PA, Anderson RJ, Potts DE, et al. Acid base disturbances in the salicylate intoxicated adult. *Arch Intern Med* 1978;138:1481.
  A retrospective study of 67 adults with salicylate toxicity focusing on acid—base disturbances. The presence of acidemia in this group correlated with neurologic symptoms.

Hall AH, Smolinske SC, Conrad FL, et al. Ibuprofen overdose: 126 cases. *Ann Emerg Med* 1986;15:1308.
  A retrospective review of 126 ibuprofen overdose cases in adults and children. Ibuprofen toxicity in most cases was benign, but two children had seizures and one child died.

Hill JB. Experimental salicylate poisoning: observations on the effects of altering blood pH on tissue and plasma salicylate concentrations. *Pediatrics* 1971;47:658.
  An experimental model that demonstrated the importance of acid—base on the distribution of salicylates. Acidemia facilitates salicylate distribution into the brain.

Johnson D, Eppler J, Giesbrecht E, et al. Effect of multiple-dose activated charcoal on the clearance of high-dose intravenous aspirin in a porcine model. *Ann Emerg Med* 1995;26:569.
  An animal model showing no benefit of multiple-dose activated charcoal in the clearance of high-dose aspirin.

Linden CH, Townsend PL. Metabolic acidosis after acute ibuprofen overdosage. *J Pediatr* 1987;111;922.
  Two case reports and a discussion of the increased anion gap after acute ibuprofen overdose.

McGuigan MA. A two-year review of salicylate deaths in Ontario. *Arch Intern Med* 1987; 147:510.
  A retrospective study of salicylate deaths that demonstrated specific management difficulties, such as establishing the diagnosis, administering activated charcoal, and using hemodialysis.

Notarianni L. A reassessment of the treatment of salicylate poisoning. *Drug Saf* 1992; 7:292.
  A review article focusing on the recent developments in salicylate toxicity, including the discouragement of forced diuresis to enhance elimination.

Smith M. The metabolic basis of the major symptoms in acute salicylate intoxication. *Clin Toxicol* 1968;1:387.
  The classic paper on the effects of salicylates on metabolism and the clinical symptoms.

Smolinske SC, Hall AH, Vandenberg SA, et al. Toxic effects of nonsteroidal anti-inflammatory drugs in overdose: an overview of recent evidence on clinical effects and dose-response relationships. *Drug Saf* 1990;5:253.

The clinical effects and toxicity of 26 different nonsteroidal antiinflammatory drugs are discussed.

Veltri JC, Rollins DE. A comparison of the frequency and severity of poisoning cases for ingestion of acetaminophen, aspirin, and ibuprofen. *Am J Emerg Med* 1988; 6:104.
Data from the American Association of Poison Control Centers regarding exposure to analgesics revealed that the majority of patients had a low rate of serious effects.

Wortzman DJ, Grunfeld A. Delayed absorption following enteric-coated aspirin overdose. *Ann Emerg Med* 1987;16:434.
A case report of delayed toxicity following an overdose of sustained-release salicylate preparation.

I. BACKGROUND

A. Sedative-hypnotic agents are a chemically diverse group of drugs with the common feature of causing general central nervous system (CNS) depression.

B. They are used to treat a wide variety of conditions such as anxiety, insomnia, musculoskeletal disorders, seizures, and withdrawal states, and for anesthesia.

C. The major drug classes are benzodiazepines (BZD), barbiturates, and nonbenzodiazepine-nonbarbiturate sedative-hypnotics (Table 111-1).

D. Acute intoxication leads to generalized CNS depression. Respiratory depression is variable depending on the agent. Other effects include hypotension and myocardial depression.

E. Tolerance develops with chronic administration. Cross tolerance may also occur between different sedatives. Withdrawal symptoms including agitation, anxiety, hypertension, and seizures may develop with abstinence after chronic use (see Chapter 112).

II. PATHOPHYSIOLOGY

A. Pharmacology

1. BZD bind to BZD receptors (omega 1, 2, or 3) in the CNS. This receptor is part of the γ-aminobutyric acid-A (GABA-A) receptor complex. Binding facilitates GABA neurotransmission by increasing the frequency of Cl⁻ ion influx through the receptor channel causing net CNS depression.

2. Barbiturates bind to the GABA-A receptor complex, causing the ion channel to remain open longer and thereby facilitating Cl⁻ flux and GABA-mediated CNS depression.

3. Nonbenzodiazepine-nonbarbiturate agents are chemically distinct and diverse but pharmacologically similar. Many act through facilitation of GABA-A neurotransmission (chloral hydrate, meprobamate, methaqualone, zolpidem, GHB). Baclofen is a GABA-B agonist. γ-Hydroxybutyric acid (GBH) binds to GHB receptors associated with the GABA complex as well as GABA-B receptors. Buspirone has serotonergic and dopaminergic as well as GABAergic activity.

B. Pharmacokinetics

1. Gastrointestinal (GI) absorption of most agents is rapid. Exceptions are glutethimide, which has erratic absorption; meprobamate and carisoprodol, which may form bezoars; and sustained-release meprobamate.

2. The onset and duration of clinical effects are partly determined by lipophilicity. More lipophilic drugs rapidly partition into the CNS gray matter and then redistribute to other tissues, leading to a rapid onset and brief duration of action. Other factors include prolonged elimination phase and active metabolites (many BZD, chloral hydrate).

3. Most sedatives are metabolized via the hepatic CYP450 enzyme system. Exceptions include chloral hydrate (alcohol dehydrogenase metabolism), baclofen (mostly renal elimination), and GHB (precursor 1,4-BD is metabolized by alcohol dehydrogenase to GHB, which is metabolized via succinate semialdehyde).

4. Protein binding is extensive for most drugs in the class, with the exception of chloral hydrate, meprobamate, and the longer acting barbiturates (phenobarbital).

III. DIAGNOSIS

A. Clinical manifestations of overdose and poisoning

1. Features common to all agents include ataxia, nystagmus, slurred speech, and CNS depression ranging from lethargy to coma. With deep coma, depression of

TABLE 111-1	Sedative-Hypnotic Agents Available in the United States

Benzodiazepines	Miscellaneous
Alprazolam	Alpidem[a]
Bromazepam[a]	Baclofen
Brotizolam[a]	Buspirone
Chlordiazepoxide	Chloral hydrate
Clobazam[a]	Chlormethiazole[a]
Clorazepate	Ethinamate
Diazepam	Ethchlorvynol
Estazolam	Glutethimide
Flunitrazepam	Meprobamate
Flurazepam	Methaqualone
Halazepam	Methyprylon
Lorazepam	Paraldehyde
Midazolam	Zolpidem
Nitrazepam	
Oxazepam	
Quazepam	
Triazolam	
Barbiturates	
Amobarbital	
Aprobarbital	
Butalbital	
Mephobarbital	
Pentobarbital	
Phenobarbital	
Secobarbital	
Thiopental	

From Irwin RS, Rippe JM, eds. *Irwin and Rippe's intensive care medicine*, 5th ed. Philadelphia: Lippincott Williams & Wilkins, 2003, p. 1596.
[a]Investigational in the United States.

respiratory, cardiovascular, and thermoregulatory centers in the brainstem can lead to apnea, hypotension, myocardial depression, hypothermia, and shock with cardiogenic or noncardiogenic pulmonary edema.

2. Unique findings include:
   a. BZD. Deep coma is unusual and occurs only with massive overdose of short-acting agents such as temazepam and triazolam or when coingested with alcohol or other CNS depressants. Paradoxical agitation and anxiety may occur.
   b. Barbiturates. Coma can be rapid in onset (particularly with short-acting agents such as amobarbital, butalbitol/butabarbital, pentobarbital, and secobarbital), prolonged (particularly with phenobarbital), and profound. Bullous skin lesions over pressure points and rhabdomyolysis can occur with prolonged coma.
   c. Chloral hydrate. This substance was added to ethanol in the "Mickey Finn." Lethal adult dose is 5 to 10 g, but significant toxicity may occur with doses of as little as 1.25 g. Symptoms include GI irritation with nausea and vomiting and cardiac dysrhythmias including ventricular tachycardia due to myocardial sensitization to endogenous catecholamines. Chloral hydrate may be seen as radiopaque material in the GI tract on plain film of the abdomen.
   d. Ethchlorvynol. Similar to phenobarbital. Half-life is prolonged with overdose leading to prolonged coma. The aromatic (new plastic shower curtain) odor of the compound may be detected on the patient's breath.

e. Glutethimide. Similar to phenobarbital. Active metabolite, which has a long duration of action and is more potent than the parent drug, leads to prolonged coma. Fluctuating level of consciousness (due to erratic absorption, redistribution from adipose tissue) and anticholinergic symptoms may be seen.

f. Methyprylon. Similar to phenobarbital. Adverse effects include nausea, vomiting, GI irritation, headache, rash, diarrhea, esophagitis, neutropenia, and thrombocytopenia.

g. Meprobamate and carisoprodol. Meprobamate is the metabolite of carisoprodol. Toxicity of both is similar to glutethimide. Prolonged and erratic absorption (due to bezoars and sustained-release preparations) can result in fluctuating level of consciousness.

h. Baclofen. GABA-B agonism produces a distinct toxicity that includes hypertension (or hypotension), bradycardia (or tachycardia), hyperreflexia, myoclonus, and seizures as well as deep coma.

i. Buspirone. Similar to benzodiazepines, but experience is limited. Serotonin syndrome (see Chapter 108) can occur when administered with other serotonergic agents.

j. Zolpidem and zaleplon. Similar to benzodiazepines.

k. GHB. Similar to baclofen but with rapid onset (minutes) and short duration (several hours). Can produce euphoria and hallucinations as well as coma. Most users take a precursor drug (1,4-butanediol), which is converted by alcohol dehydrogenase to GHB. Coingestion with ethanol, which competes for metabolism, may delay toxicity. Another precursor γ-butyrolactone does not require enzymatic conversion.

B. Differential diagnosis. Other causes of CNS depression include hypoglycemia, CNS infection, hemorrhage, or tumor, and toxicity from ethanol, anticonvulsants, antidepressants, antihistamines, antipsychotics, and opiates.

C. Evaluation

1. Vital signs should include a rectal temperature in patients with coma because hypothermia may be overlooked.

2. Patients with coma should also have arterial blood gas analysis, complete blood count (CBC), electrolytes, blood urea nitrogen (BUN), creatinine, glucose, creatine phosphokinase (CPK; looking for possible rhabdomyolysis), electrocardiogram (ECG), and chest radiograph.

3. Check acetaminophen and salicylate concentrations, particularly with Fioricet and Fiorinal ingestions, which contain acetaminophen and aspirin, respectively, as well as butalbital. Carisoprodol is also formulated with aspirin (Soma compound).

4. Urine drugs of abuse (immunoassay) screens detect most barbiturates, a minority of BZD, and no other sedative-hypnotics.

5. Quantitative serum levels are not routinely available or clinically useful except for phenobarbital (therapeutic level 10 to 40 µg/mL) and perhaps other barbiturates.

IV. TREATMENT

A. Advanced life support measures should be instituted as necessary. Particular attention should be paid to protecting the airway and assisting ventilation via endotracheal intubation in patients with coma.

B. All patients should initially have continuous pulse oximetry and cardiac monitoring along with IV access.

C. GI decontamination with activated charcoal should be considered for recent ingestions along with whole bowel irrigation for sustained release meprobamate overdose (see Chapter 105).

D. Hypotension should initially be treated with several liters of intravenous saline. Vasopressors (e.g., dopamine, norepinephrine) should be used for refractory hypotension.

E. Ventricular tachyarrhythmias from chloral hydrate should be treated with γ-blockers, lidocaine, and BZD, as for other chlorinated hydrocarbons.

F. Bradydysrhythmias should be treated according to advanced cardiac life support (ACLS) guidelines, but epinephrine should be avoided in chloral hydrate poisoning (unless the patient is pulseless).

G. Seizures from baclofen or GHB can be treated with BZD if prolonged or recurrent.

H. Rewarming measures should be instituted as needed for hypothermia.

I. Intravenous flumazenil, a competitive inhibitor of BZD at central BZD receptors, can reverse CNS depression due to BZD, zolpidem, and zaleplon.

    1. For oral BZD overdose, the recommended dose is 0.2 mg, followed by 0.3 mg, then 0.5 mg doses to a maximum of 3 mg, each dose administered over 30 seconds and waiting 30 seconds for a response before giving the next dose. For partial responders, an additional 2 mg can be administered in increments of 0.5 mg.

    2. Since flumazenil can precipitate BZD withdrawal, an initial dose of 0.1 mg is prudent if chronic BZD use or tolerance is suspected.

    3. Relative contraindications include conditions where BZD may be therapeutic (e.g., coingestion of agents known to cause seizures, epilepsy).

    4. For reversal of BZD-induced procedural sedation, initial and subsequent doses of 0.2 mg (0.01 mg/kg, up to 0.2 mg per dose in children), up to a maximum of 1 mg are recommended.

    5. Because abrupt reversal of BZD sedation can cause seizures in the absence of tolerance, administering doses more slowly than recommended (i.e., over 1 minute) may also be prudent.

J. Multidose activated charcoal and alkaline diuresis (see Chapter 105) can enhance the elimination of phenobarbital.

K. Hemodialysis can enhance the elimination of some agents and should be considered in patients with cardiovascular instability due to barbiturates, chloral hydrate, and meprobamate/carisoprodol who fail to respond to other measures. A rebound in blood levels may occur after hemodialysis as a result of drug redistribution.

V. COMPLICATIONS

A. Most patients do well with aggressive supportive care.

B. Complications include pressure-induced blisters, sores, and rhabdomyolysis; pulmonary edema; and anoxia- or shock-induced multiple-organ dysfunction.

Selected Readings

Berg MJ, Berlinger WG, Goldberg MJ, et al. Acceleration of the body clearance of phenobarbital by oral activated charcoal. *N Engl J Med* 1982;307:642–644.
Demonstrates the utility of activated charcoal for "gut dialysis" in the enhancement of phenobarbital clearance.

Spivey WH. Flumazenil and seizures: analysis of 43 cases. *Clin Ther* 1992;14:292.
This review of flumazenil-induced seizures highlights the need for cautious use in the reversal of benzodiazepine overdose, particularly in patients who coingest agents known to cause seizures or patients who have BZD tolerance.

I. GENERAL PRINCIPLES

A. Withdrawal syndromes consist of a constellation of clinical findings in patients who either abruptly discontinue, or significantly decrease, the dose or frequency of a drug. By definition reinstatement of the drug alleviates the withdrawal syndrome.

B. Withdrawal may develop with many drug classes, including ethanol, benzodiazepines (BZD), barbiturates, other sedative-hypnotics, opioids, γ-hydroxybutyric acid (GHB), antidepressants, and many other agents including antihypertensives, caffeine, and nicotine.

C. Tolerance is a decreased physiologic response to a given dose of drug after chronic administration. Patients who display tolerance are at risk for withdrawal if the drug is discontinued. Other factors increasing the risk, severity, and duration of withdrawal include use of drugs with short duration of effect, high frequency of administration, and long duration of use.

D. Cross-tolerance occurs when the chronic ingestion of one substance decreases the response to another substance. Ethanol, barbiturates, BZD, and nonbarbiturate-nonbenzodiazepine sedative-hypnotics display cross-tolerance.

II. PATHOPHYSIOLOGY

A. Ethanol

1. During periods of chronic ethanol consumption central nervous system (CNS) sympathetic pathways may counterregulate the sedative effects of ethanol.

2. Cessation of drinking may result in unopposed sympathetic compensatory mechanisms, leading to sympathomimetic excess.

3. Abrupt withdrawal of GABA-potentiating effects of ethanol leads to disinhibition of neural pathways in the CNS.

4. Upregulation of *N*-methyl-D-aspartate (NMDA) receptors, which occurs with chronic intoxication, may contribute to CNS excitation.

B. Sedative-hypnotics

1. BZD tolerance appears to be due to the upregulation of BZD receptors. The abundance of unoccupied receptors with drug cessation leads to decreased GABAergic neurotransmission and net CNS excitation.

2. Similar mechanisms likely exist for other sedative-hypnotic drugs including GHB.

3. Intrathecal baclofen infusion probably results in upregulation of spinal cord GABA-B receptors.

C. Opioids

1. Stimulation of opioid receptors reduces the firing rate of locus ceruleus noradrenergic neurons, resulting in the inhibition of catecholamine release.

2. Chronic use may produce adrenergic receptor upregulation, leading to increased sympathetic tone with abstinence.

D. Antidepressants.
The mechanism of withdrawal is unknown but may involve a rapid decline in serotonergic (and adrenergic) neurotransmission.

III. DIAGNOSIS

A. Clinical syndromes

1. Ethanol

a. Withdrawal produces a hyperadrenergic state characterized by intense sympathetic nervous system activation. Manifestations include tachycardia, hypertension, tremors, seizures, and delirium.

b. Tremors occur early and are signs of mild to moderate withdrawal. This begins 6 to 8 hours after a reduction in ethanol intake and may occur despite detectable serum ethanol concentrations of 100 mg/dL. Other symptoms in this phase include nausea, vomiting, anorexia, anxiety, and insomnia, which peak between 24 and 36 hours. Recovery occurs within a few days. About 20% to 25% of these patients progress to more serious symptoms.

c. Most ethanol withdrawal seizures occur between 7 and 48 hours of cessation or relative abstinence. They may occur after the onset of mild withdrawal symptoms or herald the onset of withdrawal. They are short, generalized, tonic-clonic seizures. Forty percent are isolated. If they recur it is generally within a few hours of the first seizure. Status epilepticus is rare. The occurrence of seizures does suggest a higher incidence of severe withdrawal, including delirium tremens.

d. The hallmark of delirium tremens is a significant alteration of sensorium associated with dramatic autonomic and CNS hyperactivity. This is rarely seen before 48 to 72 hours after cessation of ethanol and may be delayed up to 5 to 14 days. Patients are disoriented and display global confusion, hallucinations, delusions, mumbling speech, and psychomotor agitation. Tachycardia, hypertension, hyperpyrexia, diaphoresis, and mydriasis are present.

e. Alcoholic hallucinosis occurs in a small subset of patients and consists of hallucinations, typically disabling auditory hallucinations, in the absence of tremor or autonomic findings. It occurs within 8 to 48 hours of cessation, generally lasting 1 to 6 days. Rare cases persist for months.

2. Benzodiazepines
   a. Signs of BZD withdrawal are similar to those from ethanol.
   b. Unlike ethanol, the time of symptom onset depends on the particular medication. Short-acting drugs such as alprazolam cause symptom onset within hours of discontinuation, whereas diazepam withdrawal may not develop for days.

3. Barbiturate and nonbenzodiazepine-nonbarbiturate sedative-hypnotics
   a. Withdrawal is generally similar to that from ethanol.
   b. Chronic delivery of baclofen via intrathecal pump for spastic neuromuscular disorders may be interrupted when the infusion becomes disconnected or the medication runs out. Marked muscle rigidity is seen with this scenario. Withdrawal from orally dosed baclofen is uncommon.

4. GHB
   a. Withdrawal is generally similar to that from ethanol.
   b. Users of GHB typically dose the drug every 1 to 2 hours, including awakening at night for administration. Therefore, symptom onset is much more rapid than with other sedatives.

5. Opioids
   a. Early signs of opioid withdrawal include mydriasis, lacrimation, rhinorrhea, diaphoresis, yawning, piloerection, anxiety, and restlessness. This may progress to mild elevation of pulse and blood pressure as well as the development of myalgias, vomiting, diarrhea, anorexia, abdominal pain, and dehydration. Intense drug craving is unique to opioid withdrawal.
   b. Heroin withdrawal begins within 4 to 8 hours of the last dose, whereas withdrawal from methadone occurs after 36 to 72 hours.
   c. Unlike with ethanol and sedative withdrawal, opioid withdrawal is not life-threatening because patients do not have altered mental status, hyperthermia, and seizures. The exception is neonatal withdrawal, which may involve seizures and is life-threatening.

6. Antidepressants
   a. Withdrawal from any antidepressant, but particularly from short-acting selective serotonin reuptake inhibitors (paroxetine), may cause symptoms of nausea, headaches, restlessness, and fatigue.
   b. Signs and symptoms are not life-threatening.

B. Evaluation
1. Perform a complete physical examination.
2. Check vital signs for hyperpyrexia, tachycardia, and hypertension.
3. Examine for signs of trauma, infection, and focal neurologic deficits.
4. Evaluate for metabolic derangements, particularly with alcoholics.
   a. Obtain complete blood count (CBC), electrolytes (including Ca^{2+}, Mg^{2+}, Phos), blood urea nitrogen (BUN), creatinine, CPK, glucose, and liver function tests.
   b. Consider cranial computed tomography (CT) and lumbar puncture (LP) to rule out CNS trauma or infection.
C. Differential diagnosis
1. The differential for withdrawal includes all other causes of a hyperadrenergic state, including hypoglycemia, sympathomimetic drugs such as amphetamines, serotonin syndrome, neuroleptic malignant syndrome, as well as underlying metabolic, infectious, or traumatic disorders.
2. Consider the possibility of intracranial hemorrhage, meningitis, encephalitis, hypoxia, sepsis, thiamine deficiency, thyroid storm, pheochromocytoma, and hepatic encephalopathy.

IV. TREATMENT
A. General principles
1. Anticipation and recognition of early signs of ethanol and sedative-hypnotic withdrawal allow timely treatment and prevent the development of serious manifestations such as seizures, hyperthermia, and delirium.
2. In general, treatment relies on replacement therapy with cross-tolerant drugs, which alleviate symptoms and can be tapered.
3. Tapering should generally occur over 2 to 4 weeks (e.g., by decreasing the dose 10% to 20% every 3 days).
4. Management includes treatment of coexisting medical problems.
B. Ethanol
1. Utilize withdrawal assessment tools to grade severity and guide therapy.
2. The Clinical Institute Withdrawal Assessment (CIWA) scale provides a numbered grading system based on the patient's mental status (e.g., reported anxiety, hallucinations, disorientation). Scores are used to determine the need for sedation with BZD.
3. Achievement of adequate sedation (sleeping, yet arousable) is the cornerstone of therapy. BZD have proved the most effective.
   a. Long-acting BZD with active metabolites (diazepam or chlordiazepoxide) offer a prolonged therapeutic effect without the need for frequent dosing.
   b. Intravenous therapy can be followed with oral dosing.
   c. Initial doses of 5 to 20 mg intravenous diazepam every 5 minutes are given until sleep is induced.
   d. Some patients require very high doses (up to 1,000 mg diazepam in 24 hours).
4. Barbiturates act synergistically with BZD at GABA receptors.
   a. Pentobarbital in increments of 100 mg can be given orally or intravenously for severe withdrawal unresponsive to BZD.
   b. Barbiturates have a poor safety profile in nonintubated patients because of the risk of respiratory depression.
5. In intubated patients, intravenous propofol (direct GABA effect) can also be used for severe withdrawal unresponsive to BZD.
6. Phenothiazines (prochlorperazine, chlorpromazine) and butyrophenones (haldol) lower the seizure threshold, induce hypotension, impair thermoregulation, and should be avoided.
7. Other therapies include initial administration of thiamine 100 mg, folate 1 mg, and a multivitamin. Alert patients may take these orally. Magnesium replacement is also warranted because many alcoholics have low Mg^{2+} stores.

C. Sedative-hypnotics

1. Dose requirements for patients with physical dependence on BZD and barbiturates are generally far less than for alcohol withdrawal.
2. Reinstituting the withdrawn medication at previously used doses is generally sufficient to alleviate symptoms.
3. Cross-tolerant medications may be used (e.g., BZD for barbiturate withdrawal).
4. As with ethanol withdrawal, neuroleptic medications have no role in therapy.
5. GHB withdrawal may also be treated with BZD, although there is evidence that barbiturates are more effective. Initial doses of a short-acting barbiturate such as pentobarbital can be given intravenously (50 to 150 mg every 15 minutes) until mild sedation is achieved. This can be followed by oral dosing with a long-acting barbiturate such as phenobarbital (one third the effective dose of intravenous pentobarbital—usually 30 to 60 mg) every 8 hours.
6. Baclofen withdrawal should be treated by reinstituting the prior dose of baclofen.

D. Opioids

1. Withdrawal may be treated either with long-acting opioids (e.g., sustained-release oxycodone or methadone) or medications that blunt the sympathetic response to withdrawal (e.g., clonidine).
   a. An initial dose of 20 mg methadone by mouth daily will generally relieve most symptoms but may not curb drug cravings.
   b. Clonidine 0.2 to 0.3 mg orally three times a day may alleviate some of the autonomic symptoms but not drug craving.
   c. Dosing of opioids or clonidine can be tapered over several days.
2. In the United States, treatment of opioid addiction with methadone requires that the facility be licensed for such treatment by the U.S. Food and Drug Administration (FDA), the Drug Enforcement Administration (DEA), and designated state authorities. This does not preclude nonlicensed facilities from treating opioid withdrawal in patients who are admitted for other reasons.

E. Antidepressants

1. Reinstituting the previous dosage of the withdrawn agent is sufficient to alleviate symptoms.
2. The medication can then be tapered over 2 to 3 weeks.

V. COMPLICATIONS include those related to withdrawal (e.g., dehydration, electrolyte disturbances, hyperthermia, rhabdomyolysis, seizures, aspiration), to its treatment (e.g., CNS and respiratory depression, aspiration), and to underlying illness (e.g., infection, nutritional deficiencies, trauma).

Selected Readings

Ritson B, Chick J. Comparison of two benzodiazepines in the treatment of alcohol withdrawal: effects in symptoms and cognitive recovery. *Drug Alcohol Depend* 1986;18:329.
This article discusses the preferential use of long-acting benzodiazepines with active metabolites (diazepam), rather than short-acting, without active metabolites (lorazepam) in the treatment of ethanol withdrawal.

Sivilotti ML, Burns MJ, Aaron CK, et al. Pentobarbital for severe gamma-butyrolactone withdrawal. *Ann Emerg Med* 2001;38(6):660–665.
This is a case series that illustrates the features of GHB withdrawal and demonstrates the effectiveness of barbiturates compared with benzodiazepines for treating symptoms.

Surgical Problems in the Intensive Care Unit

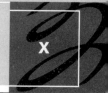

X

I. GENERAL PRINCIPLES
   A. Epistaxis is a common clinical problem that is usually mild and self-limited. However, epistaxis can become a severe and life-threatening emergency.
   B. Understanding the blood supply to the nose is essential to rendering appropriate management.

II. ANATOMY
   A. The internal and external carotid arteries supply blood to the nose.
   B. The internal carotid gives rise to the anterior and posterior ethmoidal arteries. These intracranial vessels pierce the cribriform plate to supply blood to the superior nasal passages.
      1. The anterior ethmoidal artery supplies the anterior superior septum and the anterolateral nasal wall.
      2. The posterior ethmoidal artery supplies the posterior–superior and the posterolateral nasal wall.
   C. The external carotid artery gives rise to the facial and internal maxillary arteries, which supply the cutaneous and mucosal surfaces of the nasal passage.
      1. The superior labial artery, as a terminal branch of the facial artery, supplies the nasal floor and inferior septum.
      2. Most nasal blood flow is derived from the terminal branches of the internal maxillary artery. The sphenopalatine artery perfuses the posterior septum and the lateral nasal walls.
   D. Anterior bleeding is most common and usually originates from Kisselbach's plexus, the anastamosis of the internal and external blood supply.
   E. Posterior epistaxis usually originates from the sphenopalatine artery.

III. ETIOLOGY
   A. Blunt trauma is the most common cause of epistaxis. Iatrogenic injury is common in the intensive care setting.
      1. Feeding and nasogastric tubes abrade and irritate the nasal passages.
      2. Nonhumidified oxygen delivered through a nasal cannula dries the mucosa.
      3. Primary and secondary coagulopathies are also important considerations in the pathogenesis of epistaxis.
   B. Preexisting conditions can increase the risk of epistaxis.
      1. Abuse of cocaine and nasal decongestants desiccates the mucosa.
      2. Preexisting bony or cartilaginous deformities (e.g., severe septal deviation) cause airflow turbulence and irritation.
      3. Minor trauma and dryness in patients with atherosclerosis or hypertension results in brisk, persistent bleeding that is difficult to control.
         a. The systolic pressure is elevated and the diseased vessels are noncompressible.
         b. The incidence of posterior epistaxis is higher in these patients.

IV. DIAGNOSIS
   A. A distinction between anterior and posterior epistaxis must be established by physical diagnosis to provide appropriate management.

B. In stable patients with epistaxis, a careful history and a thorough physical examination should be performed.
   1. Include any previous episodes of epistaxis, coagulopathy, and use of anticoagulants.
   2. Examine under good lighting with a nasal speculum and suction.
   3. Posterior bleeding may require nasal endoscopy for adequate visualization.
C. Visualization can be enhanced by using the vasoconstrictors topical cocaine or neosynephrine with lidocaine.

V. TREATMENT

A. Prevention is important.
   1. Rotate and inspect nasal tubes regularly.
   2. Humidified oxygen is essential to prevent mucosal desiccation.
   3. Hypertension and coagulopathies should be treated immediately.
B. The airway is a priority in unstable patients and intubation may be required.
C. Monitor vital signs and check blood count and coagulation studies.
D. Gastric decompression will minimize aspiration of blood.
E. The mainstay of treatment for direct control of bleeding is cautery and nasal packing.
   1. In most cases, external digital pressure for 5 to 10 minutes can achieve hemostasis.
   2. Cautery is also a reasonable way to achieve hemostasis. Care must be taken not to perforate the septum.
   3. If cautery is insufficient to achieve hemostasis, then packing is necessary.
   4. Packing should be placed anteriorly or posteriorly with respect to the location of the bleeding.
   5. Commercial nasal packing impregnated with vasoconstrictive agents or hemostatic agents is widely available. Petroleum gauze is a satisfactory alternative.
   6. Posterior bleeding presents a challenge with respect to effective packing.
      a. A Foley catheter is a reasonable alternative to posterior packing.
      b. Apply local anesthesia, insert the catheter into the nose, inflate the balloon in the posterior nasal cavity with 10 to 20 mL of saline. Secure the catheter to the ala with an umbilical clamp.
      c. Packing can be removed when coagulation defects or other causes of bleeding have been addressed.
F. If epistaxis is recurrent or long-term hemostasis is not achieved with sufficient packing, arterial ligation or embolization is necessary.
   1. Posterior nasal bleeding is controlled by ligation of the internal maxillary artery.
   2. Anterior bleeding is abated by the ligation of the ethmoidal arteries.
   3. In the case of diffuse bleeding, both the internal maxillary artery and the ethmoidal artery should be ligated.
   4. Angiographic embolization of the internal maxillary is an alternative to ligation.
   5. The ethmoidal arteries arise from the internal carotid, and embolization should not be attempted.
   6. Either procedure requires a stable patient and the appropriate ancillary staff.

Selected Readings

Elahi MM, Parnes LS, Fox AJ, et al. Therapeutic embolization in the treatment of intractable epistaxis. *Arch Otolarngol Head Neck Surg* 1995;121:65.
   This reference provides a review of arterial embolization.

Strong EB, Bell DA, Johnson LP, et al. Intractable epistaxis: transantral ligation vs. embolization: efficacy review and cost analysis. *Otolarngol Head Neck Surg* 1995;113:674.
   This reference provides insight into the cost-effectiveness of ligation and embolization.

Viducich RA, Blanda MP, Gerson LW. Posterior epistaxis: clinical features and acute complications. *Ann Emerg Med* 1995;25:592.
   This reference provides a review of posterior epistaxis and its complications.

ESOPHAGEAL PERFORATION AND ACUTE MEDIASTINITIS

114

Olga Ivanov, Fred A. Luchette, and Robert M. Mentzer

I. ESOPHAGEAL PERFORATION

A. Definitions. Esophageal perforation can be a result of multiple pathophysiologic stresses:
   1. Spontaneous perforation due to increased wall tension
   2. Penetrating injuries
      a. due to intraluminal causes
      b. due to extraluminal causes

B. Etiology
   1. Spontaneous rupture
      a. Due to intraluminal pressure increase that is greater than tolerated by esophagus (i.e., Boerhaave's syndrome, blunt trauma)
      b. Esophageal cancer perforation from the intrinsic necrosis
      c. Inflammatory esophageal lesions: tuberculosis, Barrett's esophagus, idiopathic eosinophilic esophagitis
   2. Extraluminal perforation
      a. Penetrating trauma from stabs or gunshot wounds
      b. Primary esophageal surgery: resection or esophagomyotomy
      c. Adjacent surgical procedures: cervical procedures, pneumonectomy, echoendoscopy, laparoscopic Nissen fundoplication, aortic surgery, and tube thoracostomy
   3. Intraluminal perforation
      a. Instrumentation
         (1) Leading edge of a stricture is a point most likely to rupture
         (2) More common with rigid rather than flexible endoscopy
      b. Esophageal stent placement, especially in cases of prior radiation and chemotherapy
      c. Congenital anomalies (esophageal atresia) from nasogastric (NG) tube placement
      d. Transesophageal echocardiography—very rare
      e. Endotracheal intubation
      f. Ingested foreign bodies
      g. Chemical burns from alkali or strong acids, resulting in mucosal damage and stricture

C. Clinical presentation
   1. Tachycardia—earliest sign of mediastinitis
   2. Tachypnea and shallow respirations
   3. Emphysema of soft tissues of the face and chest
   4. Pain: precordial, epigastric, or scapular due to diaphragmatic irritation
   5. Fever
   6. Dysphagia and odynophagia
   7. Hoarseness and cervical tenderness in cervical esophageal perforations

D. Diagnosis
   1. Chest radiography (CXR): mediastinal air, hydropneumothorax
   2. Barium esophagram—most sensitive diagnostic test; avoid water-soluble contrast due to pulmonary complications
   3. Computed tomography (CT) scan: extraluminal air, periesophageal fluid, wall thickening, extraluminal contrast

E. Treatment
1. Early— (i.e., less than 12 hours from the time of perforation):
   a. Primary closure and with subsequent drainage of the region
   b. Reinforcement of repair with a flap of parietal pleura, intercostal muscle flap, or an omental patch
2. Late— (i.e., greater than 12 hours or extensive inflammation):
   a. Esophageal diversion
   b. Generous drainage
   c. Broad-spectrum antibiotics
3. Perforations limited to the mediastinum. Antibiotics, nasogastric (NG) drainage, and total parenteral nutrition (TPN)
4. Persistent esophagomediastinal fistulas. Controlled with esophageal stents or fibrin glue.

II. ACUTE MEDIASTINITIS
A. Etiology
1. Associated with sternotomy and intrathoracic procedures.
2. Predisposing factors include advanced age, severe obesity, emergency surgery, lower preoperative ejection fraction, prolonged cardiopulmonary bypass, postoperative bleeding and need for reoperation, diabetes mellitus, use of bilateral internal mammary artery grafts, and immunosuppression as seen in heart transplant recipients.
3. Rarely could be due to spread of periodontal disease to mediastinum
4. Cervical and thoracic esophageal perforation
5. Extension of primary pulmonary infections into the mediastinal planes
6. Complications from central lines
7. Bacteriology
   a. If secondary to esophageal perforation, then organisms are typical of oral flora, especially anaerobes
   b. If secondary to surgery, *Staphylococcus aureus* and gram-negative bacilli, including *Pseudomonas aeruginosa*
   c. Lemierre's syndrome: affects young, healthy individuals following a primary oropharyngeal infection due to *Fusobacterium necrophorum*; characterized by trismus, tenderness and swelling along the angle of the mandible, and sternocleidomastoid muscle with subsequent thrombophlebitis of the internal jugular vein
8. Morbidity and mortality of mediastinitis
   a. Poststernotomy mediastinitis is seen in 1% of patients; first year postcoronary artery bypass graft survival rate of 78% with mediastinitis and 95% without it
   b. Threefold increase in mortality in patients with mediastinitis
   c. Up to 5% mediastinitis rate in post–heart transplant patients

B. Clinical presentation
1. Fever
2. Pain localized to the chest or radiating to the neck
3. Tachycardia
4. Subcutaneous emphysema
5. Postoperative infection
   a. Occurs 3 days to 4 weeks after resection
   b. Characterized by tachycardia, leukocytosis, increasing sternal pain, and sternal drainage with sternal instability

C. Diagnosis
1. CXR: air tracking in the mediastinum, retrosternally or between the leaves of the sternum
2. CT scan: diagnostic only after 2 weeks postsurgery due to disruption of natural tissue planes by surgical dissection and presence of air after any recent sternotomy

D. Treatment
1. Obtain blood and mediastinal fluid cultures

2. Broad-spectrum antibiotics
3. Resuscitate to maintain adequate cardiac output and oxygen delivery
4. Drain or débride fluid collections or necrotic tissue
5. Open-window thoracostomy for bronchopleural or esophagopleural fistulas
6. Irrigation and sternal débridement with rewiring for early exploration
7. Irrigation catheter in cases of gross purulence
8. Unilateral or bilateral pectoralis major, omental, or rectus femoris flap closure after radical sternal débridement for postoperative infections

E. Complications

1. Late failure of internal mammary arterial bypass graft in postoperative mediastinitis
2. Significant risk for redo surgery after reconstruction with thoracoabdominal muscle flaps
3. Free right ventricular wall rupture on sternal mobilization during delayed closure or on spontaneous cough or movement
4. Prolonged ventilator support, hospitalization, and death

Selected Readings

Bauwens K, Gellert K, Hanack U, et al. Open window thoracostomy in the treatment of esophageal or bronchopleural fistula with advanced mediastinitis and septic shock. *Thorac Cardiovasc Surg* 1996;44:308.
Review of open window thoracostomy as a procedure of choice in critically ill patients with bronchopleural or esophagopleural fistulas in whom primary therapy fails to control the septic focus.

Braxton J, Marrin CA, McGrath PD, et al. Mediastinitis and long-term survival after the coronary artery bypass graft surgery. *Ann Thorac Surg* 2000;70:2004.
Retrospective review of 15,406 patients undergoing CABG demonstrates a marked increase in mortality in patients with mediastinitis.

Brunet F, Brusset A, et al. Risk factors for deep sternal wound infections after sternotomy: a prospective, multicenter study. *J Thorac Cardiovasc Surg* 1996;111:1200.
Retrospective review assessing independent risk factors for deep sternal wound infections after CABG.

Cumberbatch GI, Reichl M. Oesophageal perforation: a rare complication of minor blunt trauma. *J Accid Emerg Med* 1996;13:295.
Review of published reports of esophageal perforations due to blunt trauma.

Hultmann CS, Culbertson JH, Jones GE, et al. Thoracic reconstruction with the omentum: indications, complications, and results. *Ann Plast Surg* 2001;46(3):242.
Retrospective analysis of 60 patients who underwent thoracic reconstruction with the omentum.

Jolles H, Henry DA, Roberson JP, et al. Mediastinitis following median sternotomy: CT findings. *Radiology* 1996;201:463.
Retrospective review of specificity of CT scans diagnosis of mediastinitis in patients who underwent median sternotomies.

Lee S, Mergo PJ, Ross PR. The leaking esophagus: CT patterns of the esophageal rupture, perforation, and fistulization. *Crit Rev Diagn Imaging* 1996;37:461.
Excellent review of various etiologies and CT findings of esophageal perforations.

Levashev YN, Akopov AL, Mosin IV. The possibilities of greater omentum usage in thoracic surgery. *Eur J Cardiothorac Surg* 1997;67:133.
Series of 68 patients treated with omental patch demonstrates it to be an excellent choice of repair for various thoracic procedures.

Okten I, Cangir AK, Ozdemir N, et al. Management of esophageal perforation. *Surg Today* 2001;31:36.
Retrospective review of 31 patients treated surgically or nonoperatively for esophageal perforations.

Schroder J, Siemann M, Vogel I, et al. Sepsis syndrome induced by tuberculosis perforation of the esophagus. *Infection* 1996;24:162.
Case review of TB-induced spontaneous esophageal perforation treated endoscopically and medically.

Slim K, Elbaz V, Pezet D, et al. Non-surgical treatment of the thoracic esophagus. *Presse Med* 1996;25:154.
Series of six patients, all treated successfully for esophageal perforations with nonoperative approach.

DIAGNOSIS AND MANAGEMENT OF INTRAABDOMINAL SEPSIS

Margaret Wolfe, Joseph Solomkin, and Fred A. Luchette

115

I. GENERAL PRINCIPLES

A. Intraabdominal infections are commonly encountered in the intensive care unit (ICU) setting. The presentation and causes are varied.

  1. The largest group of patients is those who have undergone a recent procedure or intervention in whom abscess must be ruled out.

  2. A second group of patients is that resident in the ICU with clinical findings suggestive of infection without obvious source.

    a. Prophylactic antibiotic usage is decreasing the occurrence of postoperative infections

    b. May be unrelated to primary problem

    c. May present as ileus without signs of infection elsewhere. Can include causes such as bowel ischemia, cholecystitis, pseudomembranous colitis, pancreatitis, or diverticulitis.

II. ETIOLOGY

A. Pathogenesis is secondary to spontaneous causes or to contamination of the peritoneal cavity by perforated viscus, which causes breakdown of peritoneal defense mechanisms.

B. Peritoneal defense mechanisms provide a system for rapid clearance of foreign particulates and solutes from the intraperitoneal space.

  1. Resident peritoneal macrophages, neutrophils, and monocytes ingest microorganisms and secrete proinflammatory molecules.

  2. Lymphatic channels provide entry of peritoneal fluid with bacteria and proinflammatory mediators into the venous system.

  3. Inspiration, especially positive pressure ventilation, causes a pressure gradient favoring fluid movement out of the abdomen.

  4. Entry of proinflammatory substances into the vascular space would be expected to produce many of the hemodynamic and respiratory findings of severe sepsis.

C. Pathogens include mixed flora—aerobic, anaerobic, and facultative gram-negative enteric bacilli are common pathogens (Table 115-1).

  1. Facultative and aerobic gram-negative organisms release endotoxin and endotoxin-associated proteins.

  2. Cytokines and leukocyte-derived inflammatory mediators give rise to systemic response, including tachycardia, fever, peripheral vasodilatation, hypotension, and decreased cardiac output.

  3. Host defenses can be suppressed by bacterial synergy, which inhibits complement activation and leukocyte migration.

III. DIAGNOSIS

A. The initial therapeutic goal should focus on resuscitation, diagnosis, and control of contamination.

B. History and physical examination are key to the diagnosis of intraabdominal sepsis in the ICU patient.

  1. Timing and evolution of symptoms—fever, localized abdominal pain/tenderness, hypotension

  2. Laboratory tests—leukocytosis, electrolyte abnormalities, increased liver, amylase

TABLE 115-1	Bacteria Commonly Encountered in Intraabdominal Infections	
Facultative gram-negative bacilli	**Obligate anaerobes**	**Facultative gram-positive cocci**
Escherichia coli	*Bacteroides fragilis*	Enterococci
Klebsiella species	*Bacteroides* species	*Staphylococcus* species
Proteus species	*Fusobacterium* species	*Streptococcus* species
Morganella morganii	*Clostridium* species	
Other enteric gram-negative bacilli	*Peptococcus* species	
Aerobic gram-negative bacilli	*Peptostreptococcus* species	
Pseudomonas aeruginosa	*Lactobacillus* species	

   C. Radiology
     1. Plain radiographs
        a. Perforation/pneumoperitoneum
        b. Bowel obstruction
        c. Pneumatosis cystoids intestinalis
        d. Pneumonia
        e. Portal venous air
     2. Ultrasound
        a. Noninvasive and can be done at bedside to localize extraluminal fluid collection
        b. Can be used for drainage
        c. Limited by body habitus, bowel gas, retroperitoneum
     3. CT
        a. Noninvasive identification of pathology not identified on physical examination, plain radiographs, or ultrasound
        b. Can be used to drain abscess

IV. TREATMENT
   A. Resuscitation
     1. Rapid volume expansion to counter vasodilatation should be done before surgical or radiologic intervention and should continue during radiologic diagnostic and therapeutic efforts are undertaken.
     2. Once patients have undergone intervention, resuscitation should be maximized, using pressors to increase cardiac output or high inspired oxygen concentrations to maintain adequate arterial oxygen saturation.
   B. Institution of appropriate antibiotics should be done as soon as diagnosis of intraabdominal sepsis is made to hasten the elimination of infecting microorganism, minimize the risk of recurrent intraabdominal infection, and shorten the clinical manifestations of infection.
     1. Appropriate coverage must anticipate pathogens most likely to be encountered at the site of infection.
     2. Initial empiric antibiotics should cover enteric gram-negative facultative and obligate anaerobic bacilli.
     3. Proximal small bowel has gram-positive aerobic and gram-negative anaerobic organisms that are generally susceptible to β-lactam antibiotics.
     4. Distal small bowel and colon perforations cause contamination with gram-negative facultative organisms and obligate anaerobes, which should be covered with broad-spectrum antibiotics. Carbapenems, cephalosporins, penicillins plus β-lactamase inhibitors, and quinolones.
     5. Reevaluation of antibiotic coverage is imperative after culture results are conclusive.

C. Percutaneous drainage can be used if there is no sign of diffuse peritonitis. Percutaneous drainage is preferable to open surgical intervention when feasible because of the initial deterioration that almost always occurs following operative manipulation of intraabdominal infection.
  1. Ultrasound guided: portable but has limitations
  2. Computed tomography (CT) guided: best modality for patients who are hemodynamically stable
D. Surgery is indicated if perforation or diffuse peritonitis exists. Operative management involves immediate evacuation of all purulent collections, débridement of necrotic tissue and control of source.
  1. Bowel resections should be done, with end colostomy if necessary.
  2. Primary closure of the wound is controversial and must take into consideration abdominal wall edema and aggressive resuscitation to avoid abdominal compartment syndrome.
  3. Second-look laparotomy may be necessary to achieve complete evacuation of infection. Fascial prostheses can be used for wound closure with planned relaparotomy and definitive closure of the abdomen once edema resolves.

V. SPECIFIC INFECTIONS
  A. Acute pancreatitis
  1. Infections superimposed on acute pancreatitis are among the most difficult intraabdominal infections to manage.
  2. When pancreatic necrosis exists, current surgical therapy consists of repetitive scheduled débridement at 48-hour intervals.
  3. A bilateral subcostal incision is used, lesser sac is entered, and blunt dissection is used to remove necrotic pancreas and loculated abscesses.
  4. Three or four reexplorations suffice to remove necrotic tissue, and patients should be monitored for recurrent infection.
  5. Localized fluid collection may be drained by percutaneous drainage. Pancreatic duct fistulas are common and may increase risk of recurrent pancreatic fluid collection.
  B. Biliary infections
  1. Ascending cholangitis is biliary obstruction with secondary bacterial infection that presents with Charcot triad of abdominal pain, fever, and jaundice.
    a. Ultrasound or CT diagnosis shows biliary ductal dilatation, wall thickening, pericholecystic fluid, and stones.
    b. Laboratory findings include hyperbilirubinemia, leukocytosis, elevated alkaline phosphatase.
    c. Treatment includes antibiotics, endoscopic retrograde cholangiopancreatography (ERCP)/percutaneous transhepatic cholangiography (PTC)
  2. Acute cholecystitis
    a. Acalculous cholecystitis is most common in ICU secondary to microvascular and mucosal dysfunction and presents as occult sepsis with or without right upper quadrant tenderness
    b. Ultrasound/CT shows wall thickening, pericholecystic fluid, sludge
    c. Treatment includes antibiotics and percutaneous cholecystostomy tube for high-risk patients who do not respond to antibiotic therapy.
  C. Intestinal ischemia
  1. Arterial or venous occlusion or low flow states are causative factors.
  2. Plain radiographs to evaluate for severe ischemia in form of pneumatosis, portal venous gas.
  3. Angiography to identify site and cause of ischemia.
  4. CT is useful to evaluate patients with less specific symptomatology and early changes such as bowel dilatation; transmural thickening with inflammatory changes in the perienteric fat can be seen. CT can also identify strangulation of closed-loop obstruction or perforation with abscess formation.

D. Postoperative intraabdominal infections
   1. Postoperative peritonitis generally due to anastomotic leak/dehiscence.
   2. It must be considered in patients with signs of sepsis who have undergone gastrointestinal anastamosis or who manifest diffuse abdominal tenderness.
   3. Ultrasound/CT will reveal fluid, which should lead to aspiration of fluid for diagnostic purposes.
   4. Surgical treatment should include resection with reanastamosis or end colostomy.
E. Enteric fistulas
   1. Small intestine is most common source, followed by colon, stomach, duodenum, biliary tract, and pancreas.
   2. Recognition of fistula is key to management because only 26% of fistulas were identified at the time of initial drainage.
   3. Fistulas can present as occult sepsis or sudden change in character or amount of drainage from wound.
   4. Fistulogram or other study must be performed to demonstrate and evaluate fistula.
   5. Management includes control by adequate drainage, skin protection, nutritional support, and formation of a mature tract formation and exclusion of downstream obstruction.
   6. Proximal diversion may be necessary for high output fistulas.

Selected Readings

Cerra FB. Multiple organ failure syndrome. *Dis Mon* 1992;26:816.
   Multiple-organ system failure as a result of intraabdominal sepsis.

Johnson WC, Gerzof SG, Robbins AH, et al. Treatment of abdominal abscesses: comparative evaluation of operative drainage versus percutaneous catheter drainage guided by computed tomography or ultrasound. *Ann Surg* 1981;194:510.
   Drainage methods and their efficacy.

Lee MI, Saini S, Brink JA. Treatment of critically ill patients with sepsis of unknown cause: value of percutaneous cholecystotomy. *Am J Surg* 1991; 156:1163.
   Management and treatment of acalculous cholecystitis.

Onderdonk AB, Bartlett JG, Louie T, et al. Microbial synergy in experimental intraabdominal abscess. *Infect Immunol* 1976;13:22.
   Discusses microbial synergy in intraabdominal infections.

Van Sonneneburg E, Wittich GR, Goodacre BW, et al. Percutaneous abscess drainage: update. *World J Surg* 2001;25:362.
   Discusses efficacy of percutaneous abscess drainage.

ACUTE PANCREATITIS

Olga Ivanov, Michael L. Steer, and Fred A. Luchette

116

I. DEFINITIONS

A. Clinically acute pancreatitis: process of rapid onset associated with pain and alterations in exocrine function

B. Clinically chronic pancreatitis: repeated episodes of pain associated with diminished exocrine function

C. Morphologically acute pancreatitis: occurs in a gland that was and will be functionally normal before and after the attack

D. Morphologically chronic pancreatitis: involves the pancreas that was morphologically or functionally abnormal before the attack and may remain abnormal after the attack

E. Pathologically acute pancreatitis

    1. Mild: associated with interstitial edema, intrapancreatic or peripancreatic acute necrosis

    2. Severe: associated with focal or diffuse acinar cell necrosis, thrombosis of intrapancreatic vessels, intraparenchymal hemorrhage, and abscess formation

F. Pathologically chronic pancreatitis: associated with scarring, fibrosis, and acinar tissue atrophy

II. ETIOLOGY

A. Biliary tract stone disease

    1. Along with ethanol abuse accounts for 60% to 80% of patients with acute pancreatitis

    2. Demographic distribution: affluent groups have more attacks due to stones, poorer patients due to ethanol abuse

    3. Three theories of gallstone pancreatitis

        a. "Common channel"—stones create a common biliopancreatic channel proximal to the stone-induced obstruction and allows bile to reflux into the pancreatic ducts, triggering pancreatitis

        b. "Duodenal reflux"—incompetent sphincter of Oddi due to the stone passage permits reflux of duodenal juice containing activated digestive enzymes into the pancreas

        c. "Pancreatic duct obstruction"—the only theory currently supported by clinical models—after duct obstruction lysosomal hydrolases activate digestive enzymes within pancreatic acinar cells, leading to their injury

B. Ethanol abuse

    1. Mean ethanol consumption is 150 to 175 g per day for 18 years for men and 11 years for women before the first attack

    2. Mechanism for acute or chronic pancreatitis is not clear

C. Drugs

    1. Most commonly seen in patients with acquired immunodeficiency syndrome (AIDS) receiving dideoxyinosine and pentamidine or transplant or inflammatory bowel disease (IBD) patients receiving azathioprine

    2. Historically, diuretics: thiazides, ethacrynic acid, and furosemide have high association with pancreatitis

    3. H_2-blockers and steroids are not currently believed to be capable of causing acute pancreatitis

  D. Pancreatic duct obstruction
   1. Tumors: duodenal, ampullary, biliary tract, or pancreatic
   2. Inflammatory lesions: peptic ulcer, duodenal Crohn disease, periampullary diverticulitis
   3. Pancreatic cysts, pseudocysts, and periampullary diverticula
   4. Ductal strictures
   5. Parasites: *Ascaris* and *Clonorchis*
  E. Miscellaneous causes of acute pancreatitis
   1. Traumatic
   2. Postoperative: duct exploration, sphincteroplasty, distal gastrectomy, endoscopic retrograde cholangiopancreatography (ERCP)
  F. Idiopathic pancreatitis
   1. Affects 5% to 10% of population
   2. Possible etiologies are: biliary sludge, familial (mutation on chromosome 7), non-classic cystic fibrosis mutations

III. CLINICAL PRESENTATION
  A. Symptoms: epigastric abdominal pain of rapid onset, nausea, vomiting that may result in Mallory-Weiss syndrome
  B. Physical examination
   1. Tachycardia, tachypnea, diaphoresis, hyperthermia, restlessness, and jaundice (20% incidence)
   2. Abdominal tenderness with voluntary and involuntary guarding, rebound, distention, epigastric mass, and diminished or absent bowel sounds
   3. Flank ecchymoses (Grey Turner sign) or other evidence of retroperitoneal bleeding (Cullen sign)

IV. DIAGNOSIS
  A. Routine blood tests
   1. Increased hemoglobin, hematocrit (HCT), blood urea nitrogen (BUN), creatinine, bilirubin, white blood cells, glucose, and triglycerides
   2. Decreased calcium, albumin
   3. In severe cases—thrombocytopenia, decreased fibrinogen levels, and prolonged prothrombin time and partial thromboplastin time
  B. Amylase
   1. May be normal in 10% of patients with lethal pancreatitis
   2. Levels increase 2 to 12 hours after attack onset, normalize after 3 to 6 days
  C. Other enzyme assays and blood tests: urine amylase and serum lipase may remain elevated for days after the attack
  D. Routine radiography
   1. Chest radiograph: left pleural effusion, basal atelectasis
   2. Plain frontal supine radiograph of the abdomen: pancreatic calcifications in chronic pancreatitis, ileus, retroperitoneal air if pancreatic abscess is formed
  E. Ultrasonography: detection of gallbladder stones or bile duct dilatation, or both
  F. Computed tomography (CT)
   1. Mild pancreatitis—normal or slightly swollen pancreas with streaking of retroperitoneal or transverse mesocolic fat
   2. Severe pancreatitis—peripancreatic or intrapancreatic fluid collections
   3. Dynamic CT—areas of pancreatic necrosis that fail to enhance with contrast administration
  G. Differential diagnosis
   1. Perforated hollow viscus
   2. Cholecystitis/cholangitis
   3. Bowel obstruction
   4. Mesenteric ischemia/infarction

V. PROGNOSIS

  A. Mild self-limited pancreatitis in 90% to 95% of patients
  B. Approximately 5% to 10% will have severe attack associated with 40% morbidity and mortality
  C. Ranson's prognostic signs
      1. On admission: age greater than 55 years; WBC greater than 16,000/mm^3; glucose greater than 200 mg/dL; lactate dehydrogenase (LDH) greater than 350 IU/L; glutamic-oxaloacetic transaminase (GOT) greater than 250 U/dL
      2. During initial 48 hours: HCT decrease more than 10%; BUN rise greater than 5 mg/dL; serum calcium less than 8 mg/dL; PaO$_2$ less than 60 mm Hg; base deficit greater than 4 mEq/L; fluid sequestration greater than 6 L
      3. Less than three criteria—mild pancreatitis—1% mortality
      4. Seven or eight criteria—severe pancreatitis—90% mortality
  D. APACHE-2—another useful system to evaluate severity of an attack
  E. Peripancreatic fluid collections on computed tomography (CT) scan
      1. Two or more fluid collections—61% incidence of late pancreatic abscess
      2. One fluid collection—12% to 17% incidence of pancreatic abscess
      3. Pancreatic enlargement only—zero incidence of pancreatic abscess

VI. TREATMENT OF ACUTE PANCREATITIS

  A. Initial management
      1. Sometimes impossible to establish diagnosis without exploratory laparotomy
      2. However, laparotomy may increase incidence of septic complications
  B. Treatment of pain. Demerol is the drug of choice; it relaxes the sphincter of Oddi, whereas morphine contracts it
  C. Fluid and electrolyte replacement
      1. Initially—hypochloremic alkalosis due to vomiting and decreased fluid intake
      2. Later—metabolic acidosis due to hypovolemia and poor tissue perfusion
      3. Hypomagnesemia and hypoalbuminemia due to preexisting malnutrition in chronic alcoholics
      4. Hypocalcemia may lead to tetany and carpopedal spasm.
      5. Hemodynamics in severe attacks resemble shock: increased heart rate, cardiac output, C.I., arterial-venous oxygen difference; decreased PVR; hypoxemia
  D. Other treatments
      1. Imipenem may be of benefit in patients with severe gallstone-induced pancreatitis.
      2. Fluconazole decreases the emergence of resistant fungi.
      3. Unclear value of nasogastric suction and agents that reduce pancreatic function, inhibit inflammatory or cytotoxic responses, or inhibit digestive enzymes
  E. Role of surgery and endoscopy in gallstone pancreatitis
      1. Mild pancreatitis—no early surgical or endoscopic intervention
      2. Severe gallstone pancreatitis—early surgical or endoscopic intervention warranted
      3. Recurrent attacks of gallstone pancreatitis should be prevented by cholecystectomy combined with surgical or endoscopic duct clearance.

VII. TREATMENT OF SYSTEMIC COMPLICATIONS

  A. Aggressive fluid and electrolyte therapy may be the most effective method of preventing pulmonary and renal failure.
  B. Pulmonary toilet and monitoring of pulmonary function with arterial blood gas measurements
  C. Prophylaxis with either antacids or H$_2$-blockers may prevent stress-induced bleeding of gastroduodenal lesions

VIII. LOCAL COMPLICATIONS OF PANCREATITIS

A. Definitions

1. Acute pancreatic and peripancreatic fluid collections. Occur early, in or near the pancreas, lack of wall.
2. Pancreatic necrosis. Either sterile or infected area of nonviable pancreatic tissue, diffuse or focal, associated with peripancreatic fat necrosis
3. Pancreatic pseudocyst
    a. Occurs 4 to 6 weeks after the attack, nonepithelialized wall of fibrous or granulation tissue enclosing a collection of pancreatic juice rich in digestive enzymes
    b. Leakage into peritoneal cavity or chest leads to pancreatic ascites or pancreatic-pleural fistula, respectively.
4. Pancreatic abscess. Circumscribed intraabdominal collection of pus close to the pancreas without necrosis

B. Diagnosis

1. Dynamic contrast-enhanced CT—identifies and quantitates areas of pancreatic necrosis or abscess based on extraintestinal gas, poor enhancement, or Gram stain of CT-guided fine-needle aspirate
2. ERCP—determines communication of fluid collections with the main pancreatic duct and/or localizes the point of duct rupture

C. Management

1. Acute fluid collections—resolve spontaneously, no treatment
2. Sterile pancreatic necrosis—mostly nonoperative management, unless clinical deterioration despite aggressive nonoperative treatment
3. Infected necrosis—aggressive and repeated surgical débridement and drainage and antibiosis; 100% mortality if untreated.
4. Pseudocysts—treat only if symptomatic, regardless of size, with internal surgical drainage (cystogastrostomy, cystoduodenostomy, Roux-en-Y cystojejunostomy), endoscopic drainage (cystogastrostomy, cystoduodenostomy), or percutaneous drainage with or without administration of somatostatin.
5. Pancreatic ascites or pancreatic-pleural fistula—bowel rest, total parental nutrition, somatostatin; most will require ERCP for identification of ductal disruption with subsequent distal pancreatectomy or Roux-en-Y pancreatojejunostomy
6. Pancreatic abscess—percutaneous or surgical drainage

Selected Readings

Fan ST, Lai ECS, Mok FPT, et al. Early treatment of acute biliary pancreatitis by endoscopic papillotomy. *N Engl J Med* 1993;328:228.
A prospective randomized trial of emergent ERCP versus conservative treatment and selective ERCP in patients with ampullary and common bile duct stones.

Kelly TR, Wagner DS. Gallstone pancreatitis: a prospective randomized trial of the timing of surgery. *Surgery* 1988;104:600.
An excellent randomized study of 165 patients and their outcomes based on early versus delayed surgical intervention for gallstone pancreatitis.

Kivisarri LZ, Somer K, Standertskjoold-Nordenstam C-G, et al. A new method for the diagnosis of acute hemorrhagic-necrotizing pancreatitis using contrast-enhanced CT. *Gastrointest Radiol* 1984;9:27.
A retrospective review of clinical outcomes of patients with pancreatitis with CT scans demonstrating low versus high enhancement values of pancreatic parenchyma.

Lambert JS, Seidlin M, Reichman RC, et al. 2'3'-Dideoxyinosine (ddI) in patients with the acquired immunodeficiency syndrome of AIDS-related complex. A phase I trial. *N Engl J Med* 1990;322:1333.
This article points toward ddI as a causative agent for pancreatitis.

Larvin M, McMahon MJ. APACHE-2 score for assessment and monitoring of acute pancreatitis. *Lancet* 1989;2:201.
A review of multiple scoring systems as successful predictors of outcome in patients with acute pancreatitis.

Ranson JHC, Balthazar E, Caccavale R, et al. Computed tomography and the prediction of pancreatic abscess in acute pancreatitis. *Ann Surg* 1985;201:656.
A retrospective review of 83 patients with acute pancreatitis demonstrating relationship of early CT findings to late pancreatic sepsis.

Ranson JHC, Lackner H. Coagulopathies. In Bradley EL, ed. *Complications of pancreatitis.* Philadelphia: WB Saunders, 1982, p. 154.

Ranson JHC. Prognostication in acute pancreatitis. In Glazer G, Ranson JHC, eds. *Acute pancreatitis.* London: Bailliere Tindall, 1988, p. 303.

Sarles H. Chronic pancreatitis: etiology and pathophysiology. In Go VLW, Gardner JD, Brooks EP, et al, eds. *The exocrine pancreas: biology, pathology, and diseases.* New York: Raven Press, 1986, p. 37.

Sarner M, Cotton PB. Classification of pancreatitis. *Gut* 1984;25:756.
Review of definitions for the updated classification of pancreatitis.

Steer ML. Etiology and pathophysiology of acute pancreatitis. In Go VLW, Gardner JD, Brooks EP, et al., eds. *The exocrine pancreas: biology, pathobiology, and diseases.* New York: Raven Press, 1986, p. 465.

Steer ML. The early intraacinar cell events which occur during acute pancreatitis. The Frank Brooks Memorial Lecture. *Pancreas* 1998;17:31.

117 MESENTERIC ISCHEMIA
Jateen Patel, Peter E. Rice, and Fred A. Luchette

I. GENERAL PRINCIPLES
  A. Circulation-insufficiency event that can occur suddenly or over a few weeks.
  B. Gut is essentially deprived of oxygen and blood, leading to acidosis, metabolic derangement, and tissue death and ultimately causing multisystem organ failure.
  C. Mortality ranges from 60% to 100%, depending on the source of occlusion.
  D. Risk factors include advanced age, atherosclerosis, and severe cardiovascular disease.
  E. The majority of events are occlusive; 20% to 30% of acute mesenteric ischemia is from nonocclusive events.
  F. Classically see pain out of proportion to examination, although this may not be seen when the patient is sedated or septic.

II. ETIOLOGY
  A. Embolism is seen in 50% of acute mesenteric ischemia, thrombosis in 25%, and venous thrombosis is the cause in 5% to 15% of cases. Nonocclusive mesenteric ischemia is seen in less than 5% of cases.
  B. The superior mesenteric artery is the source in almost all cases of occlusive disease, although usually the individual has underlying disease of the celiac or inferior mesenteric arteries.
  C. Emboli are typically found 3 to 8 cm from the origin of the superior mesenteric artery (SMA) (usually at or before a bifurcation or the takeoff of the middle colic artery). Of patients with emboli, typically 25% to 40% have a history of embolism.
  D. Thrombosis usually develops at the origin of vessels or areas of concurrent atherosclerotic stenoses.
  E. Acute venous thrombosis occurs spontaneously or as a consequence of an underlying condition (Table 117-1).
  F. Nonocclusive mesenteric ischemia is caused by a low-flow state in the vascular bed. It is usually an exacerbation in a critically ill patient with persistent vasoconstriction, vasospasm, and intestinal hypoxia.

III. PATHOPHYSIOLOGY
  A. Due to excellent collateral circulation of the gut, patients can have either single main artery occlusion or several stenoses in smaller vessels and rarely present with acute mesenteric ischemia at normotensive pressures.
  B. Reduced blood flow in a stenotic bed can produce bowel ischemia and subsequent infarction.
  C. Prolonged ischemia time can lead to bowel necrosis complicated by perforation, sepsis, and death from multisystem organ failure (MSOF).
  D. Occlusive ischemia usually results from emboli or thrombosis.
    1. Emboli usually arise from cardiac sources
      a. Atrial fibrillation
      b. Valvular disease
      c. Myocardial infarction
      d. Cardiomyopathy
    2. Thrombosis is usually associated with a systemic abnormality (e.g., diabetes, hypercoagulable state)
  E. Nonocclusive ischemia occurs from changes on a more microvascular level. Hence, these patients may demonstrate normal pulses in the major mesenteric vessels.

TABLE 117-1	Causes of Acute Mesenteric Ischemia

Venous obstruction
1. Hypercoagulable state: cancer, infection, splenomegaly, cirrhosis, trauma, diverticular disease
2. Portal hypertension, Budd-Chiari syndrome
3. Congestive heart failure, shock

Arterial obstruction
1. Dissection or trauma
2. Compression of the superior mesenteric artery by the median arcuate ligament or adhesive bands
3. Cancer: sigmoid colon, carcinoid, or tumor embolus
4. Medications: birth control pills, diuretics, cocaine, pseudoephedrine
5. Connective tissue disorders
6. Disseminated intravascular coagulation
7. Crohn disease
8. Atrial fibrillation, recent myocardial infarction, cardiopulmonary bypass
9. Vasculitis
10. Diabetes mellitus

1. Severe cardiac failure or dysfunction can lead to vasospasm of mesenteric vessels as a result of excess catecholamine release and a state of increased sympathetic tone.
2. Many medications (e.g., β-blockers, α-adrenergic agents, digitalis) or inflammatory mediators of sepsis, shock can lead to similar vasoconstriction of the mesenteric vasculature.
3. Ischemia is usually subclinical, but mortality can approach 70% in severe cases.
F. In general, acute mesenteric ischemia causes hypoxia and reduced blood flow to the bowel.
   1. Acidosis results from lactate metabolism.
   2. Reperfusion injury can occur from the release of accumulated toxins and inflammatory mediators.
   3. Sepsis and MSOF result from systemic effects of cytokines and inflammatory mediators.

IV. DIAGNOSIS
   A. Clinical presentation
      1. Patients classically complain of pain out of proportion to examination.
      2. Vomiting and/or defecating (suggestive of intestinal emptying)
      3. Examination demonstrates tenderness and/or hypoactive bowel sounds; distention seen later. Hard clinical signs usually occur with progression of the disease into infarction.
      4. Early diagnosis is key to facilitate early revascularization. High index of suspicion in cardiac patients and critically ill patients with sepsis, trauma, burns.
   B. Laboratory
      1. Electrolyte derangements from dehydration and acidosis often seen at much later stages of infarction.
      2. Elevated serum lactate; may see elevated liver enzymes from hepatic necrosis.
   C. Imaging
      1. Plain radiographs. Useful for demonstrating sequelae of bowel infarction: free air, pneumatosis intestinalis
      2. Duplex ultrasound. Elevated peak systolic velocity (PSV) at the superior mesenteric artery (SMA) and celiac arteries (CA) has been correlated with a greater than 50% stenosis of these vessels.

3. Computed tomography
4. Angiography
    a. Gold standard
    b. Time-consuming and too expensive for screening; most utility is with a high clinical suspicion.

V. TREATMENT
A. SMA embolism
    1. Arteriotomy with embolectomy, sometimes patch angioplasty required for larger explorations
    2. Bowel resection usually required with infarction, second-look procedure within 48 hours can be performed to reassess bowel viability.
    3. Endovascular approaches are usually reserved for high-risk patients in the elective setting.
B. SMA thrombosis
    1. Antegrade (proximal aortic inflow) or retrograde (iliac artery inflow) reconstructions with either native vein or prosthetic grafts.
    2. Thrombolytics rarely employed but can be an option if no evidence of bowel compromise.
C. Mesenteric venous thrombosis
    1. Anticoagulation is the mainstay.
    2. Surgery for complications (e.g., intestinal infarction).

Selected Readings

Kazmers A. Operative management of chronic mesenteric ischemia. *Ann Vasc Surg* 1998; 12:299–308.
An overview of the management of mesenteric ischemia.

Mansour MA. Management of acute mesenteric ischemia. *Arch Surg* 1999;134(3):328–330.
A great and quick review of the topic.

Nicoloff AD, Williamson WK, Moneta GL, et al. Duplex ultrasonography in evaluation of splanchnic artery stenosis. *Surg Clin North Am* 1997;77:339–355.
Analyzes the use of noninvasive testing in cases of mesenteric ischemia.

COMPARTMENT SYNDROME OF THE ABDOMINAL CAVITY

Gerard J. Abood, Dietmar H. Wittmann, and Fred A. Luchette

118

I. GENERAL PRINCIPLES

A. Overview

   1. Abdominal cavity considered single compartment enclosed by apeuronotic envelope with limited compliance.

   2. Elevated intraabdominal pressure (IAP) can impair blood flow and normal organ function.

   3. Once critical threshold volume reached, small increments in tissue volume lead to exponential increases in intraperitoneal pressure. May result in multiorgan failure and death if not reversed promptly.

B. Definitions

   1. Compartment syndrome: increased pressure in confined anatomic space that adversely affects function and viability of tissue within compartment.

   2. Abdominal compartment syndrome (ACS): sustained increased pressure within abdominal wall, pelvis, diaphragm, and retroperitoneum adversely affecting function of organs and tissue within and adjacent to abdominal cavity. Usually requires operative decompression

   3. Abdominal hypertension (AH): sustained (greater than 6 hours) increase in IAP that may or may not require operative decompression.

     a. Normal abdominal pressure: 10 mm Hg

     b. Mild AH: 10 to 20 mm Hg; usually not clinically significant.

     c. Moderate AH: 21 to 35 mm Hg; operative intervention may be required.

     d. Severe AH: sustained pressures greater than 35 mm Hg; operative decompression always warranted.

II. PATHOPHYSIOLOGY

A. Causes. Most abdominal hypertension caused by peritoneal, mesenteric, or retroperitoneal edema impinging on fascial envelope of abdominal compartment

   1. Total surface area of peritoneum is 1.8 m², which is approximately equal to entire surface area of skin. Theoretically, 1 mL of peritoneal thickening may contain 15 to 18 liters of fluid.

   2. Expanding edema can quickly exceed compensatory elasticity of abdominal fascia and diaphragm and lead to compromise.

B. Table 118-1 lists variety of causes of IAP.

III. DIAGNOSIS

A. Clinical presentation

   1. Patients typically present with tense abdominal wall, shallow respirations, low urinary output, and increased central venous pressure.

   2. Ventilated patients have increased airway pressures.

   3. Physiologic impairments in all systems observed.

     a. Cardiac output initially rises as result of increased venous return from intraabdominal veins but diminishes as pressure rises above 10 mm Hg.

       (1) Decreased preload result of pooling in lower extremities and functional narrowing of vena cava.

       (2) Afterload increased and ventricular function decreased as cardiac compliance and filling pressures negatively affected by increased IAP

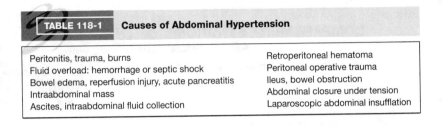

TABLE 118-1	Causes of Abdominal Hypertension
Peritonitis, trauma, burns	Retroperitoneal hematoma
Fluid overload: hemorrhage or septic shock	Peritoneal operative trauma
Bowel edema, reperfusion injury, acute pancreatitis	Ileus, bowel obstruction
Intraabdominal mass	Abdominal closure under tension
Ascites, intraabdominal fluid collection	Laparoscopic abdominal insufflation

    b. Pulmonary: decrease in diaphragmatic excursion resulting in atelectasis, pneumonia, and ventilation-perfusion mismatch. Positive end-expiratory ventilation to maintain alveolar patency worsens intrathoracic pressure and cardiac output.

    c. Renal: impaired as result of decreased cardiac output, compression of both renal inflow and outflow, and direct compression of kidney parenchyma; development of "renal compartment syndrome."

    d. Hepatic: reduction in blood flow affecting production of acute-phase proteins, immunoglobulin, and factors of the other host defense system.

    e. GI: splanchnic hypoperfusion possibly affecting mucosal pH, bacterial translocation, bowel motility.

B. Measurement of intraabdominal pressure

    1. Direct method: intraperitoneal catheter connected to a pressure transducer to take direct measurements. Preferred method for most experimental studies.

    2. Indirect method: less invasive, rely on pressure transduction to inferior vena cava, stomach, or, most commonly, the bladder. Transvesical technique: bladder behaves as passive diaphragm when volume is between 50 and 100 mL; abdominal pressure can be measured transvesically.

        a. Instill 50 to 100 mL of sterile saline into empty bladder through Foley catheter. Tubing drain clamped and 16-gauge needle advanced through aspiration port and connected to pressure transducer or manometer.

        b. Recordings correlated with direct measurements in range of 5 to 70 mm Hg.

IV. TREATMENT

A. Decompression

    1. Nonoperative decompression reserved for distention caused by ascites.

    2. Operative decompression: opening abdominal cavity in operating room or intensive care unit once intravascular fluid deficits, temperature, and coagulation abnormalities are corrected.

        a. Postdecompression compensation has been reported: systemic vascular resistance falls markedly after decompression, surpassing the increase in cardiac output.

        b. Careful monitoring, volume resuscitation prior to decompression, and judicious use of vasoconstrictors postoperatively may be of most benefit.

B. Closure

    1. Abdomen can be reapproximated by variety of methods.

    2. Type of closure dependent on degree of decompression; abdomen can be reclosed when fascia can be reapproximated without undue tension.

        a. Leaving fascia open and closing only skin with sutures or towel clips to protect bulging viscera has been recommended; moist dressings should be applied to prevent both wound desiccation and bacterial proliferation.

        b. Synthetic fascial materials that are sutured to the fascial edges, which can be approximated slowly, offer another reliable option; all meshes help to decompress the abdomen.

Selected Readings

Burch JM, Moore EE, Moore FA, et al. The abdominal compartment syndrome [review]. *Surg Clin North Am* 1996;76:833.
Concise review of the abdominal compartment syndrome.

Kron IL, Harman PK, Nolan AP. The measurement of intraabdominal pressure as a criteria for abdominal re-exploration. *Ann Surg* 1984;199:28.
One of the first articles to advocate intervention for intraabdominal pressure above 25 mm Hg.

Smith PC, Tweddell JS, Bessey PQ. Alternative approaches to abdominal wound closure in severely injured patients with massive visceral edema. *J Trauma* 1992;32:16.
Review of alternative approaches to interim closure.

Wittmann, DH, Aprahamian C, Bergstein JM. A burr-like device to facilitate temporary abdominal closure in planned multiple laparotomies. *Eur J Surg* 1993;159:75.
A practical technique for temporary closure of the abdominal wound.

119

NECROTIZING FASCIITIS AND OTHER SOFT TISSUE INFECTIONS

Julie L. Barone, David H. Ahrenholz, and Fred A. Luchette

I. OVERVIEW

A. General principles

1. Skin provides a barrier to infection; therefore, any break in skin allows bacteria to invade.
2. Risk factors for infection include trauma, edema, hematoma, ischemia, foreign body.
3. Virulent infections occur when host defenses are weak (i.e., diabetes, cancer, malnutrition, immunosuppression, advanced age, major trauma).

B. Pathophysiology

1. Group A β-hemolytic *Streptococcus pyogenes*: highly virulent; cellulitis; erysipelas with demarcated borders; ecthema contagiosum; streptococcal lymphangitis; seen in necrotizing fasciitis; exotoxins result in cytokine release causing hypovolemia (toxic shock syndrome)
2. *Staphylococcus aureus*: most common cause of skin infections; purulence; folliculitis (dermis); superficial abscess (soft tissue); carbuncle (burrowing infection); pyomyositis (hematogenous spread to intramuscular hematoma); seen in necrotizing fasciitis
3. *Clostridium perfringens*, *C. novyi*, and *C. septicum*: gram-positive, spore-forming obligate anaerobes; most common in ischemic muscle; exotoxins cause myonecrosis and sepsis
4. *Eikenella corrodens*: human bite wounds; treat with cephalosporins or penicillin
5. *Pasteurella multocida*: animal bite or scratches; treat with cephalosporins, penicillin, or tetracycline
6. *Vibrio vulnificus*: aggressive disease; seen in alcoholics; due to immunologic defect
7. *Escherichia coli, Klebsiella*: abscesses of perineal area; usually arising from infected pilonidal cyst, break in rectal mucosa causing a perirectal abscess

II. CELLULITIS AND SUBCUTANEOUS INFECTIONS

A. Etiology

1. Most common organisms: *S. aureus* and group A streptococci causing a cutaneous diffuse infection; nonpyogenic; starts with a minor break in skin, such as insect bite, puncture limited to skin and subcutaneous tissue; spread of infection through tissue facilitated by toxins and enzymes
2. In the extremity; presents with lymphadenitis or lymphangitis
3. High-risk cellulitis if involving face or extremities of immunocompromised patients
4. Folliculitis: nontoxic pyodermas centered in hair follicles
5. Subcutaneous abscess (complicated cellulitis): most common soft tissue infection
6. *Hydradenitis suppurativa*: chronic burrowing infection of groin or axilla; involving infected hair follicles; more commonly seen in diabetic or very obese patients

B. Diagnosis

1. Presents with progressive erythema and edema; may cause tenderness over the involved area
2. Low diagnostic yield on culturing tissue or aspirate

C. Treatment
   1. Uncomplicated cellulitis: treat with antibiotics and elevation; surgery not indicated unless joints or tendon sheaths involved
   2. Complicated cellulitis: treat with incision and drainage; if poorly localized infection, antibiotics are indicated

III. NECROTIZING FASCIITIS
   A. Definition
   1. A severe and progressive infection that spreads rapidly along fascia planes with minimal cutaneous signs
   2. Typically occurs after trauma or surgery in compromised patients (i.e., those with peripheral vascular disease, diabetes, or malignancy)
   3. Fournier's gangrene: rapidly spreading scrotal skin infection
   4. Requires prompt surgical débridement and parenteral antibiotics; if not treated aggressively can result in death

   B. Etiology
   1. β-Hemolytic streptococcus (90%), anaerobic gram-positive cocci, aerobic gram-negative bacilli and bacteriodes; often a combination of bacteria; most commonly occurs in immunocompromised patients or those who have atherosclerotic vascular disease, diabetes, or malignancy; begins at site of minor wound or contaminated abdominal wounds after primary closure; enteric organisms common in perineum
   2. Hematogenous seeding of contusion after blunt trauma
   3. Varicella infection in children can be complicated by streptococcal skin infection leading to necrotizing fasciitis

   C. Diagnosis
   1. Pain, edema, fever, leukocytosis with a left shift
   2. Erythema and dermal necrosis rare
   3. Streptococcocal necrotizing fasciitis: typical symptoms plus tachycardia, localized erythema, edema, and watery drainage; positive blood cultures; blistering of skin, which turns dusky after cutaneous vascular thrombosis
   4. Gold standard: surgical exploration; plain radiographs/computed tomography (CT) scan may show gas/fluid but can be misleading because may show only tissue edema

   D. Treatment
   1. Surgical débridement after fluid resuscitation; preoperative antibiotics to cover facultative and anaerobic organisms (cefoxitin, cefotetan, ampicillin/sulbactam, ticaricillin/clavulanate, piperacillin/tazobactam, imipenem/cilastatin)
   2. Intraoperative cultures to determine postoperative course of antibiotics
   3. Pack wound with antiseptic-soaked gauze after débriding viable tissue
   4. Wound can then heal by secondary intention or be skin grafted
   5. Amputation of extremity is sometimes necessary to control spreading infection
   6. Intravenous immunoglobulins for streptococcal toxic shock syndrome
   7. Diverting colostomy to reduce perineal soiling, but is not mandatory
   8. Aggressive nutritional support: treat similarly to patient with a burn 1.5 × BME
   9. Whirlpool débridement with daily dressing changes; vacuum-assisted closure on clean tissue to promote wound granulation

   E. Complications
   1. Delayed diagnosis or incomplete débridement resulting in profound sepsis
   2. Intraabdominal sepsis following postoperative necrotizing fasciitis
   3. Overall mortality 38%; worse prognosis with increasing age, female, delay in first débridement; elevated serum lactate level, organ failure

IV. NONCLOSTRIDIAL MYONECROSIS
   A. Etiology: same as necrotizing fasciitis; rarely *Aeromonas hydrophila* or *Bacillus cereus*
   B. Diagnosis: presents similarly to patient with necrotizing fasciitis; radiographs show gas outlining muscles; débridement reveals muscle and fascia necrosis; differs from clostridial myonecrosis as mixed organism on Gram stain and fewer systemic effects

   C. Treatment: Excision of all necrotic tissue including muscle, fascia, and skin
   D. Complications: mortality 76%; worse prognosis, same factors as for necrotizing fasciitis

V. CLOSTRIDIAL MYONECROSIS
A. Definition
   1. Necrotizing muscle infection often with *Clostridium perfringens* exotoxins; requires débridement and sometimes amputation
   2. Gas gangrene: term for clostridial myonecrosis; gas also seen in clostridial abscess and nonclostridial myonecrosis
B. Etiology
   1. Associated with war injuries, farm machinery accidents, or any deep tissue wounds exposed to soil organisms
   2. Also surgical manipulation, irrigation with pressure devices, injection of air, and disruption of the esophagus or trachea
   3. Occurs when wound is inadequately débrided; inoculation into surgical wounds after gastrointestinal or biliary tract surgery; *C. perfringens* most common toxin
C. Diagnosis
   1. Severe systemic toxicity; mental status changes, woody edema, gram-positive rods; cardiovascular collapse secondary to exotoxins
   2. Dermal necrosis: ischemic dermal necrosis (dry gangrene); ulcerating skin lesions (Meleney cutaneous gangrene); also seen in disseminated intravascular coagulation after septicemia (purpura fulminans), streptococcal necrotizing fasciitis
D. Treatment.
Surgical emergency; wide débridement of nonviable fascia and muscle; leave wounds packed open; penicillin G 12 to 20 million units per day or clindamycin; hyperbaric oxygen for suppressing toxin formation; amputation if necessary
E. Complications:
with hyperbaric oxygen treatment, 22% to 25%; worse if hematuria present

Selected Readings
Ahrenholz DH. Necrotizing soft tissue infections. *Surg Clin North Am* 1982;68:199.
   A comprehensive review of the diagnosis and treatment of soft tissue infections.

Eke N. Fournier's gangrene: a review of 1726 cases. *Br J Surg* 2000;87:718.
   A review of necrotizing fasciitis of the perineum.

Elliot DC, Kufera JA, Meyers RA. Necrotizing soft tissue infections. Risk factors for mortality and strategies for management. *Ann Surg* 1996;224:672.
   A review of management and outcome of various soft tissue infections.

Lewis RT. Soft tissue infections. *World J Surg* 1998;22:146–151.
   A review article that classifies soft tissue infections by their degree of localization.

Urschel JD. Necrotizing soft tissue infections. *Postgrad Med J* 1999;75:645–649.
   A review of common treatment principles for necrotizing fasciitis.

120

PRESSURE SORES: PREVENTION AND TREATMENT

Kara Criswell, John Kitzmiller, and Fred A. Luchette

I. EPIDEMIOLOGY
   A. In an acute care setting, pressure sores account for 3% to 11% of admissions.
   B. Residents in chronic care facilities are the group at highest risk for the development of pressure sores.
   C. Patients with spinal cord injury and patients in the intensive care unit often have multiple risk factors for the development of this problem.

II. PATHOPHYSIOLOGY
   A. Pressure sores form as the end result of unrelieved pressure exerted on tissue over bony prominences.
   B. Normal arterial capillary blood pressure closes at 32 mm Hg and weight-bearing prominences (sacrum, buttocks, heels, and occiput) are subject to this critical pressure while a patient is in the supine position.
   C. Prolonged exposure to ischemia results in tissue necrosis; however, differing tissues exhibit different sensitivities to ischemia.
      1. Muscle has much poorer tolerance to pressure than does skin or subcutaneous tissue.
      2. Muscle and subcutaneous tissue infarction without skin necrosis is the "tip of the iceberg" phenomenon.
      3. Studies have shown that ischemic necrosis can be prevented with intermittent restoration of blood flow.
      4. Complicating the ischemic skin breakdown in critically ill patients are other factors such as malnutrition, hypotension, impaired mobility and sensation, and fecal or urinary incontinence.

III. PREVENTION. Prevention of pressure sores begins with education and dedicated care.
   A. The tenets of prevention include pressure reduction over bony prominences, alteration of weight-bearing surfaces, good skin hygiene, and adequate nutrition.
   B. Pressure dispersion techniques include foam mattress, air mattress, low air loss beds, air-fluidized beds, and oscillating support surfaces.
   C. Patients with acute traumatic injuries and a decreased level of consciousness should be removed from backboards and cervical collars as soon as safely possible.

IV. WOUND CLASSIFICATION
   A. Grade 1: Nonblanchable erythema of the skin with the lesion being limited to the epidermis and dermis
   B. Grade 2: Full-thickness ulceration of the skin extending through to the subcutaneous adipose tissue
   C. Grade 3: Ulceration extending to the underlying muscle
   D. Grade 4: Ulceration extending through muscle and involving bone

V. WOUND MANAGEMENT
   A. Management strategies entail identification, débridement, wound dressings, pressure dispersion, and maximization of overall health status
      1. Most grade 1 and 2 ulcers respond well to these measures.
      2. For grade 3 and 4 ulcers, wet to moist dressings are initially recommended to provide optimal wound environment for healing.

3. An occlusive hydrocolloid dressing can be used as an alternative in a well-débrided wound with minimal dead space.
4. Deeper ulcers also respond better if air-fluidized pressure dispersion is used.

B. With appropriate care, up to 80% of pressure sores heal without surgery.
C. Operative treatment is reserved for patients whose wounds have plateaued in healing despite maximal conservative (including nutritional) therapy.
1. Surgery is almost never necessary for the ambulatory patient.
2. At operation, all devitalized tissue is removed and bony prominences reduced.
3. A variety of muscular advancement flaps are used, depending on the wound location.
4. Care is taken to avoid hematoma formation and tension on the closure.

D. Postoperatively, it is critical to avoid compression on the flap vascular pedicle and to minimize tension or shearing forces.
1. A special air or fluid mattress is important for the first 3 weeks.
2. Gradually, a program of weight bearing is used for the following 6 to 8 weeks.
3. The greatest challenge is to minimize future risks of pressure sore development.

Selected Readings

Dansereau JG, Conway H. Closure of decubitus in paraplegics. *Plast Reconstr Surg* 1964;33:474.
   An early article with sound principles that still apply.

Inman KJ, Sibbald WJ, Rutledge FS, et al. Clinical utility and cost-effectiveness of an air suspension bed in the prevention of pressure ulcers. *JAMA* 1993;269:1139.
   Provides a solid argument for the cost-effectiveness of air mattress technology.

National Pressure Ulcer Advisory Panel. *Pressure ulcer treatment: clinical practice guideline.* Bethesda, MD: U.S. Department of Health and Human Services, 1994:15.
   The government's approach to pressure ulcer management with useful statistics.

PAIN MANAGEMENT IN THE CRITICALLY ILL

Paul Schalch, Donald S. Stevens, and Fred A. Luchette

121

I. OVERVIEW. Pain is a major problem for critically ill patients. Effectiveness of analgesia is related to correct usage of drugs, rather than to their analgesic properties. Fears of depressing spontaneous ventilation, inducing opioid dependence, and precipitating cardiovascular instability are frequent causes for inadequate relief of pain. Appropriate pain resolution facilitates recovery. The clinician should not judge the appropriateness of pain, because it is a subjective phenomenon.

II. GENERAL PRINCIPLES. Successful management of pain is based on:
   A. Identifying the correct etiology of pain, and determining a baseline before starting treatment.
   B. Understanding other components such as anxiety, ethnocultural factors, situational meaning, prior experience.
   C. Establishing and maintaining drug levels at active sites for appropriate analgesia and anxiolysis and determining the end point of treatment so as to know when to stop management.
   D. Understanding that therapy is an iterative process in which measurements are made, therapeutic actions are taken, effectiveness is reevaluated, and the action is repeated until the desired clinical outcome is reached.

III. DEFINITIONS AND PATHOGENESIS
   A. *Pain* is an unpleasant sensory and emotional experience that can be associated with actual or potential tissue damage. *Pain-related behavior* is the only manifestation that can make the observer conclude that pain is being experienced. *Acute pain* has an identifiable temporal and causal relationship to an injury, in contrast to *chronic pain,* which persists beyond the healing process and that may not have an identifiable cause. *Nociception* is the detection and signaling of the presence of a noxious stimulus.
   B. Acute pain begins with damage to skin and/or deeper tissues. Locally produced and released algogens (prostaglandins, small peptides) sensitize or stimulate peripheral nociceptors, whose fibers propagate the signal into the dorsal horn of the spinal cord or the sensory nuclei in the brainstem. Before reaching pain-specific areas in deep brain structures or cortex, the signal is modulated (amplified or attenuated), which can increase or decrease the response to painful stimuli. These responses are either beneficial (e.g., withdrawal from noxious stimulus) or deleterious (e.g., sympathetic discharge that increases oxygen consumption from elevated muscle tone or spasm and tachycardia and increased cardiac work). Reflex hypothalamic stimulation leads to increased release of catabolic stress hormones and decreased anabolism, which may prolong or worsen the postsurgical catabolic state.

IV. DIAGNOSIS
   A. Location: it should be determined whether the location is appropriate with the type of injury sustained or the surgery performed or whether it is entirely different. Look for unrecognized sources of pain, such as missing injuries. Pain can be neuropathic in nature, or it might be chronic or to the result of malpositioning during surgery.
   B. Intensity: visual or verbal analogue scales aid the patient in quantifying her or his own pain, thus providing a baseline for the evaluation of the response to treat-

ment. In patients who are unable to communicate (e.g., are intubated), markers of sympathetic activity such as restlessness, sweating, tachycardia, lacrimation, pupillary dilation, and hypertension can be graded as signs of pain intensity.

C. Quality of sensation: pain can be sharp if it is due to direct nociception (e.g., incision), dull or aching if it arises from deeper structures, or pulling or tugging in nature if it is related to the presence of sutures or visceral stimulation. Pain manifested as tingling, stinging, or buzzing sensations is usually related to abnormal neural function, secondary to either recovery from regional anesthesia or reestablishment of neural function after neural compression. Painful dysesthesias occur in conjunction with peripheral neuropathy.

V. TREATMENT. Different techniques can be used to interfere at various levels of the pain pathway.

A. Periphery: nonsteroidal antiinflammatory drugs (NSAIDs), local anesthetic infiltration, peripheral nerve blockade. NSAIDs interfere with the production of prostaglandins, which produce hyperalgesia and induce an inflammatory response. Ketorolac is the only intravenous (IV) NSAID available in the United States. It has been shown to provide additional analgesia when used in conjunction with opioid analgesics, without compromising respiratory drive. Side effects of ketorolac include nausea, peptic ulceration, and inhibition of platelet function. Severe bronchospasm can occur in patients with asthma, nasal polyposis, and allergy to NSAIDs. Ketorolac is contraindicated in acute or chronic renal failure and in the presence of hypovolemia. It should not be given for more than 5 days, and the renal function should always be monitored. Local infiltration with anesthetics is useful in the management of postoperative pain. Studies show that the analgesic effect persists for at least 48 hours. This prolonged effect is termed *preemptive analgesia*, and it was shown to be superior to spinal or general anesthesia in the control of postoperative pain after hernia repair. Repeated intermittent intercostal nerve blocks have been used to provide analgesia for thoracic injuries and surgery. Nerve blocks provide analgesia without sedation or respiratory depression. The need for repeated injections, the risk for pneumothorax, and the risk for systemic toxicity are disadvantages of this procedure. Paravertebral nerve blockade provides analgesia over several dermatomes by bathing several intercostal nerves with anesthetic, either with a single injection or by continuous infusion through a catheter. Intrapleural analgesia with bupivacaine is useful for analgesia in the thorax and upper abdomen. Unfortunately, this technique loses effectiveness in the presence of a thoracostomy tube (anesthetic is drained out of the pleural space) or if the pain is bilateral (increased absorption and toxicity and bilateral sympathetic blockade). Contraindications to this technique include fibrosis of the pleura, inflammation/infection with or without blood or fluid in the pleural space, and anticoagulation or infection at the site of injection. Other regional blocks include brachial plexus blocks and femoral nerve or lumbar plexus blocks for the upper and lower extremities.

B. Spinal cord (first integration): epidural and intrathecal infusions of local anesthetics or opioids, transcutaneous electrical nerve stimulation (TENS). By means of high-frequency (80 to 100 Hz), low-intensity stimulation through sterile skin electrodes, and in combination with other methods of analgesia, TENS downmodulates the afferent nociceptive signal at the spinal cord and brainstem levels, thereby controlling postoperative (periincisional) pain. It is associated with reduced rates of complications (nausea, vomiting, atelectasis, ileus). Afferent conduction can be blocked at the nerve root or spinal cord level with local anesthetics, and nociceptive signals can be downmodulated centrally by intraspinal opioids acting on specific opioid receptors in the dorsal horn. Regional analgesia techniques include subarachnoid and epidural administration of local anesthetics, opioids, or mixtures thereof, with intermittent dosing or continuous infusion. Continuous subarachnoid analgesia with local anesthetics is used to manage postoperative pain. However, it requires continuous monitoring at bedside because of the potential for profound sympathectomy and hemodynamic instability. It has been associated with central nervous system infection, but current techniques are safe for at least 48 hours. Continuous epidural infusion of local anesthetics allows for prolonged analgesia, frequently associated, however, with hypotension due to sympathetic blockade. This side effect can usually be managed with intravascular volume expansion or small doses of an α-adrenergic agent. The opioid most commonly used for epidural blockade is morphine, which, because of its low lipid solubility, tends to stay dissolved in the cerebrospinal fluid. Systemic absorption and rostral spread after administration may be responsible for side effects such as nausea, pruritus, urinary retention, and early (1 hour after administration) or late respiratory depression (6 to 12 hours), which is usually preceded by progressive sedation rather than decreased respiratory rate. Naloxone is used in divided doses to treat significant respiratory depression. Epidural catheters usually remain in place for 2 to 3 days, at which time patients can take oral pain medications. They can, however, be left in place indefinitely as long as there are no signs of infection or inflammation. Newer approaches recommend the use of combinations of local anesthetics with opioids for continuous epidural infusion because of fewer side effects and increased effectiveness in postoperative pain management.

C. Higher orders of integration throughout the nervous system: systemic opioids by depot injections (intramuscular [IM] or subcutaneous [SC]), transdermal delivery systems, bolus or continuous IV infusions, or patient-controlled analgesia (PCA). Inhaled anesthetic agents have a limited role in critically ill patients because of complications resulting from prolonged exposure, such as toxicity and bone marrow suppression. They are useful only during short, painful procedures such as dressing changes in burn patients. Sedatives such as benzodiazepines, barbiturates, phenothiazines, and butyrophenones are given in conjunction with opioids and are used for anxiolysis, sedation, and production of amnesia. These medications have the potential for depressing consciousness and respiratory effort. They are useful in patients who need prolonged mechanical ventilation and in patients who require sedation for the first 24 to 48 hours postoperatively. Systemic opioid analgesia is usually given via IM or SQ injections. It, however, has limited use in intensive care unit (ICU) patients due to extreme delay in attaining therapeutic drug levels. Small IV doses are more effective. An alternative is the use of a transdermal fentanyl patch. These patches have various rates of delivery and have a delayed onset of action of 12 to 16 hours. The potential complications with this technique come from choosing the wrong dose, particularly in opioid naïve patients. The effects will gradually worsen and will persist longer than expected, depending on skin blood flow. Continuous IV infusion of opioids is a relatively simple technique, as long as the loading dose and the rate of infusion are calculated correctly to maintain therapeutic levels. Most opioids have a half-life of 3 hours. The dose required to maintain a level of analgesia is one half the loading dose used to achieve analgesia in the first place. This is divided by 3 to calculate the hourly requirements. When patients experience breakthrough pain, it must be addressed as new-onset pain and the new infusion rate titrated to effect. PCA is a technique for the administration of small doses of opioid IV on a demand basis. When establishing the upper limit for PCA (1- to 4-hour dosage limit), a fivefold increase in need during the early postoperative period must be considered, from what was originally calculated for an hourly requirement. Maintenance doses should generally not exceed 0.02 mg of morphine per kg, or 1.5 mg per dose in most adults. The lockout interval (5 to 10 min) accounts for the time required for an adequate concentration of the opioid to be established at the active site before another dose is given. PCA is useful for maintaining established analgesia but not for establishing it in the first place. Overdose with PCA is rare because patients tend to titrate themselves into the therapeutic range. Most patients actually choose not to eliminate pain entirely. Overdose is a significant risk if a basal infusion rate is administered. Accumulation tends to occur if the rate is set too high. Basal rate should not exceed half the estimated hourly requirement. Lack of adequate analgesia results from inadequate dosing secondary to the patient failing to understand the technique or equipment malfunction/programming errors. An unusual problem is parent- or spouse-controlled PCA. PCA requires that patients are awake and cooperative. PCA has also been used to give epidural medications (PCEA) with considerable safety and efficacy.

Selected Readings

Edwards WT. Optimizing opioid treatment of postoperative pain. *J Pain Symptom Manage* 1990;5:S24.
This article provides useful guidelines for the use of opioid analgesia.

Ready LB, Edwards WT. IASP Task Force on Acute Pain. In: *The management of acute pain: a practical manual.* Seattle: IASP Publications, 1992.
This reference provides an excellent review of postoperative pain management.

Ready LB, Oden R, Chadwick HS, et al. Development of an anesthesiology-based postoperative pain management service. *Anesthesiology* 1988; 68:100.
This article provides a comprehensive set of guidelines on postoperative pain management.

Stevens DS, Edwards WT. Management of pain in the critically ill. *J Intensive Care Med* 1990;5:258.
This article provides a focused approach on pain management in critically ill patients.

OBSTETRIC PROBLEMS IN THE INTENSIVE CARE UNIT

Ata Mazaheri, Jonathan Critchlow, and Fred A. Luchette

I. OVERVIEW

A. Over the past 45 years in the United States, pregnancy-associated mortality rates have declined from 50/100,000 live births to less than 10/100,000 live births. This is due to a decline in deaths from direct obstetric causes—eclampsia, hemorrhage, infection, and cardiac disease.

B. The most prevalent causes of death now are due to trauma, pulmonary embolism (PE), and poor antenatal care.

II. MATERNAL/FETAL PHYSIOLOGY

A. Cardiac output increases during the first trimester and peaks in the second trimester to almost 50% above normal.

B. Blood volume increases in the first trimester and peaks at 140% of the nonpregnant state by the third trimester.

C. Red cell mass and total blood volume increase; however, red cell mass doesn't increase at the same rate as plasma volume, which causes a modest dilutional anemia.

D. Respiratory rate and tidal volume increase in the second and third trimesters.

E. Total lung capacity and functional residual capacity (FRC) decrease in pregnancy.

F. Fetal oxygen delivery is a function of arterial O_2 content. Uterine blood flow is directly related to maternal blood pressure.

G. Blood flow to the placenta is adversely affected by alkalosis, diminished maternal cardiac output, uterine contractions, or increased sympathetic tone.

III. GENERAL CONSIDERATIONS IN DIAGNOSIS AND THERAPY

A. Monitoring

1. Cardiac pressures during pregnancy are in the range of those in the nonpregnant state.

2. Consider pulmonary artery catheterization for patients with cardiac failure, refractory pulmonary edema, severe underlying cardiac or pulmonary disease, nonhemorrhagic shock, and acute respiratory distress syndrome.

3. After trauma, continuous fetal monitoring should be used throughout resuscitation.

4. Tocographic monitoring is helpful after trauma to demonstrate premature contractions (warns of premature labor).

B. Radiation exposure

1. The risks to the fetus of death, malformation, or later childhood cancers depend on the gestational age of the fetus and the amount of radiation delivered.

2. First weeks of pregnancy, 10 cGy of radiation dose causes fetal death.

3. First 12 weeks of pregnancy, the fetus is vulnerable to developmental abnormalities (5 to 10 cGy of radiation is a cause for concern).

4. Plain films necessary for diagnosis and safe care of the pregnant patient should be obtained without undue concern over fetal exposure.

5. Computed tomography (CT) scans deliver between 5 and 10 cGy to the fetus (safe to use in third trimester).

C. Cardiopulmonary resuscitation

1. For closed-chest compression, the uterus should be shifted off the inferior vena cava (IVC) by tilting the abdomen to the left or with manual pressure. If no response, depending on fetal gestational age, downtime, and signs of life, proceed with cesarean section.

2. C-section should be performed within 5 minutes of the arrest and it should be undertaken only late in pregnancy.

D. Intubation and mechanical ventilation
   1. The indications for mechanical ventilation and intubation are the same as those for nonpregnant adults.
   2. A smaller endotracheal tube is used, and nasotracheal intubation should be avoided or performed with great care secondary to increase in blood flow and congestion of mucous membranes.

E. Drugs
   1. Analgesics and anxiolytics: Morphine and related opiates are safe to use in pregnancy (may lead to fetal withdrawal).
   2. Antibiotics
      a. Aminoglycosides are restricted to severe infections. Streptomycin and kanamycin can cause ototoxicity to the fetus.
      b. Penicillins and cephalosporins are safe to use.
      c. Sulfonamides are contraindicated near term; increase the risk of neonatal kernicterus.
      d. Chloramphenicol in large doses may cause gray syndrome.
      e. Tetracycline causes problems with bone and teeth.
      f. Clindamycin and vancomycin are safe to use.
   3. Anticoagulants
      a. Heparin is safe to use.
      b. Warfarin causes a distinct syndrome of developmental defects.
   4. Antihypertensives
      a. Hydralazine, alpha methyldopa, and nitroglycerin may be used in pregnancy.
      b. Sodium nitroprusside is unsafe due to elevated fetal cyanide levels.
   5. Vasoconstrictor and inotropic agents
      a. Ephedrine seems to best preserve the uterine blood flow.
      b. Phenylephrine is used to treat hypotension due to spinal or epidural anesthesia.

IV. NUTRITION

A. Nutritional support should commence early; enteral route is preferred.

B. Total parenteral nutrition if indicated may be used also.
   1. Keep blood glucose less than 120 mg/dL.
   2. Large quantities of IV lipid (>40% of calories) should be avoided (fatty infiltration of the placenta).

V. HYPERTENSIVE DISORDERS OF PREGNANCY

A. Chronic essential hypertension affects pregnancy only if severe.

B. Preeclampsia
   1. Definition: hypertension that occurs after the 20th week of pregnancy with proteinuria (greater than 2 g per day) and peripheral edema. It is often seen in nulliparous women, occurs in 10% of all pregnancies, and is associated with end organ failure.
   2. Pathogenesis: Arteriolar vasospasm seems to be the cause. Inciting factors: failure of prostacycline-mediated uterine vasodilatation, high thromboxane levels from endothelial damage, and increased sensitivity to angiotensin II.
   3. Laboratory testing: standard blood tests, urinalysis, renal and hepatic function tests, coagulation profile, and blood smear.
   4. Treatment: In delivery, majority of patients must be stabilized and have delivery afterward. Bed rest and vigorous IV fluids should be ordered.
   5. Control blood pressure with hydralazine, alpha methyldopa, or labatalol.

C. Eclampsia
   1. Definition: onset of seizures that are unrelated to a known seizure disorder or anatomic focus in hypertensive patients.
   2. Treatment: IV magnesium

D. HELLP syndrome
   1. Definition: Preeclamptic mothers with *h*emolysis, *e*levated *l*iver function, and *l*ow *p*latelets.
   2. Presentation: weight gain, malaise, and right upper quadrant pain
   3. Pathogenesis: vasospasm, which triggers endothelial cell damage and microangiopathic hemolysis.
   4. Diagnosis: lactate dehydrogenase (LDH) levels greater than 600 U/L, elevated liver function test values (alanine aminotransferase greater than 70 IU/L), and a platelet count less than 100, 000 cells/mm^3.
   5. Management
      a. Fetus greater than 35 weeks or with mature lungs should be prepared for delivery (can be accomplished vaginally in most cases). Steroids may be given for lung maturity if necessary.
      b. For immature fetus: bed rest, IV fluids, and antihypertensive therapy are the mainstay of treatment.
      c. For patient with ruptured subcapsular hematoma in shock, immediate operation.

VI. ANTEPARTUM HEMORRHAGE
   A. Placenta previa
   1. Definition: Areas of the placenta overlie the cervical os and may bleed through the cervix.
   2. Presentation: Painless bleeding that occurs as multiple sporadic bleeds from the lower uterine segment through the os.
   3. Diagnosis: History, ultrasound, and digital examination (if needed). Digital examination should be done in the operating room.
   4. Management
      a. With severe hemorrhage, immediate cesarean section is indicated.
      b. For a fetus beyond 35 weeks, if bleeding is not severe but continues delivery should be performed without delay.
      c. For a less mature fetus, allow fetal maturation. Manage the patient with bed rest, IV fluids, and blood as needed.
      d. The mode of delivery, vaginal or C-section, is controversial.
   B. Abruptio placentae
   1. Definition: Premature separation of the placenta from the uterus. Occurs in up to 1 in 100 pregnancies.
   2. Presentation: Pain that increases with contractions. External bleeding may be present or absent; therefore, the degree of maternal volume depletion may not correlate with observed blood loss.
   3. Diagnosis: History and physical examination. Ultrasound may miss the diagnoses of abruption.
   4. Treatment: IV fluids and blood as needed, fetal monitoring, and at times invasive monitoring to assess the degree of blood loss. Definitive treatment is delivery. A mother with mild blood loss and a term fetus without distress may be induced for vaginal delivery. For maternal and fetal distress, emergent C-section is indicated.

VII. POSTPARTUM HEMORRHAGE
   A. Definition: Vaginal delivery with blood loss in excess of 500 mL or C-section with blood loss in excess of 1,000 mL.
   B. Pathogenesis: Caused by conditions that don't allow adequate uterine contraction. These include clots or fragments, uterine overdistention, lacerations, idiopathic uterine atony, and the use of certain drugs such as terbutaline or MgSO$_4$.
   C. Management
   1. Medical treatment: Improving uterine contraction and improving coagulopathy. Compression or massage of the uterus may stimulate contraction. If not effective, use oxytocin (20 U/L) as a continuous infusion to increase contractions.

Prostaglandin $F_{2\alpha}$ and intramuscular injection of ergonovine may be used as well. Ergonovine may cause intracerebral hemorrhage.

2. Surgical treatment: If postpartum hemorrhage is not corrected by oxytocic therapy, surgery is indicated. Surgical options include curettage to remove retained placenta, hypogastric artery ligation, and hysterectomy.

3. Angiographic embolization.

VIII. TRAUMA

A. Trauma complicates 6% to 7% of all pregnancies; however, less than 1% of all pregnant women require hospitalization. In several studies trauma has been implicated as the most common cause of maternal death. Most maternal injuries during pregnancy are due to blunt trauma; automobile accidents are the most common (majority of deaths secondary to head injury and hemorrhagic shock). Maternal injury is associated with increased incidence of premature labor, spontaneous abortion, abruptio placentae, fetomaternal hemorrhage, and uterine fetal demise. In late pregnancy, significant abdominal injury may cause uterine rupture. Fetal loss is almost universal and maternal mortality approaches 10%. The incidence of fetal death exceeds that of maternal death threefold to ninefold in trauma.

B. Moderate decrease in maternal cardiac output and blood pressure (insufficient to cause maternal shock) may be detrimental to the fetus. Assessment of fetomaternal hemorrhage by the Kleihauer-Betke assay should be considered in all pregnancies complicated by trauma.

C. Resuscitation and assessment

1. The initial resuscitation and primary survey of the injured pregnant women follows the guidelines of the American College of Surgeons Committee on Advanced Trauma Life Support Program. The ABCs are first priority.

2. Standard fluid and blood resuscitation should be used.

3. Transport and care for the patient lying on the left side to improve venous return to the heart.

4. The pneumatic antishock garment should not be used.

5. The secondary survey should follow.

6. For diagnostic peritoneal lavage (DPL) the incision should be well above the fundus with an open technique.

7. Perform a formal examination of the uterus and vagina.

8. Fetal assessment includes evaluation of fetal movement, Doppler for fetal heart tones, and tocographic monitoring.

9. Obtain essential radiographs.

10. Blood should be drawn for standard tests, as well as blood typing, Rh screening, and the Kleihauer-Betke test.

11. Rh immunization should be given within 72 hours to Rh-negative mothers.

12. Ultrasonography may be used.

13. Mother and fetus require continuous monitoring.

14. Increased uterine contraction (greater than eight contractions per hour) is an early warning sign for impending placental abruption.

15. The definitive therapy for a pregnant trauma patient should mirror that given to a patient who is not pregnant.

16. With fetal distress and refractory maternal shock secondary to abruption, consideration should be given to cesarean section.

Selected Readings

Barton JR, Sibai BM. Care of the pregnancy complicating HELLP syndrome. *Obstet Gynecol Clin North Am* 1991;18(2):165.
  This review addresses the management of pregnancies complicated by HELLP syndrome.

Berkowitz RL. The management of hypertensive crisis during pregnancy. In: Berkowitz RL, ed. *Critical care of the obstetric patient.* New York: Churchill Livingstone, 1983, p. 299.

Berkowitz RL. The Swan-Ganz catheter and colloid osmotic pressure determinations. In: Berkowitz RL, ed. *Critical care of the obstetric patient.* New York: Churchill Livingstone, 1983, p. 1.

Brent RL. The effects of embryonic and fetal exposure to x-ray, microwaves and ultrasound: counseling the pregnant and non-pregnant patient. *Semin Oncol* 1989;16:347.
This review shows that medically indicated diagnostic radiographs are safe for pregnant women.

Briggs CG, Freeman RK, Yaffee SJ. *Drugs in pregnancy and lactation.* Baltimore: Williams and Wilkins, 1986.

Chow AW, Jewesson RJ. Pharmacokinetics and safety of antimicrobial agents in pregnancy. *Rev Infect Dis* 1985;7:278.
This review addresses the safety and efficacy of antimicrobial agents during pregnancy.

Committee on Trauma, American College of Surgeons. *Advanced trauma life support program for physicians.* Chicago: American College of Surgeons, 1997.

Cunningham FG, Pritchard JA. How should hypertension in pregnancy be managed? *Med Clin North Am* 1984;68:505.
This study, derived from observation of more than 20,000 pregnancies, describes the management plan of pregnancy-induced hypertension.

Hoff WS, D'Amelio LF, Tinkoff GH. Maternal predictors of fetal demise in trauma during pregnancy. *Surg Gynecol Obstet* 1991;172(3):175.
This study analyzed the incidence of fetal demise as a function of maternal characteristics determined within the first 24 hours after trauma.

Hurd WW, Miodovnik M, Hertzberg V, et al. Selective management of abruption placentae: a prospective study. *Obstet Gynecol* 1983;61:467.
This study investigates the management of abruptio placentae in women delivering vaginally and by cesarean section.

Kalter H, Warkany J. Congenital malformations. *N Engl J Med* 1983;309:1282.

Kaunitz AM, Hughes JM, Grimes D, et al. Causes of maternal mortality in the United States. *Obstet Gynecol* 1985;65:605.
This study reviewed causes of maternal death between 1974 and 1978 in the United States.

Mabie WC, Gonzalez AR, Sibai BM, et al. A comparative trial of labetalol and hydralazine in the acute management of severe hypertension complicating pregnancy. *Obstet Gynecol* 1987;70:328.
This study found that labetalol is a safe and effective alternative to hydralazine for treating hypertension in the peripartum period.

Machida H. Influence of progesterone on arterial blood and CSF acid-base balance in women. *J Appl Physiol* 1981;51:1433.
Fifty-nine pregnant and 36 nonpregnant women were studied to determine the mechanism of action of pulmonary ventilation during pregnancy and arterial and cerebral spinal fluid acid–base parameters.

Pearlman MD, Tintinalli JE, Lorenz RP. Blunt trauma during pregnancy. *N Engl J Med* 1990;323(23):1609.
This review discusses blunt trauma in pregnancy.

Sibai BM. Pitfalls in diagnosis and management of pre-eclampsia. *Am J Obstet Gynecol* 1988;159:1.
This review documents the lack of benefit in prenatal outcome from the use of antihypertensive therapies in patients with preeclampsia.

Varner MW. Maternal mortality in Iowa from 1952 to 1986. *Surg Gynecol Obstet* 1989;168:555.
This article documents the decrease in maternal death and highlights that trauma is a persistent cause of preventable maternal death.

Shock and Trauma XI

I. GENERAL PRINCIPLES

A. Definition

Shock is a multifactorial syndrome leading to systemic and localized tissue hypoperfusion and resulting in cellular hypoxia and multiple organ dysfunctions.

B. Description

1. Perfusion may be decreased systemically with obvious signs such as hypotension.
2. Perfusion may be decreased because of maldistribution as in septic shock where systemic perfusion may appear elevated
3. Signs of malperfusion may be subtle and lead to significant organ damage.
4. Prognosis is determined by degree of shock, duration of shock, number of organs affected, previous organ dysfunction, and possibly some genetic predisposition.

II. ETIOLOGY; CLASSIFICATION OF SHOCK

A. Hypovolemic shock

1. Loss of circulating intravascular volume and decrease in cardiac preload.
2. May be from hemorrhage such as with trauma, gastrointestinal bleeding, nontraumatic internal bleeding (e.g., aneurysm, ectopic rupture), or vaginal bleeding.
3. May be from nonhemorrhagic fluid loss from the gastrointestinal tract (vomiting, diarrhea, fistula), urinary losses (hyperglycemia with glucosuria), evaporative loss (fever, hyperthermia), or internal fluid shifts (third spacing as with a bowel obstruction).
4. Most common form of shock.
5. All forms of shock have some component of decreased preload.
6. Clinical signs depend on volume lost (Table 123-1). Symptoms include tachycardia, hypotension, decreased urine output, mental status changes, and tachypnea.
7. Treatment is with volume resuscitation with crystalloid solution, and in addition blood if from hemorrhage. Colloid infusion has no value in hypovolemic shock.

B. Obstructive shock

1. Caused by a mechanical obstruction to normal cardiac output with a decrease in systemic perfusion.
2. Two causes are cardiac tamponade and tension pneumothorax. Clinical signs of these include jugular venous distension, muffled heart sounds (tamponade), decreased breath sounds unilaterally (pneumothorax).
3. Other causes are massive pulmonary embolism and air embolism.
4. Treatment is maximizing preload and relief of the obstruction.

C. Cardiogenic shock

1. Caused by pump failure.
2. Most common cause is extensive myocardial infarction.
3. Other causes are reduced contractility (cardiomyopathy, sepsis induced), aortic stenosis, mitral stenosis, atrial myxoma, acute valvular failure, and cardiac dysrhythmias.
4. Treatment is maximizing preload and cardiac performance and reducing afterload.

D. Distributive shock

1. Caused by systemic vasodilatation from an inciting cause (infection, anaphylaxis), resulting in systemic hypotension and increased or decreased cardiac output.

TABLE 123-1	Classification of Hypovolemic Shock

Hypovolemic shock (based on a 70-kg patient)	Class I	Class II	Class III	Class IV
Blood loss (mL)	Up to 750	750–1,500	1,500–2,000	>2,000
% Blood volume	Up to 15	15–30	30–40	>40
Pulse rate	<100	>100	>120	>140
Blood pressure	Normal	Normal	Decreased	Decreased
Capillary refill	Normal	Decreased	Decreased	Decreased
Respiratory rate	Normal	20–30	30–40	Distress
Urinary output (mL/hr)	>30	20–30	5–15	<10
Mental status	Mild anxiety	Anxiety	Confused	Lethargic
Fluid replacement	Crystalloid	Crystalloid	Crystalloid + Blood	Crystalloid + Blood

2. Most common cause is sepsis, and used to be classified as "septic shock." Sepsis, which is caused by a systemic infection, typically is characterized by high cardiac output with systemic hypotension.
3. Distributive shock is enhanced by the inflammatory response. Despite a high cardiac output, there is cellular hypoxia likely from disruption of mitochondrial function.
4. The systemic inflammatory response syndrome (SIRS) may produce a distributive shock, which can be caused by etiologies other than infection (e.g., pancreatitis).
5. Other causes of distributive shock are anaphylaxis, severe trauma, severe liver dysfunction, and neurogenic shock. Neurogenic shock results from cervical spinal cord injury with loss of sympathetic vascular tone. There is no inflammatory response. The patient has hypotension, bradycardia, and warm extremities. Treatment is with volume and a vasoconstrictor.
6. Treatment of sepsis and SIRS, *when shock is evident,* is with massive volume to supplement preload, augmentation of blood pressure with vasoconstrictors as necessary, and treatment of underlying cause if it can be identified.

E. Endocrine shock
   1. Caused by hypothyroidism, hyperthyroidism with cardiac collapse, and adrenal insufficiency. Treatment is cardiovascular support while treating the underlying cause.
   2. Adrenal insufficiency may be a contributor to shock in critically ill patients. Patients who are unresponsive to treatment should be tested for adrenal insufficiency.

III. PATHOPHYSIOLOGY
A. The result of shock is decreased tissue perfusion and *cellular hypoxia.*
B. Cellular hypoxia leads to cellular ischemia. Ischemic cells are primed by alterations of calcium and adenosine 3',5'-cyclic monophosphate (cAMP) and creation of superoxide radicals.
C. Endothelial cells under hypoxic conditions will have enhanced vascular permeability and less control over membrane transport functions.
D. Reperfusion will result in release of superoxide radicals that cause further cell damage.
E. These processes activate neutrophils and the release of proinflammatory cytokines.

F. The inflammatory response results in further cellular damage, third spacing of fluids, and activation of the coagulation system, leading to microcirculatory thrombosis, collapse, and further ischemia

G. In septic shock and SIRS, the initial event is the inflammatory response.

H. Microcirculatory collapse leads to multiple-organ failure.

IV. DIAGNOSIS

A. Vital signs. Heart rate, blood pressure, temperature, urine output, and pulse oximetry. The traditional measures to determine shock are still regularly used in the clinical setting. Of patients with normal or near normal vital signs, 50% to 85% are still in shock.

  1. Heart rate

   a. Tachycardia is an early sign of significant volume loss in shock.

   b. The heart rate of young patients or those on β-blockers may not increase.

   c. Bradycardia after prolonged hypotension precludes cardiovascular collapse.

  2. Blood pressure (BP)

   a. Hypotension and narrowing pulse pressure are a sign of severe volume loss and shock.

   b. Mean arterial pressure (MAP) is a better guide to therapy than systolic BP.

  3. Temperature

   a. Hyperthermia, normothermia, or hypothermia may be present in shock.

   b. Hypothermia is a sign of severe hypovolemic and septic shock.

  4. Urine output

   a. Early guide of hypovolemia and end organ response (renal) to shock.

   b. This is a delayed vital sign because 1 to 2 hours are needed to obtain an accurate measure.

  5. Pulse oximetry. Continuously measured and early indicator of hypoxemia but may be invalid in hypothermic patient.

B. Invasive hemodynamic monitoring

  1. Indwelling arterial catheters give continuous blood pressure measurements.

  2. A central venous catheter gives continuous central venous pressure (CVP) measurements.

  3. Pulmonary arterial catheters (PACs) can measure CVP, right atrial pressure, pulmonary artery pressure, pulmonary arterial occlusion pressure (frequently called wedge pressure), and cardiac output. PACs will help guide aggressive resuscitation in patients with severe shock. Hemodynamic variables are listed in Table 123-2.

C. Cardiac preload. Left ventricular end-diastolic volume (LVEDV) is proportional to left ventricular end-diastolic pressure (LVEDP). Increasing LVEDV (preload) will increase myocardial fiber length and therefore increase cardiac output to a patient-specific optimal level (Frank-Starling law). Pulmonary artery occlusion pressure (PAOP) will reflect LVEDP in a patient without mitral valve disease and with stable ventricular compliance. Ventricular compliance is not stable in patients with severe shock; therefore, for patients in shock, the measured PAOP is not accurate, but the trend of PAOP will suggest the ideal preload for optimal cardiac function. Hence, measurement of PAOP will guide resuscitation and volume status.

D. Cardiac flow variables

  1. Cardiac output (CO) or cardiac index (CI) reflects cardiac function and can be directly measured by a PAC. Some PACs measure CO continuously. Optimizing CI is a goal of resuscitation. CI can be increased by increasing preload, increasing contractility, or decreasing afterload.

  2. Systemic vascular resistance index (SVRI) can be derived from the PAC measurements of CO (CI) and MAP. The SVRI, cardiac afterload, will help guide therapy. Patients with hypovolemic, obstructive, cardiogenic shock *and end-stage sepsis* have a high SVRI and a low CI. Patients with early septic shock have a low SVRI and a high CI.

TABLE 123-2	Hemodynamic Variables	

Variable (abbreviation)	Unit	Normal range
Measured variables		
Systolic blood pressure (SBP)	mm Hg	90–140
Diastolic blood pressure (DBP)	mm Hg	60–90
Systolic pulmonary blood pressure (PAS)	mm Hg	15–30
Diastolic pulmonary blood pressure (PAD)	mm Hg	4–12
Pulmonary artery occlusion pressure (PAOP)	mm Hg	2–12
Central venous pressure (CVP)	mm Hg	0–8
Heart rate (HR)	Beats/min	50–100
Cardiac output (CO)	L/min	4–6
Right ventricular ejection fraction (RVEF)	Fraction	0.4–0.6
Calculated variables		
Mean arterial pressure (MAP)	mm Hg	70–105
Mean pulmonary artery pressure (MPAP)	mm Hg	9–16
Cardiac index (CI)	L/min/m^2	2.8–4.2
Stroke volume (SV)	ML/beat	varies
Stroke volume index (SVI)	mL/beat/m^2	30–65
Systemic vascular resistance index (SVRI)	dynes $\times$ sec/cm^{-5}	1,600–2,400
Pulmonary vascular resistance index (PVRI)		250–340
Left ventricular stroke work index (LVSWI)	g $\times$ m/m^2	45–62
Right ventricular stroke work index (RVSWI)	g $\times$ m/m^2	7–12
Right ventricular end-diastolic work index (RVEDWI)	mL/m^2	60–100
Body surface area (BSA)	m^2	Varies

3. Left ventricular stroke work index (LVSWI) can be derived by the change in pressure × the change in volume and will also reflect the response to therapy. LVSWI = (MAP − PAOP) × stroke volume index (SVI = CI/HR) (0.0136).

4. Specialized PACs measure right ventricular ejection fraction (RVEF), which can calculate right ventricular end-diastolic volume (RVEDVI). (RVEDVI = SVI/RVEF). RVEDVI is a more accurate measure of true volume status.

5. Methods for measuring CO, other than with a PAC, have been devised, though without universal acceptance. Examples are analysis integration of the area beneath the arterial waveform, and noninvasive chest impedance.

E. Oxygen transport assessment (Because shock is a decrease of tissue oxygen perfusion, the delivery of oxygen to the tissues is inadequate to meet the cellular/tissue oxygen demand.)

1. Oxygen delivery index (DO_2) is the arterial oxygen content × the cardiac index. [$DO_2 = CaO_2 \times CI \times 10$ dL/L]

2. Arterial oxygen content is % saturated Hgb × the binding coefficient (1.34) and the oxygen dissolved in the plasma (a clinically insignificant amount and is disregarded). [$CaO_2 = (1.34 \times Hgb \times SaO_2) + (PaO_2 \times 0.003$]

3. Venous oxygen content is the % saturated venous Hgb × 1.34 + oxygen dissolved. [$CvO_2 = (1.34 \times Hgb \times SvO_2) + (PvO_2 \times 0.003)$]

4. Oxygen consumption index (VO_2) is the ($CaO_2 − CvO_2$). [$\dot{V}O_2 = (1.34 \times Hgb \times SaO_2 − SvO_2) \times CI \times 10$ dL/L]

5. Oxygen extraction ratio (OER) is the $\dot{V}O_2/DO_2$ and normally that is about 25%.

6. Continuous measurement of SvO_2 (available with a specialized PAC) will detect early increases of $\dot{V}O_2$ (a low SvO_2) and perhaps the need to increase the oxygen-carrying ability with transfusion or increasing the CI. A high SvO_2 is

indicative of early sepsis, SIRS, and/or cirrhosis and does not reflect the derangement of O_2 utilization at the cellular (mitochondrial) level.

F. Resuscitation end points
  1. Lactic acid production
    a. Cells with inadequate oxygen will switch to anaerobic metabolism. Lactic acid is a byproduct of anaerobic metabolism. Elevation of serum lactate is an indicative of the severity of shock; however, elevated lactate is a global measure of hypoperfusion and may not be elevated with regional hypoperfusion.
    b. Lactate may be elevated in liver or kidney diseases and may be of little value 2 or 3 days after the shock insult.
    c. The *rate of clearance of lactate* is a better marker of adequate resuscitation, rather than the absolute value.
  2. Base deficit
    a. Base deficit is the amount of base required to titrate whole blood to a normal pH. The presence of an elevated base deficit correlates with the severity of shock.
    b. Base deficit is easily obtained with an arterial blood gas.
    c. The correction of the base deficit is a guide to further resuscitation.
  3. Intramucosal pH monitoring
    a. With the mesenteric hemodynamic response to shock, the mesenteric organs will have earlier and greater hypoperfusion than other organ systems.
    b. Gastric tonometry measures intramuscular pH and is an early indicator of hypoperfusion in shock and correlates with mortality. Technical difficulties with this form of monitoring have mitigated its usage.

V. TREATMENT

A. Rapid recognition and restoration of perfusion is the key to preventing multiple-organ dysfunction and death. In all forms of shock, rapid restoration of preload with infusion of fluids is the first treatment. Crystalloid is first infused and then blood is infused if shock is secondary to hemorrhage. Treatment of shock usually precedes the diagnosis of the etiology. Early diagnosis of the etiology is essential, and further treatment of the shock depends on its etiology.

B. Hypovolemic shock
  1. Rapid infusion of multiple liters of crystalloid is the treatment for hypovolemic shock. Large-bore venous access is needed, and central access may be necessary as well. If the cause is hemorrhage, then after 2 to 3 liters of fluid, blood is transfused. Concomitantly, the source of bleeding needs to be controlled.
  2. Resuscitation is not complete until the base excess or serum lactate has decreased to an acceptable level. Patients with severe hypovolemic shock will third space fluids with resuscitation.
  3. Vasoconstrictors are rarely needed with pure hypovolemic shock.
  4. A PAC may be helpful in guiding resuscitation in patients with severe shock.

C. Obstructive shock. The cause of the obstructive shock must be identified and relieved early.
  1. Pericardiocentesis or pericardiotomy for a cardiac tamponade
  2. Needle decompression or tube thoracostomy, or both, for tension pneumothorax
  3. Ventilatory and cardiac support, possibly thrombolytics, and possibly interventional radiology procedures for pulmonary embolism

D. Cardiogenic shock
  1. Optimize preload with infusion of fluids.
  2. Optimize contractility with inotropes as needed, balancing cardiac oxygen demand. Refer to the cardiac section of this book. Consider dobutamine, amrinone, and other vasoactive drugs.
  3. Adjust afterload to maximize CO. This may involve using a vasoconstrictor if a patient is hypotensive with a low SVR. Patients with cardiogenic shock may need vasodilatation to decrease their SVR, the resistance to flow from a weak heart. Refer to the cardiac section of this book. Consider nitroprusside and nitroglycerin.

   4. Diuresis may be indicated in patients with heart failure.
   5. A PAC is recommended to guide therapy in these patients.
   6. The underlying cardiac cause needs to be identified and treated.
 E. Distributive shock
   1. In SIRS and sepsis, when shock is present it is due to toxin- or mediator-induced vasodilatation. Treatment is with immediate fluid resuscitation, and once adequate volume status is established, pressors should be considered to augment optimal MAP. Frequently, pressors are started before an adequate preload has been established. Tissue perfusion and cellular oxygenation will not be optimized unless aggressive, optimal preload augmentation is achieved.
   2. Dopamine, norepinephrine, and vasopressin should be considered.
   3. A PAC catheter is highly recommended for patients with shock and SIRS.
   4. Identification of the underlying cause of the distributive shock is essential, and removal of the cause, if possible, is essential. Many clinical trials have been conducted to identify pharmaceuticals to interrupt the inflammatory response. Activated protein C has been approved for treatment for patients with septic shock. In theory, it interrupts the microcirculatory thrombosis.

Selected Readings

Bernard GR, Vincent JL, Laterre PF, et al. Efficacy and safety of recombinant human activated protein C for severe sepsis. *N Engl J Med* 2001;344:699–709.
   Clinical trial supporting potential benefits of activated protein C for septic shock.

Cheatham ML, Block EFJ, Promes JT, et al. Shock: an overview. In: Irwin RS and Rippe JM, eds. *Irwin and Rippe's Intensive Care Medicine*, 5th ed. Philadelphia: Lippincott Williams & Wilkins.
   Good reference.

Choi PTL, Yip G, Quinonez LG, et al. Crystalloids vs. colloids in fluid resuscitation: a systematic review. *Crit Care Med* 1999;27:200–210.
   Review of literature on what to use for resuscitation: crystalloid.

Committee on Trauma of the American College of Surgeons. Advanced trauma life support program for physicians. Chicago: American College of Surgeons, 1997.
   Fundamental teaching on diagnosis and treatment of hemorrhagic shock.

Cooper MS, Stewart PM. Corticosteroid insufficiency in acutely ill patients. *N Engl J Med* 2003;348:727–734.
   Good review of the literature on steroid insufficiency and its role in shock.

Davis JW, Shackford SR, Mackersie RC, et al. Base deficit as a guide to volume resuscitation. *J Trauma* 1988;28:1464–1467.
   Excellent reference on using base deficit as an end point of resuscitation.

De Backer D, Creteur J, Silva E, et al. Effects of dopamine, norepinephrine and epinephrine on the splanchnic circulation in septic shock: which is best? *Crit Care Med* 2003;31:1659–1667.
   Good discussion on choices of vasopressors to use in patients in shock who are volume resuscitated.

Dellinger RP, Carlet JM, Masur H, et al. Surviving sepsis campaign guidelines for management of severe sepsis and septic shock. *Crit Care Med* 2004;32:858–873.
   Excellent review of the literature on sepsis with graded references to develop guidelines for the management of septic shock as well as shock in general.

Hebert PC, Wells G, Blajchman MA, et al. A multicenter, randomized controlled clinical trial of transfusion in critical care. *N Engl J Med* 1999;340:409–417.
   Significant clinical trial challenging transfusion practices in critical care patients.

Hinshaw LB, Cox BG. The fundamental mechanisms of shock. New York: Platinum Press, 1972.
   The original classifications of shock.

Ivatory RR, Simon RJ, Havrilak D, et al. Gastric mucosal pH and oxygen delivery and oxygen consumption indices in assessment of adequacy of resuscitation after trauma: a prospective, randomized study. *J Trauma* 1995;39:128–136.
Good study on measuring organ-specific tissue perfusion values to determine the end points of resuscitation.

Mizock BA, Falk JL. Lactic acidosis in critical illness. *Crit Care Med* 1992;20:80–93.
Good reference on the relationship of lactic acidosis and shock.

Rivers E, Nguyen B, Havstad S, et al. Early goal-directed therapy in the treatment of severe sepsis and septic shock. *N Engl J Med* 2001;345:1368–1377.
Important clinical trial that confirmed the need for aggressive, early large-volume resuscitation in septic shock.

Sharshar T, Blanchard A, Pallard M, et al. Circulating vasopressin levels in septic shock. *Crit Care Med* 2003;31:1526–1531.
One of the latest references outlining the current discussion for using vasopressin in patients with septic shock, when all else fails.

Shoemaker WC, Appel PL, Kram HB, et al. Prospective trial of supranormal values of survivors as therapeutic goals in high-risk surgical patients. *Chest* 1988;94:1176–1186.
The original work on supranormal oxygen delivery and its effect on survival.

Swan HJC, Ganz W, Forrester J, et al. Catheterization of the heart in man with use of a flow-directed balloon-tipped catheter. *N Engl J Med* 1970;283:447–451.
The original work for the pulmonary artery catheter.

Waxman K. Shock: ischemia, reperfusion, and inflammation. *New Horizons* 1996;4(2):153–160.
This entire journal is a good review of the pathophysiology of shock.

124

HEMORRHAGE AND RESUSCITATION
Christopher P. Michetti

I. GENERAL PRINCIPLES
A. Definition
1. Shock is a condition in which the amount of oxygen delivered to tissues is inadequate to maintain normal cellular function (i.e., aerobic metabolism).
2. Hemorrhagic shock (HS) results from tissue hypoperfusion due to hypovolemia from blood loss.

B. Epidemiology
1. Hemorrhage is second only to brain injury as a cause of early death after traumatic injury.
2. Trauma is the leading cause of death of individuals in the United States from ages 1 to 44 years.

C. Outcome
1. Outcome is proportional to the duration and severity of shock.
2. Rapid identification of shock and initiation of treatment before hypotension occurs is essential to minimize morbidity.
3. Trauma patients with HS have improved outcomes when treated at a level I trauma center (highest level) as soon as possible after injury.

II. PATHOPHYSIOLOGY
A. Physiologic alterations
1. Hypoperfusion after hemorrhage leads to tissue ischemia, a shift from aerobic to anaerobic metabolism, production of lactate and inorganic phosphates, and metabolic acidosis. Depletion of adenosine 5′-triphosphate (ATP), oxygen radical formation, and other processes of anaerobic metabolism result in cellular injury and eventually in cell death.
2. The hypothalamic-pituitary-adrenal axis is activated by shock and results in release and elevation of several hormones.
   a. Increased cortisol leads to hyperglycemia and insulin resistance, muscle breakdown, and lipolysis.
   b. Release of vasopressin causes sodium and water retention.
   c. Activation of the renin-angiotensin system produces angiotensin II, a vasoconstrictor.
3. Activation of the systemic inflammatory response results in release of proinflammatory mediators that can cause cell and organ dysfunction.
   a. Ischemia and reperfusion of tissues, especially gut, activate systemic inflammatory response.
   b. Cytokines such as tumor necrosis factor and interleukins-1 and -6 are released.
   c. The complement system is activated.
   d. Endothelial cells allow adhesion of activated neutrophils and their transmigration into tissues, where they cause tissue injury by releasing oxygen radicals and proteolytic enzymes.

B. Fluid shifts
1. Triphasic response
   a. Initial phase: Response to bleeding is fluid shift from the interstitial space into capillaries to compensate for lost intravascular volume. Lasts from start of bleeding until bleeding is controlled.

    b. Second phase: With resuscitation, fluid shifts from the intravascular space back to the interstitial space (the "third space").

      (1) Lasts 1 to several days.

      (2) Interstitial space sequesters large amounts of fluids ("capillary leak" phenomenon).

      (3) Patients become severely edematous and simultaneously intravascularly depleted.

      (4) Fluid intake markedly exceeds output.

      (5) Fluid sequestration and resultant edema are obligatory and necessary in resuscitation from HS.

    c. Third phase: A natural diuresis occurs as fluid moves from the interstitial space to the intravascular space and is filtered through the kidneys.

      (1) starts 3 to 5 days after injury

      (2) key sign of recovery from shock

  2. A common mistake among those inexperienced in shock resuscitation is to misinterpret the edema and highly positive fluid balance of shock patients as signs of increased hydrostatic pressure from congestive heart failure.

    a. Fluid intake/output balance is irrelevant in acute HS resuscitation.

    b. Tissue edema and increased body water are the natural result of successful HS resuscitation.

    c. Forced diuresis exacerbates tissue hypoperfusion by depleting intravascular volume.

III. DIAGNOSIS

A. Classifications of hemorrhagic shock

  1. Class I

    a. loss of up to 15% of total blood volume (0 to 750 mL in 70-kg person)

    b. characterized by normal vital signs and urine output, slight tachypnea, slight anxiety

  2. Class II

    a. loss of 15% to 30% of total blood volume (750 to 1500 mL)

    b. characterized by normal blood pressure, heart rate (HR) greater than100, respiration rate (RR) of 20 to 30, decreased urine output, mild anxiety

  3. Class III

    a. loss of 30% to 40% of total blood volume (1,500 to 2,000 mL)

    b. characterized by decreased blood pressure, HR greater than 120, RR 30 to 40, decreased urine output, anxiety and confusion

  4. Class IV

    a. loss of more than 40% of total blood volume (>2,000 mL)

    b. characterized by decreased blood pressure, HR greater than 140, RR greater than 35, negligible urine output, lethargy

  5. Note that blood pressure is normal until significant blood loss occurs (Class III)

  6. Tachycardia is the earliest reliable sign of shock.

B. Sources of hemorrhage

  1. There are only five locations of blood loss that can result in HS.

    a. Thorax

      (1) For example, hemothorax

      (2) Diagnosis by chest radiograph or computed tomography (CT) scan.

      (3) Of thoracic bleeding, 90% can be treated with thoracostomy tube.

    b. Abdomen

      (1) Usually due to liver or spleen injury.

      (2) Gastrointestinal bleeding is a common nontraumatic etiology.

      (3) Diagnosis is by ultrasound, CT scan, or diagnostic peritoneal lavage or visible gastrointestinal bleeding.

      (4) Physical examination is not adequate to exclude bleeding in the abdomen. Significant injuries and hemoperitoneum may be present with a normal abdominal examination.

    c. Pelvis and retroperitoneum

      (1) Exsanguination can result from pelvic fractures, especially posterior fractures.

      (2) Renal or major vascular injuries or ruptured aortic aneurysms can result in significant retroperitoneal blood loss.

      (3) Diagnosis of fractures by pelvic radiograph; CT scan best test for retroperitoneum

    d. Long-bone fractures

      (1) Can lose up to 1,500 mL of blood in each thigh from femur fractures.

      (2) Can lose up to 750 mL of blood from humerus or tibia fracture.

      (3) Diagnosis is by radiography.

    e. External sites

      (1) Bleeding from scalp lacerations, deep soft tissue wounds, or major vascular injuries can result in HS.

      (2) Diagnosis is by history (from scene) and physical examination of all wounds.

      (3) Wounds should be carefully explored and never blindly probed (to avoid dislodging a hemostatic clot and rebleeding).

  2. Intracranial bleeding or brain injuries do not cause shock.

IV. TREATMENT

A. Resuscitation

  1. The first priority for any bleeding patient is to ensure a patent, secure airway. The second priority is to ensure adequate breathing and ventilation. Hemostasis and fluid resuscitation are the third priority. In clinical practice, all of these are assessed and treated nearly simultaneously.

  2. Resuscitation from HS includes stopping the bleeding and replacing the volume loss.

    a. Direct localized pressure should be applied to any visible bleeding points.

      (1) Use of tourniquets is discouraged because of global ischemia distal to tourniquet.

      (2) Direct pressure allows hemostasis with preserved collateral flow.

    b. Resuscitation encompasses replacing volume loss and restoration of normal end-organ perfusion.

  3. Fluid resuscitation

    a. Warm lactated Ringer's or normal saline (crystalloid) solution are the preferred resuscitation fluids for HS, with initial rapid bolus of 2 liters.

    b. If hypotension persists after 2-liter bolus of crystalloid, packed red blood cells should be transfused and crystalloid infusion continued.

    c. Crystalloid should be infused to replace the volume lost and also to resuscitate the *interstitial space fluid deficit* resulting from HS.

      (1) General rule of HS resuscitation is to replace three times the volume of blood lost with crystalloid (e.g., 1 liter of blood loss should be replaced with 3 liters of crystalloid).

        (a) The 3-to-1 rule stems from classic experiments in 1960s and 1970s in dogs, in which HS was noted to result in large extracellular fluid deficit.

        (b) Mortality for resuscitation with shed blood alone was 80%, shed blood plus plasma was 70%, and lactated Ringer's plus shed blood (in a 3:1 ratio) 30%.

      (2) Replacement of hemorrhage with blood only, or less than the required ratio of crystalloid to blood loss, results in persistent hypoperfusion and acidosis and increased mortality.

      (3) Fluid resuscitation of the interstitial space is *obligatory* in HS. The resultant edema and fluid retention are the desired result, not a harmful side effect, of proper HS resuscitation. Because this space needs to be filled to several times its original volume, a larger volume of fluid than the original volume lost must be infused (3:1 rule).

4. Response to resuscitation
  a. Rapid response
    (1) "Responders" become hemodynamically normal after the initial fluid bolus and remain so without continued boluses.
    (2) Early surgical consultation is necessary because of the possible need for operative intervention.
  b. Transient response
    (1) These patients respond to the initial fluid bolus, but again become hemodynamically unstable or show signs of decreased perfusion. Continued fluid infusion and blood transfusion are required to maintain normal hemodynamics.
    (2) These patients most often require rapid surgical intervention.
  c. No response
    (1) Patients who show no response to fluid boluses and blood transfusion have continued hemorrhage and require immediate surgical intervention to stop bleeding.
    (2) Keep in mind the nonhemorrhagic causes of shock, such as tension pneumothorax, cardiac tamponade, spinal cord injury, or pump failure from blunt cardiac injury.
5. End points of resuscitation
  a. The goal of HS resuscitation is restoration of end-organ perfusion.
  b. Traditional end points (normalization of blood pressure, heart rate, urine output, capillary refill) are inadequate.
    (1) Blood pressure (BP) does not equal cardiac output (CO) and therefore may not reflect normal perfusion.
    (2) Increased systemic vascular resistance (SVR) may raise BP, with no change in perfusion.
    (3) Patients with shock but normal BP are referred to as being in "compensated shock," because they are able to maintain BP despite bleeding and hypoperfusion
      (a) Even experienced practitioners can be fooled by patients in compensated shock.
      (b) Failure to recognize compensated shock can result in underresuscitation and its sequelae.
  c. Normalization of acidosis and oxygen consumption are best current indicators of adequate resuscitation at cellular level.
    (1) Base deficit (on arterial blood gas) and lactate level are good indicators of tissue perfusion.
    (2) Oxygen delivery and consumption calculated using pulmonary artery catheter.

B. Pitfalls in resuscitation
  1. Albumin and other colloids
    a. Colloids have no benefit over crystalloids in outcome or complication rate in resuscitation and may be harmful when used in HS.
    b. In normal volunteers, colloids remain in intravascular space and increase colloid oncotic pressure, drawing fluid into intravascular space and raising BP. This physiology is not applicable to patients with HS, in which colloids leak into the interstitial space, retain fluid, and increase organ edema.
    c. Lower-volume resuscitation, a proposed benefit of colloid use, opposes the physiologic need for resuscitation of the interstitial space with fluid according to the 3:1 rule.
    d. Albumin has been shown to decrease glomerular filtration and urine output, increase sodium retention, worsen oxygenation, and increase coagulopathy when used for HS.
    e. The U.S. Food and Drug Administration in 1996 warned of potential harm of albumin solutions.

       f. Colloid use in HS or critical care is hard to justify considering lack of evidence for benefit and its high cost.

  2. Vasopressors

       a. Vasopressors increase SVR and raise BP, according to the formula BP = CO × SVR. However, increased BP does not mean increased perfusion. Because normal tissue perfusion is the goal of shock resuscitation, vasopressors may have the opposite effect of worsening perfusion through vasoconstriction.

       b. Ensure adequate intravascular volume status prior to vasopressor therapy.

  3. Diuretics

       a. Well-resuscitated patients mobilize third-space fluids naturally 3 to 5 days after resuscitation.

       b. Induced diuresis (e.g., with furosemide) is unnecessary and may be harmful if it reduces intravascular volume and perfusion.

       c. Because normal edema resulting from proper shock resuscitation is the result of an inflammatory response (not cardiogenic failure) and is obligatory, it is not reversible in the early stages of shock.

       d. Analogy: one could not prevent or treat edema in a sprained ankle (result of inflammation) with diuretics, but could do so for ankle edema from congestive heart failure (result of increased hydrostatic pressure).

  4. Bicarbonate

       a. Bicarbonate combines with hydrogen ion to form water and carbon dioxide. CO_2 diffuses into cells and worsens intracellular acidosis

       b. It is not indicated for lactic acidosis from HS.

       c. The best treatment of acidosis from HS is restoring perfusion to ischemic tissues.

C. Investigational strategies

  1. These strategies for HS resuscitation have been well tested in animals, but less so in controlled clinical human trials. None have proved superiority over the standard treatment described earlier and are not considered standard of care, but may be used by experienced practitioners in specific circumstances.

  2. Hypertonic saline

       a. Provides restoration of BP with low volume

       b. Has antiinflammatory properties

       c. Sometimes used in prehospital setting or in hypotensive brain-injured patients

  3. Hypotensive resuscitation

       a. Entails limiting fluids and accepting low BP until definitive control of hemorrhage achieved, to avoid disrupting hemostatic plugs with normal BP

       b. Only one prospective human trial involving only penetrating chest and abdominal trauma

       c. Used only in patients planned for immediate surgery

       d. Contraindicated in brain injuries; unproved in blunt trauma

  4. Hemoglobin-based oxygen carriers

       a. Solution of polymerized or cross-linked hemoglobin molecules

       b. Able to carry and deliver oxygen

       c. Universally compatible

       d. Decreased immunomodulatory and infectious risks compared to blood

       e. May decrease need for blood transfusion

V. COMPLICATIONS

  1. Multiple organ failure (MOF)

       a. Patients who survive HS but die in the hospital later usually die of MOF or sepsis.

       b. MOF results from the systemic inflammatory response.

       c. Duration and severity of HS correlate with incidence of MOF.

       d. Patients who get more than 6 units of packed red blood cells in the first 12 hours of HS resuscitation have a higher risk of MOF.

2. Coagulopathy
   a. Hypothermia
      (1) Most common cause of coagulopathy in HS.
      (2) Significant coagulopathy begins at core body temperature lower than 34°C.
      (3) Undetectable on laboratory tests of coagulation; blood warmed to 37°C before testing.
      (4) Treat with warmed fluids and external rewarming.
   b. Platelet dysfunction and deficiency
      (1) Second most common cause of coagulopathy in HS.
      (2) Hypothermia causes platelet dysfunction.
      (3) Thrombocytopenia common with massive HS.
      (4) Degree of thrombocytopenia does not correlate directly with volume of blood loss.
      (5) Platelet transfusion indicated for platelet dysfunction (presence of microvascular bleeding or diffuse oozing) or platelet count less than 100,000/mm^3 with active bleeding.
      (6) Platelet transfusion not based on number of blood transfusions given.
   c. Factor dysfunction and deficiency
      (1) Factor dysfunction in HS is usually due to hypothermia (slows enzymatic reactions of coagulation).
      (2) Dilution of factors is possible with massive resuscitation.
      (3) Treat with normalizing body temperature, and fresh frozen plasma transfusion if prothrombin time is abnormal

Selected Readings

Cochrane Injuries Group Albumin Reviewers. Human albumin administration in critically ill patients: systematic review of randomized controlled trials. *BMJ* 1998;317:235–240.

Committee on Trauma of the American College of Surgeons. *Advanced Trauma Life Support course for doctors*, 7th ed. Chicago: American College of Surgeons, 2004, pp. 69–102.
Standard reference on the initial diagnosis and management of hemorrhagic shock.

Davis JW, Shackford SR, Mackersie RC, et al. Base deficit as a guide to volume resuscitation. *J Trauma* 1988;28:1464–1467
Reference on base deficit as an end point in resuscitation.

Forsythe SM, Schmidt GA. Sodium bicarbonate for the treatment of lactic acidosis. *Chest* 2000;117:260–267.
Review on rationale for lack of efficacy of sodium bicarbonate use in lactic acidosis.

Lucas CE. The water of life: a century of confusion. *J Am Coll Surg* 2001;192:86–93.
An excellent brief review of hemorrhagic shock pathophysiology and fluid shifts.

Moore, EE. Blood substitutes: the future is now. *J Am Coll Surg* 2003;196:1–17.
Excellent reference on pathophysiology, development, and uses of hemoglobin-based oxygen carriers.

The SAFE Study Investigators. A comparison of albumin and saline for fluid resuscitation in the intensive care unit. *N Engl J Med* 2004;350:2247–2256.
A prospective randomized blinded trial in almost 7,000 patients showing no difference in outcomes between saline and albumin in critically ill patients.

Velanovich V. Crystalloid versus colloid fluid resuscitation: a meta analysis of mortality. *Surgery* 1989;105:65–71.
Two of the eight meta-analyses on fluids and mortality.

125   TRAUMA: AN OVERVIEW
Kevin Dwyer and Arthur L. Trask

I. HISTORICAL PERSPECTIVE

A. Trauma derives from the Greek meaning "bodily injury."

B. The Roman army had areas to treat injured soldiers.

C. The history of trauma care follows the methods for care of the wounded soldier.

D. The first organized battlefield trauma delivery system functioned during the Napoleonic Wars with the advent of medical teams bringing care to injured soldiers under the direction of Jean Dominique Larrey,

E. Survival from battlefield injury greatly improved during the twentieth century with the advent of blood transfusion, the understanding of resuscitation of hemorrhagic shock, methods of hemorrhage control, and early transport of the patient to definitive care.

F. The deficiency of the health care system's response to the trauma patient was outlined in the 1966 National Research Council/National Academy of Sciences publication: "Accidental Death and Disability: the Neglected Disease of Modern Society."

G. Congress enacted the National Traffic and Motor Vehicle Safety Act and the Highway Safety Act in 1966 in response to that publication, and the National Highway Traffic Safety Administration was established to develop emergency medical services (EMS) and safety programs.

H. The EMS Systems Act of 1973 helped develop the lead agency for nationwide EMS development and contributed substantial federal funds to implement the initial EMS.

I. The American College of Surgeons (ACS) had taken a leading role in the delivery of quality care for the trauma patient. The origins of the ACS Committee on Trauma (COT) reach back to 1922. The ACS COT first published the guide "Optimal Hospital Resources for Care of the Injured Patient" in 1976 and have continued to update this document as trauma systems and care of the trauma patient has changed and improved.

J. The ACS COT also developed the Advance Trauma Life Support Course (ATLS) that teaches initial assessment and management of trauma patients. The course is an essential requirement for surgical and emergency medicine training programs as well as for in-practice physicians who treat trauma patients.

K. The ACS COT has a trauma center/system consultation/verification program, which was developed as an external review program for hospitals that desire verification of their trauma center status based on the objective criteria listed earlier. This program has helped states develop trauma systems with designated trauma centers,

L. The Trauma Care Systems Planning and Development Act of 1990 established the Department of Trauma and Emergency Medical Systems (DTEMS). DTEMS published the Model Trauma Care System Plan in 1992, which give guidelines for establishing regional trauma care systems for both urban and rural America.

M. The current guide for trauma systems/center development can be found in the 1999 ACS COT document, "Resources for Optimal Care of the Injured Patient."

II. DESCRIPTION

A. Mechanisms of injury are divided into blunt and penetrating trauma.

    1. Blunt trauma involves mechanisms of injury with blunt force, such as car crashes, falls from a height, pedestrian stuck by a car, and so forth

    2. Penetrating trauma is caused by a penetrating force such as a gunshot wound or stabbing.

B. The injury severity score (ISS) is a sum of an anatomic injury scoring (AIS) system that is a posttreatment measure of the severity of injury. Patients with an ISS greater than 15 are considered severely injured and should have been triaged to a trauma center.

C. Severely injured patients have three peaks of mortality. Greater than 50% will die immediately at the scene of the trauma, 20% to 30% will die within the first 2 to 24 hours, and the rest will die usually in intensive care from multiple-organ failure in the future.

1. The patients who die immediately die from brain or spinal cord (CNS) injury, or hemorrhage. *Only injury prevention can reduce these injuries.*

2. The patients who die within a few hours also die of the same types of injuries. These patients have an increased chance of survival if they are taken to a trauma center.

3. The mortality of the third group of patients is also reduced in a center dedicated to taking care of the critically injured and critically ill.

III. TRAUMA CENTERS

A. Individual states usually designate trauma centers as centers of excellence for a dedicated response to caring for severely injured patients.

B. Levels of trauma centers

1. Level I centers are designed for the most serious injuries of all types. They must have all subspecialties represented, with the immediate response of a complete trauma team. They are required to also have a prominent role in education and research and trauma prevention.

2. Level II centers are similar to level I centers except they may be missing a few of the subspecialty areas and are not required to fulfill the education and research tasks. They are to have an immediate response of the trauma team but have a lesser role for injury prevention in their community.

3. Level III centers are designed to act as a point of entry for critically ill trauma patients, to allow immediate stabilization of the ABCs and then transfer to a higher-level trauma center for definitive care. They often care for the single system injuries that don't need higher-level care.

IV. TRAUMA SYSTEMS

A. A comprehensive trauma system encompasses all aspects of care of the injured patient. This includes injury prevention, prehospital care, acute care facilities (hospitals and trauma centers), and posthospital care to include inpatient and outpatient rehabilitation and nursing care.

B. Trauma registry is a data collection tool essential to any trauma system and the trauma centers within the system. National, state, regional, and trauma center registries collect comprehensive data on the mechanisms of injury, types of injuries, outcomes, and adverse events of the trauma patients. This data is essential to trauma research, education, injury prevention, and performance improvement.

C. Injury prevention at all levels—state, region, and system—is mandatory. The injury patterns for that state/region will be identified through the trauma registries. Strategies for prevention of injury should be developed through research and legislation to decrease mortality and morbidity from injury.

D. Performance improvement, "QI" as it used to be called, is another integral part of any trauma system/center. Each trauma center needs to have an active performance improvement program and be able to demonstrate performance improvement initiatives that elevate the quality of care of the trauma patients. In mature trauma systems, this performance improvement program must include regional prehospital, and posthospital facilities and nontrauma acute-care hospitals as well as the trauma centers.

V. DISASTER PREPAREDNESS

A. A regional disaster plan must include all prehospital units and acute-care hospitals as well as specialized trauma centers within a region.

B. With the possibility of massive injuries and mortality from weapons of mass destruction, the disaster plan must include expanded regional capabilities as well as decontamination resources.

C. A disaster plan would fit well into a mature regional trauma system because the triage plan should be well established and monitored.

D. The trauma system response should be the key element to a disaster plan.

E. The entire plan should rely on an effective communication system with backup, an authoritative incident command center, and a quality scene triage team who are readily dispatched to a disaster scene.

VI. TREATMENT PRINCIPLES

A. The severely or potentially severely injured trauma patient should be taken quickly to the closest appropriate trauma center.

B. Securing a definitive airway is the only intervention that may be necessary to increase survival in the prehospital arena for the comatose patient. All other interventions should be avoided if they will delay transfer of the patient to a trauma center.

C. The patient needs to be transported with spinal immobilization.

D. The trauma patient needs to undergo initial assessment and resuscitation by Advanced Trauma Life Support (ATLS) principles (ABCDE).

E. More definitive management of specific injuries and principles of resuscitation can be found in other chapters in this section of the manual.

Selected Readings

Committee on Trauma of the American College of Surgeons. Advanced Trauma Life Support program for physicians. Chicago: American College of Surgeons, 1997.
Fundamental course on the initial assessment and management of trauma patients. The new version is due in early 2005.

Committee on Trauma, American College of Surgeons. Resources for Optimal Care of the Injured Patient: 1999. Chicago: American College of Surgeons, 1999.
The ultimate resource for trauma center design, with guidelines for system development. A new version is due soon.

Health Resources and Services Administration. Model Trauma Care System Plan. Rockville, MD: Health Resources and Services Administration, 1992.
Well-done assessment and guidelines for trauma systems.

Mann N, Mullins R. Research recommendations and proposed action items to facilitate trauma system implementation and evaluation. *J Trauma* 1999;47(3):S75–78.
An outline of research on trauma systems.

National Research Council. Accidental death and disability: the neglected disease of modern society. Washington, DC: National Academy of Sciences, 1966.
The landmark study that led to the development of NHTSA and emergency medical services (EMS) in response to civilian trauma.

I. OVERVIEW. Traumatic brain injury (TBI) is a leading cause of death and disability in children and adults. Nearly 1.6 million head injuries occur every year in the United States, and more than 250,000 individuals will require hospitalization. There are approximately 60,000 deaths from TBI, and 80,000 patients are left with permanent neurologic disabilities. The economic burden is $100 billion annually. Motor vehicle crashes (MVC) are the most common cause of TBI and are especially common in young adults and teens; alcohol use has been shown to be a factor in 40% of TBI. Falls are the second most common cause and are seen mostly in the extremes of age.

II. PATHOPHYSIOLOGY

  A. *Primary brain injury* is a direct, immediate result of a traumatic insult and can be thought of as being either a *focal* or a *diffuse* lesion.

  B. *Secondary brain injury* occurs after the primary injury and most often results from hypotension (shock) or hypoxemia, or a combination of both.

  C. Systemic effects and consequences of TBI

    1. Diabetes insipidus (DI). The supraoptic and paraventricular nuclei of the hypothalamus produce arginine vasopressin, which acts on the kidney to increase urine osmolality. Damage to these hypothalamic nuclei and their axons within the pituitary stalk or the neurohypophysis results in polyuria, an inability to concentrate the urine, and elevated serum osmolality.

    2. Seizure disorders. Seizures following head injury are divided into early (less than 1 week from injury) and late (greater than 1 week from injury).

    3. Coagulopathies. Trauma to the head and brain, as with all trauma, usually results in a hypercoagulable state. With severe TBI, hypocoagulopathy may occur as a result of increased fibrinolysis or increased release of tissue factor, resulting in a disseminated intravascular coagulopathy (DIC).

    4. Syndrome of inappropriate antidiuretic hormone (SIADH). The inappropriate secretion of ADH results in water retention with the dilution of the serum electrolytes, most notably sodium ion.

    5. Cerebral salt-wasting syndrome (CSWS) is thought to be caused by a brain-secreted naturetic peptide. The difference between SIADH and CSWS can usually be elicited by measuring urine sodium levels, which are inappropriately elevated in CSWS. In contrast to SIADH, hypovolemia occurs along with hyponatremia.

    6. Immune system compromise is present in many major TBI patients but is not well understood.

    7. Other effects may include excessive excretion of endogenous catecholamines that may affect cardiac and pulmonary function. The mechanism for this effect is yet to be determined.

  D. High intracranial pressures (ICP) and brain herniation are the result of a mass effect or swelling inside the skull.

    1. The Monroe-Kellie hypothesis states that the skull is a rigid compartment filled to capacity with essentially noncompressible contents. If volume rises in one compartment, there must be a decrease of volume in one of the remaining compartments for pressure to remain unchanged (Fig. 126-1).

    2. Brain herniation occurs when the ICP reaches a point where brain contents herniate through the tentorial opening (incisura) either from the cranial vault downward or upward from the posterior fossa.

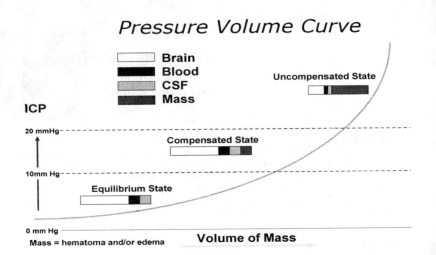

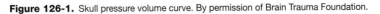

Figure 126-1. Skull pressure volume curve. By permission of Brain Trauma Foundation.

E. Brain death definition. An individual with *irreversible* cessation of all functions of the entire brain, including the brainstem. This is manifested by total absence of blood flow to all parts of the brain.

III. DIAGNOSIS

A. History of a traumatic event

B. The physiologic score (Glasgow Coma Scale score [GCS]) decreased; GCS of 8 or lower is considered coma.

C. Neurologic examination

    1. examination of pupil size and reactivity

    2. examination for skull fractures and leakage of cerebrospinal fluid from wounds, nares, or ears

    3. motor and sensation examination

    4. peripheral and central reflexes, as well as rectal tone

D. In the multiply injured patient, prioritizing the most life-threatening injuries first is essential.

E. Other tests, such as magnetic resonance imaging (MRI), transcranial Doppler (TCD), angiogram, pupillometry, and others, are usually not indicated during the early care of TBI patients.

F. Specific injuries: skull fractures, epidural hematomas (EDH), subdural hematomas (SDH), subarachnoid hemorrhage (SAH), contusions, diffuse axonal injuries (DAI). See Selected Readings for further details on diagnosis and specifics of these injuries.

G. ICP monitoring

H. Brain herniation criteria are a GCS of 3 or 4 *and* either bilateral dilated, nonreactive pupils or a single dilated nonreactive pupil.

IV. TREATMENT

A. Prevent/avoid secondary injury caused from hypotension or hypoxia or the combination of both.

B. Moderate to minor brain injuries require a different strategy beyond the scope of this chapter.

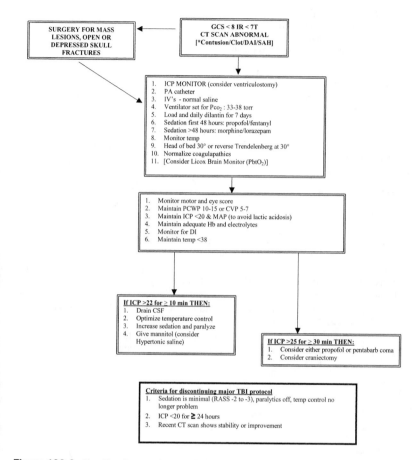

Figure 126-2. Algorithm for severe traumatic brain injury (TBI) management. CVP, central venous pressure; DAI, diffuse axonal injuries; DI, diabetes insipidus; GCS, Glasgow coma scale score; ICP, intracranial pressure; MAP, mean arterial pressure; PCWP, pulmonary capillary wedge pressure; SAH, subarachnoid hemorrhage.

- **C.** Those who, by serial examinations and computed tomography (CT) scan have a major brain/head injury are managed by a strategy that is outlined in Figure 126-2
- **D.** *Urgent surgery* is performed to remove significant SDH, EDH, elevate depressed skull fractures and washout open skull fractures. The emphasis is on *URGENT* because studies have shown sooner is better than later.

V. COMPLICATIONS
- **A.** The most significant complication is brain herniation, which if not managed immediately will result in brain death.
- **B.** Anticipate and prevent
  - **1.** Seizures
  - **2.** DI
  - **3.** SIADH
  - **4.** CSWS

5. Coagulopathies
6. Cardiac and pulmonary complications
7. Immune deficiency
   a. Ventilator-associated pneumonia (VAP)
   b. Sepsis

VI. PROGNOSIS

A. "No head injury is so serious that it should be despaired of nor so trivial that it can be ignored."
B. The long-term outcome for serious/major TBI has improved significantly following implementation of the guidelines developed by the Brain Trauma Foundation in association with the American Association of Neurologic Surgery.
C. Physiatrists and TBI rehabilitation programs have also added to the positive progress for major TBI patients.

Selected Readings

Jane J, Francel P. Age and outcome of head injury. In: *Narayan RK*, ed. *Neurotrauma*. New York: McGraw-Hill, 1996, pp. 793–804.

Management and prognosis of severe traumatic brain injury. A Joint project of the Brain Trauma Foundation and American Association of Neurological Surgeons, 2000.
   An excellent resource. Look for an update soon.

Manley G, Knudson M, et al. Hypotension, hypoxia and head injury: frequency, duration and consequences. *Arch Surg* 2001;136:1118–1123.
   Good discussion of secondary injury.

Marik P, Varon J, Trask T. Management of head trauma. *Chest* 2002;122:699–711.
   Good overview.

Marion D. Pathophysiology of cranial trauma. In: Batjer HH, Loftus CM, eds. *Textbook of neurosurgery: principles and practices.* Philadelphia: Lippincott Williams & Wilkins, 2003.

I. GENERAL PRINCIPLES

A. Complete spinal cord injury
1. No preservation of motor function and/or sensation three spinal segments below level of injury
2. Complete injuries above T6 usually associated with spinal shock
   a. Hypotension from interruption of sympathetics
   b. Bradycardia from unopposed vagal (parasympathetic) output
   c. Hypothermia
   d. Transient loss of all neurologic function resulting in a flaccid paralysis and areflexia
B. Incomplete spinal cord injury
1. Any preservation of motor and/or sensory function three spinal segments below level of injury, including sphincter function and/or perianal sensation
2. Specific incomplete spinal cord injury syndromes
   a. Central cord syndrome
      (1) Occurs in two patient populations: young athletes with congenital cervical stenosis and the elderly with acquired cervical stenosis from spondylosis
      (2) Hyperextension injury
      (3) Upper extremity weakness out of proportion to lower extremity weakness
      (4) No evidence of cervical spine fracture
   b. Brown-Sequard syndrome
      (1) Spinal cord hemisection
      (2) Loss of contralateral pain and temperature sensation, ipsilateral proprioception and vibratory sensation, and ipsilateral motor function
   c. Anterior cord syndrome
      (1) Spinal cord infarction in distribution of anterior spinal artery (anterior two thirds of cord)
      (2) Complete loss of motor function and loss of pain and temperature sensation but preserved posterior column function (proprioception and vibratory sensation)
   d. Conus medullaris syndrome
      (1) Associated with thoracolumbar junction fracture
      (2) Early loss of sexual and sphincter function
      (3) Symmetric "saddle" loss of motor and/or sensory function in lower extremities
C. American Spinal Injury Association (ASIA) impairment scale
1. A—Complete: no sensory or motor function preserved in sacral segments S4 to S5
2. B—Incomplete: sensory, but not motor, function preserved below neurologic level and extends through sacral segments S4 to S5
3. C—Incomplete: motor function preserved below neurologic level with muscle grade less than antigravity strength
4. D—Incomplete: motor function preserved below neurologic level with muscle grade greater than or equal to antigravity strength
5. E—Normal: sensory and motor functions normal

    D. Stability
1. Clinical instability: potential for further neurologic injury if allowed to bear normal physiologic loads
2. Radiographic instability: greater than 3.5 mm subluxation or greater than 11 degrees angulation
3. Missile injuries do not destabilize spine except in rare cases

    E. Level of injury: lowest spinal segment with completely normal function

II. PATHOPHYSIOLOGY

    A. Primary injury mechanisms
1. Impact plus persisting compression from burst fracture, fracture-dislocation, and herniated disc
2. Impact only with transient compression from hyperextension
3. Distraction from hyperflexion
4. Laceration or transection from burst fracture, laminar fracture, fracture-dislocation, or missile

    B. Secondary injury mechanisms
1. Neurogenic shock and hypoperfusion to injured spinal cord
2. Local vascular damage of the cord microcirculation
   - **a.** Disruption of capillaries and venules
   - **b.** Hemorrhage within cord parenchyma
   - **c.** Reduction of spinal cord blood flow by thrombosis, vasospasm, and mechanical compression of blood supply
   - **d.** Loss of autoregulation
3. Biochemical changes
   - **a.** Excitotoxicity
   - **b.** Neurotransmitter accumulation
   - **c.** Arachidonic acid release
   - **d.** Free radical production
   - **e.** Eicosanoid production
   - **f.** Lipid peroxidation
   - **g.** Endogenous opioids
   - **h.** Cytokines
4. Electrolyte shifts
   - **a.** Increased intracellular calcium
   - **b.** Increased extracellular potassium
   - **c.** Increased intracellular sodium
5. Edema
6. Loss of energy metabolism with decreased adenosine 5'-triphosphate (ATP) production

III. DIAGNOSIS

    A. Neurologic examination
1. Determination of completeness of injury
2. Determination of level of injury

    B. Radiographic examination
1. Plain radiograph anteroposterior (AP) and lateral views for fractures, subluxations, or dislocations
2. Computed tomography (CT) scan to further delineate fracture type at the level of injury
3. Magnetic resonance imaging (MRI) at the level of injury to determine degree of cord compression/injury and components of compression from soft tissue (e.g., herniated disc, epidural hematoma)

IV. TREATMENT

    A. Management in the field
1. As with all trauma victims, airway, breathing, and circulation (ABCs) first

2. Victims of major blunt trauma, whether conscious or unconscious, should be deemed to have spinal cord injury until proved otherwise
3. Cervical collar in combination with rigid backboard should be used to immobilize spine

B. Assessment in the hospital
  1. Degree of stability
     a. Rigid immobilization with cervical traction and kinetic treatment table or halo-vest orthosis for unstable fractures
     b. Nonrigid immobilization with cervical collar or thoracolumbosacral orthosis for stable fractures
  2. Need for neurologic decompression
     a. Closed reduction and traction for dislocation or subluxation with cord and/or root compression to restore normal alignment
        (1) Neurologic deterioration after reduction from herniated disc
        (2) Recommend MRI prior to reduction in obtunded patients
     b. Open surgical reduction and decompression for irreducible dislocation, bone fragment in the canal, herniated disc, or epidural hematoma causing persistent cord and/or root compression
  3. Timing of decompressive surgery
     a. Experimental evidence
        (1) Threshold spinal cord injury was produced in dogs with inflatable epidural balloons for varying amounts of time
        (2) Earlier decompression (within 8 hours) resulted in better neurologic recovery for the animal by minimizing secondary injury mechanisms of cord compression
     b. Clinical evidence
        (1) Results from animal experiments have not met with the same straightforward results in clinical practice.
        (2) Most spinal cord injuries suffered in humans are suprathreshold injuries with irreversible primary disruption of ascending and descending white matter tracts and neuronal death at the time of injury.
        (3) Early decompression may reverse secondary injury mechanisms but will not affect irreversible primary injury mechanisms.
        (4) Controversy in early versus delayed surgical decompression based on inability to differentiate threshold versus suprathreshold injuries on clinical or radiographic grounds.
  4. Potential for healing
     a. Fusion surgery not indicated for predominantly bony injuries with excellent potential for healing if properly immobilized
     b. Fusion surgery indicated for predominantly ligamentous injuries with poor potential for healing
     c. Soft clinical evidence that patients with early surgical fusion of unstable spine fracture do better because earlier mobilization was allowed and systemic complications from prolonged bed rest were avoided

C. Solumedrol protocol
  1. Administered as standard of care for spinal cord injury except in cases of penetrating injury because of possible visceral involvement and sepsis. Give within 8 hours of injury: 30 mg/kg intravenous (IV) methylprednisolone over 1 hour; then 5.4 mg/kg per hour for the next 23 hours.
  2. Third National Acute Spinal Cord Injury Study (NASCIS) found beneficial effects at 6 weeks and 6 months of 48 hours solumedrol regimen started 3 to 8 hours postinjury
  3. Beneficial effects of 48-hour solumedrol protocol must be weighed against increased incidence of sepsis and pneumonia when compared to 24-hour solumedrol group

D. Hypothermia
  1. Cooling protects spinal cord by decreasing its metabolic requirements and increasing its tolerance for decreased blood flow.

    2. Efficacy and safety of mild hypothermia in clinical setting is unproved at the present time.

    3. Systemic complications of hypothermia include cardiac arrhythmias, metabolic acidosis from decreased perfusion and hypoxemia to peripheral tissues, endocrine dysfunction, pancreatitis, and coagulopathy.

V. COMPLICATIONS

  A. Cardiovascular

    1. Hypotension and bradycardia from spinal shock.

    2. Symptomatic treatment with dopamine to support blood pressure and atropine to increase heart rate in period of spinal shock.

    3. Autonomic hyperreflexia occurring in patients with spinal cord injury above T6.

    4. Patients with autonomic hyperreflexia have exaggerated autonomic response, including headache, flushing, diaphoresis, and paroxysmal hypertension, to normally innocuous stimuli.

    5. Autonomic hyperreflexia can be life-threatening and requires rapid control of hypertension and elimination of offending stimuli.

  B. Pulmonary

    1. High cervical injuries above segments C3 to C5 that contribute to phrenic nerve may leave patient ventilator dependent or with weak cough mechanism to clear airway secretions or obstructions.

    2. Aggressive pulmonary toilet is required to prevent atelectasis and pneumonia.

    3. Immobilization makes patient vulnerable to deep vein thrombosis (DVT) and pulmonary embolism.

    4. DVT prophylaxis should be undertaken with subcutaneous heparin combined with sequential compression devices for lower extremities

  C. Gastrointestinal

    1. Most patients with acute spinal cord injury present with partial ileus.

    2. Nasogastric or orogastric tube should be placed to prevent gastric distention and perforation.

    3. H_2-receptor antagonist or proton pump inhibitor should be used to prevent ulcers from stress of trauma and/or use of high-dose steroids.

    4. Not all cardinal signs of acute abdomen are present in spinal cord–injured patients.

  D. Genitourinary

    1. Most spinal cord injured patients cannot void spontaneously.

    2. Indwelling Foley catheter used until patient is hemodynamically and neurologically stable.

    3. Intermittent straight catheterization used after Foley removed to decrease incidence of urinary tract infections (UTIs).

  E. Infectious disease/fever workup

    1. White blood cell count, erythrocyte sedimentation rate (ESR), and C-reactive protein (CRP) as markers of infection

    2. Chest radiograph for atelectasis or pneumonia

    3. Urinalysis and urine cultures for UTI

    4. Duplex ultrasound of lower extremities for DVT

    5. Abdominal laboratory tests, including liver function tests, total and direct bilirubin, and amylase and lipase, for hepatitis, acalculous cholecystitis, or pancreatitis

    6. Blood cultures for sepsis

    7 Inspection of skin/wound for infection

    8. Bone scan and plain radiographs for heterotopic bone formation

  F. Cutaneous

    1. Decubitus ulcers from prolonged positioning on pressure points

    2. Prevention with frequent turning protocol, daily bathing and lotion application, and careful skin inspection

3. Superficial wounds treated with daily sterile occlusive dressings
4. Deep, infected, or devascularized wounds treated with débridement and/or grafting
G. Musculoskeletal
1. Development of contractures and spasticity may be slowed by aggressive range-of-motion exercises
2. Heterotopic bone formation may be halted with etidronate sodium

Selected Readings

Allen AR. Surgery of experimental lesions of the spinal cord equivalent to crush injury of fracture dislocation of the spinal column. A preliminary report. *JAMA* 1911;57:878–880.
Part of series of landmark papers describing primary and secondary spinal cord injury mechanisms.

Allen BL, Ferguson RL, Lehmann TR, et al. A mechanistic classification of closed, indirect fractures and dislocations of the lower cervical spine. *Spine* 1982;7:1–27.
Classic paper describing primary spinal cord injury mechanisms.

Atkinson PP, Atkinson JLD. Spinal shock. *Mayo Clin Proc* 1996;71:384–389.
Comprehensive paper describing syndrome of spinal shock and its pathophysiology.

Bracken MB, Shepard MJ, Holford TR, et al. Administration of methylprednisolone for 24 or 48 hours or tirilazad mesylate for 48 hours in the treatment of acute spinal cord injury. Results of the third national acute spinal cord injury randomized controlled trial. *JAMA* 1997;277:1597–1604.
Important paper defining administration of solumedrol in spinal cord injury as standard of care.

Brown-Sequard CE. Transmission croissee des impressions sensitives par la moelle epiniere. *CR Seances Soc Biol Fil* 1850;2:70.
Initial paper describing Brown-Sequard syndrome.

Burns AS, Rivas DA, Ditunno JF. The management of neurogenic bladder and sexual dysfunction after spinal cord injury. *Spine* 2001;26:S129–136.
Comprehensive discussion of management of bladder and sexual dysfunction after spinal cord injury.

Denis F. The three column spine and its significance in the classification of acute thoracolumbar spinal injuries. *Spine* 1983;8:817.
Classic paper introducing three-column model of spine stability.

Frankel HL, Mathias CJ. Cardiovascular aspects of autonomic dysreflexia since Guttman and Whitteridge (1947). *Paraplegia* 1979;17:46–51.
Comprehensive description of autonomic hyperreflexia and its management in spinal cord–injured patients.

Green BA, Eismont FJ, O'Heir JT. Pre-hospital management of spinal cord injuries. *Paraplegia* 1987;25:229.
Descriptive paper on the management of spinal cord injury in the field.

Green BA, Green KL, Klose KJ. Kinetic therapy for spinal cord injury. *Spine* 1983;8:722.
Useful paper describing the prevention of decubitus ulcers.

Green D, Lee MY, Ito VY. Fixed- vs. adjusted-dose heparin in the prophylaxis of thromobembolism in spinal cord injury. *JAMA* 1988;260:1255–1258.
Important paper illustrating risk of DVT/PE and its prevention in spinal cord injury.

Gore R, Mintzer R, Galenoff L. Gastrointestinal complications of spinal cord injury. *Spine* 1981;6:538.
Descriptive review of gastrointestinal ailments specific to spinal cord–injured patients.

Hurlbert RJ. The role of steroids in acute spinal cord injury: an evidence-based analysis. *Spine* 2001;26:S39–46.
Study refuting the role of solumedrol as standard of care in acute nonpenetrating spinal cord injuries.

Inamasu J, Ichikizaki K. Mild hypothermia in neurologic emergency: an update. *Ann Emerg Med* 2002;40:220–230.
Study summarizing recent developments in hypothermia, as well as therapeutic potential and limitations, in traumatic brain injury, spinal cord injury, ischemic stroke, subarachnoid hemorrhage, cardiac arrest, hepatic encephalopathy, perinatal asphyxia, and infantile viral encephalopathy

Inamasu J, Nakamura Y, Ichikizaki K. Induced hypothermia in experimental traumatic spinal cord injury: an update. *J Neurol Sci* 2003;209:55–60.
Review of laboratory investigations showing efficacy of hypothermia in improving functional outcome of mild to moderate traumatic spinal cord injury

Jacobs RR, Asher MA, Snider RK. Thoracolumbar spinal injuries: a comparative study of recumbent and operative treatment in 100 patients. *Spine* 1980;5:463.
One of few studies attempting to address question of early versus delayed surgery in clinical practice.

Kane T, Capen DA, Waters R, et al. Spinal cord injury from civilian gunshot wounds: the Rancho experience 1980–88. *J Spinal Disord* 1991;4:306–311.
Landmark study discussing stability of the spine after penetrating missile injury.

Levi L, Wolf A, Rigamonti D, et al. Anterior decompression in cervical spine trauma: does the timing of surgery affect the outcome? *Neurosurgery* 1991;29:216–222.
One of few studies attempting to address question of early versus delayed surgery in clinical practice.

Nesathurai S. The role of methylprednisolone in acute spinal cord injuries. *J Trauma* 2001;51:421–423.
Paper disputing the beneficial effects of solumedrol in acute spinal cord injuries.

Reyes O, Sosa I, Kuffler DP. Neuroprotection of spinal neurons against blunt trauma and ischemia. *PR Health Sci J* 2003;22:277–286.
Review of experimental evidence neuroprotection afforded by hypothermia in ischemic spinal cord.

Rimoldi RL, Zigler JE, Capen DA, et al. The effect of surgical intervention on rehabilitation time in patients with thoracolumbar and lumbar spinal cord injuries. *Spine* 1992;17:1443.
One of few studies attempting to address question of early versus delayed surgery in clinical practice.

Robertson PA, Ryan MD. Neurologic deterioration after reduction of cervical subluxation: mechanical compression by disc material. *J Bone Joint Surg* 1992;72B:224–227.
Paper describing significant complication of intervertebral disc rupture after closed reduction and traction.

Schneider RC. The syndrome of acute central cervical spinal cord injury. *J Neurosurg* 1954;11:546.
Classic paper describing central cord syndrome.

Schneider RC. The syndrome of acute anterior spinal cord injury. *J Neurosurg* 1955;12:95–122.
Paper with first description of anterior cord syndrome.

Schneider RC, Crosby EC, Russo RH. Traumatic spinal cord syndromes and their management. *Clin Neurosurg* 1972;20:424–492.
One of first studies attempting to address question of early versus delayed surgery in clinical practice.

Sonntag VKH, Hadley MN. Nonoperative management of cervical spine injuries. *Clin Neurosurg* 1988; 34:630–649.
One of few studies attempting to address question of early versus delayed surgery in clinical practice.

Stover SL. Heterotopic ossification. In: Block RF, Basbaum M, eds. *Management of spinal cord injuries*. Baltimore: Williams & Wilkins, 1986, p. 127.

Comprehensive description of pathophysiology and management of heterotopic ossification in spinal cord injury.

Tarlov IM. Acute spinal cord compression paralysis. *J Neurosurg* 1972;36:10–20.
Important paper discussing implications for early versus delayed surgery for decompression in threshold and suprathreshold spinal cord injuries.

Tarlov IM, Klingler H. Spinal cord compression studies. II. Time limits for recovery after acute compression in dogs. *AMA Arch Neurol Psychiatry* 1954;71:271–290.
Part of classic series of animal experiments addressing timing of cord decompression.

Tator CH. Review of experimental spinal cord injury with emphasis on the local and systemic circulatory effects. *Neurochirurgie* 1991;37:291–302.
Part of series of landmark papers describing primary and secondary spinal cord injury mechanisms.

Tator CH, Fehlings MG. Review of the secondary injury theory of acute spinal cord trauma with emphasis on vascular mechanisms. *J Neurosurg* 1991;75:15–26.
Important review of secondary injury mechanisms in spinal cord injury.

White AA, Panjabi M. *Clinical biomechanics of the spine.* Philadelphia: JB Lippincott, 1990.
Important paper defining radiographic criteria for spine stability.

128 ABDOMINAL TRAUMA
Reza Askari and Christopher P. Michetti

I. OVERVIEW
- **A.** Background
  1. The abdomen is frequently injured after blunt or penetrating trauma
  2. Abdominal trauma occurs in 20% of civilian injuries requiring operation
  3. Half of all preventable trauma deaths related to suboptimal management of abdominal trauma
  4. Physical examination inadequate to identify or exclude intraabdominal injuries
  5. Multiple factors, including mechanism of injury, body region injured, hemodynamic and neurologic status, and associated injuries, influence the diagnostic approaches used and outcome of abdominal injuries
- **B.** Etiology
  1. Blunt trauma (most common etiology) caused by motor vehicle crashes (MVCs), motorcycle crashes, falls, assaults, and pedestrians struck by vehicles
  2. Penetrating abdominal trauma usually caused by gunshot or stab wounds
  3. Almost all causes preventable
- **C.** Diagnosis
  1. History and physical examination
     - **a.** History of traumatic event important in determining likelihood of intraabdominal injury
     - **b.** Suggestive clinical findings: abdominal wall contusions, pain, tenderness, or unexplained hypotension
     - **c.** Peritoneal signs absent in 40% of patients with significant abdominal injuries
     - **d.** Physical findings unreliable for patients with abnormal sensorium secondary to head trauma, spinal cord injury, intoxication, or distracting pain from another source
  2. Plain radiographs. Chest radiograph (CXR) may reveal pneumoperitoneum, abdominal contents in the chest (ruptured diaphragm), or lower rib fractures, suggesting underlying liver or spleen injury
  3. Diagnostic peritoneal lavage (DPL)
     - **a.** Used to evaluate hemodynamically unstable patients with blunt trauma to detect gross hemoperitoneum; also used for stable patients with anterior stab wounds to determine peritoneal penetration
     - **b.** DPL for a stab wound is considered positive with 5,000 to 20,000 red blood cells per mL^3
     - **c.** High sensitivity, but poor specificity; can miss hollow viscus and diaphragmatic injuries and is not able to evaluate the retroperitoneum
  4. Computed tomography (CT)
     - **a.** Abdomen and pelvic CT is mainstay of diagnosis for abdominal and retroperitoneal injury in the hemodynamically stable patient
     - **b.** Sensitivity rates between 92% and 97.6% and specificity rates as high as 98.7% (particularly in the new fast helical scanners)
     - **c.** Unreliable in identifying hollow visceral injuries
     - **d.** Contraindicated in hemodynamically unstable patients (who would benefit from intervention, rather than diagnostic testing)
  5. Focused abdominal sonography for trauma (FAST)
     - **a.** Has gained acceptance in evaluation of abdominal trauma; used to examine the peritoneal cavity for blood

    b. Accurate in detecting intraabdominal blood (94% to 96%) in experienced hands

    c. Advantages include being rapid, portable, and noninvasive; disadvantages include low specificity for source of hemorrhage and high operator dependence

    d. Hollow viscus and retroperitoneal injuries not detected reliably by FAST

  6. Laparoscopy

    a. Use of diagnostic laparoscopy in blunt abdominal trauma is a developing field

    b. Difficult to adequately examine small bowel and retroperitoneum

    c. Accurate in determining peritoneal or diaphragmatic penetration from stab wounds or tangential gunshot wounds

  7. Nonoperative management and serial examination. Can be used for some blunt trauma and certain superficial stab wound patients with normal mental status

D. Treatment

  1. For blunt abdominal trauma, treatment dictated by the specific injuries present

  2. Abdominal exploration required in all patients with anterior abdominal gunshot wounds because of visceral injury in more than 90% of cases

  3. For stab wounds, exploration necessary in the presence of peritoneal signs, hemodynamic instability, evisceration of abdominal contents, or confirmed peritoneal penetration

  4. Unexplained hypotension with physical signs of abdominal trauma may warrant exploration

II. SPECIFIC INJURIES

A. Diaphragm

  1. Background

    a. Often caused by penetrating injuries

    b. Patients sustaining penetrating injuries between the nipple and the costal margin should be investigated to rule out diaphragmatic injury

    c. Following penetrating trauma, injury to the diaphragm involves both sides equally; in blunt trauma the left side is more frequently injured

  2. Diagnosis

    a. Radiologic modalities usually insufficient

    b. CXR abnormal in 85% of cases, yet diagnostic in only 27% of cases

    c. If diagnosis uncertain, further evaluation warranted with DPL, laparoscopy, thoracoscopy, or exploratory celiotomy

  3. Treatment

    a. Suture repair to create watertight closure

    b. Larger defects may require use of prosthetic material

  4. Complications

    a. Early recognition critical, because mortality of an untreated injury and subsequent bowel strangulation approximately 30%

    b. Small wounds usually enlarge over time due to movement of the diaphragm, so all known injuries should be repaired

B. Spleen

  1. Background

    a. Commonly injured in both blunt and penetrating trauma

    b. May result from a blow, fall, or sports injury involving the left chest, flank, or upper abdomen; side-impact MVCs a common cause

    c. Injuries graded from I (minimal) to V (most severe)

  2. Pathophysiology

    a. Produces immunoglobulin M and initiates cellular immune response

    b. Responsible for phagocytosis and clearance of bloodborne particles as well as antigen-antibody response

    c. Asplenic patients at increased risk for sudden and often lethal systemic bacterial infection, overwhelming postsplenectomy infection (OPSI)

    d. OPSI usually caused by encapsulated organisms (*Streptococcus pneumoniae, Haemophilus influenzae,* and *Neisseria meningitidis*)

  e. Incidence of OPSI 0.6% in children and 0.3% or less in adults after splenectomy for trauma; higher incidence after splenectomy for hematologic disease

  f. After splenectomy, vaccination against the three named organisms is given before discharge or 2 weeks postoperatively

  g. Use of prophylactic antibiotics in asplenic patients controversial

3. Diagnosis

  a. FAST or DPL should be considered in unstable patients

  b. CT with intravenous (IV) contrast (oral contrast unnecessary) the most sensitive and specific study for identifying and grading splenic injury

4. Treatment

  a. Nonoperative management (NOM) of blunt splenic injuries treatment of choice in hemodynamically stable patients

  b. Surgery indicated for hemodynamically unstable patients

  c. NOM of significant injuries should be done only at level I trauma centers with the experience and intensive resources required

  d. Patients undergoing NOM should be closely monitored, usually in an intensive care unit, for 48 to 72 hours with attention to vital signs, hematocrit, and abdominal examination

  e. Surgery or angiography with embolization can be considered for stable patients with extravasation of IV contrast on CT

  f. Success rate of nonoperative management approximately 90% but varies with grade of injury

  g. Surgical treatment varies depending on severity of injury, presence of shock, and associated injuries

5. Complications

  a. Recurrent or delayed bleeding

  b. Subphrenic abscess

  c. Left pleural effusion

  d. OPSI

C. Liver and porta hepatis

1. Background

  a. Most commonly injured organ in **blunt abdominal trauma**

  b. Spontaneous hemostasis observed in more than 50% of small hepatic lacerations at time of laparotomy

  c. Most liver injuries heal without intervention

  d. Overall mortality rate range 8% to 10% depending on number of associated injuries and injury severity

  e. Injuries graded from I to V, ranging from minor tears to major lobar disruptions and avulsion from the inferior vena cava

  f. Hemobilia results from erosion of an injured blood vessel into a biliary duct

  g. Traumatic injuries to the porta hepatis uncommon; most common with penetrating trauma and have 50% mortality rate from hemorrhage

2. Diagnosis

  a. Abdominal CT the most sensitive and specific study in identifying and assessing severity of injury

  b. FAST or DPL used in hemodynamically unstable patients

  c. Triad of right upper quadrant abdominal pain, jaundice, and gastrointestinal hemorrhage occurs in about one third of patients with hemobilia

3. Treatment

  a. Nonoperative management is treatment of choice in hemodynamically stable patients

  b. Angiography with embolization can be used to stop arterial hemorrhage

  c. Surgery indicated for patients who are hemodynamically unstable, develop peritonitis, or require continuous blood transfusions

    (1) Key principles in operative trauma: exposure and hemostasis

    (2) Simple lacerations managed by direct pressure, electrocautery, argon beam coagulation, and topical hemostatic agents

(3) Hepatic packing is the preferred initial technique for significant injuries with hemorrhage

(4) Compression of the portal triad (Pringle maneuver) is effective if the aforementioned techniques fail

(5) Damage control techniques (abdominal packing and temporary closure) are frequently applied to major liver injuries.

d. Gallbladder injuries treated with cholecystectomy

e. Injuries to extrahepatic bile ducts require primary repair or anastomosis to bowel

f. Bile leaks treated with closed drainage either at surgery or percutaneously with the aid of CT or ultrasound

4. Complications

a. Bleeding, hemobilia, bile leak, and intraabdominal abscess

b. Bile leak occurs in 25% of patients with major hepatic injuries

c. Abscesses occur in 10% of patients with liver injuries; likelihood of infection increases with grade of injury, number of transfusions, use of sump drains, concomitant bowel injury, and perihepatic packing

D. Small intestine

1. Background

a. Most commonly injured organ in **penetrating abdominal trauma**

b. Blunt small bowel injury (SBI) extremely rare, with an incidence of 1.2% of all trauma admissions; one quarter of all SBI are perforated

2. Diagnosis

a. *Difficult in cases of blunt trauma*

b. Physical findings may be delayed until patient is septic or has peritonitis

c. Presence of abdominal wall bruising, especially from a seat belt, should raise suspicion of SBI

d. Lumbar Chance fractures are associated with small bowel (as well as pancreatic and duodenal) injuries

e. Findings of SBI on CT may include free air, free fluid without solid organ injury, thickened bowel wall, and mesenteric hematoma. Aside from free air, all other CT findings are insensitive and nonspecific for SBI

(1) Of patients with perforated SBI, 14% have a "negative" CT

(2) Oral contrast leak seen on CT in only 2.9% of perforated SBI

f. *High index of suspicion required;* for peritonitis or increasing abdominal tenderness mandates exploration

3. Treatment. Operative technique depends on severity of injury and can range from simple repair to resection with anastamosis

4. Complications

a. Intraabdominal abscess

b. Sepsis, especially if treatment delayed

c. Anastamotic leak

Selected Readings

Committee on Trauma of the American College of Surgeons. *Advanced Trauma Life Support course for doctors*, 7th ed. Chicago: American College of Surgeons, 2004, pp. 69–102.
The national standard of trauma care. The ATLS course is available to physicians worldwide through the American College of Surgeons.

Fakhry SM, Watts DD, Luchette FA. Current diagnostic approaches lack sensitivity in the diagnosis of perforated blunt small bowel injury: analysis from 275,557 trauma admissions from the EAST multi-institutional HVI trial. *J Trauma* 2003;54:295–306.
The definitive study on small bowel injury; discusses prevalence, morbidity, mortality, and diagnostic modalities.

Peitzman AB, Heil B, Rivera L, et al. Blunt splenic injury in adults: Multi-institutional study of the Eastern Association for the Surgery of Trauma. *J Trauma* 2000;49:177–187.
A large multicenter study of nonoperative management of splenic injury, including factors contributing to success or failure and failure rates by grade of injury.

Trunkey DD. Hepatic trauma: contemporary management. *Surg Clin N Am* 2004;84:437–450.

A thorough presentation of the historical and modern treatment of liver injuries, including nonoperative and operative management.

I. GENERAL PRINCIPLES. A burn is a tissue injury resulting from excessive exposure to thermal, chemical, electrical, or radioactive agents. The transfer of thermal energy over time is proportional to dermal damage.

A. Epidermis: invaluable for its barrier and immunologic functions; prevents evaporative losses and bacterial invasion

B. Dermis: provides the overall structural integrity of the skin

C. The epidermis will recover so long as viable dermis is present; therefore, the essence of burn wound care is to maintain dermal viability

II. CLASSIFICATION. It is essential to distinguish between partial thickness (second-degree) and full-thickness (third-degree) injuries of the dermis, because the latter require operative intervention.

A. Full-thickness injury: pale, leathery, and insensate skin

B. Partial-thickness injury: blistering, weeping, pink, and painful skin

C. Currently no technology supersedes clinical experience in making this distinction

D. The injury is dynamic, and partial-thickness injuries can worsen ("convert") to full-thickness injuries for various reasons

III. EPIDEMIOLOGY

A. In the United States, 60,000 to 80,000 people are hospitalized annually for burn care, but only 1,500 to 2,000 people sustain greater than 40% total body surface area (TBSA) burns.

B. Risk factors

   1. Infants and elderly

   2. Cognitive impairment

      a. Behavioral disorders

      b. Alcohol/drug impairment

      c. Prognosis markedly improved in the past 25 years

   3. Paradigm shift toward "early" (within 5 days) operative excision because it was realized that burned tissue drives burn shock

   4. Diminution of burn wound sepsis and advances in critical care borrowed from all disciplines have contributed to improved outcomes for young patients and the elderly

   5. The 50% mortality for young adults is 90% TBSA and for elderly is 40% TBSA.

   6. Clinical data points predicting mortality (mortality rates of 90% when all three are present, and 33% when two factors are present):

      a. Age greater than 60 years

      b. TBSA burned 40% or greater

      c. Inhalation injury

IV. PATHOPHYSIOLOGY

A. Burn shock

   1. Vasodilatory shock and has an astounding volume requirement

   2. Occurs in 20% or greater TBSA burns

      a. Begins with intravascular volume depletion from interstitial edema in both burned and unburned tissue

    b. Forces central shunting of blood to improve core perfusion but deprives the burn wound

    c. Great insensible evaporative water losses until wounds are closed

  3. Similar to sepsis and systemic inflammatory response syndrome (SIRS)

B. Massive edema

  1. Burn wound

  2. Nonburned tissues

    a. Results from increased vascular permeability driven by vasoactive mediators including kinins, serotonin, histamine, prostaglandins, and oxygen radicals

    b. Decreased oncotic pressure

C. Cardiovascular response

  1. Decreasing preload

  2. First 48 hours decreasing cardiac output (despite resuscitation) (myocardial depressant factor has been suggested)

    a. Decreasing compliance and contractility; worse in inhalation injury

    b. Elevated cardiac enzymes

  3. After first 48 hours hyperdynamic cardiac state develops that may last for weeks

D. Infection: increased susceptibility

  1. Lungs

    a. Pneumonia

    b. Tracheobronchitis

  2. Wound beds: devitalized full-thickness eschar

    a. First 10 days are typically gram-positive organisms

    b. Next, *Pseudomonas* is a common and a potentially lethal organism

    c. Next, fungal infections

  3. Central line sites

  4. Urinary tract

  5. Gut

    a. If patient not fed, may be source of translocation of bacteria and source of sepsis

    b. Enteral feedings can prevent gut atrophy and immunoenhancing nutritional regimens, especially those with glutamine, further resist atrophy and may afford better outcomes.

V. DIAGNOSIS

A. History

  1. The heat source and circumstances of the injury

  2. When the burn injury occurs coincidentally with blunt trauma

    a. Life-threatening injuries take precedence in early management

    b. Burn skin management is secondary

  3. If burn occurs in closed space, expect inhalation injury

B. Scalds

  1. Energy transfer of hot liquid is underappreciated and may be lethal

  2. May involve large body surface areas particularly while bathing

  3. More serious in children age 4 years or younger or in elderly, who often have other comorbid conditions

C. Electrical injuries

  1. High voltage. May present with little injury to the skin but significant injuries to the muscle, vasculature and bone underneath

  2. Low voltage. Present as thermal burns, with injuries to the tissue from the outside in

VI. PHYSICAL EXAMINATION

A. Multiples of the number 9 (the rule of nines) (Fig. 129-1A)

B. Lund-Browder scale (Fig. 129-1B)

C. For noncontiguous injuries, the palmar surface of the patient's hand can be used to estimate 1% TBSA

"RULE OF NINES"   LUND-BROWDER

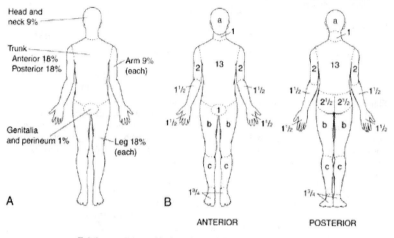

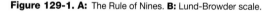

Figure 129-1. A: The Rule of Nines. B: Lund-Browder scale.

VII. TREATMENT

A. Burn shock

1. Ideal resuscitation meets the perfusion needs of the partial-thickness injury, prevents conversion to a full-thickness injury and optimizes organ function.
2. Underperfusion deprives the wound of nutrient delivery and gas exchange, leading to full-thickness conversion.
3. Excessive resuscitation adds to tissue edema, other complications, and conversion.
4. Central venous access is generally necessary and ideally, but not essentially, placed through nonburned tissue.
5. Resuscitative regimens
   a. TBSA burned and weight guide fluid management
   b. No evidence-based level I data for resuscitative fluids use
      (1) Isotonic electrolyte solutions such as lactated Ringer's solution during at least the first 12 hours of resuscitation and in most instances the first 24 hours (Table129-1)
      (2) Colloids use remains controversial
         (a) Albumin not sooner than 12 hours after injury
         (b) Fresh frozen plasma
6. May use the gut for fluid administration in burn resuscitation as long as patient is not on vasopressors
7. Consider adrenal insufficiency if patient is still hypotensive despite what appears to be adequate volume replacement
8. End points of resuscitation
   a. Urine output
      (1) Oliguria bodes poorly

TABLE 129-1	Parkland and Modified Brook Formulas	
Parkland Formula	Total fluids for 24 hours =	
	Ringer's lactate	4 mL × kg × %BSA
Modified Brooke Formula	Total fluids for 24 hours =	
	Ringer's lactate	1.5 mL × kg × %BSA
	Plasma	0.5 mL × kg × %BSA
	D5W	2,000 mL

Example: A 70-kg man with a 50% TBSA burn would thus have a total deficit of 14 L (4 mL × 70 kg × 50% BSA =14,000) in 24 hours. Half the 24-hour deficit should be replenished in the first 8 hours, due to the high risk of hypovolemic shock early in the course. In this example, that is 7 L within the first 8 hours or a rate of 875 mL per hour for the first 8 hours. It is important to note that this recommendation starts at the estimated time of injury, not simply the time care is rendered. The rate would subsequently be decreased to **438 mL per hour** for the next 16 hours.

        (2) Excessive (≥1 mL/kg/h)
           (a) Check urine electrolytes and glucose
           (b) If urinalysis normal, reduce fluid administration
    b. Base deficit/lactate levels normalized
    c. Central venous pressure and/or pulmonary artery catheter numbers suggest adequate preload and cardiac function
B. Metabolism and nutrition
  1. Metabolism
    a. Insensible fluid and protein losses from burn wounds are extreme and may result in hypothermia initially
    b. Then, as vasomotor autoregulation diminishes, significant evaporative heat loss occurs
    c. Keep the patient's room temperature over 90°F
    d. Increased muscle proteolysis, lipolysis, and gluconeogenesis occurs
    e. Hyperglycemia is common and may exacerbate muscle wasting
    f. Glucose control is essential; use insulin as needed.
    g. Hypermetabolic response that occurs after a thermal injury is greater than that observed after any other form of trauma or sepsis
    h. Protein catabolism is compounded by insensible losses through the wound bed and leaking into the interstitium, resulting in severe hypoproteinemia
  2. Nutrition
    a. Ideally, enteral nutrition should be started the day of the injury and can serve to provide volume and calories
    b. Caloric needs are — two to three times normal basal energy expenditure and require at least 2 g/kg protein with a calorie-to-nitrogen ratio approaching 100:1
    c. Total parenteral nutrition (TPN) only for patients not tolerating enteral feedings
    d. Anabolic enhancement
      (1) Recombinant human growth hormone. Caution: may cause hyperglycemia
      (2) Oxandrolone; given enterally, 10 mg twice daily
C. Infection
  1. Multiple defects in burn patient's immune system predisposes to an increased risk of infection.
  2. Burn wound sepsis
    a. Prevention of:
      (1) Topical antimicrobial agents (e.g., silver sulfadiazine or mafenide acetate). Mafenide acetate penetrates eschar and is most effective against gram-negative organisms but is known to cause metabolic acidosis as a carbonic anhydrase inhibitor.
      (2) Local wound care

b. Treatment. Urgent surgical excision and tissue coverage with autograft, skin substitute or topical antibiotics if suspect burn wound sepsis

D. Inhalation/respiratory injury

1. Restrictive respiratory failure secondary to burn eschar involving the torso requires urgent escharotomy

2. Inhalation injury

  a. Airway management, as always, is paramount

   (1) Observe for signs of upper airway obstruction, secondary to edema, which develops hours after the initial injury

   (2) Stridorous patients should be intubated urgently with an adequate endotracheal tube to allow for bronchoscopy as needed

   (3) Immediate life threats

    (a) Carbon monoxide

     i. Lethal level greater than 60% carboxyhemoglolin (COHgb)

     ii. With fraction of inspired oxygen (FiO_2) 100% (this should normalize COHgb levels)

     iii. Empirically treat all patients for 40 minutes

    (b) Hydrogen cyanide (CN-)

     i. Lethal level in serum 1 g/mL or greater

     ii. Inhibits cytochrome oxidase

     iii. Unlikely to occur without concommitant COHgb poisoning

     iv. Consider sodium thiosulphate

  b. Inhaled toxic products of combustion cause a severe inflammatory response in the bronchial pulmonary tree and systemically

   (1) Endobronchial and interstitial edema

   (2) Mucociliary dysfunction

   (3) Alveolar disruption

   (4) Functional pulmonary shunting

   (5) Decreased lung compliance

   (6) Endobronchial slough. Combines with exudates and fibrin to produce casts with increased bacterial growth and obstruction of airways

   (7) Neutrophils invade in alveolar spaces via the pulmonary vasculature and likely contribute to oxygen free radical production, promoting the inflammatory cascade and local injury

  c. Shock state is intensified with added inhalation injury often requiring up to 50% more fluid for adequate resuscitation

   (1) Mortality is greatly increased when matched to burn injuries of like size without inhalation injury

   (2) Currently, no objective scale of severity for inhalation injury

   (3) Upper airway assessment should be carried out prior to extubation by deflating cuff and noting an air leak. It is not safe to extubate if no air leak!

E. Chemical injury

1. Acids

  a. Burn by coagulation necrosis creating an eschar that limits deeper penetration

  b. Hydrofluoric acid burns carry the unique concern of calcium and magnesium chelation and risk cardiac arrest secondary to severe hypocalcemia and hypomagnesemia.

   (1) Intraarterial infusion of calcium gluconate has been met with some success and may limit digital ischemia

   (2) Calcium gluconate slurry may be massaged into the exposed area to potentiate systemic absorption

   (3) Carefully monitor ECG

2. Alkali. Burn by causing liquefaction necrosis in the subcutaneous fat, creating vascular thrombosis and subsequent dermal ischemia

F. Electrical injury

1. Life-threatening problems are dysrhythmias

2. Spinal cord injury

  a. Direct nerve/cord damage

  b. Tetany resulting in spinal column fracture and cord injury
  c. May result in respiratory problems depending on the level of injury
3. Cutaneous lesions. May be subtle and efforts should be made to find entrance and exit lesions, because these will direct the practitioner to focus on the intervening tissues
4. Compartment syndromes
  a. Myonecrosis is common, particularly in the upper extremities
  b. Myonecrosis puts the kidneys at risk for myoglobinuric renal failure
    (1) Elevations of creatinine phosphokinase into the tens of thousands are often present and maintaining a high urine output of 100 mL per hour reduces the risk of renal failure.
    (2) Mannitol may be added once resuscitation is well under way
    (3) Alkalinizing the urine is advocated by some
    (4) Consider monitoring the creatine phosphokinase (CPK) for several days to assess the amount of muscle damage and recovery; with persistent elevations suggesting need for further débridement
  c. Fasciotomy for elevated compartment pressures
  d. Débridement of nonviable or necrotic muscle and/or other tissue
5. Fluid resuscitation must be initiated quickly, with higher volumes than anticipated due to underlying tissue injury
G. Pain
  1. Rationale
    a. On a scale of 1 to 10, burns rate a 10
    b. Pain control leads to:
      (1) Patient comfort
      (2) Decreased catabolism, cardiovascular stress
      (3) Reduced risk of posttraumatic stress disorder
  2. Management
    a. Simultaneous drips of narcotic and benzodiazepines
    b. Anticipate higher than usual doses
    c. It is not prudent to reduce these medications for frequent neurologic assessment
    d. Once the patient's burn wounds have been managed adequately, a stepwise weaning of these agents is done to permit ventilator weaning and to avoid withdrawal

VIII. COMPLICATING FACTORS
A. Eschar formation. Escharotomy.
  1. Particularly for circumferential chest eschar to optimize oxygenation/ventilation
  2. For limbs to prevent compartment syndromes
B. Burn wound sepsis
  1. Early excision
    a. Has lessened this complication
    b. Nonetheless, loss of skin barrier and immune suppression may still not totally prevent burn wound sepsis
  2. Signs
    a. Diffuse or focal discoloration of the burn
    b. Purulent fluid from the wound
    c. Early eschar separation
  3. Treatment
    a. Immediate treatment or *systemic sepsis will occur*
    b. Total excision of the infected wound
    c. Systemic antibiotics covering the infective microbes
C. Abdominal compartment syndrome
  1. If allowed to occur, promotes renal failure, respiratory failure, and bowel ischemia
  2. Urinary bladder pressure measurement with transducer

3. Gives indirect measure of abdominal pressure

4. Pressure of 20 cm H_2O or greater suggests abdominal hypertension, and 30 cm H_2O or greater is generally accepted as requiring operative intervention; celiotomy and leaving the abdominal compartment open

D. Pneumonia

　　1. Increased risk because of immune compromise, immobility, and problems clearing secretions

　　2. Worse with inhalation injury (see section on inhalation injury)

　　3. Incidence increases with larger burns

　　4. Prevention

　　　　a. Good pulmonary toilet

　　　　b. Limit aspiration by keeping head of bed at 30 degrees

　　　　c. If on ventilator; lung protective ventilator management

　　　　d. Frequent surveillance

　　　　e. Prophylactic antibiotics are not recommended

　　5. Treatment. Culture-directed therapy reflecting local biograms

Selected Readings

Herndon DN, ed. *Total burn care*, 2nd ed. London: Saunders, 2002.
　A complete text regarding all aspects of burn care and management.

Ivy ME, Possenti PP, Kepros J, et al. Abdominal compartment syndrome in patients with burns. *J Burn Care Rehabil* 1999;20(5):351–353.
　An important paper on a previously under appreciated cause of mortality.

Pruitt BA. Does hypertonic burn resuscitation make a difference? *Crit Care Med* 2000;28(1):277–278.
　Deals with the ongoing research on fluid management in burns.

Rai J, Jeschke M, Barrow RE, et al. Electrical injuries: a 30-year review. *J Trauma* 1999;46(5):933–936.
　An excellent and credible review.

Ryan CM, Schoenfeld DA, Cassem EH, et al. Estimates of the probability of death from burn injuries. *N Engl J Med* 1998;338(25):1848–1850.
　A paper that shows how advances in burn care have greatly affected mortality.

Sheridan RL, Tompkins RG. What's new in burns and metabolism. *J Am Coll Surg* 2004;198(2):243–263.
　An excellent and credible review.

Thiessen JL, Herndon LD, Traber HA, et al. Smoke inhalation and pulmonary blood flow. *Prog Resp Res* 1990;26:77–84.
　Emphasizes the influence of inhalation injury on burn mortality.

130 THORACIC TRAUMA
Hani Seoudi

I. GENERAL PRINCIPLES. Chest injuries cause one of every four deaths in the United States. It is imperative that physicians who encounter trauma patients be able to assess and treat these injuries correctly and with dispatch.

II. ETIOLOGY. Motor vehicle crashes, falls, and penetrating wounds are the principal causes.

III. DIAGNOSIS
   A. Tension pneumothorax. Air enters the pleural space but does not leave because of a flap valve effect in the injured lung or from an open (sucking) chest wound. As a result, the ipsilateral lung collapses and the mediastinum is pushed toward the contralateral lung. This results in hypotension and tachycardia due to impaired venous return. These effects are particularly pronounced in children and in hypovolemic patients.
   B. Massive hemothorax. This represents a massive accumulation of more than 1,500 mL of blood within the pleural space.
   C. Flail chest. This indicates that a segment of chest wall has lost bony continuity with the remainder of the chest due to fracture of more than one rib in more than one location unilaterally or bilaterally, resulting in paradoxical movement of the flail segment during respiration. The morbidity of this condition is primarily due to the associated severe pulmonary contusion.
   D. Cardiac tamponade. This may result from either blunt or penetrating trauma. Acute accumulation of relatively small amounts of blood can result in tamponade pathophysiology. Clinical findings include hypotension, tachycardia, muffled heart sounds, distended neck veins, and pulsus paradoxus.
   E. Major airway injury. This injury is characterized by stridor and subcutaneous emphysema. Endotracheal intubation can be very difficult and a failed attempt at intubation can actually compromise the airway further. It is recommended that an emergency tracheostomy/cricothyroidotomy be performed. Urgent operative repair is needed.
   F. Penetrating chest injury. Penetrating injuries in addition to the stated problems may also result in **bronchovenous fistula,** whereby air flows from the injured bronchus into one of the pulmonary veins resulting in massive air embolism. This condition can have a delayed presentation and appear when positive pressure ventilation is initiated. The condition is rapidly fatal and requires immediate thoracotomy.

IV. IMMEDIATE LIFESAVING INTERVENTIONS
   A. Endotracheal intubation. Intubation is indicated when the airway is compromised by direct trauma, aspiration of blood/gastric contents, or a depressed level of consciousness. Oral intubation is the preferred method.
   B. Cricothyroidotomy. The practitioner must be capable of performing this procedure in a safe and swift manner. Tracheostomy is usually not performed in a lifesaving situation.
   C. Needle decompression or tube thoracostomy. Immediately on identification of a tension pneumothorax, a needle thoracostomy should be performed. This should be followed by a tube thoracostomy as quickly as possible.
   D. Thoracotomy. It is recommended that a thoracotomy be performed if the initial drainage from the tube thoracostomy is 1,500 mL or greater or when the hourly output is more than 250 mL for several hours. **Resuscitative thoracotomy:**

Generally a resuscitative thoracotomy is not performed on blunt trauma victims who are without vital signs (unless the patient loses vital signs while being examined by the resuscitating physician). For penetrating-injury patients, it may be performed when the patient is pulseless to provide access to the heart, descending aorta, and lung hilum. The success rate for this procedure is dismal.

V. DIAGNOSTIC STUDIES

A. Chest radiograph

B. Computed tomography (CT).
High-speed helical CT scanners permit rapid evaluation of chest injuries and are accurate for diagnosing lung contusions and occult hemopneumothorax and today may be diagnostic for blunt aortic injury. **Dynamic CT with contrast:** This technique is now recommended for visualizing major pulmonary emboli.

C. Angiography.
Aortography remains the gold standard for making the diagnosis of blunt aortic injury. Pulmonary angiography remains important for the diagnosis of pulmonary emboli.

D. Echocardiography.
Echocardiography is used to evaluate unstable patients for possible cardiac injury or to detect fluid or blood in the pericardium, to evaluate heart valves, and to assess ventricular function. **Transesophageal echocardiography (TEE)** is more precise than the transthoracic echo but requires special expertise and may not always be possible in the trauma patient.

VI. TREATMENT

A. Chest wall and pleural cavity injury

1. **Rib fractures.** Rib fractures need only to be treated symptomatically. Pain control can be challenging depending on the number of rib fractures. A thoracic epidural catheter may be needed if the patient is requiring large doses of narcotics for pain control. **Flail chest:** This injury is particularly challenging because patients frequently go into respiratory failure due to the severe pain, which limits respiratory effort, and the underlying pulmonary contusion. Mechanical ventilation is usually necessary.

2. **Sternal fracture.** Symptomatic treatment for this injury is appropriate.

3. **Pneumothorax.** Pneumothorax is generally treated with tube thoracostomy. A very small pneumothorax may be observed if the patient is not symptomatic. **Open pneumothorax:** The initial management includes immediately applying an occlusive dressing over the wound and insertion of a chest tube. Operative intervention is urgently needed when the assessment for other life-threatening injuries has been completed.

B. Lung

1. **Pulmonary contusion.** Treatment is supportive with supplemental oxygen. Mechanical ventilation is necessary if the patient's oxygen or ventilation is unsatisfactory.

2. **Acute respiratory distress syndrome (ARDS).** ARDS is a syndrome of diffuse inflammatory reaction in the lung as part of a systemic inflammatory response. It may occur following multiple trauma, sepsis, massive blood transfusions, and many other causes. Refer to the Chapter 43 for more details.

C. Trachea and major bronchial injuries.
After securing an airway, these injuries require immediate operative intervention.

D. Heart and great vessels

1. **Blunt cardiac injury.** This term encompasses a variety of injuries including myocardial contusion, rupture of a cardiac chamber or septum, and valve disruption.
   a. Treatment for myocardial contusion requires cardiac monitoring and supportive care.
   b. Treatment of chamber, septal, or valve injury requires urgent cardiosurgical repair.

2. **Blunt aortic injury.** Most patients with this injury die before reaching the hospital. Approximately half of those who reach the hospital will have a free rupture within the first 24 hours. Therefore, urgent surgical repair is indicated. **Nonoperative management:** Conservative supportive measures or interventional radiology procedures may be considered for the poor-risk or elderly patient.

3. **Traumatic asphyxia.** When a trauma patient is diagnosed with this problem, treatment is supportive after establishing an airway and ventilation.
4. **Diaphragm rupture.** Surgical treatment is indicated.
5. **Esophageal rupture.** Surgical treatment is indicated.

Selected Readings

Advanced trauma life support for doctors, 6th edition. Chicago: American College of Surgeons Committee on Trauma, 1997.
This is the international standard for the initial care of the trauma patient. The seventh edition will be available in 2005.

Cohn SM, Burns GA, Jaffe C, et al. Exclusion of aortic tear in the unstable trauma patient: the utility of transesophageal echocardiography. *J Trauma* 1995;39:1087–1090.
Specifies the utility of TEE for a rapid exclusion of aortic injury in the multiple-injured patient.

Dunham MB, Zygun D, et al. Endovascular stent grafts for acute blunt aortic injury. *J Trauma* 2004;56(6):1173–1178.
Reviews early results of this procedure.

Karmakar MK, Ho AM. Acute pain management of patients with multiple fractured ribs. *J Trauma* 2003;54(3):615–625.
Reviews strengths and weaknesses for each modality of pain control.

Karmy-Jones R, Nathens A, Jurkovich G, et al. Urgent and emergent thoracotomy for penetrating chest trauma. *J Trauma* 2004;56(3):664–669.
Discusses the impact of patient selection on the outcome of resuscitative thoracotomy.

Melton SM, Kerby JD, McGiffin D. The evolution of chest computed tomography for the definitive diagnosis of blunt aortic injury: a single-center experience. *J Trauma* 2004;56(2):243–250.
Identifies the improvements made in CT scans and the correct diagnosis of blunt aortic injury.

Trauma practice guidelines. Eastern Association of Trauma. www.east.org
A very useful Web site for trauma patient management.

Wahl WL, Michaels AJ, Wang SC, et al. Delayed versus early operative repair of blunt thoracic aortic injury. *J Trauma* 1998;45(6):1112.
Reviews the principles of nonoperative management of aortic injury.

Wilson RF, Steiger Z, et al. Thoracic trauma. In: Wilson RF, Walt AJ, eds. *Management of trauma: pitfalls and practice.* Baltimore: Williams & Wilkins;,1996, pp. 314–410.
Very helpful summary of thoracic trauma.

Wu CL, Jani ND, et al. Thoracic epidural analgesia versus intravenous patient-controlled analgesia for the treatment of rib fracture pain after motor vehicle crash. *J Trauma* 1999;47(3):564–567.
States that epidural analgesia provides better pain control.

I. GENERAL PRINCIPLES

A. Definition

1. The muscles of the extremities are divided into compartments, each having its own nerve and blood supply, enveloped by a tough layer of poorly compliant fascia.

2. A compartment syndrome occurs when the pressure in the myofascial compartment exceeds the intravascular capillary pressure, thereby compromising tissue perfusion within the compartment. In the majority of cases, the increased pressure is due to tissue edema or intracompartmental bleeding.

3. Extremity compartment syndrome occurs more frequently in the lower, rather than upper, extremity; it is also more common in the calf than the thigh.

B. Anatomy

1. Lower extremity

  a. Calf: There are four compartments

    (1) Anterior: most frequently involved; contains the anterior tibial artery and deep peroneal nerve

    (2) Lateral: contains the superficial peroneal nerve

    (3) Superficial posterior: contains the sural nerve

    (4) Deep posterior: contains the posterior tibial and peroneal arteries and the tibial nerve

  b. Thigh: There are three compartments

    (1) Anterior: most frequently involved; contains the quadratus femoris muscle

    (2) Posterior: contains the hamstring muscles and the sciatic nerve

    (3) Medial: contains the adductor muscles and the femoral neurovascular bundle

2. Upper extremity

  a. Forearm: There are two compartments

    (1) Volar: contains the flexors of the hand, the ulnar and radial arteries, and the median and ulnar nerves

    (2) Dorsal: contains the posterior interosseus nerve

  b. Arm: There are three compartments

    (1) Deltoid: contains the axillary nerve

    (2) Anterior: contains the brachial vessels and the musculocutaneous, median, and ulnar nerves

    (3) Posterior: contains the radial nerve

II. ETIOLOGY

A. The most common causes are:

1. Fractures

2. Ischemia from vascular occlusion followed by reperfusion

3. Vascular injury

4. Extensive soft tissue contusion/crush injuries

5. Prolonged external pressure

6. Burns/electrical injuries

7. Infiltrated infusion

III. PATHOPHYSIOLOGY

A. An initial insult produces cell damage and increases capillary permeability. Swelling of the intracompartmental tissues ensues, leading to further compression of tissues and worsening cellular ischemia.

B. On reperfusion, the sudden supply of oxygen to the ischemic tissues leads to the formation of oxygen free radicals, which in turn induce further cellular damage and capillary leak, resulting in worsening edema in the compartment.

C. Because the fascia is poorly compliant, once a pressure of 20 mm Hg is reached, very small increases in intracompartmental volume result in exponential increases in pressure.

D. Once the compartmental pressure overcomes the intravascular capillary pressure (which is 20 to 30 mm Hg), capillary perfusion stops and oxygen delivery to the compartmental tissues is impaired, despite ongoing blood flow in the higher-pressure main arteries.

E. Nervous tissue being the most sensitive to ischemia, nerve dysfunction occurs early and is less likely to be reversible after even short periods of increased compartmental pressure.

IV. DIAGNOSIS
A. Clinical presentation
  1. The signs and symptoms of compartment syndrome
   a. Pain
   b. Pressure (palpably tense compartment)
   c. Paresthesia
   d. Paralysis
   e. Pulselessness
   f. Pallor
  2. Pulse and color are maintained until late. By the time they are compromised, significant nerve damage has already likely occurred.
  3. Pain is usually severe, out of proportion to associated injuries and exacerbated by passively stretching the muscles of the involved compartment.
  4. It is important to thoroughly examine the patient, including under bandages and casts. These can potentially hide a compartment syndrome and result in a delayed or missed diagnosis.

B. Investigations
  1. Suspicion of a compartment syndrome should be raised by history (proper mechanism of injury) and physical examination. Confirmation of the diagnosis is made by direct measurement of the compartment pressures.
  2. Intracompartmental pressures are measured by introducing a needle into the compartment and connecting it to a pressure transducer.
  3. Pressures less than 20 mm Hg are unlikely to be of concern. Pressures above 30 mm Hg are clearly abnormal. Pressures between 20 and 30 mm Hg are in a "gray zone" and are potentially of concern, especially in the presence of some signs and symptoms suggestive of compartment syndrome.
  4. Diagnosis of a compartment syndrome should not be based exclusively on pressure measurement. A correlation with the patient's clinical picture is imperative for accurate diagnosis.
  5. When there is suspicion of a compartment syndrome, the pressures of all the compartments in the involved extremity should be measured.

V. TREATMENT
A. It is critical that the developing compartment syndrome be recognized early, because neuromuscular dysfunction is reversible when promptly treated.

B. Fasciotomies should be performed immediately to release the compartment pressure. All potentially constricting layers of soft tissue around the involved muscle group should be released. The fascia is the most constricting layer, and a complete incision of the fascia is the most important step.

C. Usually, two skin incisions are used to release the compartments of the calf: a medial incision, to decompress the superficial and deep posterior compartments, and a lateral incision, to decompress the anterior and lateral compartments.

D. For the thigh, the anterior and posterior compartments can be decompressed through a lateral skin incision. Because the medial compartment is rarely involved, a medial incision is usually not necessary.

E. Two skin incisions are used for forearm fasciotomies: the volar compartment is accessed through a medial incision, and the dorsal compartment through a lateral incision.

F. One medial skin incision through the biceps—triceps groove is sufficient to decompress both the anterior and posterior compartments of the arm.

G. After fasciotomy, the wounds should be left open and covered with moist, sterile dressings. The leg is elevated and passive range of motion is begun.

H. Fasciotomy wounds can usually be closed within a week, rarely primarily but more commonly with split-thickness skin graft.

VI. COMPLICATIONS
A. Ischemic neuropathy

B. Myonecrosis and fibrosis, resulting in contracture

C. Severe shock from reperfusion of ischemic tissue and free radical release

D. Myoglobinemia resulting in acute renal failure

E. Hyperkalemia, hyperphosphatemia, metabolic acidosis from rhabdomyolysis

Selected Readings
Bibbo C, Lin S, et al. Acute traumatic compartment syndrome of the foot in children, *Pediatr Emerg Care* 2000,16:244–248.
A short discussion of a less frequently seen type of compartment syndrome.

Evaluation and management of the high-risk orthopedic emergency. *Emerg Med Clin North Am* 2003;21:159–204.
An in-depth review of common pitfalls in the diagnosis of various orthopedic injuries.

Mubarak SJ, Pedowitz RA, Hargens AR. Compartment syndromes. *Curr Orthop* 1989;3: 36–40.
A good overview.

Tiwari A, Haq AI, Myint F, et al. Acute compartment syndromes. *Br J Surg* 2002; 89(4):397–412.
An excellent review of the topic.

Velmahos GC, Toutouzas KG. Vascular trauma and compartment syndromes. *Surg Clin North Am* 2002; 82(1):125–141.
A good review including common pitfalls in the diagnosis and treatment of compartment syndromes.

132

SEPSIS
Antine Stenbit and Kenneth J. Serio

I. DEFINITIONS
A. Sepsis: a complex activation of the immune system with a documented infection
B. Systemic inflammatory response syndrome (SIRS): a complex activation of the immune system regardless of etiology, infection, trauma, burns, or a sterile inflammatory process.
C. Severe sepsis: sepsis plus organ dysfunction
D. Septic shock: sepsis plus unexplained acute circulatory collapse with organ dysfunction, hypotension, and tissue hypoperfusion.

II. EPIDEMIOLOGY.
Sepsis is the tenth most common cause of death in the United States, with an increase in incidence and number of related deaths observed between 1979 and 2000. Because of the recent development of novel treatments and improved intensive medical care, sepsis mortality rate has declined to approximately 17.9%.

III. PATHOPHYSIOLOGY
A. Systemic exposure to microbial antigens, including lipopolysaccharide (LPS) from gram-negative bacteria, leads to the clinical manifestations of sepsis. Recent evidence suggests that host genetics may predict the nature of this response. The binding of LPS (and other microbial components) to Toll-like receptors (TLRs) on inflammatory cells results in a coordinated immune response, involving T-cells, macrophages, neutrophils, endothelial cells, and dendritic cells. These events lead to a subsequent alteration in expression of complement as well as fibrinolytic, coagulation, and inflammatory genes and their products.
B. Mediators implicated in the pathogenesis of sepsis include cytokines (such as IL-1, IL-6, IL-8), growth factors (such as TNFa,), high mobility group box-1 (HMGB-1), arachidonic acid metabolites, and nitric oxide. The end-organ consequences include enhanced microvascular thrombosis and permeability, vasodilatation and maldistribution of blood flow, myocardial dysfunction, altered cellular nutrient utilization, and cellular apoptosis.

IV. DIAGNOSIS
A. Initial
  1. Tachycardia
  2. Oliguria
  3. Hyperglycemia
B. Established sepsis
  1. Altered mental status
  2. Metabolic acidosis, respiratory alkalosis
  3. Hypotension with decreased systemic vascular resistance (SVR) and elevated cardiac output
  4. Coagulopathy
C. Late manifestations
  1. Organ dysfunction: acute lung injury (ALI), ARDS, acute renal failure, hepatic dysfunction
  2. Refractory shock
D. Differentiation between sepsis and SIRS
  1. Identification of an inflammatory source is crucial to abolish the inciting stimulus for the ongoing immune response. The most common sites of infection

in sepsis are the respiratory tract and the urinary tract; other sites are listed in Table 132-1. The most common etiologic microbes in sepsis have recently shifted from gram-negative to gram-positive organisms, jointly accounting for almost 90% of cases. Fungi, anaerobes, and polymicrobial infections account for the microbiologic etiology of the remaining 10% of cases. Imaging studies, as well as blood, urine, pleural, wound, and cerebrospinal fluid cultures should be performed to identify a potential organism.

2. A proposed PIRO sepsis staging system stratifies patients by the following criteria: predisposing factors to sepsis (i.e., comorbid conditions and genetic factors, which may play a role in the development and severity of sepsis); insulting infection (i.e., the site, type, and severity of infection and the organism susceptibility); response (i.e., the degree of the host response to the insult); and finally, the presence and severity of organ dysfunction. This staging system may facilitate individualization of treatment regimens, as well as aid in the prediction of outcomes and prevention of complications.

TABLE 132-1 Common Sites and Diseases Associated With Sepsis/SIRS

Organ system	Location	Disease
Respiratory	Upper respiratory tract	Sinusitis
		Mastoiditis
	Lower respiratory tract	Pneumonia
		Lung abscess
		Empyema
Gastrointestinal	Mediastinum	Esophageal rupture/perforation
	Hepatobiliary	Hepatic abscess
		Cholangitis
		Cholecystitis
	Intraabdominal	Intestinal infarction/perforation
		Pancreatitis
		Intraabdominal/diverticular abscess
Cardiovascular	Mediastinum	Postoperative mediastinitis
	Native or prosthetic cardiac valve	Endocarditis
Genitourinary	Kidney, ureter, and bladder	Perinephric abscess
		Pyelonephritis
		Cystitis
Neurologic	Brain and meninges	Meningitis
		Intracranial Abscess
Dermatologic	Traumatic wound, surgical wound, or burn site	Soft tissue abscess
		Necrotizing fasciitis
		Infected decubitus ulcer
		Full- and partial-thickness burn
Prosthetic	Central/peripheral venous catheter	Catheter infection
	Arterial catheter	
	Ventriculoperitoneal shunt	
	Dialysis catheter	
	Articular prosthetic device	Infected prosthesis
	Dialysis graft/shunt	
Other	Vascular system	Septic thrombophlebitis

V. TREATMENT. Therapy in sepsis should be targeted toward the following: specific treatment of an infectious source, optimal fluid resuscitation and pressor/inotrope use, activated protein C therapy, and adjunctive therapies.

   A. *Specific treatment of an infectious source* includes therapeutic drainage of an infected space or removal of infected tissue and may serve to both establish the diagnosis and guide early and aggressive antibiotic therapy. In most cases, a multiagent empiric antibiotic regimen is initially used, with attention paid to the degree of penetration into the suspected infection site, local microbial resistance patterns, efficacy against the most likely organisms, and risks of side effects. The antibiotic regimen should be reevaluated daily to minimize cost and potential toxicities.

   B. *Optimal fluid resuscitation*, which has been demonstrated to improve survival, should include early goal-directed fluid resuscitation (preferably via a large-bore venous catheter) initiated in the emergency department or as soon as the diagnosis is suspected. (See Selected Readings.) Although some data suggest that fluid resuscitation with colloids (such as albumin), as compared to crystalloids (such as saline), may increase mortality; recent meta-analyses do not support this contention. Although larger volumes of crystalloid are required to achieve the same end points of resuscitation, as compared to colloid, the increased cost of colloids precludes their indiscriminate use. Combined use of crystalloids and colloids is preferable and should be based on cost and potential benefit to the patient.

   C. *Pressors and inotropes* may be required prior to the achievement of full fluid resuscitation and should be targeted to restore end-organ perfusion. Neosynephrine, dopamine, and vasopressin are acceptable agents, although recent studies suggest that norepinephrine may be the preferred initial agent. Studies do not indicate that low-dose dopamine possesses any benefit in terms of renal protection. Maintenance of normal blood pH values is important, because many vasopressors are ineffective in the setting of acidemia. Inotropes, such as dobutamine, should be reserved for patients with low cardiac stroke work and low output in the face of maximal therapy.

   D. *Monitoring* of fluid resuscitation and pressor/inotrope utilization usually requires placement of an arterial line, because noninvasive blood pressure measurements are inaccurate in shock. Although pulmonary artery catheter use has been suggested to contribute to increased mortality, this concern likely reflects selection bias in the reported studies. However, the use of pulmonary artery catheters has never been shown to improve outcome, and their use should be carefully considered, given the increased cost and risks of complications. The crucial end points for the fluids, pressors, and inotrope resuscitation strategy are the optimization of oxygen delivery and the clearance of serum lactate; selected additional end points are shown in Table 132-2.

   E. *Recombinant human activated protein C* has recently been introduced and shown great promise in reducing sepsis mortality. This agent inhibits the microvascular thromboses associated with sepsis, although other mechanisms of action may also exist. However, because of the low, but defined, risk of hemorrhage and the fact that the agent has not been well studied in patients with known bleeding diatheses (such as chronic liver disease), patient selection and monitoring of therapy is crucial. (See Selected Readings.)

   F. *Other adjunctive therapies* should additionally be considered in selected patients with sepsis. Although steroid replacement in sepsis has no demonstrated benefit in unselected patient populations, studies suggest a high frequency of occult adrenal insufficiency in sepsis. Randomized trials support the efficacy and safety of replacement steroids in a subset of patients with septic shock and relative adrenal insufficiency. Although many experts advocate early enteral feeding in sepsis, recent trials indicate that this approach may not be beneficial. Intensive insulin therapy to control blood glucose has been shown to improve outcome in sepsis. (See Selected Readings.)

VI. SUMMARY. The sepsis/SIRS mortality rate has deceased, although rates remain high. Recent advances in the understanding of the host immune response, advances in disease staging, and novel therapies may further advance the treatment of this syndrome.

TABLE 132-2	End Points for Resuscitation in Sepsis

End point	Goal
Patient tolerance	Monitor patient response to resuscitation strategy (monitor for signs of fluid overload, arrhythmias, etc.)
Hemoglobin	Support with goal to optimize oxygen delivery
Cardiac output	Maximize with goal to optimize oxygen delivery
Hemoglobin Saturation (SaO$_2$)	Maximize with goal to optimize oxygen delivery
Oxygen delivery	Support the hemoglobin, cardiac output, and hemoglobin saturation to optimize the oxygen delivery
Mixed venous oxygen saturation (SvO$_2$)	Maintain SvO$_2 \geq$ 70%
Heart rate	Maintain at levels that allow adequate diastolic cardiac filling
Mean arterial pressure (MAP)	Maintain at MAP $\geq$ 65 mm Hg
Central venous pressure (CVP)	Maintain at 8–12 mm Hg (12–15 mm Hg in ventilated patients)
Serum lactate	Restore normal pH and monitor for resolution of lactic acidosis
Urine output	Maintain at urine output $\geq$ 0.5 mL/kg/h
Serum glucose	Maintain at $\leq$ 110 g/dL
Minute ventilation	Monitor arterial blood gases (ABG) closely for signs of inadequate respiratory compensation for metabolic acidosis Ventilatory support (if necessary)

Selected Readings

Annane D, Sebille V, Charpentier C, et al. Effect of treatment with low doses of hydrocortisone and fludrocortisone on mortality in patients with septic shock. *JAMA* 2002;288:862–871.
Trial demonstrating that a select group of patients benefit from steroid replacement therapy in sepsis.

Bernard GR, Vincent JL, Laterre PF, et al. Efficacy and safety of recombinant human activated protein C for severe sepsis. *N Engl J Med* 2001;344:699–709.
Landmark Prowess trial documenting the efficacy of activated protein C administration in severe sepsis.

Dellinger RP, Carlet JM, Masur H, et al. Surviving sepsis campaign guidelines for management of severe sepsis and septic shock. *Crit Care Med* 2004;32:858–873.
Most recent international consensus conference on the diagnosis and management of sepsis.

Hotchkiss RS, Karl IE. The pathophysiology and treatment of sepsis. *N Engl J Med* 2003; 348:138–150.
Excellent review of the standard of care in sepsis.

Kern JW, Shoemaker WC. Meta-analysis of hemodynamic optimization in high-risk patients. *Crit Care Med* 2002;30:1686–1692.
Meta-analysis of 21 trials demonstrating the efficacy of early hemodynamic optimization, particularly when instituted before the onset of organ failure and when the goal of increased oxygen delivery was achieved.

Levy MM, Fink MP, Marshall JC, et al. 2001 SCCM/ESICM/ACCP/ATS/SIS International Sepsis Definitions Conference. *Crit Care Med* 2003;31:1250–1256.
Most recent international consensus conference on the definitions of sepsis. The consensus group strongly considered a revision in sepsis definitions, although none was provided at this conference.

Lin MT, Albertson TE. Genomic polymorphisms in sepsis. *Crit Care Med* 2004;32:569–579.
Review of the reported polymorphisms that may define the susceptibility to sepsis.

Martin GS, Mannino DM, Eaton S, et al. 2003. The epidemiology of sepsis in the United States from 1979 through 2000. *N Engl J Med* 2003;348:1546–1554.
Review of the trends and epidemiology of sepsis over the past 20 years. This article demonstrates an increasing incidence of sepsis with a corresponding decrease in the mortality rate. The study also documents a shift in the pattern of microbes responsible for sepsis during this same period.

Rivers E, Nguyen B, Havstad S, et al. 2001. Early goal-directed therapy in the treatment of severe sepsis and septic shock. *N Engl J Med* 2001;345:1368–1377.
Article demonstrating the importance of early goal-directed therapy (initiated in the emergency department) in the treatment of sepsis leading to an improved 28-day mortality rate.

van den Berghe G, Wouters P, Weekers F, et al. Intensive insulin therapy in the critically ill patients. *N Engl J Med* 2001;345:1359–1367.
Landmark article demonstrating the efficacy of intensive insulin therapy in critically ill patients leading to an improved 28-day mortality rate.

Wilkes MM, Navickis RJ. Patient survival after human albumin administration. A meta-analysis of randomized, controlled trials. *Ann Intern Med* 2001;135:149–164.
Meta-analysis of 55 trials demonstrating that the use of albumin in fluid resuscitation does not adversely impact mortality.

MULTIPLE ORGAN DYSFUNCTION SYNDROME

133

Paola Fata and Samir Fakhry

I. BACKGROUND

A. Multiple-organ dysfunction syndrome (MODS) has been described as a "disease of medical progress" or the unwanted outcome of successful shock resuscitation.

B. Develops in approximately 15% of medical and surgical intensive care patients.

C. In the intensive care unit (ICU), the incidence of single-organ failure approaches 48%. The lung is the most common organ to develop obvious clinical failure, followed by the liver, kidney, gastrointestinal (GI) tract, and cardiovascular system.

II. DEFINITION

A. MODS refers to the presence of altered organ function in a severely ill patient so that homeostasis cannot be maintained without intervention.

B. The physiologic definition is: severe acquired dysfunction of at least two organ systems lasting at least 24 to 48 hours in the setting of sepsis, trauma, burns, or severe inflammatory conditions. Both the number of dysfunctional organs and the duration of dysfunction are critical to the definition. The mortality increases proportionally with number and duration of dysfunctions.

C. Single organ failure lasting more than 1 day results in a mortality risk of 20%; if two organs are involved, mortality increases to 40%; whereas persistent dysfunction (over 72 hours) present in three organ systems can result in a mortality risk of 80%.

III. HISTORY

A. 1973: Tilney identifies a syndrome of sequential organ failure following rupture of abdominal aortic aneurysms.

B. 1977: Eiseman first introduced the term "multiple organ failure" as a consequence of technical complications related to clinical management in almost 60% of patients.

C. 1980: Fry and colleagues proposed that infection is the probable cause for development of this syndrome.

D. 1985: Goris found in contrast, that bacterial sepsis was found in 65% of intra-abdominal sepsis patients but only in 33% of trauma patients diagnosed with multiple organ failure and therefore, sepsis is probably not the essential cause of MODS; rather an uncontrolled hyperinflammatory response is responsible.

IV. SCORING SYSTEMS

A. A number of scoring systems have been developed to predict mortality from organ dysfunction, and they are useful as a baseline severity assessment.

B. Changes in score may reflect recovery or deterioration of organ function and may be employed across ICUs as a quality performance marker.

C. Two most frequently employed clinical measurement systems are the Sepsis-related Organ Failure Assessment *(SOFA)* and the Multiple Organ Dysfunction Score *(MODS)* (Table 133-1).

V. PATHOPHYSIOLOGY. An evidence-based understanding of the pathophysiology is still pending, and various mechanisms have been proposed.

A. Uncontrolled infection

    1. Earlier reports suggested MODS was caused by occult or uncontrolled infection, commonly pneumonia or peritonitis. Infection in patients with MODS is

TABLE 133-1	Clinical Measurement Systems to Assess Organ Dysfunction				
Parameter	SOFA	Score	MODS	Score
---	---	---	---	---
Respiratory	PaO$_2$/FiO$_2$ Ventilation	0–4	PaO$_2$/FiO$_2$	0–4
Coagulation	Platelet number Cell number	0–4	Platelet number	0–4
Hepatic	Bilirubin	0–4	Bilirubin	0–4
Cardiac	Blood pressure Vasopressor use	0–4	Blood pressure Heart rate Central venous pressure	0–4
CNS	Glasgow Coma scale	0–4	Glasgow coma scale	0–4
Renal	Creatinine urine output	0–4	Creatinine urine output	0–4
Aggregate score	Add worst daily score	0–24	Add worst daily score	0–24

CNS, central nervous system; SOFA, Sepsis-related Organ Failure Assessment; MODS, Multiple Organ Dysfunction Score.

common, and nosocomial infection is rare in patients without organ dysfunction. Infection, however, is not necessarily present.

2. Endotoxin, which correlates poorly with culture-proved infection, can be absorbed through the (GI) tract or lung and has been postulated to play an important role.

B. Gut hypothesis

1. Splanchnic hypoperfusion is common in critical illness.

2. High susceptibility of the GI tract to diminished tissue perfusion and ischemia results in:

a. Mucosal atrophy with increased permeability

b. Altered immune function

c. Bacterial translocation

d. Bacteria in the systemic circulation activate the inflammatory response, resulting in organ dysfunction.

C. Tissue hypoxia. Diminished oxygen delivery at the cellular level inhibits the normal physiologic activity of the cell, which is a common pathway for organ dysfunction.

D. Microvascular coagulopathy

1. Inflammation and inappropriate activation of coagulation may be related to the development of organ dysfunction via abnormal microvascular thrombosis.

2. Endotoxin and inflammatory cytokines activate tissue factor. Tissue factor activates the coagulation pathway as well as gene expression for the proinflammatory cytokines, such as tumor necrosis factor (TNF).

3. Alterations in factor levels determining the balance between coagulation and fibrinolysis precede organ dysfunction.

E. Systemic inflammation

1. Defined as the activation of circulating leukocytes, endothelial cells, and chemical mediators, which are normally suppressed by antiinflammatory mediators.

2. When the patient's inflammatory response process is uncontrolled, MODS ensues:

a. The initiating event may be severe tissue trauma or intraabdominal sepsis, which results in massive activation of inflammatory mediators. Then systemic damage to vascular endothelia, permeability edema, and impaired oxygen availability to the mitochondria occurs (despite adequate arterial oxygen transport).

b. Increased circulating levels of cytokines TNF, IL-1, and IL-6 are associated with organ dysfunction and increased mortality.

c. Systemic inflammation seems to be the initiating event or final common pathway of the previous four hypotheses.

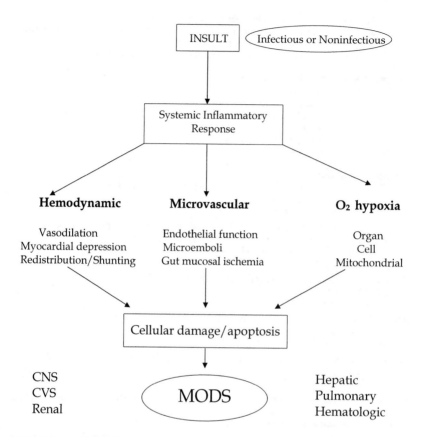

Figure 133-1. MODS etiologic factors.

F. MODS cannot be traced to a single cause for most patients. A single theory about the development is not enough to explain the clinical syndrome. Tissue hypoxia, splanchnic hypoperfusion, microvascular coagulopathy, and systemic inflammation are the integrated responses to severe injury resulting in clinical organ dysfunction (Fig. 133-1).

VI. THERAPY

A. The capacity to treat MODS when it is diagnosed is limited despite therapeutic advances in critical care. **The mortality rate remains unchanged.**

B. Multiple clinical trials have evaluated the use of antiinflammatory agents (methylprednisolone, intravenous ibuprofen, anti-TNF monoclonal antibodies), and all have thus far been ineffective. Recent data suggest that activated protein C can decrease the mortality of sepsis and MODS.

C. Selective decontamination of the digestive tract to decrease bacterial translocation has yielded varying results and remains controversial.

D. It is important to address the underlying causes in patients at risk for MODS (i.e., identify and treat infection early, aggressive shock resuscitation, damage control rather than definitive operations in emergent situations, correcting acidosis, hypothermia, and control of bleeding).

E. Supportive therapy is used to treat MODS when it is diagnosed:

1. Modern ventilation techniques for acute lung injury
2. Support of each failing organ system with the most current evidence-based strategies
3. Renal replacement therapy for kidney failure
4. Attempt to identify and remove possible precipitating causes

VII. POSSIBLE FUTURE THERAPIES
   A. Cell adhesion retardation
   B. Inflammatory mediator reduction
   C. Neutralizing antibodies directed at cytokines, vasoactive substances, complement, and mediators of coagulation
   D. Antiinflammatory protein induction
   E. Antioxidants and antiproteases.

Selected Readings

Bone RC, Grodzin CJ, Balk RA. Sepsis: a new hypothesis for the pathogenesis of the disease process. *Chest* 1997;112:235.
Another hypothesis on etiology.

Doig CJ, Sutherland LR, Sandham JS, et al. Increased intestinal permeability is associated with the development of multiple organ dysfunction syndrome in critically ill ICU patients. *Am J Respir Crit Care Med* 1998;158:444.
The gut and MODS.

Goris RJ. Multi-organ failure. Generalized autodestructive inflammation? *Arch Surg* 1985;120 (10):1109.
An early descriptor of MODS.

Johnson D, Mayers I. Multiple organ dysfunction syndrome: a narrative review. *Can J Anesth* 2001;48:5,502.
Excellent current review article.

Knaus WA, Wagner DP. Multiple systems organ failure: epidemiology and prognosis. *Crit Care Clin* 1989;5:221.
An early article on MODS.

Marshall JC, Cook DJ, Christou NV, et al. Multiple organ dysfunction score: a reliable descriptor of a complex clinical outcome. *Crit Care Med* 1995;23:1638.
Explains the rationale for the MODS.

Marshall, JC. Inflammation, coagulopathy, and the pathogenesis of multiple organ dysfunction syndrome. *Crit Care Med* 2001;29(7):S99.
In-depth article on the pathogenesis of MODS.

Matuschak GM. Multiple organ system failure: clinical expression, pathogenesis, and therapy. *Principles of Critical Care* 1998, Hall, Wood and Schmidt, McGraw-Hill.
A good review.

Vincent JL, Moreno R, Takala J, et al. The SOFA (Sepsis-related Organ Failure Assessment) score to describe organ dysfunction/failure. On behalf of the Working Group on Sepsis-Related problems of the European Society of Intensive Care Medicine. *Intensive Care Med* 1996;22:707.
Explains the rationale for the SOFA.

Neurologic Problems in the Intensive Care Unit

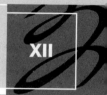

XII

134

AN APPROACH TO NEUROLOGIC PROBLEMS IN THE INTENSIVE CARE UNIT

David A. Drachman

I. GENERAL PRINCIPLES

A. Patients with neurologic problems present in the intensive care unit (ICU) as primary neurologic problems or as neurologic complications secondary to medical or surgical disorders. Only a few common neurologic *situations* occur in the ICU, although they can be caused by many *diseases*.

  1. Depressed state of consciousness, coma
  2. Altered mental function
  3. Required support of respirations or other vital functions
  4. Monitoring: increased intracranial pressure (ICP), respirations, consciousness
  5. Determination of brain death
  6. Prevention of further damage to the central nervous system (CNS)
  7. Management of seizures or status epilepticus
  8. Evaluation of a neurologic change occurring in a known medical disease
  9. Management of medical disease developing during neurologic illness

B. Primary neurologic problems in the ICU include:

  1. Myasthenia gravis
  2. Guillain-Barré syndrome
  3. Head trauma
  4. Stroke

C. Neurologic complications of medical disease are far more common than primary neurologic problems. They include:

  1. Impaired consciousness following cardiopulmonary resuscitation
  2. Development of delirium
  3. Focal neurologic deficits in a patient with multisystem disease

D. Indications for neurologic consultation in the ICU

  1. *Depressed state of consciousness.* Depressed consciousness ranges from lethargy to coma and raises many questions:
    a. Is there a focal brainstem lesion or diffuse cerebral involvement?
    b. Is there an anatomic lesion or a metabolic disorder?
    c. Have vital brainstem functions been impaired?
    d. Is intracranial pressure increased?
  2. The most common *primary neurologic causes* of depressed consciousness include:
    a. Head trauma
    b. Intracranial hemorrhage
    c. Inapparent seizures.
  3. The *secondary conditions* seen most often are:
    a. Metabolic-anoxic disorders
    b. Drug intoxications
    c. Diabetic acidosis
  4. It is crucial to establish whether depressed consciousness is the result of:
    a. Intrinsic brainstem damage
    b. Increased intracranial pressure
    c. Toxins
    d. Widespread anoxic ischemia
    e. Other, less common causes.

II. DIAGNOSIS

A. In the patient with depressed consciousness, it is particularly important to identify rapidly the component(s) that may be treatable!

1. Neurologic examination of patients with stupor or coma. Examination of the patient with depressed consciousness includes: evaluation of mental status, cranial nerve functions, motor functions and coordination, reflexes, sensation, and vascular integrity, supplemented by appropriate laboratory studies.

a. Mental status

(1) Detailed evaluation of memory and cognitive function is rarely possible in lethargic patients and is impossible when stupor or coma is present.

(2) Estimate the responsiveness of the patient, including vital functions, respiratory pattern, eye opening, response to painful stimuli, and speech.

b. Cranial nerve evaluations: vision (e.g., blink to threat), pupils (size and response), corneal reflexes, "doll's eyes" responses, and, if absent, ice water caloric response, cough, facial movements to pain, and gag reflex are tested.

c. Motor function: evaluate by observing all limbs for spontaneous movement, symmetry, and adventitious movements. Pinch or other noxious stimulus may help evaluate purposeful defensive movements.

(1) Decerebrate (four-limb extensor) or decorticate (upper limbs flexor, lower limbs extensor) rigidity is observed

(2) Tone is assessed for spasticity or rigidity.

d. Reflexes: Deep tendon reflexes; grasp, suck, snout, and plantar reflexes are evaluated.

e. Sensation: Pain is often the only testable sensation; withdrawal from pinprick in the feet must be distinguished from an extensor plantar response.

f. Vascular status: Listen for bruits over the carotid, subclavian, and vertebral arteries.

g. Interpretation: This examination reveals the patient's state of consciousness, the integrity of brainstem reflexes, and the presence of focal neurologic deficits.

2. Laboratory studies

a. Imaging studies. MRI or CT can reveal evidence of stroke, hemorrhage, trauma, tumor, and so forth, despite the difficulty of obtaining these studies.

b. Electroencephalography. This reveals seizure activity; functional state; symmetry; certain toxic-metabolic conditions; and so on. Can be performed at the bedside.

c. Metabolic studies. Electrolytes, ammonia, pH, O_2 saturation, renal function, hepatic function, toxic substances; and others.

3. Management of patients with depressed consciousness depends on determining the cause and applying the appropriate techniques for eliminating toxins, reducing intracranial pressure, and maintaining vital functions.

B. Altered Mental Function.

1. In the awake patient, disorders that affect mental function can produce patterns of: confusion, delirium, aphasia, dementia, or isolated memory impairment. Ask the following questions:

a. Is the abnormal mentation a recent change or longstanding?

b. Did the change develop abruptly after surgery or cardiac arrest?

c. Is the mental change improving, worsening, or stable?

2. Confusion and delirium: often result from *metabolic* or *toxic* disorders; they are commonly reversible.

3. Persistent aphasia and *isolated* memory impairment: suggest focal anatomic damage to the brain. Neurologic examination for localization, and imaging studies are useful.

4. Dementia/cognitive impairment: can be assessed *only* in patients with a clear sensorium; it cannot be evaluated in patients with depressed consciousness, confusion, or delirium. Cognitive impairment can indicate either *reversible* (drug-induced, depression-related) conditions or *irreversible* damage (diffuse anoxia, ischemia, strokes; or a degenerative dementia).

Recent change of mental status in the ICU requires evaluation by an experienced neurologist as early as possible.

C. Support of respiration and other vital functions

  1. Respiratory support is needed for neurologic patients with:

    a. Loss of brainstem control of respiration

    b. With impairment of effective transmission of neural impulses to respiratory muscles.

      Brainstem lesions produce characteristic respiratory patterns, depending on the site of damage (e.g., central neurogenic hyperventilation, Cheyne-Stokes or periodic breathing, apnea). Transmission of respiratory impulses can be impaired at the cervical spinal cord, anterior horn cells, peripheral nerves, neuromuscular junctions, or muscles of respiration. Traumatic cervical cord injuries, amyotrophic lateral sclerosis, the Guillain-Barré syndrome, myasthenia gravis, and muscular dystrophy interfere with breathing at different levels. Some conditions are transitory (Guillain-Barré syndrome) or treatable (myasthenia gravis), with *complete recovery* if respiration is successfully maintained.

D. Monitoring intracranial pressure and state of consciousness. Head trauma, subarachnoid hemorrhage, and stroke may require neural monitoring.

  1. Lethargic patients should be observed for increased intracranial pressure caused by cerebral edema, intracranial (subdural, epidural, intracerebral) hemorrhage, or both.

  2. Once uncal or tonsillar *herniation* with brainstem compression occurs, the secondary brain injury may far outweigh the initial damage. (Methods for monitoring ICP and assessing consciousness with the Glasgow coma scale are described elsewhere [Chapter 144 and Appendix]).

E. Determination of brain death

  1. Death of the brain and brainstem is equivalent to death of the patient.

    a. Brain death is specifically a determination that the brain *and* the brainstem are already dead—not a prediction of unlikely useful recovery.

    b. The mnemonic *CADRE* is useful to remember the criteria for brain death: **c**oma, **a**pnea, **d**ilated, fixed pupils, **r**eflex (brainstem) absence, and **e**lectroencephalographic (EEG) silence.

F. Preventing further damage to the CNS

  1. In stroke, thrombolytic treatment can reverse the ischemic process and neuroprotective agents may prevent further damage.

  2. Spinal cord compression by tumor requires radiation therapy to avoid cord transection.

  3. *Cerebral ischemia, anoxia, hemorrhage, increased ICP, spinal cord compression, and other acute neurologic disorders require prompt institution of treatment.*

G. Managing status epilepticus. Status epilepticus threatens lasting deficits or death if not controlled.

  1. Patients with *continuous* or *recurrent* seizures that cannot be promptly arrested must be treated in the ICU.

  2. Therapy ranging up to general anesthesia or artificial ventilation may be required.

H. Evaluating secondary neurologic disease in severe medical illness. Patients in the ICU with myocardial infarctions, subacute bacterial endocarditis, cardiac arrhythmias, pneumonia, renal disease, and so forth may develop neurologic changes during treatment for the medical problem. These neurologic findings may result from the underlying disease or be coincidental; a neurologist should evaluate such patients.

I. Managing secondary severe medical disease in neurologic illness. Patients with chronic neurologic disorders often develop unrelated medical illness: myocardial infarcts occurring in demented patients or septicemia in patients with multiple sclerosis. Early recognition of a change in the neurologic patient's condition is often critical to a successful outcome.

III. PROGNOSTIC AND ETHICAL CONSIDERATIONS

  A. When severe damage involves the brain, physicians and families often need guidance regarding the probable outcome. Three critical questions should be addressed:

    1. Will the patient survive?

    2. Has irreversible brain damage occurred?

    3. What is the likely degree of residual disability?

  B. The most important consideration is whether *irreversible damage* has affected crucial brain areas, rather than the level of consciousness. The probability of neurologic recovery declines with age, size and location of the lesion, and duration of the deficit. (Some reported statistical guidelines are of value in estimating recovery; see, for example, Levy D, Caronna J, Singer B, et al.)

Selected Readings

Levy D, Caronna J, Singer B, et al. Predicting outcome from hypoxic-ischemic coma. *JAMA* 1985;253:1420.

    An excellent summary of the features that predict survival and function following hypoxic-ischemic coma.

Plum F, Posner JB. *The diagnosis of stupor and coma*, 3rd edition. Philadelphia: FA Davis, 1982.

    A classic review of the neurologic aspects of impaired consciousness.

Ropper A. *Neurological and neurosurgical intensive care*, 4th edition. Philadelphia: Lippincott Williams and Wilkins, 2003.

    A multiauthor book with detailed discussions of many aspects of neurologic intensive care.

Wanzer S, Federman D, Adelstein S, et al. The physician's responsibility toward hopelessly ill patients: a second look. *N Engl J Med* 1989;320:844.

    A thoughtful approach to end-of-life issues in patients with terminal illness.

Zandbergen E, deHaan R Reitsma J, et al. Survival and recovery of consciousness in anoxic-ischemic coma after cardiopulmonary resuscitation. *Intensive Care Med* 2003;29:1911–1915.

    A recent review of recovery following anoxic-ischemic coma.

I. OVERVIEW

A. Many diseases lead to acute impairment of consciousness, including some that are potentially life threatening but treatable if recognized early, and require a systematic and complete evaluation:

1. Rapid determination of the type of mental status change

2. Administration of life support measures when needed

3. Obtaining a detailed history, physical examination, and ancillary studies

4. Initiation of definitive treatment based on this assessment

B. Pathophysiology

1. Altered sensorium (state of consciousness) results from damage to the reticular activating system in the brainstem and diencephalons, and/or their projections to *both* cerebral hemispheres.

2. Many structural/physiological disorders can affect these structures and impair consciousness (Table 135-1).

C. Prognosis. Depends on the cause of coma and any secondary complications (see later).

D. Diagnosis. Distinguish among normal sleep, coma, status epilepticus, akinetic mutism, locked-in state, and aphasia.

E. Treatment. Depends on the underlying cause and the presence or absence of cerebral edema

II. THE PATIENT WHO APPEARS UNCONSCIOUS

A. General principles. Some patients appear to be unconscious. The differential diagnosis includes the following.

1. Normal sleep (can be aroused to complete wakefulness by verbal or physical stimulation)

2. Impaired consciousness and brain death (sustained arousal by stimuli cannot be obtained)

3. Locked-in state (awake and can communicate by vertical eye movements)

4. Psychogenic coma (demonstrate clinical and electroencephalographic [EEG] evidence of wakefulness)

5. Inapparent status epilepticus (impaired consciousness with EEG evidence of continuous seizures)

B. Prognosis

1. Depressed consciousness: Prognosis depends on the underlying cause, degree of reversibility, and presence of secondary brain damage from effects of raised intracranial pressure (ICP).

2. Locked-in-state: Patients usually have permanent paralysis but can communicate though blinks. Acute locked-in state can sometimes be reversible with treatment of the underlying cause (thrombolytic therapy for a basilar artery stroke).

3. Status epilepticus: usually reversible with antiepileptic drugs but may sustain permanent damage after prolonged seizure activity.

C. Diagnosis

1. Rapid evaluation for the presence of neck rigidity (meningitis or subarachnoid hemorrhage), needle marks (drug overdose), or asymmetric dilated pupils (impending herniation) should be a priority before a more detailed examination.

TABLE 135-1	Localization of Brain Dysfunction in Patients with Apparent Change in Consciousness

Clinical state	Area of dysfunction
Depressed consciousness	Reticular activating system (RAS)
Drowsiness	Reticular activating system (RAS)
Stupor/coma	RAS and bilateral cerebral hemispheres
Acute confusional state	Bilateral cerebral hemispheres
Receptive aphasia	Dominant temporoparietal lobes
Akinetic mutism	Bilateral frontal lobes; diencephalons bilaterally
Persistent vegetative state	Bilateral cerebral hemispheres

2. Detailed history of onset, preceding events, and past medical conditions and medications and drugs is crucial to establishing the correct diagnosis.

3. In mild brain dysfunction (lethargy, hypersomnolence) mild sensory stimulation results in orientation and appropriate responses are made. In more severe brain dysfunction (obtundation and stupor) more severe and sustained sensory stimuli are required to achieve transient arousal. Patients may have purposeful movements when aroused but lack normal content of consciousness.

4. Severe brain dysfunction results in coma, from which patients cannot be aroused.

5. If spontaneous blinking is present in a paralyzed patient, appropriate responses may be elicited to questions, indicating normal cortical function (locked-in syndrome).

6. Comatose patients demonstrating active resistance, rapid closure of the eyelids, pupillary constriction to visual threat, fast phase of nystagmus on oculovestibular or optokinetic testing, and avoidance of self-injury may have psychogenic coma.

7. Nonfocal neurologic examination is suggestive of a toxic-metabolic coma, with some exceptions (meningoencephalitis, subarachnoid hemorrhage, bilateral subdural hematomas, or thrombosis of the superior sagittal sinus) (Table 135-2).

8. Presence of focal neurologic signs (cranial nerves or motor system) suggests a structural lesion as the underlying cause of coma.

9. Brain death is the irreversible destruction of the brain (total absence of all cortical and brainstem function, although spinal cord reflexes may remain).

   a. Pupils are in midposition, are round, and do not respond to light.

   b. No inspiratory effort (i.e., central apnea) even when arterial carbon dioxide tension (PCO_2) is raised to levels that should stimulate respiration. Sedating medications, drug intoxications, metabolic disturbances, hypothermia, and shock should be excluded as complicating conditions in determining brain death.

D. Ancillary tests

1. Computed tomographic (CT) or magnetic resonance imaging (MRI) scan without contrast demonstrates intracranial hemorrhage and hydrocephalus; contrast enhancement is required for infections or neoplastic masses. MRI demonstrates ischemia within minutes after stroke onset.

2. Comprehensive metabolic profile, blood gases, and toxic screen must be performed, especially if CT and MRI fail to demonstrate a structural lesion.

3. The cerebrospinal fluid must be examined if meningoencephalitis or subarachnoid hemorrhage is suspected.

4. EEG is most useful in suspected seizures, as a confirmatory test for brain death, in suspected infections (herpes encephalitis, Creutzfeldt-Jakob disease), and to demonstrate normal rhythm and reactivity in locked-in syndrome and psychogenic coma.

E. Treatment

1. Definitive treatment of altered consciousness depends on the underlying cause.

TABLE 135-2	Classification of Causes of Altered Consciousness Based on Most Common Clinical Presentation

1. Depressed consciousness or acute confusional state *without* focal or lateralizing neurologic signs and without signs of meningeal irritation.[a]
   - Metabolic disorders: hepatic failure, uremia, hypercapnia, hypoxia, hypoglycemia, diabetic hyperosmolar state, hypercalcemia, thiamine or cobalamine deficiency, hypotension
   - Drug intoxications or poisoning: opiates, alcohol, barbiturates, tricyclic antidepressants, amphetamines, anticholinergic agents, other sedatives, carbon monoxide, heavy metal toxins
   - Infectious and other febrile illnesses: septicemia, pneumonia, rheumatic fever, connective tissue diseases
   - Nonconvulsive status epilepticus or postconvulsive lethargy
   - Situational psychoses: intensive care unit, puerperal, postoperative, or posttraumatic psychoses; severe sleep deprivation can be complicating factor
   - Abstinence states (i.e., withdrawal states): alcohol (delirium tremens), barbiturates, benzodiazepines
   - Space-occupying lesions: bilateral subdural hematoma, midline cerebral tumors (e.g., lymphoma, glioma), abscess
   - Hydrocephalus
2. Altered consciousness *with* signs of meningeal irritation
   - Infectious disorders: meningoencephalitis (bacterial, viral, fungal, parasitic)
   - Subarachnoid hemorrhage: brain contusion, ruptured aneurysm, or other vascular malformation
   - Rheumatologic conditions: meningeal granulomatous disorders (e.g., sarcoid, Wegener granulomatosis)
3. Altered consciousness with *focal or lateralizing neurologic signs*
   - Space-occupying lesion: neoplasm, hemorrhage, inflammatory process (e.g., abscess, autoimmune encephalitis)
   - Cerebral ischemia or infarction: stroke, hypertensive encephalopathy

[a]Meningismus is often absent in deeply comatose patients with meningeal inflammation.

---

2. Reversal of depressed consciousness with intravenous thiamine, glucose, and naloxone often provides rapid diagnostic clues about unsuspected thiamine deficiency, hypoglycemia, or opioid overdose, respectively.

3. Fluid replacement, oxygenation, suctioning, positioning, nutrition, corneal protection, and bowel and bladder care are essential.

N.B.: Sedating drugs confound the accurate monitoring of the patient's neurologic condition and *should be avoided or minimized whenever possible*.

4. In ischemic/hypoxic cases due to cardiac arrest **induced hypothermia** may limit neurologic damage and improve outcome (refer to Chapter 137.

III. THE PATIENT APPEARS AWAKE BUT IS CONFUSED OR NONCOMMUNICATIVE

A. General principles. Patients with this clinical presentation may have acute confusional state, nonconvulsive seizures, receptive aphasia, or akinetic mutism.

1. Acute confusional state. Easily distracted, poor attention span with resultant poor recall and short-term memory

2. Delirium
   a. Behave as in acute confusional state
   b. Autonomic hyperactivity with hypervigilance
   c. Delusions and often visual hallucinations

3. Nonconvulsive status epilepticus. Signs that are suggestive of this diagnosis are episodic staring, eye deviation or nystagmoid jerks, facial or hand clonic activity, and automatisms.

4. Receptive aphasia
   a. Unable to respond to command or repeat
   b. Fluent but jargon speech with paraphasias (word substitution)
5. Akinetic mutism
   a. Brainstem function is intact and sleep—wake cycles may be present.
   b. Little evidence is seen of cognitive function. Patient may open eyes to auditory stimulation or track moving objects, but only a paucity of spontaneous movement occurs. *Persistent vegetative state* is similar but more severe and usually follows prolonged coma. Complex subcortical responses are absent, but decorticate or decerebrate posturing and other rudimentary subcortical responses (e.g., yawn, cough) are seen.

B. Diagnosis
   1. The history is critical in determining the cause of the patient's condition, and efforts to locate family members, witnesses, and medication lists are almost always fruitful.
      a. Knowledge of preexisting cerebral dysfunction (e.g., dementia, multiple sclerosis, mental retardation) is important in determining the degree of depressed consciousness or confusion expected for a specific systemic derangement (e.g., hyponatremia, sepsis, drug intoxication).
      b. A reliable account of the tempo of loss of consciousness is important. For example, truly sudden coma in a healthy person suggests drug intoxication, intracranial hemorrhage, brainstem ischemic stroke, meningoencephalitis, or an unwitnessed seizure.
   2. Focal neurologic signs suggest a structural cause of altered consciousness, although focal weakness or partial motor seizures sometimes occur in metabolic encephalopathies (e.g., hypoglycemia). Other falsely localizing signs include sixth nerve palsies caused by transmitted increased ICP and visual field cuts caused by compression of the posterior cerebral artery. Conversely, a nonfocal examination does not invariably indicate toxic-metabolic encephalopathy, although it often will cause symmetric neurologic dysfunction (see Table 135-2).
   C. Treatment. Refer earlier to treatment of impaired consciousness

Selected Readings

Adams RD, Victor M, Ropper AH. *Principles of neurology*, 6th edition. New York: McGraw-Hill, 1997.
A lucid and comprehensive review of disorders of consciousness (Chapter 17) and acute confusional states (Chapter 20).

Hayward LJ, Drachman DA. Evaluating the patient with altered consciousness in the intensive care unit. In: Irwin RS, Cerra FB, Rippe JM, eds. *Intensive care medicine*, 5th ed. Philadelphia: Lippincott, Williams & Wilkins, 2003.
The full-length version of this chapter.

Fisher CM. The neurological examination of the comatose patient. *Acta Neurol Scand* 1969;45(suppl 36):1–56.
Insightful account of important neurologic signs.

Plum F, Posner JB. *Diagnosis of stupor and coma*, 3rd ed. Philadelphia: FA Davis, 1980.
Classic monograph, with original investigations on stupor and coma.

I. BACKGROUND

A. Metabolic encephalopathy is defined as global brain dysfunction caused by a biochemical derangement.

B. There is often a fluctuating level of consciousness with nonfocal signs. Patients can present with:

    1. Delirium (confusion, sleeplessness, hallucinosis).

    2. Depressed level of consciousness (drowsiness, stupor, coma).

C. Metabolic encephalopathy is common in illnesses that cause multiorgan failure.

D. The following increase the risk of developing metabolic encephalopathy:

    1. Age greater than 60 years

    2. Systemic infection

    3. Temperature dysregulation

    4. Chronic disease of the central nervous system (CNS)

    5. Organ failure

    6. Endocrine disorders

    7. Multiple CNS-acting drugs

    8. Nutritional deficiency

    9. Alcoholism

    10. History of perinatal injury

    11. Sleep deprivation, sensory deprivation

E. In cases of a correctible metabolic disorder, prompt treatment may result in reversal of encephalopathy.

F. Progression to stupor or coma may lead to prolonged encephalopathy and complications, with a poor neurologic outcome.

II. ETIOLOGY

A. Drugs and toxins (50%)

B. Hepatic, renal, or pulmonary failure (12%)

C. Endocrine or electrolyte disturbances (8%)

D. Other causes: thiamine deficiency (exacerbated by glucose loading), prolonged hypoglycemia, hypoperfusion during cardiac bypass, hyperthermia (>105°F), hyperammonemia

III. PATHOGENESIS

A. Altered substrate (glucose/oxygen) for neurotransmitter function

B. CNS depressant drug accumulation due to abnormal volume of distribution (decreased protein, high lipophilicity)

C. Impaired cerebral blood flow

D. Abnormal cerebrospinal fluid (CSF) dynamics

E. Altered neuronal function due to temperature and or ionic changes

IV. DIAGNOSIS. Metabolic encephalopathy should be considered when a patient exhibits altered cognition or alertness. The clinical examination should include (Table 136-1):

A. General physical examination:

    1. Vital signs, breathing pattern, pulse oximetry

    2. Fundoscopy, to evaluate for papilledema (increased intracranial pressure), septic emboli

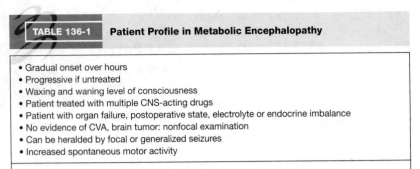

TABLE 136-1   Patient Profile in Metabolic Encephalopathy

- Gradual onset over hours
- Progressive if untreated
- Waxing and waning level of consciousness
- Patient treated with multiple CNS-acting drugs
- Patient with organ failure, postoperative state, electrolyte or endocrine imbalance
- No evidence of CVA, brain tumor: nonfocal examination
- Can be heralded by focal or generalized seizures
- Increased spontaneous motor activity

CNS, central nervous system; CVA, cerebrovascular accident.

   3. Cardiovascular examination: global cerebral hypoperfusion may result from congestive heart failure
   4. Bowel sounds: obstruction/perforation may cause agitation and changes in mental status
   5. Bladder distention: retention can lead to agitation
  B. Neurologic examination
   1. Behavioral changes: inattention, diminished speech, disorientation, impaired short-term memory, indifference, blunted affect, waxing and waning consciousness, hallucinosis
   2. Abnormal extraocular eye movements should raise suspicion of brainstem stroke or thiamine deficiency; pupils are usually small and reactive, although they may be dilated in some toxic encephalopathies related to adrenergic excess (e.g., thyroid storm, cocaine overdose)
   3. Respiratory pattern can be deranged in a variety of ways, including hyperventilation (e.g., acidosis), Cheyne-Stokes respiration, hypoventilation, gasping, apneic episodes (central or obstructive), hiccoughing.
   4. Abnormal motor activity: tremors, myoclonus, asterixis, restlessness, chorea, muscle spasms, rigidity, rigors
   5. Hyperreflexia and Babinski signs may be present.
   6. Dysautonomia with widely fluctuating blood pressure and core temperature should raise suspicion of sepsis.
  C. Metabolic encephalopathy should be distinguished from:
   1. Brainstem stroke (see Chapter 139)
   2. Increased intracranial pressure from an expanding mass lesion in the brain
   3. Meningoencephalitis (e.g., herpes)
   4. Occult head trauma
   5. Nonconvulsive status epilepticus
  D. Metabolic encephalopathy due to thiamine deficiency should be suspected in all encephalopathic patients who are malnourished and/or have a history of alcohol abuse. Patients with the syndrome can present with oculomotor paresis, nystagmus, pupillary abnormalities. Administration of glucose without parenteral thiamine can lead to severe exacerbation of encephalopathy and lead to permanent CNS injury.

V. LABORATORY STUDIES
  A. Body fluids
   1. Toxicology screen, especially in patients with history of major depression, substance abuse. Include salicylates, barbiturates, opioids, amphetamines, alcohol, benzodiazepines, caffeine, theophyllines.
   2. Drug levels: digoxin, anticonvulsants, lithium

3. Metabolic panel: blood urea nitrogen (BUN), creatinine, electrolytes, complete blood count (CBC), platelet count, thyroid-stimulating hormone (TSH), calcium, phosphate, arterial ammonia, blood gases, serum and urine osmolality, blood glucose
4. When indicated, CSF analysis for infection, inflammation, subarachnoid blood
5. Urinalysis, urine culture, blood cultures
B. Electroencephalogram (EEG): background slow wave activity or frontal triphasic waves are seen in metabolic encephalopathy. Epileptiform activity raises possibility of nonconvulsive status epilepticus.
C. Imaging studies
   1. Computed tomography (CT) or magnetic resonance imaging (MRI) scan of the brain, to evaluate for an acute structural lesion
   2. Chest radiographic films, to evaluate for occult pneumonia
   3. Abdominal radiographic films, to evaluate for bowel obstruction.

VI. TREATMENT

A. Correction of the underlying metabolic disturbance. Acute encephalopathy due to thiamine deficiency is a medical emergency. If suspected, give thiamine 100 mg intravenously daily for at least 3 days; the oral route is not suitable for rapidly repleting thiamine.
B. Improvement in cognition and arousal may lag behind the improvement in metabolic parameters by days to weeks in some cases.
   1. With underlying neurodegenerative disease, patients may not recover to their baseline level despite stabilized metabolic values.
   2. Avoid adding CNS-acting drugs, such as stimulants and sedatives, for the behavioral changes of metabolic encephalopathy before addressing the inherent causes.

VII. CONCLUSIONS

A. Metabolic encephalopathy is a common cause of altered neurologic function in the intensive care unit (ICU) setting.
B. It should be suspected when there is a fluctuating mental status, bouts of restlessness, and a nonfocal examination.
C. The causes are varied, but vigilant correction of metabolic disorders, reduction in CNS-acting drugs, and general supportive measures improve the outcome in most patients.
D. Patients in the ICU commonly have poor nutritional status and global encephalopathy. These patients should be treated empirically for acute thiamine deficiency.

Selected Readings

Adams RD, Victor M, Ropper AH. The acquired metabolic disorders of the nervous system. In: *Principles of neurology*, 6th edition. McGraw-Hill, 1997.
Barlas I, et al. Neurologic complications in intensive care. *Curr Opin Crit Care* 2001;7: 68–73.
Hung SC, et al. Thiamine deficiency and unexplained encephalopathy in peritoneal dialysis patients. *Am J Kidney Dis* 2001 38: 941–947.
Kunze K. Metabolic encephalopathies. *J Neurol* 2002;249:1150–1159.
Lewis M and Howdle PD. The neurology of liver failure. *QJM* 2003;96: 623–633.
Victor M. Neurologic disorders due to alcoholism and malnutrition. In Baker AB, Baker LH, eds. *Clinical neurology*, 2nd edition. Philadelphia: Harper and Row, 1983.

137 GENERALIZED ANOXIA/ISCHEMIA OF THE NERVOUS SYSTEM
Majaz Moonis and Carol F. Lippa

I. GENERAL PRINCIPLES
A. Failure of blood flow (cardiac arrest) or reduced oxygenation to the brain (respiratory failure, carbon monoxide or cyanide poisoning) for 4 to 5 minutes results in brain damage, since the brain tolerates oxygen deprivation poorly.

B. Anoxia resulting from respiratory failure from any cause is better tolerated than when the primary event is cardiac arrest.

II. PROGNOSIS.
Many factors determine the prognosis after anoxic brain insult. These include the cause of the anoxic/ischemic insult, effective time to establish recirculation (arrest time [AT] + CPR time), level of consciousness, age of patient and neurological signs present at 24–72 hours.

A. Favorable prognostic indicators include:
1. Retained consciousness during the anoxic/ischemic insult

2. Primary respiratory failure carries a better prognosis than primary cardiac arrest.

3. Recovery of multiple brainstem responses within 48 hours of arrest (pupillary, corneal, and oculovestibular).

4. Return of purposeful motor movements within 24 hours (localization of pain).

5. Young age (children may do well even beyond this time period).

6. Primary pulmonary event leading to the coma.

7. Hypothermia at arrest time (cold water drowning).

B. Poor prognostic indicators in patients with persistent coma after 72 hours include:
1. The absence of pupillary responses or motor response to pain at 72 hours

2. Presence of diffuse cerebral edema on CT scan

3. Certain abnormal EEG patterns including alpha coma , burst suppression or low voltage unreactive delta activity.

4. Absent cortical evoked potential N20 response after 72 hours of coma. If the cortical N20 responses can be elicited, the chances of improvement are increased to 25%.

5. CSF neuron-specific enolase greater than 24 ng/ml at 24 hour or a creatine kinase-BB greater than 50 U/L at 48 to 72 hours.

III. ETIOLOGY
A. Cardiac arrest from any cause

B. Respiratory Failure from any cause

C. Poisoning (carbon monoxide, cyanide, others)

IV. PATHOPHYSIOLOGY.
Following these injuries, excess glutamate release results in activation of the excitotoxic cascade, calcium influx into neurons and cell death.

V. DIAGNOSIS
A. History
1. Cardiac arrest

2. Respiratory failure

3. Drowning

4. Drug intoxication/ poisoning

B. Examination. Patients are comatose without focal neurological deficits. Rarely soft neurological signs have been documented

C. Imaging and Laboratory Studies

1. Computerized tomography scan to rule out structural lesions such as stroke, hemorrhage within a tumor or brain herniation.
2. Blood glucose, liver function tests including ammonia, blood urea nitrogen, and creatinine should be obtained to rule out hypoglycemia or other causes of metabolic encephalopathy.
3. Toxic screen should be obtained when the cause of coma is unknown
4. An immediate electroencephalogram (EEG) if nonconvulsive status is suspected

VI. TREATMENT

A. Adequate oxygenation (PaO_2 over 100 mm Hg) and mean arterial blood pressure (90 to 110 mm Hg) should be maintained.

B. Patients should be kept slightly hypovolemic and the head of the bed elevated to 30 degrees.

C. Underlying causes such as toxins or drug ingestion should be treated.

D. Cardiac arrhythmias should be controlled.

E. A diligent search for infections should be done and treated appropriately.

F. Patients should not be allowed to become hyperthermic.

G. All other toxic, metabolic, or structural causes of comas should be ruled out.

H. Vital signs, hematocrit, electrolytes, blood sugar, and serum osmolarity should be maintained within the normal range.

I. Seizures (25%). Fosphenytoin at 20 phenytoin equivalents/kg intravenously (IV) or intramuscularly (low risk of inducing hypotension and can be given intramuscularly if there is no IV access). Alternatively, phenytoin in the same doses can be given with careful blood pressure and cardiac monitoring. If serious acute underlying cardiac arrhythmias exist, IV phenobarbital is preferred.

J. EEG monitoring

1. If seizures are controlled, a delayed EEG is done after 48 hours.
2. Continuous EEG monitoring is required for status epilepticus.

K. Controlling brain edema

1. There is no role for the use of steroids or high-dose barbiturates, and hyperosmolar agents are seldom helpful in anoxic or hypoxic coma.
2. Controlled hyperventilation with a PCO_2 of 25 to 28 mm may be effective in the short term to avoid impending herniation.

L. Hypothermia. In two prospective trials, *induced hypothermia* (IH) with rapid cooling to 33°C for 12 to 24 hours was found to be significantly better in improving outcome after coma due to cardiac arrest compared with patients allowed to maintain normothermia. Increased vascular resistance and decreased cardiac output were significant complications. However, the incidence of cardiac arrhythmia was similar in the hypothermic and normothermic groups. Larger trials with better methods of rapid cooling should be explored; in some medical centers, IH is currently considered the standard of practice.

M. Mobilization. Once coma begins to lighten, early mobilization should be the goal to prevent other complications.

VII. COMPLICATIONS

A. Delayed brain damage. Seen rarely, 3 to 30 days after the initial recovery especially following carbon monoxide poisoning; a late functional decline occurs, with irritability, lethargy, and increased muscle tone. Pathologically, widespread demyelination is found. Most patients survive this second insult.

B. Intention myoclonus is another delayed consequence. This can be distinguished from seizures by the absence of corresponding EEG changes.

C. Persistent vegetative state. No cortical functions, although the person appears awake and retains many of the bodily functions (feeding, sleep-wake cycle).

D. Brain death. The criteria for brain death are defined in Chapters 134 and 152. Total absence of electrocerebral activity, not associated with sedative hypnotic drugs or hypothermia, is helpful in confirming brain death in difficult cases. Similarly, a brain scan showing absence of blood flow is strongly suggestive of brain death. Many institutions have specific brain death protocols that should be followed when determining brain death.

Selected Readings

Abramson NS, Safar P, Detre KM. Neurological recovery after cardiac arrest. Effect of duration of ischemia. *Crit Care Med* 1985;14:930.
A useful article that reviews the relationship between the duration of cerebral ischemia and clinical outcome in anoxic encephalopathy.

Bernard SA, Gray TW, Buist MD, et al. Treatment of comatose survivors of out-of-hospital cardiac arrest with induced hypothermia. *N Engl J Med* 2002;346:557–563.
This landmark prospective trial demonstrated that induced hypothermia improves outcome after out-of-hospital cardiac arrest and anoxic coma.

Chatrian GE. Coma, other states of altered responsiveness and brain death. In: Daly DD, Pedley AT, eds. *Current practice of clinical electroencephalography*, 2nd ed. Philadelphia: Lippincott–Raven, 1990, p. 425.
Electroencephalogram patterns and their prognostic significance in coma.

Garcia JH. Morphology of cerebral ischemia. *Crit Care Med* 1988;16:979.
A review of various sequelae of anoxic encephalopathy.

Levy DE, Bates D, Caronna JJ, et al. Prognosis in non-traumatic coma. *Ann Intern Med* 1981;94:293.
A landmark article on the prognosis in nontraumatic coma.

Plum F, Posner JB. *Multifocal, diffuse and metabolic brain diseases causing stupor and coma in the diagnosis of stupor and coma.* Philadelphia: FA Davis, 1982, p. 177.
A classic work that reviews anoxic encephalopathy.

Simon RP. Hypoxia versus ischemia. *Neurology* 1999;52:7.
A thoughtful discussion on the prognostic outcome between the two types of cerebral anoxia.

The Hypothermia After Cardiac Arrest Study Group: Mild therapeutic hypothermia to improve the neurological outcome after cardiac arrest. *N Engl J Med* 2002;346:549–556
A multicenter trial of induced hypothermia (IH) in anoxic coma where rapid external cooling to 33°C followed by delayed rewarming led to a significantly better outcome for recovery. The rationale of IH and benefits and risks are discussed.

Wijdicks EF, Parisi JE, Sharbrough FW. Prognostic value of myoclonus status in comatose survivors of cardiac arrest. *Ann Neurol* 1994;35:239.
A brief article that assesses the different types of seizure activity in anoxic encephalopathy and prognostic implications of the various seizure types.

Zandbergen EGJ, de Haan RJ, Stoutenbeek CP, et al. Systemic review of early prediction of poor outcome in anoxic-ischemic coma. *Lancet* 1998;352:1808.
A summary of the literature concerning reliable indicators of death or a vegetative state following acute anoxia.

I. DEFINITIONS
A. *Status epilepticus* is defined as:
  1. Usually, one or more epileptic seizures lasting 30 minutes or longer without recovery between attacks; or
  2. Seizure activity lasting 5 minutes or longer; or
  3. Two or more seizures with incomplete recovery of consciousness between them.
B. *Myoclonic status* is repetitive, asynchronous myoclonic jerks with variable clouding of consciousness, usually in the setting of severe encephalopathy such as cerebral anoxia; patients are usually comatose.
C. *Simple partial status* is continuous or repetitive focal seizures without loss of consciousness. This includes *epilepsia partialis continua*, with continuous localized clonic seizure activity that does not generalize and in which consciousness is maintained.
D. *Nonconvulsive status* is a confusional state of 30 minutes or more.
  1. In *absence status*, consciousness varies with subtle myoclonic facial movements and automatisms of face and hands.
  2. *Complex partial status* involves either a series of complex partial seizures, separated by a confusional state, or a prolonged state of partial responsiveness and semipurposeful automatisms.

II. ETIOLOGY
A. Symptomatic status—status caused by a neurologic or metabolic insult—is more common than idiopathic status.
B. Status can be caused by stroke (ischemic or hemorrhagic), anoxic brain injury, electrolyte disturbances (e.g., hyponatremia, hypomagnesemia, hypoglycemia, hyperglycemia, uremia, sepsis), drug or other toxicity, alcohol or other drug withdrawal, and decreasing antiepileptic medication.
C. Viral encephalitis from Epstein-Barr syndrome or herpes simplex virus can have an abrupt onset heralded by status epilepticus.

III. PROGNOSIS AND SEQUELAE
A. Overall, mortality rate is 7% to 25%. Advanced age and prolonged status are poor prognostic factors.
B. Status caused by anoxia has the highest mortality rate, followed by hemorrhage, tumor, metabolic disorders, and systemic infection. Status caused by alcohol withdrawal and antiepileptic drug discontinuation, and idiopathic status, have lower mortality rates.
C. In one study, duration greater than 60 minutes was associated with a mortality rate of 32%, compared with 3% for duration less than 60 minutes.
D. Long-term sequelae may include intellectual deterioration, permanent focal neurologic deficits, and chronic epilepsy. Aspiration pneumonia is a common complication of status.
E. Generalized tonic—clonic status epilepticus is the most common form of status with the most severe neurologic sequelae.

IV. INITIAL ASSESSMENT
A. Patients with generalized tonic—clonic status usually do not convulse continuously, and observation is necessary to determine that generalized seizures occur without recovery of consciousness.

TABLE 138-1	Management Protocol for Generalized Status Epilepticus in Adults

Minutes: 0–10
1. If diagnosis is uncertain, observe recurrence of generalized seizures without subsequent recovery of consciousness.
2. Assess cardiopulmonary status; establish airway, administer O_2, initiate cardiac monitoring.
3. Start IV line with normal saline.
4. Draw blood for complete blood count and differential, glucose, blood urea nitrogen, creatinine, electrolytes, calcium, liver function tests, antiepileptic drug levels, toxicology screen; perform bedside glucose determination.
5. Give glucose (D_{50}) 50 mL and thiamine 100 mg IV if hypoglycemia is present.
6. Monitor respirations, blood pressure, ECG, oximetry, and, if possible, EEG.
7. Give lorazepam (0.1 mg/kg) IV bolus, <2 mg/min (may use 2 to 4 mg initial dose, and complete dose as needed).

Minutes: 10–30
8. Start phenytoin or fosphenytoin (20 mg/kg) IV, ≤50 mg/min, with slower rate if hypotension develops.
9. Give additional boluses of phenytoin or fosphenytoin (5 mg/kg), to a maximum of 30 mg/kg, if patient is still having seizures.

Minutes: 30–90
10. If status continues after phenytoin infusion is completed, immediately start phenobarbital (20 mg/kg) IV ≤100 mg/min; intubation is necessary either before or during phenobarbital infusion.
11. If status persists, induce coma using one of the agents listed below (items a to c). Continuous EEG is needed to monitor seizure control and level of anesthesia. Monitor EEG hourly once burst-suppression pattern is present.
    a. Pentobarbital: 5 mg/kg IV load, given slowly; give additional 5-mg/kg boluses as necessary to produce burst-suppression pattern. Maintenance infusion of 0.5 to 5 mg/kg/h.
    b. Midazolam, 0.1 to 0.3 mg/kg IV load, infusion rate 0.05 to 2 mg/kg/h.
    c. Propofol, 1- to 5-mg/kg load, infusion rate 1 to 15 mg/kg/h.
12. Slowly withdraw medication at 12 hours; if seizures recur, resume infusion for 24 hours, then stop again; continue this process as necessary.

    B. In nonconvulsive or focal motor status, the diagnosis requires 30 minutes of continuous clinical (or electrical) seizure activity. When status epilepticus presents with a change in mental status only, an electroencephalogram (EEG) is required for confirmation.

V. INITIAL MANAGEMENT AND MEDICAL STABILIZATION
    A. Initial assessment and treatment should begin within 5 minutes of onset of seizure activity (Table 138-1).
    B. History: include information on a preexisting chronic seizure disorder and antiepileptic drug use.
    C. Examination: signs of systemic illness (e.g., uremia, hepatic disease, infection); illicit drug use; trauma; focal neurologic abnormalities.
    D. Administer glucose for hypoglycemia (hypoglycemic status is rare but easily reversible; can cause irreversible central nervous system [CNS] damage untreated). Thiamine should be given because glucose can precipitate Wernicke-Korsakoff syndrome with marginal nutrition.
    E. IV infusions should consist of saline solution, because some antiepileptic drugs precipitate in glucose solutions.
    F. Hyperthermia caused by status: treat with alcohol sponge baths, cooling blankets, or ice packs.

G. Oxygenation must be maintained.

H. Metabolic acidosis often develops early in status but usually resolves spontaneously once seizures stop; treatment with bicarbonate is usually not necessary.

I. Blood pressure must be monitored; if hypotension occurs, the brain is vulnerable to inadequate perfusion. Pharmacologic intervention for the seizures can exacerbate hypotension.

J. When a metabolic disorder causes status, pharmacologic intervention alone is not effective.

K. Exclude systemic and CNS infections; lumbar puncture (LP) is often necessary; (leukocytosis, fever, and cerebrospinal fluid pleocytosis may be caused by status itself).

L. Only short-acting paralytic agents should be used, if these agents are absolutely required; otherwise, ongoing EEG monitoring will be necessary.

M. Contrast-enhanced head computed tomography (CT) scan may demonstrate a structural cause, but scan should be done after the patient has been stabilized and the seizures controlled. Magnetic resonance imaging (MRI) is preferred but often not practical in the emergent setting.

VI. PHARMACOLOGIC MANAGEMENT OF GENERALIZED STATUS EPILEPTICUS

A. Goals: stop seizures early; prevent recurrence. Generalized convulsive status is a medical emergency.

B. A benzodiazepine drug is the initial therapy for status. Diazepam has a brief duration of action (10 to 25 minutes). Lorazepam is equally effective with a much longer duration of action (2 to 24 hours). Both benzodiazepines have essentially the same cardiac, respiratory, and CNS depressant side effects. Respiratory depression and apnea can occur abruptly with the initial doses, especially when given IV, and previous administration of sedative drugs and increasing age potentiate cardiorespiratory side effects.

   1. Lorazepam should be given 0.1 mg/kg IV at 2 mg/min; a 2- to 4-mg dose may be given initially. A total dose of up to 0.2 mg/kg may be given if necessary. The dose of diazepam is 0.15 mg/kg, with an additional 0.1 mg/kg if necessary.

   2. Hypotension may be partially caused by the propylene glycol solvent in IV diazepam and lorazepam.

   3. Rectal diazepam is an alternative. For adults, 7.5 to 10 mg of the IV preparation or 0.2 mg/kg of the rectal gel preparation, is administered per rectum (PR). The incidence of significant respiratory depression is lower with PR compared to IV administration.

   4. IM absorption of these agents is delayed and incomplete; this route is unsuitable for treating status.

   5. Midazolam can also be effective but has an extremely short duration of action and a high recurrence rate of seizures.

C. *Phenytoin* IV is very effective in status. Phenytoin should *not* be given IM. A 20-mg/kg load is given at a maximal rate of 50 mg/min, with an additional 10 mg/kg if the initial load is not effective.

   1. Hypotension, electrocardiographic (ECG) changes and respiratory depression can occur, partly from the propylene glycol diluent. Cardiac monitoring should be performed and the drug given more slowly (25 mg/min) in elderly patients or in those with a history of cardiac arrhythmias, compromised pulmonary function, or hypotension. The most common adverse effect is hypotension.

   2. Severe tissue injury can also occur if phenytoin extravasates into tissue.

D. *Fosphenytoin*: a water-soluble prodrug of phenytoin, rapidly converted to phenytoin. Fosphenytoin should be considered when IV access is not available or phenytoin infusion is poorly tolerated at the infusion site.

   1. Fosphenytoin has greater aqueous solubility than phenytoin; it may be used IV or IM, is nonirritating, and is rapidly and completely absorbed by either route.

   2. Therapeutic phenytoin concentrations are attained in 10 minutes with rapid IV infusion and in 30 minutes with slower IV infusion or IM injection.

   3. Fosphenytoin is dosed in "phenytoin equivalents" (PE) units, (same as for phenytoin [load 20 mg/kg PE]); administered at rates up to 150 mg/min PE.

   4. Cardiac monitoring is required with IV fosphenytoin.

E. Phenobarbital is as effective as the combination of benzodiazepines and phenytoin for initial therapy, but CNS depression is a major side effect.

    1. If status persists 10 minutes after phenytoin is given, IV phenobarbital should be given (10 mg/kg) as an initial dose, then repeated if seizures continue (up to 20 mg/kg).

    2. Phenobarbital can be administered up to 100 mg/min.

    3. *Respiratory depression is a major side effect,* especially if benzodiazepines have been used, and it is imperative to monitor respirations and ensure an adequate airway.

    4. In some cases, treatment of the status proceeds directly to induction of anesthesia as described below, without using phenobarbital.

F. Refractory status epilepticus. If status continues after full loading doses of phenytoin and phenobarbital, a drug-induced coma to completely suppress electrical seizure activity is indicated.

    1. Intubate patient; close hemodynamic monitoring. Pressors are frequently needed. Ileus is also common.

    2. Simultaneous EEG monitoring required to monitor electrical seizure activity, assess depth of anesthesia.

    3. Barbiturates (e.g., pentobarbital), benzodiazepines, and propofol are commonly used to achieve drug-induced coma. Phenobarbital is not used for this purpose because it causes very prolonged coma.

    4. Drug dose is increased until a burst-suppression pattern (flat background punctuated by bursts of mixed-frequency activity) is seen on the EEG. If the bursts contain electrographic seizure activity, the coma should be deepened, at times to virtual electrocerebral silence.

    5. Goal: *terminate electrical seizure activity,* not just to produce a burst-suppression pattern.

    6. Maintenance doses of phenytoin and phenobarbital are continued and serum levels followed.

    7. Drug-induced coma is continued for 12 to 24 hours, then anesthesia is slowly withdrawn. If electrical seizures recur, the process is repeated for a longer period of time.

    8. If midazolam is used to induce coma and status is not terminated within 48 hours, substitute a different drug (e.g., pentobarbital, propofol) because the effects of midazolam tolerance will complicate therapy.

VII. PHARMACOLOGIC MANAGEMENT OF PARTIAL AND ABSENCE STATUS EPILEPTICUS

    A. Absence status is not associated with the severe adverse sequelae of convulsive status, but should be treated promptly.

    B. IV lorazepam is recommended, followed by more definitive treatment for absence epilepsy.

    C. Partial status may lead to neuronal injury and should be treated aggressively, using the same protocol as for generalized status but with longer time allotments for each phase of the protocol, particularly before the induction of generalized anesthesia.

Selected Readings

DeLorenzo RJ, Towne AR, Pellock JM, et al. Status epilepticus in children, adults and the elderly. *Epilepsia* 1992;33(suppl 4):515.
Epidemiologic factors and determinants, including age, duration of status epilepticus, and cause, are reviewed in a retrospective study to predict outcome of status epilepticus at different ages.

Lowenstein DH, Alldredge BK. Status epilepticus. *N Engl J Med* 1998;338:970.
Reviews the current concepts in the definition, clinical features, pathophysiology, and management of status epilepticus.

Towne AR, Pellock JM, Ko D, et al. Determinants of mortality in status epilepticus. *Epilepsia* 1994;35:27.

Factors, including age, duration of seizure, cerebral vascular disease, discontinuation of antiepileptic drugs, alcohol withdrawal, trauma, and so on, as determinants of mortality in status epilepticus are addressed and discussed in detail.

Treiman DM, Meyers PD, Walton NY, et al. A comparison of four treatments for generalized convulsive status epilepticus. *N Engl J Med* 1998;339:792.

Comparison of lorazepam, diazepam followed by phenytoin, phenytoin, and phenobarbital in the treatment of generalized convulsive status epilepticus in a randomized double-blinded multicenter trial is evaluated, with lorazepam being the most effective.

Working Group on Status Epilepticus. Treatment of convulsive status epilepticus. *JAMA* 1993;270:854.

Guidelines for the management of status epilepticus as recommended by an expert panel of the Epilepsy Foundation of America.

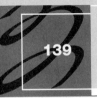

139 CEREBROVASCULAR DISEASE
Majaz Moonis, John P. Weaver, and Marc Fisher

I. GENERAL PRINCIPLES
  A. Cerebrovascular disease includes:
    1. Stroke caused by thrombotic or embolic ischemia
    2. Intracerebral and subarachnoid hemorrhage
  B. Admission to the intensive care unit (ICU) is often warranted because of the severity of the disease or institution of newer therapies.
  C. This chapter focuses on both ischemic cerebrovascular disease (ICVD) and intracerebral hemorrhage.

II. ISCHEMIC CEREBROVASCULAR DISEASE
  A. Prognosis
    1. Altered sensorium (state of consciousness), conjugate gaze paresis, and early radiologic signs of *large* infarction predict a poor outcome without intervention
    2. Lacunar stroke has a better prognosis (70% to 80% recovery).
    3. Following a transient ischemic attack (TIA), about 11% patients will have a stroke within 30 days, half of these within 48 hours with a significant mortality, suggesting the need for hospitalization of all patients presenting with a TIA.
  B. Etiology
    1. ICVD results from restriction of blood flow to the brain because of arterial occlusion.
    2. Cardioembolic stroke is due to ischemic heart disease, atrial fibrillation, or cardiomyopathy.
    3. Atherothrombotic stroke is caused by occlusion of a large intra/extracranial portion of the carotid/vertebrobasilar system from local stenosis and occlusion.
    4. Lacunar stroke is due to small blood vessel occlusion.
    5. Watershed territory strokes result from systemic hypotension, with resulting border zone infarction (areas between anterior and middle cerebral artery, or middle and posterior cerebral artery distributions).
  C. Diagnosis
    1. History. Helps to determine type of stroke:
      a. cardioembolic more common during the day with acute onset;
      b. atherothrombotic more often during sleep;
      c. intracranial hemorrhage often starts with a headache and deficit may progress for considerable time.
      d. Course: reversibility suggests TIA; coma at onset or presentation is a poor prognostic sign; lacunar stroke generally has a good prognosis.
    2. Examination
      a. Aphasia, hemiparesis or hemiparesthesia, and monocular visual loss suggest carotid system infarct.
      b. Vertigo, cerebellar ataxia, and crossed deficits (ipsilateral cranial nerve and the contralateral hemiparesis or hemiesthesia) suggest involvement of the vertebrobasilar system.
      c. Pure motor hemiparesis, pure sensory stroke, ataxic hemiparesis, and dysarthria—clumsy hand syndrome suggest the diagnosis of lacunar stroke.

3. Laboratory and radiological evaluation

   a. *Neuroimaging*: An essential procedure!

   (1) To exclude intracerebral or subarachnoid hemorrhage

   (2) To select patients for acute thrombolytic therapy.

   (3) Diffusion-weighted magnetic resonance imaging (DWI) can demonstrate ischemic lesions within minutes of onset, whereas perfusion imaging (PI) demonstrates the area at risk of eventual infarction. A DWI-PI mismatch demonstrates the penumbra (salvageable tissue). Perfusion computed tomography (CT), and CT angiography can be reasonable alternatives

   b. An *electrocardiogram* (ECG) and either telemetry or Holter monitoring should be obtained in all patients to look for rhythm disturbances or ischemic change.

   c. *Echocardiography,* preferably a transesophageal echocardiogram, should also be considered especially in younger patients with stroke.

   d. *Carotid ultrasound* provides information about extracranial vessels, and transcranial Doppler ultrasound provides information about the intracranial vessels.

   e. *Contrast-enhanced magnetic resonance angiography* (MRA) approaches angiography in defining details of carotid and vertebral artery disease.

   f. *Blood studies,* at a minimum, should include a complete blood count (CBC), erythrocyte sedimentation rate (ESR), coagulation profile, fasting lipid and blood glucose profile, and homocysteine levels. Hypercoagulable workup and anticardiolipin antibodies may be obtained in younger patients with history of venous thrombosis, recurrent abortions, thrombocytopenia and migraine (lupus anticoagulant syndrome), or unexplained stroke.

D. Treatment

1. The first step is to identify patients who are candidates for thrombolytic therapy with rt-PA. Thrombolytic therapy with rt-PA is associated with a 33% increased chance of being free of any disability after 3 months of treatment, but there is a 10-fold increased risk of intracranial bleeding—which can be reduced by careful patient selection.

   a. Patients presenting within 3 hours of onset of ischemic stroke should have an urgent CT scan to rule out hemorrhage and large infarcts (greater than one third the middle cerebral artery territory). Wherever available, a CT angiogram or preferably MRI (DWI-PI) and MR angiography should be performed.

   b. If DWI-PI mismatch is present in patients, there may be grounds to consider thrombolysis, even later than 3 hours poststroke.

   c. In large vessel stroke, nonspecialized medical centers may initiate intravenous rt-PA (two thirds of the normal 0.9-mg/kg dose) and then transfer the patient to a tertiary stroke center for an angiogram and possible additional intraarterial thrombolysis.

2. Blood pressure should be lowered to less than 185/105 mm Hg before thrombolytic therapy is initiated. For other patients, blood pressure can be observed in the absence of malignant hypertension; it should not be excessively lowered.

3. Subcutaneous heparin therapy and compression boots should be considered in immobilized patients.

4. Elevated temperature and hyperglycemia should be aggressively treated.

5. Oral feedings should be delayed until swallowing is well performed.

6. Cardioembolic stroke can be treated with delayed warfarin therapy. There is currently no clear role for the use of full intravenous heparin or heparinoids in secondary stroke prevention or to improve outcome.

7. Antiplatelet therapy should be considered in patients who do not have a clear embolic source. Extended-release dipyridamole and aspirin (ERDP/ASA; Aggrenox) is FDA approved and is 23% more effective in reducing recurrent stroke compared with aspirin.

8. Treatment with statins to reduce low-density lipoprotein (LDL) cholesterol to less than 100 mg/dL and delayed antihypertensive therapy with angiotensin-converting enzyme (ACE) inhibitors further reduce risk of recurrent stroke by 30% to 40%

9. Large strokes with worsening sensorium are treated with short-term mannitol and at times with intracranial pressure (ICP) monitoring. Neuroprotective therapy still remains a desired goal.

III. INTRACEREBRAL HEMORRHAGE

A. **General principles.** Nontraumatic intracerebral hemorrhage (ICH) often requires management in the ICU. Most cases are caused by hypertensive ICH or rupture of saccular aneurysms and arteriovenous malformations.

B. **Prognosis.** The prognosis for ICH is worse for larger lesions. Pontine ICH has the highest mortality, followed by cerebellar and then basal ganglia ICH. Lobar ICH carries the most favorable outlook for survival and functional recovery.

C. **Etiology**
   1. Hypertensive ICH results from rupture of arterial branch point acquired micro-aneurysm (Charcot-Bouchard aneurysms). Surrounding edema exerts a mass effect and blood may block ventricles, causing hydrocephalus.
   2. Nonhypertensive hemorrhage
      a. amyloid angiopathy;
      b. rupture of arteriovenous malformation (AVM)/aneurysm
      c. bleeding or coagulation disorders causing thrombocytopenia, loss of factors involved in coagulation (leukemia, idiopathic thrombocytopenia, severe liver disease, disseminated intravascular coagulation [DIC], and other rare disorders of coagulation

D. **Diagnosis**
   1. History. The presentation of ICH is abrupt and often associated with headache and progressive neurologic deficits over minutes to hours.
   2. Examination
      a. Helpful clinical hints to suggest ICH include deficits that extend beyond the distribution of a single artery and presence of altered sensorium.
      b. Localization
         (1) Putamen (hemiparesis, hemiesthesia)
         (2) Pons (hyperthermia, coma, pinpoint pupils)
         (3) Thalamus (hemiesthesia)
         (4) Cerebellum (ataxia, nystagmus, head tilt, vomiting)
         (5) Cerebral cortex. If cortical signs are present in a nonhypertensive ICH, suspect cerebral amyloid angiopathy.
   3. Radiological and laboratory tests
      a. CT scan demonstrates the site and size of the hematoma with great accuracy.
      b. Angiography should be considered if an underlying aneurysm or AVM is suspected.
      c. Lumbar puncture is contraindicated in ICH because of the risk of tentorial herniation.
      d. Coagulation profile and CBC to exclude underlying bleeding disorder.

E. **Treatment**
   1. Correct any predisposing systemic hemorrhagic factors to prevent further clinical deterioration.
   2. Lower systolic blood pressure in the acute phase of ICH to between 110 and 160 mm Hg. β-Blockers are the agents of choice. Vasodilators (e.g., Nipride) should be avoided because they can promote cerebral edema and elevate ICP.
   3. Acute increases in ICP may require hyperventilation and hyperosmolar agents, such as mannitol. Treatment of ICH with steroids can be detrimental.
   4. Elevation of ICP from hydrocephalus is treated with ventriculostomy.
   5. Surgery may be indicated for large superficial lobar ICH and cerebellar ICHs. Early surgical intervention is indicated for lesions greater than 2.5 cm or in

smaller lesions with clinical deterioration, because of a very high mortality rate in patients with untreated lesions.

6. Anticonvulsants are not routinely used in ICH.

7. Prophylaxis against venous thrombosis should be accomplished with pneumatic boots.

8. Delayed angiography may be performed in patients with no history of hypertension or if the bleeding is in an atypical location.

Selected Readings

Adams HP Jr, Adams RJ, Brott T, et al. Guidelines for the early management of patients with ischemic stroke: A scientific statement from the Stroke Council of the American Stroke Association. *Stroke* 2003;34(4):1056–1083.
Guidelines for stroke treatment offered by the stroke council of the American Stroke Association.

Bogousslavsky J, Van Melle G, Regli F. The Lausanne stroke registry. *Stroke* 1988;19:1083.
The first registry with complete computed tomography and Doppler data on all patients, allowing correlation between clinical findings, presumed cause, and stroke location.

Borges LF. Management of nontraumatic brain hemorrhage. In: Ropper AM, Kennedy SF, eds. Neurological and neurosurgical intensive care. Rockville, MD: Aspen, 1988, p. 209.
Management of intracerebral hemorrhage in a text that is essential for all intensive care units.

Chambers BR, Norris JW, Shurvell BL, et al. Prognosis of acute stroke. *Neurology* 1987;27:221.
A helpful discussion of the prognosis of acute stroke.

Clark WM, Portland OR, Warach SJ for the Citicoline Study Group. Randomized dose response trial of citicoline in acute ischemic stroke patients. *Neurology* 1996;46 (S1):A425.
Report on a trial of citicoline, an agent with minimal risks, in acute stroke.

Dewitt LD, Wechsler LR. Transcranial Doppler. *Stroke* 1988;19:915.
An important discussion of a noninvasive technique to assess intracerebral circulation.

Moonis M, Fisher M. Antiplatelet treatment for secondary prevention of acute ischemic stroke and transient ischemic attacks: mechanisms, choices and possible emerging patterns of use. *Expert Rev Cardiovasc Ther* 2003;1(4):611–615.
This is a useful article that puts into perspective antiplatelet agent use in primary and secondary stroke prevention.

Moonis M, Fisher M. Considering the role of heparin and low-molecular-weight heparins in acute ischemic stroke. *Stroke* 2002;33(7):1927–1933.
This article offers a balanced view of the current role of full-doze intravenous heparin in acute ischemic stroke.

National Institute of Neurological Disorders and Stroke rt-PA Stroke Study Group. Tissue PA for acute ischemic stroke. *N Engl J Med* 1995;333:1581.
The seminal work on tissue-type plasminogen activator in the treatment of acute stroke.

Omae T, Ueda K, Ogata J, et al. Parenchymatous hemorrhage: etiology, pathology and clinical aspects. In: Toule JF, ed. *Handbook of clinical neurology*, Vol 10. New York: Elsevier, 1989, p. 287.
An excellent review on intracerebral hemorrhage.

Ott KH, Kase CS, Ojemann RG, et al. Cerebellar hemorrhage: diagnosis and treatment—a review of 56 cases. *Arch Neurol* 1974;31:160.
An excellent review on cerebellar hemorrhage, which is important because of the differences in management between cerebellar and other types of intracerebral hemorrhage.

Poungvarin N, Bhoopat W, Viniarejakul A, et al. Effects of dexamethasone in primary supratentorial intracerebral hemorrhage. *N Engl J Med* 1987;316:1229.
An important discussion of management of intracerebral hemorrhage.

140 SUBARACHNOID HEMORRHAGE
Majaz Moonis, John P. Weaver, and Marc Fisher

I. GENERAL PRINCIPLES
  A. Frequency and morbidity of subarachnoid hemorrhage (SAH)
   1. Intracranial hemorrhage secondary to the rupture of saccular aneurysms accounts for 6% to 8% of all strokes.
   2. The mortality and morbidity associated with SAH are significant, causing disability despite modern medical or surgical management, rehabilitation, and chronic care provided in these cases.
  B. Management of SAH caused by a ruptured aneurysm includes:
   1. Early surgery to limit rebleeding
   2. A calcium antagonist to ameliorate cerebral injury secondary to vasospasm
   3. Blood volume replacement in cases of a deficit and circulatory control

II. PROGNOSIS. Prognostic indicators:
  A. Aneurysms greater than 10 mm in size and smaller aneurysms at the basilar tip are more likely to rupture as compared with smaller aneurysms in other locations.
  B. Coma at onset or decerebration (Hess and Hunt grades 3 and 4) is associated with worse outcome after SAH

III. PATHOGENESIS
  A. Saccular (berry) aneurysms are distinguished from other types of intracerebral aneurysms caused by trauma, vascular dissection, or mycotic lesions and those related to tumors.
  B. Of saccular aneurysms, 85% are located in the anterior circulation and 15% in the posterior circulation. Multiple aneurysms can occur in families or with systemic diseases such as polycystic kidney, Marfan syndrome, Ehlers-Danlos syndrome, pseudoxanthoma elasticum, fibromuscular dysplasia, and coarctation of the aorta.

IV. DIAGNOSIS
  A. History
   1. Severe headache, usually described as the worst headache ever; abrupt onset and peaks in intensity immediately
   2. Sudden loss of consciousness, nausea, vomiting
   3. Facial pain, pupillary dilation and ptosis (from oculomotor nerve compression), and visual field defects (from optic nerve or chiasm compression)
   4. A warning leak, or sentinel hemorrhage, which occurs in approximately 20% of patients, can be misdiagnosed. The physician should have a high index of suspicion for aneurysmal expansion or warning leak because such events precede major hemorrhage.
  B. Examination
   1. Neck stiffness
   2. Altered sensorium
   3. Focal signs (hemiparesis, oculomotor palsy, visual loss, paraparesis)
  C. Laboratory studies
   1. A noncontrast head computed tomography (CT) is used to identify, localize, and quantify the hemorrhage.
   2. A lumbar puncture is indicated if the CT is nondiagnostic.

3. If surgery is emergent, CT angiography is the preferred study.
4. Four-vessel cerebral angiography is necessary to localize the aneurysm(s), define the vascular anatomy, and assess vasospasm. If angiography does not reveal an aneurysm, magnetic resonance imaging (MRI) and angiography (MRA) can be performed to reveal aneurysms larger than 4 mm. If these studies are also negative, angiography is repeated in 2 to 3 weeks.

V. TREATMENT
A. Management
1. Preoperative medical management includes bed rest, head elevation to improve cerebral venous return, pulmonary toilet, thrombophlebitis prophylaxis, antiemetics, anticonvulsant prophylaxis, and pain control.
2. A systolic blood pressure over 160 mm Hg is managed with β-blocking agents, which also reduce the risks of cardiac arrhythmias.
3. Hyponatremia can develop from hypothalamic dysfunction, causing the syndrome of inappropriate antidiuretic hormone, or a salt-wasting diuresis, caused by an increase in circulating natriuretic peptide levels and iatrogenic volume expansion. Fluid balance, serum electrolytes, and osmolarity must be followed.
4. Hyponatremia after SAH is treated with normal saline to support central venous pressure (CVP). Fluid restriction is rarely needed; if used, however, CVP should be monitored to minimize hypotension. Elevated intracranial pressure (ICP) must be treated promptly with mannitol or ventricular cerebrospinal fluid (CSF) drainage.
5. Hypothalamic damage can cause cardiac dysrhythmias from excessive sympathetic stimulation; other cardiac complications can also occur with SAH.

B. Neurologic complications
1. **Rebleeding** is a serious and frequent neurologic complication of SAH, which is postulated to be caused by breakdown of the perianeurysmal clot. The peak incidence of rebleeding occurs during the first day after SAH and one half to two thirds of patients who rebleed die at the time of rebleeding. The antifibrinolytic agent epsilon aminocaproic acid (Amicar) can be used in patients not undergoing early surgery or who are at high risk of rebleeding, but it increases the risk of vasospasm.
2. **Hydrocephalus** can develop acutely within the first 24 hours after SAH because of impaired CSF resorption at the arachnoid granulations or intraventricular blood obstruction of CSF outflow. Ventricular drainage or shunting may be indicated.
3. **Cerebral vasospasm** is a major cause of morbidity and mortality. Noted angiographically in 70% of patients, vasospasm causes symptoms because of cerebral ischemia in only 36% of cases. The clinical presentation of vasospasm occurs progressively: it can be apparent as early as the third day after hemorrhage, with a peak between days 4 to 12. It occurs more frequently in patients with a poor clinical condition, thick focal blood clots, or a diffuse layer of blood in the subarachnoid space. Neurologic deficits are correlated with the areas of cerebral ischemia. Vasospasm is diagnosed by angiography or noninvasively by transcranial Doppler (TCD).
   a. **Hyperdynamic therapy.** The current mainstay of therapy for symptomatic vasospasm is hypervolemic, hypertensive, hemodilution therapy to augment cerebral blood flow (CBF). Elevation of arterial pressure increases CBF; volume augmentation provides hemodilution, decreases viscosity, and improves cerebral microcirculation. Criteria to initiate treatment include increased TCD blood flow velocity, focal neurologic deficits, or impaired consciousness without hydrocephalus. Inotropic drugs are used to keep systolic blood pressures 20 to 40 mm Hg over pretreatment levels, and plasma volume is expanded with albumin, hetastarch, or plasmanate. Hematocrit is maintained at approximately 30. Risks of therapy include myocardial infarction, congestive heart failure, dysrhythmias, hemorrhagic infarcts, rebleeding, hyponatremia, and hemothorax.

b. Calcium antagonists. The calcium antagonist nimodipine can ameliorate neurologic deficits caused by delayed vasospasm. Nimodipine exerts a beneficial effect by decreasing postinjury intracellular calcium; dilating leptomeningeal vessels; improving collateral circulation to ischemic areas; improving erythrocyte deformability; or exerting an antiplatelet aggregating effect. The only adverse effect is mild transient hypotension. Nimodipine (60 mg) is given orally every 4 hours for 21 days from the onset of SAH. If hypotension occurs, the dose is divided in half and administered every 2 hours.

C. Surgical management of ruptured aneurysm

1. Craniotomy: Current standard surgical management is craniotomy with clip occlusion of the aneurysm neck, usually within 48 hours of rupture in most noncomatose patients. The appropriate timing for surgical intervention for comatose patients is controversial. Unique problems that dictate the use of specialized techniques included vertebral-basilar system aneurysms, giant aneurysms (>25 mm), and multiple aneurysms.

2. Postoperative management

a. Angiography is performed to evaluate occlusion of the aneurysm and patency of the surrounding vessels. Treatment of intracranial hypertension may require an ICP monitor, and CVP monitoring is required for hypervolemic—hypertensive therapy. The patient may be discharged from the intensive care unit when the aneurysm has been obliterated, the risk of vasospasm has passed, and other urgent medical problems have been successfully treated.

b. Transcranial Doppler: The TCD studies performed serially as a bedside test of arterial blood flow velocity (BFV) are sensitive to the onset of cerebral vasospasm; an elevated BFV often precedes ischemic complications of vasospasm. More aggressive medical treatment aimed at increasing cerebral perfusion pressure and improving circulation rheology can be instituted before the onset of neurologic impairment.

D. Interventional neuroradiology

1. Endovascular techniques include:

a. Balloon occlusion

b. Coil technologies

c. Angioplasty

d. Intraoperative arteriographic definition of vascular reconstruction

2. These methods are used to treat aneurysms by occluding the parent artery or by selective occlusion of the aneurysm. Early clinical reports demonstrate a relatively high success rate for aneurysm obliteration and lower morbidity and mortality than either balloon or free-coil embolization. Angioplasty can be used to treat constricted arteries during cerebral vasospasm in patients with arteriographic vasospasm without infarction and with a clipped aneurysm. Most successful angioplasties are performed in the first 48 hours after onset of major symptoms, because the procedure is much less effective after cerebrovascular reserve is depleted and vascular fibrosis occurs.

Selected Readings

Biller J, Godersk JC, Adams HP. Management of aneurysmal subarachnoid hemorrhage. *Stroke* 1988;19:1300.
An excellent article describing management of SAH.

Diringer MN, Wu KC, Verbalis JG, et al. Hypervolemic therapy prevents volume contraction but not hyponatremia following subarachnoid hemorrhage. *Ann Neurol* 1992;31:543.
Fluid management following SAH.

Guglielmi G, Vinuela F, Dion J, et al. Electrothrombosis of saccular aneurysms via endovascular approach. *J Neurosurg* 1991;75:8.

Heffez DS, Passonneau JV. Effect of nimodipine on cerebral metabolism during ischemia and recirculation in the Mongolian gerbils. *J Cereb Blood Flow Metab* 1985;5:523.
Calcium antagonist treatment for ischemic neurologic deficits.

Heros RC, Kistler JP. Intracranial arterial aneurysm: an update. *Stroke* 1983;14:628.
Article associating connective tissue and familial disease with aneurysms.

Heros RC, Kistler JP. Subarachnoid hemorrhage due to a ruptured saccular aneurysm. In Ropper AH, Kennedy SF, eds. *Neurological and neurosurgical intensive care.* Rockville, MD: Aspen Publishers, 1988, p. 219.
A standard textbook of neurologic intensive care medicine.

Jakobsson KE, Saveland H, Hillman J, et al. Warning leak and management outcome in aneurysmal subarachnoid hemorrhage. *J Neurosurg* 1996;85:995.
Article documenting the frequency of missed SAH.

Kassell NF, Sasaki T, Colohan ART, et al. Cerebral vasospasm following aneurysmal subarachnoid hemorrhage. *Stroke* 1985;16:562.
Correlation between angiography and clinical presentation of vasospasm.

Newel DW, Eskridge JM, Mayberg MR, et al. Angioplasty for the treatment of symptomatic vasospasm following subarachnoid hemorrhage. *J Neurosurg* 1989;71:654.
Interventional neuroradiology techniques for treating aneurysms and complications of aneurysm rupture.

Nichols DA, Meyer FB, Piegras DG, et al. Endovascular treatment of intracranial aneurysms. *Mayo Clin Proc* 1994;69:272.

Stebbens WE. *Pathology of the cerebral blood vessels.* St. Louis: CV Mosby, 1972, p. 351.
The early definition of intracranial aneurysm anatomy and location.

West HH, Mani RI, Eisenberg RL. Normal cerebral arteriography in patients with spontaneous subarachnoid hemorrhage. *Neurology* 1972;27:592.
Diagnostic imaging following hemorrhage and early nondiagnostic studies.

Wilkins RM. Subarachnoid hemorrhage and saccular intracranial aneurysm: an update. *Surg Neurol* 1981;15:92.

141 GUILLAIN-BARRÉ SYNDROME
Isabelita R. Bella and David A. Chad

I. GENERAL PRINCIPLES
A. Until recently, the term Guillain-Barré syndrome (GBS) has been used synonymously with acute inflammatory demyelinating polyradiculoneuropathy (AIDP), an immunologically mediated disorder producing multifocal demyelination of nerve roots and cranial and peripheral nerves that occurs at all ages.

B. In recent years, the recognition of primary axonal forms of GBS has broadened the spectrum of GBS to include both the demyelinating form (AIDP) and axonal variants: acute motor axonal neuropathy (AMAN) and acute motor sensory axonal neuropathy (AMSAN).

C. All present similarly with rapidly progressive weakness, areflexia, and elevated spinal fluid protein without pleocytosis.

D. GBS is the most common cause of rapidly progressive weakness and can be fatal because of respiratory failure and autonomic nervous system abnormalities.

E. AIDP is the most common subtype in developed countries, whereas axonal forms are more common in northern China.

II. DIAGNOSIS
A. Clinical features of acute inflammatory demyelinating polyradiculoneuropathy
  1. The major clinical features of AIDP are rapidly evolving weakness (usually over days) and areflexia, heralded by dysesthesias of the feet or hands, or both.
    a. Weakness classically ascends from legs to arms but can start from the cranial nerves or arms and descend to the legs.
    b. Proximal muscle involvement is seen early in the course of the disease.
    c. In severe cases, respiratory and bulbar muscles are affected.
  2. Patients can become quadriparetic and respirator dependent within a few days or can have only mild weakness of the face and limbs.
  3. Weakness typically does not progress beyond 1 month.
    a. Progression beyond 4 weeks but arresting within 8 weeks has been termed subacute inflammatory demyelinating polyneuropathy (SIDP).
    b. Progression beyond 2 months is designated "chronic inflammatory demyelinating polyradiculoneuropathy" (CIDP), a disorder with a natural history different from GBS.
    c. A small percentage (2% to 5%) of patients have recurrent GBS.
  4. Approximately two thirds of patients have an antecedent infectious event 1 to 3 weeks prior to the onset of GBS.
    a. Often a flulike or diarrheal illness caused by a variety of infectious agents, including cytomegalovirus, Epstein-Barr and herpes simplex viruses, mycoplasma, chlamydia, and *Campylobacter jejuni.*
    b. Also associated with HIV infection, Hodgkin's disease, systemic lupus erythematosus, immunization, general surgery, and renal transplantation. Lyme disease can mimic GBS.

B. Physical examination
  1. There is symmetric weakness in both proximal and distal muscle groups associated with attenuation or loss of deep tendon reflexes
  2. Objective sensory loss is usually mild.
  3. Between 10% and 25% of patients require ventilator assistance within 18 days after onset. Patients must be followed carefully with serial vital capacity measurements until weakness has stopped progressing.

4. Mild to moderate bilateral facial weakness often occurs in addition to bulbar difficulties.

5. Ocular signs

    a. Ophthalmoparesis is unusual unless seen in the Miller Fisher variant (characterized by ophthalmoplegia, ataxia, and areflexia, with little limb weakness).

    b. Pupillary abnormalities and papilledema are rare.

6. Autonomic nervous system disturbances are seen in more than 50% of patients and include cardiac arrhythmias, orthostatic hypotension, hypertension, transient bladder paralysis, increased or decreased sweating, and paralytic ileus.

C. Clinical features in axonal forms. Patients with axonal forms, such as AIDP, present with rapidly progressive weakness, areflexia, and albuminocytologic dissociation, but they differ in the following ways:

    1. AMAN patients lack sensory abnormalities, and this form is more commonly found in northern China during summer months among children and young adults.

    2. AMSAN is generally associated with a more severe course and longer time to recovery.

D. Laboratory studies

    1. Cerebrospinal fluid

        a. An elevated cerebrospinal fluid (CSF) protein without an elevation in cells (albuminocytologic dissociation) is characteristic of GBS.

        b. CSF protein may be normal within the first 48 hours but often is elevated within 1 week of onset; rarely, it remains normal several weeks after the onset of GBS.

        c. The cell count rarely exceeds 10 cells/cm^3 and is mononuclear in nature.

        d. When GBS occurs as a manifestation of HIV infection or Lyme disease, the CSF white cell count is generally increased (25 to 50 cells).

        e. The CSF glucose is always normal.

    2. Electrodiagnostic studies in AIDP

        a. Typically disclose slowing (<80% of normal) of nerve conduction velocity, with prolonged distal motor and sensory latencies.

        b. The amplitude of the evoked motor responses may be reduced and is frequently dispersed.

        c. Early in the course of GBS, routine nerve conduction studies can be normal, with the exception of prolonged F responses or absent H reflexes; electromyography may demonstrate only decreased numbers of motor unit potentials firing on voluntary effort.

        d. Active denervation changes may be seen several weeks later if superimposed axon loss has occurred.

    3. Electrodiagnostic studies in axonal forms

        a. In AMSAN nerve conduction studies may reveal inexcitable motor and sensory nerves.

        b. In AMAN, nerve conduction studies reveal low to absent motor responses with normal sensory responses and conduction velocities.

        c. Needle examination may reveal denervation potentials in both axonal forms.

    4. Autoantibodies to glycoconjugates

        a. Approximately 90% of Miller-Fisher syndrome patients have high titers of GQ1b antibodies.

        b. Although 25% to 60% of GBS patients have been reported to have anti-GM1 antibodies, their significance is unclear. Several studies suggest they occur more frequently in the pure motor form of GBS, in axonal variants, and in those with poor prognosis, whereas others have found no relationship between the presence of antibodies and outcome or pattern of disease.

        c. IgG anti-GD1a antibodies have been strongly associated with the AMAN subtype of GBS.

III. **DIFFERENTIAL DIAGNOSIS.** A number of conditions causing rapidly progressive weakness must be differentiated from GBS.

   A. Neuromuscular junction disorders: myasthenia gravis and botulism
   B. Disorders of peripheral nerve: tick paralysis, shellfish poisoning, toxic neuropathy, acute intermittent porphyria, diphtheritic neuropathy, and critical illness polyneuropathy
   C. Motor neuron disorders: amyotrophic lateral sclerosis and poliomyelitis
   D. Disorders of muscle: periodic paralysis, metabolic myopathies, inflammatory myopathies, and myopathy if the patient is in intensive care

IV. **PATHOGENESIS**

   A. The varied presentations of GBS are all immune–mediated, but the immune response may be targeting different epitopes of peripheral nerve.
      1. The exact antigens to which the immune system response is directed have not been identified.
      2. In AIDP the immune attack appears to be directed to epitopes on the Schwann cell.
      3. In axonal variants, epitopes on the axolemma are preferentially targeted, with some evidence suggesting a GD1a-like epitope as the target of the immune attack.
   B. AIDP is thought to be produced by immunologically mediated demyelination of the peripheral nervous system. It is likely that both humoral and cellular components play a role.
   C. The concept of molecular mimicry, in which an immune attack occurs on the epitope shared by the nerve fiber and infectious organism, is thought to be a possible mechanism for *C. jejuni*—associated GBS.

V. **PATHOLOGY.** Pathologic studies in AIDP have usually shown endoneurial mononuclear cellular infiltration with a predilection for perivenular regions and segmental demyelination. The inflammatory process occurs throughout the length of the nerve (from the level of the root to distal nerve twigs).

VI. **MEDICAL MANAGEMENT**

   A. Close observation for potential respiratory and autonomic nervous system dysfunction is required, preferably in an ICU.
      1. Forced vital capacity (VC) and maximal inspiratory pressure should be followed.
      2. A baseline arterial blood gas should be obtained.
      3. Ropper and Kehne suggest intubation if any one of the following criteria is met:
         a. mechanical ventilatory failure with reduced expiratory VC of 12 to 15 mL/kg
         b. oropharyngeal paresis with aspiration
         c. falling VC over 4 to 6 hours
         d. clinical signs of respiratory fatigue at a VC of 15 mL/kg.
      4. Tracheostomy should be delayed because patients can improve rapidly.
   B. Because of potential autonomic dysfunction, careful monitoring of blood pressure, fluid status, and cardiac rhythm is essential in managing patients with GBS. Hypertension can be managed with short-acting α-adrenergic—blocking agents, hypotension with fluids, and bradyarrhythmias with atropine.
   C. Immunotherapy
      1. Patients can be treated with plasmapheresis or intravenous immunoglobulin (IVIG). Both are equally efficacious, but because IVIG is easier to administer, it is more commonly used as the initial treatment.
      2. Plasmapheresis
         a. GBS study group recommends exchanging 200 to 250 mL/kg in three to five sessions over 7 to 14 days.
         b. Requires good venous access and can induce hypotension; patients with cardiovascular disease, therefore, may not tolerate the procedure well.

3. IVIG
- **a.** Dose administered is 400 mg/kg/day for 5 consecutive days.
- **b.** Easier to administer but can produce side effects such as flulike symptoms, headache, and malaise.
- **c.** Should be avoided in patients with IgA deficiency and renal insufficiency.

4. Corticosteroids. Generally ineffective in GBS. Although a pilot study suggested treatment with IVIG and methylprednisolone may be more advantageous than treatment with IVIG alone, a recent large randomized double-blind placebo-controlled trial did not support this.

5. Addition of Interferon beta (IFNβ) to IVIG did not show any significant difference in rate of improvement from IVIG alone in a pilot study.

VII. OUTCOME

A. Most patients recover over weeks to months.

B. Approximately 15% have no residual deficits, 65% are restored to nearly normal function, and 5% to 10% are left with severe residual weakness or numbness.

C. Patients with the worst prognosis are those with severely low motor amplitudes on electrodiagnostic studies, presumably from axon loss.

D. Despite close monitoring in the ICU, mortality rates range from 3% to 8%.

E. Causes of fatal outcomes include dysautonomia, sepsis, acute respiratory distress syndrome, and pulmonary emboli.

Selected Readings

Arnason BGW. Acute inflammatory demyelinating polyradiculoneuropathy. In: Dyck PJ, Thomas PK, Griffin JW, et al, eds. *Peripheral neuropathy*. Philadelphia: WB Saunders, 1993, pp. 1437–1497.
A comprehensive chapter with a good description of the pathology.

Asbury AK, Cornblath DR. Assessment of current diagnostic criteria for Guillain-Barré syndrome. *Ann Neurol* 1990;27(suppl):S21–S24.
This article describes the clinical, laboratory, and electrodiagnostic criteria of Guillain-Barré syndrome.

Barohn R, Kissel J, Warmolts J, et al. Chronic inflammatory polyradiculoneuropathy. Clinical characteristics, course, and recommendations for diagnostic criteria. *Arch Neurol* 1989;46:878–884.
Evaluation of 60 chronic inflammatory polyradiculoneuropathy patients over a 10-year period.

Donofrio PD. Immunotherapy of idiopathic inflammatory neuropathies. *Muscle Nerve* 2003;28:273–292.
An excellent review of various treatment modalities in inflammatory neuropathies.

Fisher CM. Unusual variant of acute idiopathic polyneuritis (syndrome of ophthalmoplegia, ataxia and areflexia). *N Engl J Med* 1956;255:57–65.
This article describes the Miller Fisher variant of Guillain-Barré syndrome.

French Cooperative Group on Plasma Exchange in Guillain-Barré Syndrome. Efficiency of plasma exchange in Guillain-Barré syndrome: role of replacement fluids. *Ann Neurol* 1987;22:753–761.
This article describes the benefits of plasma exchange if given at an early stage of the disease.

Griffin JW, Li CY, Ho TW, et al. Pathology of the motor-sensory axonal Guillain-Barré syndrome. *Ann Neurol* 1996;39:17–28.
An excellent article that enlightens the pathophysiology of the various forms of Guillain-Barré syndrome.

The Guillain-Barré Syndrome Study Group. Plasmapheresis and acute Guillain-Barré syndrome. *Neurology* 1985;35:1096–1104.
This classic paper presents the benefits of plasmapheresis as seen in a large randomized trial.

Lichtenfeld P. Autonomic dysfunction in the Guillain-Barré syndrome. *Am J Med* 1971;50: 772–780.
An excellent review of autonomic nervous system findings in Guillain-Barré syndrome.

McKhann GM, Cornblath DR, Griffin JW, et al. Acute motor axonal neuropathy: a frequent cause of acute flaccid paralysis in China. *Neurology* 1993;33:333–342.
This article describes a pure motor form of Guillain-Barré syndrome.

McKhann GM, Griffin JW, Cornblath DR, et al. and the Guillain-Barré Syndrome Study Group. Plasmapheresis and Guillain-Barré syndrome: analysis of prognostic factors and the effect of plasmapheresis. *Ann Neurol* 1988;23:347–353.
This article describes the important predictive factors associated with poor outcome.

Plasma Exchange/Sandoglobulin Guillain-Barré Syndrome Trial Group. Randomised trial of plasma exchange, intravenous immunoglobulin, and combined treatments in Guillain-Barré syndrome. *Lancet* 1997;349:225–230.
A prospective trial comparing efficacy of certain treatment options in 383 patients.

Ropper AH. The Guillain-Barré syndrome. *N Engl J Med* 1992;326:1130–1136.
An excellent review of Guillain-Barré syndrome.

Ropper AH, Kehne SM. Guillain-Barré syndrome: management of respiratory failure. *Neurology* 1985;35:1662–1665.
This article suggests criteria for intubation.

Ropper AH, Wijdicks EFM, Truax BT. *Guillain-Barré syndrome.* Philadelphia: FA Davis, 1991.
An authoritative and comprehensive text on Guillain-Barré syndrome.

van der Meche FGA, Schmitz PIM, Dutch Guillain-Barré Study Group. A randomized trial comparing intravenous immune globulin and plasma exchange in Guillain-Barré syndrome. *N Engl J Med* 1992;326:1123–1129.
First large randomized trial showing comparative efficacy of intravenous immune globulin to plasma exchange.

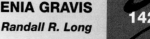
I. GENERAL PRINCIPLES

A. Myasthenia gravis (MG) is an autoimmune disorder characterized by muscle weakness and exaggerated muscle fatigue.

B. Prevalence is 1 in 20,000 with 3:2 female-to-male predominance.

C. Incidence in women peaks in the third decade; in men in the fifth to sixth decades.

D. Oculomotor and bulbar muscles are most commonly affected; proximal muscles usually are more affected than distal muscles; variability over time in both severity and distribution of weakness is common.

E. Myasthenic crisis reflects limiting bulbar and respiratory muscle weakness, constituting a medical emergency and requiring intensive care.

F. Factors commonly associated with myasthenic crisis include systemic infection, electrolyte imbalance, anesthesia, and drugs that impair neuromuscular transmission (Tables 142-1 and 142-2).

II. PATHOPHYSIOLOGY

A. Circulating autoantibodies bind with acetylcholine receptors in postsynaptic muscle membrane.

B. Receptors may be blocked, and receptor density decreases due to accelerated degradation and turnover.

C. Miniature end-plate potentials are normal in number (indicating normal quantal release of acetylcholine) but decreased in amplitude.

III. PROGNOSIS

A. Available therapies offer effective treatment for the vast majority of patients.

B. Aggressive airway management and respiratory support during myasthenic crises minimize morbidity and mortality.

C. Elective thymectomy favorably alters the natural history of the disease.

IV. DIAGNOSIS

A. Clinical presentation

1. MG should be considered in any patient with unexplained weakness, especially when weakness fluctuates or involves bulbar muscles.

2. Normal sensation, tendon reflexes, pupillary reflexes, and mental status distinguish MG from most other acute and subacute paralytic illnesses.

B. Antiacetylcholine receptor antibodies

1. 80% of patients have serum antibodies to acetylcholine receptors.

2. Among "seronegative" patients, some will have anti-MuSK antibodies to muscle-specific tyrosine kinase.

C. Tensilon (edrophonium HCl) test

1. Pretreat with 0.5 mg atropine.

2. Give 2 mg (0.2 mL) intravenous (IV) predose; monitor for bradyarrhythmia.

3. Give 8 mg (0.8 mL) IV test dose; observe for 1 to 5 minutes for transitory increase in muscle strength.

4. Equivocal result is a negative result.

5. Adjust dose in children (0.03 mg/kg).

D. Electrodiagnostic studies

1. Decrement (>15%) in compound muscle action potential amplitude with 2 to 3/sec repetitive supramaximal stimulation.

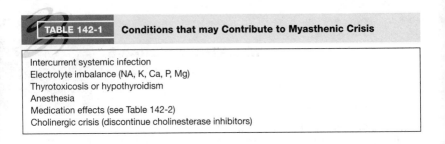

TABLE 142-1 Conditions that may Contribute to Myasthenic Crisis

Intercurrent systemic infection
Electrolyte imbalance (NA, K, Ca, P, Mg)
Thyrotoxicosis or hypothyroidism
Anesthesia
Medication effects (see Table 142-2)
Cholinergic crisis (discontinue cholinesterase inhibitors)

    2. Increased "jitter" on single-fiber electromyograph (EMG).
    3. Electrodiagnostic studies may support—but never exclude—the diagnosis of MG.
  E. Chest imaging. All patients with MG should be screened for thymic hyperplasia or thymoma.

V. TREATMENT. Immunosuppressive therapy is indicated for most patients with MG, but benefits are often delayed. Plasmapheresis and intravenous immune globulin (IVIG) offer a more rapid, but transitory, benefit. Cholinesterase inhibition is a useful adjunctive therapy.

TABLE 142-2 Medications that may Accentuate Myasthenic Weakness

Antibiotics	**Neuromuscular Blockers and Muscle Relaxants**
Amikacin	Anectine (succinylcholine)
Clindamycin	Norcuron (vecuronium)
Colistin	Pavulon (pancuronium)
Gentamycin	Tacrium (atracurium)
Neomycin	Benzodiazepines
Polymyxin	Curare
Streptomycin	Dantrium (dantrolene)
Tobramycin	Flexeril (cyclobenzaprine)
tetracyclines	Lioresal (baclofen)
trimethoprim/	Robaxin (methocarbamol)
sulfamethoxazole	Soma (carisoprodol)
	Quinine sulfate
Antiarrhythmics and antihypertensives	**Antirheumatics**
Lidocaine	Chloroquine
quinidine	D-penicillamine
procainamide	
β-blockers	
Calcium channel blockers	
Antipsychotics	**Others**
Lithium	Opiate analgesics
Phenothiazines	Oral contraceptives
Tricyclics	Antihistamines
	Anticholinergics

TABLE 142-3	Cholinesterase Inhibitors and Dose Equivalencies		
		Route and dose (mg)	
Agent	**Commercial name**	**Oral**	**Parenteral**
Pyridostigmine bromide	Mestinon	60	
Neostigmine bromide	Prostigmin	15	
Neostigmine methylsulfate	Prostigmin		0.5

A. Plasmapheresis
   1. Exchange 50 mL/kg/day for 3 to 7 days
   2. Response within 48 to 72 hours
B. IVIG
   1. 400 mg/kg/day for 5 days
   2. Response within 7 to 10 days
C. Corticosteroids
   1. Response rate greater than 80%
   2. 25 mg/day (single dose), increasing by 5 mg/day every third day to 60 mg/day.
   3. Beware of increased weakness at the outset of steroid treatment.
   4. After maximal response (2 to 3 months), gradually shift to equivalent alternate day dose; then taper slowly by decreasing alternate day dose by 5 mg each month to 25 mg every other day target.
   5. Complete discontinuation, with maintained response, is rare.
   6. Azathioprine, cyclosporine, Cellcept, and other immunosuppressants can be considered in patients who are steroid intolerant or unresponsive.
D. Cholinesterase inhibition (Table 142-3 shows dose equivalencies)
   1. Pyridostigmine (Mestinon) and neostigmine (Prostigmine) are useful adjuncts.
   2. IV neostigmine infusion can be used in patients who can take nothing by mouth; begin with an hourly rate equal to half the prior 24-hour oral dose; increase or decrease gradually according to clinical response versus cholinergic side effects (see later).
   3. Cholinergic crisis is increased weakness due to excess cholinergic stimulation; fasciculation, diaphoresis, and diarrhea are concomitants.
E. Supportive care in the ICU and recovery room
   1. Avoid incentive spirometry!
   2. Maximal inspiratory pressure (MIP), maximal expiratory pressure (MEP), and forced vital capacity (FVC) are the best indicators of respiratory muscle function; O_2 saturation is a poor indicator.
   3. Early intubation is prudent in the event of declining respiratory muscle function.
   4. Cholinesterase inhibition will increase oral and airway secretions.
F. Thymectomy. Elective thymectomy via median sternotomy is indicated for all but the most elderly, frail myasthenic patients. Results are best when done within 5 years of onset.

Selected Readings

Asura E. Experience with intravenous immunoglobulin in myasthenia gravis. *Clin Immunol Immunopathol* 1989;53:5170.
   Landmark article outlining the use of intravenous immunoglobulin in the management of myasthenia gravis.

Drachman DB, deSilva S, Ramsay D, et al. Humoral pathogenesis of myasthenia gravis. In: Drachman DB, ed. *Myasthenia gravis: biology and treatment.* New York: New York Academy of Sciences, 1987.
   Analysis of the immunology of myasthenia gravis.

Howard FM Jr, Lennon VA, Finley J, et al. Clinical correlations of antibodies that bind, block, or modulate human acetylcholine receptors in myasthenia gravis. In: Drachman DB, ed. *Myasthenia gravis: biology and treatment*. New York: New York Academy of Sciences, 1987.
Detailed characterization of the strengths and limitations of antibody testing.

Johns TR. Long-term corticosteroid treatment of myasthenia gravis. In: Drachman DB, ed. *Myasthenia gravis: biology and treatment*. New York: New York Academy of Sciences, 1987.
Overview of long-term immunosuppressive therapy in myasthenia gravis.

Perlo VP, Arnason B, Poskanzer D, et al. The role of thymectomy in the treatment of myasthenia gravis. *Ann NY Acad Sci* 1971;183:308.
Landmark article establishing the role of thymectomy in myasthenia gravis.

Perlo VP, Shahani B, Huggins C, et al. Effect of plasmapheresis in myasthenia gravis. *Ann NY Acad Sci* 1981;377:709.
Confirmation of earlier studies indicating a role for plasmapheresis in myasthenia gravis.

Pinching AJ, Peters DK, Newson-Davis J. Remission of myasthenia gravis following plasma exchange. *Lancet* 1976;2:1373.
Landmark article reporting the effectiveness of plasma exchange in myasthenia gravis.

Seybold ME, Drachman DB. Gradually increasing doses of prednisone in myasthenia gravis. *N Engl J Med* 1974;290:81.
Detailed look at problems associated with the introduction of corticosteroids in the treatment of myasthenia gravis.

I. OVERVIEW

A. Although preexisting neuromuscular disorders may cause weakness in intensive care unit (ICU) patients, two of the most common causes of *newly acquired* weakness arising in the ICU setting are:

1. Critical illness polyneuropathy

2. Critical illness myopathy

B. Etiologic factors of weakness acquired in the ICU

1. A recent large prospective cohort study found the incidence of acquired weakness in the ICU to be 25%.

2. Both critical illness *polyneuropathy* and *myopathy* are the most common causes of acquired weakness in the ICU setting. Distinguishing between them poses major challenges to the clinician.

3. The major contributor to *severe* acquired weakness, with failure to wean from ventilators, is due to critical illness myopathy; critical illness polyneuropathy plays a lesser role in the evolution of paresis in the ICU.

II. CRITICAL ILLNESS MYOPATHY

A. Diagnosis. Clinical features:

1. Weakness is typically diffuse.

2. Affects all limb muscles and neck flexors.

3. May involve facial muscles, but extraocular muscles are rarely involved,

4. Often affects the diaphragm, causing failure to wean.

5. Tendon reflexes are often depressed or absent.

B. Risk factors

1. Intravenous corticosteroids (CS) and neuromuscular blocking agents (NMBAs).

2. Develops in one third of patients treated for status asthmaticus in the ICU.

3. Described in patients who have not received CS and NMBAs, but who had severe systemic illness with multiorgan failure and sepsis.

4. Critical illness myopathy accounts for 42% of patients with weakness in the surgical and medical ICU setting.

C. Laboratory studies

1. Serum creatine kinase (CK) is elevated in 50% of patients; the rise tends to occur early in the course of the illness.

2. Electromyography (EMG)

  a. Low amplitude or absent motor responses; sensory responses relatively preserved (sensory responses may be reduced).

  b. Fibrillation potential activity in some, but not all, patients.

  c. Motor unit potentials may be short in duration and polyphasic with early recruitment.

  d. Motor unit potential analysis is difficult owing to severe weakness or encephalopathy, or both (no motor units may be available for analysis).

  e. Electrical inexcitability of muscle membrane demonstrated by direct muscle stimulation.

D. Pathophysiology

1. Loss of myosin thick filaments

2. Muscle membrane inexcitability

E. Treatment
1. Treatment is essentially symptomatic.
2. To prevent, use CS or NMBAs, or both, *as sparingly as possible!*

F. Outcome.
If patient survives systemic illness, recovery occurs over weeks to months, depending on severity of the myopathy.

III. CRITICAL ILLNESS POLYNEUROPATHY

A. Diagnosis.
Clinical features as classically described:
1. Distal more than proximal symmetrical sensory loss and weakness
2. Reflexes reduced or absent
3. Cranial nerve—innervated muscles typically spared
4. Concomitant encephalopathy

B. Risk factors
1. Sepsis and multiorgan failure
2. Of patients admitted to the ICU for at least 2-weeks, 50% show at least EMG evidence of an axon-loss polyneuropathy.

C. Laboratory studies.
Electromyography (EMG)
1. Reduced or absent sensory and motor responses
2. Nerve conduction velocities: normal or mildly reduced
3. Fibrillation potential activity with reduced recruitment of motor unit potentials

D. Pathophysiology.
Inadequate perfusion of peripheral nerves as a consequence of the systemic inflammatory response

E. Treatment is essentially symptomatic
1. Attempt to stabilize underlying critical conditions
2. Vigorous treatment of sepsis

F. Outcome.
Recovery of sensory and motor function occurs over weeks to months depending on the severity of the neuropathy.

G. Differential diagnosis
1. Guillain-Barré syndrome (see Chapter 141)
2. Acute intermittent porphyric neuropathy
   a. Generalized weakness (symmetrical or asymmetrical) in the context of abdominal pain and psychiatric disorder and prominent dysautonomia. Triggered by drugs that induce the hepatic cytochrome P-450 system (e.g., barbiturates).
   b. May be associated with respiratory failure
   c. EMG: Marked motor axon—loss polyneuropathy without conduction block
   d. Diagnosis suggested by presence of urinary porphyrin precursors, notably δ-aminolevulinic acid
   e. Respond to oral or parenteral carbohydrate loading and to IV hematin therapy
3. Prolonged neuromuscular blockade by muscle relaxants
   a. Associated with renal or hepatic failure
   b. Elevated levels of vecuronium metabolite in some instances (3-desacetylvecuronium)
   c. No sensory deficits and normal reflexes
   d. Normal sensory and motor nerve conduction studies
   e. On EMG, decremental response at slow rates of stimulation (3 Hz)
   f. Transient improvement after infusion of acetylcholinesterase inhibitors
4. Myasthenia gravis (see Chapter 142)
5. Lambert Eaton myasthenic syndrome
   a. Generalized weakness with autonomic symptoms and signs
   b. Strength may *improve* with repetitive contractions
   c. About 50% of patients have an underlying neoplasm (typically small-cell lung cancer)
   d. Presence of antibody to voltage gated calcium channels in 80% of patients
   e. EMG: very low motor amplitudes that increase after a short burst of isometric exercise; sensory studies are normal.

6. Botulism
  a. Diffuse, symmetrical weakness; proximal greater than distal muscle involvement
  b. Cranial nerve involvement:
   (1) Dysarthria and dysphagia
   (2) Ptosis and ophthalmoparesis
  c. Autonomic involvement
   (1) Dilated pupils
   (2) Bradyarrhythmias
   (3) Hypotension
   (4) Urinary retention
  d. Management is supportive care and trivalent (ABE) antitoxin.
7. Motor neuron disease
  a. Scenario: an ICU patient admitted for pneumonia and ventilator support who fails to wean.
  b. The examination classically reveals a combination of lower and upper motor neuron signs (atrophy/fasciculations and hyperreflexia/spasticity, respectively) in bulbar (especially tongue and palate) and limb muscles (often asymmetric, distal and proximal) with a normal sensory examination.
8. Muscular dystrophies
  a. Uncommon scenario, but patients with certain muscular dystrophies are prone to respiratory muscle involvement and pneumonia.
  b. These include:
   (1) Myotonic dystrophy
    (a) Percussion and grip myotonia
    (b) Frontal balding/temporalis muscle atrophy
    (c) Distal muscle weakness and wasting
    (d) Cardiac conduction defects
    (e) Central hypoventilation
   (2) Duchenne and Becker dystrophy (X-linked dystrophy—dystrophinopathy)
    (a) Calf pseudohypertrophy
    (b) Severe generalized weakness and wheelchair before age 12 (Duchenne); mild to moderate generalized weakness with ambulation to at least age 16 (Becker)
    (c) Cardiomyopathy
    (d) Elevated CK (10 to 50 times above normal)
   (3) Congenital myopathy (severe forms of nemaline rod and centronuclear)

Selected Readings

Jonghe B, Sharshar T, LeFaucheur J-P, et al. Paresis acquired in the intensive care unit. A prospective multicenter study. *JAMA* 2002;288:2859–2867.
Large prospective study using simple bedside criteria finds the incidence of acquired weakness in the ICU is 25%.

Hund E. Critical illness polyneuropathy. A review. *Curr Opin Neurol* 2001;5:649–653.
A common disorder affecting 70% to 80% of patients with severe sepsis and multiorgan failure.

Lacomis D, Petrella JT, Giuliani MJ. Causes of neuromuscular weakness in the intensive care unit: a study of ninety-two patients. *Muscle & Nerve* 1998;21:610–617.
The spectrum of neuromuscular disorders among ICU patients has shifted from traditional conditions (such as GBS and myasthenia gravis) to disorders acquired in the ICU, and acute myopathy is three times as common as acute polyneuropathy.

Lacomis D, Giuliani MJ, Van Cott A, et al. Acute myopathy of intensive care: clinical, electromyographic, and pathological aspects. *Ann Neurol* 1996;40:645–654.
A study of 14 patients who developed critical illness myopathy after organ transplantation or during treatment for severe pulmonary disorders and sepsis. Most patients received high-dose intravenous corticosteroids and neuromuscular junction blocking agents.

Rich MM, Bird SJ, Raps EC, et al. Direct muscle stimulation in acute quadriplegic myopathy. *Muscle & Nerve* 1997;20:665–673.
Critical illness myopathy may be more common than previously appreciated and the predominant contributor to severe weakness.

Trojaborg W, Weimer LH, Hays AP. Electrophysiologic studies in critical illness associated weakness: myopathy or neuropathy—a reappraisal. *Clin Neurophys* 2001;112:1586–1593.
Authors conclude that critical illness myopathy is much more commonly associated with severe weakness than is critical illness polyneuropathy.

Sander HW, Golden M, Danon MJ. Quadriplegic areflexic ICU illness: selective thick filament loss and normal nerve histology. *Muscle & Nerve* 2002;26:499–505.
The authors conclude that severe acquired weakness in the ICU is a primary myopathy and not an axon-loss polyneuropathy.

Sandrock AW, Louis DN. Case records of the Massachusetts General Hospital. Case 11–1997. *N Engl J Med* 1997;336:1079–1088.
A discussion of critical illness myopathy—case presentation and detailed description of differential diagnosis.

I. OVERVIEW. Patients with primary brain tumors, spinal cord tumors, peripheral nerve tumors, or metastatic tumors from other organs may require care in the intensive care unit (ICU) for several reasons:
- **A.** Increased intracranial pressure
- **B.** Hydrocephalus
- **C.** Postoperative complications
- **D.** Seizures
- **E.** Compression of critical neural structures (e.g., spinal cord)
- **F.** Systemic complications of brain tumors

II. ELEVATED INTRACRANIAL PRESSURE
- **A.** General principles
  - **1.** Elevated intracranial pressure (ICP) may be present at initial presentation of patient with tumor or develop postoperatively.
  - **2.** Increased volume in closed intracranial space causes increased pressure.
  - **3.** Elevated ICP may be due to circumscribed or invasive, low-grade or high-grade neoplasm.
- **B.** Pathophysiology of Elevated ICP
  - **1.** Tumor mass
  - **2.** Secondary cerebral edema
  - **3.** Hydrocephalus, due to obstruction of cerebrospinal fluid (CSF) pathways
  - **4.** Hypercarbia with decreased ventilation
  - **5.** Hemorrhage
    - **a.** Spontaneously from tumor
    - **b.** Surgical complication
  - **6.** Cerebral ischemia. Vascular compression by tumor
- **C.** Diagnosis
  - **1.** Clinical presentation
    - **a.** Headache
      - **(1)** "Bandlike" or "pressure"
      - **(2)** Worse in morning on arising
    - **b.** Vomiting
      - **(1)** Projectile
      - **(2)** Often in morning
    - **c.** Papilledema. Chronic ICP elevation finding
    - **d.** Decreased level of consciousness
    - **e.** Cognitive changes
    - **f.** Pupillary dilation when tentorial herniation develops
    - **g.** Light-near pupillary dissociation
    - **h.** Cushing triad
      - **(1)** Systolic hypertension (with wide pulse pressure)
      - **(2)** Bradycardia
      - **(3)** Respiratory depression
  - **2.** Radiologic studies
    - **a.** Computed tomography (CT) more available than magnetic resonance imaging (MRI)

  b. Findings
   (1) Tumor signal variable; may enhance with contrast
   (2) Edema surrounding tumor is hypodense
   (3) Midline shifted away from tumor
   (4) Midbrain cisterns compressed
 3. Laboratory studies
  a. Arterial blood gas for elevated pCO_2
  b. Serum sodium for hyponatremia
D. Treatment
  a. Head elevation
  b. Hyperventilation: pCO_2 less than 32 but greater than 25
  c. Fluid restriction
  d. Furosemide: 1 mg/kg single dose
  e. Mannitol: 1 g/kg initially, then 0.25 g/kg every 4 to 6 hours
  f. Dexamethasone: 10 to 20 mg initially, then 4 mg every 6 hours
  g. Ventriculostomy
   (1) CSF drainage reduces volume and pressure rapidly
   (2) Low-risk bedside surgical procedure

III. HYDROCEPHALUS

A. General principles
 1. Definition: increased ventricular size due to increased CSF volume under increased pressure
 2. Consequence of tumor or surgical complication
B. Pathophysiology/etiology
 1. Subarachnoid tumor
  a. Carcinomatous meningitis may prevent CSF absorption
   (1) Metastases
   (2) Primary tumors (aggressive/infiltrative)
  b. Cerebello-pontine angle tumors may compress fourth ventricle
 2. Intraventricular tumors may occlude CSF pathways
 3. Intraparenchymal tumors
  a. Basal ganglia and thalamic tumors may compress foramen of Monro
  b. Pineal region tumors may compress posterior third ventricle or cerebral aqueduct
  c. Brainstem or cerebellar tumors may compress fourth ventricle
C. Diagnosis
 1. Clinical presentation
  a. Symptoms and signs of elevated ICP (see earlier)
  b. Abrupt or gradual time course
  c. May occur following tumor treatment, radiation or surgery
 2. Radiologic studies
  a. MRI better anatomic detail; CT often more efficient
  b. Findings based on tumor site
   (1) Lateral ventricles enlarged, prominent temporal horns
   (2) Third ventricle round unless compressed by tumor
   (3) Fourth ventricle dilated if poor CSF absorption
   (4) Periventricular edema due to transependymal leakage
D. Treatment
 1. Dexamethasone
 2. Ventriculostomy
  a. External CSF diversion in rapidly deteriorating patient
  b. Temporary solution; risk of infection increases if catheter remains longer
 3. Tumor resection
  a. Decompresses CSF pathway
  b. Not always definitive treatment

4. Ventriculoperitoneal shunt. Permanent CSF diversion if hydrocephalus persists following treatment.

IV. SEIZURES

A. General principles. May precipitate rapid deterioration when ICP elevated
B. Pathophysiology
   1. Tumor progression
   2. Hemorrhage
   3. Hypoxia
   4. Hyponatremia
   5. Hypoglycemia
   6. Subtherapeutic anticonvulsant(s)
C. Diagnosis
   1. Clinical presentation
      a. Variety of seizure presentations
         (1) Generalized tonic–clonic activity
         (2) Focal movements
         (3) Speech arrest
         (4) Episodic numbness
         (5) Transient visual obscurations
      b. May occur shortly following postoperative emergence from anesthesia
   2. Radiologic studies; CT scan to evaluate for hemorrhage
   3. Laboratory studies
      a. Anticonvulsant level
      b. Serum Na^+
      c. Arterial blood gases
      d. Serum glucose
D. Treatment
   1. Airway management
      a. Methods to establish patent airway
         (1) Oral airway
         (2) Nasal trumpet
         (3) Endotracheal intubation
      b. Ventilate to avoid hypercarbia
   2. Anticonvulsant medications
      a. Lorazepam: 2 mg every 5 minutes (8 mg maximum) for status epilepticus
      b. Phenytoin: 15 mg/kg for seizure prophylaxis in perioperative period, or concurrent treatment with lorazepam for status epilepticus
      c. Other options
         (1) Carbamazepine: for prophylaxis but not for status (not IV)
         (2) Phenobarbital: more sedating than phenytoin

V. POSTOPERATIVE COMPLICATIONS

A. General principles
   1. Following brain tumor surgery, patient followed in ICU for possible neurologic deterioration
   2. Neurologic and medical conditions determine time frame
B. Diagnosis
   1. Clinical presentation
      a. Headache
      b. Hemiparesis
      c. Aphasia
      d. Decreased level of consciousness
      e. Excessive fatigue
      f. Polyuria/polydipsia
      g. Fever

    2. Differential diagnosis
- **a.** Intracranial hemorrhage into tumor bed, subdural or epidural space
    - **(1)** Risk factors
        - **(a)** Coagulopathy
        - **(b)** Coughing and "bucking" during anesthesia emergence
        - **(c)** Hypertension
- **b.** Cerebral edema
    - **(1)** Brain manipulation
    - **(2)** Overhydration
- **c.** Cerebral infarction
    - **(1)** Vascular injury
    - **(2)** Vasospasm
    - **(3)** Hypercoagulability
- **d.** Endocrinopathy: associated with sellar/parasellar tumors
    - **(1)** Diabetes insipidus
        - **(a)** 18 to 36 hours postoperative
        - **(b)** Greater than 200 mL urine output for 2 consecutive hours, specific gravity less than 1.005, and Na^+ greater than 147 mEq/L
    - **(2)** Hypocortisolemia: onset 1 or 2 days after stopping corticosteroids
    - **(3)** Hypothyroidism: Presents more than 1 week postoperatively
    - **(4)** Hyponatremia: syndrome of inappropriate secretion of diuretic hormone (SIADH) not infrequent in postoperative period
- **e.** Central nervous system infection
    - **(1)** Meningitis
        - **(a)** Low probability (0.8%) in clean operative field
        - **(b)** Usually 2 days to 2 weeks postoperatively
    - **(2)** Cerebral abscess: uncommon; presents weeks postoperatively
    - **(3)** Bone flap infection and empyema
        - **(a)** Presentation often months postoperatively
        - **(b)** Wound drainage frequently

    3. Radiologic studies. Head CT without and with contrast

    4. Laboratory studies
- **a.** Arterial blood gases (ABG)
- **b.** Serum Na^+
- **c.** Serum glucose
- **d.** Complete blood count (CBC), erythrocyte sedimentation rate (ESR)
- **e.** Fasting cortisol
- **f.** Thyroid-stimulating hormone (TSH), T_3 Uptake, T_4
- **g.** Urine specific gravity

C. Treatment

    1. Hemorrhage
- **a.** Correct coagulopathy
- **b.** Surgery if hemorrhage causing significant mass effect
- **c.** Maintain blood pressure below 160 systolic

    2. Cerebral edema
- **a.** Hyperventilation
- **b.** Dexamethasone
- **c.** Mannitol

    3. Infarction
- **a.** Maintain cerebral perfusion
- **b.** Treat symptomatic edema

    4. Endocrinopathy
- **a.** Hydrocortisone (adrenal insufficiency)
- **b.** Levothyroxine (hypothyroidism)
- **c.** DDAVP: 1.0 mcg bid (diabetes insipidus)

    5. Hyponatremia
- **a.** Fluid restriction for SIADH
- **b.** 3.0% NaCl if Na^+ less than 120

6. Central nervous system infections
  a. Antibiotics
  b. Remove infected bone flap
  c. Drain purulent collections

VI. SPINAL TUMORS
  A. General principles. ICU for neurologic or ventilatory issues
    1. Cervical spinal tumors
    2. Postoperative following transthoracic approaches
  B. Pathophysiology
    1. Tumor compresses spinal cord
    2. Spinal cord ischemia/infarction
      a. Tumor compresses anterior or posterior spinal arteries
      b. Blood vessels manipulated during surgery
    3. Postoperative hemorrhage
    4. Autonomic dysfunction
  C. Diagnosis
    1. Clinical presentation
      a. Respiratory insufficiency
        (1) Paralysis of intercostal muscles (lesion C6 and below)
        (2) Decreased diaphragm function (lesion above C6)
        (3) Atelectasis
      b. Ileus
      c. Urinary retention
      d. Hypotension
      e. Bradycardia
    2. Physical examination
      a. Vital capacity every 6 hours
      b. Bowel sounds: absent
      c. Abdomen: distended
      d. Vital signs
    3. Laboratory tests. Oxygen saturation: situation ominous once decline noted
  D. Treatment
    1. Intubation/ventilator if vital capacity less than 12 mL/kg body weight
    2. Nasogastric tube
    3. Foley catheter versus intermittent catheterization
    4. Pressors to keep blood pressure greater than 90 to 100 systolic
    5. Atropine versus pacemaker

VII. SYSTEMIC COMPLICATIONS OF CEREBRAL TUMORS
  A. Pathophysiology
    1. Immobility
    2. Hypercoagulability
  B. Diagnosis
    1. Clinical manifestations
      a. Deep venous thrombosis (DVT)
      b. Pulmonary embolism
      c. Systemic infections
        (1) Urinary tract infection
        (2) Pneumonia
        (3) Line sepsis
    2. Radiologic studies
      a. Venous duplex scan
      b. Ventilation/perfusion scan
      c. CT angiogram of chest
      d. Chest radiograph
    3. Laboratory studies
      a. CBC
      b. Cultures: urine, sputum, blood

    C. Treatment

       1. DVT prevention: TED hose and leg sequential compression boots

       2. Greenfield filter for DVT if less than 2 weeks postoperatively

       3. Heparin or Coumadin safe if greater than 2 weeks postoperatively

       4. Antibiotics

       5. D/C central line if line sepsis

Selected Readings

Apuzzo MLJ, ed. *Brain surgery. Complication avoidance and management.* New York: Churchill Livingston, 1993.
    A comprehensive two-volume textbook detailing, among other topics, avoidance and management of postoperative complications of surgery for a variety of brain tumors.

Kay AH, Laws ER, eds. *Brain tumors.* Hong Kong: Churchill Livingstone, 1995.
    A textbook with extensive descriptions of issues regarding care of patients with brain tumor.

Litofsky NS, Recht LD. Neuro-oncologic problems in the intensive care unit. In Irwin RS, Rippe JM, eds. *Irwin and Rippe's intensive care medicine,* 5th ed. Philadelphia: Lippincott Williams & Wilkins, 2003, pp. 1894–1902.
    A detailed chapter discussing management of patients with brain and spine tumors in the intensive care unit setting.

Posner JB. *Neurologic complications of cancer.* Philadelphia: FA Davis, 1995.
    Definitive monograph by one of the founders of the field, covering all aspects of neurooncology, with exhaustive references.

Vecht CJ, ed. *Neuro-oncology. Part III. Neurologic disorders in systemic cancer.* In Vinken PJ, Bryuyn, eds. *Handbook of clinical neurology.* Amsterdam: Elsevier, 1997.
    A multiauthored volume in a well-known handbook series addressing neurology of cancer in a comprehensive fashion.

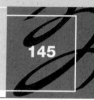

MISCELLANEOUS ICU NEUROLOGIC PROBLEMS 145
Nancy M. Fontneau and Ann L. Mitchell

I. OVERVIEW. A variety of disorders affecting the nervous system, not easily categorized otherwise, require management in the intensive care unit (ICU). These include:
- **A.** Suicidal hanging
- **B.** Electrical injuries
- **C.** Carbon monoxide poisoning
- **D.** Decompression syndrome ("the bends")
- **E.** Cerebral fat embolism
- **F.** Hiccups

II. SUICIDAL HANGING
- **A. Background.** Third most common means of committing suicide
- **B. Pathophysiology**
  1. Death usually by slow strangulation with compression of the jugular veins or carotid arteries.
  2. Interruption of blood flow for more than a few minutes results in hypoxic–ischemic injury with neuronal death, cytotoxic and vasogenic edema, increased intracranial pressure (ICP), and altered mental status.
- **C. Prognosis**
  1. Coma of greater than 24 hours' duration portends major neurologic dysfunction in survivors.
  2. Some recovery expected, but dementia, amnesia, Korsakoff syndrome, restlessness, myoclonus, and other movement disorders can result.
- **D. Management**
  1. Cardiopulmonary resuscitation.
  2. Cervical fracture should be ruled out or stabilized.
  3. Monitor for paratracheal or laryngeal trauma, or acute respiratory distress syndrome; endotracheal intubation for airway obstruction.
  4. Treat cardiac arrhythmias and seizures.
  5. Raised ICP treated with hyperventilation-induced hypocarbia, which produces reflex cerebral vasoconstriction.

III. ELECTRICAL INJURIES
- **A. Background.** In the United States there are 4,000 injuries and 1,000 deaths from electric shock annually.
- **B. Pathophysiology**
  1. Voltage related to severity of exterior burns, muscle necrosis, myoglobinuria and renal failure, closed-head injury, and fractures
  2. Ventricular fibrillation and respiratory arrest, especially from alternating current
  3. Nervous system tissues especially vulnerable to injury
     - **a.** Common neurologic injuries involve cervical spinal cord and peripheral nerves of the arm, because current most often flows through one or both arms to ground.
     - **b.** With electrical injury to brain, transient unconsciousness, seizures, confusion, cerebral edema, and brain hemorrhage.

C. Prognosis
1. Patients may recover fully from their neurologic dysfunction.
2. About 25% of patients have acute or chronic neurologic sequelae.

D. Management
1. Cardiopulmonary resuscitation.
2. Monitor for delayed cardiac arrhythmias.
3. Stabilize spine and long bone fractures.
4. Isosmotic fluid resuscitation and alkalization of the urine to prevent myoglobin nephropathy.
5. Compartment syndrome may require débridement and fasciotomy.
6. Extensive burns should be managed in burn units.
7. Tetanus prophylaxis.

IV. CARBON MONOXIDE POISONING

A. Background
1. Carbon monoxide (CO) gas is a colorless, tasteless, and odorless byproduct of incomplete combustion.
2. Atmospheric CO concentration is normally less than 0.001%; CO concentrations of 0.1% can be fatal.

B. Pathophysiology
1. Carboxyhemoglobin accumulation due to prolonged binding of CO to hemoglobin.
2. Clinical effects depend on the carboxyhemoglobin level (by percent).
   a. Less than 10: mild headache, dyspnea on exertion
   b. 10 to 20: headache, easy fatigability
   c. 20 to 30: pounding headache, impaired dexterity, blurred vision, irritability
   d. 30 to 40: weakness, nausea, vomiting, confusion, delirium, cherry red color
   e. 40 to 50: tachycardia, arrhythmias
   f. 50 to 60: seizures, respiratory insufficiency
   g. Greater than 60: coma
   h. 60 to 70: coma, death

C. Treatment
1. 100% oxygen by tight-fitting nonrebreathing face mask
2. Goal carboxyhemoglobin level of less than 5%
3. Hyperbaric oxygen therapy useful for treating cerebral edema
4. Steroids not indicated

D. Prognosis
1. Approximately 75% recover quite well.
2. About 10% to 30% develop memory impairment or extrapyramidal signs reminiscent of parkinsonism. Basal ganglia and substantia nigra neurons highly sensitive to CO exposure.

V. DECOMPRESSION SICKNESS ("THE BENDS")

A. Background. Decompression sickness can arise following:
1. rapid ascent of scuba divers or tunnel workers
2. decompression or high-altitude flying with inadequate cabin pressure
3. flying after scuba diving

B. Pathophysiology
1. Decompression sickness occurs when gases dissolved in body fluids under high atmospheric pressure come out of solution under conditions of lower pressure.
   a. Small gas bubbles form in tissues and venous blood.
   b. Bubbles coalesce, causing local tissue ischemia or venous obstruction.
2. Neurologic symptoms are seen in nearly 80% of patients.
   a. Focal or diffuse paresthesia is the most frequent symptom, affecting the skin and joints.
   b. Weakness of one limb or more.

    c. Visual disturbances, vertigo, headache, lethargy, paralysis; unconsciousness less common.

    d. Abnormal brain magnetic resonance imaging (MRI) scan, with white matter hyperintensities, even in divers who do not get typical decompression syndrome.

  3. Air embolism is a more severe and acute decompression illness.

    a. Overinflation of the lungs causes rupture and gas bubble formation in the pulmonary veins.

    b. Cerebral arterial embolism can result if a patent foramen ovale exists.

      (1) Unconsciousness and stupor are the most common symptoms.

      (2) Onset usually within 5 minutes of decompression.

      (3) Cardiopulmonary arrest can occur.

C. Treatment

  1. Recompression is the definitive treatment.

    a. Begin recompression as quickly as possible.

    b. Move patient to the nearest decompression (hyperbaric) chamber.

    c. Interim management

      (1) Place patient in the Trendelenburg position on the left side.

      (2) Administer 100% oxygen (with air breaks to avoid pulmonary oxygen toxicity).

      (3) Intubation if pulmonary edema develops.

      (4) Pneumothorax or pneumomediastinum should be treated with chest tube drainage.

      (5) Circulatory support with colloid and vasopressors may be required.

      (6) Although steroids are often used to reduce cerebral edema in decompression sickness, no role has yet been proved for them in these cases.

  2. Emergency phone numbers: The National Diving Accident Network consultation service

    a. Daytime: Duke University, (919) 684-2948

    b. 24-hour emergency line: (919) 684-8111

D. Prognosis

  1. Most patients improve when the gas bubbles redistribute to the venous circulation.

  2. Remarkable recovery can occur after recompression.

    a. Recompression treatment can be effective even after delays of up to 2 weeks.

    b. Relapse requiring repeated decompression treatment occurs in 30% to 50% of patients.

VI. CEREBRAL FAT EMBOLISM SYNDROME

A. Background

  1. Consequence of long bone fracture

    a. present in up to 2% of patients

    b. present in 5% to 10% of multitrauma patients

    c. begins 12 to 48 hours after trauma

  2. Symptoms depend on location of fat emboli:

    a. hypoxemia from pulmonary insufficiency

    b. neurologic

      (1) confusion

      (2) impaired consciousness or coma

      (3) seizures

      (4) focal neurologic signs in approximately one third of patients

    c. fever

    d. tachycardia

    e. cutaneous petechiae

    f. thrombocytopenia

    g. anemia

B. Pathology
1. Microscopic fat emboli in the gray matter
2. Perivascular hemorrhages predominantly in cerebral and cerebellar white matter
3. Cerebral edema

C. Management
1. Rapid immobilization of fractures
2. Monitor and correct oxygenation
3. Fluid resuscitation
4. Computed tomography (CT) of the brain to rule out direct traumatic brain injury as the cause of neurologic symptoms
5. Raised intracranial pressure managed initially by hyperventilation
6. Steroid therapy not proved useful

D. Prognosis
1. Mortality rate: 10% to 20%
2. Permanent neurologic deficit: 25% of patients

VII. HICCUP

A. Background
1. Hiccups are usually a benign, self-limited condition.
2. Prolonged hiccupping can produce fatigue, sleeplessness, weight loss, difficulty in ventilation, and wound dehiscence.

B. Pathophysiology
1. Troublesome hiccup most commonly associated with chest, abdomen, neck, and brainstem disorders.
2. Lateral medulla or phrenic or vagus nerve injury are usual causes.
3. Metabolic disorders (e.g., uremia) or toxins.
4. Gastroesophageal reflux disease.

C. Management
1. Find and treat underlying structural or metabolic disorder.
2. Core studies
   a. Physical examination
   b. Radiographs, CT or MRI
   c. Electrolytes, glucose, blood urea nitrogen, creatinine, and a toxic screen for alcohol and barbiturates
   d. Lumbar puncture if central nervous system infection suspected
3. Medications
   a. Chlorpromazine (25 to 50 mg) by mouth or intramuscularly (IM) three to four times a day.
   b. Intravenous infusion of chlorpromazine (25 to 50 mg in 500 mL of normal saline) if oral or IM is ineffective.
   c. Metoclopramide (10 mg) orally four times a day.
   d. Haloperidol (5 mg) given three times a day may also prove effective.
4. Mechanical treatments for hiccup alter the responsible reflex arc by direct stimulation of the posterior pharynx.
   a. red rubber catheter inserted through the nares used to tickle the posterior pharynx
   b. nasogastric intubation
   c. swallowing dry granulated sugar
5. **Refractory hiccup**
   a. surgically extirpation of phrenic nerve
   b. transcutaneous stimulation of the phrenic nerve

VIII. PERIPHERAL NERVE DISORDERS

A. Critical illness polyneuropathy (see Chapter 143)
B. Compression neuropathies
1. **Background.** Can result in significant delayed morbidity

2. **Clinical features.** Compression of the peroneal nerve at the fibular head and the ulnar nerve at the elbow most common, with weakness and numbness in nerve distributions
3. **Prevention.** Avoid compression by proper patient positioning.
4. **Treatment.** Supportive in most patients

Selected Readings

Hund E. Critical illness polyneuropathy. *Curr Opin Neurol* 2001;14:649.
A concise review of the pathophysiology, differential diagnosis, and management of critical illness polyneuropathy.

Kamenar E, Burger P. Cerebral fat embolism: a neuropathological study of a microembolic state. *Stroke* 1980;11:477.
Good neuropathologic description.

Koumbourlis AC. Electrical injuries. *Crit Care Med* 2002;30:S424.
An excellent review of electrical principles and injuries, arranged by organ system.

McHugh TP, Stout M. Near-hanging injury. *Ann Emerg Med* 1983;12:774.
A good immediate response approach.

Melamed Y, Shupak A, Bitterman H. Medical problems associated with underwater diving. *N Engl J Med* 1992;326:30.
Excellent review of underwater diving injuries.

Min SK. A brain syndrome associated with delayed neuropsychiatric sequelae following acute carbon monoxide intoxication. *Acta Psychiatr Scand* 1986;73:80.
An excellent clinical overview.

Williamson BWA, MacIntyre IMC. Management of intractable hiccup. *BMJ* 1977;2:501.
Excellent review that includes a useful treatment algorithm.

Transplantation

XIII

CRITICAL CARE OF ORGAN TRANSPLANT RECIPIENTS: OVERVIEW

146

Christoph Troppmann

I. GENERAL PRINCIPLES

A. The increased number of organ transplants during the last two decades has been paralleled by significant improvements in both patient and graft survival. These improvements can be attributed to several factors:

  1. The availability of polyclonal and monoclonal antilymphocyte antibody preparations to prevent and treat rejection episodes.

  2. The introduction in the early 1980s of a powerful immunosuppressant agent: cyclosporine, followed almost a decade later by tacrolimus and mycophenolate mofetil. More recently, several additional new drugs have become available or are in the final stages of regulatory approval (e.g., sirolimus, alemtuzumab, FTY-720), augmenting the immunosuppressive armamentarium considerably and allowing for more individualized immunosuppression of organ recipients.

  3. Improvements in organ preservation (e.g., introduction of the University of Wisconsin preservation solution in the late 1980s).

  4. Thorough preoperative patient screening.

  5. Increasing sophistication in postoperative intensive care, allowing also for transplantation of high-risk recipients with significant medical comorbidities.

  6. Availability of potent, yet nontoxic antibacterial, antifungal, and antiviral agents has allowed for more effective prevention and treatment of opportunistic infections.

  7. Refinements in surgical techniques.

B. Transplantation has thus become the treatment of choice for many patients with end-stage failure of kidneys, liver, endocrine pancreas, heart, lungs, and small bowel. Criteria for potential recipients have been expanded to include infants, children, and individuals thought to be at higher risk for complications (e.g., patients with diabetes, elderly patients).

C. Current absolute contraindications to transplantation include malignancy (untreated, metastatic, or at high risk for recurrence); uncontrolled infection; and medical-surgical contraindications to undergo, or inability to recover from, major surgery.

D. The gap between available organs and patients awaiting transplantation is widening. As a result, transplant wait list mortality is increasing.

II. THE ORGAN DONOR SHORTAGE: POTENTIAL SOLUTIONS

A. Live donors

  1. Due to the lack of deceased organ donors, and the development of a noninvasive (laparoscopic) nephrectomy technique, live donor kidney transplants have significantly increased over the past decade. In 2001, for the first time, live kidney donors outnumbered deceased kidney donors in the United States.

  2. Live donor liver, small bowel, pancreas, and lung transplants are also done, albeit in smaller numbers.

B. Deceased organ donors

  1. Donation after cardiac death (DCD) donors: an increasingly used donor type (typically, families of unconscious patients with severe, irreversible terminal brain injury who do not fulfill the formal criteria of brain death, decide to forego any further life-sustaining treatments and to donate the organs).

  2. Brain-dead donors: By far the most common deceased donor type.

3. Maximizing donation within the currently underused pool of potential brain-dead and DCD donors carries the most significant potential for increasing the number of available organs for transplant. Critical care physicians and other intensive care health personnel play a crucial role in optimizing the rate of conversion from being a potential donor to being an actual donor (see Chapter 152. Critical Care of the Deceased Organ Donor).

D. Unconventional donor organ sources (e.g., liver or heart domino transplants, reuse of already transplanted organs, paid organ donors): They cannot *significantly* increase the number of available organs. Paying live organ donors is against federal law in the United States and is not an accepted option in Western industrialized countries.

III. ORGAN-SPECIFIC CONSIDERATIONS

A. Kidney transplantation
   1. Treatment of choice for nearly all patients of all ages with advanced chronic kidney failure and end-stage renal disease.
   2. Kidney transplants do not only improve quality of life, but also prolong life.
   3. Less expensive from a socioeconomic standpoint than chronic hemodialysis.

B. Liver transplantation
   1. Treatment of choice for patients with acute and chronic end-stage liver disease.
   2. Dramatic improvement in graft survival after introduction of cyclosporine in the late 1970s. Currently, no reliable means exists to substitute for a failing liver other than with a transplant.
   3. Recent attempts to alleviate the severe donor shortage include the increased use of marginal donors and innovative surgical techniques (e.g., living donor and split liver transplants).

C. Pancreas and islet transplantation
   1. Indications: Most pancreas transplants are done for selected, medically suitable patients with type I diabetes who have developed significant secondary diabetic complications or have poor quality of life (e.g., due to severe hypoglycemic unawareness).
   2. At present, pancreas transplantation is the only effective option to consistently restore normal glucose homeostasis and normalize glycosylated hemoglobin (HbA1c) levels.
   3. Successful pancreas transplants significantly improve quality of life and decrease incidence and severity of secondary diabetic complications.
   4. Most pancreas transplants are performed simultaneously with a kidney transplant in preuremic patients with significant renal dysfunction, or in uremic patients with end-stage diabetic nephropathy.

D. Small bowel transplantation
   1. Indications: Congenital or acquired short bowel syndrome, especially if liver dysfunction occurs because of long-term parenteral nutrition or if establishing or maintaining central venous access becomes difficult.
   2. In patients who have also advanced liver disease, a combined liver–small bowel transplant may be indicated.
   3. With refinement of surgical techniques, more specific immunosuppression, and better postoperative monitoring for rejection, graft survival has considerably improved over the past decade and approaches that of other solid organ grafts (e.g., lung transplants).

E. Heart transplantation
   1. Treatment of choice for patients with end-stage congenital and acquired parenchymal and vascular diseases of the heart after exhaustion of all conventional medical and surgical options.
   2. Considerably improved results since introduction of cyclosporine in the early 1980s and refinements in diagnosing and treating rejection episodes.
   3. Mechanical devices (e.g., total artificial heart, ventricular assist device) can serve as a temporary bridge between heart failure and transplant.

F. Heart-lung and lung transplantation
   1. Effective treatment for patients with advanced pulmonary parenchymal or vascular disease with or without primary or secondary cardiac involvement.
   2. Increase in lung transplants (most frequently done as single or bilateral single lung transplants) is in large part due to technical improvements, resulting in fewer surgical complications, and to advances in perioperative and postoperative care.
   3. Mechanical ventilation or extracorporeal membrane oxygenation (ECMO) can be a temporary bridge to transplant.
G. Hematopoietic cell transplantation——see Chapter 153.

IV. FUTURE CHALLENGES IN ORGAN TRANSPLANTATION
   A. Increase number of available donor organs.
   B. Minimize rates of chronic graft failure (e.g., secondary to chronic rejection, graft atherosclerosis).
   C. Develop immunosuppressive drugs and protocols that have fewer side effects and further improve long-term graft survival.
   D. Develop tolerance-promoting protocols, which would obviate need for chronic immunosuppression beyond the induction phase.

Selected Readings
Auchincloss H Jr. In search of the elusive Holy Grail: the mechanisms and prospects for achieving clinical transplantation tolerance. *Am J Transplant* 2001;1:6–12.
A didactic review of the history of transplantation tolerance and current tolerance concepts.

Balsam LB, Yuh DD, Robbins RC, et al. Heart-lung and lung transplantation. In: Cohn LM, Edmunds LH Jr, eds. Cardiac surgery in the adult, 2nd edition. New York: McGraw-Hill, 2004, pp. 1461–1490.
An up-to-date comprehensive overview of the field of heart-lung and lung transplantation.

Bethea BT, Yuh DD, Conte JV, et al. Heart transplantation. In: Cohn LM, Edmunds LH Jr, eds. Cardiac surgery in the adult, 2nd edition. New York: McGraw-Hill, 2004, pp. 1427–1459.
An up-to-date comprehensive overview of cardiac transplantation.

Fishbein TM. The current state of intestinal transplantation. *Transplantation* 2004;78:175–178.
A comprehensive review of the surgical, immunosuppressive, and medical progress and of the challenges ahead.

Gridelli B, Remuzzi G. Strategies for making more organs available for transplantation. *N Engl J Med* 2000;343:404–410.
A comprehensive review of current and potential strategies to increase the number of donor organs.

Robertson RP, Davis C, Larsen J, et al. Pancreas and islet transplantation for patients with diabetes. *Diabetes Care* 2000; 23:112–116.
A concise report on rationale and patient selection criteria for pancreas transplantation.

Starzl TE, Iwatsuki S, Van Thiel DH, et al. Evolution of liver transplantation. *Hepatology* 1982;2:614–636.
A historical overview by a pioneer of the field.

Wolfe RA, Ashby VB, Milford EL, et al. Comparison of mortality in all patients on dialysis, patients on dialysis awaiting transplantation, and recipients of a first cadaveric transplant. *N Engl J Med* 1999;341:1725–1730.
A landmark study on the life-prolonging effect of kidney transplantation.

147 REJECTION, INFECTION, AND MALIGNANCY IN SOLID ORGAN TRANSPLANT RECIPIENTS
Brian J. Gallay

I. GENERAL PRINCIPLES. Immunosuppressive therapy must be balanced to prevent transplant rejection and minimize risk of infection and malignancy. The level of immunosuppression required varies depending on risk of rejection of the transplanted organ. Although the risk of complications varies among organ types, all transplants share characteristic features of rejection, infection, and malignancy.

II. REJECTION
  A. The alloimmune response
  1. Highly polymorphic human leukocyte antigens (HLA) are expressed on cell surfaces in different individuals.
  2. Foreign HLA molecules expressed on transplants are recognized by recipient helper and cytotoxic T lymphocytes, B lymphocytes, and natural killer cells.
  3. T lymphocytes are central to alloimmunity as well as immunity to viruses and malignant cells.
  4. B lymphocytes produce anti–donor HLA antibodies. Sensitization to donor HLA may occur in recipients with repeated exposures from previous transplant, multiple blood transfusions, or multiple pregnancies.
  5. Immunosuppression targets T lymphocytes. Dual or triple maintenance therapy permits lower drug doses while providing synergy.
    a. Corticosteroids inhibit lymphocyte activation and are cytolytic at high doses (side effects include fluid retention, psychosis, hyperlipidemia, weight gain).
    b. Antimetabolites (azathioprine, mycophenolate mofetil) inhibit lymphocyte proliferation (side effects include neutropenia, anemia; adjust dose to maintain peripheral leukocyte count >3,000/mm^3).
    c. Calcineurin inhibitors (cyclosporine, tacrolimus) inhibit production of interleukin-2 (IL-2), a critical signal for T lymphocyte activation (side effects include acute and chronic nephrotoxicity, hypertension, neurotoxicity [e.g., seizures, tremor]).
    d. mTOR inhibitors (sirolimus, everolimus) prevent entry of lymphocytes into the cell cycle after activation (side effects include thrombocytopenia, anemia, leukopenia, delayed wound healing, hyperlipidemia).
    e. Induction immunosuppression depletes T lymphocytes (OKT-3, antithymocyte globulin; side effects include aseptic meningitis [OKT-3]; fever, myalgia, pulmonary edema [cytokine release syndrome]; neutropenia and thrombocytopenia [antithymocyte globulin]) or inhibits their activation by blocking the IL-2 receptor (basiliximab, daclizumab).
  B. Acute rejection
  1. General: Transplant dysfunction is the most common presentation, but often subclinical rejection is identified on biopsy. Systemic inflammatory symptoms are less common. Acute cellular rejection is characterized histologically by lymphocytic cellular infiltrate with active parenchymal injury. Humoral rejection is characterized by vascular endothelial cell injury with intravascular antibody deposition, fibrin formation, and complement activation. Biopsy is essential to confirm presence and severity of rejection. Therapy with high-dose corticosteroids or antilymphocyte antibody is required.
  2. Kidney: Acute rise of serum creatinine. Rule out drug nephrotoxicity, pyelonephritis, systemic infection, urologic obstruction, intravascular volume depletion, and vascular compromise.

3. Liver: Acute rise in serum transaminases. Rule out recurrent disease, biliary complications, hepatic artery thrombosis, and drug toxicity.

4. Heart: Acute decrease in left ventricular ejection fraction, or rejection identified on routine endomyocardial biopsy. Rule out infection.

5. Pancreas: Acute serum amylase elevation and decreased urinary amylase excretion (bladder-drained pancreas grafts). Hyperglycemia is a late manifestation. Rule out arterial graft thrombosis, impaired exocrine drainage, drug toxicity, or infection.

6. Lung: Acute decrease in ventilation and oxygenation, or rejection identified on routine bronchoscopic biopsy. Rule out infection, airway or vascular anastomotic complications, malignancy, and recurrent disease.

C. Chronic rejection occurs as coronary artery disease in heart, bronchiolitis obliterans in lung, or ischemia and fibrosis in kidney, pancreas, and liver grafts. Both immunologic and nonimmunologic risk factors are important, including frequency and severity of acute rejection, recurrence of original disease, drug toxicity, and infection. Therapy includes increased immunosuppression, avoidance of drug toxicity, or treatment of recurrent disease.

III. INFECTION

A. General

1. Because immunosuppression targets T lymphocytes, risk of opportunistic infection by pathogens controlled by T cell immunity is increased.

2. Risk decreases over time with immunosuppression intensity.

a. Peritransplant infection due to nosocomial infection as in other postoperative patients.

b. Opportunistic infection most common 3 to 6 months after transplant.

c. Later infection generally community-acquired or persistent opportunistic infection.

3. Antimicrobial prophylaxis and empiric therapy are guided by time after transplant and level of immunosuppression, but a wide differential diagnosis and rapid identification of pathogens are always required.

B. Bacterial

1. Peritransplant nosocomial infection: pneumonia, catheter infection, superficial or deep wound infection, or urinary tract infection.

2. Community-acquired respiratory and urologic tract pathogens predominate later.

3. Consider Nocardia or Legionella in pneumonia.

4. Consider Listeria in acute meningitis.

5. Tuberculosis may occur at any time and often presents as disseminated disease.

C. Viral

1. Cytomegalovirus (CMV)

a. Active infection occurs by reactivation of latent virus or by *de novo* infection with transplant (CMV-negative recipients of CMV-position donor organs at highest risk).

b. Highest incidence in the first 6 months: pneumonitis, esophagitis, gastritis, colitis, hepatitis, nephritis, bone marrow infection, or febrile syndrome. Diagnosis is confirmed by presence of viremia or biopsy.

c. Prophylaxis with oral ganciclovir or valganciclovir is maintained for at least 3 months, especially in high-risk recipients.

1. Epstein-Barr virus (EBV) is associated with posttransplant lymphoproliferative disease (PTLD). It may cause acute hepatitis or infectious mononucleosis.

2. Pneumonitis due to adenovirus, respiratory syncytial virus, and influenza virus requires rapid bronchoscopic diagnosis and specific antiviral therapy.

4. Hepatitis B and C viruses are most commonly acquired before transplant, but *de novo* infection at transplant can cause acute hepatitis and fulminant liver failure.

D. Fungal

1. Pneumocystis pneumonia presents as acute pneumonitis in the first 6 months after transplant. Prophylaxis with trimethoprim-sulfamethoxazole is highly effective.

2. Aspergillosis is often disseminated and associated with high mortality.
3. Cryptococcosis must be considered in meningitis.
4. Coccidiomycosis, histoplasmosis, and blastomycosis should be considered after careful demographic evaluation to determine exposure risk. Meningitis, pneumonitis, and dermatitis are common presentations.
5. Candidiasis may present as disseminated infection, urinary tract infection, or intraabdominal abscess.

E. Parasitic
1. Parasitic infection should be suspected in the setting of eosinophilia.
2. Strongyloidiasis may present in the first 6 months with abdominal symptoms, systemic inflammatory symptoms, or pneumonitis in patients harboring the organism at time of transplant.
3. Toxoplasmosis may present in the first 2 months with systemic inflammation, meningoencephalitis, pneumonitis, pericarditis, myocarditis, or retinitis. Prophylaxis with trimethoprim-sulfamethoxazole is effective.

IV. MALIGNANCY

A. Skin cancer is the most common malignancy in all transplant recipients. Risk increases with levels of sun exposure and immunosuppression. Squamous cell carcinoma is most common. Melanoma may present as metastatic disease with an unidentified primary lesion. Kaposi's sarcoma is common in patients of Mediterranean origin.

B. Solid organ cancers
1. Recurrent disease is possible, especially colon, breast, and melanoma.
2. May present as metastatic disease, but a primary lesion is commonly identified.
3. Risk is increased approximately threefold over that for the general population.
4. Risk factors are similar to those for nonimmunosuppressed patients.

C. Post transplant lymphoproliferative disease
1. Presents typically as polymorphic non-Hodgkin B cell lymphoma, commonly associated with EBV infection. The primary lesion may arise in the small bowel, central nervous system, or allograft. Lymphadenopathy is easily identified on physical examination or radiologic imaging.
2. PTLD usually presents within 1 year after transplant but may also occur later. Risk is 2% for renal transplant recipients to 10% for heart and lung recipients.
3. Therapy
   a. Reduce or discontinue immunosuppression.
   b. Cytotoxic chemotherapy or therapy with anti-CD20 antibody (rituximab) targeting B lymphocytes.
   c. Antiviral (anti-EBV) therapy with acyclovir or ganciclovir (limited evidence-based support).
   d. Consider surgical resection in cases with isolated, limited involvement (e.g., allograft, gastrointestinal lymphoma).
   e. Radiation most effective for central nervous system PTLD.

Selected Readings

Delves PJ, Roitt IM. The immune system: first of two parts. *N Engl J Med* 2000;343:37–49;The immune system: second of two parts. *N Engl J Med* 2000; 343:108–117.
An excellent, well-written, and clear description of immune system function.

Euvrard S, Kanitakis J, Claudy A. Skin cancers after organ transplantation. *N Engl J Med* 2003; 348:1681–1691
Thorough review of all skin malignancy manifestations in organ recipients.

Fishman JA, Rubin RH. Infection in organ-transplant recipients. *N Engl J Med* 1998;338:1741–1751.
A recent comprehensive review of early and late infectious complications.

Krensky AM. Immune response to allografts. In: Norman DJ, Turka LA, eds. *Primer on transplantation*, 2nd ed. American Society of Transplantation, 2001, pp, 16–25.
Summarizes the central components of the alloimmune response.

Olyaei AJ, de Mattos AM, Bennett WM. Pharmacology of immunosuppressive drugs. *Drugs Today (Barc.)* 1998;34:463–479.
Description of current immunosuppressive agents by leaders in the field of transplant pharmacology.

Patel R. Infection in recipients of kidney transplants. *Infect Dis Clin N Am* 2001;15:901–952.
An in-depth review focused on renal transplant infections.

Penn I. Post-transplant malignancy: the role of immunosuppression. *Drug Saf* 2000; 23: 101–113
A comprehensive review of the relationship of level of immunosuppression to risk of malignancy.

Pizzo PA. Fever in immunocompromised patients. *N Engl J Med* 1999;341:893–900
Overview of how to evaluate patients as they present with infection or malignancy.

Villacian JS, Paya CV. Prevention of infections in solid organ transplant recipients. *Transpl Infect Dis* 1999;1:50–64.
Describes strategies for prophylaxis of all common infections.

148 CRITICAL CARE OF KIDNEY TRANSPLANT RECIPIENTS
Brian J. Gallay

I. GENERAL PRINCIPLES. Renal transplant is the most common solid organ transplant. It improves quality of life and survival compared to dialysis therapy for patients with chronic kidney disease. Diabetic and hypertensive nephropathy are the most common causes of chronic kidney disease leading to transplant. Underlying disease and its pathophysiology must be considered in pretransplant evaluation and postoperative management.

II. PRETRANSPLANT EVALUATION. Chronic kidney disease is a risk factor for cardiovascular disease and infection. Special attention must be paid to these as well as acute metabolic abnormalities.

  A. Cardiovascular
    1. Assessment: History of coronary artery disease, symptoms of angina or congestive heart failure, recent change in exercise tolerance, new ischemic changes on ECG. Decreased pulse or bruit on peripheral vascular examination, new murmur on cardiac examination.
    2. Prevention: Preoperative and postoperative β-blocker therapy (atenolol 5 mg intravenously preoperatively and 50 to 100 mg orally daily for at least the first postoperative week), with careful monitoring for hyperkalemia, bradycardia, and hypotension. Consider continuing or starting aspirin for patients with multiple risk factors.

  B. Infection
    1. Assessment: Signs or symptoms of active infection. Careful assessment of indwelling hemodialysis or peritoneal dialysis catheters and hemodialysis access grafts. Culture and cell count of peritoneal fluid from Tenckhoff catheter.
    2. Prevention: Postpone transplant until active infection has been treated. Cephalosporin therapy for perioperative antibacterial prophylaxis.

  C. Preoperative dialysis
    1. Assessment of hypervolemia by physical examination. Determine pretransplant daily urine output to facilitate interpretation of urine output after transplant. Laboratory assessment for hyperkalemia or severe metabolic acidosis.
    2. Acute dialysis treatment to correct electrolyte abnormalities and volume status, avoiding excessive volume removal.

III. INTRAOPERATIVE CARE
  A. Careful attention to volume status is critical to avoid hypovolemia that will impair renal perfusion and contribute to delayed graft function (need for dialysis therapy during the first week after transplant, a risk factor for acute rejection).
  B. Intravascular volume status should be maintained at adequate central venous pressure without predisposing to pulmonary edema. Central venous pressure monitoring is recommended to maintain pressure approximately between 5 and 10 cm H_2O.
  C. Consider pulmonary artery catheterization to assess hemodynamics in patients with significantly decreased left ventricular function.

IV. POSTOPERATIVE CARE
  A. Postoperative management is determined by initial allograft function. Chest radiograph and frequent electrolyte monitoring, including sodium, potassium, calcium, and magnesium levels are essential to help assess volume and metabolic status.

794

B. Oliguria (urine output <20 mL/h) requires careful attention to intravascular volume status. If euvolemic or hypervolemic, then aggressive fluid resuscitation should be avoided and complications such as urinary obstruction, vascular thrombosis, and acute tubular necrosis must be considered. Hyperkalemia must be identified and treated.

C. With immediate graft function, urine output can reach 1 L/h. Careful fluid and electrolyte replacement is required to avoid hypovolemia and electrolyte depletion.

V. POSTOPERATIVE CONSIDERATIONS

A. Surgical complications

1. Hemorrhage

    a. Risk of occurrence 1.9% to 12%.

    b. Increased risk for patients requiring preoperative reversal of chronic Coumadin anticoagulation.

    c. Frequently due to vascular anastomotic bleeding, but in half of cases no obvious source is identified.

2. Allograft thrombosis

    a. Risk factors

        (1) Hypotension and hypovolemia

        (2) Hypercoagulable state (antiphospholipid antibody syndrome; factors C, S, or antithrombin III deficiency; factor V Leiden mutation; acute humoral rejection).

        (3) Severe peripheral vascular disease (increased risk of intimal flap and other anastomotic complications).

        (4) Multiple small renal arteries

    b. Presentation, diagnosis, and treatment

        (1) Sudden oligoanuria (arterial thrombosis), gross hematuria, allograft pain and swelling (venous thrombosis).

        (2) Doppler ultrasound including visualization of flow in renal artery and vein confirms diagnosis.

        (3) Almost always requires allograft nephrectomy.

    c. Prevention

        (1) Maintain adequate blood pressure and intravascular volume.

        (2) Aspirin for severe peripheral vascular disease.

        (3) IV heparin for hypercoagulable state. No definitive evidence-based guidelines are available, but therapeutic target partial thromboplastin time (PTT) of 1.5 to 1.9 times the upper limit of normal PTT range has been suggested with low risk of bleeding.

3. Urologic

    a. Significant hematuria with passage of clots may require continuous bladder irrigation. Avoid excessively high intravesical pressures that can lead to rupture of the ureteroneocystotomy.

    b. Urinary leak

        (1) Occurs at the ureteroneocystostomy due to anastomotic complication or distal ureteral ischemia and necrosis. Patient may present with sudden oligoanuria or significant increase in wound drainage.

        (2) Ultrasound may identify perigraft fluid collection (urinoma), nuclear medicine scan may identify extravasation of tracer from ureter, and increased creatinine level of wound drainage (when compared to serum creatinine) will confirm urine leak.

        (3) In some cases, replacement of Foley catheter with bladder decompression is sufficient. Surgical reexploration with ureteral reimplantation and stent placement may be required.

4. Wound

    a. Infection and dehiscence are infrequent complications (less than 5%). Risk is increased with obesity (body mass index >30) and combined use of sirolimus and steroids for immunosuppression, which both impair wound healing.

b. Lymphoceles requiring therapy occur in approximately 5%. Patients present with ureteral or venous obstruction of the graft, which are often associated with ipsilateral lower extremity edema. Definitive treatment most often requires laparoscopic internal drainage through a peritoneal window. External drainage and sclerotherapy are less effective.

B. MEDICAL COMPLICATIONS

1. Cardiovascular

    a. Because of the increased risk of myocardial infarction in patients with end-stage renal disease (ESRD), a high index of suspicion is required, especially with prolonged intraoperative hypotension or postoperative pulmonary edema.

    b. Pericarditis occurs in approximately 2%. Causes include uremia and infection, especially cytomegalovirus (CMV; unusual in the immediate postoperative period).

2. Metabolic

    a. Hyperkalemia can occur with delayed graft function. Immediate therapy is required with calcium chloride, insulin and dextrose, and bicarbonate. Kayexalate or dialysis is required if diuresis to eliminate potassium cannot be induced.

    b. Hypokalemia may occur with large-volume diuresis early postoperatively, requiring frequent monitoring and repletion.

    c. Hypocalcemia, hypophosphatemia, and hypomagnesemia can occur with large-volume diuresis and early renal tubular dysfunction. Frequent electrolyte monitoring (at least every 12 hours) and repletion are required.

3. Infection in the early postoperative period is due to bacterial etiology similar to that for other surgical patients. Risk is greatest in patients with diabetes or those over 60 years old. Prophylactic antibiotic therapy with cephalosporins is required.

4. Neurologic

    a. Stroke is a rare early postoperative complication. Risk is greatest in patients with any significant vascular disease. Stroke should be considered in the setting of a postoperatively unexplained altered level of consciousness or with other neurologic changes.

    b. New onset seizure is also uncommon. Uremia in the setting of delayed graft function, stroke, or drug toxicity with OKT-3 is a common cause.

Selected Readings

Amante AJ, Kahan BD. Technical complications of renal transplantation. *Surg Clin North Am* 1994;74(5):1117–1131.
A comprehensive review of surgical complications of renal transplantation.

Brennan DC. Immediate postoperative management of the kidney transplant recipient. In: Norman DJ, Turka LA, eds. *Primer on transplantation*, 2nd edition. American Society of Transplantation, 2001, pp. 440–447.
A concise overview of early surgical and medical complications.

Bruno A, Adams H. Neurologic problems in renal transplant recipients. *Neurol Clin* 1988;6:305–325.
An excellent review of neurologic complications in kidney transplant recipients.

Fishman JA, Rubin RH. Infection in organ-transplant recipients. *N Engl J Med* 1998; 338(24):1741–1751.
A recent comprehensive review of early and late infectious complications.

Humar A, Kerr SR, Ramacharan T, et al. Peri-operative morbidity in kidney transplant recipients: incidence and risk factors. *Clin Transplant* 2001;15:154–158.
An excellent study of perioperative cardiovascular complications and risk factors.

Mangano DT, Layug EL, Wallace A, et al. Effect of atenolol on cardiovascular mortality after noncardiac surgery. *N Engl J Med* 1996;335(23):713–720.
This original study outlines the benefit of perioperative β-blocker therapy in patients with high risk of cardiovascular complications undergoing transplant surgery.

Naraghi RM, Jordan ML. Surgical complications. In Shapiro R, Simmons RL, Starzl TE, eds. *Renal transplantation*. Stamford, CT: Appleton and Lange, 1997, pp. 269–297.
Excellent review of surgical complications with good discussion of radiologic procedures used in diagnosis.

Shapiro R. The transplant procedure. In: Shapiro R, Simmons RL, Starzl TE, eds. *Renal transplantation*. Stamford, CT: Appleton and Lange, 1997, pp. 103–140.
A comprehensive review of surgical techniques that provides a basis for understanding postoperative complications.

149 CRITICAL CARE OF PANCREAS TRANSPLANT RECIPIENTS
Christoph Troppmann

I. GENERAL PRINCIPLES
  A. Currently, pancreas transplantation is the only diabetes treatment that consistently normalizes glycosylated hemoglobin (HbA1c) levels, positively influences the progression of secondary diabetic complications, significantly ameliorates quality of life, and may prolong life. Most pancreas transplants are done for selected, medically suitable patients with type I diabetes. Type II diabetes is a relatively infrequent indication (<10% of all pancreas transplants).

  B. Depending on the kidney status, pancreas transplants are performed in three recipient categories:
    1. Simultaneous pancreas-kidney transplants (SPK) in preuremic and uremic patients
    2. Pancreas after kidney transplants (PAK) in posturemic recipients of a previous kidney transplant (from a deceased or a live donor)
    3. Pancreas transplants alone (PTA) in nonuremic recipients with extremely labile diabetes but adequate native renal function

  C. Pancreas graft survival rates have significantly improved over the past decade, and now exceed 95% at 1 year and 70% at 5 years (SPK).

II. PRETRANSPLANT EVALUATION.
Patients admitted to the hospital for pancreas transplantation must be evaluated for the following risk factors for adverse perioperative outcomes:

  A. Coronary artery disease. High incidence of coronary artery disease in diabetics (with and without end-stage renal disease [ESRD]). In the course of their transplant workup, prospective recipients will have been screened for coronary artery disease by noninvasive tests or coronary angiography. Immediately preoperatively, particular attention must be paid to new symptoms of angina, congestive heart failure, recent changes in exercise tolerance, and new, possibly ischemic, changes on the ECG.

  B. Peripheral vascular disease. Decreased peripheral pulses or new bruits on peripheral vascular examination, when compared to baseline. Infected diabetic foot ulcers are generally a contraindication to transplantation. Check also for new signs and symptoms of stroke and ischemic cerebrovascular disease.

  C. Infectious disease. Diabetes in combination with uremia is a significant risk factor for infection. Preoperatively, chest radiograph, urinalysis, and careful assessment of indwelling catheters and catheter exit sites (hemodialysis catheters, peritoneal dialysis catheters [including a peritoneal fluid culture]) and of vascular access grafts, are mandatory. Active infection is a contraindication to transplantation.

  D. Metabolic and fluid status. Hyperkalemic uremic patients admitted for transplant may need therapy before the transplant operation (e.g., oral sodium polystyrene sulfonate [Kayexalate], intravenous [IV] insulin and glucose, dialysis). Hypervolemic recipients may need preoperative dialysis. Hyperglycemia with metabolic acidosis requires preoperative correction.

  E. Absolute contraindications to transplantation
    1. Active sepsis
    2. Active viral infection
    3. Acquired immunodeficiency syndrome (AIDS)
    4. Malignancy (except if treated, nonmetastatic, without recurrence, and with sufficient posttreatment follow-up)

III. INTRAOPERATIVE CONSIDERATIONS

A. Operative technique

  1. Nearly all pancreas transplants currently performed are from deceased donors and entail transplantation of the entire organ with an attached segment of duodenum that serves as conduit for the exocrine secretions.

  2. Management of pancreatic exocrine secretions. The exocrine secretions of most pancreas transplants are drained enterically via an anastomosis of the graft's duodenal segment to the recipient's small intestine. For PAK and PTA recipients, bladder drainage (creation of a duodenocystostomy) can provide a useful additional means to monitor for rejection (by measuring urinary amylase).

  3. Venous pancreas graft drainage. The venous effluent of the pancreas graft can be drained systemically, into an iliac vein, or portally, into the superior mesenteric vein. Portal drainage has theoretical, but clinically to date unproved advantages (host tolerance facilitation by portally delivered graft antigen; avoidance of potential systemic hyperinsulinemia sequelae).

B. Cardiovascular care and monitoring

  1. Recipients benefit from perioperative cardioprotection with β-blockers (e.g., atenolol, 5 to 10 mg IV started preoperatively, repeat every 12 hours, and then 50 to 100 mg by mouth every day for at least the first postoperative week).

  2. Hemodynamic monitoring: central venous pressure (CVP) catheter and arterial line; pulmonary artery catheter if indicated (e.g., presence of left ventricular dysfunction).

  3. Maintain adequate intravascular volume status, avoiding high CVPs that can predispose pancreas grafts with systemic venous drainage to edema, while providing adequate preload for optimal perfusion of the kidney graft (SPK recipients). Judicious fluid management to avoid fluid overload and acute myocardial strain is paramount.

C. Foley catheter, nasogastric tube

D. Metabolic care. Frequent (at least hourly) intraoperative monitoring of blood glucose levels is important, because the pancreas graft often begins to function immediately postreperfusion, resulting in decreasing blood glucose levels and no further need for exogenous insulin.

IV. POSTOPERATIVE CARE

A. General: Immediate postoperative chest radiograph and frequent electrolyte monitoring; daily serum amylase and lipase levels.

B. Metabolic

  1. In the few grafts that have delayed function, temporary administration of exogenous insulin may be necessary (initially, most easily by IV insulin infusion with hourly blood glucose monitoring).

  2. Bladder-drained recipients must be monitored closely for fluid and electrolyte losses from the exocrine pancreas, which can result in dehydration and metabolic acidosis. Urine is collected over an 8-hour period on each postoperative day, and hourly urinary amylase production (expressed as amylase U/hr) is determined. With normal pancreas graft recovery from preservation and reperfusion injury, urinary amylase excretion should increase daily before reaching its baseline, usually after discharge of the recipient from the hospital.

C. Kidney graft monitoring and management (see Chapter 148).

D. Provision of adequate immunosuppression

  1. Immunosuppression may include a combination of any of the following: polyclonal or monoclonal anti-T-cell antibodies for induction therapy during the first week (e.g., antithymocyte globulin, alemtuzumab [Campath]), steroids, calcineurin inhibitors (tacrolimus, cyclosporine), mycophenolate mofetil, mTOR inhibitors (sirolimus, everolimus).

  2. Solitary pancreas transplants (PAK and PTA) are more immunogenic and do not have a kidney from the same donor (as SPK recipients do) that would easily allow for rejection monitoring (i.e., by checking serum creatine levels). They therefore require closer surveillance for rejection and often more immunosuppression.

E. Antimicrobial prophylaxis
   1. IV broad-spectrum antibiotics for 3 to 5 days.
   2. Antifungal prophylaxis with fluconazole for 7 to 14 days.
   3. Cytomegalovirus (CMV) prophylaxis for 1 to 6 months (depending on donor–recipient CMV serostatus).
   4. *Pneumocystis jiroveci* prophylaxis with trimethoprim-sulfamethoxazole (Bactrim).
F. Graft thrombosis prophylaxis
   1. No prospective data are available to support current empiric practices.
   2. Some centers partially anticoagulate recipients perioperatively for the first 3 to 7 days (e.g., heparin infusion at 300 to 700 U/h IV).
   3. Many transplant programs start recipients perioperatively on oral acetylsalicylic acid, which is continued indefinitely.

V. POSTOPERATIVE CONSIDERATIONS
A. Surgical complications
   1. Postoperative bleeding
      a. Diagnosis: by serial hemoglobin/hematocrit levels; hemodynamic changes (hypotension, tachycardia, decreased CVP, decreased left ventricular filling pressures).
      b. Most common bleeding sources: free intraabdominal bleeding from the graft itself or the vascular anastomoses; intravesical bleeding with massive hematuria (from the duodenovesical anastomosis in bladder-drained grafts); gastrointestinal bleeding manifesting as lower GI bleeding (from the duodenoenteric anastomosis in enteric-drained grafts).
      c. Check platelets, prothrombin time (PT), and partial thromboplastin time (PTT). Replace coagulation factors and platelets as indicated.
      d. For ongoing intraabdominal bleeding, relaparotomy for hemostasis and evacuation of hematoma may be necessary.
   2. Pancreas graft thrombosis
      a. Most frequent serious surgical complication (incidence: 5% to 10%); results nearly always in graft loss.
      b. Symptoms. Sudden onset of otherwise unexplained hyperglycemia (arterial and/or venous thrombosis); graft tenderness and enlargement (venous thrombosis); dark, massive hematuria (venous thrombosis of bladder-drained pancreas grafts); markedly decreased or absent urinary amylase on spot urinary amylase check (bladder-drained grafts).
      c. Diagnosis
         (1) Imaging studies: Doppler duplex ultrasonography, magnetic resonance angiography, computed tomographic angiography, conventional angiography.
         (2) Diagnosis made during exploratory relaparotomy.
      d. Treatment: Transplant pancreatectomy.
   3. Surgical wound infection
      a. Superficial wound infection
         (1) Symptoms: fever, wound drainage, cellulitis, leukocytosis.
         (2) Treatment: IV antibiotics and local incision and drainage; open wound care with daily dressing changes.
      b. Deep wound infection (intraabdominal abscess)
         (1) Occurs usually within the first 30 days posttransplant; bacterial abscesses are diagnosed earlier than fungal abscesses. Of all intraabdominal infections, 50% are diffuse and 50% are localized; 30% are associated with a leak.
         (2) Clinical presentation: ranges from nonspecific abdominal complaints to diffuse peritonitis, fever, ileus, nausea, vomiting, leukocytosis, hyperglycemia, and sepsis.
         (3) Risk factors: include donor age greater than 45 years, retransplant, pretransplant peritoneal dialysis, graft pancreatitis.
         (4) Diagnosis: abdominal CT with oral and IV contrast (for bladder-drained grafts also with retrograde bladder contrast to rule out leak).

(5) Treatment:

   (a) Percutaneous catheter drainage is appropriate as first line treatment in stable recipients with localized intraabdominal abscess.

   (b) For unstable recipients and those with diffuse peritonitis, relaparotomy and open abscess drainage. If leak is present, relaparotomy in enteric drained recipients is mandatory, but in stable bladder-drained recipients, conservative treatment (prolonged Foley catheterization and percutaneous drainage of localized abscesses) may be attempted.

   (c) IV antibiotics; bowel rest and nasogastric tube if ileus is present.

4. Leaks

   a. Enteric drained grafts

   (1) Incidence 5 to 10%

   (2) Symptoms: abdominal pain, peritonitis, ileus, fever, leukocytosis, hyperamylasemia

   (3) Diagnosis

   (a) Abdominal computed tomography (CT) with oral contrast

   (b) Diagnosis made at exploratory relaparotomy

   (4) Treatment: relaparotomy is mandatory (anastomotic revision or transplant pancreatectomy)

   b. Bladder-drained grafts

   (1) Incidence: 10% to 15%

   (2) Early leaks (<4 weeks posttransplant) usually at the duodenocystostomy anastomosis, late leaks (>4 weeks posttransplant) typically from the graft duodenum (e.g., duodenal ulceration or perforation, CMV infection).

   (3) Symptoms: abdominal pain, distention, fever, vomiting, decreased urine output, peritonitis, improvement after Foley catheter placement. Differential diagnosis must include early ureteral anastomotic leak of a simultaneously transplanted kidney (SPK).

   (4) Diagnosis

   (a) Low-pressure cystography

   (b) CT with retrograde bladder contrast (most accurate)

   (5) Treatment

   (a) Early leaks: prolonged bladder decompression using Foley catheterization, percutaneous drainage of all intraabdominal fluid collections.

   (b) Infected leaks with peritonitis: relaparotomy and direct leak repair or transplant pancreatectomy.

   (c) Late leaks: usually require conversion from bladder to enteric drainage, irrespective of etiology

5. Graft pancreatitis

   a. Prolonged posttransplant hyperamylasemia observed in up to 35% of all pancreas transplant recipients.

   b. Risk factors: donor quality (e.g., obesity, age, excessive inotropic requirements), prolonged preservation time (ischemia-reperfusion pancreatitis), pancreatic duct outflow impairment, bladder drainage ("reflux pancreatitis").

   c. Complications: (peri-)pancreatic abscess, pancreatic necrosis (sterile and infected), pancreatic fistula, pseudocyst.

   d. Symptoms: abdominal pain, graft tenderness, nausea, vomiting, ileus. Serum amylase and lipase levels may be elevated but correlate poorly with severity of pancreatitis. Endocrine secretory capacity often is only mildly impaired, even with severe pancreatitis.

   e. Diagnostic studies: CT with appropriately timed IV contrast bolus to assess pancreatic parenchymal viability and need for débridement of pancreatic necrosis.

   f. Treatment

   (1) Moderate and severe pancreatitis: nasogastric tube, bowel rest, total parenteral nutrition.

   (2) Reflux pancreatitis in bladder-drained recipients: insertion of a Foley catheter not only is diagnostic but also constitutes effective treatment.

Repetitive episodes of reflux pancreatitis usually require conversion from bladder to enteric drainage.

(3) Mechanical pancreatic duct obstruction: relaparotomy to address underlying surgical-technical problem.

(4) No definitive data available on the utility of the somatostatin analogue octreotide for prevention and treatment of established pancreatitis.

6. Hematuria (bladder-drained recipients)

a. Early postoperative hematuria: usually anastomotic and self-limited. Severe cases must be treated by continuous bladder irrigation and normalization of coagulation parameters.

b. Late hematuria: frequently associated with duodenal pathology (e.g., CMV infection). Cystoscopy and graft duodenal segment biopsy may be required. Depending on pathology, conversion to enteric drainage and antiviral treatment may be necessary.

B. Medical complications

1. Rejection

a. Acute rejection

(1) Symptoms may include: hyperamylasemia, fever, graft tenderness, decreasing urinary amylase; serum creatinine elevation in recipients of a simultaneously transplanted kidney (SPK). Hyperglycemia is a late symptom, usually indicative of an advanced rejection process with irreversible graft injury.

(2) Diagnosis confirmation: percutaneous graft biopsy (gold standard).

(3) Treatment

(a) High-dose IV steroids

(b) Anti-T-cell therapy

b. Chronic rejection

(1) Associated with graft fibrosis and graft vasculopathy; irreversible.

(2) Symptoms: decreasing glucose tolerance, hyperglycemia, increasing HbA1c levels; decreasing or absent urinary amylase (bladder-drained grafts).

(3) Treatment

(a) Symptomatic: oral antidiabetic agents, return to exogenous insulin therapy

(b) Pancreas retransplantation

(c) Graft pancreatectomy usually not necessary

2. Acute perioperative myocardial ischemia: diagnosed on postoperative ECG and by elevated troponin and CK-MB levels. Treatment of acute myocardial ischemia as in any nontransplant patient.

3. Metabolic complications

a. Hyperkalemia (in SPK recipients) can be encountered with delayed kidney graft function and may, depending on severity, require IV calcium chloride, insulin and dextrose, and bicarbonate. Potassium excretion can be augmented by IV loop diuretics; if diuresis cannot be induced, oral Kayexalate and dialysis may become necessary.

b. Hypokalemia, hypocalcemia, hypophosphatemia, and hypomagnesemia all can occur as the consequence of large-volume diuresis of a simultaneous kidney graft (SPK). Monitor at least every 12 hours; substitute electrolytes as indicated.

c. Hyperglycemia may reflect transient delayed graft function (rare) and may require temporary exogenous insulin.

4. Infectious complications. Most early posttransplant infections are bacterial or fungal. Viral and parasitic infections begin to emerge after 6 weeks posttransplant.

5. Neurologic complications

a. Seizures. Overall rare; rule out electrolyte abnormalities, drug side effects (e.g., muromonab-CD3 [Orthoclone OKT3], tacrolimus), central nervous system infection (may require lumbar puncture).

b. Acute cerebrovascular events: must be considered in all patients with new onset of seizures or otherwise unexplained postoperatively altered level of consciousness or new onset of other neurologic symptoms.

6. Immunosuppressive drug side effects
   a. Hematologic: leukopenia or thrombocytopenia (e.g., secondary to anti-T-cell therapy with antithymocyte globulin, alemtuzumab; mycophenolate mofetil, sirolimus). Adjust or hold drug doses as necessary.
   b. Acute nephrotoxicity (calcineurin inhibitors [cyclosporine, tacrolimus]).
   c. Neurologic: seizures, tremor, peripheral neuropathic symptoms (calcineurin inhibitors), aseptic meningitis and seizures (Orthoclone OKT3).
   d. Pulmonary: pulmonary edema (cytokine release syndrome associated with polyclonal or monoclonal anti-T-cell therapy), interstitial pulmonary fibrosis (sirolimus).
   e. Hyperlipidemia: associated with steroids, cyclosporine, tacrolimus, and sirolimus.
7. Posttransplant malignancies: posttransplant lymphoproliferative disease; increased incidence of skin cancers.

Selected Readings

Bilous RW, Mauer SM, Sutherland DE, et al. The effects of pancreas transplantation on the glomerular structure of renal allografts in patients with insulin-dependent diabetes mellitus. *N Engl J Med* 1989; 321:80–85.
An important study that demonstrates the beneficial effects for kidney grafts of restoring glucose homeostasis by pancreas transplantation.

Fioretto P, Steffes MW, Sutherland DE, et al. Reversal of lesions of diabetic nephropathy after pancreas transplantation. *N Engl J Med* 1998;339:69–75.
A landmark publication demonstrating the positive impact of long-term pancreas graft function on diabetic nephropathy in native kidneys.

Gruessner RWG. Immunosuppression in pancreas transplantation—maintenance therapy. In: Gruessner RWG and Sutherland DER, eds. *Pancreas transplantation* New York: Springer, 2004, pp. 301–347.
A comprehensive state-of-the-art review of maintenance immunosuppression for pancreas transplants.

Kaufman DB. Immunosuppression in pancreas transplantation—induction therapy. In: Gruessner RWG and Sutherland DER, eds. *Pancreas transplantation.* New York, NY. Springer, 2004, pp. 267–300.
An up-to-date extensive review of current immunosuppressive practices for induction therapy.

Navarro X, Sutherland DER, Kennedy WR. Long-term effects of pancreatic transplantation on diabetic neuropathy. *Ann Neurol* 1997;42:727–736.
A large long-term study on the beneficial impact of pancreas transplantation on diabetic neuropathy.

Robertson RP, Davis C, Larsen J, et al. Pancreas and islet transplantation for patients with diabetes. *Diabetes Care* 2000;23:112–116.
A concise report on rationale and patient selection criteria for pancreas transplantation.

Smets YFC, Westendorp RGJ, van der Pijl JW, et al. Effect of simultaneous pancreas-kidney transplantation on mortality of patients with type-1 diabetes mellitus and end-stage renal failure. *Lancet* 1999;353:1915–1919.
A large population-based study on the impact of pancreas transplantation on survival of diabetic patients.

Troppmann C, Gruessner AC, Benedetti E, et al. Vascular graft thrombosis after pancreatic transplantation: univariate and multivariate operative and nonoperative risk factor analysis. *J Am Coll Surg* 1996;182:285–316.
A thorough analysis of the most frequent serious posttransplant complication.

Troppmann C. Surgical complications. In: Gruessner RWG and Sutherland DER, eds. *Pancreas transplantation.* New York: Springer, 2004, pp. 206–237.
A comprehensive, up-to-date review of posttransplant surgical complications, their diagnosis, and management.

150

CRITICAL CARE OF LIVER TRANSPLANT RECIPIENTS

Ty Dunn and Rainer W. G. Gruessner

I. GENERAL PRINCIPLES. Liver transplantation has become the accepted treatment of choice for acute and chronic end-stage liver disease, selected hepatomas, early cholangiocarcinoma, and some liver-based metabolic disorders. Depending on the patient's condition and organ availability, options include whole-organ deceased donor, split-liver deceased donor, and living donor transplantation. Liver transplantation currently affords patients a survival posttransplant of greater than 85% at 1 year and greater than 70% at 5 years.

II. PRETRANSPLANT EVALUATION. The pretransplant evaluation has several purposes and should be systematic, covering all organ systems to ensure that no major problems are overlooked.
  A. Determine the etiology of liver disease and identify patients with decompensated liver cirrhosis:
    1. Spontaneous hepatic encephalopathy
    2. Refractory ascites
    3. Hepatorenal syndrome
    4. Hepatopulmonary syndrome
    5. Recurrent or refractory variceal bleeding
    6. Recurrent infections such as cholangitis or spontaneous bacterial peritonitis
    7. Intractable pruritus
    8. Severe malnutrition
  B. Identify underlying medical problems that should be dealt with to optimize the candidate's overall condition before transplant
  C. Identify and address psychiatric, chemical dependency, and compliance issues and how they impact a potential candidate's appropriateness for, and timing of, transplant
  D. Identify absolute contraindications:
    1. Active extrahepatic sepsis
    2. Extrahepatic malignancy
    3. Acquired immune deficiency syndrome
    4. Advanced cardiopulmonary disease
  E. For patients with hepatic malignancy, order preoperative imaging to detect extrahepatic spread
  F. For acute (fulminant) liver failure (ALF) patients (generally more ill than those with chronic failure), refer them early to a transplant center
    1. Poor prognostic indicators for spontaneous recovery from ALF:
      a. Factor V level less than 30%
      b. pH less than 7.3
      c. International normalized ratio (INR) greater than 6.5
      d. Stage 3 or 4 encephalopathy
      e. Lack of response to medical therapy within 24 to 48 hours
    2. More severe hepatic parenchymal dysfunction, manifested by coagulopathy, hypoglycemia, and lactic acidosis
    3. More infectious complications
    4. Higher incidence of renal failure
    5. Higher incidence of cerebral edema and neurologic complications
      a. Some centers use intracranial pressure monitoring to monitor cerebral edema.

   b. Mannitol, hyperventilation, and thiopental have been used to prevent elevated intracranial pressure (>15 mm Hg).
   6. Multiple-organ dysfunction syndrome

III. INTRAOPERATIVE CARE

   A. Venous and arterial monitoring catheters and large-volume infusion lines are placed in the operating room and can be a source of immediate morbidity (pneumothorax or hemothorax, pericardial tamponade, arterial pseudoaneurysm, air embolism) and hemorrhage in the coagulopathic patient.
   B. The transplant operation is divided into three phases:
   1. Pre-anhepatic (mobilizing the recipient's diseased liver in preparation for its removal)
   2. Anhepatic, characterized by coagulopathy and decreased venous return to the heart because of occlusion of the inferior vena cava and portal vein
      a. Many centers routinely use a venous bypass system during this time.
      b. After the native liver is removed, the donor liver is anastomosed to the appropriate structures to place the new liver in an orthotopic or piggyback (using a side-to-side cavoplasty technique) position.
   3. Post-anhepatic, beginning after reperfusion. Hemodynamic instability on reperfusion can result in hypotension and serious arrhythmias due to acidosis, electrolyte abnormalities, air embolus, and cardiac strain.

IV. POSTOPERATIVE CARE.
The postoperative course can range from smooth to extremely complicated, depending mainly on the patient's preoperative status and the development of any complications. Initial posttransplant care should be in a critical care unit with continuous invasive hemodynamic monitoring and mechanical ventilation as needed.
   A. Stabilization and recovery of major organ systems functions
   B. Evaluation for continual improvement in graft function
   1. Normalizing mental status
   2. Normalizing coagulation profile
   3. Resolution of hypoglycemia
   4. Clearance of serum lactate
   5. Serum transaminase levels usually rise during the first 24 to 48 hours secondary to reperfusion and preservation injury and then fall rapidly over the next 48 to 72 hours. Serum bilirubin and alkaline phosphatase levels may take several days longer to normalize.
   C. Provision of adequate immunosuppression
   D. Prevention along with vigilant monitoring for, and expeditious management of, complications in the immediate posttransplant period, to minimize morbidity and mortality
   1. Avoid oversedation with benzodiazepines or morphine.
   2. Avoid hypotension (systolic blood pressure below 100 mm Hg) to avoid renal dysfunction and graft thrombosis. Provision of adequate preload is paramount.
   3. Limit central venous pressure to 8 to 12 cm H_2O to
      a. optimize portocaval pressure gradient and graft perfusion
      b. minimize liver graft congestion/edema and bleeding risk from caval anastomoses

V. POSTOPERATIVE COMPLICATIONS
   A. Surgical complications
   1. Hemorrhage. Bleeding is common and can be compounded by deficits in coagulation factors, fibrinolysis, and platelet function. Blood loss should be monitored by serial measurements of hemoglobin and detection of changes associated with acute hypovolemia (e.g., decreased central venous pressure and urine output). If bleeding persists despite correction of coagulation deficiencies, surgical exploration is indicated.

2. Vascular complications. The overall incidence of vascular complications is reported to be 8% to 12%. Thrombosis is the most common early event; stenosis and pseudoaneurysm formation occur later. Doppler ultrasound evaluation is the initial investigation of choice, with more than 90% sensitivity and specificity for thrombosis.

   a. Hepatic artery thrombosis (HAT) has a reported incidence of approximately 2% in adults and 10% in children. If detected early, up to 70% of grafts can be salvaged with urgent exploration, thrombectomy, or revision of the anastomosis. HAT can also present in a less dramatic fashion with common bile duct ischemia resulting in a bile leak at the anastomosis or a more chronic, diffuse biliary stricture. Overall, about 50% of patients with HAT require retransplantation.

   b. Thrombosis of the portal vein or hepatic veins is far less frequent. Liver dysfunction, tense ascites, and variceal bleeding can occur. If thrombosis is diagnosed early, operative thrombectomy and revision of the anastomosis may be successful. If thrombosis occurs late, liver function is frequently preserved because of the collateral veins; a retransplant is usually not necessary: attention is focused on relieving left-sided portal hypertension.

3. Biliary complications. Biliary complications occur in 15% to 35% of cases.

   a. Leak (early)

      (1) Clinical symptoms: fever, abdominal pain, and peritoneal irritation.

      (2) Diagnosis: Bilious output from surgical drains; ultrasound may demonstrate a fluid collection; hepatobiliary scintigraphy (e.g., HIDA [hepatobiliary iminodiacetic acid] scan) may demonstrate extravasation of radioactive tracer; *cholangiography* (PTCA [percutaneous transluminal coronary angioplasty] or ERCP [endoscopic retrograde cholangiopancreatography]) is often required for definitive diagnosis.

      (3) Management: Endoscopic stent placement and biloma drainage, or operative repair (if the patient is systemically ill or unresponsive to stent placement) by revision of the anastomosis (if not done already at transplantation; frequently requires creation of a Roux-en-Y hepaticojejunostomy).

   b. Stricture (later), most common at the anastomotic site, likely related to local ischemia

      (1) Clinical symptoms: cholangitis or cholestasis, or both

      (2) Diagnosis: Ultrasound, magnetic resonance cholangiopancreatography, cholangiography

      (3) Management: balloon dilatation or stent placement across the stricture, or both. Surgical revision is reserved for endoscopic and interventional radiologic treatment failures.

4. Wound complications

   a. Superficial wound infection, hematoma, and seroma (early)

      (1) Diagnosis: drainage, increasing pain, erythema, fluctuance

      (2) Management: (Re)incision and drainage, allowing for healing by secondary intention (serial open wound dressing changes). If significant cellulitis or systemic symptoms are present, intravenous antibiotics should be administered.

   b. Incisional hernias (later), associated with malnutrition, attenuated fascia, and immunosuppression

5. Primary nonfunction

   a. Incidence: 3% to 5%

   b. Mortality rate is more than 80% without a retransplant

   c. Definition: poor or no hepatic function from the time of transplant

   d. Associated donor factors.

      (1) Donor age greater than 49 years

      (2) Macrosteatosis greater than 30%

      (3) Donor intensive care unit stay greater than 3 days

      (4) Cold ischemia time greater than 18 hours

(5) Reduced-size grafts

e. Diagnosis: rule out HAT, severe preservation injury, accelerated acute rejection, and severe infection, because they can mimic primary nonfunction. The diagnosis is usually based on clinical parameters; graft biopsy may be helpful in some cases.

f. Treatment

(1) Intravenous prostaglandin E_1

(2) Early relisting for retransplantation

B. Medical complications. Potential complications are numerous, and every major organ system can be affected.

1. Neurologic, most commonly related to drugs or a poorly functioning graft

a. Symptoms:

(1) Decreased level of consciousness

(2) Seizures

(3) Focal neurologic deficits

b. Other neurologic complications:

(1) Hypoxic ischemic encephalopathy

(2) Central pontine myelinolysis

(3) Cerebral edema

(4) Intracranial hematomas

2. Pulmonary, in up to 75% of recipients

a. Noninfectious complications (first postoperative week):

(1) Pulmonary edema

(2) Pleural effusions

(3) Atelectasis

(4) Acute respiratory distress syndrome (ARDS)

(a) incidence less than 5%, but mortality greater than 80%

(b) most common when underlying bacterial infection is present, but other risk factors include multiple transfusions, hypertension, aspiration, and antilymphocyte therapy

b. Infectious complications (after the first week):

(1) Bacterial

(2) Fungal

(3) Viral

3. Renal, affecting almost all liver recipients. Renal failure increases the mortality rate. Causes of renal failure:

a. Pretransplant

(1) Hepatorenal syndrome

(2) Acute tubular necrosis

b. Postoperative

(1) Hypovolemia

(2) Ischemic acute tubular necrosis

(3) Drug nephrotoxicity (calcineurin inhibitors)

(4) Preexisting subclinical or overt renal disease (e.g., diabetic nephropathy, hepatitis C–associated membranous or membranoproliferative glomerulonephritis)

4. Immunosuppressive:

a. Posttransplant diabetes

b. Hyperlipidemia

c. Viral and fungal infections

d. Squamous and basal cell skin cancers and lymphoma

5. Recurrence of primary liver disease (may require treatment and can significantly impact graft and patient survival).

a. Hepatitis B (Highly effective peritransplant and posttransplant long-term prophylaxis protocols that include lamivudine and/or hepatitis B immune globulin [HBIg] prevent hepatitis B recurrence.)

b. Hepatitis C (~20% cirrhosis rate from recurrent hepatitis C at 5 years posttransplant; no evidence-based recommendations on posttransplant treatment and efficacy of prophylaxis with pegylated interferon and ribavirin available)

c. Autoimmune liver diseases (Recurrence rates of clinically significant autoimmune hepatitis, primary sclerosing cholangitis, and primary biliary cirrhosis are low and controversial; long-term posttransplant immunosuppression that includes steroids may offer theoretical [but not evidence-based] added benefits with regard to autoimmune disease recurrence prevention.)

Selected Readings

Dee GW, Kondo N, Farell ML, et al. Cardiovascular complications following liver transplantation. *Clin Transplant* 1995;9:463.
A good review of cardiovascular complications.

Gonwa TA, Klintmalm GB, Levy M, et al. Impact of pretransplant renal function on survival after liver transplantation. *Transplantation* 1995;59:361.
A good study of the negative impact of renal failure on survival.

Langnas AN, Marujo W, Stratta RJ, et al. Vascular complications after orthotopic liver transplantation. *Am J Surg* 1991;161:76.
A comprehensive review of vascular complications.

McGilvray ID, Greig PD. Critical care of the liver transplant patient: an update. *Curr Opin Crit Care* 2002;8(2):178–182.
A good summary of the intensive care problems encountered in liver transplant recipients.

O'Connor TP, Lewis WD, Jenkins RL. Biliary tract complications after liver transplantation. *Arch Surg* 1995;130:312.
A comprehensive review of biliary complications.

Pokorny H, Langer F, Herkner H, et al. Influence of cumulative number of marginal donor criteria on primary organ dysfunction in liver recipients. *Clin Transplant* 2005;19:532–536.

Saner FH, Kavuk I, Lang H, et al. Intensive care management of acute liver failure. *Eur J Med Res* 2004;9(5):261–266.
A good overview of special considerations in the management of acute liver failure.

Stange BJ, Glanemann M, Nuessler NC, et al. Hepatic artery thrombosis after adult liver transplantation. *Liver Transpl* 2003;9(6):612–620.
Current data on HAT and management strategies.

Stein DP, Lederman RJ, Vogt DP, et al. Neurological complications following liver transplantation. *Ann Neurol* 1992;31:644.
A good review of neurologic complications.

I. CARDIAC TRANSPLANT RECIPIENTS

A. General principles

1. **Objective.** The primary initial critical care management objective is to optimize cardiopulmonary function with inotropic support, afterload reduction, and judicious fluid management.

2. **Monitoring**

   a. Arterial and central venous monitoring lines and pulse oximetry. Pulmonary arterial catheters are frequently helpful early postoperatively to aid in maximizing cardiac output with inotropic support, IV fluids, and vasodilators and are essential when the recipient has known pulmonary hypertension, donor right ventricular dysfunction.

   b. Foley bladder catheter with temperature probe for urine output and core temperature.

   c. Temporary epicardial pacing wires placed intraoperatively are routinely connected to a backup setting at 60 beats per minute (bpm) for patients with adequate intrinsic cardiac graft rhythm.

   d. Mediastinal and pleural drains are placed to 20 cm of underwater seal suction to monitor postoperative thoracic hemorrhage.

B. Pathophysiology

1. **Cardiac allograft denervation**

   a. Autonomic regulation via antagonistic sympathetic and parasympathetic mechanisms is interrupted with transection of these pathways during allograft procurement.

      (1) Without this autonomic input, the sinoatrial node of the allograft fires at an increased intrinsic resting rate of 90 to 110 bpm.

      (2) Denervation also affects therapeutic interventions mediated by autonomic mechanisms. For example, carotid sinus massage, Valsalva maneuvers, and atropine no longer affect sinoatrial node firing or atrioventricular node conduction.

   b. The allograft relies on adrenergic mechanisms (chronotropic and inotropic, primarily endogenous catecholamine production) for its functional regulation. The allograft physiologic response to stress (e.g., hypovolemia, hypoxia, anemia) is delayed until circulating catecholamines can exert their positive chronotropic effects.

2. **Early allograft failure**

   a. Early cardiac allograft dysfunction accounts for up to 25% of perioperative deaths. The most common etiologies include pulmonary hypertension, myocardial injury due to prolonged ischemia or inadequate preservation, and acute rejection.

   b. Initial depletion of myocardial catecholamine stores resulting from donor inotropic support frequently triggers need for early posttransplant inotropic allograft support.

   c. *Right ventricular failure.* Early right ventricular failure is a leading cause of early mortality and is almost always associated with moderate to severe pulmonary hypertension stemming from chronic left ventricular failure in the recipient.

(1) Right ventricular failure manifests as a hypokinetic, dilated right ventricular cavity and left ventricular underfilling on echocardiography and elevated central venous pressures (CVP) (15 to 25 mm Hg) with low cardiac outputs.

(2) Initial management involves employing pulmonary vasodilators, including inhaled nitric oxide, nitroglycerin, and milrinone. Pulmonary hypertension refractory to these vasodilators often responds to prostaglandin E_1 (PGE_1).

(3) Right ventricular failure refractory to these measures may require temporary right ventricular assist device (RVAD) support. The Abiomed BVS 5000 (Abiomed; Danvers, MA) is a frequently used device in this setting.

d. *Left ventricular failure.* Left ventricular failure is less frequently encountered than right ventricular failure.

(1) Left ventricular failure manifests as a hypokinetic, dilated left ventricular cavity on echocardiography and elevated left ventricular end diastolic pressures (LVEDP) with low cardiac output and systemic hypotension.

(2) Primary treatment centers on intravenous inotropic support (i.e., epinephrine, dobutamine, dopamine, milrinone), afterload reduction (i.e., nipride, milrinone), and preload management, avoiding overfluid resuscitation.

(3) Left ventricular failure refractory to pharmacologic support may require temporary intraaortic balloon counterpulsation (IABP) or a left ventricular assist device (LVAD).

3. Dysrhythmias

a. *Bradycardia.* Sinus or junctional bradycardia in more than 50% of heart recipients. Primary risk factor for sinus node dysfunction: prolonged preservation; mechanical trauma during implantation (putative). Most bradyarrhythmias resolve over 1 to 2 weeks; recovery may be further prolonged in recipients receiving amiodarone preoperatively.

(1) Because cardiac output is primarily rate dependent after transplantation, the heart rate should be maintained between 90 and 110 bpm with parenteral inotropic agents or temporary atrial (DOO) or atrioventricular (DDD) epicardial pacing for the first several days.

(2) Isoproterenol (Isuprel) is an effective chronotrope.

(3) Thereafter, the cardiac allograft is permitted to contract at intrinsic rates between 70 and 90 bpm.

(4) Theophylline may help to achieve adequate heart rates during this early transitional period.

(5) In rare cases of persistent bradycardia, permanent pacemakers may be employed.

b. *Atrial fibrillation.* Atrial fibrillation or flutter is treated with digoxin at higher doses than used with innervated hearts. Such arrhythmias may serve as markers for acute allograft rejection.

c. *Ventricular arrhythmias.* Ventricular arrhythmias, primarily premature ventricular contractions (PVCs) and nonsustained ventricular tachycardia, have been reported in up to 60% of recipients. In these cases, underlying etiologies should be aggressively discerned. Potential causes include acute rejection, electrolyte disturbances, and acidosis.

4. Coagulopathy

a. Heart recipients are frequently coagulopathic early postoperatively. Predisposing factors include: preoperative warfarin therapy, cardiopulmonary bypass, hepatic failure, and chronic renal insufficiency.

b. Immediately postoperatively, check prothrombin time (PT)/partial thromboplastin time (PTT), platelet count, and fibrinogen levels. Therapy as indicated with fresh frozen platelets (FFP), platelets, cryoprecipitate, and/or protamine.

C. Management issues
1. Inotropic and fluid management
   a. *Preload optimization.* Intravenous fluids (crystalloids or colloids) should be judiciously administered while continuously monitoring for adequacy of systemic perfusion.

      (1) Clinical parameters include palpable distal pulses, warm extremities, adequate urine output (>0.5 mL/kg/h) without diuretics, normal acid—base balance, and cardiac index greater than 2.0 L/min/m^2.

      (2) A central venous pressure (CVP) of 8 to 12 mm Hg and/or pulmonary capillary wedge pressures of 15 to 20 mm Hg in the setting of systemic vascular resistance between 1,000 to 1,400 dynes/sec/cm^5 are indicative of adequate fluid resuscitation.

   b. *Inotropic support.* Indicated if in the presence of adequate preload, the cardiac index remains below 2.0 L/min/m^2 with 1 or more β-adrenergic agents. The phosphodiesterase inhibitor milrinone can dramatically improve myocardial function, particularly for the right ventricle and in recipients with high systemic afterload or pulmonary hypertension.

   c. *Afterload management.* Mean arterial pressures in excess of 80 mm Hg should be treated to avoid excessive ventricular wall stress in the allograft.

      (1) Early postoperatively, IV sodium nitroprusside or nitroglycerin is administered. Nitroglycerin is associated with less intrapulmonary shunting due to relative preservation of the pulmonary hypoxic vasoconstrictor reflex.

      (2) Afterload reduction should be titrated to achieve mean arterial pressures between 65 and 80 mm Hg and/or a calculated systemic vascular resistance between 1,000 and 1,400 dynes/sec/cm^5.

      (3) If hypertension persists, an oral antihypertensive can be added to permit weaning of parenteral agents. β-Blockers are generally avoided in heart recipients early postoperatively.

      (4) Transient vasodilation with systemic hypotension, frequently seen early after cardiopulmonary bypass in patients previously taking angiotensin-converting—enzyme inhibitors, is usually effectively managed with inotropes containing an α-adrenergic component, such as epinephrine or norepinephrine.

2. Respiratory management.
The respiratory management of the cardiac transplant recipient follows the same principles used following routine cardiac operations.

   a. Initial ventilator parameters on arrival in the intensive care unit (ICU): tidal volume of 10 mL/kg, ventilatory rate of 10 breaths per minute, positive end-expiratory pressure (PEEP) of 5 cm H$_2$O, and fraction of inspired oxygen (FiO$_2$) of 1.0.

   b. Goal is to reduce the FiO$_2$ to 0.4, maintaining oxygen saturation greater than 90%, with an arterial oxygen tension (paO$_2$) greater than 70 mm Hg.

   c. Ventilatory rate and tidal volume are adjusted to achieve partial arterial pressure (paCO$_2$) between 30 and 40 mm Hg and normal pH (7.35 to 7.45).

3. Electrolyte balance and renal function
   a. Management of fluid and electrolytes homeostasis of the cardiac transplant recipient follows the same principles used after routine cardiac operations.

   b. Serum electrolytes are checked frequently. Maintaining normal K$^+$, Mg^{++}, and Ca^{++} levels is particularly important to reduce the frequency of arrhythmias.

   c. Serum glucose is monitored every 6 hours. Hyperglycemia is commonly observed, particularly in the first 24 to 48 hours after surgery due to physiologic stress, inotropic support, and glucocorticoid administration. Insulin (subcutaneous or continuous IV infusion) is titrated to maintain serum glucose levels between 100 and 150 mg/dL.

   d. A daily fluid restriction of 2,000 mL is maintained for the first 3 to 4 days, depending on the recipient's preoperative fluid status and postoperative renal function.

e. On initiation of immunosuppressant therapies, particularly cyclosporine, serum creatinine is followed closely to monitor for early nephrotoxicity.

f. Diuresis with furosemide is usually initiated 24 to 48 hours postoperatively and continued to eventually achieve euvolemia, often indicated by a return to preoperative body weight.

4. Perioperative infection prophylaxis

a. First-generation cephalosporins are given perioperatively.

b. Routine strict isolation is no longer employed. Hand washing, gloves, and gowns are used to avoid infectious cross-transmission.

c. Trimethoprim-sulfamethoxazole (TMP/SMX), or aerosolized pentamidine if TMP/SMX is not tolerated, is used as prophylaxis against *Pneumocystis jiroveci* pneumonia, *Toxoplasma gondii*, Listeria, Legionella, and possibly Nocardia infections.

d. Nystatin or clotrimazole is usually used as prophylaxis for mucocutaneous candidiasis. Fluconazole is indicated for candidiasis refractory to these topical antifungal agents or involving the esophagus.

e. Routine low-dose acyclovir to reduce frequency and severity of herpes simplex and varicella-zoster infections.

f. Recipients with a positive PPD skin test should be considered for isoniazid (rifampin) prophylaxis.

g. Cytomegalovirus (CMV) is the most common causative pathogen in cardiac transplant recipients and is thought to play a role in chronic allograft rejection. Routine prophylaxis with intravenous ganciclovir for 1 to 2 weeks followed by oral maintenance dosing for 3 months is recommended, particularly for a CMV seronegative recipient/seropositive donor combination.

5. Immunosuppression

a. The primary objectives of immunosuppressive therapy include:

(1) the selective modulation of the immune response to prevent allograft rejection

(2) maintaining immunocompetence to prevent infection and neoplasia

(3) minimizing during toxicity

b. The choice and combinations of immunosuppressive agents, doses, and schedules vary significantly among transplantation centers. Most centers employ triple immunosuppressive therapy consisting of cyclosporine, corticosteroids, and azathioprine or mycophenolate mofetil. An example of such a regimen is outlined in Table 151-1. Such multidrug regimens are designed to exploit synergism between the different mechanisms of action, permitting lower doses of each component and reduced toxicities.

II. HEART-LUNG AND LUNG TRANSPLANT RECIPIENTS

A. General principles

1. Objectives

a. Early postoperative care is based on judicious fluid and ventilatory management.

b. The primary objectives during this period are to maintain adequate perfusion and gas exchange while minimizing IV fluids, cardiac work, and barotrauma.

2. Monitoring

a. Arterial and central venous monitoring lines; pulse oximetry.

b. Pulmonary arterial catheters are frequently helpful early postoperatively period to aid in maximizing cardiac output with inotropic support, IV fluids, and vasodilators and are essential when the recipient has known pulmonary hypertension, donor right ventricular dysfunction.

B. Pathophysiology

1. Lung allograft denervation

a. Denervation of the lungs diminishes cough reflex and impairs mucociliary clearance. Therefore, lung recipients require aggressive postoperative pulmonary toilet.

TABLE 151-1	**Immunosuppressive Regimen for Heart Transplantation at the Johns Hopkins Hospital**

Preoperative preparation
  Cyclosporine: 4–10 mg/kg PO (dosage based on serum creatinine)
Intraoperative management
  Methylprednisolone: 500 mg IV (after administration of protamine)
Immediate postoperative therapy
  Methylprednisolone: 125 mg/kg IV for 3 doses
  Prednisone: 1 mg/kg PO Qd tapered to 0.4 mg/kg by 2 wks
  Cyclosporine: 0.5 mg/kg/day IV until taking PO then
    5–10 mg/kg/day PO
Postoperative maintenance therapy
  Prednisone: 0.2 mg/kg PO Qd
  Mycophenolate mofetil: 1 g PO/IV B.I.D.
  Cyclosporine: 5 mg/kg PO Qd (dose adjusted to maintain
    serum levels between 200–350 mg/mL)*

*Cyclo Trac SP[125] I RIA Kit, INCSTAR, Stillwater, MN.
Reproduced with permission from Bethea BT, Yuh DD, Conte JV, Baumgartner WA. Heart transplantation. In: Cohn LM, Edmunds LH Jr., eds. *Cardiac surgery in the adult, 2nd edition*. New York: McGraw-Hill, 2004, pp. 1427–1459.

    b. Early pulmonary allograft function is impacted by ischemia, reperfusion injury, and disrupted pulmonary lymphatics, all leading to increased vascular permeability, interstitial edema, and elevated arterial-alveolar gradients.
  2. Early allograft failure
    a. *Cardiac allograft dysfunction*
      (1) As in cardiac transplant recipients, early cardiac dysfunction may develop in heart-lung recipients due to prolonged ischemia, inadequate preservation, or catecholamine depletion.
      (2) Hypovolemia, tamponade, sepsis, and bradycardia may contribute to this early dysfunction and should be treated expediently if present. Otherwise, management of early cardiac dysfunction in heart-lung transplant recipients is as described with isolated cardiac transplant recipients.
    b. *Lung allograft dysfunction*
      (1) Early lung graft dysfunction manifests as persistently marginal gas exchange (i.e., hypoxia, hypercarbia) and pulmonary hypertension in the absence of infection or rejection.
      (2) Occurring in less than 15%, primary graft failure is usually caused by ischemia-reperfusion injury and results in pulmonary capillary leak causing alveolar edema, impaired lung compliance, and elevated pulmonary vascular resistance shortly after ICU admission.
        (a) Particularly severe cases of pulmonary hypertension can lead to right ventricular failure.
        (b) This syndrome resembles ARDS with a severe arterial-alveolar gradient (PaO_2:FiO_2 ratio <150 mm Hg), diffuse interstitial infiltrates on early postoperative chest radiographs, and diffuse alveolar damage on histology.
        (c) The degree of pulmonary edema has been observed to be inversely related to the quality of preservation, although the development of severe ischemia-reperfusion injury is still largely unpredictable.
      (3) Early lung graft dysfunction is managed by increased FiO_2, PEEP, sedation, neuromuscular blockade, and careful diuresis to maintain fluid balance and reduce pulmonary edema.

(4) In cases of persistently severe graft dysfunction refractory to standard ventilatory and medical management, extracorporeal membrane oxygenation (ECMO) and inhaled nitric oxide may be used to stabilize gas exchange.

(a) Nitric oxide acts to relax preconstricted pulmonary vascular smooth muscle and is justified in recipients with pulmonary infiltrates, poor oxygenation, and mild to moderate pulmonary hypertension early postoperatively.

(b) Redistribution of pulmonary flow with nitric oxide was shown to decrease the intrapulmonary shunt fraction in patients after transplantation.

(c) Nitric oxide therapy should be initiated at 10 to 20 ppm for 12 to 24 hours. Toxicity is monitored by methemoglobin levels. Nitric oxide is rapidly inactivated by hemoglobin, producing methemoglobin, which can impair oxygen delivery at high levels.

(d) If oxygenation and pulmonary infiltrates improve, nitric oxide may be weaned over 6 to 12 hours to 5 ppm, after which a slower wean, even over several days, is initiated; more profound hemodynamic consequences of weaning from 5 ppm to 0 ppm than from 20 ppm to 5 ppm have often been observed. Right heart failure, manifested by a rise in CVP and fall in cardiac output, is monitored for during nitric oxide weaning.

3. Dysrhythmias (see Cardiac transplant recipients)

C. Management issues

1. Inotropic and fluid management

2. Respiratory management

a. After ICU admission: anteroposterior chest radiograph; initial ventilator settings: FiO_2 of 50%, tidal volume of 10 to 15 mL/Kg, assist-control rate of 10 to 14 breaths per minute, and PEEP of 3 to 5 cm H_2O. Initial tidal volumes and flow rates are adjusted to limit peak airway pressures to less than 40 cm H_2O, to minimize barotrauma and high airway pressures, which may compromise bronchial mucosal blood flow.

b. Arterial blood gases 30 minutes after each ventilator setting change to achieve a paO_2 greater than 75 mmHg on an FiO_2 of 0.4, a $paCO_2$ between 30 and 40 mmHg, and a pH between 7.35 and 7.45.

c. Weaning to extubation is initiated after the patient is stable, awake, and alert. Generally, weaning is conducted through successive decrements in the intermittent mandatory ventilation (IMV) rate, followed by a sustained trail of continuous positive airway pressure (CPAP). Extubation is often possible within the first 24 hours posttransplant.

d. Subsequent pulmonary management comprises diuresis, supplemental oxygen to maintain adequate oxygen saturations, bronchodilators, aggressive pulmonary toilet and incentive spirometry, and frequent interval chest radiographs.

(1) Albuterol and ipratropium bromide (Atrovent) inhaled therapy is helpful in cases of bronchospasm in the native lung, due to underlying disease, and/or in the lung allograft due to mild ischemia-reperfusion injury.

(2) Due to pulmonary airway denervation, pulmonary toilet with frequent endotracheal suctioning is necessary to avoid the development of mucous plugs and atelectasis. Care should be taken during deep suctioning to avoid unnecessary trauma to the tracheal or bronchial anastomoses.

3. Coagulopathy (see Cardiac Transplant Recipients)

4. Electrolyte and renal dysfunction (see Cardiac transplant recipients)

5. Perioperative infection prophylaxis (see Cardiac transplant recipients)

6. Immunosuppression (see Cardiac transplant recipients)

Selected Readings

Adatia I, Lillehie C. Arnold JH, et al. Inhaled nitric oxide in the treatment of postoperative graft dysfunction after lung transplantation. *Ann Thorac Surg* 1994; 57:1311.

An excellent guide toward the use of inhaled nitric oxide in the treatment of pulmonary allograft dysfunction.

Armitage JM, Hardy RL, Griffith BP. Prostaglandin E₁: an effective treatment of right heart failure after orthotopic heart transplantation. *J Heart Transplant* 1987; 6:348.
A good review of the use of prostaglandin in the treatment of right heart failure in the cardiac transplant recipient.

Balsam LB, Yuh DD, Robbins RC, et al. Heart-lung and lung transplantation. In: Cohn LM, Edmunds Jr. LH, eds. *Cardiac surgery in the adult*, 2nd edition. New York: Mc-Graw-Hill, 2004, pp. 1461–1490.
An up-to-date comprehensive overview of the field of heart-lung and lung transplantation coauthored by the originator of heart-lung transplantation.

Baumgartner WA, Reitz BA, Oyer PE, et al. Cardiac transplantation. Curr Probl Surg 1979; 16:6.
A classic overview of cardiac transplantation written by many of the field's early pioneers.

Bethea BT, Yuh DD, Conte JV, et al. Heart transplantation. In: Cohn LM, Edmunds Jr. LH, eds. Cardiac Surgery in the Adult 2/e. New York, NY, McGraw-Hill, 2004, pp. 1427–1459.
An up-to-date comprehensive overview of cardiac transplantation.

Chan GLC, Gruber SA, Skjei KL, et al. Principles of immunosuppression. *Crit Care Clin* 1990;6:841.
A good discussion of the concepts behind pharmacologic immunosuppression.

Christie JD, Bavaria JE, Palevsky HI, et al. Primary graft failure following lung transplantation. *Chest* 1998;114:51.
An excellent discussion of the causes of primary graft failure after lung transplantation.

Little RE, Kay GN, Epstein AE, et al. Arrhythmias after orthotopic cardiac transplantation: prevalence and determinants during initial hospitalization and late follow-up. *Circulation* 1989;80:III-140.
An excellent review of arrhythmias encountered after cardiac transplantation.

Moon MR, Barlow CW, Robbins RC. Early postoperative care of lung and heart-lung transplant recipients. In: Baumgartner WA, Reitz BA, Kasper E, Theodore J, eds. Heart and lung transplantation, 2ⁿᵈ edition. Philadelphia: WB Saunders, 2002, pp. 225–232.
An excellent textbook with detailed discussion on the postoperative management of heart, lung, and heart-lung transplant recipients.

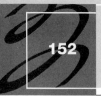

152 | CRITICAL CARE OF THE DECEASED ORGAN DONOR
Christoph Troppmann

I. GENERAL PRINCIPLES
  A. The gap between available donor organs and those waiting for transplants is widening, and wait list mortality is increasing.
  B. Critical care physicians and other health-care personnel play a key role in early identification of potential organ donors; early referral to organ procurement organizations; in a coordinated approach to the potential donor families for obtaining consent; and maintaining and optimizing organ function and viability for transplantation.
  C. Predicted annual number of brain-dead potential organ donors ranges between 10,500 and 13,800, but in 2003, organs were recovered from only 5,630 deceased organ donors (Sheehy, 2003).

II. DONOR CLASSIFICATION
  A. Donation after cardiac death (DCD) donors.
    1. Currently less than 10% of all deceased organ donors, but number is increasing.
    2. Usually time and place of death are controlled (e.g., families of unconscious patients with severe irreversible terminal brain injuries, who do not fulfill the formal criteria of brain death, decide to forgo any further life-sustaining treatment and wish to donate the organs).
    3. The prospective donor is brought to the operating room, life-supporting treatment is discontinued, and organ procurement is initiated once death has been pronounced by a physician not belonging to the organ recovery and transplant team.
  B. Brain-dead deceased donors.
    1. The most common deceased donor type.
    2. Unequivocal diagnosis of brain death is required before proceeding with organ procurement.

III. ORGAN DONOR SCREENING (DONATION AFTER CARDIAC DEATH DONORS AND BRAIN-DEAD DECEASED DONORS)
  A. Age 0 to 90 years
  B. Patient's death imminent
  C. Near brain death, brain-dead, or impending withdrawal of support in patients with severe irreversible terminal brain injury
  D. Contraindications
    1. Current untreated severe viral, bacterial, fungal, or protozoan infection
    2. Evidence of systemic sepsis syndrome
    3. Viral encephalitis with severe systemic viral infection
    4. HIV-positive serology
    5. Malignancy (except nonmelanoma skin cancers, primary brain tumors with little propensity to disseminate)
  E. After identification of any potential donor, federal required-request legislation mandates that hospitals notify their local organ procurement organization (OPO) in a timely manner.
  F. If local OPO address is unknown, a 24-hour access number to the United Network for Organ Sharing (UNOS) is available for further referral information: 1-800-292-9537.
  G. The OPO will assist in completing preliminary screening of the potential donor and consult with the transplant team regarding use of marginal donors.

IV. BRAIN DEATH DIAGNOSIS

A. "An individual who has sustained either irreversible cessation of circulatory and respiratory function, or irreversible cessation of all functions of the entire brain, including the brainstem, is dead. A determination of death must be made in accordance with accepted standards" (President's Commission for the Study of Ethical Problems in Medicine *Uniform Determination of Death Act*, 1981).

B. The clinical diagnosis of brain death rests on three criteria:

  1. Irreversibility of the neurologic insult

  2. Absence of clinical evidence of cerebral function

  3. Most important, absence of clinical evidence of brainstem function

C. Clinical brain death examination and apnea test are outlined in Table 152-1.

D. Spinal reflexes can be preserved and do not exclude the diagnosis of brain death.

TABLE 152-1 **Brain Death Criteria and Clinical Diagnosis of Brain Death**

1. Irreversible, well-defined etiology of unconsciousness
   a. Structural disease or metabolic cause.
   b. Exclusion of hypothermia; hypotension, severe electrolyte, endocrine, or acid–base disturbance; drug or substance intoxication.
   c. Sufficient observation period (at least 6 h) between two brain-death examinations.
2. No clinical evidence of cerebral function
   a. No spontaneous movement, eye opening, or movement or response after auditory, verbal, or visual commands.
   b. No movement elicited by painful stimuli to the face and trunk (e.g., sternal rub, pinching of a nipple or fingernail bed) other than spinal cord reflex movements.
3. No clinical evidence of brainstem function
   a. No pupillary reflex: pupils are fixed and midposition; no change of pupil size in either eye after shining a strong light source in each eye sequentially in a dark room.
   b. No corneal reflex: no eyelid movements after touching the cornea (not the conjunctiva) with a sterile cotton swab or tissue.
   c. No gag reflex: no retching or movement of the uvula after touching the back of the pharynx with a tongue depressor or after moving the endotracheal tube.
   d. No cough reflex: no coughing with deep tracheal irrigation and suctioning.
   e. No oculocephalic reflex (doll's eyes reflex): no eye movement in response to brisk turning of the head from side to side with the head of the supine patient elevated 30 degrees.
   f. No oculovestibular reflex (caloric reflex): no eye movements within 3 minutes after removing earwax and irrigating each tympanic membrane (if intact) sequentially with 50 mL ice water for 30 to 45 seconds while the head of the supine patient is elevated 30 degrees.
   g. No integrated motor response to pain: no localizing or withdrawal response, no extensor or flexor posturing.
4. Apnea testing
   a. Patient is preoxygenated with FiO_2 of 1.0 for 10 to 15 minutes while adjusting ventilatory rate and volume so that paCO2 reaches about 40 to 45 mm Hg.
   b. Obtain arterial baseline blood gas, disconnect patient from the ventilator, deliver O_2 at 6 to 8 L/min through a cannula advanced 20 to 30 cm into the endotracheal tube (cannula tip at the carina).
   c. Use continuous pulse oxymetry for early detection of desaturation.
   d. If brain-dead, a paO_2 >60 mm Hg is achieved within 3 to 5 minutes after withdrawal of ventilatory support; at this point the patient should be reconnected to the ventilator (or earlier, should hemodynamic instability, desaturation, or spontaneous breathing movements occur).
   e. Arterial blood gas sampling immediately before reinstitution of mechanical ventilation to confirm the $paCO_2$ rise to >60 mm Hg.
   f. Criteria for positive apnea test: No evidence of spontaneous respirations before reinstitution of mechanical ventilation in the presence of $paCO_2$ >60 mm Hg or $paCO_2$ increase of >20 mm Hg from the normal baseline value.

TABLE 152-2	Pitfalls in Clinical Brain Death Testing and Potential Remedial Measures

Pitfalls	Remedial measure(s)
Hypotension, shock	Institute fluid resuscitation, use pressor agents
Hypothermia	Use warmed fluids, heated ventilator gases
Intoxication or drug overdose	If measurable, check drug levels and toxicology screens, or increase waiting time between brain death examinations
Neuromuscular and sedative drugs, which can interfere with elicitation of motor responses	Discontinue muscle relaxants and mood- or consciousness-altering medications, increase waiting time between brain death examinations
Pupillary fixation, which may be caused by anticholinergic drugs (e.g., atropine given during a cardiac arrest), neuromuscular blocking agents, or preexisting disease	Discontinue anticholinergic medications and muscle relaxants, increase waiting time between brain death examinations, obtain careful patient history
Corneal reflexes absent due to overlooked contact lenses	Remove contact lenses before brain death examination
Oculovestibular reflexes diminished or abolished after prior use of ototoxic drugs (e.g., aminoglycosides, loop diuretics, vancomycin) or agents with suppressive side effects on the vestibular system (e.g., tricyclic antidepressants, anticonvulsants, and barbiturates) or due to preexisting disease	Obtain careful medication history and patient history

5. Confirmatory tests should be used when the observation period needs to be shortened (e.g., unstable donors); in equivocal situations (including age younger than 1 year); or if one of the potential pitfalls (Table 152-2) cannot be ruled out. Tests must demonstrate absence of intracranial circulation by angiographic contrast or radioisotopic flow studies, transcranial Doppler ultrasonography, or electrocerebral silence documented by an electroencephalogram. Pursue donation after cardiac death if patient is unconscious, has suffered significant irreversible brain injury, but does not fulfill all formal criteria for brain death.

V. OBTAINING CONSENT FOR ORGAN DONATION
A. Early involvement of the OPO in the organ donation and consent process is crucial.
B. Consent rates are highest when a hospital-based health-care professional (but not a physician) broaches the possibility of organ donation with the family, followed by a meeting with an OPO staff person.
C. Other important factors affecting the decision to donate include level of public education, understanding and awareness of the irreversibility of severe brain injury (DCD donors) and of brain death, amount of time spent by the organ procurement organization representative with the family, and covering discussion topics of importance to donor families (e.g., costs, funeral, choices regarding amount of tissue/organs donated) (Siminoff, 2001).

VI. PERIOPERATIVE CARE OF THE DONATION AFTER CARDIAC DEATH (DCD) DONOR
A. Preoperative care of potential DCD donors (prior to obtaining consent for organ donation)
1. The therapy remains primarily aimed at treating the underlying pathology (e.g., head trauma, cerebrovascular accident)

B. Preoperative care of actual DCD donors (after having obtained consent for organ donation)

    1. The focus switches from cerebral protection to preservation of organ function and optimization of peripheral oxygen delivery.

    2. Maintenance therapy end points in DCD donors are identical to those described below (VII.B.2.a-h) for brain-dead organ donors.

C. Intraoperative care of DCD donors

    1. Maintenace therapy as outline above (VI.B.) is continued until support is withdrawn and the patient is extubated.

    2. Any additional premortem interventions (e.g., surgical: insertion of femoral cannulas in preparation of organ recovery; pharmacologic: administration of intravenous herapin, opioids, and phentolamine) must occur in strict accordance with local OPO/hospital DCD protocols and policies.

    3. Death is pronounced by a physician not belonging to the organ recovery and transplant team (usually the patient's intensive care physician).

    4. After an additional postmortem waiting time (minutes) specified by the local OPO/hospital DCD protocol, surgical organ recovery begins.

    5. Disposition of the patient, if death does not occur within a specified postwithdrawal of support waiting time, is determined by the local protocol (e.g., return patient to a non–intensive care hospital floor for comfort care only).

VII. PERIOPERATIVE CARE OF THE BRAIN-DEAD ORGAN DONOR

A. General considerations

    1. Once consent for organ donation is obtained, the focus switches from cerebral protection to preservation of organ function and optimization of peripheral oxygen delivery.

    2. Inadequate brain-dead donor management may result in loss of transplantable organs or even (in up to 15% of all cases) loss of the organ donor altogether.

    3. Pathophysiology of brain-death maintenance phase

        a. Hypothermia

        b. Hypotension due to complete arterial and venous vasomotor collapse.

        c. Abolition of resting vagal tone secondary to destruction of the nucleus ambiguus, eliminating all chronotropic effects of atropine.

        d. Absence of pituitary hormones (including vasopressin).

        e. Upregulation of proinflammatory and immunoregulatory pathways.

B. Management principles

    1. Monitoring

        a. Core temperature, central venous pressure (CVP), systemic arterial blood pressure (arterial line), pulmonary artery (PA) catheter in selected donors, pulse oximetry.

        b. Foley catheter (urine output).

        c. Frequent determination of electrolytes and arterial blood gases.

        d. Regular monitoring (every 12 hours) of blood urea nitrogen (BUN) and creatinine level, liver enzymes, amylase, cipase, and coagulation tests to help assess organ status and function.

    2. Maintenance therapy end points in brain-dead organ donors

        a. Systolic blood pressure 100 to 120 mm Hg, mean arterial pressure (MAP) greater than 60 mm Hg.

        b. CVP 8 to 10 mm Hg.

        c. Systemic vascular resistance (SVR) 800 to 1,200 dyne·sec·cm^{-5}

        d. Dopamine less than 10 μg/kg per minute

        e. Urine output 100 to 300 mL per hour

        f. Core temperature >35°C.

        g. paO_2 80 to 100 mm Hg, SaO_2 >95%, pH 7.37 to 7.45.

        h. Hemoglobin 10 to 12 g/dL, hematocrit 30% to 35%.

    3. Cardiovascular support. Hypotension most common, usually due to hypovolemia, but there is a wide array of other differential diagnoses (Table 152-3).

        a. If hypotension persists despite euvolemia, use dopamine or α-adrenergic agents (e.g., phenylnephrine).

TABLE 152-3	Differential Diagnosis of Hypotension in the Brain-Dead Organ Donor

Hypovolemia

Hypothermia

Cardiac dysfunction
  Arrhythmia (ischemia, catecholamines, hypokalemia, hypomagnesemia)
  Acidosis
  Hypooxygenation
  Excessive positive end-expiratory ventilatory pressure
  Congestive heart failure due to excessive fluid administration
  Hypophosphatemia
  Hypocalcemia
  Causes related to the injury that caused brain death (cardiac tamponade, myocardial contusion)
  Myocardial sequelae of autonomic storm during brain herniation
  Preexisting cardiac disease

Pneumothorax (traumatic or iatrogenic)

Drug side effect or overdose (e.g., long-acting beta-blocker, calcium-channel antagonist, antihypertensive agent)

  b. Treat hypertension with short-acting vasodilatory agents (e.g., sodium nitroprusside) or short-acting β-blockers.
  c. Use of low-dose arginine vasopressin and T_3 (see dosages later under "Hormonal/endocrine support") may further reduce inotropic requirements.
4. Respiratory maintenance
  a. Vigorous tracheobronchial toilet with frequent suctioning; aspiration precautions.
  b. Positive end-expiratory pressure (PEEP) at 5 cm H_2O, tidal volumes 10 to 12 mL/kg, peak airway pressures less than 30 cm H_2O. For potential lung donors. CVP should be kept at 6 to 8 mm Hg, pulmonary artery balloon occlusion pressure at 8 to 12 mm Hg.
  c. Steroid bolus treatments during the maintenance phase may exert potential beneficial effects (improved oxygenation and increased donor lung recovery rates; see dosage later under "Hormonal/endocrine support").
5. Renal function and electrolyte management
  a. Goals (for potential kidney donors)
    (1) Maintain adequate systemic arterial perfusion pressure.
    (2) Maintain brisk urine output (>1 to 2 mL/kg/h).
    (3) Minimize use of vasopressors to maximize posttransplant graft function.
    (4) Insufficient urine production (less than 1 mL/kg/h) after adequate resuscitation: give loop or osmotic diuretics (furosemide, mannitol).
    (5) Avoid nephrotoxic drugs.
  b. Polyuria
    (1) Frequently observed in brain-dead donors.
    (2) Etiologies
      (a) Osmotic diuresis (induced by mannitol administered to decrease intracranial pressure (ICP) during pre–brain death phase, or hyperglycemia).
      (b) Hypothermia
      (c) Diabetes insipidus
        i. Diagnosis
          • Urine volumes greater than 300 mL per hour (or >5 mL/kg/h) with hypernatremia (serum sodium >150 mEq/L), elevated serum osmolality (>310 mOsm/kg), and low urinary sodium concentration
          • Not infrequently associated with other electrolyte abnormalities: hypokalemia, hypocalcemia, hypomagnesemia.

      ii. Treatment.
- Vasopressin or vasopressin analogues (indicated once urine output exceeds 300 mL/h). Desmopressin (desamino-8-D-arginine vasopressin [DDAVP]) has a long duration of action and high antidiuretic–pressor ratio, reducing undesirable splanchnic vasoconstrictor effects of arginine vasopressin. Dosage: 1 to 2 µg desmopressin are administered IV every 8 to 12 hours to titrate urine output to values of 100 to 300 mL per hour.
- Correct hypernatremia: Use infusion solutions with low or no sodium content (e.g., D5W solution [free water]). Take into consideration sodium content of other IV fluids (e.g., of 5% albumin solutions).
- Adjunct measures: discontinue mannitol, correct coexisting hypovolemia and hyperglycemia.

6. Hypothermia
    a. After brain death, when the body becomes poikilothermic because of the loss of central temperature control mechanisms, hypothermia is further aggravated by peripheral vasodilatation. Hypothermia is observed in up to 80% of brain-dead bodies.
    b. Adverse effects: Decreased myocardial contractility, hypotension, cardiac arrhythmias, cardiac arrest, hepatic and renal dysfunction, acidosis, and coagulopathy.
    c. Therapy: Maintain donor core temperature at > 35°C using warmed IV fluids and blood products, warming blankets, heated ventilator gases.

7. Coagulation system.
    a. Coagulopathy and disseminated intravascular coagulation are common findings in brain-dead donors, particularly after head injury.
    b. Clinical findings: pathologic bleeding, abnormal prothrombin time (PT)/international normalized ratio (INR), thrombocytopenia, hypofibrinogenemia, increased fibrin/fibrinogen degradation products.
    c. Treat coagulopathy using blood products as indicated by specific findings. Correct underlying pathophysiology (e.g., hypothermia, acidosis).

8. Hormonal/endocrine support
    a. Hyperglycemia
      (1) Frequent in brain-dead donors
      (2) Etiology
        (a) Increased catecholamine release
        (b) Altered carbohydrate metabolism
        (c) Steroid administration for treatment of cerebral edema
        (d) Infusion of large amounts of dextrose-containing IV fluids
        (e) Peripheral insulin resistance
      (3) Treatment: insulin (subcutaneously or continuous IV infusion) to maintain glucose levels 100 to 150 mg/dL.
      (4) Good glycemic control also prevents ketoacidosis and osmotic diuresis and may be beneficial for pancreas graft function in recipients.
    b. Recently published retrospective clinical evidence suggests that hormonal support may stabilize and improve cardiac function in brain-dead donors and may result in increased probability of kidney, heart, liver, lung, and pancreas recovery and transplantation (awaits confirmation in prospective controlled trials). Recommended doses (based on American Society of Transplant Surgeons and American Society of Transplantation 2002 Consensus Conference Recommendations):
      (1) Triiodothyronine (T_3: 4 µg bolus, 3 µg/h continuous IV infusion): (effects: reversal of myocardial dysfunction, improved arterial pressure, decreased central venous pressure, significant reduction of inotropic requirements)
      (2) Methylprednisolone: 15 mg/kg/bolus IV (repeat every 24 hours) (effects: improved oxygenation and increased donor lung recovery; putative beneficial effects in the donor and the organ recipient from attenuation of the effects

of proinflammatory cytokines released as a consequence of brain death).

(3) Arginine vasopressin: one unit bolus, followed by 0.5 to 4.0 unit per hour IV continuous infusion (titrate SVR to 800 to 1,200 dyne·sec·cm^{-5} if PA catheter in place) (effects: treatment of diabetes insipidus, reduces inotropic requirements; better kidney, liver, and heart graft function; beneficial effects are present even in unstable donors who do *not* have diabetes insipidus).

C. Intraoperative care

1. In brain-dead donors, full cardiovascular and ventilatory support is maintained throughout the donor operation until the start of the organ flush phase.

2. Maintain hemodynamic stability and ensure adequate fluid resuscitation, particularly in thoracic and abdominal organ donors when both body cavities are open and significant evaporative and massive third space fluid losses can occur.

3. Maintain normothermia

Selected Readings

Chen JM, Cullinane S, Spanier TB, et al. Vasopressin deficiency and pressor hypersensitivity in hemodynamically unstable organ donors. *Circulation* 1999; 100(suppl II):II-244–II-246.
Clinical study that provides a rationale for use of low-dose vasopressin in brain-dead donors.

Pratschke J, Wilhelm MJ, Kusaka M, et al. Brain death and its influence on donor organ quality and outcome after transplantation. *Transplantation* 1999;67:343–348.
An overview of the impact of brain death on organ physiology, function, and morphology in the donor and recipient.

Report of the Quality Standards Subcommittee of the American Academy of Neurology. Practice parameters for determining brain death in adults (summary statement). *Neurology* 1995;45:1012–1014.
Summary statement issued by the American Academy of Neurology.

Rosendale JD, Chabalewski FL, McBride MA, et al. Increased transplanted organs from the use of a standardized donor management protocol. *Am J Transplant* 2002;2:761–768.
Important results of a national pilot study on the beneficial effect of instituting a critical pathway for organ recovery rates.

Rosendale JD, Kauffman HM, McBride MA, et al. Aggressive pharmacologic donor management results in more transplanted organs. *Transplantation* 2003;75:482–487.
Large retrospective study that suggests a beneficial impact of hormonal resuscitation on organ recovery rates.

Rosengard BR, Feng, S, Alfrey EJ, et al. Report of the Crystal City meeting to maximize the use of organs recovered from the cadaver donor. *Am J Transplant* 2002;2:701–711.
Broadly supported consensus conference recommendations on maximizing organ recovery from deceased donors.

Sheehy E, Conrad SL, Brigham LE, et al. Estimating the number of potential organ donors in the United States. *N Engl J Med* 2003;349:667–674.
A current estimate of the number of potential organ donors and of the lost opportunities due to lack of obtaining consent.

Siminoff LA, Gordon N, Hewlett J, et al. Factors influencing families' consent for donation of solid organs for transplantation. *JAMA* 2001;286:71–77.
An important study on factors affecting families' decision to donate.

Troppmann C, Dunn DL. Management of the organ donor. In: Irwin RS, Rippe JM, eds. *Irwin and Rippe's intensive care medicine,* 5th edition. Philadelphia: Lippincott Williams & Wilkins, 2003, pp. 1973–1992.
An extensive review of medical, legal, and practical-clinical aspects concerning organ donation and the brain-dead donor.

Wijdicks EFM. The diagnosis of brain death. *N Engl J Med* 2001;344:1215–1221.

I. GENERAL PRINCIPLES

A. Definition. Hematopoietic cell transplantation (HCT) is a potentially curative treatment for malignant and nonmalignant diseases, including leukemia, lymphoma, multiple myeloma, aplastic anemia, hemoglobinopathies, and congenital immune deficiencies. HCT may have a role in the treatment of certain solid tumors such as renal cell carcinoma, germ cell tumors, and breast cancer. High-dose chemoradiation is typically used to eradicate the underlying disease and is followed by intravenous infusion of the stem cell graft. Among other cells, the graft contains the stem cells that reconstitute the ablated hematopoietic system of the patient. Immunosuppressive therapy is required after allogeneic HCT to prevent graft-versus-host disease (GVHD) and graft rejection.

B. Classification. HCT can be categorized according to the source of stem cells, the type of donor, and the intensity of the preparative regimen. Determining the type of HCT to be used in an individual patient is a complex decision based on patient's age, diagnosis, donor availability, and presence of comorbidities:

1. **Stem cell source**
   a. **Bone marrow.** Marrow is harvested from the iliac crest under general anesthesia.
   b. **"Mobilized" peripheral blood.** Growth factors are frequently used alone (e.g., granulocyte colony-stimulating factor, or G-CSF) or in combination with chemotherapy (in autologous HCT) for "mobilization" of hematopoietic stem cells, which are collected by blood leukapheresis. "Mobilized" blood cells engraft faster than marrow-derived cells.
   c. **Cord blood.** Collected from the umbilical cord after delivery of a baby. Engraftment takes longer compared with other sources of stem cells.

2. **Donor type**
   a. **Autologous.** Using one's own stem cells.
   b. **Syngeneic.** Identical twin (no genetic disparity between donor and recipient).
   c. **Allogeneic.** Donor with similar human leukocyte antigen (HLA) type.
      (1) Sibling donor. The statistical likelihood that a sibling is fully HLA-matched with the patient is 25%. The likelihood of identifying an HLA-matched sibling increases with the number of available siblings.
      (2) Unrelated donor. HLA-matched volunteer donor who was identified through a database search.

3. **Intensity of the preparative regimen**
   a. **Myeloablative.** The preparative regimen ablates the hematopoietic system of the patients and leads to transient but profound myelosuppression with pancytopenia.
   b. **Nonmyeloablative.** The preparative regimen is mainly immunosuppressive and aimed at preventing graft rejection. The underlying disease is eliminated through ensuing immunologic graft-versus-tumor effects. Toxicity from the preparative regimen is considerably milder compared with myeloablative HCT. Many patients receive the transplant in an outpatient setting. The onset of typical post-HCT complications such as GVHD and infections is delayed.

C. Epidemiology. Current estimates of annual numbers of HCT are 45,000 to 50,000 worldwide. Approximately two thirds of patients have autologous HCT and one third have allogeneic HCT.

D. Risk factors. The likelihood of developing transplant-related complications depends on patient age, intensity of the preparative regimen, type and stage of the underlying disease, and presence of comorbidities. Also, allogeneic HCT recipients have a greater risk of transplant-related morbidity and mortality than autologous HCT recipients. HLA disparity between donor and recipient further increases the risk owing to the greater likelihood of developing GVHD and graft rejection.

E. Prognosis. Prognosis after HCT is highly variable and is influenced by numerous factors that predict for mortality related to the transplant procedure itself and to recurrent malignancy after surviving the transplant. Patients with chronic myelogenous leukemia (CML) in chronic phase who have HCT from an HLA-identical sibling, for example, have a greater than 80% to 90% chance of long-term survival. In contrast, less than 50% of patients with more advanced leukemia at the time of HCT will be cured.

II. TRANSPLANT-RELATED COMPLICATIONS. The problems after HCT that typically cause procedure-related morbidity and mortality can broadly be categorized into five groups: hemolysis, toxicity of the preparative regimen, infection, bleeding, and GVHD.

A. Hemolysis

1. **General principles.** The inheritance of blood group antigens (e.g., ABO, Rh, Jk) is independent of that of the HLA antigens. ABO incompatibility between donor and recipient, however, is not a barrier to successful allogeneic HCT. Acute or delayed immunohemolytic complications due to ABO incompatibility should be distinguished from anaphylactic reactions precipitated by infusion of foreign proteins.

2. **Etiology/pathophysiology.** Acute (at the time of infusion) or delayed (5 to 15 days after HCT) immunohemolytic complications due to ABO incompatibility occur in patients with *minor* ABO-incompatibility (donor-derived isohemagglutinins directed against recipient red blood cells [RBCs]). Immediate hemolysis occurs if the graft contains preexisting isohemagglutinins that lyse recipient RBCs. Delayed hemolysis is due to generation of "new" isohemagglutinins by "passenger lymphocytes" in the graft. Delayed hemolysis due to minor ABO incompatibility is a rare complication but can be dramatic and life-threatening. *Major* ABO incompatibility (recipient-derived isohemagglutinins directed against donor RBCs) may lead to chronic hemolysis and pure red cell anemia (PRCA).

3. **Diagnosis**
   a. **Clinical presentation.** Mild hemolysis due to major ABO incompatibility may be associated with prolonged RBC transfusion requirements (PRCA). Delayed hemolysis due to minor ABO incompatibility may cause rapid lysis of all recipient RBCs over a few days. This may lead to acute renal failure or pulmonary edema and may be fatal. Plasma exchange in the recipient and plasma removal or RBC removal from the graft are standard procedures that minimize the risk of preventable hemolytic complication after ABO-mismatched HCT.

   b. **Laboratory and radiologic studies.** Emergence of donor-derived RBC and isohemagglutinin titers should be monitored after allogeneic HCT. Serum levels of (indirect) bilirubin and lactate dehydrogenase (LDH), reticulocyte counts, and the direct agglutinin test (DAT) are useful markers of hemolysis.

   c. **Differential diagnosis.** Parvovirus 19 infection may cause PRCA after HCT. Non–ABO-related Coombs-positive autoimmune hemolytic anemia (AIHA) may develop late after HCT. Drugs such as fluarabine or infections with mycoplasm may also produce hemolysis. Thrombotic microangiopathy (TM) is frequently related to cyclosporine or tacrolimus and associated with RBC fragmentation (schistocytes). Hyperbilirubinemia after HCT may have many other causes (e.g., sinusoidal obstruction syndrome[SOS] of the liver; drug effects). Dimethylsulfoxide (DMSO), a cryoprotectant used to store autologous stem cells, may cause anaphylactic and nonallergic reactions (e.g., hypotension, dyspnea, flushing, diarrhea) during infusion of thawed stem cell products.

4. **Treatment.** Chronic hemolysis due to major ABO incompatibility is usually self-limited. Patients with refractory or more acute immune hemolysis may require interventions aimed at suppressing ongoing donor-directed isohemag-glutinin production (corticosteroids, donor lymphocyte infusion, rituximab) or removal of the offending antibody (plasma exchange). Supportive care measures to maintain renal function are critical.

B. **Toxicity of the preparative regimen.** Cytotoxic chemotherapy with or without total body irradiation (TBI) may compromise the function of the lungs, heart, kidneys, nervous system, and gastrointestinal tract including the liver. This type of toxicity occurs predominantly within the first 3 to 4 weeks after HCT and is considerably more severe after myeloablative HCT than after nonmyeloablative HCT.

1. **Lung**

a. **Etiology/pathophysiology.** Idiopathic pneumonia syndrome (IPS), a noninfectious inflammatory lung process that may be triggered by TBI and chemotherapeutic drugs (e.g., BCNU, busulfan), occurs with a median onset of 2 to 3 weeks after HCT. Contributing factors to IPS lung injury may be release of inflammatory cytokines due to alloreactivity and/or sepsis. The role of possible latent infections is controversial. Other common noninfectious pulmonary problems that may occur within 30 days from the transplant include pulmonary hemorrhage, edema syndromes resulting from excessive fluid administration or cyclophosphamide-induced cardiomyopathy, and sepsis with acute respiratory distress syndrome (ARDS).

b. **Diagnosis**

(1) **Clinical presentation.** Fever, nonproductive cough, tachypnea, hypoxemia. Hemoptysis is an infrequent symptom of IPS or DAH.

(2) **Laboratory and radiologic studies.** Diffuse or multifocal intraalveolar or interstitial infiltrates on chest radiography. Computed tomography (CT) of the lung improves the imaging resolution and frequently reveals additional lesions. An increased alveolar-arterial oxygen gradient, a new restrictive pattern, or a diffusion capacity abnormality is evidence of abnormal pulmonary physiology. CT of the head prior to attempted biopsy for focal lung lesion is recommended owing to the high prevalence of disseminated fungal disease. Measurements of pulmonary artery wedge pressure or echocardiography may be useful to rule out cardiogenic pulmonary edema.

(3) **Differential diagnosis.** It is paramount to distinguish noninfectious (e.g., IPS) from infectious (e.g., CMV, bacterial, fungal) causes of diffuse pulmonary infiltrates. The diagnosis of IPS requires a negative bronchoalveolar lavage or lung biopsy with examination of stains and cultures for bacteria, fungi, and viruses. Localized parenchymal lung disease is usually due to infection. Bronchiolitis obliterans with organizing pneumonia (BOOP) can be related to chronic GVHD. Patients may also relapse in the lung with their underlying malignancy, particularly with lymphoma.

(4) **Treatment.** Treatment of IPS consists of supportive care and prevention of secondary infection. Empiric broad-spectrum antibiotics and a trial of diuretics should be instituted. The antibiotic coverage should be narrowed in case an infectious etiology is identified. Bleeding disorders should be corrected. Although no prospective trials support the use of high-dose corticosteroids, a small percentage of IPS patients do respond to doses of 1 to 2 mg/kg per day. Preemptive antifungal therapy (e.g., itraconazole, voriconazole) should be given to patients on high-dose steroids. Patients with BOOP frequently respond to corticosteroid therapy (1 mg/kg per day).

(5) **Prognosis.** The mortality associated with diffuse IPS after myeloablative HCT is 50% to 70%. Approximately 6% of patients who require mechanical ventilation after HCT survive for 30 days after extubation and are discharged; half of these survivors live for more than 2 years. The presence of either hemodynamic instability or sustained hepatic and renal failure makes survival of ventilated patients with IPS extremely unlikely.

However, improvements in supportive care and evolution of nonmyeloablative transplant protocols may improve the prognosis of HCT recipients who require mechanical ventilation. Therefore, treatment decisions have to be individualized. Aggressive management, including initiation of mechanical ventilation to identify and treat reversible causes of respiratory failure, is a reasonable approach for most HCT recipients with diffuse or multifocal pulmonary infiltrates. Evidence-based guidelines for the withdrawal of mechanical ventilation may be appropriate in specific situations.

2. Gastrointestinal tract

a. Etiology/pathophysiology. Oral mucositis, esophagitis/gastritis, and diarrhea are commonly associated with chemoradiation and can be worsened by methotrexate given for prophylaxis against GVHD. Breakdown of mucosal barriers causes pain, swelling, and sloughing of the oropharyngeal epithelium, and involvement can extend into the hypopharynx and esophagus. This constellation places patients at a high risk for aspiration and facilitates translocation of intestinal bacteria with sepsis.

b. Diagnosis

(1) Clinical presentation. Dysphagia, odynophagia, mucosal ulcerations and hemorrhage, oropharyngeal hypersecretion, anorexia, nausea, vomiting, diarrhea, dyspnea, signs of upper airway compromise.

(2) Laboratory and radiologic studies. Usually noncontributory.

(3) Differential diagnosis. Mucosal inflammation and ulceration may be associated with infections (herpes simplex virus [HSV], cytomegalovirus [CMV], varicella-zoster virus [VZV], or fungal) and GVHD. Anorexia, nausea, vomiting, and diarrhea persisting beyond 3 weeks from allogeneic HCT may be caused by GVHD and/or herpesvirus infection, or medications.

(4) Treatment. Supportive care, opioid analgesia, and institution of parenteral nutrition. Severe oropharyngeal mucositis with impending airway compromise may require intubation for airway protection. Mucosal regeneration has usually occurred by day 16 after HCT.

3. Liver

a. Etiology/pathophysiology. Jaundice, hepatomegaly, and abnormal liver tests within the first 2 months post-HCT may have many causes, including toxicity from the preparative regimen. A total bilirubin of greater than 4 mg/dL, regardless of its etiology, is a powerful predictor for transplant-related mortality. Sinusoidal obstruction syndrome (SOS), also referred to as venoocclusive disease (VOD), occurs in 0% to 50% of myeloablative HCT recipients. Cyclophosphamide and TBI (>1,200 cGy) used in the preparative regimen and preexisting chronic liver disease are risk factors for the development of SOS.

b. Diagnosis

(1) Clinical presentation. Tender hepatomegaly, renal sodium retention with weight gain, and jaundice following the preparative regimen in the absence of other explanations for these signs and symptoms are suggestive of SOS. The severity of these signs/symptoms is predictive for mortality. The typical onset is 10 to 20 days after a cyclophosphamide-based regimen.

(2) Laboratory and radiologic studies. Total serum bilirubin is sensitive but nonspecific. Aspartate aminotransferase (AST) greater than 750 U/L is one marker of a poor prognosis. Hepatomegaly, ascites, and attenuated hepatic venous flow by ultrasound and venous duplex are consistent with SOS; biliary dilatation or infiltrative lesions should be excluded. Measurement of the hepatic venous pressure gradient with biopsy may be useful in patients in whom the cause of liver dysfunction is unclear.

(3) Differential diagnosis. Other causes of post-HCT jaundice seldom lead to renal sodium avidity, rapid weight gain, and hepatomegaly before the onset of jaundice. Combinations of illnesses that may mimic SOS are: sepsis with renal insufficiency and cholestasis, cholestatic liver disease with hemolysis and congestive heart failure, and GVHD and sepsis syndrome.

Hepatic VZV infection may occur in VZV-seropositive patients who are not on prophylactic acyclovir (transaminases typically >1,000 U/mL). Empiric acyclovir should be given until VZV hepatitis has been ruled out.

c. Treatment. Ursodeoxycholic acid (ursidiol) has been reported to reduce the severity of post-HCT SOS in two randomized trials. Because 70% to 85% of patients recover spontaneously, supportive management of sodium and water balance for ascites associated with discomfort (sodium restriction, diuretics, paracentesis) or pulmonary compromise is important. Anticoagulation with heparin and thrombolytic therapy (tissue plasmin activator [TPA]) may be a consideration in patients with a high (>20%) estimated risk of fatality. Uncontrolled trials with defibrotide have been promising.

4. Heart

a. Etiology/pathophysiology. The major dose-limiting toxicity of high-dose cyclophosphamide (doses above 200 mg/kg), a component of many preparative regimens, is cardiac injury with hemorrhagic myocardial necrosis. Risk factors for cyclophosphamide cardiotoxicity include diagnosis of lymphoma, prior radiation to the mediastinum or left chest wall, older age, and prior abnormal cardiac ejection fraction. Patients who had a cumulative anthracyclin dose exceeding 550 mg/m^2 (doxorubicin) as part of preceding chemotherapy are at an increased risk for developing heart failure.

b. Diagnosis

(1) Clinical presentation. Signs and symptoms of congestive heart failure occurring within a few days of receiving cyclophosphamide. Anthracyclin-related cardiomyopathy may have a delayed onset.

(2) Laboratory and radiologic studies. Voltage loss on **electrocardiogram** (ECG); arrhythmia; ECHO shows signs of systolic dysfunction. Pericardial effusion/tamponade may be present.

(3) Differential diagnosis. Congestive heart failure due to fluid overload; malignant effusion; infectious perimyocarditis.

c. Treatment. Management of fluid and sodium balance, afterload reduction, inotropes. Even though cyclophosphamide cardiotoxicity is rare, it has a high case mortality rate.

5. Kidney

a. Etiology/pathophysiology. Severe renal dysfunction (doubling of serum creatinine) is more frequent after allogeneic compared with autologous HCT (58% vs. 7%). Many of the drugs used in transplant patients may affect renal function. The most common agents are cyclosporine, tacrolimus, amphotericin, and aminoglycosides. Of allogeneic HCT recipients, 6% to 10% develop a TM, which is the result of endothelial injury by chemotherapy, irradiation, and cyclosporine or tacrolimus. The overall mortality of acute renal failure post-HCT requiring dialysis has been reported to exceed 80%.

b. Diagnosis

(1) Clinical presentation. Post-HCT patients with medication-related renal toxicity are usually asymptomatic. The minority of HCT patients with TM will show several of the symptoms associated with classic thrombotic thrombocytopenic purpura (TTP): thrombocytopenia, fragmentation hemolysis, neurologic abnormalities, fever, and renal insufficiency.

(2) Laboratory studies. Serum creatinine elevation. Cyclosporine and amphotericin use may lead to renal potassium and magnesium wasting. The hallmark of TM is RBC fragmentation (schistocytes) associated with increased RBC turnover (increased reticulocytes; elevations of serum LDH and indirect bilirubin) without evidence for either immune-mediated hemolysis or disseminated intravascular coagulation (DIC).

(3) Differential diagnosis. Liver disease (SOS) may cause renal dysfunction (hepatorenal syndrome) associated with increased sodium avidity. Also consider prerenal mechanisms (heart failure, hypotension, volume depletion), sepsis, and tumor lysis syndrome.

c. Treatment. Careful assessment of volume status. Discontinuation of the likely offending agent and/or adjustment of cyclosporine/tacrolimus serum levels. The efficacy of substituting tacrolimus for cyclosporine is controversial. As compared with classic TTP, TM after HCT is usually not responsive to plasma exchange (differences in disease mechanism).

6. Central nervous system

    a. Etiology/pathophysiology. Neurologic complications after HCT can result from infectious, cerebrovascular, metabolic, toxic, and immune-mediated causes. The time of their occurrence after HCT may provide important information with regard to their differential diagnosis.

        (1) During or shortly after conditioning therapy. *Chemotherapeutic drugs* such as high-dose busulfan (4 mg/kg per day for 4 days) and carmustine (BCNU) may cause encephalopathy and seizures and prophylactic anticonvulsant treatment (phenytoin) has been recommended. Central nervous system (CNS) toxicity manifested as coma has been reported with use of ifosfamide, even in conventional doses. High-dose cytarabine may cause cerebellar dysfunction, encephalopathy, and seizures. Fludarabine, which is frequently used in nonmyeloablative preparative regimens, may cause an encephalopathy.

        (2) Preengraftment (during pancytopenia). Intracranial *hemorrhage* is a frequently fatal complication in patients with refractory thrombocytopenia. Subdural hematomas have a more favorable prognosis. Metabolic encephalopathy is most often related to gram-negative sepsis, the use of sedative-hypnotic drugs, and *hepatic* encephalopathy due to SOS. Bacterial meningitis may be encountered occasionally. Human herpesvirus 6 (HHV-6) encephalitis, although rare, may typically be encountered during the first 30 days after HCT.

        (3) Postengraftment (during GVHD-related immunosuppression). Host immunosuppression associated with GVHD and its treatment predisposes patients to a variety of opportunistic infections. *Aspergillus* spp. account for 30% to 50% of CNS infections in autopsy series. Given the available prophylaxis with trimethoprim-sulfamethoxazole and acyclovir, *Toxoplasma gondii*, herpes simplex, and varicella zoster encephalitis are rarely seen in HCT recipients. *Cyclosporine* causes more neurologic problems in HCT patients than any other drug; seizures and encephalopathy are the most common serious complications. *Corticosteroid* administration may be associated with psychosis, mania, or delirium in a dose-dependent fashion. *Hypoxic* encephalopathy (due to idiopathic pneumonia syndrome) and *hepatic* encephalopathy due to GVHD occur most likely during this period.

    b. Diagnosis

        (1) Clinical presentation. Focal symptoms are more indicative of infectious or cerebrovascular mechanisms, whereas diffuse symptoms such as delirium or coma may have metabolic causes. Fever is not necessarily associated with CNS infections.

        (2) Laboratory and radiologic studies. Neurologic symptoms occurring in an HCT patient should prompt a thorough workup, including magnetic resonance imaging (MRI) or CT imaging, followed by lumbar puncture for cerebrospinal fluid (CSF) analysis if an infection is suspected. Appropriate cultures, stains, and viral (HHV-6) PCR studies should be ordered. Patients with cyclosporine neurotoxicity may have T2 and FLAIR sequence abnormalities on MRI, with multifocal areas of signal hyperintensity, most often in the occipital lobe white matter.

    c. Treatment. Post-HCT CNS infections have a poor prognosis, and treatment should be based on a multidisciplinary approach (e.g., medical oncology, infectious diseases, neurosurgery). Treatment of metabolic encephalopathies should be directed at the underlying problem, and offending drugs have to be discontinued. In patients with cyclosporine neurotoxicity, temporary discontinuation of the drug and the restarting at a lower dose are usually successful. Short-term phenytoin for seizure prophylaxis may be indicated.

C. Infection

1. General principles. Infections are frequent complications after autologous and allogeneic HCT. Their pattern of occurrence is determined by a number of factors, including the recipient's pretransplant history and underlying disease, the intensity of the preparative regimen, the regimen used for infection prevention, the microbiological flora of the patient and of the individual transplant unit, and the degree of immunosuppression after transplant (activity of GVHD). The recovery of the hematopoietic system and nonhematologic organs after HCT can broadly be categorized into three phases. Each phase is characterized by a spectrum of opportunistic infections:

a. Preengraftment (less than 30 days posttransplant)

(1) This period is characterized by neutropenia and oral/gastrointestinal mucosal damage. The most common infections are bacterial and fungal. The most likely viral infection early after HCT is HSV. Thus, many transplant centers use a prophylactic regimen of antibiotics (e.g., levofloxacin), antifungals (e.g., fluconazole), and antivirals (e.g., acyclovir). With the use of indwelling central venous catheters, the risk of gram-positive infections with *staphylococci* and *streptococci* is greater compared to gram-negative infections with *Eschericia coli* and *Pseudomonas* spp. Possible fungal infections that may occur during this period may present with skin lesions (*Candida*), sinus involvement (*Aspergillus* and mucor), lung lesions (*Aspergillus*), or hepatitis (*Candida*).

(2) Workup and treatment. Fever should be treated immediately as a presumptive infection. The fever workup should consist of a careful history and physical examination, blood cultures for bacteria and fungi, urine culture, and a chest radiographic study. Antibiotics to treat gram-positive and gram-negative infections, including pseudomonas, should be started promptly. A common regimen is ceftazidime, with or without an aminoglycoside. If fever persists an additional 48 hours or if the central line site is red or tender, additional coverage for gram-positive infections (e.g., vancomycin) should be added. If fever persists an additional 2 to 4 days or clinical suspicion of fungus exists, antifungal agents as empiric coverage should be considered. *Clostridium difficile* colitis can be a common infection in transplant patients, particularly those in intensive care units. *C. difficile* infection should be considered in patients with diarrhea and can be treated with oral metronidazole.

b. Postengraftment (30 to 100 days posttransplant)

(1) This period is characterized by skin and mucosal damage and compromised cellular immunity related to GVHD and its treatment. Viral (e.g., CMV) and fungal (e.g., *Aspergillus*, *P. jiroveci*) infections predominate during this period. Gram-negative bacteremias related to GVHD-associated mucosal damage and gram-positive infections due to indwelling catheters may occur. Other causes of fever of unknown origin after engraftment include occult sinusitis, hepatosplenic candidiasis, and pulmonary or disseminated *Aspergillus* infection.

(2) Workup and treatment. Transplant patients with pulmonary infiltrates should undergo bronchoscopy to establish a diagnosis. Serial blood cultures and sinus CT may be indicated. CMV reactivation and infection are typically treated with ganciclovir (myelosuppressive). Intravenous immunoglobulin (IVIG) is added in patients with CMV pneumonia. *P. carinii* pneumonia is treated with trimethoprim-sulfamethoxazole, dapsone, or pentamidine. Removal of the central venous catheter is occasionally required. Aspergillus infections are treated with amphotericin B (or liposomal derivatives) or voriconazole.

c. Late phase (greater than 100 days posttransplant)

(1) This period is characterized by a persistently decreased cellular immunity in patients with chronic GVHD. Patients with chronic GVHD are highly susceptible to recurrent bacterial infections, especially from encapsulated bacteria, including *Streptococcus pneumonia, Haemophilus influenzae,* and *Neisseria meningitidis* (functional asplenia). Bronchopulmonary infections, septicemia, and ear, nose, and throat infections occur. Common nonbacterial infections at this time include varicella zoster, CMV, *P. jiroveci,* and Aspergillus.

(2) **Workup and treatment.** Patients with active chronic GVHD should receive prophylaxis with penicillin and trimethoprim-sulfamethoxazole. Late sinopulmonary infections can be successfully treated with a variety of antibiotics, including penicillin, trimethoprim-sulfamethoxazole, cephalosporins, and new-generation macrolides. Herpes zoster is treated with high-dose intravenous acyclovir. Immunoglobulin deficiency should be ruled out and treated if there is a history of recurrent infections.

D. Bleeding

1. **Etiology/pathophysiology.** Bleeding can occur as a result of thrombocytopenia or coagulopathy. Breakdown of mucosal barriers as a result of regimen-related toxicity and/or GVHD increases the likelihood of hemorrhage. CNS hemorrhage can be rapidly fatal. High-dose cyclophosphamide and BK virus infection are causes of hemorrhagic cystitis.

2. **Diagnosis.** Oropharyngeal bleeding and epistaxis are obvious. Endoscopic evaluation (colonoscopy, esophagogastroduodenoscopy, bronchoscopy) or CNS imaging may be indicated according to the clinical picture.

3. **Treatment.** A platelet count below 10,000/mm^3 increases the risk of spontaneous bleeding and should be treated prophylactically with platelet transfusion. The decision to transfuse platelets above the "prophylactic" threshold of 10,000/mm^3 should be guided by the clinical situation. Patients who have received multiple transfusions can become alloimmunized and demonstrate poor response to platelet transfusion. Transfusion of unpooled (single-donor) or HLA-matched platelets may be helpful. All transplant patients should receive either CMV-negative or leukocyte-reduced (leukocytes harbor CMV) blood products to reduce the risk of primary CMV infection. All patients should receive irradiated blood products to reduce the risk of transfusion-associated GVHD. Diffuse alveolar hemorrhage is in the differential diagnosis of pulmonary infiltrates. Bleeding can be seen on bronchoscopy. The treatment consists of high doses of corticosteroids (e.g., 1 g per day for 3 days).

E. Graft-versus-host disease

1. **General principles.** GVHD is a major cause of morbidity and mortality after allogeneic HCT. Patients who develop GVHD, however, have lower relapse rates than patients without GVHD, which can be explained by an immunologic graft-versus-tumor effect that helps eradicate the underlying malignancy.

2. **Etiology/pathophysiology.** The GVHD syndrome is caused by donor T cells that are activated by immunologically disparate HLA or non-HLA antigens in the recipient, resulting in an inflammatory immune response. Older patient age, HCT from a mismatched and/or unrelated donor, and a female donor increase the risk of developing GVHD.

3. **Diagnosis**

   a. **Clinical presentation.** Acute GVHD (defined as occurring before posttransplant day 100) tends to have a more sudden onset and may involve the skin, gastrointestinal tract, and liver. Signs and symptoms include an erythematous rash, nausea, vomiting, diarrhea, and liver function abnormalities. Clinical features of chronic GVHD (defined as occurring after posttransplant day 100), which typically has a more insidious onset, may involve the skin, eyes, joints, and liver and are reminiscent of autoimmune diseases such as systemic sclerosis. Obstructive lung disease may occur in patients with chronic GVHD (bronchiolitis obliterans with organizing pneumonia [BOOP]). Although the *Glucksberg* grading system describes the severity of acute GVHD (grades I to IV), chronic GVHD is categorized according to the need for systemic immunosuppressive therapy (limited versus extensive chronic GVHD). GVHD may occur weeks to months later after nonmyeloablative HCT compared with myeloablative HCT.

b. **Laboratory and radiologic studies.** Skin punch biopsy, gastrointestinal endoscopy with biopsy, and liver biopsy confirm the diagnosis in the appropriate clinical setting. Cholestatic jaundice is the hallmark of liver involvement. Pulmonary function test and lung biopsy in patients with presumed BOOP to rule out infectious etiologies.

c. **Differential diagnosis.** Drug rash, peptic ulceration, and viral or mycotic enteritis should be ruled out. In patients with liver function abnormalities, drug toxicities (e.g., cyclosporine), sepsis (cholangitis lenta), biliary sludge syndrome, viral infections (CMV, EBV, hepatitis B), and concurrent hemolysis should be considered.

4. **Treatment.** Despite prophylaxis against GVHD (e.g., cyclosporine plus methotrexate), 40% to 80% of allogeneic HCT recipients develop this complication. Corticosteroids are standard first-line therapy of GVHD (e.g., prednisone 2 mg/kg per day; slow taper after 2 weeks). Immunosuppressive treatment of GVHD with corticosteroids contributes to the increased susceptibility of patients with GVHD to a variety of bacterial, viral, and fungal infections. Steroid-refractory patients require second-line immunosuppressive therapy and usually have a poor prognosis.

Selected Readings

Bearman SI. Veno-occlusive disease of the liver. *Curr Opin Oncol* 2000;12:103–109.
Review of sinusoidal obstruction syndrome occurring after allogeneic hematopoietic cell transplantation (HCT).

Boeckh M, Marr K. Infections in hematopoietic stem cell transplantation. In: Rubin R, Young LS, eds. *Clinical approach to infection in the compromised host*, 4th edition. New York: Plenum Medical Book Co., 2002, pp. 527–572.
Approach to diagnosis and treatment of infections occurring after HCT.

Chao NJ, Duncan SR, Long GD, et al. Corticosteroid therapy for diffuse alveolar hemorrhage in autologous bone marrow transplant recipients. *Ann Intern Med* 1991;114:145–146.
A small series showing improved survival with the use of high doses of steroids.

Clark JG, Hansen JA, Hertz MI, et al. NHLBI workshop summary. Idiopathic pneumonia syndrome after bone marrow transplantation. *Am Rev Respir Dis* 1993;147:1601–1606.
Review of idiopathic pneumonia syndrome (IPS) after myeloablative HCT.

Fukuda T, Hackman RC, Guthrie KA, et al. Risks and outcomes of idiopathic pneumonia syndrome after nonmyeloablative and conventional conditioning regimens for allogeneic hematopoietic stem cell transplantation. *Blood* 2003;102:2777–2785.
IPS after nonmyeloablative HCT is compared with the experience after ablative HCT.

Groeger JS, Lemeshow S, Price K, et al. Multicenter outcome study of cancer patients admitted to the intensive care unit: a probability of mortality model. *J Clin Oncol* 1998;16:761–770.
This study corroborates earlier data from Rubenfeld and Crawford (1996).

Hansen JA, Gooley TA, Martin PJ, et al. Bone marrow transplants from unrelated donors for patients with chronic myeloid leukemia. *N Engl J Med* 1998;338:962–968.
This paper shows the excellent outcome in patients with CML who have transplants from well-matched unrelated donors.

Hogan WJ, Maris M, Storer B, et al. Hepatic injury after nonmyeloablative conditioning followed by allogeneic hematopoietic cell transplantation: a study of 193 patients. *Blood* 2004;103:78–84.
The prognostic value of serum bilirubin elevations for survival after nonmyeloablative HCT is compared with the experience after ablative HCT.

Lee JL, Gooley T, Bensinger W, et al. Veno-occlusive disease of the liver after busulfan, melphalan, and thiotepa conditioning therapy: incidence, risk factors, and outcome. *Biol Blood Marrow Transplant* 1999;5:306–315
Review of sinusoidal obstruction syndrome occurring after autologous HCT.

Mielcarek M, Martin PJ, Leisenring W, et al. Graft-versus-host disease after nonmyeloablative versus conventional hematopoietic stem cell transplantation. *Blood* 2003;102: 756–762.
Graft-versus-host disease after nonmyeloablative HCT is compared with the experience after ablative HCT.

Mielcarek M, Storb R. Non-myeloablative hematopoietic cell transplantation as immunotherapy for hematologic malignancies. *Cancer Treat Rev.* 2003;29:283–290.
Review of non-myeloablative hematopoietic cell transplantation (HCT).

Parikh CR, McSweeney PA, Korular D, et al. Renal dysfunction in allogeneic hematopoietic cell transplantation. *Kidney Int.* 2002;62:566–573.
A description of types and severity of renal dysfunction encountered after HCT.

Rowley SD. Hematopoietic stem cell transplantation between red cell incompatible donor-recipient pairs. *Bone Marrow Transplant.* 2001;28:315–321.
Review of hemolytic complications due to ABO-incompatibility occurring after HCT.

Rubenfeld GD, Crawford SW. Withdrawing life support from mechanically ventilated recipients of bone marrow transplants: a case for evidence-based guidelines. *Ann Intern Med* 1996;125:625–633.
The study provides survival estimates for patients requiring mechanical ventilation after HCT.

Schriber JR, Herzig GP. Transplantation-associated thrombotic thrombocytopenic purpura and hemolytic uremic syndrome. *Semin Hematol* 1997;34:126–133.
Review of TTP occurring after HCT.

Wingard JR, Sostrin MB, Vriesendorp HM, et al. Interstitial pneumonitis following autologous bone marrow transplantation. *Transplantation* 1988;46:61–65.

Wingard JR. Fungal infections after bone marrow transplant. *Biol Blood Marrow Transplant* 1999;5:55–68.

Rheumatologic and Immunologic Problems in the Intensive Care Unit

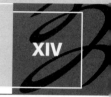

XIV

I. OVERVIEW. This chapter reviews the important rheumatic diseases most likely to be encountered in the intensive care unit (ICU). Brief descriptions and treatment options are discussed with a constant emphasis on the ongoing risk of infectious complications that may lead to critical illness.

II. RHEUMATOID ARTHRITIS
   A. General principles. A chronic inflammatory disorder affecting the synovial lining of joints, tendons, and bursae in addition to a large variety of extraarticular structures. The etiology of rheumatoid arthritis (RA) is unknown. Patients may require ICU admission because of disease complications or complications of therapy, typically infection.
   B. Treatment. Table 154-1 details current treatment. When infection is suspected in critically ill patients, strong consideration is given to holding medications for RA.
   C. System-specific considerations in RA
      1. Pulmonary
         a. Pleural disease
            (1) Pleural inflammation/effusions occur frequently.
            (2) May be asymptomatic or lead to large symptomatic effusions.
            (3) Effusions require aspiration to rule out infection or other causes.
            (4) Effusions are transudative with low cell counts and low glucose levels.
         b. Parenchymal lung involvement
            (1) Bronchiolitis obliterans with organizing pneumonia (BOOP)
            (2) Interstitial lung disease
            (3) Lung toxicity from medications, principally methotrexate-induced pneumonitis
            (4) Infection due to immunocompromised state, including tuberculosis
            (5) Pulmonary rheumatoid nodules
         c. Diagnosis
            (1) Presence of ground glass and reticular changes on high-resolution CT scanning.
            (2) Bronchosopy and bronchoalveolar lavage (BAL) are useful to rule out opportunistic infection.
            (3) Open lung biopsy or video-assisted thoracic surgery (VATS) is reserved for cases where there is diagnostic confusion or in patients who have failed to respond to initial treatment.
         d. Treatment
            (1) BOOP and acute methotrexate toxicity tend to be steroid responsive and usually do not require other immunosuppressive agents.
            (2) Interstitial lung disease (ILD) treatment in RA is controversial. Corticosteroids and cyclophosphamide have been used in rapidly advancing disease
      2. Neurologic involvement
         a. Spinal cord compression due to cervical vertebral instability is one of the most common neurologic sequelae of long-standing severe RA.
         b. Synovitis damages the transverse ligament leading to subluxation of the odontoid peg of C2, compressing the spinal cord and brainstem. This area is particularly vulnerable during endotracheal intubation or endoscopy

TABLE 154-1   **Current Treatment in Rheumatoid Arthritis**

	Dose/ administration	Class	Adverse reactions	Special considerations
Methotrexate	7.5 to 25 mg q week PO/SC/IM	Dihydrofolate reductase inhibitor	Hepatotoxicity, bone marrow suppression, pulmonary fibrosis, decreased resistance to infection	
Leflunomide (Arava)	10 to 20 mg q.d. PO	Pyrimidine synthesis inhibitor	Diarrhea, alopecia, rash, hepatotoxicity, decreased resistance to infection; increases hepatotoxicity of other drugs	Metabolized via enterohepatic circulation with half-life of greater than 90 days Urgent elimination requires treatment with cholestyramine
Etanercept (Enbrel)	50 mg q week SC in single or divided doses	TNF receptor blocker	Sepsis	Caution in CHF Avoid live vaccines Contraindicated in serious infections
Adalimumab (Humira)	40 mg q 2 weeks SC	Monoclonal anti-TNF antibody	Sepsis, reactivation of TB	Caution in CHF Avoid live vaccines Contraindicated in serious infections
Anakinra (Kineret)	100 mg q.d. SC	IL-1 receptor antagonist	Diarrhea, increased risk of infection	Avoid live vaccines
Infliximab (Remicade)	3 to 5 mg/kg q 4 to 8 weeks via IV infusion	Monoclonal anti-TNF antibody	Sepsis, infusion reactions	Caution in CHF Avoid live vaccines Contraindicated in serious infections

TNF, tumor necrosis factor; CHF, congestive heart failure; TB, tuberculosis; IL-1, interleukin-1; PO, by mouth; IM, intramuscularly; SC, subcutaneously; q.d., every day.

    c. Patients with long-standing RA should ideally be screened with flexion and extension imaging of the cervical spine prior to any intubation.

    d. If instability is present or even suspected, endoscopic intubation following neck stabilization should be undertaken.

III. CRYSTAL ARTHROPATHY

    A. Gout. Acute attacks represent an inflammatory reaction to the crystalline form of uric acid when it precipitates in joints and/or soft tissues. Attacks may involve one or more joints, typically the first metatarsophalangeal (MTP) joint, ankle, knee, or wrist.

      1. Pathogenesis

        a. Sudden fluxes in serum uric acid levels facilitate uric acid crystallization in joints.

    b. Uric acid levels are sensitive to the use of IV fluids, dietary changes and the use of a variety of medications.

  2. General principles

    a. Acute attacks lead to the sudden onset of severe pain and tenderness, with erythema and warmth over the affected joint, which can include nearly any joint.

    b. Low-grade fever is common, especially if more than one joint is involved.

  3. Diagnosis

    a. Diagnosed by demonstrating the presence of intracellular monosodium urate crystals on polarized microscopy of synovial fluid.

    b. Synovial fluid white blood cell (WBC) counts may vary from 5,000 to 80,000/mm^3.

  4. Treatment. See Table 154-2.

B. Pseudogout

  1. General

    a. Caused by the presence of intraarticular calcium pyrophosphate crystals.

    b. Typically affects knees or hands.

TABLE 154-2   **Treatment of Gout**

Drug	Dosage	Adverse reactions	Special considerations
Colchicine	0.6 mg tid PO or 0.6 mg hourly for total of 10 doses	GI toxicity (nausea, diarrhea), bone marrow suppression (granulocytopenia)	Dosage needs to be adjusted for renal function; IV dosing is rarely used and is reserved for the experienced prescriber.
Corticosteroids Prednisone	20 to 40 mg qd PO for 2 to 3 days then taper over 1 week	Immune suppression hyperglycemia	PO route is usually not appropriate in ICU patients.
ACTH	40 to 80 units im May need to repeated once or twice at 12 hourly intervals		Caution in anticoagulated patients
Intraarticular steroid	Dose varied depending on joint involved	If high suspicion of joint infection, wait for Gram stain result	
	Methylprednisolone 15 to 80 mg		
	Triamcinolone 10 to 40 mg		
NSAIDs	Indomethacin is most commonly used. Start at maximum daily dose, reduce as symptoms subside and continue for 48 hours after symptoms resolve	GI toxicity, renal toxicity, platelet dysfunction	Usually not appropriate for ICU patients

GI, gastrointestinal; ICU, intensive care unit; ACTH, adrenocorticotropic hormone; NSAIDs, nonsteroidal antiinflammatory drugs; tid, three times a day; PO, by mouth; q.d., every day.

     c. Clinical appearance is identical to that of gout.

  2. Diagnosis. Synovial fluid aspiration shows the presence of intracellular weakly positively birefringent rhomboid crystals. Plain radiographs may show chondrocalcinosis indicates chronic calcium pyrophosphate within the joint.

  3. Treatment
    a. Identical to that for gout.
    b. Joint aspiration may be sufficient to resolve some cases.
    c. Colchicine is less effective as in gout.

C. Other crystal arthritidies. Rarer forms of crystal arthropathy include those caused by calcium oxalate and calcium hydroxyapatite, which tend to occur in individuals on dialysis.

IV. SEPTIC ARTHRITIS

A. General principles
  1. Bones, joints, and bursae may be infected with a large variety of microorganisms.
  2. *Staphylococcus aureus* is the most common cause of musculoskeletal infection.
  3. Other microorganisms are increasing in prevalence.
  4. Most cases are acute with swelling, pain, surrounding erythema, and loss of joint function.
  5. Monoarticular involvement is most common, but several joints may be affected with hematogenous spread.
  6. Fever is usually present but is not invariable.

B. Diagnosis
  1. Immediate joint aspiration is imperative in any suspected case.
  2. Synovial fluid should be sent for:
    a. Gram stain
    b. Cell count and differential cell count
    c. Culture and sensitivity
    d. Polarized microscopy for crystals
  3. Cell count may vary but is usually greater than $50,000/mm^3$
  4. The presence of crystals does not out rule the possibility of infection.

C. Treatment
  1. Repeated daily aspirations or surgical washout is essential.
  2. Empiric antibiotic therapy should be initiated following a stat Gram stain and antibiotics adjusted once cultures become available (see table 154-3).
  3. The joint should be rested with physical therapy referral to prevent contractures.
  4. Baseline radiographs should be obtained to follow progress.
  5. Baseline C-reactive protein (CRP) may be helpful in monitoring longer-term therapeutic response.
  6. Fungal joint infection is rare, more indolent in presentation, and occurs usually in immunocompromised patients.
  7. Fungal components are normally visible on Gram stain, allowing for early initiation of antifungal therapy.

V. ANTIPHOSPHOLIPID ANTIBODY SYNDROME.
Defined as recurrent arterial or venous thrombosis often associated with fetal losses in the presence of anticardiolipin antibodies or lupus anticoagulant. It may be primary or may be associated with another connective tissue disease.

A. Diagnosis. Clinical features include:
  1. One or more episodes of arterial or venous thrombosis or both.
  2. Fetal death or recurrent spontaneous abortion.
  3. Other features include thrombocytopenia, livedo reticularis, cardiac valvular lesions, migraine headaches, chorea, and leg ulcers.
  4. Presence of either anticardiolipin antibody IgM or IGG in medium or high titer or lupus anticoagulant on two occasions at least 6 weeks apart.

B. Treatment
  1. Anticoagulation with heparin followed by lifelong warfarin is indicated.

TABLE 154-3	Antibiotics in Septic Arthritis	
Clinical setting	**Top three microorganisms**	**Empiric antibiotic choice**
Nonimmunocompromised, Non sexually active	1) *Staphylococcus aureus* 2) *Streptococcus* 3) Gram-negative bacilli	3rd-generation cephalosporin with nafcillin or vancomycin (depending on risk of Staph resistance)
Non immunocompromised, sexually active	1) *Neisseria gonorrheae*	Gram stain negative – 3rd generation cephalosporin
	2) *S. aureus* 3) *Streptococci*	Gram stain showing gram-positive cocci in clusters – nafcillin or oxacillin
Prosthetic joints	1) *Staphylococcus epidermidis* 2) *S. aureus* 3) *Enterobacteriaceae*	Vancomycin and ciprofloxacin

   2. The catastrophic antiphospholipid antibody defines a syndrome involving widespread thrombosis with life-threatening illness. Treatment may include corticosteroids, cyclophosphamide, and plasmapheresis in addition to antico-agulation.

VI. IDIOPATHIC INFLAMMATORY MYOSITIS.
Polymyositis and dermatomyositis are inflammatory muscle diseases characterized by proximal muscle weakness, elevated muscle enzymes, and characteristic cutaneous features.
   A. Diagnosis. Clinical features include:
   1. Proximal girdle and shoulder weakness
   2. Skin involvement includes Gottron's papules; erythema of the neck, chest, and forehead; heliotrope rash; and periungual erythema.
   3. Dysphagia and aspiration pneumonia
   4. Interstitial lung disease, especially in patients who are Jo-1 antibody–positive
   5. Cardiomyopathy, arrhythmias, and congestive heart failure
   B. Treatment
   1. High-dose corticosteroids with consideration for an additional agent such as methotrexate
   2. In progressive ILD, high-dose steroids with cyclophosphamide are indicated.

VII. SYSTEMIC LUPUS ERYTHEMATOSUS (SLE)
   A. General principles. An inflammatory disorder of unknown etiology character-ized by antibody production, immune complex deposition and a wide variety of organ and system involvement. Diagnosis is based on the presence of characteristic clinical features and laboratory findings, including decreased complement levels, cytopenias, and typical autoantibody profiles.
   B. Renal involvement. Occurs in 50% of patients. Treatment protocols exist, depend-ing on the histologic classification on renal biopsy, with active nephritis requiring treatment with corticosteroids and cyclophosphamide.
   C. Pulmonary involvement
   1. Pleuritis is the most common pulmonary manifestation of SLE, affecting about 50% of SLE patients.
   2. Pulmonary hemorrhage is a rare but serious complication of SLE.
      a. Patients, frequently young females, present with severe hypoxia, patchy in-filtrates, and hemoptysis.

   b. Treatment is with high-dose corticosteroids and immunosuppressive agents with a potential role for plasmaphoresis.

D. Hematologic
   1. Autoimmune hemolytic anemias respond well to high-dose steroids; heavier immunosuppressants and splenectomy are an option for unresponsive cases.
   2. Idiopathic thrombocytopenic purpura (ITP) can also occur; treatment is with high-dose oral or intravenous steroids and if needed intravenous immunoglobulin.

E. Neurologic
   1. Neuropsychiatric lupus is the name given to the large variety of neurologic presentations seen in SLE.
   2. These include seizure disorders, stroke disease, demyelinating disorders, psychosis, transverse myelopathy, peripheral neuropathy, and headache.

VIII. SCLERODERMA

A. General principles. Multisystem disease characterized by tissue inflammation and fibrosis with vascular involvement leading to episodic vasospasm and tissue ischemia.

B. Interstitial lung disease. Frequent complication and the leading cause of death.
   1. Diagnosis is based on the presence of ground glass changes on high-resolution CT images.
   2. BAL shows an elevated neutrophil and eosinophil count; pulmonary function tests show a restrictive pattern.
   3. Treatment includes cyclophosphamide combined with corticosteroids.

C. Pulmonary hypertension
   1. Complication of typically long-standing limited scleroderma.
   2. Diagnosis is based on echocardiography and confirmed on right heart catheterization.
   3. Treatment with intravenous prostacyclins and endothelin antagonists increases survival.

D. Renal scleroderma
   1. Renal crisis is a syndrome of rapidly progressive hypertensive renal failure.
   2. Accompanied by microvascular hemolysis.
   3. The associated hyperreninemic state drives the process and treatment is therefore with urgent administration of high-dose angiotensin-converting enzyme inhibitors.
   4. Rarely, normotensive renal crisis can occur.

E. Gastrointestinal
   1. Constipation due to decreased peristalsis.
   2. Diarrhea due to bacterial overgrowth.
   3. Enteral nutrition should be maintained when possible in the ICU setting.

Selected Readings

Asherson RA. The catastrophic syndrome, 1998. A review of the clinical features, possible pathogenesis and treatment. Lupus 1998;7:S55.
   Reviews the concept of the catastrophic antiphospholipid syndrome.

Aranow C, Ginzler EM. SLE. In: Hochberg M, et al., eds. Rheumatology, 3rd edition. Edinburgh: Mosby, 2002.
   Excellent chapter review of management of SLE.

Goldenberg DL. Septic arthritis. *Lancet* 1998;351(9097):197.
   An update on the treatment and causes of septic arthritis.

Goldenberg DL, Cohen AS, et al. Treatment of septic arthritis: comparison of needle aspiration and surgery as initial modes of joint drainage. *Arthritis Rheum* 1975;18:83.
   Compares surgical versus needle drainage in the treatment of septic arthritis.

Latsi PI, Wells AU. Evaluation and management of alveolitis and interstitial lung disease in scleroderma. *Curr Opin Rheumatol* 2003;15(6):748.
   Excellent review on the management of ILD in scleroderma.

Marie I, Hachulla E, Cherin P, et al. Interstitial lung disease in polymyositis and dermato-myositis. *Arthritis Rheum* 2002;47(6).614.
An excellent review of a large cohort of patients with polymyositis/dermatomyositis.

Olsen NJ, Stein CM. New drugs for rheumatoid arthritis. *N Engl J Med* 2004;350(21): 2167.
A great update on the use of biologic agents in inflammatory arthritis.

Preston IR, Hill NS. Evaluation and management of pulmonary hypertension in systemic sclerosis. *Curr Opin Rheumatol* 2003:15(6):761.
A thorough reference on the pathogenesis, treatment, and potential treatments for pul-monary hypertension.

Rott KT, Agudelo CA. Gout. *JAMA* 2003:289(21):2857.
Excellent review.

155 ANAPHYLAXIS
Helen M. Hollingsworth and Nereida A. Parada

I. GENERAL PRINCIPLES
A. A severe and potentially fatal form of immediate hypersensitivity.

B. An *anaphylactoid reaction* differs from anaphylactic reactions only because mast cell/basophil activation is through a mechanism other than IgE recognition of antigen.

C. In this chapter, IgE-mediated and non—IgE-mediated reactions are referred to as *anaphylactic reactions.*

II. PATHOPHYSIOLOGY
A. Binding of allergenic antigen (Table 155-1) to adjacent IgE molecules on sensitized mast cells/basophils activates synthesis and secretion of mediators of anaphylaxis, such as histamine, leukotrienes (LTC4, LTD4, and LTE4), and cytokines.

B. Mast cell and basophil activation also occur through a variety of non—IgE-mediated mechanisms (Table 155-2).

III. CLINICAL FEATURES
A. The major clinical features of anaphylaxis are urticaria, angioedema, respiratory obstruction (stridor, wheezing, breathlessness), and vascular collapse (dizziness, loss of consciousness), with urticaria being the most common.

B. Additional clinical manifestations include: a sense of impending doom, rhinorrhea, generalized pruritus and swelling, dysphagia, vomiting, and abdominal pain.

C. **Physical examination** of a patient with anaphylactic shock often reveals a rapid, weak, irregular, or unobtainable pulse; tachypnea, respiratory distress, cyanosis, hoarseness, or stridor; diminished breath sounds, wheezes, and hyperinflated lungs; urticaria; angioedema, or conjunctival edema. Only a subset of these may occur in any given patient.

D. **Laboratory findings** include elevation of blood histamine and tryptase levels, low complement levels, and disseminated intravascular coagulation (DIC). No diagnostic blood test is currently available.

E. Arrhythmias may occur.

IV. DIAGNOSIS
A. The rapid onset and progression of typical symptoms to a severe and sometimes fatal outcome after exposure to a typical antigen are characteristic of anaphylaxis.

B. Mild systemic reactions often last for several hours, rarely more than 24 hours.

C. Severe manifestations (e.g., laryngeal edema, bronchoconstriction, hypotension), if not fatal, can persist or recur for several days but sometimes resolve within minutes of treatment.

V. TREATMENT: GENERAL CARDIOPULMONARY SUPPORTIVE MEASURES
A. Oxygen saturation, blood pressure, and cardiac rate and rhythm should be monitored closely and supplemental oxygen administered.

B. Intubation and assisted ventilation may be necessary for laryngeal edema or severe bronchoconstriction.

C. Occasionally, cricothyroidotomy is necessary.

D. One characteristic of patients with biphasic or protracted anaphylaxis is oral ingestion of the offending antigen. Enteral administration of activated charcoal and sorbitol may reduce absorption and duration of exposure to the antigen.

TABLE 155-1   Causes of IgE-mediated Anaphylaxis

Type	Agent	Example
Proteins	Allergen extracts	Pollen, dust mite, mold
	Enzymes	Chymopapain, streptokinase, L-asparaginase
	Food	Egg white, legumes, milk, nuts, celery, shellfish, psyllium, wheat
	Heterologous serum	Tetanus antitoxin, antithymocyte globulin, snake antivenom
	Hormones	Insulin, ACTH, TSH, progesterone, salmon calcitonin
	Vaccines	Influenza
	Venoms	Hymenoptera
	Others	Heparin, latex, thiobarbiturates, seminal fluid
Haptens	Antibiotics	β-Lactams, ethambutol, nitrofurantoin, sulfonamides, streptomycin, vancomycin
	Disinfectants	Ethylene oxide
	Local anesthetics[a]	Benzocaine, tetracaine, xylocaine, mepivacaine
	Others	Cisplatin, carboplatin

[a]Precise mechanism not established.
ACTH, adrenocorticotropic hormone; TSH, thyroid-stimulating hormone.

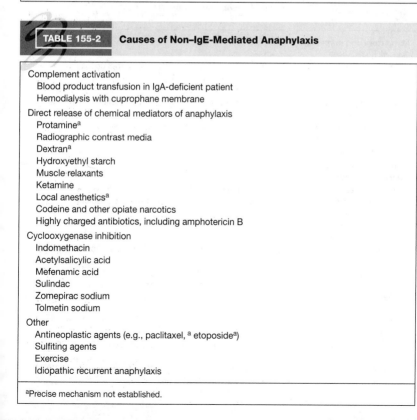

TABLE 155-2   Causes of Non–IgE-Mediated Anaphylaxis

Complement activation
  Blood product transfusion in IgA-deficient patient
  Hemodialysis with cuprophane membrane
Direct release of chemical mediators of anaphylaxis
  Protamine[a]
  Radiographic contrast media
  Dextran[a]
  Hydroxyethyl starch
  Muscle relaxants
  Ketamine
  Local anesthetics[a]
  Codeine and other opiate narcotics
  Highly charged antibiotics, including amphotericin B
Cyclooxygenase inhibition
  Indomethacin
  Acetylsalicylic acid
  Mefenamic acid
  Sulindac
  Zomepirac sodium
  Tolmetin sodium
Other
  Antineoplastic agents (e.g., paclitaxel,[a] etoposide[a])
  Sulfiting agents
  Exercise
  Idiopathic recurrent anaphylaxis

[a]Precise mechanism not established.

VI. TREATMENT: PHARMACOLOGIC (Table 155-3).

A. β-Adrenergic agents

1. Epinephrine hydrochloride should be given promptly to treat all initial manifestations of anaphylaxis.
2. A delay in administration of epinephrine may be fatal.
3. Epinephrine delays antigen absorption when infiltrated locally into an injection or sting site.

B. Antihistamines

1. H_1 receptor—blocking antihistamines reverse histamine-induced vasodilatation, tachycardia, and bronchoconstriction, as well as cutaneous manifestations.
2. The H_2 blocker cimetidine has been reported to reverse refractory systemic anaphylaxis.

C. Glucocorticosteroids

1. Systemic glucocorticosteroids increase tissue responses to β-adrenergic agonists and inhibit generation of LTC4, LTD4, and LTE4.
2. Despite the general sense that glucocorticosteroids prevent late recurrences of anaphylaxis, biphasic anaphylaxis may occur in 20% of anaphylactic reactions despite glucocorticosteroid therapy.

VII. PREVENTION OF ANAPHYLACTIC REACTIONS

A. Obtaining and recording a careful history identifying possible precipitants of anaphylaxis at the time of presentation is crucial.

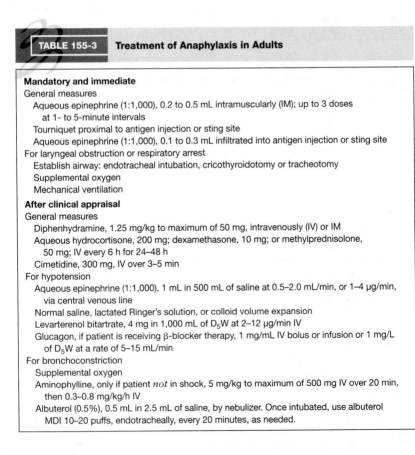

TABLE 155-3   Treatment of Anaphylaxis in Adults

Mandatory and immediate
General measures
    Aqueous epinephrine (1:1,000), 0.2 to 0.5 mL intramuscularly (IM); up to 3 doses at 1- to 5-minute intervals
    Tourniquet proximal to antigen injection or sting site
    Aqueous epinephrine (1:1,000), 0.1 to 0.3 mL infiltrated into antigen injection or sting site
For laryngeal obstruction or respiratory arrest
    Establish airway: endotracheal intubation, cricothyroidotomy or tracheotomy
    Supplemental oxygen
    Mechanical ventilation

After clinical appraisal
General measures
    Diphenhydramine, 1.25 mg/kg to maximum of 50 mg, intravenously (IV) or IM
    Aqueous hydrocortisone, 200 mg; dexamethasone, 10 mg; or methylprednisolone, 50 mg; IV every 6 h for 24–48 h
    Cimetidine, 300 mg, IV over 3–5 min
For hypotension
    Aqueous epinephrine (1:1,000), 1 mL in 500 mL of saline at 0.5–2.0 mL/min, or 1–4 μg/min, via central venous line
    Normal saline, lactated Ringer's solution, or colloid volume expansion
    Levarterenol bitartrate, 4 mg in 1,000 mL of D_5W at 2–12 μg/min IV
    Glucagon, if patient is receiving β-blocker therapy, 1 mg/mL IV bolus or infusion or 1 mg/L of D_5W at a rate of 5–15 mL/min
For bronchoconstriction
    Supplemental oxygen
    Aminophylline, only if patient *not* in shock, 5 mg/kg to maximum of 500 mg IV over 20 min, then 0.3–0.8 mg/kg/h IV
    Albuterol (0.5%), 0.5 mL in 2.5 mL of saline, by nebulizer. Once intubated, use albuterol MDI 10–20 puffs, endotracheally, every 20 minutes, as needed.

B. Patients should be encouraged to wear a MedicAlert (MedicAlert Foundation, 2323 Colorado Ave., Turlock, CA 95382 or www.medicalert.org) or similar identifying bracelet.

C. Patients should carry two epinephrine devices for intramuscular injection (e.g., EpiPen or EpiPen, Jr.).

D. β-Blocking medication may increase the risk and make anaphylaxis more refractory to treatment, so β-blocking medication should be avoided if possible in patients at risk for recurrent anaphylaxis.

VIII. MANAGEMENT OF ANAPHYLAXIS TO SPECIFIC PRECIPITANTS

A. β-Lactam antibiotic anaphylaxis.

1. Approximately 10% of allergic reactions to β-lactams are life threatening: Of these, 2% to 10% are fatal.

2. Skin testing that includes both major and minor antigenic determinants detects IgE-mediated sensitivity but is not currently commercially available.

3. Skin testing does not evaluate other types of sensitivity, such as serum sickness reactions, morbilliform rashes, and interstitial nephritis.

4. Cross-reactivity occurs infrequently between penicillin and cephalosporins (5.4% to 16.5%) but frequently between penicillins and carbapenems (e.g., imipenem).

5. Monobactams (e.g., aztreonam) do not show cross-reactivity with penicillins but do cross-react with the cephalosporins.

6. For less severe reactions and when no alternative agent is available, desensitization may be attempted in the intensive care unit (ICU) setting. Five of six tenfold dilutions of the target concentration are administered in sequence, starting with the most dilute and progressing to the next stronger concentration every 15 to 20 minutes.

B. Stinging insect venom anaphylaxis

1. Patients should be referred to an allergist for skin testing and possible desensitization.

2. Specific venom desensitization provides greater than 95% protection against anaphylaxis on subsequent stings.

C. Food anaphylaxis

1. Eggs, milk, peanuts, soy, tree nuts, wheat, fish, and shellfish are the foods that most commonly cause severe reactions.

2. Fatal anaphylaxis from food occurs most commonly in patients with asthma, in a public setting rather than at home, and when administration of epinephrine is delayed.

3. Strict avoidance of implicated foods is essential.

D. Radiographic contrast media anaphylaxis

1. In patients with a history of a previous radiocontrast media anaphylactic reaction, the repeat reaction rate is reported to be 35% to 60%.

2. Patients with a general history of allergies, whether to inhalant allergens, foods, or medications, have an increased reaction rate compared with nonallergic individuals.

3. Low ionic contrast or alternative radiographic studies (e.g., computed tomography with gadolinium, magnetic resonance imaging, or ultrasound) should be considered.

4. Pretreatment with corticosteroids (50 mg prednisone, 13 hours, 7 hours, and 1 hour prior to administration) and diphenhydramine (50 mg orally or intramuscularly 1 hour prior to administration) with or without ephedrine (25 mg orally 1 hour prior to administration) may reduce the reaction rate.

5. For an emergent procedure, hydrocortisone (200 mg) can be given intravenously (IV) immediately and repeated every 4 hours until the procedure with diphenhydramine (50 mg IV) immediately prior to the procedure.

E. Latex-induced anaphylaxis

1. Patients with spina bifida or a history of multiple surgeries and health-care workers are at increased risk for latex anaphylaxis.

   2. Latex is found in a wide spectrum of medical products.
   3. Serum radioallergosorbent testing (CAP-Pharmacia) is helpful in diagnosis but may have false-negative results (50% to 60% sensitivity).
   4. Standardized skin testing is not commercially available.
   5. Patients with latex allergy should be cared for in latex-free operating rooms, ICUs, and hospital rooms.

F. Angiotensin-converting enzyme inhibitor anaphylaxis

   1. Severe, potentially life-threatening facial and oropharyngeal angioedema can occur in individuals with sensitivity to angiotensin-converting enzyme (ACE) inhibitors and angiotensin receptor blockers (ARBs).
   2. Onset of angioedema usually starts within the first several hours or up to a week after beginning therapy but may be delayed for months to years.
   3. Cross-reactivity does occur among the different ACE inhibitors but usually not between ACE inhibitors and ARBs.
   4. Epinephrine is not always helpful: endotracheal intubation or cricothyroid-otomy may be necessary to maintain an airway. Angioedema may take 1 to 3 days to resolve.

G. Hereditary angioedema

   1. Individuals with absent or inactive C1 esterase inhibitor can develop life-threatening angioedema of the upper respiratory tract.
   2. Urticaria is generally not present, but a history of recurrent abdominal pain from intestinal angioedema may be elicited.
   3. Acutely, complement C2 and C4 levels are low; C1q is normal in the hereditary form and low in the acquired form.
   4. C1 esterase inhibitor is either low or nonfunctional.
   5. Angioedema is frequently refractory to epinephrine, necessitating: intubation or cricothyroidotomy.
   6. Stanazol 4 mg orally every 4 hours for four doses shortens the duration of symptoms.

Selected Readings

Borish L, Tamir R, Rosenwasser LJ. Intravenous desensitization to beta-lactam antibiotics. *J Allergy Clin Immunol* 1987;80:314.
   Outlines desensitization protocol for β-lactam antibiotics.

Crnkovich DJ, Carlson RW. Anaphylaxis: an organized approach to management and prevention. *Journal Critical Illness* 1993;8:3,332.
   A succinct review of the pathophysiology and treatment of anaphylaxis.

Greenberger PA, Patterson R. The prevention of immediate generalized reactions to radiocontrast media in high-risk patients. *J Allergy Clin Immunol* 1991;87:867.
   Details the preventive management of contrast media use in emergent situations in patients with previous anaphylaxis reactions.

Gruchalla RS. Drug allergy. *J Allergy Clin Immunol* 2003;111:S548.
   Excellent review of penicillin, cephalosporin, and sulfonamide allergy.

Kemp SF, Lockey RF. Anaphylaxis: a review of causes and mechanisms. *J Allergy Clin Immunol* 2002;110:341.
   A review article that includes mechanisms, epidemiology, clinical features, and approaches to anaphylaxis prevention and therapy.

Little FF, Hollingsworth HM. Anaphylaxis. In: Irwin RS, Rippe JM, eds. *Intensive care medicine*, 5th edition. Philadelphia: Lippincott Williams & Wilkins, 2003, p.2113.
   An in-depth discussion of critical care management of anaphylaxis.

Neugut AI, Ghatak AT, Miller RL. Anaphylaxis in the United States: an investigation into its epidemiology. *Arch Intern Med* 2001;161:15–21.
   Reviews relative frequency of different causes of anaphylaxis in the United States.

Nichlas RA, Bernstein IL, Li JT, et al. The diagnosis and management of anaphylaxis. *J Allergy Clin Immunol* 1998;101:6.

A comprehensive document that provides consensus summary statements for the treatment and management of anaphylaxis.

Roberts JR, Wuerz RC. Clinical characteristics of angiotensin-converting enzyme inhibitor-induced angioedema. *Ann Emerg Med* 1991;20:555.
Details the clinical allergic reactions to angiotensin-converting enzyme inhibitors.

Salkind AR, Cuddy PG, Foxworth JW. Is this patient allergic to penicillin? An evidence-based analysis of the likelihood of penicillin allergy. *JAMA* 2001;285(19):2498.
ANOTATION TO COME.

Sampson HA, Mendelson L, Rosen JP. Fatal and near-fatal anaphylactic reactions to food in children and adolescents. *N Engl J Med* 1992;327:380.
A review of common food allergens and clinical manifestations.

Toogood JH. Risk of anaphylaxis in patients receiving beta-blocker drugs. *J Allergy Clin Immunol* 1988;81:1.
Describes the risks of β-blocker use in patients undergoing anaphylaxis and treatment strategy.

Valentine MD. Insect venom allergy: diagnosis and treatment. *J Allergy Clin Immunol* 1984;73:299.
A comprehensive review of venom allergy and immunotherapy.

Wong S, Dykewicz MS, Patterson R. Idiopathic anaphylaxis. *Arch Intern Med* 1990;150:1323.
A retrospective evaluation of 175 patients with idiopathic anaphylaxis.

Zaloga GP, Delacey W, Holmboe E, et al. Glucagon reversal of hypotension in a case of anaphylactoid shock. *Ann Intern Med* 1986;105:65.
Details an anaphylaxis clinical case with response to glucagon.

156 VASCULITIS IN THE INTENSIVE CARE UNIT
Paul F. Dellaripa

I. OVERVIEW. A group of disorders in which inflammation and necrosis of blood vessels leads to organ dysfunction due to the development of thrombosis or hemorrhage. Mimics of vasculitis include subacute bacterial endocarditis, atrial myxoma, antiphospholipid syndrome, and cholesterol embolism.

II. WEGENER GRANULOMATOSIS

A. General principles
1. Characterized by granulomatous inflammation of the upper and lower respiratory tract, segmental necrotizing glomerulonephritis and small vessel inflammation of other organs systems.
2. Reasons for intensive care unit (ICU) admission for Wegener granulomatosis (WG) and all of the vasculitidies include respiratory failure due to alveolar hemorrhage, rapidly progressive renal failure, and infections due to immunosuppressive treatment of disease. Stridor due to subglottic stenosis is rare in WG.

B. Pathogenesis
1. There is no known etiologic agent for WG.
2. Antineutrophilic cytoplasmic antibodies (ANCA) are present in more than 90% of cases of WG. C-ANCA (with specificity to PR3 antigen) seen in 10% and P-ANCA (with specificity to myeloperoxidase [MPO]) seen in a minority of cases.

C. Diagnosis
1. Clinical presentation typically includes sinusitis, rhinitis, epistaxis, otitis media, and hearing loss.
2. Lower respiratory tract is involved frequently, with cough, dyspnea, hemoptysis, and progressive respiratory failure due to alveolar hemorrhage. Pulmonary infiltrates or nodules may be diffuse or cavitary. Lung biopsy may be necessary to confirm diagnosis and eliminate the possibility of mycobacterial or fungal disease.
3. Renal involvement may be rapidly progressive leading to dialysis. Rarely, ANCA-associated vasculitis coexists with antiglomerular basement antibodies. Diagnosis is confirmed based on clinical findings, presence of ANCA, and tissue biopsy.

D. Treatment
1. In the setting of respiratory failure, alveolar hemorrhage, and progressive renal failure, therapy should include cyclophosphamide and high-dose corticosteroids. Intravenous (IV) methylprednisolone in doses of 1,000 mg per day for 3 days may be considered.
2. Oral dosing of cyclophosphamide (CYC) is 2 mg/kg, but in renal failure it is as follows: 1.5 mg/kg per day if creatinine clearance (CrCl) is 50 to 99; 1.2 mg/kg per day if CrCl is 25 to 49; 1.0 mg/kg per day if CrCl is 15 to 24; and 0.8 mg/kg per day if CrCl is less than 15 or dialysis.
3. In the setting of critical illness and potential variability of gastrointestinal (GI) absorption, IV CYC (0.5 g/m^2 to 1 g/m^2) is indicated.
4. Pneumocystis pneumonia (PCP) prophylaxis should be offered.
5. Plasmapheresis and intravenous immunoglobulin may be useful in severe or refractory WG and severe alveolar hemorrhage with or without anti-GBM antibodies.
6. The presence of worsening pulmonary infiltrates in those treated with CYC and steroids raises the suspicion of fungal infections and PCP, warranting early bronchoscopy or biopsy and early consideration for antifungal and PCP therapy.

III. MICROSCOPIC POLYANGIITIS
A. General principles
1. Small and medium vessel necrotizing vasculitis presenting with pauciimmune segmental necrotizing glomerulonephritis and pulmonary capillaritis with alveolar hemorrhage.
2. ANCA, (P-ANCA with MPO specificity) is positive in 70% of cases.
3. Clinical presentation can overlap with WG, though pathologically there is lack of granulomas
B. Diagnosis.
Biopsy of appropriate tissue, typically kidney, lung, or nerve in conjunction with ANCA positivity
C. Treatment.
Treatment is similar to that for WG.

IV. CHURG STRAUSS SYNDROME (CSS)
A. General principles
1. Characterized by eosinophilic infiltrates and granulomas in the respiratory tract in the setting of a history of asthma and eosinophilia.
2. Peripheral neuropathy, mesenteric ischemia, cardiac, and central nervous system (CNS) involvement may occur. Renal involvement and alveolar hemorrhage are rare.
B. Diagnosis.
ANCA is positive in 60% of patients, mostly MPO pattern. Biopsy of suspected organs shows granulomas and fibrinoid necrosis.
C. Treatment
1. Corticosteroids in milder presentation, with CYC in more severe disease.
2. Five-factor score (proteinuria greater than 1 g per day, azotemia, GI or CNS dysfunction, cardiomyopathy) helps to determine prognosis and level of treatment.

V. POLYARTERITIS NODOSA (PAN)
A. General principles.
Systemic necrotizing vasculitis involving small and medium muscular arteries.
B. Etiology.
The etiology of PAN is unknown, though rarely the presence of circulating hepatitis B surface antigen in vessel walls is noted.
C. Diagnosis
1. Presents with a prodrome of malaise, fatigue fever, and weight loss.
2. Vasculitic lesions may result in mononeurtis multiplex, cutaneous lesions, intestinal ischemia, myocardial infarction, and congestive heart failure.
3. Laboratory findings include anemia and elevated sedimentation rate. ANCA is absent.
4. Diagnosis is confirmed by tissue biopsy or evidence of microaneurysms on mesenteric angiogram.
D. Treatment
1. High-dose corticosteroid therapy orally or intravenously with pulse methylprednisolone at 1 g per day for 3 days; CYC used in severe cases.
2. In cases associated with hepatitis B, antiviral agents used early in conjunction with corticosteroids and plasmapheresis.

VI. CRYOGLOBULINEMIC VASCULITIS
A. General principles.
Cryoglobulins are immunoglobulins that precipitate in the cold. There are three types, with types II and III closely, though not exclusively, associated with hepatitis C infection.
B. Diagnosis
1. Findings include palpable purpura, peripheral neuropathy, and infrequently life-threatening renal, GI, and pulmonary involvement including pulmonary hemorrhage.
2. Laboratory values include low complement levels (C4), abnormal liver enzymes, positive rheumatoid factor.
C. Treatment
1. Treatment consist of high-dose corticosteroid and adding CYC in cases of renal failure or mononeuritis multiplex
2. Plasmapheresis or cryofiltration may be beneficial in severe cases.

VII. VASCULITIS OF THE CENTRAL NERVOUS SYSTEM

   A. General principles. Heterogeneous group of neurologic disorders divided into primary (granulomatous and nongranulomatous) and secondary forms.

   B. Diagnosis
   1. Granulomatous angiitis of the central nervous system (GACNS): usually a slow, progressive process characterized by headache, focal deficits, and changes in higher cortical function.
      a. Lumbar puncture reveals mononuclear pleocytosis and elevated protein.
      b. MRI shows abnormal multifocal vascular lesions and leptomeningeal enhancement.
      c. Angiography is nonspecific or normal in up to 60% of cases.
      d. Biopsy of the cortex and leptomeninges showing granulomas and giant cells is diagnostic procedure of choice.
   2. Nongranulomatous angiitis of the CNS may share clinical features with GACNS or may present with a more rapid course and variable, and sometimes normal, spinal fluid.
   3. Benign angiopathy of the CNS (BACNS)
      a. Typically in young women with severe-onset headache or focal neurologic deficit in a monophasic pattern
      b. CSF analysis is normal, and angiography is frequently consistent with vasoconstriction or spasm. Biopsy may be necessary if angiographic features are not conclusive.

   C. Treatment. CNS vasculitis is treated with corticosteroids and CYC, with the exception of BACNS, which may be treated with shorter courses of steroids alone.

Selected Readings

Calabrese LH, Duna GF, Lie JT. Vasculitis in the central nervous system. *Arthritis Rheum* 1997;40:1189.
   Classic review on this complicated topic.

Falk RJ, Jennette JC. ANCA Small vessel vasculitis. *J Am Soc Nephrol* 1997;8:314.
   An excellent review focusing on the pulmonary renal syndromes.

Guillevin L, Lhote F, Gayraud M, et al. Prognostic factors in *Polyarteritis nodosa* and Churg-Strauss syndrome. *Medicine* 1996;75(1):17.
   Largest and most complete prospective evaluation and assessment of prognosis in these two rare diseases.

Guillevin L, Pagnoux C. Indications of plasma exchange for systemic vasculitides. *Ther Apher Dial* 2003;2:155.
   Reviews major indications for plasmapheresis in various vasculitic syndromes

Hochberg MC, Silman AJ, Smolen JS, et al, ed. The vasculities. In: *Rheumatology*, 3rd edition. Edinburgh: Mosby, 2002, p. 1583.
   Excellent chapter reviews within a general rheumatology text.

Hoffman GS, Weyand CM. Inflammatory diseases of blood vessels. New York: Marcel Dekker, 2002.
   Superb text devoted to chapter reviews of all the vasculitic syndromes.

Jayne D. Evidence based treatment of systemic vasculitis. *Rheumatology* 2000;39:585.
   Review of all the major treatment trials in vasculitis.

Klemmer PJ, Chalermskulrat MD, Reif MS, et al. Plasmapheresis therapy for diffuse alveolar hemorrhage in patients with small vessel vasculitis. *Am J Kidney Dis* 2003;42:1149.
   Retrospective review of the effect of apheresis in alveolar hemorrhage.

Schmitt WH, Gross WL. Vasculitis in the seriously ill patient: diagnostic approaches and therapeutic options in ANCA associated vasculitis. *Kidney Int* 1998:53(64):S39.
   Excellent review of treatment in seriously ill ANCA-associated diseases.

Soding PF, Lockwood CM, Park GR. The intensive care of patients with fulminant vasculitis. *Anaesth Intens Care* 1994:22:81.
   A practical case-based presentation of treatment strategies in fulminant disease.

Psychiatric Issues in Intensive Care

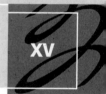

XV

157

DIAGNOSIS AND TREATMENT OF AGITATION AND DELIRIUM IN THE INTENSIVE CARE UNIT PATIENT

John Querques, Theodore A. Stern, George E. Tesar, and Stephan Heckers

I. GENERAL PRINCIPLES

A. Description

1. Agitation and delirium are common problems in the intensive care unit (ICU) that warrant evaluation and treatment of metabolic abnormalities, drug toxicity, withdrawal states, and other potentially reversible conditions.
2. Agitation is manifested by behavioral dyscontrol (e.g., restlessness, thrashing in bed, removing indwelling catheters and tubes).
3. Also called acute confusional state or encephalopathy, delirium is characterized by an altered level of consciousness, cognitive deficits, and either psychomotor agitation or retardation. It is acute in onset and usually reversible within days or weeks, although some cases result in permanent cognitive dysfunction.

B. Epidemiology

1. The frequency of delirium depends on patient demographics, the nature and severity of the patient's medical or surgical conditions, and the treatments for these conditions.
2. Delirium is most prevalent in surgical ICUs, followed by medical ICUs, coronary care units, and general medical and surgical wards.

C. Risk factors.
Apart from severe medical illness, risk factors for delirium include older age, male gender, dementia, depression, immobility, alcoholism, and sensory impairment.

II. ETIOLOGY

A. Agitation can be caused by:

1. Panic-level anxiety. Anxiety is a prominent and expected reaction to many conditions that require intensive care, including the process of weaning from mechanical ventilation. When anxiety is the cause of agitation, education and reassurance may be beneficial; when severe, anxiolytic medications are necessary.
2. Pain. Often undetected because of the patient's inability to communicate effectively and undertreated for fear of promoting addiction, pain can precipitate considerable agitation.
3. Personality style. Patients with rigid, obsessive, compulsive, and controlling characteristics experience the greatest difficulty coping with an ICU stay. Intolerable frustration can lead to agitation and a demand to leave the hospital against medical advice.
4. Poor comprehension or sensory impairment. Mental retardation, dementia, a language barrier, or a visual or hearing impairment can compromise a patient's understanding of the need for ICU care and, thereby, precipitate agitation.
5. Delirium

B. Delirium
can be caused by a panoply of anatomical and physiologic disturbances that cluster into four groups (Table 157-1); life-threatening causes of delirium should be excluded first (Table 157-2). In ICUs, where patients are commonly prescribed numerous medications affecting multiple organ systems, pharmacologic agents—alone or in combination—frequently precipitate delirium (Table 157-3).

III. PATHOGENESIS

A. The pathogenesis of delirium is unknown.

B. One leading theory posits that dopamine excess or acetylcholine deficiency in the brain—or a combination of both—provides the pathogenetic substrate for delirium.

TABLE 157-1	Etiologies of Delirium
Problem	**Etiologic factors**

Primary intracranial disease	Infection
	  HIV
	  Meningitis/encephalitis
	  Neurosyphilis
	Neoplasm
	Seizure
	  Complex partial seizures
	  Postictal state
	Vascular
	  Hypertensive encephalopathy
	  Stroke
	  Vasculitis
	Normal pressure hydrocephalus

Systemic diseases that secondarily affect the brain	Cardiopulmonary
	  Cardiac arrest
	  Shock
	  Congestive heart failure
	  Respiratory failure
	Endocrine/metabolic
	  Acid–base disorder
	  Fluid/electrolyte derangement
	  Diabetic ketoacidosis
	  Hypoglycemia
	  Parathyroid dysfunction
	  Thyroid dysfunction
	  Hepatic failure
	  Renal failure
	Infection
	  Sepsis
	  Subacute bacterial endocarditis
	Neoplasm
	  Paraneoplastic syndromes
	Nutritional deficiency
	  Folic acid
	  Vitamin B_{12} (pernicious anemia)
	  Thiamine (Wernicke encephalopathy)

Exogenous toxic agents	Drugs of abuse
	  Alcohol
	  Amphetamines
	  Cocaine
	  Lysergic acid diethylamide
	  Phencyclidine
	Nonmedicinal substances
	  Carbon monoxide
	  Heavy metals
	Medications (see Table 157-3)

Drug withdrawal	Alcohol
	Propanediols
	  Chloral hydrate
	  Meprobamate
	Sedative-hypnotic agents
	  Benzodiazepines
	  Barbiturates
	  Narcotics

Adapted from Lipowski ZJ. Delirium in the elderly patient. *N Engl J Med* 1989;320:578–582; and Ludwig, AM. *Principles of clinical psychiatry*. New York: Free Press, 1980.

TABLE 157-2	Life-Threatening Causes of Delirium: WWHHHIIMMP

Wernicke encephalopathy
Withdrawal from drugs
Hypertensive encephalopathy
Hypoglycemia
Hypoxia
Intracerebral hemorrhage
Infection
Meningitis/encephalitis
Metabolic derangements
Poisoning

Adapted from Tesar GE, Stern TA. Evaluation and treatment of agitation in the intensive care unit. *J Intensive Care Med* 1986;1:137–148.

IV. DIAGNOSIS

A. Clinical features

1. Agitated patients are often unable to cooperate with necessary procedures and interventions. At worst, agitation may result in combativeness or a demand to leave the hospital.

2. Delirious patients can be restless and agitated, or they can be so quiet and slowed (i.e., psychomotorically retarded) that they are thought to have a depressive disorder. Regardless of their behavioral state, by definition delirious patients exhibit inattentiveness (i.e., an inability to focus on a given task or to shift focus from a previous task to a later one). Disorientation and short-term memory impairment frequently result from such inattention; alterations in perception (i.e., illusions and hallucinations) and in thought (i.e., delusions, often

TABLE 157-3	Selected Common Delirium-inducing Drugs Used in the ICU

Drug group	Agent
Antiarrhythmic agents	Lidocaine
	Mexiletine
	Procainamide
	Quinidine
Antibiotics	Penicillin
Anticholinergics	Atropine
Antihistamines	Nonselective
	Diphenhydramine
	Selective histamine-2 blockers
	Cimetidine
	Ranitidine
Beta-Blockers	Propranolol
Narcotics	Meperidine
	Morphine
	Pentazocine

Adapted from Tesar GE, Stern TA. Evaluation and treatment of agitation in the intensive care unit. *J Intensive Care Med* 1986;1:137–148.

persecutory) also occur. These behavioral and cognitive disturbances fluctuate throughout the day and are often worse at night.

B. Differential diagnosis

    1. Agitation and delirium must be distinguished from dementia, depression, psychosis, mania, dissociative disorders, and severe personality disturbance (e.g., borderline personality disorder).

    2. If a patient is not fully awake, alert, and attentive, delirium rises to the top of the differential. The patient may have one of these conditions in addition to delirium (e.g., a demented patient can be delirious); however, discernment of these other diagnoses is often difficult, if not impossible, in a delirious patient.

    3. The importance of prompt recognition, evaluation, and treatment of delirium nearly uniformly trumps these other considerations, which can be addressed after the delirium resolves.

V. TREATMENT

    A. The cornerstone of management of the agitated or delirious patient is specific treatment for the underlying disorder(s) considered to be the causative culprit(s) (e.g., correction of metabolic abnormalities, treatment of drug withdrawal, alleviation of pain or anxiety).

    B. Other steps, which can be instituted concurrently with these treatments or when a specific cause for delirium cannot be identified or corrected, include use of mechanical restraints and pharmacologic management with antipsychotics, benzodiazepines, and other medications.

    C. In addition to narcotics, propofol, and nondepolarizing muscle relaxants, the pharmacologic methods used to control agitation and to treat delirium include the following agents:

        1. Haloperidol

            a. Oral haloperidol. In stable patients, the starting dose of this high-potency butyrophenone neuroleptic is often 2 to 5 mg two or three times daily. A lower initial dose (e.g., 0.5 mg two or three times daily) and gradual upward titration are advised in patients with advanced age, hemodynamic instability, or evidence of neurologic dysfunction in addition to delirium (e.g., stroke, dementia). Observation of haloperidol's effect should guide the adjustment of dosage and the frequency of administration.

            b. Parenteral haloperidol. When intense agitation requires rapid treatment, administer haloperidol by the intramuscular (IM) or intravenous (IV) route. The initial dose is 2 to 5 mg, depending on age, hemodynamic instability, and severity of agitation. If a calming effect does not occur within 20 minutes, the next dose should be doubled. This process of systematic dose escalation (i.e., doubling successive doses every 20 minutes) should be reserved for the IV route and can be continued until the patient is calm. When agitation returns, the dose that ultimately tranquilized the patient should be repeated.

            c. Side effects. In the ICU, side effects of haloperidol, whether administered orally or parenterally, are usually mild and inconsequential.

                (1) Extrapyramidal effects. The use of IV haloperidol in critically ill patients has been associated with fewer extrapyramidal effects (e.g., akathisia, dystonia, parkinsonism) than its use IM or orally.

                (2) Cardiovascular effects. Although haloperidol typically has trivial effects on the cardiovascular system, two potential complications can be life-threatening. First, in combination with haloperidol, propranolol has been reported to cause cardiopulmonary arrest and hypotension. Second, cardiac-conduction prolongation, premature ventricular contractions, ventricular tachycardia, torsades de pointes, and asystole can occur in some patients after the administration of haloperidol. Therefore, the corrected QT interval and serum levels of potassium, calcium, and magnesium must be monitored and normalized during high-dose haloperidol treatment.

| TABLE 157-4 | Pharmacologic Properties of Commonly Used Antipsychotics |

Drug	Route	Onset (min)	Peak effect (min)	Metabolites	Starting dose
Haloperidol	IM, IV[a]	5–20	15–45	Several (? active)	2–5 mg
	PO	30–60	120–240	0.5–5 mg BID–TID	
Droperidol[b]	IM, IV	3–10	15–45	Inactive	2.5–10 mg
Chlorpromazine	IM, IV[c]	5–40	10–30	Active and inactive	25 mg
	PO	30–60	120–240		
Olanzapine	PO, SL, IM	20–60	60–120	Inactive	2.5–5 mg

[a] Intravenous haloperidol is not approved for routine use by the U.S. Food and Drug Administration. Permission for its use should be requested from the hospital's formulary.
[b] A "black box" warning in the *Physicians Desk Reference* advises that continuous electrocardiographic monitoring be employed due to the risk of conduction disturbances and ventricular arrhythmia.
[c] Intravenous administration of chlorpromazine is more likely to cause cardiovascular disturbances (e.g., hypotension) than is intramuscular administration.
BID, two times daily; IM, intramuscular; IV, intravenous; PO, oral; SL, sublingual (orally disintegrating wafer); TID, three times daily.
Adapted from Tesar GE, Stern TA. Rapid tranquilization of the agitated intensive care unit patient. *J Intensive Care Med* 1988;3:195–201.

2. Combination of haloperidol and a benzodiazepine. Use of a benzodiazepine in addition to haloperidol often promotes further calming. Lorazepam has been used more often than other agents for this purpose, but diazepam and midazolam are preferred when agitation is explosive.

3. Other antipsychotic agents. If IV haloperidol alone or in combination with a benzodiazepine is ineffective, use of a more sedating neuroleptic (e.g., droperidol or chlorpromazine) may be helpful. Table 157-4 summarizes the pharmacologic properties of commonly used antipsychotic drugs. More recently, a bevy of atypical antipsychotic agents (including risperidone, olanzapine, quietapine, and ziprasidone), available for use by several routes of administration, have proved efficacious in the treatment of agitation and delirium.

    a. Compared with haloperidol, droperidol is more likely to produce sedation and hypotension. However, one should be mindful of the "black box" warning in the *Physicians Desk Reference* (PDR) regarding conduction disturbances and ventricular arrhythmia.

    b. Chlorpromazine can cause severe orthostatic hypotension, and its quinidine-like properties can increase the likelihood of cardiac arrhythmias. The risk of serious side effects is less with oral and IM administration than with IV use.

4. Benzodiazepines. A benzodiazepine alone is the treatment of choice when panic and severe anxiety account for agitated behavior. After continuous infusion of midazolam over a prolonged period, a gradual tapering should follow. Benzodiazepine monotherapy can worsen delirium and should be avoided.

Selected Readings

Alexander HE, McCarty K, Giffen MB. Hypotension and cardiopulmonary arrest associated with concurrent haloperidol and propranolol therapy. *JAMA* 1984;252:87–88.
   A report of a single case of cardiopulmonary arrest and hypotension in a woman with schizophrenia and hypertension treated with this combination of neuroleptic and β-blocker.

American Psychiatric Association. Practice guideline on delirium. *Am J Psychiatry* 1999;156 (suppl):1–20.
  A monograph covering all aspects of the diagnosis and treatment of the delirious patient.

Burns A, Gallagley A, Byrne J. Delirium. *J Neurol Neurosurg Psychiatry* 2004;75:362–367.
  A recent review of the terminology, clinical features, epidemiology, risk factors, etiologies, pathophysiology, patient experience, management, and prevention of delirium.

Cassem NH, Murray GB, Lafayette JM, et al. Delirious patients. In: Stern TA, Fricchione GF, Cassem NH, et al., eds. *Massachusetts General Hospital handbook of general hospital psychiatry*, 5th edition. Philadelphia: Mosby, 2004, pp. 119–134.
  A comprehensive review of the psychiatric manifestations of delirium and a guide to differential diagnosis and effective management.

Diagnostic and statistical manual of mental disorders, 4th edition. Washington, DC: American Psychiatric Association, 1994.
  Known as DSM-IV, this "bible" of psychiatry enumerates the diagnostic criteria for the gamut of psychiatric maladies.

Hunt N, Stern TA. The association between intravenous haloperidol and torsades de pointes. *Psychosomatics* 1995;36:541–549.
  A report of three cases of torsades de pointes in patients receiving intravenous haloperidol, as well as a review of the literature on ventricular arrhythmias associated with use of this neuroleptic.

Lipowski ZJ. Delirium (acute confusional states). *JAMA* 1987;258:1789–1792.
  A review of the clinical features, etiology, pathogenesis, and treatment of delirium.

Lipowski ZJ. Delirium in the elderly patient. *N Engl J Med* 1989;320:578–582.
  A review of the clinical features, differential diagnosis, organic causes, and treatment of delirium, with special emphasis on the geriatric population.

Lipowski ZJ. Transient cognitive disorders (delirium, acute confusional states) in the elderly. *Am J Psychiatry* 1983;140:1426–1436.
  A discussion of the clinical features, etiology, pathogenesis, diagnosis, and treatment of delirium and related transient disorders of cognition in the elderly.

Ludwig, AM. *Principles of clinical psychiatry.* New York: Free Press, 1980.
  This textbook of psychiatry contains a helpful chapter on organic brain syndromes, which the author refers to as the clouding-delirium-dementia-coma complex.

Tesar GE, Stern TA. Evaluation and treatment of agitation in the intensive care unit. *J Intensive Care Med* 1986;1:137–148.
  A comprehensive review of the evaluation and management of the agitated intensive care unit patient.

Tesar GE, Stern TA. Rapid tranquilization of the agitated intensive care unit patient. *J Intensive Care Med* 1988;3:195–201.
  A comprehensive discussion of the pharmacologic management of agitation in the intensive care unit and of the risks and benefits of neuroleptics, benzodiazepines, narcotics, and nondepolarizing muscle relaxants.

DIAGNOSIS AND TREATMENT OF ANXIETY IN THE INTENSIVE CARE UNIT PATIENT

John Querques, Theodore A. Stern, Lawrence A. Labbate, and Mark H. Pollack

158

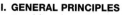

I. GENERAL PRINCIPLES

A. Although anxiety in the intensive care unit (ICU) can be expected as a normal, transient response to the stress of critical illness, pathologic anxiety has a negative impact on morbidity, mortality, and treatment compliance and merits timely evaluation and treatment.

B. Pathologic anxiety:

1. Is a distressing experience of foreboding that is autonomous and persistent

2. Causes a level of distress beyond the patient's capacity to bear it and results in impaired functioning or abnormal behavior (e.g., avoidance or withdrawal)

II. DIAGNOSIS

A. Clinical features

1. Anxiety is manifested by physical, affective, behavioral, and cognitive symptoms and signs.

a. Physical: Autonomic arousal, including tachycardia, hypertension, tachypnea, diaphoresis, lightheadedness, and mydriasis

b. Affective: Ranges from mild edginess to terror and panic

c. Behavioral: Avoidance (e.g., refusal of medical procedures) and withdrawal (e.g., refusal to speak to family and medical staff, demands to leave the hospital)

d. Cognitive: Worry, apprehension, and thoughts about emotional or bodily damage

B. Differential diagnosis

1. Anxiety in the ICU patient can be caused by a medical illness or its treatment, a primary psychiatric syndrome, a failure of psychological coping mechanisms, or fear.

a. Medical causes

(1) Anxiety that occurs in the absence of a psychologically charged situation or in conjunction with discrete physical events (e.g., supraventricular tachycardia) should trigger a search for an organic etiology.

(2) Attention should first be paid to the patient's known medical illness, its complications, and its treatment.

(3) Anxiety can be a manifestation of delirium (see Chapter 157).

b. Psychiatric causes

(1) When primary psychopathology is the cause of anxiety in the ICU patient, the acute medical condition hinders access to substances to which the patient may be addicted, exacerbates a premorbid psychiatric condition or its treatment, or provokes an initial episode of anxiety or panic.

(2) The differential diagnosis includes:

(a) Substance withdrawal

(b) Schizophrenia

(c) Bipolar disorder

(d) Akathisia, an internal sense of restlessness, sometimes caused by antipsychotic therapy

(e) A primary anxiety disorder (e.g., panic disorder, generalized anxiety disorder, simple phobia, social phobia, posttraumatic stress disorder, or obsessive-compulsive disorder)

    c. Failure of psychological coping mechanisms

        (1) Patients deal with the stress of hospitalization with a variety of coping strategies (e.g., rationalization, reassurance, religion, family support).

        (2) Even in patients without a history of anxiety, these mechanisms can be overwhelmed in the ICU when patients regress or feel alone, the illness is sudden, or social supports are unavailable.

III. TREATMENT. Management of the anxious patient in the ICU involves correction of underlying medical factors and use of both pharmacologic and nonpharmacologic interventions.

  A. Pharmacologic interventions

    1. Benzodiazepines. These agents are generally considered the mainstays of anxiolytic pharmacotherapy in the ICU because of their relative safety and rapid therapeutic effects. Drug selection is determined by the clinical situation and the pharmacokinetic properties of the agent. For example, an acutely anxious patient requires a drug with a rapid onset of action (e.g., diazepam or midazolam). Table 158-1 summarizes important pharmacologic properties of some commonly used benzodiazepines.

      a. Dose. For many patients, it is reasonable to initiate treatment with a low dose of a shorter-acting, easily metabolized agent on a fixed-dose (not as-needed) schedule (e.g., lorazepam 1 mg three or four times daily). The dosage can then be titrated to anxiolytic effect. Dosages in elderly patients should be roughly half those used in younger patients. Patients with impaired hepatic function should receive agents that have shorter half-lives and fewer (or no) active metabolites (e.g., lorazepam) to minimize drug accumulation.

      b. Route of administration. Benzodiazepines should be administered parenterally when immediate relief of anxiety is necessary or when the oral route is unavailable. Intravenous (IV) administration of diazepam and chlordiazepoxide is preferred to the intramuscular (IM) route because IM absorption of these agents is erratic. Lorazepam, on the other hand, is well absorbed after IM administration; it can also be given sublingually to achieve a quicker onset of action than the oral route provides. Hypotension and respiratory depression are potential risks of IV administration of benzodiazepines.

TABLE 158-1	Pharmacologic Properties of Benzodiazepines Commonly Used in the ICU				
Drug	**Route**	**Onset (min)**	**Peak effect (min)**	**Active metabolites**	**Starting dose**
Chlordiazepoxide	IV	2–10	60–120	Several	25–50 mg
	PO	30–60	120–240		5–25 mg
Diazepam	IV	2–5	5–30	Nordiazepam,[a] oxazepam	2–5 mg
	PO	10–60	30–180		
Lorazepam	IM, IV	2–20	60–120	None	1–2 mg
	SL	2–20	20–60		0.5–1 mg
	PO	20–60	20–120		0.5–1 mg
Midazolam	IM, IV	1–2	30–40	1- and 4-hydroxy-midazolam	0.05–0.15 mg/kg

[a] The half-life of nordiazepam (desmethyldiazepam) is 60 to 100 hours.
IM, intramuscular; IV, intravenous; PO, oral; SL, sublingual.
Adapted from Tesar GE, Stern TA. Rapid tranquilization of the agitated intensive care unit patient. *J Intensive Care Med* 1988;3:195–201.

    2. Antipsychotics. When the patient is unable to think clearly, becomes transiently psychotic, or is fearful, antipsychotics (e.g., haloperidol) are preferred over benzodiazepines.

   B. Nonpharmacologic interventions. Clarification; education; appropriate reassurance; hypnosis; behavioral strategies (e.g., relaxation techniques); and the support of clergy, friends, and family can all be an important part of the management of the anxious patient.

Selected Readings

Geringer ES, Stern TA. Anxiety and depression in critically ill patients. *Problems in Critical Care* 1988;2:35–46.

   A practical review of the manifestations, differential diagnosis, and treatment of depression and anxiety in patients with critical illness.

Pollack MH, Otto MW, Bernstein JG, et al. Anxious patients. In: Stern TA, Fricchione GF, Cassem NH, et al., eds. *Massachusetts General Hospital handbook of general hospital psychiatry*, 5th edition. Philadelphia: Mosby, 2004, pp. 175–201.

   A comprehensive review of the manifestations of anxiety, and a guide to differential diagnosis and effective management in the general hospital.

Tesar GE, Stern TA. Rapid tranquilization of the agitated intensive care unit patient. *J Intensive Care Med* 1988;3:195–201.

   A comprehensive discussion of the pharmacologic management of agitation in the intensive care unit and of the risks and benefits of antipsychotics, benzodiazepines, narcotics, and nondepolarizing muscle relaxants.

159 DIAGNOSIS AND TREATMENT OF DEPRESSION IN THE INTENSIVE CARE UNIT PATIENT

John Querques, Theodore A. Stern, and Edith S. Geringer

I. GENERAL PRINCIPLES

A. Major depressive disorder is a psychiatric condition that affects mood and neuro-vegetative functions (e.g., sleep, appetite, concentration).

1. It is never a normal or appropriate reaction to a stressful situation.

2. Left untreated, major depression decreases survival in general and increases morbidity and mortality from cardiac conditions.

B. Definition

1. Major depressive disorder is a syndrome characterized by five of the symptoms listed in Table 159-1 for 2 weeks or more.

2. One of the five symptoms must be either depressed mood or anhedonia (i.e., a decrease in one's interests or drives in life).

3. The mnemonic SIG: E CAPS (i.e., label: energy capsules) is a helpful guide to remember these defining criteria (Table 159-1).

II. DIAGNOSIS

A. Clinical features. The manifestations of depression include affective, behavioral, and cognitive abnormalities (i.e., the ABCs of depression) (Table 159-2).

B. Differential diagnosis. Depression in the intensive care unit (ICU) can occur as a primary affective disorder (e.g., major depressive disorder), a mood disorder associated with a specific medical condition or its treatment, or a psychological reaction to an acute medical illness.

1. Medical causes. Various medical conditions (Table 159-3) and medications (Table 159-4) can cause depression. Laboratory testing should be guided by results of a comprehensive history and physical examination.

2. Psychological reaction. Critical illness often threatens a patient's sense of physical integrity and autonomy and can remind some patients of either personal or family histories of similar life-threatening circumstances.

III. TREATMENT. Management of depression includes pharmacologic treatment, psychological interventions, and electroconvulsive therapy (ECT).

A. Pharmacologic treatment. In the ICU, medications are used most frequently. An antidepressant medication is selected based on side-effect profile and rapidity of onset of action.

1. Psychostimulants

a. Dextroamphetamine and methylphenidate work within days.

b. Can cause tachycardia, hypertension, arrhythmias, and coronary spasm, but rarely at the low doses (5 to 20 mg per day) usually used.

c. Bupropion has a stimulantlike effect.

2. Selective serotonin reuptake inhibitors (SSRIs) (see Table 159-5)

a. Exert their therapeutic effect within 4 to 6 weeks.

b. Can cause agitation, irritability, insomnia, tremulousness, diaphoresis, anorexia, nausea, vomiting, diarrhea, and sexual dysfunction.

c. Have fewer cardiovascular effects than TCAs and do not commonly cause orthostatic hypotension.

d. Extensively metabolized by the hepatic cytochrome P-450 system.

e. All of them, except citalopram and escitalopram, inhibit this enzymatic pathway and raise serum levels of co-administered drugs (See Table 159-6).

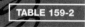 **TABLE 159-1**   **Mnemonic for the Diagnostic Criteria for a Depressive Episode**

Depressed mood
Sleep (increased or decreased)
Interest (decreased)
Guilt (or worthlessness)
Energy (decreased)
Concentration (decreased)
Appetite (increased or decreased) or weight gain or loss
Psychomotor agitation or retardation
Suicidal thinking or thoughts of death

Adapted from Geringer ES, Stern TA. Recognition and treatment of depression in the intensive care unit patient. In: Irwin RS, Rippe JM, eds. *Intensive care medicine*, 5th edition. Philadelphia: Lippincott Williams and Wilkins, 2003, pp. 2170–2184.

TABLE 159-2   **Affective, Behavioral, and Cognitive Features of Depression—the ABCs**

Affective symptoms
Depressed mood
Hopelessness
Crying
Irritability
Anger
Decreased interest

Behavioral symptoms
Insomnia
Anorexia
Apathy
Increased sleep
Increased appetite
Decreased energy
Psychomotor agitation
Psychomotor retardation
Noncompliance
Deliberate self-harm
Impulsivity
Poor eye contact
Increased or intractable pain

Cognitive symptoms
Guilty rumination
Decreased concentration
Suicidal thinking or thoughts of death
Confusion
Dementia-like symptoms
Somatic preoccupation

Adapted from Geringer ES, Stern TA:. Recognition and treatment of depression in the intensive care unit patient. In: Irwin RS, Rippe JM, eds. *Intensive care medicine*, 5th edition. Philadelphia: Lippincott Williams and Wilkins, 2003, pp. 2170–2184.

TABLE 159-3   **Selected Medical Conditions Associated with Depression**

Cardiovascular
Congestive heart failure
Hypertensive encephalopathy

Collagen-vascular
Systemic lupus erythematosus

Endocrine
Diabetes mellitus
Hypo- and hyperadrenalism
Hypo- and hyperparathyroidism
Hypo- and hyperthyroidism

Infectious
Hepatitis
HIV infection
Mononucleosis

Metabolic
Acid—base disorders
Hypokalemia
Hypo- and hypernatremia
Renal failure

Neoplastic
Carcinoid syndrome
Pancreatic carcinoma
Paraneoplastic syndromes

Neurologic
Brain tumor
Multiple sclerosis
Parkinson disease
Complex partial seizures
Stroke
Subcortical dementia

Nutritional
Vitamin B_{12} deficiency (pernicious anemia)
Thiamine deficiency (Wernicke encephalopathy)

Adapted from Geringer ES, Stern TA. Recognition and treatment of depression in the intensive care unit patient. In: Irwin RS, Rippe JM, eds. *Intensive care medicine*, 5th edition. Philadelphia: Lippincott Williams and Wilkins, 2003, pp. 2170–2184.

---

3. Other, newer agents (see Table 159-5)
   a. Venlafaxine
      (1) A norepinephrine and serotonin reuptake inhibitor
      (2) Can cause a dose-dependent increase in supine diastolic blood pressure
      (3) Does not inhibit the P-450 system
   b. Mirtazapine
      (1) Enhances sleep and appetite
      (2) Available in an orally disintegrating formulation that is useful in patients who cannot swallow pills
4. Tricyclic antidepressants
   a. Can cause sedation, confusion, blurred vision, dry mouth, constipation, orthostatic hypotension, and disturbances of cardiac conduction and rhythm (See Tables 159-7 and 159-8)

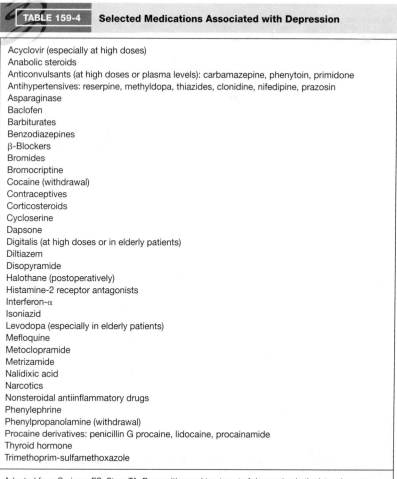

TABLE 159-4   **Selected Medications Associated with Depression**

Acyclovir (especially at high doses)
Anabolic steroids
Anticonvulsants (at high doses or plasma levels): carbamazepine, phenytoin, primidone
Antihypertensives: reserpine, methyldopa, thiazides, clonidine, nifedipine, prazosin
Asparaginase
Baclofen
Barbiturates
Benzodiazepines
β-Blockers
Bromides
Bromocriptine
Cocaine (withdrawal)
Contraceptives
Corticosteroids
Cycloserine
Dapsone
Digitalis (at high doses or in elderly patients)
Diltiazem
Disopyramide
Halothane (postoperatively)
Histamine-2 receptor antagonists
Interferon-α
Isoniazid
Levodopa (especially in elderly patients)
Mefloquine
Metoclopramide
Metrizamide
Nalidixic acid
Narcotics
Nonsteroidal antiinflammatory drugs
Phenylephrine
Phenylpropanolamine (withdrawal)
Procaine derivatives: penicillin G procaine, lidocaine, procainamide
Thyroid hormone
Trimethoprim-sulfamethoxazole

Adapted from Geringer ES, Stern TA. Recognition and treatment of depression in the intensive care unit patient. In: Irwin RS, Rippe JM, eds. *Intensive care medicine*, 5th edition. Philadelphia: Lippincott Williams and Wilkins, 2003, pp. 2170–2184.

TABLE 159-5   **Selective Serotonin Reuptake Inhibitors and Other, Newer Agents**

Agent	Usual starting dose[a] (mg/d)
Fluoxetine	5–10
Sertraline	25–50
Paroxetine	5–10
Citalopram	5–10
Escitalopram	5–10
Venlafaxine	37.5–75
Mirtazapine	7.5–15

[a] In critically ill patients.

TABLE 159-6	Selected Substrates and Inhibitors of Cytochrome P-450 Isoenzymes

	1A2	2C	2D6	3A3/4
Substrates	Acetaminophen	Barbiturates	Codeine	Amiodarone
	Aminophylline	Diazepam	Encainide	Calcium channel blockers
	Haloperidol	Omeprazole	Flecainide	Diazepam
	TCAs	Phenytoin	Haloperidol	Disopyramide
	Theophylline	Propranolol	Hydrocodone	Lidocaine
		TCAs	Metoprolol	Macrolide antibiotics
			Propranolol	Omeprazole
			TCAs	Quinidine
			Timolol	Steroids
				TCAs
Inhibitors	Fluoxetine	Fluoxetine[a]	Fluoxetine[a]	Fluoxetine
	Paroxetine	Sertraline	Paroxetine[a]	Nefazodone[a]
			Sertraline	Sertraline

[a] Strong inhibitor.
TCA, tricyclic antidepressant.
Adapted from Geringer ES, Stern TA: Recognition and treatment of depression in the intensive care unit patient. In: Irwin RS, Rippe JM, eds. *Intensive care medicine*, 5th edition. Philadelphia: Lippincott Williams and Wilkins, 2003, pp. 2170–2184.

   b. Should be used with great caution in patients:
      (1) With pre-existing conduction delays
      (2) With a corrected QT interval (QT_c) of >440 msec
      (3) Who are taking other drugs that also have type I antiarrhythmic effects
   5. Monoamine oxidase inhibitors. Phenelzine and tranylcypromine are not useful in the ICU because of the profound hypertensive crises that might result when these agents are combined with pressors.

TABLE 159-7	Comparative Properties of Tricylic Antidepressants

Drug	ACh effects	Sedative effects	OH	Target dose range (mg/d)	Comments
Tertiary amines					
Amitriptyline	+++	+++	+++	≥150	Most anticholinergic
Doxepin	++	+++	++	≥200	
Imipramine	++	++	+++	≥200	
Secondary amines					
Desipramine	+	+	+++	≥150	
Nortriptyline	++	++	+	≥100	Least OH; safest in cardiac disease
Protriptyline	+++	+	++	≥30	

ACh, anticholinergic; OH, orthostatic hypotension; +++, high; ++, moderate; +, low.
Adapted from Geringer ES, Stern TA: Recognition and treatment of depression in the intensive care unit patient. In: Irwin RS, Rippe JM, eds. *Intensive care medicine*, 5th edition. Philadelphia: Lippincott Williams and Wilkins, 2003, pp. 2170–2184.

| | TABLE 159-8 | The Use of TCAs in Patients with Selected Cardiovascular Conditions | |

Cardiac status	Comments	TCA of choice (based on available data)
Bundle-branch block	• Caution advised • All TCAs prolong HV interval • Pretreatment ECG recommended in patients >50 years • Hospitalization/telemetric monitoring suggested at start of treatment • Maintain lowest effective plasma level	Nortriptyline ? Doxepin
Ventricular arrhythmia	• TCAs possess type-I (quinidine-like) effects • PVCs may improve on TCAs • Antiarrhythmic dosage may require a decrease • Holter monitor suggested	Imipramine Desipramine
Orthostatic hypotension	• All TCAs can produce further orthostatic changes that can be predicted (to some degree) by orthostatic changes before TCA initiation • Effect can occur independent of plasma levels • Symptoms may be minimal despite significant decrease in blood pressure • Symptoms may decrease over time	Nortriptyline
Left ventricular	• Impairment of contractility is uncommon dysfunction/CHF • CHF is very rare; it may occur secondary to heart rate increases from anticholinergic effects	All TCAs
Recent acute myocardial infarction	• Delay use of TCAs for several weeks because of hypotension, tachycardia, and systemic effects	None
Atrial fibrillation	• Avoid TCAs unless concurrently treated with digoxin	None
Prolonged QT$_c$	• Use with caution because of risk of sudden death when QT$_c$ >440 msec	Nortriptyline ? Doxepin

TCAs, tricyclic antidepressants; HV, His-ventricular; ECG, electrocardiogram; PVC, premature ventricular contraction; CHF, congestive heart failure; QTc, corrected QT interval.
Adapted from Dec GW, Stern TA. Tricyclic antidepressants in the intensive care unit. *J Intensive Care Med* 1990;5:69–81.

B. Psychological. Patients often benefit from information, clarification, reassurance, and support. Asking about patients' families, work, hobbies, and interests helps restore their sense of identity.

C. Electroconvulsive therapy (ECT). ECT is reserved for patients with severe or delusional depression and for those who cannot tolerate, or have failed to respond to, pharmacologic and talking therapies.

Selected Readings

Cassem NH, Papakostas GI, Fava M, Stern TA. Mood-disordered patients. In: Stern TA, Fricchione GL, Cassem NH, et al., eds. *Massachusetts General Hospital handbook of general hospital psychiatry*, 5th edition. Philadelphia: Mosby, 2004, pp. 69–92.
A comprehensive review of the characteristics of depressive disorders, their differential diagnosis, and their treatment in the context of comorbid medical illness.

Dec GW, Stern TA. Tricyclic antidepressants in the intensive care unit. *J Intensive Care Med* 1990;5:69–81.
A review of the pharmacology of tricyclic antidepressants, their major cardiovascular and neurologic effects, and the management of tricyclic antidepressant overdose.

Diagnostic and statistical manual of mental disorders, 4th ed. Washington, DC: American Psychiatric Association, 1994.
Known as DSM-IV, this bible of psychiatry enumerates the diagnostic criteria for the gamut of psychiatric maladies.

Ellison JM, Milofsky JE, Ely E. Fluoxetine-induced bradycardia and syncope in two patients. *J Clin Psychiatry* 1990;51:385–386.
A report of two cases of bradycardia—one with syncope, one with faintness—during treatment with fluoxetine.

Glassman AH, O'Connor CM, Califf RM, et al. Sertraline treatment of major depression in patients with acute MI or unstable angina. *JAMA* 2002;288:701–709.
A randomized, double-blind, placebo-controlled trial of 369 patients with major depressive disorder and either acute MI or unstable angina, which showed that sertraline is a safe and effective treatment for recurrent depression in patients with unstable ischemic cardiac disease—the first published evidence that antidepressant drugs are safe and efficacious in this population.

Kaufmann MW, Murray GB, Cassem NH. Use of psychostimulants in medically ill depressed patients. *Psychosomatics* 1982;23:817–819.
A report of the beneficial and safe use of methylphenidate and dextroamphetamine in medically ill patients with comorbid depression.

Matthews J, Papakostas G. Mood disorders: depression. In: Stern TA, Herman JB, eds. *Psychiatry update and board preparation*, 2nd ed. New York: McGraw-Hill, 2004, pp. 103–112.
A concise review of depressive disorders and their pharmacologic and nonpharmacologic treatments.

Roose SP, Glassman AH, Giardina EGV, et al. Tricyclic antidepressants in depressed patients with cardiac conduction disease. *Arch Gen Psychiatry* 1987;44:273–275.
A prospective study that compared the risk of cardiac complications of imipramine and nortriptyline in depressed patients with and without cardiac conduction delays.

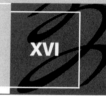

John J. Paris, Gregory Webster, and Frank E. Reardon

I. BACKGROUND

A. Medical ethics applies moral principles to choices made in a medical context.

B. Major principles in bioethics are

  1. Autonomy

    a. The dignity of every human allows the competent individual to make personal choices regarding medical treatment.

    b. An individual without decision-making capacity also has the right of choice with regard to medical decisions.

      (1) Exercised by a surrogate or designated proxy.

      (2) Decisions are to be based on the patient's personal values. If these are not known, decision is made in the best interests of the patient.

  2. Beneficence. Physician has a fiduciary duty to act for the patient's well-being.

  3. Nonmalifiance. Physician must seek to avoid harm to the patient. The guiding principle of physician interaction with the patient is: "First do no harm."

  4. Justice

    a. Individual justice. Provide each person with what is due to the individual within the circumstances of the situation.

    b. Social justice. Concerned with the impact of individual decisions on the community as a whole. The common good as well as individual benefit must be considered.

  5. Truth telling. Requires the physician be open and honest with the patient.

  6. Promise keeping. Physician owes a duty of loyalty to the patient.

  7. Confidentiality

    a. The physician keeps secret those things revealed by the patient in the physician—patient relationship.

    b. Two exceptions:

      (1) There is a "duty to warn" if danger of significant harm to a third party. Gun shot wounds and suspected child abuse have mandatory reporting requirements.

      (2) Communicable diseases such as tuberculosis or smallpox must be reported to public health authorities.

II. DECISION-MAKING PROCESS

A. The age of physician paternalism—"The doctor knows best"—is over.

B. Good medical decision making is not one-dimensional. At a minimum, it must consider three factors: physician, patient, and society.

  1. Physician

    a. Diagnosis: determination of the patient's medical condition.

    b. Prognosis: assessment of implications of the diagnosis based on medical training and experience.

    c. Recommendation: Physician has a positive duty to propose a treatment regimen to the patient.

    d. Action: Physician has a duty to carry out agreed-upon treatments.

  2. Patient. Assesses the physician's recommendation based on individual psychosocial values. Entire range of factors such as cost, burden, pain, anticipated outcome, dislocation, family structure, and personal plans are to be considered. Patient (or proxy) then decides to:

    a. Accept proposed treatment.

    b. Negotiate with the physician for a different, but medically acceptable course.

    c. Reject the proposed treatment.

       (1) Seeks alternative or nonconventional modalities.

       (2) Utilizes no intervention.

  3. Society

    a. Protects individual from undertreatment or neglect.

    b. Intervenes to prevent overtreatment.

       (1) Unwanted—Court rulings from Quinlan (1976) to Cruzan (1990) establish that both competent and noncompetent patients have a right to refuse unwanted medical interventions.

       (2) Wanted by patient (or proxy) but believed by physician to be:

          (a) Overly burdensome.

          (b) Medically unwarranted.

       (3) Wanted by the patient and offers benefit, but believed to be overly expensive by:

          (a) Insurance plan

          (b) Health maintenance organization (HMO)

          (c) Medicare/Medicaid

             (i) Noncovered treatment

             (ii) Rationing by price

  c. Courts should be the place of last resort to resolve utterly irreconcilable clashes.

    (1) Costly

    (2) Cumbersome

    (3) Adversarial

    (4) Unpredictable

       (a) Almost always support requests for life-sustaining treatment.

       (b) Set standards that then govern medical practice.

III. RESPONSIBILITY FOR DECISION. Judgments concerning burden and benefit to the patient are moral choices.

  A. Belong to patient or those responsible for the welfare of an incompetent patient.

  B. Disputes between physician and patient (or proxy). Best resolved by negotiation between physician and patient or involvement of an ethics committee.

    1. Substitution of physician assessment for patient values clashes with prevailing standards of both ethics and the law.

      a. Patient preferences with regard to recommended treatment should prevail.

      b. Patient or proxy may request, but cannot compel, treatment not recommended by physician.

    2. Physicians considering withholding or withdrawing life-sustaining treatment over the patient or family objections should not act unilaterally.

      a. American Medical Association (AMA) guidelines advise a procedural, rather than a substantive, approach. Decision should be:

         (1) Made in consultation with specialists.

         (2) Supported by data from literature.

         (3) Approved by an ethics committee.

         (4) Patient (proxy) given opportunity for outside second opinion.

         (5) Patient (proxy) given opportunity of a transfer.

      b. Once these steps are taken, AMA guidelines indicate treating physician has no further obligation to follow family demands.

IV. DO NOT RESUSCITATE ORDERS. Despite strong agreement in ethical literature and judicial rulings that patient preferences on forgoing aggressive medical interventions should be respected, the SUPPORT Study reveals that physicians are reluctant to honor such requests. Particularly true of do not resuscitate (DNR) orders.

  A. One third of patients preferred cardiopulmonary resuscitation (CPR) be withheld.

    1. Only 47% of physicians accurately reported that preference.

    2. Of those patients, 49% did not have a written DNR order.

B. Blackhall notes, "Physicians have no obligation to provide, and patients and families no right to demand, medical treatment that is of no demonstrable benefit."

    1. In such cases, patient or family desire for CPR is irrelevant.

    2. Assessment of anticipated medical benefit is a decision entirely within the physician's technical expertise.

        a. Physician's duty is to explain to the family that the patient's physical condition is such that no intervention will reverse the dying process.

        b. When cardiac arrest occurs during the final phase of the dying process, CPR will not be attempted.

C. Appropriateness of CPR when resuscitation is physically possible is a decision to be made by the patient or family based on assessment of the patient's present or future quality of life. That subjective choice belongs to the patient.

D. Decision making on CPR for the elderly dying patient with no family or friends should be done as it customarily has been done in hospitals—by the attending physician with the concurrence of another physician or an institutionally designated patient advocate. These decisions are well within the scope of common medical practice.

    1. They should not be elevated to the role of moral dilemma.

    2. They should not be perceived as a judicial problem.

    3. Patients should not be subjected to aggressive attempts at resuscitation without a reasonable expectation of successful outcome.

V. BRAIN DEATH. Though philosophical debate continues on the meaning of death, as a practical matter every jurisdiction recognizes medically determined cessation of electrical activity in the whole brain, including the brainstem, as death.

A. The brain-dead patient is dead.

B. Other than for potential organ donation, there is no legal or medical rationale to oxygenate the cadaver.

C. No family permission is required to cease ventilation of the corpse; none should be requested.

    1. Physician should inform the family that the patient is dead.

    2. Physician should request organ donation.

    3. If declined, the physician should inform—not ask—the family that all medical interventions will be withdrawn.

VI. WITHHOLDING AND WITHDRAWAL OF MEDICAL INTERVENTIONS. Once it is agreed that a particular intervention is not appropriate—because the patient refuses it or it proves ineffective—it may be withheld or withdrawn.

A. Same justification that applies to withholding applies to withdrawal.

    1. No legal difference between withholding/withdrawal.

    2. No ethical difference between withholding/withdrawal.

    3. Psychologically easier not to start than to stop.

B. Moral issue in withholding/withdrawal is to ensure patient comfort. Too-rapid withdrawal produces air hunger, gagging, gasping, struggle in patient.

    1. Premedicate patient

        a. morphine to alleviate dyspnea

        b. benzodiazepine for anxiety

        c. titrate to patient's comfort

    2. Do not institute neuromuscular blocking agents at time of disconnecting ventilator.

        a. Blur difference between allowing to die and actively causing patient's death

        b. Have no analgesic or sedative properties

    3. If neuromuscular agents are already in use:

        a. Attempt to reverse paralysis.

        b. If effect cannot be expeditiously reversed, do not compel the patient and family to wait days or weeks until paralysis is reversed before withdrawal of ventilator.

            (1) Write a clear note in chart on rationale for withdrawal despite presence of paralytic agent.

            (2) Provides explanation that withdrawal is not a means of achieving euthanasia.

VII. ADVANCE DIRECTIVES. The federal Patient Self-Determination Act of 1990 mandates that all medical facilities notify patient of right to decline unwanted medical interventions.

A. Living will

1. Written statement of patient's wishes regarding utilization of medical therapies should patient lose decision-making capacity.

2. Tend to be written in broad terms. Unless very specific these are not very helpful in making nuanced or difficult decisions for the patient.

B. Durable power of attorney designates a proxy who is authorized to make medical decisions for the incompetent patient.

1. Proxy has the same decision-making role as the patient.

   a. Acts on known values of patient.

   b. Is able to adjust decisions to changing clinical situation.

2. Existence of a proxy does not absolve medical staff of responsibility to ensure that decisions are made in the patient's best interests.

Selected Readings

American Thoracic Society. Withholding and withdrawal of life-sustaining therapy. *Am Rev Respir Dis* 1991;144:726–731.
Official guidelines on end-of-life care by the professional association of physicians who treat patients with respiratory diseases.

Angus D, Barnato AE, Linde-Zwirble, et al. Use of intensive care at the end of life in the United States: an epidemiologic study. *Crit Care Med* 2004;32:638–643.
One in five Americans currently dies while in an ICU. The authors explore the implications of this reality for a society whose population of persons over 65 will double by the year 2030.

Blackhall L. Must we always use CPR? *N Engl J Med* 1987;317:1281.
A landmark article on limits for use of cardiopulmonary resuscitation.

Curtis JR, Rubenfeld GD. Managing death in the intensive care unit: the transition from cure to comfort. New York: Oxford University Press, 2001.
A comprehensive review of ICU care at the end of life. Has specific recommendations on transition from attempts at cure to provision of comfort care only.

Fetters MD, Churchill L, Denis M. Conflict resolution at the end of life. *Crit Care Med* 2001;29:921–925.
Discussion of the way physicians handle requests for treatment deemed nonbeneficial by either the physician or family.

Luce JM. Physicians do not have a responsibility to provide futile or unreasonable care if a patient or family insists. *Crit Care Med* 1995;23:760.
A forceful statement by one of the nation's leading physicians on the limits of a patient's right to demand medical interventions.

Luce JM, Alpers A. End-of-life care: what do the American courts say? *Crit Care Med* 2001;29(2 supp):N40–N45.
A clear and easy-to-understand guide through court rulings on end-of-life decisions.

Nyman DJ, Sprung CL. End-of-life decision making in the intensive care unit. *Intensive Care Med* 2000;26:1414–1420.
Excellent review of issues confronting physicians in ICUs.

Paris JJ, Crone RK, Reardon FE. Physician refusal of requested treatment: the case of Baby L. *N Engl J Med* 1990;322:1012.
First reported case of physician refusal to provide a life-sustaining intervention.

Paris JJ, Schreiber MD, Statter M, et al. Beyond autonomy: physician refusal of life-prolonging ECMO. *N Engl J Med* 1991;325:511.
First reported case of physician refusal to continue life-prolonging technology.

The Society of Critical Care Medicine Ethics Committee. Attitudes of critical care medicine professionals concerning distribution of intensive care resources. *Crit Care Med* 1994;22:358.
A survey of attitudes of critical care providers on distribution or resources.

Spring CL, Cohen SL, Sjokvist P, et al. End-of-life practices in European intensive care units: the ethics study. *JAMA* 2003;290:790–797.
A review of practice patterns in 37 ICUs across 17 European countries reveals that physician biases as well as medical status influence end-of-life decisions.

The SUPPORT Principal Investigators. A controlled trial to improve care for seriously ill hospitalized patients: the study to understand prognosis and preferences for outcomes and risks of treatments (SUPPORT). *JAMA* 1995;274:1591.
A landmark study of physician behavior in critical care medicine.

Thurow L. Learning to say "no." *N Engl J Med* 1984;311:1569.
A superb essay by an economist concluding that in the absence of agreed-on societal values the marketplace will determine what medicine will be provided.

Treece P, Engelberg RA, Crowley L, et al. Evaluation of a standardized order form for withdrawal of life support in the intensive care unit. *Crit Care Med* 2004;32:1141–1148.
A helpful mechanism for consistent application of appropriate sedation without hastening death in ICU.

Truog RD, Burns JP, Mitchell C, et al. Pharmacologic paralysis and withdrawal of mechanical ventilation at the end of life. *N Engl J Med* 2000;342:508–511.
A careful analysis of appropriate medication to accompany withdrawal of ventilatory support.

Truog RD, Cist AFM, Bracket SE, et al. Recommendations for end-of-life care in the intensive care unit: The Ethic Committee of the Society of Critical Care Medicine. *Crit Care Med* 2001;29:2332–2348.
Well-considered recommendations by the professional society of critical care physicians.

Veatch RM, Spicer CM. Medically futile care: the role of the physician in setting limits. *Am J Law Med* 1992;18:15.
The best statement of the position that patient autonomy is the overriding principle in medical ethics.

Wenrich MD, Curtis JR, Shannon S, et al. Communicating with dying patients within the spectrum of medical care from terminal diagnosis to death. *Arch Intern Med* 2001;161:868–874.
A sensitive and thoughtful exploration of communication skills in delivering bad news.

APP

CALCULATIONS COMMONLY USED IN CRITICAL CARE

 A. FAHRENHEIT AND CELSIUS TEMPERATURE CONVERSIONS

°C	°F
45	113.0
44	111.2
43	109.4
42	107.6
41	105.8
40	104.0
39	102.2
38	100.4
37	98.6
36	96.8
35	95.0
34	93.2
33	91.4
32	89.6
31	87.8
30	86.0
29	84.2
28	82.4
27	80.6
26	78.8
25	77.0

°C to °F: °F = (°C × 9/5) + 32
°F to °C: °C = (°F − 32) × 5/9

B. HEMODYNAMIC CALCULATIONS

MEAN ARTERIAL BLOOD PRESSURE (mm Hg)
= MAP
= [systolic BP + (2 diastolic BP)]/3
= diastolic BP + 1/3 (systolic BP − diastolic BP)
Normal range: 85–95 mm Hg

FICK EQUATION FOR CARDIAC INDEX (L/min/m²)
= CI
= CO/BSA
= oxygen consumption/(arterial O_2 content − venous O_2 content)
= [10 × $\dot{V}O_2$ (mL/min/m²)]/[Hgb (g/dL) × 1.34 × (arterial % saturation − venous % saturation)]
Normal range: 2.5–4.2 L/min/m²

SYSTEMIC VASCULAR RESISTANCE (dyne·sec·cm⁻⁵)
= SVR
= [80 × (MAP − right atrial mean BP)]/CO (L/min)
Normal range: 770–1,500 dyne·sec·cm⁻⁵

PULMONARY VASCULAR RESISTANCE (dyne·sec·cm^{-5})
$$= PVR$$
$$= [80 \times (\text{pulmonary artery mean BP} - \text{pulmonary capillary wedge pressure})]$$
$$/CO \text{ (L/min)}$$
Normal range: 20–120 dyne·sec·cm^{-5}

C. PULMONARY CALCULATIONS

ALVEOLAR GAS EQUATION (mm Hg)
$$P_{A}O_2 = PIO_2 - (Paco_2/R)$$
$$= [FIO_2 \times (P_{atm} - P_{H_2O})] - (Paco_2/R)$$
$$= 150 - (Paco_2/R) \text{ (on room air, at sea level)}$$
Normal value: ~100 mm Hg (on room air, at sea level)

ALVEOLAR–ARTERIAL OXYGEN TENSION GRADIENT (mm Hg)
$$= A - a \text{ gradient}$$
$$= PAo_2 - Pao_2$$
Normal values (upright): $2.5 + (0.21 \times \text{age})$

ARTERIAL BLOOD OXYGEN CONTENT (mL/dL)
$$= Cao_2$$
$$= \text{oxygen dissolved in blood} + \text{oxygen carried by hemoglobin}$$
$$= [0.003 \text{ (mL } O_2/dL) \times Pao_2] + [1.34 \times Hgb \text{ (g/dL)} \times \% \text{ Hgb saturated with } O_2]$$
Normal range: 17.5–23.5 mL/dL

COMPLIANCE (mL/cm H_2O)
$$= \Delta\text{Volume}/\Delta\text{Pressure}$$
On Mechanical Ventilation:
Static respiratory system compliance $= C_{st} = $ Tidal volume/$(P_{plateau} - P_{end exp})$
Dynamic effective compliance $= C_{dyn} = $ Tidal volume/$(P_{peak} - P_{end exp})$

D. ELECTROLYTE AND RENAL CALCULATIONS

ANION GAP (mEq/L)
$$= [Na^+] - ([Cl^-] + [HCO_3^-])$$
Normal range: 9–13 mEq/L

EXPECTED ANION GAP IN HYPOALBUMINEMIA
$$= 3 \times [\text{albumin (g/dL)}]$$

CALCULATED SERUM OSMOLALITY (mOsm/kg)
$$= (2 \times [Na^+]) + ([\text{glucose}]/18) + ([\text{BUN}]/2.8)$$
Normal range: 275–290 mOsm/kg

OSMOLAR GAP (mOsm/kg)
$$= \text{Measured serum osmolality} - \text{Calculated serum osmolality}$$
Normal range: 0–5 mOsm/kg

Na^+ CORRECTION FOR HYPERGLYCEMIA
Increase $[Na^+]$ by 1.6 mEq/L for each 100 mg/dL increase in [glucose] above 100 mg/dL

Ca^{2+} CORRECTION FOR HYPOALBUMINEMIA
Increase $[Ca^{2+}]$ by 0.8 mg/dL for each 1.0 gm/dL decrease in [albumin] from 4 g/dL

WATER DEFICIT IN HYPERNATREMIA (L)
$$= [0.6 \times \text{body weight (kg)}] \times \{([Na^+]/140) - 1\}$$

Na^+ DEFICIT IN HYPONATREMIA (mEq)
$$= [0.6 \times \text{body weight (kg)}] \times (\text{desired plasma } [Na^+] - 140)$$

FRACTIONAL EXCRETION OF SODIUM (%)
$$= F_ENa$$
$$= \{(\text{excreted } [Na^+])/(\text{filtered } [Na^+])\} \times 100$$
$$= \{(\text{urine } [Na^+])/(\text{serum } [Na^+])\}/\{(\text{urine } [Creat])/(\text{serum } [Creat])\} \times 100$$

CREATININE CLEARANCE (mL/min)
 = (urine [Creat]) × (urine volume over 24 hours)
 = {(urine [Creat (gm/dL)]) × {[urine volume (mL/d)]/1440 (min/day)]}
   /serum [Creat] (mg/dL)
Estimated for males = {(140 − age) × [lean body weight (kg)]}
                     /{serum [Creat] (mg/dL) × 72}
Estimated for females = 0.85 × (estimate for males)
Normal range: 74–160 mL/min

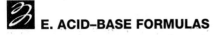 **E. ACID–BASE FORMULAS**

HENDERSON'S EQUATION FOR [H$^+$]
 [H$^+$] (nm/L) = 24 × {Paco$_2$/[HCO$_3^-$]}
Normal values: [H$^+$] is 40 nm/L at pH of 7.40 and each 0.01 unit change in pH corre-
              sponds to an approximate opposite deviation of [H$^+$] of 1 nm/L (over the
              pH range of 7.10–7.50)

METABOLIC ACIDOSIS
Bicarbonate deficit (mEq/L) = 0.5 × body weight (kg) × (24 − [HCO$_3^-$])
Expected Paco$_2$ compensation = (1.5 × [HCO$_3^-$]) + 8 ± 2

RESPIRATORY ACIDOSIS
Acute = Δ[H$^+$]/ΔPaCO$_2$ = 0.8
Chronic = Δ[H$^+$]/ΔPaCO$_2$ = 0.3

RESPIRATORY ALKALOSIS
Acute = Δ[H$^+$]/ΔPaCO$_2$ = 0.8
Chronic = Δ[H$^+$]/ΔPaCO$_2$ = 0.17

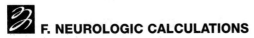 **F. NEUROLOGIC CALCULATIONS**

GLASGOW COMA SCALE
 = eye score (1–4) + motor score (1–6) + verbal score (1–5)

Specific Components of the Glasgow Coma Scale:

Component	Score
Eye opening	
spontaneous	4
to speech	3
to pain	2
none	1
Motor response	
obeys commands	6
localizes	5
withdraws	4
exhibits abnormal flexion	3
exhibits abnormal extension	2
none	1
Verbal response	
oriented	5
confused, conversant	4
uses inappropriate words	3
incomprehensible sounds	2
none	1

Normal total value: 15 (range 3–15)

G. PHARMACOLOGIC CALCULATIONS

DRUG ELIMINATION CONSTANT
   = Ke
   = fractional elimination of drug per unit time
   = $\{\ln ([\text{peak}]/[\text{trough}])/(t_{\text{peak}} - t_{\text{trough}})\}$

DRUG HALF-LIFE
   = $t^{1/2}$
   = 0.693/Ke

VOLUME OF DISTRIBUTION (L/kg)
   = Vd
   = [(dose) × (fraction of active drug in circulation)]
      /[(area under single dose curve) × Ke]

DRUG CLEARANCE
   = Vd × Ke

DRUG LOADING DOSE
   = Vd × [target peak]

DRUG DOSING INTERVAL
   = $\{-\text{Ke}^{-1} \times \ln ([\text{desired trough}]/[\text{desired peak}])\}$ + infusion time (h)

H. NUTRITIONAL CALCULATIONS

BODY MASS INDEX
   = BMI
   = weight (kg)/[height (cm)]^2

RESPIRATORY QUOTIENT
   = R
   = CO_2 production (mL/min)/O_2 consumption (mL/min)
Normal value: 0.8

HARRIS-BENEDICT EQUATION OF RESTING ENERGY EXPENDITURE (kcal/day)
Males = 66 + [13.7 × weight (kg)] + [5 × height (cm)] − (6.8 × age)
Females = 655 + [9.6 × weight (kg)] + [1.8 × height (cm)] − (4.7 × age)

Note: Page numbers followed by f indicate illustrations; those followed by t indicate tables.